Catheter Ablation of
Cardiac Arrhythmias

Catheter Ablation of Cardiac Arrhythmias

Edited by

Shoei K. Stephen Huang, M.D.
Professor of Medicine, Dean, College of Medicine, China Medical University;
Vice-Superintendent, China Medical University Hospital, Taichung, Taiwan

Mark A. Wood, M.D.
Professor of Medicine, Assistant Director, Cardiac Electrophysiology Laboratory,
Virginia Commonwealth University Medical Center, Richmond, Virginia

Foreword by

Melvin M. Scheinman, M.D.
Professor of Medicine, University of California, San Francisco, California

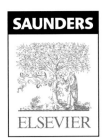

SAUNDERS

ELSEVIER

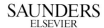

1600 John F. Kennedy Blvd.
Ste 1800
Philadelphia, PA 19103-2899

CATHETER ABLATION OF CARDIAC ARRHYTHMIAS   ISBN-13: 978-1-4160-0312-0
Copyright © 2006, Elsevier Inc.   ISBN-10: 1-4160-0312-6

Notice

Knowledge and best practice in this field are constantly changing. As new research and experience broaden our knowledge, changes in practice, treatment and drug therapy may become necessary or appropriate. Readers are advised to check the most current information provided (i) on procedures featured or (ii) by the manufacturer of each product to be administered, to verify the recommended dose or formula, the method and duration of administration, and contraindications. It is the responsibility of the practitioner, relying on their own experience and knowledge of the patient, to make diagnoses, to determine dosages and the best treatment for each individual patient, and to take all appropriate safety precautions. To the fullest extent of the law, neither the Publisher nor the Editors assume any liability for any injury and/or damage to persons or property arising out of or related to any use of the material contained in this book.

Library of Congress Cataloging-in-Publication Data
Catheter ablation for cardiac arrhythmias / [edited by] Shoei K. Stephen Huang, Mark A.
    Wood.–1st ed.
        p. ; cm.
    Includes bibliographical references and index.
    ISBN 1-4160-0312-6
    1. Catheter ablation. 2. Arrhythmia—Surgery. I. Huang, Shoei K. II. Wood, Mark A.
    [DNLM: 1. Tachycardia–therapy. 2. Arrhythmia—therapy. 3. Catheter Ablation—
methods. WG 330 C3623 2006]
    RD598.35.C39C36 2006
    617.4'12—dc22

                                                                    2005050030

Acquisitions Editor: Susan Pioli
Publishing Services Manager: Mary Stermel
Design Direction: Gene Harris
Cover Designer: Gene Harris

Printed in China

Last digit is the print number: 9 8 7 6 5 4 3 2 1

Working together to grow
libraries in developing countries

www.elsevier.com | www.bookaid.org | www.sabre.org

ELSEVIER   BOOK AID International   Sabre Foundation

To all cardiac electrophysiology colleagues, physicians, fellows, and friends
who are dedicated to the care of patients with cardiac arrhythmias

and

To my wife, Su-Mei, for her continued inspiration and support;
my children, Priscilla, Melvin, and Jessica for the encouragement;
my late parents, Yu-Shih (father) and Hsing-Tzu (mother) for their illumination.

Shoei K. Stephen Huang, M.D.

To my wife, Helen, for all of her patience and love and to our new daughter,
Lily, who has come so far to be with us

Mark Wood, M.D.

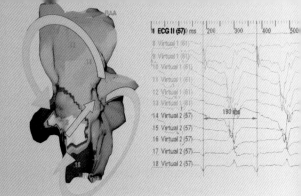

Contents

Part I
Fundamental Concepts of Trans-Catheter Energy Applications

Part II
Cardiac Mapping and Imaging

Part III
Catheter Ablation of Atrial Tachycardia and Flutter

Part IV
Catheter Ablation for Atrial Fibrillation

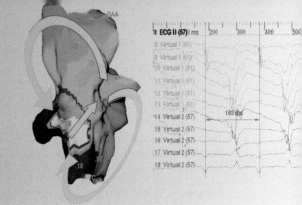

Contributing Authors

Amin Al-Ahmed, M.D. Clinical Instructor, Cardiac Electrophysiology, Department of Medicine, Division of Cardiovascular Medicine, Stanford University School of Medicine and Stanford University Hospitals and Clinics, Stanford, California

Robert H. Anderson, BSc, MD, FRCPath Joseph Levy Professor of Pediatric Cardiac Morphology, Cardiac Unit, Institute of Child Health, University College; Honorary Consultant, Great Ormond Street Hospital for Children, London, United Kingdom

Rishi Arora, M.D. Assistant Professor of Medicine, Medicine/Cardiology/Cardiac Electrophysiology, Northwestern University, Feinberg School of Medicine; Attending Physician, Medicine/Cardiology/Cardiac Electrophysiology, Northwestern Memorial Hospital, Chicago, Illinois

Samuel J. Asirvatham, M.D. Assistant Professor of Medicine, Department of Cardiology, Mayo School of Medicine; Consultant, Cardiac Electrophysiology and Pacing, Mayo Clinic, Rochester, Minnesota

Deepak Bhakta, M.D. Assistant Professor of Medicine, Department of Medicine, Krannert Institute of Cardiology, Indiana University School of Medicine, Indianapolis, Indiana

JA Cabrera, M.D. Director of Cardiac Electrophysiology, Cardiology Unit, Fundación Jiménez Díaz, Madrid, Spain

Jose Manuel Rubio Campal, M.D., Ph.D. Department of Cardiology, Fundacion Jimenez Diaz, Madrid, Spain

Hugh Calkins, B.S. Professor of Medicine, Johns Hopkins University; Director of Electrophysiology, Johns Hopkins Hospital, Baltimore, Maryland

David John Callans, M.D. Professor of Medicine, Department of Cardiology, University of Pennsylvania; Director, Electrophysiology Laboratory, Department of Cardiology, Hospital of the University of Pennsylvania, Philadelphia, Pennsylvania

Kuan-Cheng Chang, M.D. Assistant Professor of Medicine, Department of Medicine, China Medical University; Attending Physician, Division of Cardiology, Department of Medicine, China Medical University Hospital, Taichung, Taiwan, ROC

Henry Albert Chen, M.D. Fellow, Cardiac Electrophysiology, Department of Cardiovascular Medicine, Stanford University School of Medicine; Clinical Fellow, Department of Medicine, Division of Cardiovascular Medicine, Stanford University Hospital and Clinics, Stanford, California

Jan-Yow Chen, M.D. Lecturer, School of Medicine, China Medical University; Cardiologist, Division of Cardiology, Department of Medicine, China Medical University, Taichung, Taiwan

Shih-Ann Chen, M.D. Professor of Medicine, National Yang Ming University; Director of Cardiac Electrophysiology, Taipei Veterans General Hospital, Taipei, Taiwan

Tayseer H. Chowdhry, B.S. Research Fellow, Electrophysiology, Johns Hopkins, Baltimore, Maryland

Jacques Clementy, M.D. Professor, Department of Cardiology, Universite Victor Segalen; Medecin-Chef de Service, Department of Cardiology, Hopital Haut Leveque, Bordeaux, France

Mithilesh Kumar Das, M.D., MRCP, FACC Assistant Professor of Medicine, Department of Medicine, Division of Cardiology, Indiana School of Medicine, Indiana Universitya and Krannert Institute of Cardiology; Chief of Cardiac Arrhythmia Service, Department of Medicine, Division of Cardiology, Roudebush VA Medical Center, Indianapolis, Indiana

Deeptankar Demazumder, Ph.D Post Doctoral Research Associate and Medical Student (class of 2006), School of Medicine, Virginia Commonwealth University Medical Center. Richmond, Virginia

Sanjay Dixit, M.D. Assistant Professor, Division of Cardiology, University of Pennsylvania School of Medicine; Director, Electrophysiology Laboratories, Cardiology Section, Philadelphia Veterans Affairs Medical Center, Philadelphia, Pennsylvania

Shepal Doshi, M.D. Director, Cardiac Electrophysiology and Pacing, Saint Johns Health Center; Director, Cardiac Electrophysiology Research, Pacific Heart Institute, Santa Monica, California

Marc Dubuc M.D., FRCPC Associate Professor of Medicine, Faculty of Medicine, University of Montreal; Associate Professor of Medicine, Electrophysiology Service, Department of Medicine, Montreal Heart Institute, Montreal, Quebec, Canada

Kenneth A. Ellenbogen, M.D. Kontos Professor of Medicine, Division of Cardiology, Director, Electrophysiology and Pacing, VCU School of Medicine; Virginia Commonwealth University, Richmond, Virginia

Jerónimo Farré M.D, Ph.D., FESC Professor of Cardiology and Chairman, Department of Cardiology, Fundación Jiménez Díaz, Universidad Autónoma de Madrid, Madrid, Spain

Gregory K. Feld, M.D. Professor of Medicine, Department of Medicine, University of California, San Diego; Director, Electrophysiology Laboratory, Department of Cardiology, University of California San Diego Medical Center, San Diego, California

Westby G. Fisher, M.D., FACC Assistant Professor of Medicine, Feinberg School of Medicine, Northwestern University; Director, Cardiac Electrophysiology, Department of Medicine, Evanston Northwestern Healthcare, Evanston, Illinois

Mario D. Gonzalez, M.D., Ph.D. Associate Professor of Medicine, Division of Cardiovascular Medicine, University of Florida; Director, Electrophysiology Laboratory, Division of Cardiovascular Medicine, Shands Hospital, Gainesville, Florida

David E. Haines, M.D. Director of Heart Rhythm Center, Cardiology Division, William Beaumont Hospital, Royal Oak, Michigan

Michel Haïssaguerre, M.D. Professor of Cardiology, University of Bordeaux II and Hôpital Cardiologique du Haut-Lévêque, Bordeaux, France

Satoshi Higa, MD, PhD Instructor, Second Department of Internal Medicine, Faculty of Medicine, University of the Ryukyus and Hospital, University of Ryukyus, Okinawa, Japan

Siew Yen Ho, Ph.D, FRCPath Reader, National Heart and Lung Institute, Imperial College; Honorary Consultant, Cardiac Morphology, Pediatrics, Royal Brompton and Harefield NHS Trust, London, United Kingdom

Méléze Hocini, M.D. Assistant Professor, Clinical Cardiology, Universite Victor Segalen, Bordeaux II; Assistant Professor, Permanent Staff, Electrophysiology Department, Hôpital Cardiologique due Haut-Lévèque, Bordeaux-Pessac, France

Bobbi L. Hoppe, M.D. Cardiovascular Consultants, Ltd, Minneapolis, Minnesota

Li-Fern Hus, MBBS, MRCP Doctor, Service du Rythmologie, Hopital Cardiolgique du Haut-Leveque, Bordeaux, France; Doctor, Department of Cardiology, National Heart Center, Singapore, Malaysia

Shoei K. Stephen Huang, M.D. Professor of Medicine, Dean, College of Medicine, China Medical University; Vice-Superintendent, China Medical University Hospital, Taichung, Taiwan

Pierre Jais, M.D. Universite Victor Segalen Bordeux II; Hopital Haut Leveque, Bordeaux, France

Alan Kadish, M.D. Professor of Medicine, Department of Medicine, Northwestern University; Medical Director of Electrophysiology, Associate Chief, Division of Cardiology, Department of Medicine, Northwestern Memorial Hospital, Chicago, Illinois

Jonathan Kalman, MBBS, PhD Professor of Medicine, Department of Medicine, University of Melbourne; Director of Cardiac Electrophysiology, Department of Cardiology, Royal Melbourne Hospital, Melbourne, Australia

G. Neal Kay, M.D. Professor of Medicine, Division of Cardiovascular Diseases, University of Alabama at Birmingham, Birmingham, Alabama

David Keane, M.D., Ph.D. Cardiac Electrophysiologist, Cardiac Arrhythmia Service, St James's Hospital, Dublin, Ireland

George J. Klein, M.D., FRCP(C) Professor of Medicine, Division of Cardiology, Department of Medicine, University of Western Ontario and University Hospital, London, Ontario, Canada

Andrew D. Krahn, M.D. Professor, Division of Cardiology, Department of Medicine, University of Western Ontario, London, Ontario, Canada

Ling-Ping Lai, M.D., Ph.D. Associate Professor, Institute of Pharmacology, National Taiwan University; Visiting Staff, Department of Internal Medicine, National Taiwan University Hospital, Taipei, Taiwan

David Lin, M.D. Assistant Professor of Medicine, Department of Medicine, University of Pennsylvania; Attending Phyisican, Medicine/Cardiac Electrophysiology, Hospital of the University of Pennsylvania, Philadelphia, Pennsylvania

Jiunn-Lee Lin, M.D., Ph.D. Professor of Medicine, Department of Internal Medicine, National Taiwan University Hospital College of Medicine; Director of Cardiac Electrophysiology and Pacing Service, Division of Cardiology, Deputy Chairman, Department of Internal Medicine, National Taiwan University Hospital, Taipei, Taiwan, Republic of China

Yu-Chin Lin, M.D. Staff Cardiologist, Division of Cardiology, Department of Medicine, China Medical University Hospital, Taichung, Taiwan, Republic of China

Byron K. Lee, M.D. Assistant Professor of Medicine, Division of Cardiology, Cardiac Electrophysiology, University of California School of Medicine and University of California Medical Center, San Francisco, California

Bruce B. Lerman, M.D. Hilda Altschul Master Professor of Medicine and Chief, Division of Cardiology, Department of Medicine, Cornell University Medical College; Director, Cardiac Electrophysiology Laboratory, Cornell University Medical Center, New York, New York

Francis E. Marchlinski, M.D. Professor of Medicine, University of Pennsylvania School of Medicine; Director of Electrophysiology, Hospital of the University of Pennsylvania, Philadelphia, Pennsylvania

Steven M. Markowitz, M.D. Associate Professor of Medicine, Department of Medicine, Cornell University Medical Center, New York, New York

Hugh Thomas McElderry Jr., M.D. Assistant Professor of Medicine, Division of Cardiovascular Disease, University of Alabama at Birmingham, Birmingham, Alabama

John M. Miller, M.D. Professor of Medicine, Department of Medicine, Cardiology Division, Indiana University School of Medicine; Director, Clinical Cardiac Electrophysiology; Clarian Health System, Indianapolis, Indiana

Joseph Morton, MBBS, PhD Senior Fellow, Department of Medicine, University of Melbourne; Cardiologist, Department of Cardiology, Royal Melbourne Hospital, Melbourne, Australia

Chrishan Joseph Nalliah, BSc (Adv) Research Student, Service de Rythmologie, Hôpital Cardiologique du Haut-Lévêque, Bordeaux-Pessac, France

Om Narayan MBBS (Hons) BmedSci Final Year Medical Student, The University of Melbourne and St. Vincent's Hospital, Melbourne, Australia

Akihiko Nogami, M.D. Clinical Associate Professor, Department of Cardiology, Tokyo Medical and Dental University, Bunkyo, Tokyo; Director of Clinical Cardiac Electrophysiology and Pacemaker Services, Department of Cardiology, Yokohama Rosai Hospital, Yokohama, Kanagawa, Japan

Paul Novak, M.D., FRCPC Fellow in Electrophysiology, Electrophysiology Service, Department of Medicine, Montreal Heart Institute, Montreal, Quebec, Canada

Jeffrey Olgin, M.D. Associate Professor in Residence, Chief Cardiac Electrophysiology, Cardiac Electrophysiology, Division of Cardiology, Department of Medicine, University of California San Francisco, San Francisco, California

Carlo Pappone, M.D., FACC Professor of Cardiology, Director of Research, Cardiology and Cardiac Surgery, University San Raffaele; Chief of Electrophysiology and Cardiac Pacing Unit, San Raffaele Hospital, Milan, Italy

Basilios Petrellis, MB, BS, FRACP Consultant, Arrhythmia Service, Division of Cardiology, University of Toronto, St. Michael's Hospital, Toronto, Ontario, Canada

Vivek Y. Reddy, M.D. Harvard Medical School; Director, Experimental Electrophysiology Laboratory, Cardiac Arrhythmia Service, Massachusetts General Hospital, Boston, Massachusetts

Jaime Rivera, M.D. Research Electrophysiology Fellow, Division of Cardiovascular Medicine, University of Florida, Gainesville, Florida

Alexander S. Ro, M.D. Clinical Instructor, Electrophysiology, Northwestern University; Director, Cardiac Device Therapies, Department of Electrophysiology, Evanston Northwestern Healthcaer, Evanston, Illinois

Thomas Rostock, M.D. Service de Rythmologie Hopital Cardiologique du Haut Leveque, Bordeaux-Pessac, France

Martin Rotter, M.D. Service de Rythmologie Hopital Cardiologique du Haut Leveque, Bordeaux-Pessac, France

Frederic Sacher Universite Bordeaux II, Hopital Cardiologique, Bordeaux-Pessac, France

Damian Sanchez-Quintana Professor of Human Anatomy, Department of Human Anatomy and Cell Biology, Faculty of Medicine, University of Extremadura, Badajoz, Spain

Vincenzo Santinelli, M.D. Professor of Cardiology, Scientific Director of Electrophysiology, Department of Cardiology and Cardiac Surgery, University San Raffaele; Cardiology, Electrophysiology, Cardiac Pacing Unit, San Raffaele Hospital, Milan, Italy

J. Philip Saul, M.D., FACC Professor of Pediatrics; Chief, Pediatric Cardiology, Department of Pediatrics, Medical University of South Carolina, Charleston, South Carolina

Prashanthan Sanders, MBBS (Hons.), PhD, FRACP W.H. Knapman, National Heart Foundation of Australia Chair of Cardiology Research, Deparment of Medicine, University of Adelaide; Director, Cardiac Electrophysiology, Department of Cardiology, Royal Adelaide Hospital, Adelaide, South Australia, Australia; Clinical and Research Associate, Sevice de Rythmologie, Hopital Cardiologique du Haut-Leveque, Bordeaux-Pessac, France

Mauricio Scanavacca, M.D., Ph.D. Assistant Professor, Department of Cardiology, Sao Paulo Medical School University; Electrophysiology Laboratory Supervisor, Department of Cardiology, Heart Institute, Sao Paulo Medical School, Sao Paulo, Brazil

David Schwartzman, M.D. Associate Professor of Medicine, Cardiovascular Institute, University of Pittsburgh, Pittsburgh, Pennsylvania

Allan Skanes, M.D., FRCPC Associate Professor of Medicine, University of Western Ontario; Director, Electrophysiology Laboratory, Division of Cardiology, London Health Sciences Center, London, Ontario, Canada

Eduardo Sosa, M.D. Associate Professor and Director of Clinical Arrhythmia and Pacemaker Unit, Clinical Division, Heart Institute—InCor-HC.FMUSP, Sao Paulo, Brazil

Uma N. Srivatsa, M.D. Assistant Professor of Medicine, Division of Cardiology, University of California Davis Medical Center, Sacramento, California

Ching-Tai Tai, M.D. Professor, Department of Medicine, Division of Cardiology, Yang-Ming University School of Medicine; Attending Physician, Department of Medicine, Division of Cardiology, Taipei Veterans General Hospital, Taipei, Taiwan

Yoshihide Takahashi, M.D. Universite Victor Segalen Bordeaux 2; Clinical Research Fellow, Service de Rythmologie, Hopital Cardiologique du Haut-Leveque, Pessac-Bordeaux, France

George F. Van Hare, M.D. Professor, Department of Pediatrics, Stanford University; Director, Pediatric Arrhythmia Center, Lucile Packard Children's Hospital, Palo Alto; Director, Pediatric Arrhythmia Center, University of California San Francisco Children's Hospital, San Francisco, California

Edward P. Walsh, M.D. Associate Professor, Department of Pediatrics, Harvard Medical School; Chief, Electrophysiology Division, Department of Cardiology, Children's Hospital, Boston, Massachusetts

Paul J. Wang, M.D. Professor of Medicine, Cardiovascular Medicine, Stanford University School of Medicine; Director, Cardiac Arrhythmia Service and Cardiac Electrophysiology Laboratory, Stanford University Medical Center, Stanford, California

David Wilber, M.D. George M. Eisenberg Professor of Cardiovascular Sciences, Loyola Stritch School of Medicine; Director, Division of Cardiology and Cardiovascular Institute, Loyola University Medical Center, Maywood, Illinois

Mark A. Wood, M.D. Professor of Medicine, Co-Director, Cardiac Electrophysiology Service, Virginia Commonwealth University Medical Center, Richmond, Virginia

Anil V. Yadav, M.D., FACC Assistant Professor of Clinical Medicine, Department of Medicine, Indiana University, Indianapolis, Indiana

Raymond Yee, M.D. Professor, Department of Medicine, University of Western Ontario; Director, Department of Cardiology, Arrhythmias Services, London Health Sciences Center, UC, London, Ontario

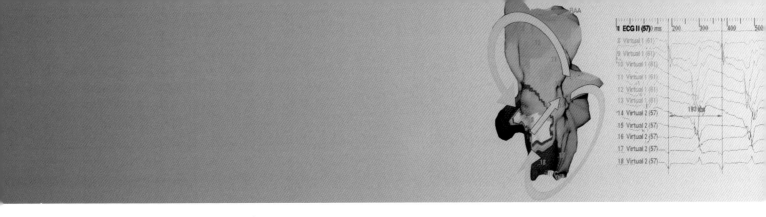

Preface

It has been over 20 years since the introduction of catheter ablation techniques for curative approaches to cardiac arrhythmias, first with direct-current, later with radiofrequency and most recently with cryo energy. There were some other energy sources (such as microwave, ultrasound, and laser, etc.) that had been applied in experimental use. New knowledge and ablation techniques have evolved in the past two decades. As such, we believe that a contemporary and comprehensive textbook is needed at this time as an accessible resource and reference for everyday use in the electrophysiology laboratory or office setting. Our goal is to produce a book that clinical electrophysiologists, trainees, and industry personnel will use as a practical guide to assist in patient care, to aid teaching, and to prepare for board examination in clinical cardiac electrophysiology.

To achieve our goal, we have designed the book in a unique chapter format that distinguishes itself from all the previously published books on catheter ablation. We strived for consistent organization of the content of each chapter. For chapters covering specific arrhythmia ablation (chapters 10-31), we include the topics from anatomy, pathophysiology, mapping, differential diagnosis to ablation techniques, and troubleshooting the difficult cases. In such chapters, we also use consistent tables to outline certain important information for quick reference. These tables include the key points, diagnostic criteria, target sites for ablation, and troubleshooting problems, and their solutions. Numerous color illustrations and high-quality figures are utilized to achieve the state-of-the-art publication that is unmatched among publications in the field. Our book is published in full color and in letter-sized page.

The book is divided into several parts. Part I (chapters 1-5) is devoted to the fundamental concepts of energy applications, including biophysics and monitoring system of radiofrequency ablation, updated reviews of catheter irrigation system and cryo energy ablation, and introduction of alternative energy sources, such as ultrasound, microwave and laser. A thorough understanding of these basic concepts is a prerequisite for appropriate clinical practice. Part II (chapters 6-9) introduces contemporary cardiac mapping and imaging techniques including advanced catheter mapping and navigation systems and intracardiac echocardiography to assist accurate diagnosis and ablation. Parts III-VII (chapters 10-31) provide the most important and practical approaches to the ablation of specific cardiac arrhythmias: atrial tachycardia and flutter, atrial fibrillation (this section is specifically expanded), atrioventricular nodal reentrant tachycardia, tachycardias related to accessory atrioventricular connections, and ventricular tachycardia. The final part (chapters 32-34) addresses special issues of patient safety, complications, transseptal catheterization, and ablation for pediatric patients.

Each chapter is written by experienced and recognized experts with hopes to provide the most comprehensive and detailed ablation text published to date. We wish that this book will become a standard reference text in many years to come. With your continued encouragement, we seek to publish future editions to provide updated information in the field of catheter ablation for treating cardiac arrhythmias.

Shoei K. Stephen Huang, M.D.
Mark A. Wood, M.D.

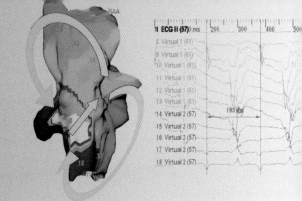

Acknowledgments

We are in debt to all of the contributing authors, many of whom are the leading experts in this field. We thank our colleagues at our respective institutions for their encouragement and support during the preparation of this book. Special thanks are owed to Ms. Anne Lenehan (former cardiology publisher) and Vera Ginsburgs of Elsevier, who accepted our initial proposal and worked diligently with us toward the publication of this book. We are equally grateful to Susan Pioli, the cardiology publisher of Elsevier, for her continued support, encouragement and faith in this project. Additional thanks should be given to everyone at Elsevier, who devoted their time and efforts in an incredibly professional manner to bring this book to successful completion.

Shoei K. Stephen Huang, M.D.
Mark A. Wood, M.D.

Foreword

It is indeed both fitting and desirable to review the current status of catheter ablation for cardiac arrhythmias approximately 25 years after it was introduced into clinical medicine. I very much enjoyed and learned a great deal from my review of this excellent textbook edited by two pre-eminent authorities in this area. Although the work uses multiple authors, consistent themes are found within each chapter. This includes a view of: key points before each chapter, basic physiology, use of special equipment or techniques, clinical results and emphasis on troubleshooting practical problems arising in the course of ablation. The latter is particularly valuable for the practicing "clinical ablators."

I was particularly pleased by the authors' consistent ability to meld pathophysiology with appropriate diagnostic techniques in an effort to make the ablative procedures both comprehensible and easy to follow. The ability of the text to integrate recent advances in technology was exceptional. Discussed are the uses of newer mapping techniques including anatomic mapping, and non-contact mapping, as well as indications for navigational and/or robotic catheter systems. In addition, discussed in each of the sections and where appropriate in separate chapters are updated reviews of newer energy systems including use of both internal as well as external catheter-saline irrigation systems and use of cryo energy for ablation. Especially appreciated is the attention devoted to indications for use of epicardial ablation approaches for care of difficult cardiac arrhythmias.

Each of the chapters are written by recognized experts and the literature review is both extensive and complete, making it easy for one to check the relevant newer contributions for each of the arrhythmias. The text is very complete in terms of exploring use of ablative techniques for both common as well as unusual cardiac arrhythmias. The authors very nicely supplement the text with figures that are clear and practical.

In summary, I am indeed pleased to highly commend the authors for an excellent and important contribution to the area of catheter ablation. This text should find a welcome home both for those beginning their cardiac electrophysiology training as well as for more experienced clinicians. We hope that the contributions over the next 25 years will be equally productive.

—*Melvin M. Scheinman, M.D.*

Fundamental Concepts of Trans-Catheter Energy Applications

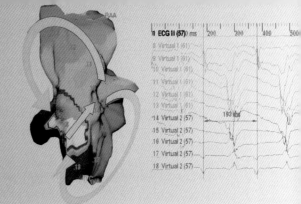

1

Biophysics of Radiofrequency Lesion Formation

David E. Haines

Key Points

- Radiofrequency (RF) energy induces thermal lesion formation through resistive heating of myocardial tissue. Tissue temperatures of 50°C or higher are necessary for irreversible injury.

- Under controlled conditions, RF lesion size is directly proportional to delivered power, electrode-tissue interface temperature, electrode diameter, and contact pressure.

- Power density declines with the square of distance from the source and tissue temperature declines inversely with distance from the heat source.

- The ultimate RF lesion size is determined by the zone of acute necrosis as well as the region of microvascular injury.

- Electrode cooling reduces the efficiency of tissue heating. For a fixed energy delivery, blood flow over the electrode-tissue interface reduces lesion size by convective tissue cooling. Cooled ablation increases lesion size by increasing the power that can be delivered before limiting electrode temperatures are achieved.

When Huang et al. first introduced radiofrequency (RF) catheter ablation in 1985 as a potentially useful modality for the management of cardiac arrhythmias, few would have predicted its meteoric rise. In the past two decades, it has become one of the most useful and widely employed therapies in the field of cardiac electrophysiology. RF catheter ablation has enjoyed a high efficacy and safety profile, and indications for its use continue to expand. Improvements in catheter design have continued to enhance the operator's ability to target the arrhythmogenic substrate, and modifications to RF energy delivery and electrode design have resulted in more effective energy coupling to the tissue. It is likely that most operators view RF catheter ablation as a "black box" in that, once the target is acquired, they need only push the button on the RF generator. However, gaining insight into the biophysics of RF energy delivery and the mechanisms of tissue injury in response to this intervention will help the clinician optimize catheter ablation and ultimately may enhance its efficacy and safety.

Biophysics of Tissue Heating

RF energy is a form of alternating electrical current that generates a lesion in the heart by electrical heating of the myocardium. A common form of RF ablation found in the medical environment is the electrocautery employed for tissue cutting and coagulation during surgical procedures. The goal of catheter ablation with RF energy is to effectively transform electromagnetic energy into thermal energy in the tissue, destroying the arrhythmogenic tissues by heating them to a lethal temperature. The mode of tissue heating by RF energy is resistive (electrical) heating. As electrical current passes through a resistive medium, the voltage drops and heat is produced (similar to the heat that is created in an incandescent light bulb). The RF electrical current is typically delivered in a unipolar fashion, with completion of the circuit via an indifferent electrode placed on the skin. Typically, an oscillation frequency of 500 kHz is selected. Lower frequencies are more likely to stimulate cardiac muscle and nerves, resulting in arrhythmia generation and pain sensation. Higher frequencies result in tissue heating, but in the MHz range, the mode of energy transfer changes from electrical (resistive) heating to dielectric heating (as observed with microwave energy). With very high frequencies, conventional electrode catheters become less effective at transferring the electromagnetic energy to the tissue, and complex and expensive catheter "antenna" designs must be employed.[1]

Resistive heating of tissue is proportional to the RF power density, which, in turn, is proportional to the square of the current density. When RF energy is delivered in a unipolar fashion, the current distributes radially from the source. The current density decreases in proportion to the square of the distance from the RF electrode source. Thus, direct resistive heating of the tissue decreases proportionally with the distance from the electrode raised to the fourth power (Fig. 1–1). As a result, only the narrow rim of tissue in close contact with the catheter electrode (2 to 3 mm) is heated directly. All heating of deeper tissue layers occurs passively through heat conduction.[2] If higher power levels are used, the depth of direct resistive heating is increased, and the size and radius of the virtual heat source are increased as well. Key equations related to the biophysics of RF ablation are listed in Table 1–1.

Most of the tissue heating that results in lesion formation during RF catheter ablation occurs as a result of thermal conduction from the direct resistive heat source. Transfer of heat through tissue follows basic thermodynamic principles and is represented by the bioheat transfer equation.[3] The tissue temperature change with increasing distance from the heat source is called the *radial temperature gradient*. The steady-state relationship of tissue temperature to distance from the electrode is described in equation 4 of Table 1–1. At onset of RF energy delivery, the temperature is very high at the source of heating and falls off rapidly over a short distance. As time progresses, more thermal energy is transferred to deeper tissue layers by means of thermal conduction. The rise of tissue temperature at any given distance from the heat source increases in a monoexponential fashion

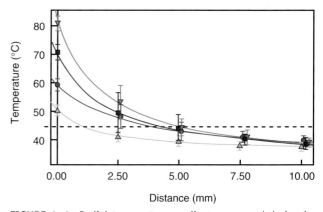

FIGURE 1–1. Radial temperature gradients measured during in vitro catheter ablation with source temperatures varying from 50° C to 80° C. The tissue temperature falls in inverse proportion to distance from the electrode. The dashed line represents the 50° C isothermal line. The point at which the radial temperature gradient crosses the 50° C isotherm determines the boundary of the lesion. A higher source temperature results in a greater lesion depth.

TABLE 1–1	
Equations Describing Biophysics of Radiofrequency Ablation	
$V = IR$	Ohm's Law: V, voltage; I, current; R, resistance
$Power = VI (\cos \dot{\alpha})$	Cos $\dot{\alpha}$ represents the phase shift between voltage (V) and current (I) in alternating current
$Current\ Density = I/4\pi r^2$	I, total electrode current; r, distance from electrode center
$H \approx pI^2/16\pi^2 r^4$	H, heat production per unit volume of tissue; p, tissue resistivity; I, current; r, distance from the electrode center
$r/r_i = (t_0 - T)/(t - T)$	Relationship between tissue temperature and distance from heat source in an ideal system: r, distance from center of heat source; r_i, radius of heat source; t_0, temperature at electrode tissue interface; T, basal tissue temperature; t, temperature at radius r*

*From Haines DE, Watson DD, Verow AF: Electrode radius predicts lesion radius during radiofrequency energy heating: Validation of a proposed thermodynamic model. Circ Res 67:124-129, 1990, with permission.

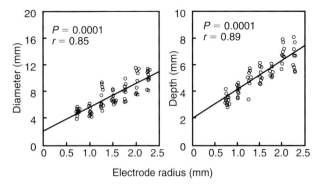

FIGURE 1–2. Lesion depth and diameter are compared with electrode radius in temperature-feedback power-controlled radiofrequency ablation. A larger-diameter ablation electrode results in higher power delivery and a proportional increase in lesion dimension. *(From Haines DE, Watson DD, Verow AF: Electrode radius predicts lesion radius during radiofrequency energy heating: Validation of a proposed thermodynamic model. Circ Res 67:124-129, 1990, with permission.)*

over time. Sites close to the heat source have a rapid rise in temperature (a short half-time of temperature rise), whereas sites remote from the source heat up more slowly.[4] Eventually, the entire electrode-tissue system reaches steady state, meaning that the amount of energy entering the tissue at the thermal source equals the amount of energy that is being dissipated at the tissue margins beyond the lesion border. At steady state, the radial temperature gradient becomes constant. If RF power delivery is interrupted before steady state is achieved, the tissue temperature will continue to rise in deeper tissue planes due to thermal conduction from more superficial layers that are heated to higher temperatures. In one study, the duration of continued temperature rise at the lesion border zone after a 10-second RF energy delivery was 6 seconds. The temperature rose an additional 3.4°C and remained above the temperature recorded at the termination of energy delivery for longer than 18 seconds. This phenomenon, termed *thermal latency,* has important clinical implications, because active ablation, with beneficial or adverse effects, continues for a period of time despite cessation of RF current flow.[5]

Because the mechanism of tissue injury in response to RF ablation is thermal, the final peak temperature at the border zone of the ablative lesion

should be relatively constant. Experimental studies predict this temperature with hyperthermic ablation to be approximately 50°C.[1] This is called the isotherm of irreversible tissue injury. The point where the radial temperature gradient crosses the 50°C isothermal line defines the lesion radius in that dimension. One can predict the three-dimensional (3-D) temperature gradients with thermodynamic modeling and finite element analysis and by doing so can predict the anticipated lesion dimensions and geometry with the 50°C isotherm. In an idealized medium of uniform thermal conduction without convective heat loss, a number of relationships can be defined using boundary conditions when a steady-state radial temperature gradient is achieved. In this theoretical model, it is predicted that the radial temperature gradient is inversely proportional to the distance from the heat source. The 50°C isotherm boundary (lesion radius) increases in distance from the source in direct proportion to the temperature at that source. It was predicted, then demonstrated experimentally, that, in the absence of significant heat loss due to convective cooling, the lesion depth and diameter are best predicted by the electrode-tissue interface temperature.[2] In the clinical setting, however, the opposing effect of convective cooling by circulating blood flow diminishes the value of temperature monitoring to assess lesion size. The thermodynamic model also predicted, and then demonstrated, that the radius of the lesion is directly proportional to the radius of the heat source (Fig. 1–2).[6] If one considers the virtual heat source radius as the shell of direct resistive heating in tissue contiguous to the electrode, it is not surprising that larger electrode diameter, length, and contact area all result in a larger source radius and larger lesion size, and that this may result in enhanced procedural success. Higher power delivery not only increases the source temperature but also increases the radius of the heat source, thereby increasing lesion size in two ways. These theoretical means of increasing efficacy of RF catheter ablation have been realized in the clinical setting with large-tipped catheters and cooled-tip catheters.[7-9]

The relationship between the distance of the ablation catheter from the ablation target and the power requirements for clinical effect were tested in a Langendorff-perfused canine heart preparation. Catheter ablation of the right bundle branch was attempted at varying distances, while delivered power was increased in a step-wise fashion. The RF power required to block right bundle branch conduction increased exponentially with increasing distance from the catheter. At a distance of 4 mm, most RF energy deliveries reached the threshold of impedance rise before block was achieved. When pulsatile flow was streamed past the ablation electrode, the power required to cause the block increased fourfold.[10] The efficiency of heating diminished with cooling from circulating blood, and small increases in distance from the ablation target corresponded with large increases in ablation power requirements, emphasizing the importance of optimal targeting for successful catheter ablation.

In a uniform medium of a heat-resistant material, the steady-state radial temperature gradient should continue to shift deeper into the medium as the source temperature increases. A very high source temperature should, theoretically, yield a very deep $50°C$ isotherm temperature. Unfortunately, this process is limited in the biologic setting by the formation of coagulum and char at the electrode-tissue interface if temperatures exceed $100°C$. At $100°C$, blood literally begins to boil. As the blood and tissue in contact with the electrode catheter desiccate, the residue of denatured proteins adheres to the electrode surface. These substances are electrically insulating and result in a smaller electrode surface area available for electrical conduction. This concentrates the same magnitude of power over a smaller surface area, and the power density increases. With higher power density, the heat production increases and more coagulum forms. Thus, in a positive feedback fashion, the electrode becomes completely encased in coagulum in 1 to 2 seconds, ending effective power delivery and lesion formation. In a study testing ablation with a 2-mm-tip electrode in vitro and in vivo, a measured temperature of $100°C$ or higher correlated closely with a sudden rise in electrical impedance (Fig. 1–3).[11] Modern RF energy ablation systems all have an automatic energy cut-off if a rapid rise in electrical impedance is observed. Some experimenters have described soft thrombus that accumu-

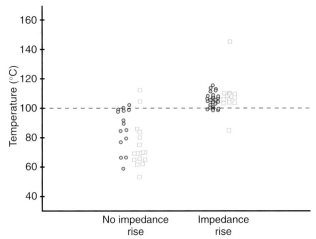

FIGURE 1–3. The association of measured electrode-tip temperature and sudden rise in electrical impedance is shown in this study of radiofrequency catheter ablation with a 2-mm-tip ablation electrode in vitro *(circles)* and in vivo *(squares)*. The peak temperature recorded at the electrode-tissue interface is shown. Almost all ablations without a sudden rise in electrical impedance had a peak temperature of $100°C$ or less, whereas all but one ablation manifesting a sudden rise in electrical impedance had a peak temperature greater than $100°C$. *(From Haines DE, Verow AF: Observations on electrode-tissue interface temperature and effect on electrical impedance during radiofrequency ablation of ventricular myocardium. Circulation 82:1038, 1990, with permission.)*

lates when temperatures exceed $80°C$.[12] This is probably caused by blood protein denaturation and accumulation, but fortunately it appears to be more of a laboratory phenomenon than one observed in the clinical setting. When high temperatures and sudden rises in electrical impedance are observed, there is concern about the accumulation of char and coagulum, with the subsequent risk of char embolism. Anticoagulation and antiplatelet therapies have been proposed as preventive measures,[13] but avoidance of excessive heating at the electrode-tissue interface remains the best strategy to avoid this risk.

The major thermodynamic factor opposing the transfer of thermal energy to deeper tissue layers is convective cooling. Convection is the process whereby heat is distributed through a medium rapidly by active mixing of that medium. In the case of RF catheter ablation, the heat is produced by resistive heating and transferred to deeper layers by thermal conduction. Simultaneously, the heat is conducted back into the circulating blood pool and to the metal electrode tip. Heating of the electrode is therefore passive. Because the blood is moving rapidly past the electrode and over the endocardial surface, and because water (the main constituent of blood) has a high heat capacity, a large amount of the heat produced at the site of ablation can be carried away by the blood. Convective cooling is such an important factor that it dominates the thermodynamics of catheter ablation.[14] Efficiency of energy coupling to the tissue can be as low as 10% depending on electrode size, catheter stability, and catheter position relative to intracavitary blood flow.[15] In the clinical ablation setting, tip cooling may be accomplished in several ways. Unstable, sliding catheter contact results in significant tip cooling and decreased efficiency of tissue heating.[16] This is most often observed with ablation along the tricuspid or mitral valve annuli.

Investigators have taken advantage of the convective cooling phenomenon to increase lesion size. As noted earlier, maximum power delivery is limited by the occurrence of boiling and coagulum formation at the electrode tip. If the tip is cooled, a higher amplitude of power may be delivered without a sudden rise in electrical impedance. The higher amplitude of power increases the depth of direct resistive heating and, in turn, increases the radius of the effective heat source. In addition, higher temperatures are achieved 3 to 4 mm below the surface, and the entire radial temperature curve over greater tissue depths is shifted to a higher temperature. The result is a greater 50°C isotherm radius and a greater depth and diameter of the lesion. Nakagawa et al.[17] demonstrated this phenomenon in a blood-superfused exposed thigh muscle preparation. In this study, intramural tissue temperatures 3.5 mm from the surface averaged 95°C with an irrigated-tip catheter despite a mean electrode-tissue interface temperature of 69°C. Lesion depths were 9.9 mm, compared with 6.1 mm in a comparison group treated with temperature-feedback power-controlled delivery and no electrode irrigation (Fig. 1–4). An important finding of this study was that 6 of 75 lesions had a sudden rise in electrical impedance associated with an audible pop. In these cases, the intramural temperature exceeded 100°C, resulting in sudden steam formation and a steam pop. The clinical concern about "pop lesions" is that sudden steam venting to the endocardial or epicardial surface (or both) can potentially cause perforation and tamponade.[17]

The observation of increasing lesion size with ablation tip cooling holds true as long as the ablation is not power limited. If only limited power is applied, however, convective cooling dissipates a greater proportion of energy, and less of the available RF energy is converted into tissue heat. The resulting lesion may be smaller than it would have been had there been no convective cooling. Convective electrode tip cooling can lead to paradoxical observations. For example, it has been demonstrated that lesion size may be inversely related to the electrode-tissue interface temperature if the ablation is not power

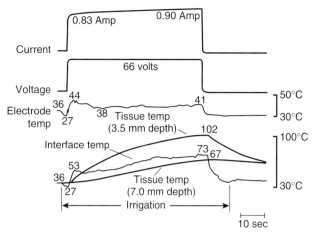

FIGURE 1–4. Current, voltage, and temperature values measured during radiofrequency catheter ablation with a perfused-tip electrode catheter in a canine exposed thigh muscle preparation. Temperatures were recorded within the electrode, at the electrode-tissue interface, and within the muscle below the ablation catheter at depths of 3.5 and 7 mm. Because the electrode-tissue interface is actively cooled, high current and voltage levels can be employed. This results in an increased depth of direct resistive heating and superheating of the tissue below the surface of ablation. In this example, the peak temperature was 102°C at a depth of 3.5 mm, and 67°C at 7 mm, indicating that the 50°C isotherm defining the lesion border was significantly deeper than 7 mm. *(From Nakagawa H, Yamanashi WS, Pitha JV, et al.: Comparison of in vivo tissue temperature profile and lesion geometry for radiofrequency ablation with a saline-irrigated electrode versus temperature control in a canine thigh muscle preparation. Circulation 91:2264-2273, 1995, with permission.)*

limited.[18] However, if the power level is fixed, then lesion size increases in proportion to the electrode-tissue interface temperature even in the setting of significant convective cooling (Fig. 1–5).[19]

Electrode tip cooling can be achieved passively or actively. Passive tip cooling occurs when the circulating blood flow cools the mass of the ablation electrode and cools the electrode-tissue interface. This can be enhanced by use of a large-tip ablation electrode.[20] Active tip cooling can be realized with a closed or open perfused-tip system. In each case, circulating saline from an infusion pump actively cools the electrode tip. One design recirculates the saline through a return port; another infuses the saline through weep holes in the electrode into the blood stream. Both designs are effective and result in larger lesions and greater procedure efficacy than with standard RF catheter ablation.[21-23] The tip cooling or perfusion has the apparent advantage of reducing the prevalence of coagulum and char formation. However, because the peak tissue temperature is shifted from the endocardial surface to deeper intramyocardial layers, there is the risk of excessive intramural heating and "pop" lesions. Cooling at the

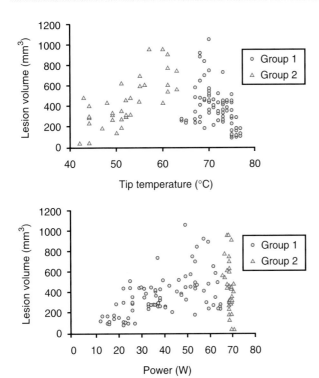

FIGURE 1–5. Temperatures measured at the tip of the electrode during experimental radiofrequency ablation and power were compared with the resulting lesion volumes in this study. A maximum power of 70 W was employed. If lesion creation was not power limited (group 1), then lesion volume was a function of the delivered power. But if lesion production was limited by the 70 W available power maximum (group 2), then the temperature measured at the electrode tip correlated with lesion size. *(From Petersen HH, Chen X, Pietersen A, et al.: Lesion dimensions during temperature-controlled radiofrequency catheter ablation of left ventricular porcine myocardium: Impact of ablation site, electrode size, and convective cooling. Circulation 99:319-325, 1999, with permission.)*

electrode-tissue interface limits the value of temperature monitoring to prevent excess power delivery and steam pops, but if temperatures are maintained below 45°C, these may be avoided.[24]

One of the great advantages of conventional RF ablation since its inception has been its excellent safety profile. This undoubtedly has been a result of the relatively shallow depth of lesion production. Despite the routine positioning of ablation catheters in close proximity to coronary arteries, there have been few coronary arterial complications with this procedure. As new catheter technologies designed to increase the depth of the ablative lesion are employed, it is expected that complications due to collateral damage will increase. For example, left atrial ablation with large-tip ablation catheters has resulted in sporadic cases of esophageal injury, perforation, and death. The blood flow within the coronary artery is rapid, and the zone of tissue around the artery is convectively cooled by this blood flow. Fuller and Wood[25] tested the effect of flow rate through a marginal artery of Langendorff-perfused rabbit hearts. RF ablation with an electrode-tissue interface temperature of 60°C or 80°C was performed on the right ventricular free wall with two lesions straddling the artery, and conduction through this region was monitored. They observed that arterial flow rates as low as 1 mL/min through these small (0.34 ± 0.1 mm diameter) arteries prevented complete transmural ablation and conduction block.[25] This heat sink effect is especially protective of the vascular endothelium. But with higher power output and new ablation technologies, the convective cooling of the arterial flow may be overwhelmed and there may be increased risk of vascular injury. With greater destructive power possible, operators need to be mindful to use only enough power to achieve complete ablation of the targeted tissue in order to safely accomplish the goal of arrhythmia ablation.

Current Distribution and Tissue Heating

Catheter ablation depends on the passage of RF electrical current through tissue. Tissue contact can be assessed by measuring baseline system impedance. In one clinical study,[26] a very small (10 μA) current was passed through the ablation catheter, and the efficiency of heating was measured to assess tissue contact. A significant positive correlation between preablation impedance and heating efficiency was observed. As tissue is heated, there is a temperature-dependent fall in the electrical impedance. In this same study, a significant correlation was also observed between heating efficiency and the maximum drop in impedance during energy delivery.[26] When electrode-tissue interface temperature monitoring is unreliable due to high-magnitude convective cooling, the slow impedance drop is a useful indicator that tissue heating is occurring. With the progressive fall in impedance during ablation, the delivered current increases along with tissue heating.[27]

As previously described, the magnitude of tissue heating is proportional to the square of the power density, or the current density to the fourth power. Therefore, the distribution of the RF field around the electrodes in unipolar, bipolar, or phased RF energy delivery determines the distribution of tissue heating. If energy is delivered in a unipolar fashion in a uniform medium from a spherical electrode to an indifferent electrode with infinite surface area, then current density around the electrode should be entirely uniform. Standard 4-mm electrode tips are small enough so that heating around the tip is fairly uniform, even with varying tip contact angle to the tissue. One study showed that temperature monitoring with a thermistor located at the tip of a 4-mm-tip electrode underestimated the peak electrode-tissue interface temperature recorded from multiple temperature sensors distributed around the electrode in only 4% of the applications. In RF applications in which high power was employed and a sudden rise in electrical impedance occurred, the peak temperature recorded from the electrode tip was lower than 95°C in only 1 of 17 cases.[28] However, present-day electrode geometries vary considerably. Also, tissue characteristics and placements of indifferent electrodes affect tissue heating. Surface temperature recordings routinely underestimate peak subendocardial tissue temperatures. An understanding of the pattern of the RF current field in vivo is needed to comprehend all of the factors that affect formation of the final ablative lesion.

The power dissipated in the complete circuit is proportional to the voltage drop and impedance for each part of the series circuit. The inherent resistance of the ablation system and transmission lines is low, so most of the delivered power is dissipated in the body. The site of greatest impedance, voltage drop, and power dissipation is at the electrode-tissue interface. However, a significant amount of power is also lost due to electrical conduction through the body and into the dispersive electrode. The return path of current to the indifferent electrode certainly affects the current density near that indifferent electrode, but its placement (anterior versus posterior, high versus low on the torso) has only a small effect on the distribution of RF current field lines within millimeters of the electrode in most cases. Therefore, lesion geometry should not be affected greatly by dispersive electrode placement. However, the proportion of RF energy that contributes to lesion formation will be reduced if a greater proportion of that energy is dissipated in a longer return pathway to the dispersive electrode. This is particularly the case if RF energy delivery is power limited. In an experiment that compared placement of the dispersive electrode directly opposite the ablation electrode with placement at a more remote site, lesion depth was increased by 26% with optimal placement.[29] When the ablation is power limited, it is advantageous to minimize the proportion of energy that is dissipated along the current pathway at sites other than the electrode-tissue interface in order to achieve the greatest magnitude of tissue heating and the largest lesion. Vigorous skin preparation to minimize impedance at the interface of skin with the dispersive electrode,

closer placement of the dispersive electrode to the heart, and use of multiple dispersive electrodes to increase skin contact area all increase tissue heating in a power-limited energy delivery. Nath et al.[30] reported that in the setting of a system impedance greater than 100 ohms, adding a second dispersive electrode increased the peak electrode-tip temperature during clinical catheter ablation (Fig. 1–6).

It is not surprising that electrical field lines are not entirely uniform around the tip of a unipolar ablation electrode. The distribution of field lines from an electrode source is affected by changes in geometry. At points of geometric transition, the field lines become more concentrated. This so-called edge effect can result in significant non-uniformity of heating around electrodes. The less symmetrical the electrode design (such as is found with long electrodes), the greater the degree of non-uniform heating. McRury et al.[31] tested ablation with electrodes of 12.5 mm. They found that a centrally placed temperature sensor significantly underestimated the peak electrode-tissue interface temperature. Finite element analysis demonstrated a concentration of electrical current at each of the electrode edges (Fig. 1–7). When dual thermocouples were placed on the edge of the electrode, the risk of coagulum formation and

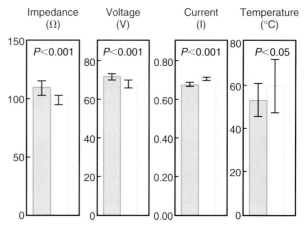

| Single dispersive electrode | Double dispersive electrode |

FIGURE 1–6. Impedance, voltage, current, and catheter-tip temperature readings during radiofrequency catheter ablation in a subset of patients with a baseline system impedance greater than 100 ohms. Ablations using a single dispersive electrode were compared with those using a double dispersive electrode. A lower system impedance was observed with addition of the second dispersive patch. This resulted in greater current delivery and higher temperatures measured at the electrode-tissue interface. Values shown are means and standard deviations. *(From Nath S, DiMarco JP, Gallop RG, et al.: Effects of dispersive electrode position and surface area on electrical parameters and temperature during radiofrequency catheter ablation. Am J Cardiol 77:765-767, 1996, with permission.)*

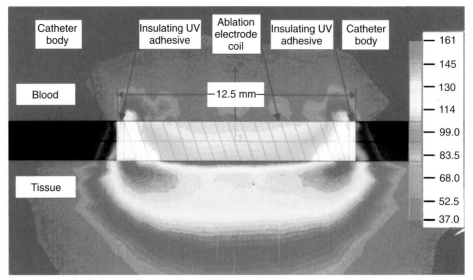

FIGURE 1–7. Steady-state temperature distribution derived from a finite element analysis of radiofrequency ablation with a 12-mm-long coil electrode. In this analysis, the temperature at the center of the electrode was maintained at 71° C. The legend of temperatures is shown at the right of the graph and ranges from the physiologic normal temperature, 37° C *(violet)*, to the maximum tissue temperature, 161° C *(red)*, located below the electrode edges. There is a significant gradient of heating between the peak temperatures at the electrode edges and the temperature at the center of the electrode. *(From McRury ID, Panescu D, Mitchell MA, Haines DE: Nonuniform heating during radiofrequency catheter ablation with long electrodes: Monitoring the edge effect. Circulation 96:4057-4064, 1997, with permission.)*

impedance rise was significantly reduced during ablation testing in vivo.[31] Despite the fact that temperature monitoring during catheter ablation enhances the safety of this procedure and provides some feedback to the operator about adequacy of electrode contact with the tissue and efficiency of tissue heating, there are enough variables affecting the measured temperature that one cannot rely solely on this measurement to assess ablation efficacy.

Tissue Pathology and Response to Radiofrequency Ablation

The endocardial surface in contact with the ablation catheter shows pallor and sometimes a small depression due to volume loss of the acute lesion. If excessive power has been applied, there may be visible coagulum or char adherent to the ablation site. On sectioning, the gross appearance of the acute lesion produced by RF energy is characterized by a central zone of pallor and tissue desiccation. There is volume loss, and the lesion frequently has a teardrop shape, with a narrower lesion width in the immediate subendocardial region and a wider width 2 to 3 mm below the endocardial surface. This occurs because of

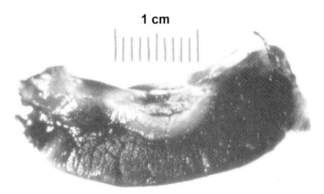

FIGURE 1–8. Typical appearance of radiofrequency catheter ablation lesion. There is a small central depression with volume loss, surrounded by an area of pallor, and then a hemorrhagic border zone. The specimen has been stained with nitro blue tetrazolium to differentiate viable from nonviable tissue.

surface convective cooling by the endocardial blood flow. Immediately outside the pale central zone is a band of hemorrhagic tissue. Beyond that border, the tissue appears relatively normal. The acute lesion border, as assessed by vital staining, correlates with the border between the hemorrhagic and normal tissue (Fig. 1–8). The histologic appearance of the lesion is consistent with coagulation necrosis. Contraction bands in the sarcomeres, nuclear pyknosis, and basophilic stippling consistent with intracellular calcium overload are present.[32]

The temperature at the border zone of an acute hyperthermic lesion assessed by vital staining with nitro blue tetrazolium (NBT) is 52°C to 55°C.[1] However, it is likely that the actual isotherm of irreversible thermal injury occurs at a lower temperature boundary, outside the lesion boundary, that cannot be identified acutely. Coagulation necrosis is a manifestation of thermal inactivation of the contractile and cytoskeletal proteins in the cell. Changes in the appearance of vital stains are caused by loss of enzyme activity, as is the case with NBT staining and dehydrogenase activity.[33] Therefore, the acute assessment of the lesion border represents the border of thermal inactivation of various proteins, but the ultimate viability of the cell may depend on the integrity of more thermally sensitive organelles such as the plasma membrane (see later discussion). In the clinical setting, recorded temperature does correlate with response to ablation. In patients with manifest Wolff-Parkinson-White syndrome, reversible accessory pathway conduction block was observed at a mean temperature of 50°C ± 8°C, whereas permanent block occurred at a temperature of 62°C ± 15°C.[34] In a study of electrode-tip temperature monitoring during atrioventricular (AV) junctional ablation, an accelerated junctional rhythm was observed at a mean temperature of 51°C ± 4°C. Permanent complete heart block was observed at ablation temperatures of 60°C ± 7°C.[35] Because the targeted tissue was probably millimeters below the endocardial surface, the temperatures recorded by the catheter were most likely higher than those achieved intramurally at the critical site of ablation.

The subacute pathology of the RF lesion is similar to what is observed with other types of injury. The appearance of typical coagulation necrosis persists, but the lesion border becomes more sharply demarcated with infiltration of mononuclear inflammatory cells. A layer of fibrin adheres to the lesion surface, coating the area of endothelial injury. After 4 to 5 days, the transition zone at the lesion border is lost and the border between the RF lesion and surrounding tissue becomes sharply demarcated. The changes in the transition zone within the first hours and days after ablation probably account for the phenomena of early recurrence of arrhythmia (injury with recovery)[36] and delayed cure (progressive injury due to the secondary inflammatory response).[37] The coagulation necrosis in the body of the lesion shows early evidence of fatty infiltration. By 8 weeks after ablation, the necrotic zone has been replaced with fatty tissue, cartilage, and fibrosis and may be surrounded by chronic inflammation.[38] The chronic RF ablative lesion evolves to uniform scar. The uniformity of the healed lesion accounts for the absence of any proarrhythmic effect of RF catheter ablation, unless multiple lesions with gaps are made. As with any fibrotic scar, there is significant contraction of the scar with

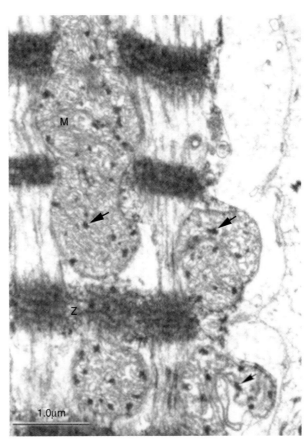

FIGURE 1–9. Electron micrograph of a myocardial sample 3 mm outside the border zone of acute injury created by radiofrequency catheter ablation. There is severe disruption of the sarcomere, with contracted Z bands, disorganized mitochondria (M), and basophilic stippling *(arrows)*. Bar scale is 1.0 μm. (33,000×) *(From Nath S, Redick JA, Whayne JG, Haines DE: Ultrastructural observations in the myocardium beyond the region of acute coagulation necrosis following radiofrequency catheter ablation. J Cardiovasc Electrophysiol 5:838-845, 1994, with permission.)*

healing. Relatively large and wide acute linear lesions have the final gross appearance of narrow lines of glistening scar when examined 6 months after the ablation procedure.[39]

The ultrastructural appearance of the acute RF lesion offers some insight into the mechanism of tissue injury at the lesion border zone. In cases of experimental RF ablation in vivo,[40] ventricular myocardium was examined in a band 3 mm from the edge of the acute pathologic lesion as defined by vital staining (Fig. 1–9). It showed marked disruption in cellular architecture characterized by dissolution of lipid membranes and inactivation of structural proteins. The plasma membranes were severely disrupted or missing. There was extravasation of erythrocytes and complete absence of basement membrane. The mitochondria showed marked distortion of architecture with swollen and discontinuous cristae membranes. The sarcomeres were extended with loss of myofilament structure or severely contracted. The T-tubules and sarcoplasmic reticulum were absent or severely disrupted. Gap junctions were severely distorted or absent. Therefore, despite the fact that the tissue examined was outside of the border of the acute pathologic lesion, the changes were profound enough to conclude that some progression of necrosis would occur within this border zone. The band of tissue 3 to 6 mm from the edge of the pathologic lesion was examined and manifested significant ultrastructural abnormalities, but not as severe as those described closer to the lesion core. Severe abnormalities of the plasma membrane were still present, but gap junctions and mitochondria were mainly intact. The sarcomeres were variable in appearance, with some relatively normal and some partially contracted. Although ultrastructural disarray was observed in the 3- to 6-mm zone, the myocytes appeared to be viable and would most likely recover from the injury.[40]

In addition to direct injury to the myocytes, RF-induced hyperthermia has an effect on the myocardial vasculature and on myocardial perfusion. Impairment of the microcirculation could contribute to lesion formation by an ischemic mechanism. A study examined the effects of microvascular perfusion during acute RF lesion formation.[41] In open-chest canine preparations, the left ventricle was imaged with ultrasound from the epicardial surface, and a myocardial echocardiographic contrast agent was injected into the left anterior descending artery during endocardial RF catheter ablation. After ablation, the center of the lesion showed no echo contrast, consistent with severe vascular injury and absence of blood flow to that region. In the border zone of the lesion, a halo effect of retained myocardial contrast was observed. This suggested marked slowing of the contrast transit rate through these tissues. The measured contrast transit rate at the boundary of the gross pathologic lesion was $25\% \pm 12\%$ of that in normal tissue. In the band of myocardium 3 mm outside the lesion edge, the contrast transit rate was $48\% \pm 27\%$ of normal, and in the 3- to 6-mm band it was $82\% \pm 28\%$ of normal ($P < .05$ for all comparisons). The ultrastructural appearance of the arterioles demonstrated marked disruption of the plasma membrane and basement membrane and extravasation of red blood cells in these regions of impaired myocardial perfusion. The relative contribution of microvascular injury and myocardial ischemia to ultimate lesion formation is unknown, but these mechanisms may play a role in lesion extension during the early postablation phases.[41]

The effect of RF heating on larger arteries is a function of the size of the artery, the arterial flow rate, and the proximity to the RF source. In one study,[25] the flow rate through a marginal artery (or intramural perfusion cannula) in an in vitro rabbit heart preparation was varied between 0 and 10 mL/min. A pair of epicardial ablations was produced with epicardial RF energy applications. Even at low flow rates, there was substantial sparing of the artery and the surrounding tissue due to the heat sink effect of the arterial flow (Fig. 1–10). However, if 45 W of power was applied along with RF electrode tip cooling, complete

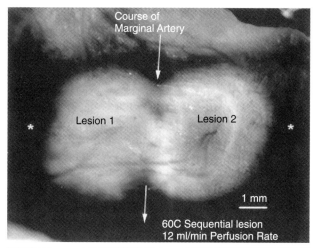

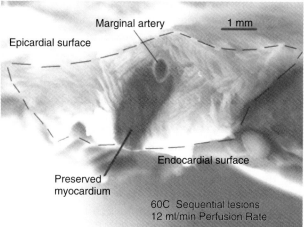

FIGURE 1–10. Top panel: Epicardial view of two radiofrequency lesions created during perfusion of a penetrating marginal artery. The lesions show central pallor that is apparent after vital staining. The course of the artery is marked *(arrows)*. The asterisks mark the line used for perpendicular sectioning of the lesion. **Bottom panel:** Cross-section through the middle of a lesion perpendicular to a marginal artery. The broken lines outline the lesion boundary. A region of preserved myocardium adjacent to the penetrating marginal artery *(labeled)* is apparent. Electrical conduction was present through this bridge of viable myocardium after ablation. *(From Fuller IA, Wood MA: Intramural coronary vasculature prevents transmural radiofrequency lesion formation: Implications for linear ablation. Circulation 107:1797-1803, 2003, with permission.)*

ablation of the tissue contiguous to the intramural perfusion cannula was achieved.[25] Although this may be a desirable effect in the setting of small perfusing arteries through a region of conduction critical for arrhythmia propagation, it is not desirable if the vessel is a large epicardial artery that happens to be contiguous to an ablation site, as is sometimes the case with accessory pathway or slow atrioventricular nodal pathway ablation or with ablation in the tricuspid-subeustachian isthmus for atrial flutter. Cases of arterial injury have been reported, particularly with the use of large-tip catheters or tip-cooling technologies that allow for application of high RF powers.[42,43] In particular, if high-power ablation is required within the coronary sinus or great cardiac vein, it is prudent to define the course of the arterial anatomy to avoid unwanted arterial thermal injury.

The injury to targeted myocardium is usually achieved if effort is made to optimize electrode-tissue contact. To ensure procedural success, particularly with ablation of more complex substrates such as that found with atrial fibrillation, operators have employed a number of large-lesion RF technologies such as cooled-tip, perfused-tip, or large-tip catheters. With deep lesions sometimes comes unintended collateral injury to contiguous structures. An understanding of the anatomic relationships and careful titration of RF energy delivery can avoid adverse consequences of ablation in most cases. One such unintended complication of ablation of atrial fibrillation has been pulmonary vein stenosis.[44] The target for pulmonary vein isolation has been the myocardial sleeve tissue that surrounds the base of the vein and sometimes extends 3 to 4 cm into the vein. If the temperature of the ablated tissue is too high, irreversible changes in the collagen and elastin of the vein wall occur. In vitro heating of pulmonary vein rings showed a 53% reduction in circumference and a loss of compliance with hyperthermic exposure at 70°C or higher; the histologic examination showed loss of the typical collagen structure, presumably due to thermal denaturation of that protein.[45] There are anecdotal reports of severe esophageal injury after RF ablation with a large-tip catheter in the posterior left atrium, emphasizing the importance of collateral injury.

Cellular Mechanisms of Thermal Injury

The therapeutic effect of RF catheter ablation results from electrical heating of tissue and thermal injury. The field of hyperthermia is broad, and the effects of long-duration exposures to mild and moderate hyperthermia have been well characterized in the oncology literature. Thermal injury is both time and temperature dependent. For example, if human bone marrow cells in culture are exposed to a temperature of 42°C, cell survival is 45% at 300 minutes. But if those cells are heated to 45.5°C, survival at 20 minutes is only 1%.[46] Data regarding the effects of brief exposure of myocardium to higher temperatures, as is the case during catheter ablation, are more limited and are reviewed in this section. The central zone of the ablation lesion reaches high temperatures and is simply coagulated. Lower temperatures are reached during the ablation in the border zones of the lesion. The responses of the various cellular components to low and moderate hyperthermia determine the pathophysiologic response to ablation. The thermally sensitive elements that are involved in the overall thermal injury to the myocyte include the plasma membrane with its integrated channel proteins, the nucleus, and the cytoskeleton. Changes in these structures that occur during hyperthermic exposure all contribute to the ultimate demise of the cell.

The plasma membrane is very thermally sensitive. A pure phospholipid bilayer undergoes phase transitions from a relatively solid form to a semiliquid form. Addition of integral proteins and the varying composition of the phospholipids with regard to saturation of the hydrocarbon side chains affect the degree of membrane fluidity in eukaryotic cells. In one study,[47] cultured mammalian cell membranes were found to have a phase transition at 8°C, and a second transition between 22°C and 36°C. No phase changes were seen in the 37°C to 45°C range, but studies have not been performed examining this phenomenon in sarcomeres, or at temperatures greater than 45°C.[47] Regarding the function of integral plasma membrane proteins during exposure to heating, both inhibition and accentuation of protein activity have been observed. Stevenson et al.[48] reported an increase in intracellular K^+ uptake in cultured Chinese hamster ovary (CHO) cells during heating to 42°C. This was blocked by ouabain, indicating an increased activity of the sodium-potassium adenosine triphosphatase (Na^+-K^+ ATPase) pump. Nath et al.[49] examined action potentials in vitro in a superfused guinea pig papillary muscle preparation. In the low hyperthermic range between 38°C and 45°C, there was an increase in the maximum rate of voltage rise (dV/dt) of the action potential, indicating enhanced sodium channel kinetics. In the moderate hyperthermia range from 45°C to 50°C, the maximum dV/dt decreased to less than baseline values. The mechanism of this sodium channel inhibition was hypothesized to be either partial thermal inactivation of the sodium channel or, more likely, voltage-dependent sodium channel inactivation resulting from thermally mediated cellular depolarization[49] (see later discussion).

The cytoskeleton is composed of structural proteins that form microtubules, microfilaments, and intermediate filaments. The microfilaments coalesce into stress filaments. These comprise the proteins actin, actinin, and tropomyosin and form the framework to which the contractile elements of the myocyte attach. The cytoskeletal elements may have varying degrees of thermal sensitivity depending on the cell type. For example, in human erythrocytes, the cytoskeleton is composed predominantly of the protein spectrin. Spectrin is thermally inactivated at 50°C. When erythrocytes are exposed to temperatures greater than 50°C, the erythrocytes rapidly lose their biconcave shape.[50] There is no scientific literature reporting the inactivation temperature of the cytoskeletal proteins in myocytes. However, electron micrographs of the border zone of RF lesions show significant disruption in the cellular architecture with loss of the myofilament structure.[40] In the central portion of the RF lesion, thermal inactivation of the cytoskeleton contributes to the typical appearance of coagulation necrosis.

The eukaryote nucleus shows evidence of thermal sensitivity in both structure and function. Nuclear membrane vesiculation, condensation of cytoplasmic elements in the perinuclear region, and a decrease in heterochromatin content have been described.[51,52] The nucleolus appears to be the most heat-sensitive component of the nucleus. Whether or not hyperthermia induces DNA strand breaks is controversial. One reproducible finding after hyperthermic exposure is the elaboration of nuclear proteins called heat shock proteins (HSP). The function of HSP has not been entirely elucidated, but they appear to exert a protective effect on the cell. It is hypothesized that HSP 70 facilitates the effective production and folding of proteins and assists their transit among organelles.[53]

Hyperthermia leads to dramatic effects on the electrophysiology of myocardium. The thermal sensitivity of myocytes has been tested in a variety of experimental systems, and the mechanisms of the electrophysiologic responses to catheter ablation have been elucidated. In one series of in vitro experiments,[49] isolated superfused guinea pig papillary muscles were subjected to 60 seconds of exposure to hyperthermic superfusate at temperatures varying from 38°C to 55°C. Action potentials were recorded continuously during and after the hyperthermic pulse. If resting membrane potential was not restored after return to normothermia, the muscle was discarded and testing proceeded with a new tissue sample. The resting membrane potential was assessed in unpaced preparations, and the action potential amplitude, duration, dV/dt, and excitability were tested during pacing. The preparations maintained a normal resting membrane potential in the low hyperthermic range (<45°C). In the intermediate hyperthermic range (45°C to 50°C), the myocytes showed a temperature-dependent depolarization that was reversible on return to normothermic superfusion. Finally, experiments in the high hyperthermic range (>50°C) typically resulted in irreversible depolarization, contracture, and death (Fig. 1–11). There was a temperature-dependent decrease in action potential amplitude between 37°C and 50°C, as well as an inverse linear relationship between temperature and action potential duration. With increasing temperatures, the dV/dt increased, but at temperatures greater than 46°C this measurement began to decrease in preparations that had a greater magnitude of resting membrane potential depolarization. Spontaneous automaticity was observed in both paced and unpaced preparations at a median temperature of 50°C, compared with 44°C in preparations without automaticity. The occurrence of automaticity in unpaced preparations in the setting of hyperthermia-induced depolarization suggested abnormal automaticity as the mechanism. Beginning at temperatures greater than 42°C, loss of excitability to external field stimulation was seen in some paced preparations and was dependent on the resting mem-

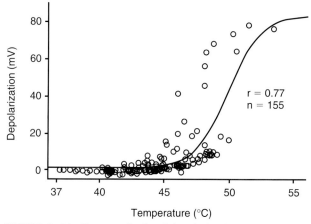

FIGURE 1–11. The magnitude of depolarization of guinea pig papillary muscle cells exposed to 1-minute pulses of hyperthermic perfusate versus perfusate temperature. At temperatures lower than 45°C, little depolarization is seen. The cells show progressive depolarization between 45°C and 50°C. At temperatures greater than 50°C, few recordings are made because most cells have undergone irreversible contracture and death. *(From Nath S, Lynch C III, Whayne JG, Haines DE: Cellular electrophysiological effects of hyperthermia on isolated guinea pig papillary muscle: Implications for catheter ablation. Circulation 88:1826-1831, 1993, with permission.)*

brane potential. Mean resting membrane potential observed with loss of excitability was –44 mV, compared with –82 mV for normal excitability. The superfusate temperature measured during reversible loss of excitability was 43°C to 51°C, but irreversible loss of excitability (cell death) occurred only at temperatures 50°C or greater.[49] Therefore, it appeared from these experiments that there was increased cationic entry into the hyperthermic cell, and that the resultant depolarization led to loss of excitability and cell death.

In a preparation similar to that just described, Everett et al.[54] further elucidated the specific mechanisms for cellular depolarization and death in response to hyperthermia. Isolated superfused guinea pig papillary muscles were attached to a force transducer to assess the pattern of contractility with varying hyperthermic exposure. Consistent with the observations of resting membrane potential changes during heating, there was a reversible increase in tonic resting muscle tension at temperatures between 45°C and 50°C. With temperatures greater than 50°C, the preparations showed evidence of irreversible contracture. This suggested that hyperther-

mia was causing calcium entry into the cell and, ultimately, calcium overload. This hypothesis was confirmed with calcium-sensitive Fluo-3 AM dye. Hyperthermic increases in papillary muscle tension correlated well with Fluo-3 AM luminescence. To elucidate the mechanism of calcium entry into the cell and its role in cellular injury, preparations were pretreated with either a calcium channel blocker (cadmium or verapamil) or an inhibitor of the sarcoplasmic reticulum calcium pump (thapsigargin). Preparations heated to 42°C to 44°C showed no significant changes in tension at baseline or with drug treatment. With exposure to 48°C, treatment with calcium channel blockers did not reduce the increase in resting tension or Fluo-3 AM fluorescence, suggesting that the increase in cytosolic calcium was not the consequence of channel-specific calcium entry into the cell. In contrast, thapsigargin treatment led to irreversible papillary muscle contracture at lower temperatures (45°C to 50°C) than observed without this agent. For preparations heated to 48°C, there was a greater increase in muscle tension and Fluo-3 AM fluorescence in the thapsigargin group, compared with controls (Fig. 1–12). The authors concluded that

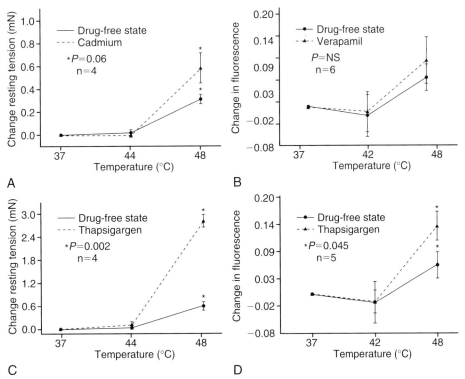

FIGURE 1–12. The effects of hyperthermic exposure on calcium entry into cells was tested in isolated perfused guinea pig papillary muscles. Change in resting tension was used as a surrogate measure for cytosolic calcium concentration (**A, C**), and change in Fluo-2 fluorescence was used as a direct measure of free cytosolic calcium (**B, D**). With exposure to mild hyperthermia (42°C to 44°C), little change in calcium levels was observed. With moderate hyperthermia (48°C), both muscle tension and Fluo-3 fluorescence increased significantly. This increase was not channel specific, because calcium channel blockade with cadmium or verapamil did not alter this response (**A, B**). The response was accentuated by thapsigargin (**C, D**), an agent that blocks calcium reuptake by the sarcoplasmic reticulum. *(From Everett TH, Nath S, Lynch C III, et al.: Role of calcium in acute hyperthermic myocardial injury. J Cardiovasc Electrophysiol 12:563-569, 2001, with permission.)*

hyperthermia results in significant increases in intracellular calcium, probably due to nonspecific transmembrane transit through thermally induced sarcolemmal pores. With increased intracellular calcium entry, the sarcoplasmic reticulum acts as a protective buffer against calcium overload, unless this function is blocked with an agent such as thapsigargin. In that case, cell contracture and death occurs at lower temperatures than expected.[54]

Simmers et al.[55] examined the effects of hyperthermia on impulse conduction in vitro in a preparation of superfused canine myocardium. Average conduction velocity at baseline temperatures of 37°C was 0.35 m/sec. When the superfusate temperature was raised, conduction velocity increased to supranormal values, reaching a maximum (114% of baseline) at 42.5°C. At temperatures greater than 45.4°C, conduction velocity slowed. Transient conduction block was observed at temperatures between 49.5°C and 51.5°C; above 51.7°C, permanent block was observed (Fig. 1–13).[55] These findings are exactly concordant with the temperature-related changes in cellular electrophysiology described earlier. In a related experiment,[56] the authors assessed myocardial conduction across a surgically created isthmus during heating with RF energy. The temperatures recorded during transient conduction block (50.7°C ± 3.0°C) and permanent conduction block (58.0°C ± 3.4°C) were almost identical to those temperature ranges recorded in the experiments performed with hyperthermic perfusate. The authors concluded that the sole effects of RF ablation on the electrophysiologic properties of the myocardium were hyperthermic,

and that there was no additional pathophysiologic response that could be attributed to direct effects of passage of electrical current through the tissue.[56-57]

Determinants of Lesion Size

The success of catheter ablation is dependent on a number of factors (Table 1–2). The first and foremost factor is optimal targeting of the arrhythmogenic substrate. It is intuitive that increasing the size and depth of an ablative lesion will not improve ablation success if the ablation site selection is poor. In order to optimize site selection, it is necessary to understand the physiology and anatomy of the arrhythmia in its entirety. The chapters describing clinical arrhythmia syndromes in this text provide critical information to help the catheter ablation operator position the ablation electrode at the optimal location for ablation success. Once the desired ablation target is elucidated, the catheter must be maneuvered to the proper location. This has traditionally been achieved with steerable electrode catheters and fluoroscopic guidance. In the past decade, several global positioning systems for catheter manipulation in the heart have been developed. These systems employ magnetic, electrical, or ultrasound fields to triangulate the position of the ablation electrode in the heart. The next generation of these systems will employ image fusion to project catheter positions and mapping electrograms on 3-D anatomic images derived from magnetic resonance imaging, computer tomographic imaging, or intracardiac echocardiography. Ultimately, these images may be fused with 4-D images that show the movement of the cardiac structures in a looping cardiac cycle. The penultimate system would incorporate real-time 3-D imaging with magnetic resonance imaging in the procedure lab, or real-time intracardiac echocardiography that continuously updates the background 4-D looping image. To assist the operator with maneuvering the electrode catheter to the optimal site in the highly processed 3-D or 4-D image, work is underway to incorporate automated catheter manipulation systems. One system being used presently employs a large external magnetic field and manipulates a magnetic-tipped catheter by altering the field. Another approach employs a sheath-within-a-sheath design with a motorized drive system that is controlled by a computer and 3-D joystick. In any case, whether it is an experienced operator with a thumbwheel-driven ablation catheter or a multimillion-dollar computer-driven system that is used to approximate the ablation target, target selection and the proximity of the

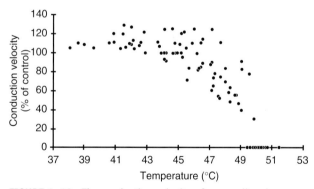

FIGURE 1–13. The conduction velocity of myocardium in superfused canine myocardium in vitro versus the temperature of the superfusate. A mild augmentation of conduction velocity due to an increase in rate of phase & depolarization is observed at temperatures up to 45°C. Between 45°C and 50°C, conduction velocity falls, and at temperatures greater than 50°C, conduction is blocked. *(From Simmers TA, de Bakker JM, Wittkampf FH, Hauer RN: Effects of heating on impulse propagation in superfused canine myocardium. J Am Coll Cardiol 25:1457-1464, 1995, with permission.)*

TABLE 1–2	
Factors Influencing Radiofrequency Lesion Size	
Factor	**Effect on Lesion Size**
Power	Directly proportional to lesion size
Ablation electrode temperature	Directly proportional to lesion size
Duration of energy delivery	Monoexponential relation to lesion size with half-time lesion formation of 5-10 sec
Ablation circuit impedance	Direct effects from altering delivered power
Electrode-tissue contact pressure	Directly proportional to lesion size
Electrode radius	Directly proportional to lesion size
Electrode geometry	Affects lesion size and shape by concentrating current density at electrode edges and asymmetries

Blood flow
   Over electrode-tissue interface
   Intramyocardial
	
	 With fixed energy delivery, reduces lesion size; with unlimited energy, increases lesion size
	 Has potential to prevent transmural lesion formation

Remote electrode size and position	Direct effects from altering system impedance
Tissue properties	Smaller lesion sizes in scar

Radiofrequency characteristics
   Pulsed
   Phased
   Frequency
	
	 May increase lesion size by allowing electrode cooling
	 Increases continuity of linear lesions formed with multielectrode arrays
	 Reduced heating efficiency at higher (MHz) frequencies

Electrode material	Higher heat-conductive materials increase lesion size by electrode cooling

electrode to that target are the most important factors for ablation success.

Ultimately, lesion size is a function of tissue heating, and tissue heating is a function of the magnitude of RF power that is converted into heat in the tissues. Therefore, higher power yields larger lesions. The success of cooled-tip catheters in clinical catheter ablation relates directly to the ability to deliver higher power to the ablation electrode without fear of overheating the electrode-tissue interface and causing a sudden rise in electrical impedance. Because of variable electrode-tissue contact and varying efficiency of energy transfer to tissue, high-power delivery always favors larger lesion formation and improved procedural success. However, high-power delivery is also associated with a higher procedural risk due to collateral damage of contiguous structures such as the esophagus, coronary arteries, and nontargeted components of the cardiac conduction system.

Myocardial ablation is achieved with thermal injury, and the thermodynamic properties of conductive heating in myocardium are highly predictable. If intramural tissue temperature could be reliably measured, it would be the most accurate and useful measure of lesion formation. Power could be titrated

to achieve the desired temperature gradient, and lesion size and geometry would be highly predictable and reproducible. However, the dominant factors determining temperature at the electrode tip are the magnitude of local blood flow and the stability of the electrode tip, in addition to power magnitude. Most temperature sensors that are economically feasible to include with catheter ablation systems measure temperature within the electrode tip or on the electrode surface. Nevertheless, temperature monitoring does allow the operator to titrate power to high levels and minimize the risk of boiling with associated coagulum, char, and steam pops. As a result, most present-day ablation catheters employ some form of temperature-feedback power control. Even if tip cooling is employed to increase lesion size, temperature-feedback power control with a lower set temperature (usually 40°C to 45°C) results in the maximum safe delivery of power.

The greater the magnitude of power delivered to the tissue, the greater the lesion size. Convective cooling at the electrode-tissue interface allows the operator to safely increase the power amplitude. However, if the ablation is power limited (i.e., the maximum available power is delivered throughout the ablation), then greater degrees of convective cooling will result in a lower fraction of delivered power being converted to tissue heat and a smaller lesion size. The two factors that affect passive cooling at the electrode-tissue interface are the magnitude of regional blood flow and the stability of the electrode catheter on the tissue surface. Sites of catheter ablation such as those on the tricuspid or mitral valve annuli have a high volume of regional blood flow. Because the endocardium is smooth and the contour is convex, catheter stability is often poor. The difficulty in achieving close coupling of energy delivery to the myocardium at these types of sites may translate into dissipation of the majority of ablation energy into the circulating blood pool and, consequently, smaller lesion size. Fortunately, most ablation targets along the valve annuli, such as accessory pathways, are relatively superficial and can usually be effectively treated with conventional ablation tools. In contrast, electrode placement in trabeculated myocardium or under valve leaflets produces highly efficient energy transfer to the tissue. Higher-power delivery in these cases usually results in excessive surface heating with an associated rise in electrical impedance. To maximize the size and depth of the ablative lesion, active cooling of the electrode tip is usually required. Thus, factors that stabilize tip contact on the target also increase lesion size and ablation success, particularly if coupled with techniques or technologies to maximize the delivered power amplitude.

If the goal is to maximize lesion size, larger electrodes are always better than smaller electrodes. Larger electrodes increase the surface area and allow the operator to deliver higher total power without excessive current density at the electrode-tissue interface. In this way, coagulum formation with a sudden rise in electrical impedance can be avoided despite high total power delivery. The higher-power delivery to the tissue increases the depth of direct volume heating, which in turn increases the size of the virtual heat source. This translates directly into a larger lesion. As with cooled electrodes, a large electrode results in larger lesion formation only if it is accompanied by higher power delivery. If a large electrode is employed with lower power, a larger endocardial surface area may be ablated, but the lesion will not be as deep. RF energy delivery to multiple electrodes simultaneously may also produce a large lesion, but other issues, such as catheter and target geometry, may limit energy coupling to the tissue if the electrode-tissue contact is poor.

Conclusion

RF catheter ablation remains the dominant modality for ablative therapy of arrhythmias. This technology is simple and has a high success rate and a low complication rate. Despite the fact that new ablation technologies (e.g., ultrasound, laser, microwave, cyrothermy) are being tested and promoted as easier, safer, or more efficacious methods, they are unlikely to supplant RF energy as the first choice for ablation of most arrhythmias. An appreciation of the biophysics and pathophysiology of RF energy heating of myocardium during catheter ablation helps the operator to make the proper adjustments to optimize ablation safety and success. A tissue temperature of 50°C must be reached to achieve irreversible tissue injury. This most likely occurs as a result of sarcolemmal membrane injury and intracellular calcium overload. The 50°C isotherm determines the boundary of the lesion. Greater lesion size is achieved with higher-power delivery and higher intramural tissue temperatures. Monitoring of surface temperatures is useful to help prevent boiling of blood with coagulum formation and a sudden increase in electrical impedance. The appropriate selection of a standard versus cooled-tip catheter; 4-mm versus 5-, 8-, or 10-mm electrode tip size; maximum power delivered; and maximum electrode tip temperature targeted may be achieved with a full understanding of the biophysics of catheter ablation. Finally, a complete understanding of the anatomy and physiology of the arrhythmogenic substrate allows the operator to select the optimal ablation approach.

References

1. Whayne JG, Nath S, Haines DE: Microwave catheter ablation of myocardium in vitro: Assessment of the characteristics of tissue heating and injury. Circulation 89:2390-2395, 1994.
2. Haines DE, Watson DD: Tissue heating during radiofrequency catheter ablation: A thermodynamic model and observations in isolated perfused and superfused canine right ventricular free wall. Pacing Clin Electrophysiol 12:962-976, 1989.
3. Erez A, Shitzer A: Controlled destruction and temperature distributions in biological tissues subjected to monoactive electrocoagulation. J Biomech Eng 102:42-49, 1980.
4. Haines DE: Determinants of lesion size during radiofrequency catheter ablation: The role of electrode-tissue contact pressure and duration of energy delivery. J Cardiovasc Electrophysiol 2:509-515, 1991.
5. Wittkampf FH, Nakagawa H, Yamanashi WS, et al.: Thermal latency in radiofrequency ablation. Circulation 93:1083-1086, 1996.
6. Haines DE, Watson DD, Verow AF: Electrode radius predicts lesion radius during radiofrequency energy heating: Validation of a proposed thermodynamic model. Circ Res 67:124-129, 1990.

7. Schreieck J, Zrenner B, Kumpmann J, et al.: Prospective randomized comparison of closed cooled-tip versus 8-mm-tip catheters for radiofrequency ablation of typical atrial flutter. J Cardiovasc Electrophysiol 13:980-985, 2002.

8. Tsai CF, Tai CT, Yu WC, et al.: Is 8-mm more effective than 4-mm tip electrode catheter for ablation of typical atrial flutter? Circulation 100:768-771, 1999.

9. Kasai A, Anselme F, Teo WS, et al.: Comparison of effectiveness of an 8-mm versus a 4-mm tip electrode catheter for radiofrequency ablation of typical atrial flutter. Am J Cardiol 86:1029-1032, A10, 2000.

10. Simmers TA, de Bakker JM, Coronel R, et al.: Effects of intracavitary blood flow and electrode-target distance on radiofrequency power required for transient conduction block in a Langendorff-perfused canine model. J Am Coll Cardiol 31:231-235, 1998.

11. Haines DE, Verow AF: Observations on electrode-tissue interface temperature and effect on electrical impedance during radiofrequency ablation of ventricular myocardium. Circulation 82:1034-1038, 1990.

12. Demolin JM, Eick OJ, Munch K, et al.: Soft thrombus formation in radiofrequency catheter ablation. Pacing Clin Electrophysiol 25:1219-1222, 2002.

13. Wang TL, Lin JL, Hwang JJ, et al.: The evolution of platelet aggregability in patients undergoing catheter ablation for supraventricular tachycardia with radiofrequency energy: The role of antiplatelet therapy. Pacing Clin Electrophysiol 18:1980-1990, 1995.

14. Jain MK, Wolf PD: A three-dimensional finite element model of radiofrequency ablation with blood flow and its experimental validation. Ann Biomed Eng 28:1075-1084, 2000.

15. Strickberger SA, Hummel J, Gallagher M, et al.: Effect of accessory pathway location on the efficiency of heating during radiofrequency catheter ablation. Am Heart J 129:54-58, 1995.

16. Kalman JM, Fitzpatrick AP, Olgin JE, et al.: Biophysical characteristics of radiofrequency lesion formation in vivo: Dynamics of catheter tip-tissue contact evaluated by intracardiac echocardiography. Am Heart J 133:8-18, 1997.

17. Nakagawa H, Yamanashi WS, Pitha JV, et al.: Comparison of in vivo tissue temperature profile and lesion geometry for radiofrequency ablation with a saline-irrigated electrode versus temperature control in a canine thigh muscle preparation. Circulation 91:2264-2273, 1995.

18. Mukherjee R, Laohakunakorn P, Welzig MC, et al.: Counter intuitive relations between in vivo RF lesion size, power, and tip temperature. J Interv Card Electrophysiol 9:309-315, 2003.

19. Petersen HH, Chen X, Pietersen A, et al.: Lesion dimensions during temperature-controlled radiofrequency catheter ablation of left ventricular porcine myocardium: Impact of ablation site, electrode size, and convective cooling. Circulation 99:319-325, 1999.

20. Otomo K, Yamanashi WS, Tondo C, et al.: Why a large tip electrode makes a deeper radiofrequency lesion: Effects of increase in electrode cooling and electrode-tissue interface area. J Cardiovasc Electrophysiol 9:47-54, 1998.

21. Dorwarth U, Fiek M, Remp T, et al.: Radiofrequency catheter ablation: Different cooled and noncooled electrode systems induce specific lesion geometries and adverse effects profiles. Pacing Clin Electrophysiol 26:1438-1445, 2003.

22. Spitzer SG, Karolyi L, Rammler C, Otto T: Primary closed cooled tip ablation of typical atrial flutter in comparison to conventional radiofrequency ablation. Europace 4:265-271, 2002.

23. Atiga WL, Worley SJ, Hummel J, et al.: Prospective randomized comparison of cooled radiofrequency versus standard radiofrequency energy for ablation of typical atrial flutter. Pacing Clin Electrophysiol 25:1172-1178, 2002.

24. Watanabe I, Masaki R, Min N, et al.: Cooled-tip ablation results in increased radiofrequency power delivery and lesion size in the canine heart: Importance of catheter-tip temperature monitoring for prevention of popping and impedance rise. J Interv Card Electrophysiol 6:9-16, 2002.

25. Fuller IA, Wood MA: Intramural coronary vasculature prevents transmural radiofrequency lesion formation: Implications for linear ablation. Circulation 107:1797-1803, 2003.

26. Ko WC, Huang SK, Lin JL, et al.: New method for predicting efficiency of heating by measuring bioimpedance during radiofrequency catheter ablation in humans. J Cardiovasc Electrophysiol 12:819-823, 2001.

27. Jain MK, Wolf PD: Temperature-controlled and constant-power radiofrequency ablation: What affects lesion growth? Trans Biomed Eng 46:1405-1412, 1999.

28. McRury ID, Whayne JG, Haines DE: Temperature measurement as a determinant of tissue heating during radiofrequency catheter ablation: An examination of electrode thermistor positioning for measurement accuracy. J Cardiovasc Electrophysiol 6:268-278, 1995.

29. Jain MK, Tomassoni G, Riley RE, Wolf PD: Effect of skin electrode location on radiofrequency ablation lesions: An in vivo and a three-dimensional finite element study. J Cardiovasc Electrophysiol 9:1325-1335, 1998.

30. Nath S, DiMarco JP, Gallop RG, et al.: Effects of dispersive electrode position and surface area on electrical parameters and temperature during radiofrequency catheter ablation. Am J Cardiol 77:765-767, 1996.

31. McRury ID, Panescu D, Mitchell MA, Haines DE: Nonuniform heating during radiofrequency catheter ablation with long electrodes: Monitoring the edge effect. Circulation 96:4057-4064, 1997.

32. Huang SK, Bharati S, Graham AR, et al.: Closed chest catheter desiccation of the atrioventricular junction using radiofrequency energy: A new method of catheter ablation. J Am Coll Cardiol 9:349-358, 1987.

33. Butcher RG: The measurement in tissue sections of the two formazans derived from nitroblue tetrazolium in dehydrogenase reactions. Histochem J 10:739-744, 1978.

34. Langberg JJ, Calkins H, el Atassi R, et al.: Temperature monitoring during radiofrequency catheter ablation of accessory pathways [see comment]. Circulation 86:1469-1474, 1992.

35. Nath S, DiMarco JP, Mounsey JP, et al.: Correlation of temperature and pathophysiological effect during radiofrequency catheter ablation of the AV junction. Circulation 92:1188-1192, 1995.

36. Langberg JJ, Calkins H, Kim YN, et al.: Recurrence of conduction in accessory atrioventricular connections after initially successful radiofrequency catheter ablation. J Am Coll Cardiol 1992; 19(7):1588-1592.

37. DeLacey WA, Nath S, Haines DE, et al.: Adenosine and verapamil-sensitive ventricular tachycardia originating from the left ventricle: Radiofrequency catheter ablation [see comment]. Pacing Clin Electrophysiol 15:2240-2244, 1992.

38. Huang SK, Bharati S, Lev M, Marcus FI: Electrophysiologic and histologic observations of chronic atrioventricular block induced by closed-chest catheter desiccation with radiofrequency energy. Pacing Clin Electrophysiol 10:805-816, 1987.

39. Avitall B, Urbonas A, Urboniene D, et al.: Time course of left atrial mechanical recovery after linear lesions: Normal sinus rhythm versus a chronic atrial fibrillation dog model [see comment]. J Cardiovasc Electrophysiol 11:1397-1406, 2000.

40. Nath S, Redick JA, Whayne JG, Haines DE: Ultrastructural observations in the myocardium beyond the region of acute coagulation necrosis following radiofrequency catheter ablation. J Cardiovasc Electrophysiol 5:838-845, 1994.

41. Nath S, Whayne JG, Kaul S, et al.: Effects of radiofrequency catheter ablation on regional myocardial blood flow: Possible mechanism for late electrophysiological outcome. Circulation 89:2667-2672, 1994.

42. Duong T, Hui P, Mailhot J: Acute right coronary artery occlusion in an adult patient after radiofrequency catheter ablation of a posteroseptal accessory pathway. J Invasive Cardiol 16:657-659, 2004.

43. Sassone B, Leone O, Martinelli GN, Di Pasquale G: Acute myocardial infarction after radiofrequency catheter ablation of typical atrial flutter: Histopathological findings and etiopathogenetic hypothesis. Ital Heart J 5:403-407, 2004.

44. Saad EB, Marrouche NF, Saad CP, et al.: Pulmonary vein stenosis after catheter ablation of atrial fibrillation: Emergence of a new clinical syndrome [see comment]. [Summary for patients in Ann Intern Med 138:1, 2003; **??huh??**PMID: 12693916]. Ann Intern Med 138:634-638, 2003.

45. Kok LC, Everett TH, Akar JG, Haines DE: Effect of heating on pulmonary veins: How to avoid pulmonary vein stenosis. J Cardiovasc Electrophysiol 14:250-254, 2003.

46. Bromer RH, Mitchell JB, Soares N: Response of human hematopoietic precursor cells (CFUc) to hyperthermia and radiation. Cancer Res 42:1261-1265, 1982.

47. Lepock JR: Involvement of membranes in cellular responses to hyperthermia. Radiat Res 92:433-438, 1982.

48. Stevenson AP, Galey WR, Tobey RA, et al.: Hyperthermia-induced increase in potassium transport in Chinese hamster cells. J Cell Physiol 115:75-86, 1983.

49. Nath S, Lynch C III, Whayne JG, Haines DE: Cellular electrophysiological effects of hyperthermia on isolated guinea pig papillary muscle: Implications for catheter ablation. Circulation 88:1826-1831, 1993.

50. Coakley WT: Hyperthermia effects on the cytoskeleton and on cell morphology [review—83 refs]. Symp Soc Exp Biol 41:187-211, 1987.

51. Warters RL, Henle KJ: DNA degradation in Chinese hamster ovary cells after exposure to hyperthermia. Cancer Res 42:4427-4432, 1982.

52. Warters RL, Roti Roti JL: Hyperthermia and the cell nucleus. Radiat Res 92:458-462, 1982.

53. Warters RL, Brizgys LM, Sharma R, Roti Roti JL: Heat shock (45 degrees C) results in an increase of nuclear matrix protein mass in HeLa cells. Int J Radiat Biol 50:253-268, 1986.

54. Everett TH, Nath S, Lynch C III, et al.: Role of calcium in acute hyperthermic myocardial injury. J Cardiovasc Electrophysiol 12:563-569, 2001.

55. Simmers TA, de Bakker JM, Wittkampf FH, Hauer RN: Effects of heating on impulse propagation in superfused canine myocardium. J Am Coll Cardiol 25:1457-1464, 1995.

56. Simmers TA, de Bakker JM, Wittkampf FH, Hauer RN: Effects of heating with radiofrequency power on myocardial impulse conduction: Is radiofrequency ablation exclusively thermally mediated? J Cardiovasc Electrophysiol 7:243-247, 1996.

57. Haines DE, Verow AF: Observations on electrode-tissue interface temperature and effect on electrical impedance during radiofrequency ablation of ventricular myocardium. Circulation 82:1038, 1990.

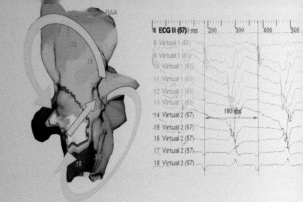

2

Titration of Radiofrequency Energy During Endocardial Catheter Ablation

Deeptankar Demazumder • David Schwartzman

Key Points

- All methods of radiofrequency (RF) energy titration are flawed. Common methods include changes in ablation electrode temperature (T_E), changes in ablation circuit impedance, electrogram amplitude reduction (EAR), and fixed power.

- T_E tracks myocardial temperature with varying accuracy. The presence and magnitude of inaccuracy is difficult to predict in current standard ablation practice. Induced change in ablation circuit impedance is similarly afflicted.

- A frequently observed phenomenon is the "irrigation effect," whereby flowing blood cools the electrode, permitting delivery of high RF power. This results in myocardial boiling despite low T_E and in the absence of impedance rise. This phenomenon is probably common in current clinical practice.

- EAR provides direct tissue information as to the status of ablation but results in smaller lesions and can be used only in certain regions.

- Stable catheter-tissue contact is important to achieve safe and effective RF ablation but is poorly assessed by fluoroscopy, physician "feel," or electrogram characteristics.

- Myocardial overheating and "boiling" is probably under-recognized in clinical procedures due to limitations in methods of titrating RF energy.

Percutaneous, endocardially based, under-blood ablation of myocardium using radiofrequency (RF) energy is an effective technique for management of many arrhythmias. Although this technique is associated with high rates of safety, its complications are well described.[1-4] These are particularly prominent during procedures involving the left side of the heart or a large lesion burden, or both. It is our thesis that complications are related, in part, to specific methods of titration of RF. This chapter examines methods for RF titration, emphasizing practical biophysical relationships including electrode and myocardial temperature, ablation circuit impedance, and electrogram amplitude. Key elements are demonstrated in vitro, with their importance illustrated in vivo.

In Vitro Studies

METHODS

Ablation System

The details of this system were reported previously.[5] In brief, bovine myocardium from freshly killed animals was mounted on an isolated ground plate at the base of a tank circulating bovine heparinized whole blood (10 to 12 L) at 37°C. Thermocouples (T-type; 0.3-mm diameter; measurement accuracy, ± 2°C; Omega Engineering, Stamford, Conn.) were inserted at depths of 0 (electrode-endocardial interface), 1, 3, and 5 mm; these were labeled T_0, T_1, T_3, and T_5, respectively. Each thermocouple was electrically insulated and aligned so that its leads were perpendicular to the applied RF field, to minimize nonthermal artifacts and prevent fluctuations of averaged temperatures greater than 0.5°C root-mean-square. The electrode was mounted on a force-transducer (AccuForce; Acme Scale, San Leandro, Calif.) and locked into position such that it was aligned perpendicular to the tissue, in direct contact with T_0 and directly above T_3, and T_5. Force was varied to achieve the following magnitudes of electrode surface area in direct contact with myocardium: 0% (blood contact only), 25%, 60%, or 95%. Blood flow was directed to the electrode-endocardial interface with the use of a pulsatile flow pump (Masterflex; Cole Parmer, Vernon Hills, Ill.) set to a rate of 30 pulses per minute. When activated, the pump delivered blood in such a way as to achieve a peak velocity of 0.26 m/sec (mean velocity, 0.20 m/sec) at the electrode-endocardial interface on the side of the electrode adjacent to the blood flow source. This is in the range of velocities commonly measured along the atrial endocardial surface in humans. While the pump was inactivated, interfacial flow velocity was negligible. The interface was imaged with the use of a multiplane phased-array echocardiographic transducer mounted into the tank (ATL, Bothell, Wash.). Two-dimensional imaging was performed at a frequency of 5 MHz. A time calibration was employed to permit synchronization of echocardiography with temperature and impedance measurements. RF was applied continuously in a unipolar fashion between the ablation electrode and the ground plate, using a commercial generator (EP Technologies, Sunnyvale, Calif.) operating at approximately 550 kHz. This was the frequency at which circuit impedance (Ω) was measured. In addition, power, voltage, and current were measured, and energy was calculated. Biophysical and temperature data were measured continuously during RF application with sampling at 200 Hz by means of a commercial data acquisition system (Superscope II; GW Instruments, Somerville, Mass.). A commercial, standard-shaped platinum electrode of 2.3 mm diameter and 4.5 mm length was used (Biosense Webster, Diamond Bar, Calif.). The electrode incorporated a thermistor located adjacent to the electrode tip (Fig. 2–1). RF was titrated to achieve and maintain an electrode temperature (T_E) of 70°C.

Pathology

After each RF application, the electrode and contiguous myocardium were examined visually. The lesion was then sectioned coronally and stained with 1% triphenyl tetrazolium chloride. This dye stains intracellular dehydrogenase, which distinguishes viable and necrotic tissue. Evidence of necrosis by this method was observed when myocardial temperature exceeded 55°C for at least 10 seconds. Lesion volume was calculated by assuming that the lesion was an oblate ellipsoid and subtracting the estimated volume extending above the surface of the tissue (Figs. 2–2 and 2–3).

Analytical Methods

At least 10 repetitions were performed for each set of experimental parameters. Continuous variables were compared with the use of Student's t test, and categorical variables were compared with a chi-square test. Correlations were performed by the Spearman method. For each statistical technique, significance was demarcated by a P value less than .05. Data are expressed as mean ± standard deviation, unless otherwise stated (Table 2–1).

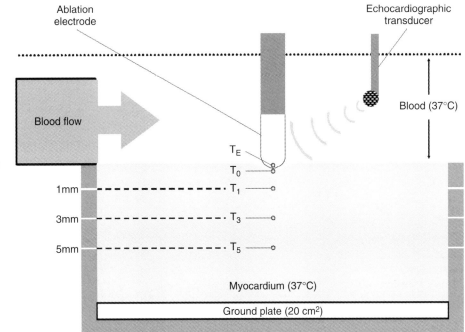

FIGURE 2–1. In vitro ablation apparatus.

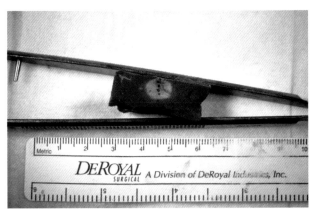

FIGURE 2-2. Typical tetrazolium-stained myocardium in region of radiofrequency energy application, shown in cross-section. Ablated territory appears light, viable myocardium red. Holes in the myocardium demarcate locations of thermocouples.

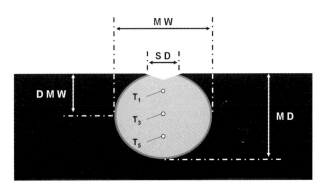

FIGURE 2-3. Lesion sizing schematic. Markings defining maximum lesion width (MW), maximum depth (MD), depth at which lesion width was maximum (DMW), and lesion width at the endocardial surface (SD) are demonstrated.

In the absence of electrode-myocardial contact (0%), the introduction of flow markedly increased the RF requirement, compared with no flow. This had a small effect on myocardial temperature; no lesion was observed in either case. At 25% contact, in the absence of blood flow, electrode and interfacial temperatures were similar; as expected, intramyocardial temperature diminished as a function of distance from the interface (Fig. 2–4).

The introduction of flow changed these relationships: in association with a marked increase in RF power required to achieve and maintain the goal T_E, interfacial temperature markedly exceeded T_E, as did some intramyocardial temperatures (Fig. 2–5). Despite the fact that the interfacial temperature reached the boiling point (100°C), there was no significant rise in impedance nor attenuation of energy delivery, so lesion growth continued unimpeded. Despite identical electrode-myocardial contact, T_E, and RF duration, the lesion volume in the setting of blood flow was markedly larger than that observed in its absence. The approach of myocardial temperature to the boiling point was associated with the elaboration of echogenic "bubbles" from the

TABLE 2–1

*Summary of In Vitro Data**

Parameters of RF Application	CONTACT							
	0%		25%		60%		95%	
Peak blood flow velocity (m/sec)	0	0.26	0	0.26	0	0.26	0	0.26
T_E (°C)	70	70	70	70	70	70	70	70
T_0 (°C)	55 ± 0.5	**42 ± 5**	75 ± 1	**103 ± 1**	71 ± 1	**85 ± 1**	60 ± 1	62 ± 1
T_1 (°C)	42 ± 0.3	**45 ± 0.7**	65 ± 1	**99 ± 4**	63 ± 1	**76 ± 2**	60 ± 1	61 ± 1
T_3 (°C)	37	37	50 ± 2	**78 ± 6**	44 ± 1	**61 ± 3**	40 ± 1	42 ± 1
T_5 (°C)	37	37	40 ± 1	**61 ± 4**	37	**49 ± 2**	37	37
Baseline Z	76 ± 1	78 ± 1	86 ± 2	82 ± 5	91 ± 1	93 ± 2	132 ± 9	111 ± 2
ΔZ (Ω)	11 ± 2	11 ± 1	10 ± 3	12 ± 2	10 ± 1	9 ± 2	12 ± 2	10 ± 1
Maximum power applied (W)	7.7 ± 0.8	**31 ± 2**	6.0 ± 0.7	**23 ± 2**	2.9 ± 0.2	**9.5 ± 0.6**	0.9 ± 0.1	**3.5 ± 0.8**
Cumulative energy delivered (J)	457 ± 47	**1883 ± 90**	358 ± 60	**1375 ± 122**	190 ± 27	**611 ± 52**	59 ± 5	**225 ± 40**
Volume of ablation lesion (cc)	0	0	25 ± 7	**144 ± 41**	20 ± 6	**58 ± 16**	15 ± 4	15 ± 4
Echo bubbling	N	N	N	**Y**	N	N	N	N
Coagulum (endocardial surface)	N	N	N	**Y**	N	N	N	N
Coagulum (electrode)	N	N	N	N	N	N	N	N

*Data in bold were significantly different from data obtained under the same conditions during 0 m/sec flow. See text for details.

Baseline Z, impedance of RF circuit while electrode is in contact with myocardium and blood before RF application; Echo bubbling, elaboration of echogenic bubbles from electrode-endocardial interface during RF application; RF, radiofrequency energy; T_E, maximum electrode temperature; T_0, maximum electrode-endocardial interfacial temperature; T_x, maximum intramyocardial temperature at x mm depth; ΔZ, minimum impedance value during RF application.

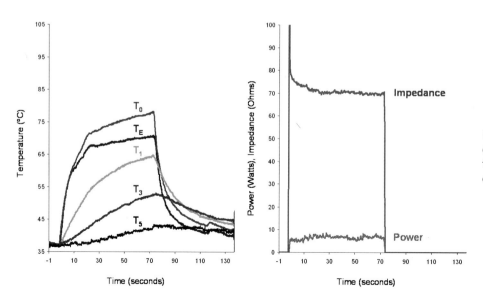

FIGURE 2–4. Typical example of data output from in vitro system for 25% contact with blood flow of 0 m/sec. See text for details.

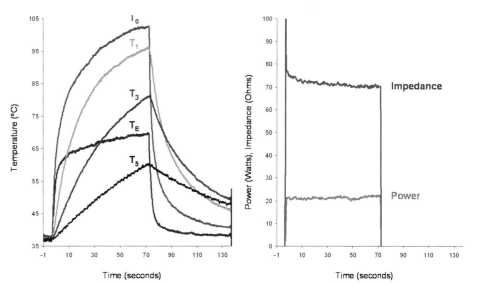

FIGURE 2–5. Typical example of data output from in vitro system for 25% contact and blood flow of 0.26 m/sec. See text for details.

electrode-endocardial interface zone; for faster rates of rise of temperature, this event could be explosive. (Faster rates of temperature rise were observed during lesion applications in which RF was increased at a faster rate; this situation was typical of the servotitration algorithms common to commercial ablation software.) Adherent endocardial coagulum, a product of boiling, was sometimes seen in association with lesions during which interfacial boiling had occurred (Fig. 2–6); coagulum was not observed on the electrode. Lesions for which explosive bubbling was observed sometimes evidenced focal barotrauma (disruption or tearing) of the endocardium.

At 60% contact, similar phenomena were observed, but they were muted in comparison with the effects of 25% contact. Specifically, the difference in maximum RF power with blood flow (versus no blood flow) was smaller. Although interfacial temperature exceeded T_E (as did the more superficial intramyocardial temperatures), these temperatures did not approach boiling, no echocardiographic bubbling was observed, lesion volumes were smaller than for 25% contact, and there was no endocardial coagulum.

With near-complete electrode-myocardial contact (95%), blood flow had a minimal impact on RF requirement, myocardial temperature, and lesion volume. T_E exceeded all myocardial temperatures.

Note that, at baseline, ablation circuit impedance increased in direct relation to the degree of myocardial contact. Despite variation in myocardial temperatures seen across these experiments, the maximum decrease in ablation circuit impedance during RF application remained relatively constant. Therefore, the best impedance-temperature correlation was with the T_E.

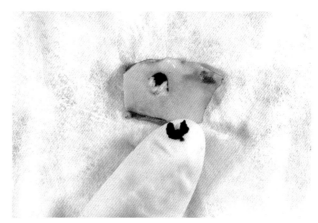

FIGURE 2–6. Endocardial coagulum, some of which has been removed onto gloved fingertip.

DISCUSSION

These data demonstrate that T_E portrays myocardial temperature with varying accuracy, influenced by the degree of electrode-myocardial contact and regional blood flow. Despite a fixed T_E, lesion volume varied markedly. Blood flow produced electrode cooling, which increased the RF requirement to achieve the targeted T_E. The additional RF did not simply offset the cooling effect of blood; it also yielded markedly higher myocardial temperatures and greater lesion volume. This "irrigation effect" of flowing blood was proportional to the area of the interface between blood and the electrode surface. This effect is identical to that exerted by artificial electrode irrigation.[5,6]

Under certain conditions, boiling at the electrode-endocardial interface was observed despite continued RF application and lesion growth. This phenomenon was not betrayed by T_E or ablation circuit impedance but was associated with the elaboration of echogenic bubbles from the interface. As we previously demonstrated,[5] the primary mechanism by which irrigation increases lesion volume is not prevention of interfacial boiling; rather, it is prevention of impedance rise in the setting of continued higher RF application.

Given the higher resistivity of myocardium relative to blood, it was not surprising that ablation circuit impedance at baseline was correlated with the magnitude of electrode-myocardial contact. Note that this relationship is best described by an exponential function, and that the difference between 0% contact and 25% contact was relatively small. The observation that the change (decrease) in ablation circuit impedance during RF application correlated best with T_E suggests that utilization of this value to guide to RF titration would be beset by similar inaccuracy.

In Vivo Animal Studies

METHODS

Animal Model

Forty-five large (35 to 60 kg), healthy pigs were studied. It was previously demonstrated that atrial chamber dimensions, blood flow velocities, and atrial wall thicknesses in this model are similar to those of the human adult.[7] Access to the right atrium was gained via the femoral vein. Access to the left atrium (LA) was gained via atrial transseptal puncture. Each animal was in sinus rhythm and systemically heparinized for the duration of the procedure. Atrial endocardial anatomy was divided into smooth and trabeculated regions.

Imaging

Intracardiac echocardiography (ICE) was used to image the electrode-endocardial interface at each ablation site (UltraICE 9F/9MHz, Boston Scientific, Natick, Mass.).[8] It was used to ensure stable ablation electrode-endocardial contact at each ablation site during RF application and to monitor the ablation electrode-endocardial interface throughout the RF application, similar to the manner in which echocardiographic imaging was used in vitro (described earlier). We previously showed that ICE imaging of the interface during its approach to boiling demonstrates the elaboration of bubbles; if formation is rapid enough, bubble release can be explosive.[9,10]

Ablation

Single RF applications were made at discrete endocardial sites. A commercial ablation catheter (Navi-Star, Biosense Webster) was used. The ablation electrode was identical to that used for the in vitro experiments. A 2-mm-length ring electrode was located just proximal to the ablation electrode, and the adjacent edge-to-edge interelectrode distance was 1 mm. The distal electrode incorporated a thermocouple embedded near its tip. RF was applied via a commercial generator (Radionics, Burlington, Mass.) in unipolar fashion, between the distal electrode of the ablation catheter and a cutaneous ground pad placed on the thorax or abdomen. During each RF application, maximum power, T_E, and ablation circuit impedance were recorded continuously. The maximum decrease in circuit impedance relative to baseline (measured with a small, nonheating current passed through the ablation circuit) was also recorded. The generator was set to automatically shut off if T_E exceeded 90°C. The ablation electrode was visually inspected after each lesion.

Electrogram Recording

Electrograms were sampled at a rate of 2 kHz using a band-pass filter setting of 10 to 400 Hz. The following recordings were made before and continuously during each RF application: (1) ablation electrode unipolar (U_{ABL}) electrogram and (2) ablation electrode–ring electrode bipolar (BI) electrogram.

Pathology

Animals were euthanized within 2 hours after RF application. The heart and contiguous tissues were first inspected in situ. The heart was then removed for further assessment. The atrial epicardium was inspected for evidence of ablation damage. The atria were then incised, and each lesion was assessed for evidence of endocardial coagulum or barotrauma. After gross inspection, hearts were immersed in 1% triphenyl tetrazolium chloride for 30 minutes. Atrial wall thickness and lesion dimensions were measured with a caliper. Lesions that spanned endocardium to epicardium were defined as transmural.

Experimental Groups

Two different RF titration techniques were compared. In group 1, RF titration was guided by T_E, with a goal of 60°C for 15 seconds. If an impedance rise (defined as >5Ω) was observed, the application was immediately terminated. In group 2, RF titration was guided by electrogram amplitude reduction (EAR), a method we reported previously,[9] with a goal of greater than 90% reduction in the amplitude of U_{ABL} or BI (or both) for 15 seconds.

Analytical Methods

Data are reported as mean ± standard deviation. A chi-square test or McNemar's test was performed for proportions and a paired or unpaired t test for continuous variables. Correlations were assessed by the Spearman method. For each test, a P value of less than .05 was considered significant (Table 2–2).

Group 1 (T_E Guided): Smooth Endocardial Regions

A total of 26 lesions were evaluated. Consistent with our observations in vitro, T_E was significantly correlated with maximal decrease in ablation circuit impedance (ΔZ; $r = .86$; $P < .001$).

(Baseline Z was the same whether the ablation electrode was floating in the cavity or in firm and stable contact, as determined echocardiographically. In addition, there were small oscillations in the value, with frequencies consistent with heart and ventilation rates. These data suggest that baseline Z is not a sensitive method to assay electrode-endocardial contact in smooth endocardial regions, and that even with firm contact a large portion of the electrode surface is in contact with blood. It is likely that the oscillations denote movement of the electrode sufficient to allow at least intermittent blood contact to the entire surface. These observations are consistent with the profound irrigation effect noted during ablation in these regions.)

Endocardial coagulum (Fig. 2–7) accompanied some lesions; for all of these lesions, interfacial bubbling was observed during deployment. The sensitivity of bubbling for endocardial coagulum was 100%, its specificity was 60%, and its positive predictive value was 65%.

Endocardial barotrauma (Fig. 2–8) was evident at sites at which application of RF was associated with

TABLE 2–2

Summary of Data for Radiofrequency Titration Techniques Compared in the Animal Model*

Parameters of RF Application	RF TITRATION METHOD			
	T_E = 60°C		EAR	
Endocardial region type	Smooth	Trabeculated	Smooth	Trabeculated
Sample size (no.)	26	6	29	17
Power (W)	67 ± 20	26 ± 16	**31 ± 11**	**35 ± 11**
T_E (°C)	61 ± 7	61 ± 1	**51 ± 6**	**88 ± 8**
ΔZ (Ω)	9 ± 3	8 ± 1	**5 ± 2**	**13 ± 3**
↓BI amplitude (%)	96 ± 4	47 ± 10	**87 ± 8**	52 ± 14
↓U_{ABL} amplitude (%)	95 ± 2	65 ± 15	**88 ± 9**	72 ± 17
Impedance rise (%)	19	0	**0**	12
ICE bubbling (%)	77	0	7	10
ICE explosion (%)	62	0	0	0
Lesion transmurality (%)	100	—	82	—
Lesion diameter (mm)	8.9 ± 2.1	—	**7.3 ± 3.2**	—
Electrode coagulum (%)	19	0	0	0
Endocardial coagulum (%)	42	0	3	12
Endocardial barotrauma (%)	46	0	0	0

*Data in bold obtained during EAR-guided RF titration were significantly different from data obtained under the same conditions during T_E-guided RF titration. See text for details.

↓BI, reduction in bipolar electrogram recorded from ablation catheter; EAR, electrogram amplitude reduction; ICE, intracardiac echocardiography; RF, radiofrequency energy; T_E, maximum electrode temperature; ↓U_{ABL} amplitude, reduction in unipolar electrogram recorded using the ablation electrode; ΔZ, minimum impedance value during RF application.

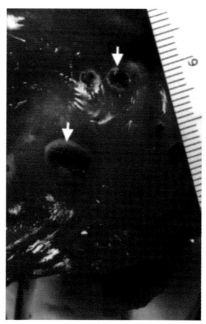

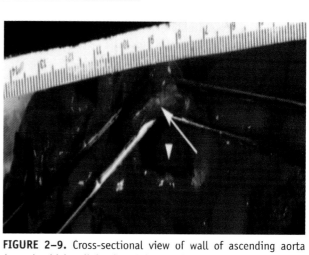

FIGURE 2–9. Cross-sectional view of wall of ascending aorta (arrow) which adjoined a right atrial endocardial site (arrowhead) at which radiofrequency (RF) energy was applied. The tissue has been stained with tetrazolium to demonstrate evidence of RF damage to the media.

FIGURE 2–7. *En face* view of atrial endocardium after tetrazolium staining, demonstrating coagulum *(arrows)* overlying lesions.

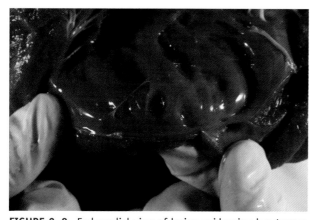

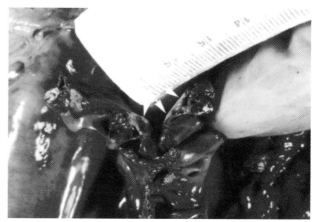

FIGURE 2–10. Cross-sectional view of trabeculated atrial myocardium (epicardial surface adjacent to ruler). The tissue has been stained with tetrazolium to demonstrate the presence of lesion *(arrows)* that involve the subepicardial surface and adjacent trabecular regions but spare the cavitary aspects of the trabeculae *(en face)*.

FIGURE 2–8. Endocardial view of lesion evidencing barotrauma (endocardial tear).

explosive bubble release. The sensitivity of explosive bubble release for evidence of barotrauma at pathologic analysis was 100%; specificity was 33% and positive predictive value was 52%.

All lesions were transmural, with a maximal diameter exceeding 5 mm. Damage to contiguous extra-atrial structures was also observed (Fig. 2–9). Despite the frequent ICE and pathologic evidence of endocardial boiling, impedance rise was observed infrequently during these applications. Electrode coagulum was also infrequently observed, and only in association with impedance rise.

Group 1 (T_E Guided): Trabeculated Endocardial Regions

A total of six lesions were evaluated. T_E was again significantly correlated with $\Delta Z (r = .92; P < .05)$. During lesion deployment, there was no evidence of bubbling. Lesions were free of coagulum and barotrauma. No damage to contiguous extra-atrial structures was observed. Given the complex topography, it was not possible to characterize lesion dimensions. However, morphology was notable for the absence of lesion on the cavitary surface of trabeculae (Fig. 2–10).

Group 2 (EAR Guided): Smooth Endocardial Regions

A total of 29 lesions were evaluated. Maximum RF power was markedly lower than that observed during T_E-guided applications. T_E was again significantly correlated with $\Delta Z (r = .74; P < .001)$. ICE bubbling was observed only in regions where myocardial thickness exceeded 4 mm; these were also the only regions where endocardial coagulum was observed. At pathologic analysis, there was no endocardial barotrauma, no electrode coagulum, and no evidence of damage to contiguous extra-atrial structures. However, approximately 25% of the lesions were not transmural.

Group 2 (EAR Guided): Trabeculated Endocardial Regions

A total of 17 lesions were evaluated. Sufficient EAR could not be reached in 11 applications because T_E in excess of 90°C prevented upward power titration. T_E was again significantly correlated with $\Delta Z (r = .86; P < .05)$. Despite the high T_E, evidence of lesion formation on the cavitary surface of the pectinate bundles was almost never observed, as for T_E-guided lesions in these regions. Endocardial coagulum was observed in two lesions; electrode coagulum was never observed, nor was barotrauma or damage to contiguous extra-atrial structures.

DISCUSSION

In smooth endocardial regions, where, despite firm endocardial contact, electrode surface interface with blood remained, RF power titration guided by T_E was associated with frequent myocardial boiling. This is clear evidence of the irrigation effect and also demonstrates in vivo how T_E can be misleading as a surrogate for maximal myocardial temperature. The consistent, excellent correlation between T_E and ΔZ demonstrated that RF titration guided by changes in ablation circuit impedance would be similarly susceptible to misrepresentation of myocardial temperature. In contrast, EAR-guided ablation used much less power and was largely without evidence of myocardial boiling, except in thicker areas where lesion transmurality most likely necessitated interfacial boiling. Overall, lesion dimensions were significantly smaller than during T_E-guided ablation. It is important to note the marked discrepancy in power and lesion pathology between the two techniques, despite the rather small difference in T_E (60°C versus a mean of 51°C). This is a demonstration of the remarkably potent "thermal homeostasis" of (liquid) flowing blood in the region of the electrode, a property not shared by (solid) myocardium, which accumulates heat. These data support the utility of EAR-guided power titration in smooth endocardial regions and the potential danger of thermometry-guided ablation. Unlike "ablation electrode–based" RF titration techniques such as those guided by T_E or by induced changes in ablation circuit impedance, EAR gauges the power requirement by response of the tissue. In return for a higher level of safety, however, the EAR technique is associated with a smaller lesion and therefore may necessitate a larger number of lesions for a given procedure.[10]

Another important phenomenon observed during ablation in smooth endocardial regions was the presence of endocardial coagulum despite the absence of an ablation circuit impedance rise during lesion application. Impedance rise is caused by the accumulation of gas (an electrical insulator) along the electrode surface, which is supported by the presence of a solid interface (e.g., myocardium) but diminished by the presence of a fluid interface (e.g., blood).[5] Unless a sufficient proportion of the electrode surface has a solid interface such as myocardium or coagulum (to confine the elaborated gas) or the rate of gas production is fast and sustained enough to exclude blood from the electrode surface, a parallel current pathway exists and overall circuit impedance may change little or not at all despite myocardial boiling. (Part of the issue here is the low acquisition rate and high frequency at which commercial RF generators measure and report impedance; this subject is beyond the scope of this chapter.) Endocardial coagulum is caused by boiling (denaturation) of blood in the region of the electrode-endocardial interface, which is then "annealed" to the endocardium. The absence of electrode coagulum is evidence of the cooling effect of flow in regions of the electrode surface that are in direct contact with blood. If electrode coagulum is observed, it is usually at the margin of myocardial contact, where temperatures are high and the presence of the electrode impedes blood flow, or at the proximal edge of the electrode, where a high current density produces a discrete region of high temperature.[11] Note that, in the presence of a high proportion of electrode-blood contact, the formation of coagulum on the electrode is necessary but not sufficient to produce an impedance rise: this substance is not an insulator, but, as noted earlier, it acts to promote accumulation of gas at the electrode interface by excluding blood flow, similar to myocardium. This is why an electrode with coagulum permits continued ablation while acting as if it had a diminished surface area or a higher proportion of myocardial contact (e.g., lower peak power to achieve a given T_E).

In trabeculated endocardial regions, the ablation electrode usually abutted a thin epimyocardial layer, wedged between pectinate muscle bundles. The electrode surface probably had minimal contact with flowing blood. As demonstrated in vitro, in this setting T_E provides a much more accurate estimate of maximal myocardial temperature. This is why peak power during T_E-guided ablation was markedly lower than in smooth endocardial regions. Low power was associated with a small lesion; in addition, access of flowing blood to the cavitary aspects of the pectinate bundles most likely explained the absence of ablation in these areas. During EAR-guided ablation, power titration sufficient to achieve the desired goal was not possible, because the peak permitted RF power was insufficient to ablate the adjacent thick, blood-protected pectinate muscle bundles. These observations are consistent with observations during clinical ablation in trabeculated regions, such as the cavotricuspid isthmus. In these relatively uncommon situations, induction of flow at the ablation electrode-endocardial interface, such as that achieved with the use of artificial irrigation, may be needed to permit application of power sufficient to achieve the lesion goal. However, it is important to recognize the potential danger of this approach. With electrode irrigation or the use of electrodes with large surface areas, T_E may be unable to report (prevent) even extreme tissue heating. Given the high degree of myocardial contact, boiling would probably be reported as an impedance rise, but this would occur after the fact and therefore would not prevent the occurrence of barotrauma. This sequence is particularly likely if a fixed-power RF titration approach is used. We believe that it underlies some of the morbid events recently reported during ablation procedures. Even generally smooth endocardial regions have areas of "pitting" or trabeculation that can confine an electrode, unbeknownst to an operator. For this reason, we believe that, particularly at high RF powers (e.g., >25 W), a fixed-power RF titration technique should never be used in the absence of direct, continuous, real-time imaging of the ablation electrode-endocardial interface, such as that provided by ICE.

In Vivo Human Studies

METHODS

Patients

Twenty-five consecutive patients with intrusive, drug-resistant atrial fibrillation were referred for ablation targeting the posterior LA, a topographically complex region comprising generally smooth, angu-lated endocardium; high regional blood flow velocities; ridges; and orifices.[12,13] None of these patients had had prior LA ablation. There were 22 men, ages 37 to 69 years, all with LA volume less than 150 mL, preserved left ventricular systolic function, and pulmonary vein flow velocities in normal range. All patients were in sinus rhythm during ablation.

Operative Preparation

Patients underwent induction of general anesthesia including endotracheal intubation and full paralysis. High-frequency jet ventilation was used to eliminate respiration-induced cardiac motion. Access to the central circulation was gained via right and left femoral veins. Access to the LA was gained via dual atrial septal puncture.

Imaging

As in the animal model, ICE (UltraICE 9F/9 MHz, Boston Scientific) was used to visualize the ablation electrode and endocardium. Before ablation procedure, the catheter operator was permitted to manipulate the catheter so as to achieve "stable" ablation electrode-endocardial contact at two distinct sites (in the regions of the left and right pulmonary veins, respectively), based on "feel," single-plane (left anterior oblique) fluoroscopy, and electrogram amplitude/morphologic stability; during this phase, the operator was blinded to the ICE image. During the ablation procedure, ICE was used to guide the ablation electrode into firm and stable endocardial contact before RF application and to monitor the electrode-endocardial interface continuously during energy delivery. ICE bubbling was characterized as in the animal study reported earlier. If it was observed, RF was discontinued immediately.

Ablation Technique

The ablation electrode was the same as that used in vitro and in the animal model. RF was applied in unipolar fashion via a commercial generator (EP Technologies) using dual cutaneous (posterior thorax) ground pads. RF power was titrated in 5-W steps at 5-second increments until an EAR criterion (bipolar amplitude reduction greater than 90%) was met, after which the power was increased an additional 5 W for 15 seconds. T_E was not permitted to exceed 60°C. Individual lesions were applied in contiguity so as to encircle each pulmonary venous vestibule.[14] After the lesion was completed, electrical isolation of the subtended myocardium was documented using entrance and exit conduction block criteria.[15]

Analytical Methods

Data are presented as mean ± standard deviation, unless otherwise noted. An unpaired *t* test was used to compare continuous variables; a *P* value of less than .05 was considered significant (Table 2–3).

Fifty sites designated by the catheter operator as "stable" were imaged with ICE. Stability, as defined by ICE, was genuine at only 27 (54%) of these sites. Instability, characterized echocardiographically by frank noncontact, intermittent contact (bouncing), or movement with continuous contact (sliding), was observed in the remainder, per protocol unassociated with significant differences in mean impedance (97 ± 14 Ω for stable contact sites versus 95 ± 18 Ω for unstable contact sites—values not significantly different from those measured when the electrode was floating in the LA cavitary blood and not in myocardial contact [94 ± 15 Ω], impedance flux, electrogram amplitude/morphology, or fluoroscopic stability.

A total of 2574 RF applications were analyzed, 1127 in the left and 1447 in the right vestibule. Despite a T_E that rarely exceeded 50°C, ICE bubbling was observed during a significant minority of applications, and bubbling occasionally was explosive. Bubbling was not associated with an obvious deflection in the impedance or T_E readout from the RF generator. Interestingly, the bipolar electrogram recorded from the ablation and contiguous ring electrode evidenced a high-frequency artifact that correlated with ICE bubbling (Fig. 2–11).

ICE evidence of endocardial coagulum was observed only rarely after RF application, and only at sites where bubbling had been observed. Explosive bubbling was usually mild and almost never associated with echocardiographic evidence of endocardial barotrauma. One notable exception involved a lesion application along the septal aspect of a right vestibule lesion, during which, in retrospect, RF was overtitrated due to confusion stemming from voltage

TABLE 2–3

*Summary of Data for Radiofrequency Applications in Patients**

Parameters of RF Application	No Bubbling	Nonexplosive Bubbling	Explosive Bubbling
No. of lesions (%)	2257 (88)	286 (11)	31 (1)
T_E (range) (°C)	48 ± 12 (41-57)	51 ± 9 (42-59)	49 ± 6 (41-57)
RF duration (sec)	67 ± 12	**42 ± 15**	**47 ± 8**
Maximum power (range) (W)	27 ± 8 (10-50)	31 ± 6 (20-40)	29 ± 11 (25-40)

*Data in bold are significantly different from data obtained during RF applications during which no ICE bubbling was observed. See text for details. ICE, intracardiac echocardiography; RF, radiofrequency energy; T_E, maximum electrode temperature.

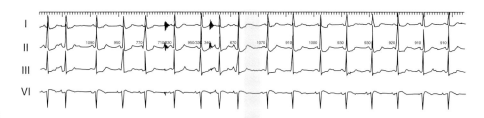
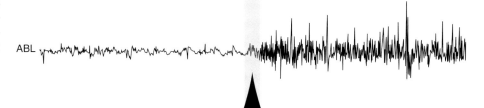

FIGURE 2–11. Surface *(top)* and intracardiac electrograms recorded bracketing an intracardiac echocardiography (ICE) bubbling event, the moment of which is demarcated by the *arrow*.

generated by contiguous right atrial myocardium. Sudden, unheralded, explosive bubbling was observed at an RF power of 30 W and a T_E of 46°C. It was associated with a small, discrete impedance "bump" that occurred at the moment of the explosion but was not sustained, which was succeeded seconds later by an abrupt rise in T_E in association with bubbles enveloping the electrode (Fig. 2–12); RF was immediately terminated. Subsequently, we observed a transmural tear with bleeding into the interatrial connective tissue region, which was self-contained. The postoperative course of this patient was uneventful, except for the development of severe Dressler's syndrome. Although we have had no other occurrences of Dressler's syndrome after this procedure, evidence of pericarditis is common on the first few postoperative days. This is further testimony to the transmural heating of a thin-walled target, even with our "gentle" power titration technique. Two patients (0.3%) experienced thromboembolic complications, each within 24 hours after the procedure. In each of these patients, several lesions had been observed during which there was ICE bubbling (none explosive). Neither of these patients demonstrated ICE evidence of endocardial coagulum, which is rarely observed. The incidence of bubbling in these patients was not significantly higher than in the remaining cohort. Neither endocardial nor electrode coagulum was observed in either patient.

DISCUSSION

Despite an operative preparation that eliminated muscular motion and respiration-induced cardiac motion, impedance, electrographic data, fluoroscopy, and "feel" were often inaccurate in predicting electrode-endocardial contact stability in this region of the heart. There were various patterns of instability, which were not necessarily cyclic. Contact instability introduces an additional dimension of complexity to RF titration, because it alters the relationships among power, T_E, and myocardial temperature, which cannot be adequately monitored using electrode-based data. In this setting, an "empiric" RF titration technique (e.g., fixed power, targeted T_E) would most likely result in a spectrum of lesion pathology. EAR-guided titration might also be unreliable.

During RF applications in which stable electrode-endocardial contact was assured, the irrigation effect was evident: transmural lesion formation was associated with low T_E. This is consistent with observations in the animal model. Interfacial boiling (ICE bubbling) was observed in a substantial number of applications. The observation that the T_E during applications that demonstrated bubbling was not significantly different from the T_E in those that did not suggests that T_E had a varying relationship with myocardial temperature. Accepting ICE bubbling (with or without explosion) as proof of myocardial boiling, by inference the magnitude of inaccuracy of T_E for myocardial temperature could exceed 50°C. As demonstrated both in vitro and in the animal model, interfacial boiling was invisible to impedance and temperature monitoring. In one case, explosion produced barotrauma with clinical repercussions. Had this been a free-wall region, we have no doubt that this patient would have fared worse; such sequences have been reported.[4] It is unclear whether and how the early postoperative embolic events observed were related to endocardial sites at which boiling had occurred.

Despite our conservative RF titration method, evidence of myocardial boiling occurred with a substantial frequency. It is likely that in current common clinical practice, in which power is fixed or adjusted to achieve or maintain a T_E of 50°C to 60°C, boiling is more common. In addition, as noted earlier, the high rate at which commercial software drives power elevation is particularly conducive to barotrauma. It is likely that overtitration of power has played a role in the complications observed during under-blood, endocardium-based catheter ablation, which have included cardiac perforation, pericarditis, pulmonary

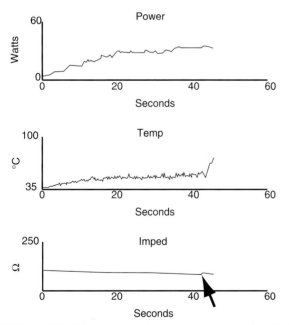

FIGURE 2–12. Data recorded during lesion application that resulted in a transmural left atrial tear (see text). At the moment of sudden, explosive release of intracardiac echocardiography bubbles, a small, nonsustained "bump" in impedance was observed. A few seconds later *(arrow)*, electrode temperature rose abruptly in association with bubbles engulfing the ablation electrode.

vein stenosis, cardioembolism, and esophageal fistulization. In view of the echocardiographic observations made here, the excellent record of safety associated with ablation is amazing to us; it is testimony to the resilience of the human body, our poor ability to detect pathologic events, and the low number of lesions needed for most arrhythmia targets. Serendipitous support in this area has also undoubtedly come from the limitation of most commercial RF generators to 50W. In this regard, recent availability of higher peak-power RF generators is of major concern.

It is interesting that the high success rates of ablation procedures that target discrete arrhythmogenic foci has most likely occurred in the setting of the irrigation effect and myocardial boiling. If power were to be more conservatively titrated, procedural success or lesion number (or both) might be significantly affected.

Additional Notes

We and others have attempted to use ICE to guide RF titration, rather than as a technique (as in the experiments reported earlier), to observe phenomena occurring in association with other RF titration methods. As demonstrated by ICE imaging, RF delivery without myocardial boiling results in myocardial swelling (due to edema) and, at clinical imaging frequencies (5 to 10MHz), rather mild associated changes in echogenicity.[16,17] The magnitude of swelling increases with time and is an imprecise measure of lesion volume and transmurality, particularly when multiple lesions are placed in contigu-

ity.[17] Boiling, as demarcated by ICE bubbling (with or without explosion) results in more marked changes in echogenicity, particularly in the endocardial and subendocardial regions at the ablation electrode (Fig. 2–13); it is our thesis that this effect results from destruction of tissue architecture, a feature not observed immediately after ablation in the absence of boiling. Some have used bubbling to modify or terminate RF energy[18,19]; as emphasized earlier, the risk of lesion complications limits the desirability of this approach.

Recently, Lardo et al.[20] reported a technique using magnetic resonance imaging for visualization of RF lesion formation in real time. RF application resulted in a hyperintensity signal, the volume of which could be assayed in three dimensions. There was excellent

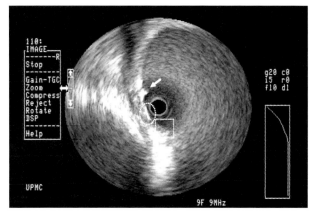

FIGURE 2–13. Postablation intracardiac echocardiography image demonstrating regions where boiling occurred, showing hyperdensity of the subendocardial regions *(oval)* in comparison with an adjacent ablated region in which boiling did not occur *(square)*. The arrow shows endocardial coagulum associated with another region where boiling occurred.

TABLE 2–4			
Summary of Radiofrequency Titration Techniques			
Method	**Commonly Used Target Parameters**	**Advantages**	**Disadvantages**
Ablation electrode temperature (T_E)	4-mm electrode: 55-65°C 8-mm electrode: ≤50°C Irrigated electrode: <40–45°C	Easy to apply; facilitated by commercial software	Variable/unpredictable accuracy for myocardial temperature and lesion size; risk of lesion complications
Change in ablation circuit impedance	5-10 Ω decrease	Can be used with any electrode	Variable/unpredictable accuracy for myocardial temperature
Electrogram amplitude reduction (EAR)	>90% reduction in bipolar electrogram	Direct (tissue) information; may be safer	May be less effective (smaller lesions); limited to certain myocardial territories
Fixed power	Variable	Easy to apply	Variable/unpredictable lesion size; risk of complications

correlation between the image and pathologic lesion morphology and dimensions. Data such as these, when combined with the potential utility of this technology for navigation, give magnetic resonance imaging great promise for future clinical application. The various RF titration techniques are summarized in Table 2–4.

References

1. Packer D, Keelan P, Munger T, et al.: Clinical presentation, investigation, and management of pulmonary vein stenosis complicating ablation for atrial fibrillation. Circulation 111:546-554, 2005.

2. Pappone C, Oral H, Santinelli V, et al.: Atrio-esophageal fistula as a complication of percutaneous transcatheter ablation of atrial fibrillation. Circulation 109:2724-2726, 2004.

3. Epstein M, Knapp L, Martindill M, et al.: Embolic complications associated with radiofrequency catheter ablation. Am J Cardiol 77:655-658, 1996.

4. Hsu L, Jais P, Hocini M, et al.: Incidence and prevention of cardiac tamponade complicating ablation for atrial fibrillation. Pacing Clin Electrophysiol 28:S106-S109, 2005.

5. Demazumder D, Mirotznik M, Schwartzman D: Biophysics of radiofrequency ablation using an irrigated electrode. J Interv Card Electrophysiol 5:377-389, 2001.

6. Demazumder D, Mirotznik M, Schwartzman D: Comparison of irrigated electrode designs for radiofrequency ablation of myocardium. J Interv Card Electrophysiol 5:391-400, 2001.

7. Ren J, Schwartzman D, Lighty G, et al.: Multiplane transesophageal and intracardiac echocardiography in large swine: Imaging technique, normal values, and research applications. Echocardiography 14:135-147, 1997.

8. Ren J, Schwartzman D, Callans D, Marchlinski F: Intracardiac echocardiography (9 MHz) in humans: Methods, imaging views and clinical utility. Ultrasound Med Biol 25:1077-1086, 1999.

9. Schwartzman D, Michele J, Trankiem C, Ren J: Electrogram-guided radiofrequency ablation of atrial tissue: Characterization of a new method and comparison with thermometry-guided ablation. J Interv Card Electrophysiol 5:253-266, 2001.

10. Schwartzman D, Parizhskaya M, Devine W. Linear ablation using an irrigated electrode: electrophysiologic and histologic lesion evolution; comparison with ablation utilizing a non-irrigated electrode. J Interv Card Electrophysiol 5:17-26, 2001.

11. Mirotznik M, Schwartzman D: Inhomogenous heating patterns of commercial electrodes for radiofrequency catheter ablation. J Cardiovasc Electrophysiol 7:1058-1062, 1996.

12. Bazaz R, Nosbisch J, Schwartzman D: Insights gained into form and function of the posterior left atrium. Pacing Clin Electrophysiol 26:1386-1406, 2003.

13. Schwartzman D, Lacomis J, Wigginton W: Characterization of left atrium and distal pulmonary vein morphology using multidimensional computed tomography. J Am Coll Cardiol 41:1349-57, 2003.

14. Schwartzman D: Catheter ablation to suppress atrial fibrillation: Evolution of technique at a single center. J Interv Card Electrophysiol 9:295-300, 2003.

15. Gerstenfeld E, Dixit S, Callans D, et al.: Utility of exit block for identifying electrical isolation of the pulmonary veins. J Cardiovasc Electrophysiol 13:971-979, 2002.

16. Callans D, Ren J, Schwartzman D, et al.: Narrowing of the superior vena cava-right atrium junction during radiofrequency catheter ablation for inappropriate sinus tachycardia: Analysis with intracardiac echocardiography. J Am Coll Cardiol 33:1667-1670, 1999.

17. Schwartzman D, Ren J, Devine W, Callans D: Cardiac swelling associated with linear radiofrequency ablation in the atrium. J Interv Card Electrophysiol 5:253-266, 2001.

18. Marrouche N, Martine D, Wazni O, et al.: Phased array intracardiac echocardiography monitoring during pulmonary vein isolation in patients with atrial fibrillation: Impact on outcome and complications. Circulation 107:2710-2716, 2003.

19. Wood M, Shafer K, Ellenbogen A, Ownby E: Microbubbles during radiofrequency ablation: Composition and formation. Heart Rhythm (in press).

20. Lardo A, McVeigh E, Jumrussirikul P: Visualization and temporal/spatial characterization of cardiac radiofrequency ablation lesions using magnetic resonance imaging. Circulation 102:698-705, 2000.

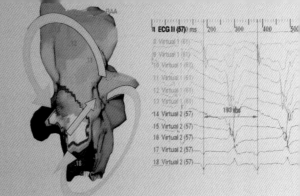

3

Irrigated and Cooled-tip Radiofrequency Catheter Ablation

Kuo-Hung Lin • Jan-Yow Chen • Yu-Chin Lin
Kuan-Cheng Chang • Shoei K. Stephen Huang

Key Points

- Cooled ablation circumvents the limitations on power delivery imposed by excessive electrode temperatures and char formation with standard radiofrequency (RF) ablation.

- Cooled RF ablation increases lesion size by increasing power delivery.

- Ablation electrode cooling may be passive (large electrode size) or active (irrigated electrode).

- Cooled ablation improves the efficacy of ablation for ventricular tachycardia, atrial flutter, and atrial fibrillation in the clinical setting.

Radiofrequency (RF) ablation has become a standard form of therapy for most cases of supraventricular tachycardia[1-6] and some ventricular tachycardias (VT).[7-9] More recently, RF ablation has also been used increasingly for the treatment of more complicated arrhythmias, particularly VT associated with structural heart disease,[10,11] atrial flutter,[12-14] and atrial fibrillation.[15,16] Although the results have been promising, RF current delivered through a standard 7 French (7F), 4-mm-tip electrode catheter has been limited for ablation of arrhythmogenic tissue located within a few millimeters of the ablation electrode. The overall success rate may be improved if the lesion size created by RF ablation can be increased. In 1% to 10% of patients with accessory pathways[17-19] and 30% to 50% of patients with nonidiopathic VT,[10,20-22] the arrhythmogenic tissue cannot be destroyed with a conventional ablation electrode. There is a need to create deeper lesions for ablation of VT originating from midmyocardial or epicardial ventricular sites and for creation of continuous linear and transmural lesions across trabeculated or thickened atrial myocardium.

Reduction of the temperature of the tip of the ablation catheter has proved to be a solution for increasing the RF application duration and thereby developing a larger and deeper lesion.[23,24] The aim of this chapter is to review current understanding of the mechanism of irrigated and cooled-tip catheter ablation as well as the results of studies and clinical trials that have employed this technology.

Biophysics of Cooled Radiofrequency Ablation

During RF application, delivery of RF current through the tip of the catheter results in a shell of resistive heating. This layer of resistive heating serves as a heat source that conducts heat to the myocardium surrounding the electrode tip (Fig. 3–1). The shell of resistive heating is thought to be thin and within a diameter only somewhat greater than the diameter of the electrode tip. Conductive heat is responsible for further thermal injury up to several millimeters away.[25,26] For any given electrode size and tissue contact area, RF lesion size is a function of RF power level and exposure time.[27,28] At higher power, however, the exposure time is frequently limited by an impedance rise that occurs when the temperature at the electrode-tissue interface reaches 100°C,[29,30] because tissue desiccation, steam, and coagulum formation occur at this temperature. Attempts to increase RF current delivery further are limited by the develop-

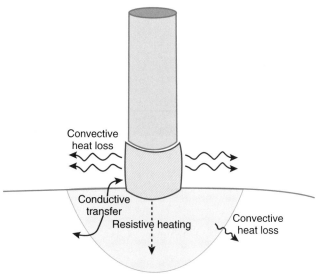

FIGURE 3–1. Schematic drawing of radiofrequency catheter ablation on the endocardium demonstrating zones of resistive and conductive heating and convective heat loss into the blood pool and coronary arteries. Superficial myocardium near the catheter is ablated via resistive heating, and deeper myocardium is heated via conductive heating. From EP Lab Digest, with permission.

ment of steam and coagulum that form around the electrode tip. The impedance rise limits the duration of RF current delivery, the total amount of energy delivered, and the size of the lesion generated.

Although currently used temperature-controlled[25,26,31-35] RF delivery systems are able to minimize the incidence of coagulum formation and impedance rise, the power applied is usually decreased and the lesion size becomes limited. During temperature-controlled RF ablation, the tip temperature, tissue temperature, and lesion size are affected by the electrode-tissue contact and by cooling effects resulting from blood flow. With good contact between catheter tip and tissue and low cooling of the catheter tip, the target temperature can be reached with little power, resulting in fairly small lesions even though a high tip temperature is being measured. In contrast, a low tip temperature can be caused by a high level of convective cooling, which results in high power consumption to reach the target temperature, yielding a relatively large lesion.

Two methods have been used to cool the catheter tip, prevent the impedance rise, and maximize power delivery. In one approach, larger ablation electrodes (8F, 8 to 10mm in length) are used.[26,35,36] The larger electrode-tissue contact area results in a greater volume of direct resistive heating. In addition, the larger electrode surface area exposed to blood results in greater convective cooling of the electrode by the blood. This cooling effect helps to prevent an impedance rise, allowing longer application of RF current

Comparison between cooled tip and standard RF ablation

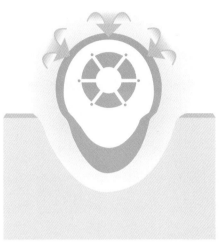

FIGURE 3–2. Comparison between cooled-tip and standard radiofrequency (RF) ablation. **A,** Cross-section of cooled tip showing effect of saline envelope. **B,** Cross-section of standard RF tip showing heat dissipation above ablation site. Courtesy of Boston Scientific Electrophysiology, San Jose, CA, USA.

Cross section of cooled tip
Showing effect of saline envelope

Cross section of standard RF tip
Showing heat dissipation above ablation site

at higher power, which produces a larger, deeper lesion.

An alternative approach, described by Wittkampf et al.[23] in 1988, is to irrigate the ablation electrode with saline to cool down the electrode-tissue interface temperature and prevent an impedance rise.[23,24,37-41] This approach allows cooler saline to internally or externally bathe the ablation electrode, dissipating heat generated during RF ablation (Fig. 3–2). It decreases the electrode-myocardial interface temperature and allows for a larger amount of RF current to be passed before heating of tissue that results in the development of impedance rises and "pops."[42] Compared with conventional RF ablation, cooled ablation allows passage of both higher powers and longer durations of RF current with less likelihood of impedance rises. In addition, because convective cooling from the blood stream in not required, an irrigated electrode may be capable of delivering higher RF power at sites of low blood flow, such as within a ventricular trabecular crevasse.[43]

During cooled ablation, as the RF current is passed through the electrode to the myocardium, resistive heating still occurs at the electrode-myocardial interface. However, unlike with standard RF ablation, the area of maximum temperature with cooled ablation is within the myocardium rather than at the electrode-myocardial interface. Nakagawa et al.[41] demonstrated that the maximum temperature generated by cooled RF ablation will be several millimeters away from the electrode-myocardial interface due to the active electrode cooling. In the study by Dorwarth et al.,[44] the "hottest point" extended from the electrode surface to 3.2 to 3.6 mm within the myocardium from the electrode-tissue interface for

cooled ablation modeled with a catheter cooled by internal perfusion of saline. Therefore, tissue temperature generated during cooled RF ablation increases from the electrode tip to a maximum temperature a couple of millimeters within the myocardium. The current density and the width of the shell of resistive heating are increased around the electrode-myocardial interface, resulting in a larger effective radiant surface diameter and larger lesion depth, width, and volume.

Because the catheter tip is cooled actively, the temperature at the tip-tissue interface during cooled RF application is unreliable as a marker for determining the duration of RF application. Limiting tip temperature to less than 100°C prevents almost all impedance rises with conventional RF ablation. However, because the maximum tissue temperature is several millimeters away from the catheter tip during cooled ablation, the maximum tissue temperature may not be accurately monitored by a tip thermistor or thermocouple. Although RF current is increased with cooled RF ablation, intramyocardial tissues could be heated to 100°C, which would result in intramyocardial steam and crater formation. The maximum temperature may now be intramyocardial and surrounded by cooler areas of tissue.[44] The development of intramyocardial steam may result in explosions with resultant formation of a deep crater, possibly associated with dissection, perforation, and thrombus formation. Some animal studies suggest that the optimal powers to avoid large craters are no greater than 50 W for an internally cooled catheter or 20 W for an irrigated catheter.[45-47] For the same reason, because cooling is adequate, the target tip temperature for predicting impedance rises due to tissue

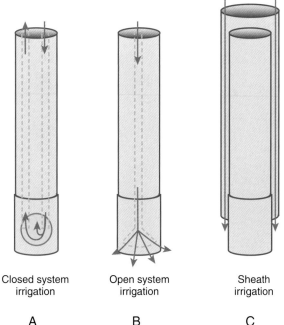

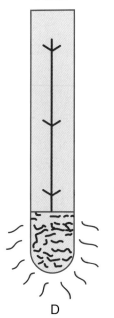

FIGURE 3–3. Schematic drawings of four different methods of cooling: internal saline irrigation (**A**), opened showerhead or sprinkler type (**B**), external sheath irrigation (**C**), and porous irrigated-tip catheter (**D**). From EP Lab Digest, with permission.

overheating should not be 100°C. Wharton et al.[48] demonstrated that impedance rises may be minimized to less than 6.3% if tip temperatures are maintained at less than 45°C. Nibley et al.[38] also showed that a constantly maintained power of 50 W for the internally cooled catheter tip may deliver the maximum energy. Further studies are needed to expand these observations over a range of catheter types and clinical conditions in order to better understand how to limit power in cooled RF ablation in humans to prevent crater formation.

Design of Irrigated and Cooled-tip Radiofrequency Catheters

Cooling of the catheter tip during RF ablation is achieved by circulating saline through or around the tip of the ablation catheter while RF current is being delivered. Four different cooled catheters have been designed, as shown in Figure 3–3. The internally cooled catheter (Boston Scientific Electrophysiology, San Jose, Calif.) has an internally cooled (or chilled) tip electrode that is perfused with room-temperature, saline (see Fig. 3–3A). With this closed loop system, saline perfuses the tip of the catheter via a conduit in the catheter shaft and returns back via a second conduit in the catheter. Saline is not infused into the body (Fig. 3–4). The second approach uses an externally irrigated (or opened) system, in which saline is infused into the body after irrigating the tip of the

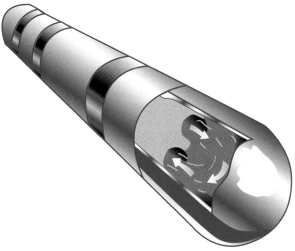

FIGURE 3–4. Schematic drawing of the Chilli® cooled-tip catheter. Courtesy of Boston Scientific Electrophysiology, San Jose, CA, USA.

electrode. The saline irrigation sprinkler catheter system (Medtronic CardioRhythm, San Jose, Calif.) is a showerhead-type catheter with 13 holes (approximately 0.010-inch diameter) distributed over the electrode surface, including one at the tip and four near the proximal edge of the electrode (see Fig. 3–3B). Another opened irrigated catheter design infuses saline through a long sheath surrounding the tip (see Fig. 3–3C). The third externally irrigated system (see Fig. 3–3D) uses a catheter tip made of porous metal (Angeion, Minneapolis, Minn.). Saline is taken to the tip of the catheter via a conduit in the catheter shaft and then extruded through multiple pores at the tip of the catheter.

Many other designs have been investigated in vivo and in vitro. A screw-tip needle electrode, through which saline and contrast material could be infused during RF ablation, has been demonstrated to create a larger lesion in canines.[49] This technology may create significantly deeper but narrower lesions without evidence of tissue boiling. A newly developed, long irrigated ablation catheter (tripolar; 7F; length of each electrode, 22 mm; interelectrode distance, 2 mm; helix radius, 9 and 10 mm), covered by a porous membrane to provide continuous irrigation, could create long and deeper lesions in vivo.[50] The ability to create a long linear lesion without gap could be applied to pulmonary vein isolation and cavotricuspid isthmus ablation.

Both internally cooled and externally irrigated catheter systems have been proven to increase the RF lesion size compared with standard ablation catheter in investigation models. Demazumder et al.[51] reported that the internally cooled model led to a somewhat smaller lesion when compared with the showerhead or sheath approach. This is probably a result of the greater cooling of the electrode-myocardial interface afforded by external irrigation.

The Chilli® Cooled Radiofrequency Ablation System (Boston Scientific) (see Fig. 3–4) is approved by the U.S. Food and Drug Administration for use in patients with nonidiopathic VT. In clinical application, cooling is achieved by pumping 0.6 mL/sec of saline to the tip of the catheter during RF application. RF energy is generated titrated to achieve an electrode temperature between 40°C to 50°C, to a maximum 50 W.

The other cooled RF ablation system that has been used is a showerhead-type irrigated-tip catheter (Cordis-Webster, Medtronic). Cooling is achieved with saline infused at a rate of 17 mL/min during RF application and 3 mL/min during all other times. Both systems have been employed in clinical trials recently.

Results of Animal Studies

Some authors have demonstrated on animal and experimental models that lesions caused by cooled RF catheter ablation are larger and deeper than lesions caused by conventional ablation.

Nibley et al.[38] conducted a canine study in which RF current was delivered via an internally cooled tip. Energy delivery duration could be prolonged with the use of the cooled-tip catheter, and impedance rise was delayed for longer periods. Ruffy et al.[40] reported an ovine study in which RF lesions

were created through a closed internal saline-cooled ablation catheter at 30 W and compared with standard RF. The mean power delivered with the cooled electrode was 22.04 ± 4.51 W, versus 6.10 ± 2.47 W with standard RF ablation ($P < .001$). Mean lesion volume was 436.07 ± 177.00 mm^3 versus 1247.78 ± 520.51 mm^3 ($P < .001$).

Nakagawa et al.[41] evaluated cooled ablation in the canine thigh muscle in vivo. They used a 7F, 5-mm-tip electrode catheter having a central lumen with six irrigation holes and an internal thermistor, which was positioned perpendicular to the thigh muscle. Using thermal probes inserted at the electrode surface and at depths of 3.5 and 7.0 mm within the muscle, this study demonstrated that the maximum tissue temperature (94.7°C) during cooled ablation occurred 3.5 mm from the tip of the electrode. In comparison, conventional fixed-voltage (66 V) and temperature-controlled (85°C) RF without irrigation showed temperatures that were maximal at the electrode interface and decreased with further distance from the electrode tip. Therefore, saline irrigation maintains a low electrode-tissue interface temperature during RF application at high power, which prevents an impedance rise and produces a deeper and larger lesion. A higher temperature in the tissue (3.5 mm deep) than at the electrode-tissue interface indicates that direct resistive heating occurred deeper in the tissue, rather than heating by conduction from the surface (Fig. 3–5). Of note, with saline irrigation the maximum width of the ablation lesion was at intramyocardial sites, not at the myocardial surface. This reflects the fact that the cooling effect decreases lesion expansion along the myocardial surface.

Mittleman and Huang et al.[39] also demonstrated the use of a luminal electrode catheter with an end hole and two side holes (Bard Electrophysiology, Haverhill, Mass.) for infusion of saline during RF ablation. Application of power for 60 seconds at either 10 or 20 W could produce a significantly larger lesion than that produced with a standard catheter in canine myocardium in vivo and was effective in preventing impedance rise (Figs. 3–6 and 3–7).

Dorwarth et al.[44] compared various cooled and noncooled catheter systems in terms of specific lesion geometry, incidence of impedance rise, and crater and coagulum formation. The study investigated myocardial lesion generation of three actively cooled-catheter systems (7F, 4-mm tip): one with a showerhead-type (sprinkler) electrode tip one with a porous metal tip, and one internally cooled catheter. Noncooled catheters (7F) had electrodes with either a large tip (8 mm) or a standard tip (4 mm). RF energy was delivered on isolated porcine myocardium superfused with heparinized pig blood (37°C) at power settings of 10 to 40 W. Both irrigated systems

RF Lesion Dimensions

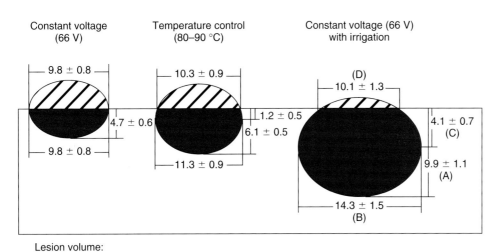

Lesion volume:
135 ± 33 mm³   275 ± 55 mm³   700 ± 217 mm³

FIGURE 3–5. Diagram of lesion dimensions for the three groups studied. Values are expressed in millimeters (mean ± standard deviation). A indicates maximal lesion depth; B, maximal lesion diameter; C, depth at maximal lesion diameter; and D, lesion surface diameter. Lesion volume was calculated by use of the formula for an oblate ellipsoid, by subtracting the volume of the "missing cap" *(hatched area).* From reference 41, figure 9, with permission.

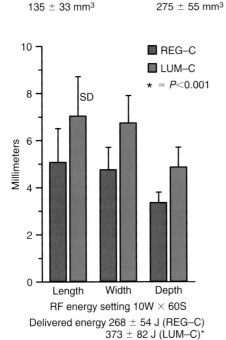

RF energy setting 10W × 60S
Delivered energy 268 ± 54 J (REG–C)
              373 ± 82 J (LUM–C)*

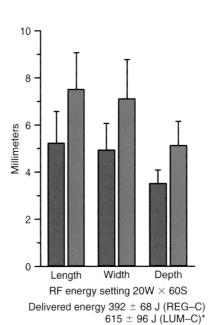

RF energy setting 20W × 60S
Delivered energy 392 ± 68 J (REG–C)
              615 ± 96 J (LUM–C)*

FIGURE 3–6. Dimensions of lesions (mean ± standard deviation) created at two set energy levels (10 W × 60 seconds and 20 W × 60 seconds). REG-C, standard electrode catheter; LUM-C, saline-infused electrode catheter. *, p < 0.001 versus standard catheter. From reference 39, figure 2, with permission.

were characterized by a large lesion depth (8.1 ± 1.6 mm) and a large lesion diameter (13.8 ± 1.6 mm). Lesions created by the internally cooled catheter showed a similar lesion depth (8.0 ± 1.0 mm) but a significantly smaller lesion diameter (12.3 ± 1.2 mm; *P* = .04). Compared with the irrigated systems, lesions created by the large-tip noncooled catheters had a similar lesion diameter (14.5 ± 1.6 mm) but a significantly smaller lesion depth (6.3 ± 1.0 mm; *P* = .002). However, lesion volume was not significantly different between the three cooled catheters and the large-tip catheter. The lesion volume increased as power delivery increased initially, but above a certain power setting lesion volume decreased or remained unchanged as a result of intramyocardial overheating and impedance rise. Maximum lesion volume was induced at a power setting of 30 W for the two open-

irrigation catheter systems and 20 W for the internally cooled catheter.

Larger electrode diameter or length during conventional RF ablation may generate larger lesions.[36] However, Nakagawa et al.[52] demonstrated an inverse relationship between electrode size and lesion size during RF ablation with active electrode cooling with the electrodes perpendicular to the tissue. A 2-mm electrode delivered 49% more heating power to the tissue than a 5-mm electrode did; the latter lost more current to the surrounding blood, decreasing the effective RF current. Tissue temperature at depths of 3.5 and 7 mm and lesion size were measured. In the perpendicular electrode-tissue orientation, RF applications at 50 V resulted in lower power with the 2-mm electrode compared with the 5-mm electrode (26 versus 36 W, respectively) but higher tissue tempera-

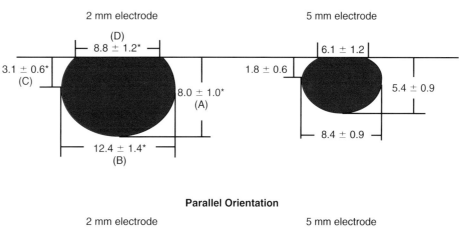

FIGURE 3–7. Examples of lesion created with either a saline-infused catheter *(left)* or with a standard catheter *(right)*, in the anterior and posterior wall of the left ventricle, respectively. The lesion on the left is bigger and exhibits a larger area of pitting and more extensive necrosis. The energy level for both lesions was 20 W for 60 seconds. Ruler divisions are at 1-mm intervals. From reference 39, figure 3, with permission.

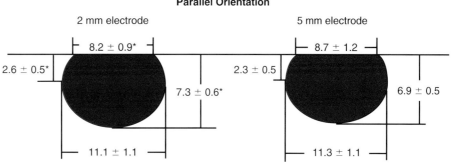

FIGURE 3–8. Diagram of lesion dimensions for two groups studied. Values are expressed in millimeters (mean ± standard deviation). A indicates maximal lesion depth; B, maximal lesion diameter; C, depth at maximal lesion diameter; and D, lesion surface diameter. *, $P < .05$ between 2-mm and 5-mm ablation electrodes within same electrode-tissue orientation. From reference 52, figure 5, with permission.

tures, larger lesion depth (8.0 versus 5.4 mm), and greater diameter (12.4 versus 8.4 mm). With the electrodes parallel to the tissue, overall power was lower with the 2-mm electrode (25 versus 33 W), but tissue temperatures were higher and lesions were deeper (7.3 versus 6.9 mm). Lesion diameter was similar (11.1 versus 11.3 mm) for both electrodes. Therefore, if the cooling is adequate, the smaller actively cooled electrode transmitted a greater fraction of the RF power to the tissue and resulted in higher tissue temperature and larger lesions (Fig. 3–8).

Flow rates of saline infusion may also affect the size of a lesion created by cooled ablation.[53] A higher flow rate might cause a greater cooling effect to the catheter tip, which could potentially generate a larger lesion but which also could waste more RF current due to overcooling. In contrast, a lower flow rate might result in a lesion size approaching that of conventional RF ablation. Weiss et al.[54] investigated the impact of various irrigation catheter flow rates on the development of lesion dimension and thrombus formation. Three flow rates (5, 10, and 20 mL/min) were used for RF ablation on sheep thigh muscle preparations. With high-flow irrigation (20 mL/min), the surface diameter was significantly smaller (0.63 ± 0.1 cm) than with rates of 5 mL/min (0.88 ± 0.2 cm) or 10 mL/min (1 ± 0.1 cm) (Table 3–1). Thrombus formation was not observed during any RF application. It was demonstrated that, with sufficient cooling of the ablation electrode, a tip temperature of 40°C is provided even with flow rates of 5 mL/min. In cases of high flow rates (20 mL/min), the lesion diameters at the surface were reduced due to increased cooling of the superficial muscle layers. However, the power delivery to deeper tissue layers was not influenced, and the measured tissue temperature at 7 mm and the corresponding lesion depth were not significantly different from those of lesions achieved with lower flow rates. Further, decreasing the irrigation flow rate to less than 5 mL/min may lead to a loss of sufficient electrode cooling. This study also demonstrated that increased catheter contact pressure results in a deeper lesion with an increased risk of steam pops.[54] Tight contact may inhibit the cooling effect below the catheter.

Temperature monitoring during cooled RF application may be an unreliable marker because the actual surface temperature is underestimated. In the design of longer catheter tip (6 to 10 mm) for increased convective cooling of the catheter tip, Petersen et al.[47] found a negative correlation between tip temperature reached and lesion volume for applications in which maximum generator output was not achieved, whereas delivered power and lesion volume correlated positively. They also directly examined the tissue temperatures and lesion volumes formed by a showerhead-type cooled tip in the setting of either temperature control or power control. Power-controlled RF ablation at 40 W generated lesions that were similar to those achieved with temperature control at both 80°C and 70°C; lesions formed with temperature control at 60°C were significantly smaller. Importantly, positive correlations between lesion volume and real tissue temperature did not appear at the peak electrode-tip temperatures.

For monitoring of internal tissue temperatures, Thiagalingam et al.[49] designed an intramural needle ablation catheter with an internally cooled 1.1-mm-diameter straight needle that could be advanced up to 12 mm into the myocardium. This catheter could create deeper ablation lesions than a conventional irrigated-tip catheter (5-mm electrode; Thermocool D curve system, Cordis Webster). The irrigation rate, target temperature, and maximum power were 10 mL/min, 85°C, and 20 W for the intramural needle catheter and 20 mL/min, 50°C, and 50 W for the irrigated-tip catheter. Cooled intramural needle ablation created significantly deeper and more transmural lesions without evidence of tissue boiling (Table 3–2).

We might expect RF ablation efficiency with active cooling to be even greater on the epicardial surface because of (1) the lack of convective cooling of the ablation catheter in pericardial space, which would cause the impedance to rise rapidly and reduce the duration of RF energy delivery, and (2) the varying presence of epicardial adipose tissue interposed between the ablation electrode and the target site.

D'Avila et al.[55] examined the dimensions and biophysical characteristics of RF lesions generated by either standard or cooled-tip ablation catheters deliv-

TABLE 3–1

Temperatures During Radiofrequency Application with Various Irrigation Flow Rates

Parameters of RF Application	IRRIGATION FLOW RATE (ML/MIN)		
	5 (n = 15)	10 (n = 14)	20 (n = 14)
Total power	929 ± 12	939 ± 12	935 ± 5
Maximum impedance (Ω)	133 ± 13	125 ± 12	113 ± 12
Maximum catheter tip temperature (°C)	43 ± 3	39 ± 3	37 ± 3
Maximum tissue temperature (°C)			
At 3.5 mm	79 ± 8*	67 ± 5	57 ± 4
At 7.0 mm	57 ± 4	67 ± 5	58 ± 6
Audible pops	0	0	0
Thrombus formation	0	0	0

*$P < .01$ versus 10 and 20 mL/min. All RF applications were achieved with a 30-W power output and a 30-second pulse duration.
RF, radiofrequency.
From reference 54, table 1, with permission.

FIGURE 3–9. A and **B,** Cooled-tip and standard radiofrequency (RF) epicardial ablation lesions. **A,** The smallest epicardial lesion was generated with standard RF energy *(yellow arrow);* the other five lesions on this heart were created with cooled-tip RF application. **B,** Contour of cooled-tip epicardial lesions on normal epicardial surface and on fat *(black arrow).* **C** and **D,** Histopathologic slides of epicardial lesions. Epicardial fat interposed between the tip of the ablation catheter and epicardium prejudiced creation of deep epicardial RF lesions. **C,** Lesion created with standard RF application shows a distinct border at the beginning of the epicardial fat layer. **D,** Significant attenuation toward the area covered by epicardial fat in a lesion created by cooled-tip RF application. From reference 55, figure 1, with permission.

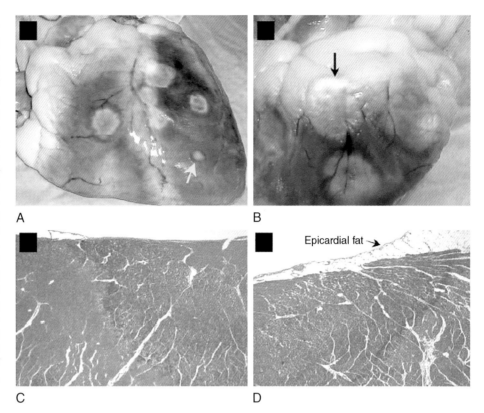

A

B

Epicardial fat →

C

D

TABLE 3–2					
Comparison of the Lesion Size Between Intramural Needle Ablation Catheter and Irrigated-tip Catheter					
Catheter	Power (W)	Lesion Depth (mm)	Lesion Width (mm)	Transmural (>90% of tissue depth)	Lesion Volume (mm³)
Intramural needle	20 ± 3.0*	12.5 ± 3.0*	3.9 ± 1.1*	22%(34%)	172 ± 120*
Irrigated tip	43 ± 3.7*	8.3 ± 2.1*	11.5 ± 2.0*	16%(16%)	420 ± 256*

*Significance: $p < 0.01$ with correction for repeated measures.
From reference 49, table 1, with permission.

ered to normal and infarcted epicardial ventricular tissue. The study used 10 normal goats and 7 pigs with healed anterior-wall myocardial infarction in which nonsurgical subxiphoid pericardial access was achieved. A 4-mm cooled-tip RF ablation catheter with continuous saline circulation at 0.6 mL/sec (Chilli®, Boston Scientific) was used to deliver epicardial ventricular lesions. Lesions created on normal epicardial tissue with standard and cooled-tip RF ablation were 3.7 ± 1.3 mm and 6.7 ± 1.7 mm in depth, respectively. On scar tissue, lesions made by the cooled-tip catheter were 14.6 ± 2.7 mm in length, 11.8 ± 2.9 mm in width, and 5.6 ± 1.2 mm in depth. Lesions located at the right ventricular boundary of the scar were consistently transmural (ranging from 4 to 5 mm in depth). During cooled-tip RF ablation, 35.6 ± 7.1 W of power was required to achieve a temperature of 41.4°C ± 2.2°C. The presence of epicardial fat

interposed between the catheter tip and myocardial tissue prevented lesion formation with standard RF ablation and also attenuated the efficacy of cooled-tip ablation (4.1 ± 2 mm in depth) (Fig. 3–9). This study raised the possibility that midmyocardial and even endocardial VT circuits may be eliminated by cooled-tip RF ablation from the pericardial space.

Clinical Studies

COOLED RADIOFREQUENCY ABLATION FOR NONIDIOPATHIC VENTRICULAR TACHYCARDIA

A clinical trial was conducted by Calkins et al.[56] (Cardiac Pathways, Inc.) to survey catheter ablation of VT using a cooled-tip catheter. This prospective study enrolled 146 consecutive patients at 18 institutions between 1995 and 1997. The Chilli® cooled RF system, with a 7F quadripolar catheter containing a deflectable 4-mm electrode tip, was used. Cooling was achieved by pumping 0.6 mL/sec of saline to the tip of the catheter through two internal cooling channels during RF application. RF energy of 25 W was delivered initially, with further increases to achieve an electrode temperature between 40°C and 50°C. Maximum output of 50 W for 60 to 180 seconds was delivered. Delivery of RF energy was terminated if impedance rose to greater than 250 Ω or electrode temperatures to greater than 65°C. All patients presented with a structural heart disease: ischemic heart disease was present in 119 patients (82%), and 107 patients (73%) had an ejection fraction (EF) of 35% or less, with a mean of 31% ± 13%. The primary end point for the study was the elimination of all mappable VT or all hemodynamically stable VT; this was accomplished in 75% of all the mappable VT (n = 106), but only 41% of the 146 enrolled patients were completely noninducible after ablation. Some VT or ventricular fibrillation recurred at follow-up (4% of the patients); the mean time to recurrence was 24 days, and the 1-year recurrence rate was 56%. The frequency of VT episodes was reduced by 75% at 2 months after ablation in 81% of the patients. Multivariate analysis was performed to determine factors that were predictive of success. Major complications occurred in 12 patients (8%), and there were 4 deaths (2.7%) from stroke, tamponade, valve injury, and myocardial infarction. No "pop" was heard during any RF delivery. The percentage of patients experiencing major complications was not significantly greater than that reported previously in various series, which averaged from 5% to 12%. Because this trial did not randomly assign patients to cooled versus standard RF ablation, it is not possible to precisely define the magnitude of benefit achieved by use of the cooled RF ablation system.

Reddy et al.[57] evaluated the safety and acute procedural efficacy of a combined electrophysiologic and anatomic approach to ablate all inducible VT during sinus rhythm using an irrigated-tip RF ablation catheter. The RF ablation lesions were placed in a linear fashion traversing the border zones of infarcted and normal tissue (mean of 3.4 linear lesions per patient). The majority of RF lesions were placed with the use of a saline-irrigated 3.5-mm-tip ablation catheter (Navi-Star, Biosense Webster). This catheter is equipped with a central lumen and a showerhead-type configuration at the catheter tip. To actively cool the ablation electrode, saline solution (0.45% to 0.9%) was infused through the catheter at 2 mL/min during catheter manipulation and at 15 to 30 mL/min during RF delivery. The RF lesions were

placed in 60-second intervals under power control (25 to 50 W) with impedance monitoring. The target VT was eliminated in 9 (82%) of 11 patients. Furthermore, when all inducible monomorphic VTs were targeted, complete procedural success was achieved in 7 (64%) of 11 patients. During the follow-up period (mean, 13.1 ± 1.9 weeks), spontaneous VT was noted only in the two patients with no acute procedural benefit.

Soejima et al.[58] compared the efficacy of VT termination using standard versus cooled-tip RF application. Cooled-tip RF terminated VT more frequently at isthmus sites where an isolated potential was present (89%, versus 54% with standard RF; $P = .003$), at isthmus sites without an isolated potential (36% versus 21%; $P = .04$), and at inner loop sites (60% versus 22%; $P = .04$). Termination rates were similarly low for cooled versus standard RF at bystander sites (14% versus 9%; $P = .56$) and at outer loop sites (13% versus 11%; $P = .93$). The termination rate at isthmus sites was significantly higher in the cooled RF group, suggesting that these reentry circuit isthmuses often exceed the width and depth of a standard RF lesion.

COOLED RADIOFREQUENCY ABLATION FOR ATRIAL FLUTTER

The most common type of atrial flutter is isthmus-dependent atrial flutter, in which reentry is confined to the right atrium with the wavefront progressing in a counterclockwise or clockwise direction across the cavotricuspid isthmus. Because of the pouches, recesses, ridges, and trabeculations that may occur in the isthmus, it often is advantageous to create lesions that are larger than those created with conventional 4-mm-tip ablation catheters. RF ablation catheters have an 8-mm distal electrode or a cooled- or irrigated-tip electrode to allow the creation of larger lesions in both high- and low-flow regions. Several studies have demonstrated that complete isthmus block is more reliably achieved with a cooled- or irrigated-tip catheter than with a conventional ablation catheter.[59-64] Cooled-tip ablation has proved to be as safe as standard RF ablation and may achieve isthmus block more expeditiously during atrial flutter ablation.

Jais et al.[59] compared conventional and irrigated-tip catheter ablation of typical atrial flutter using a showerhead-type system (Thermocool D curve system, Cordis Webster). Temperatures were maintained at 50°C with a power limit of 50 W for 60 seconds. Cooling was achieved with saline pumped at a rate of 17 mL/min during RF application and 3 mL/min during all other times. Of the 26 patients, 22 (85%) in the conventional catheter group achieved successful creation of bidirectional isthmus block and flutter termination, as did all patients (100%) in the irrigated-tip catheter group. The four patients who failed conventional flutter ablation were then crossed over to the irrigated-tip group and were all treated successfully. No neighboring coronary artery (right coronary artery) damage was found by coronary angiograms performed on the first 30 enrolled patients. After a mean follow-up of 5 ± 2 months, no recurrences of flutter were noted, except in one patient in the conventional arm who required additional ablation 2 days after the initial procedure. No procedural complications resulting from flutter ablation were noted in either group. In addition to a high success rate, significantly fewer RF applications were required to achieve bidirectional block in the irrigated-tip group (5 ± 3, compared with 13 ± 10 for the conventional group; $P = .0003$). The mean procedure time was significantly less in the cooled-tip group (27 ± 16 versus 53 ± 41 minutes; $P < .0008$). The total x-ray exposure time was also decreased in the cooled-tip group 9 ± 6 versus 27 ± 16 minutes; $P = .01$). In another study, Jais et al.[60] recruited those patients who failed in conventional atrial flutter ablation due to gaps within the isthmus line. Using the same irrigated-tip catheter system, complete block was achieved in 12 (92%) of the 13 patients; 6 patients required only a single additional cooled RF application, and 6 had two to six additional applications. Both studies showed that cooled RF ablation in atrial flutter is as safe as conventional RF ablation and may be more effective in creating complete bidirectional block along the isthmus while decreasing procedural times and x-ray exposure.

Atiga et al.[61] also investigated the benefit of cooled-tip catheter ablation in patients with type I atrial flutter. One group of patients underwent standard RF ablation, and a second group underwent cooled-tip ablation with the Chilli® system initially. They crossed over two groups if bidirectional isthmus block could not be achieved in 12 attempts at catheter ablation. The end point was either successful bidirectional isthmus block or a total of 24 RF applications in all groups. After the initial six RF applications, 25% of the patients in the cooled-tip group and 23% of those in the conventional group achieved bidirectional isthmus block. After 12 total RF applications, a significantly greater number of patients in the cooled-tip group achieved bidirectional block (79% versus 55%). As in the studies by Jais et al., no major complications (e.g., death, tamponade, pericardial effusion) occurred in either group. In a randomized study that compared the 8-mm-tip and cooled-tip catheters by Scavee and Jais et al.,[62] complete isthmus block was achieved in 99% of 100 patients, with the efficacy of the two catheters being equally high.

An increasing number of clinical studies of irrigated- and cooled-tip catheter ablation in isthmus-dependent atrial flutter have shown remarkable results with the same safety as in standard RF ablation.[63,64] However, the clinical use of cooled-tip RF ablation in non–isthmus-dependent atrial flutter still needs further investigation.

COOLED RADIOFREQUENCY ABLATION FOR ATRIAL FIBRILLATION

In the past several years, the most exciting developments in catheter ablation of supraventricular arrhythmias have occurred in the field of atrial fibrillation. The landmark study by Haissaguerre et al.[15] in 1998 focused attention on the importance of the pulmonary veins in the generation of atrial fibrillation. This observation led to the technique of focal ablation within the pulmonary veins to eliminate the triggers of atrial fibrillation. Pulmonary vein isolation has been performed with conventional 4-mm-tip catheters, 8-mm-tip catheters, and saline-cooled or irrigated-tip catheters.[65,66] In a study that compared the three types of catheters, the best results were obtained with the 8-mm-tip catheter.[66] However, other researchers achieved pulmonary vein isolation reliably with a conventional 4-mm-tip catheter.[67] It is possible that the deeper lesions created with an 8-mm-tip catheter increase the risk of pulmonary vein stenosis, and the type of ablation catheter that is associated with the most favorable risk-to-benefit ratio is unclear. If a cooled-tip catheter or an 8-mm-tip catheter is used, monitoring of microbubble formation by intracardiac echocardiography during applications of RF energy may reduce the risk of pulmonary vein stenosis and improve efficacy.[68]

COOLED RADIOFREQUENCY ABLATION FOR ATRIOVENTRICULAR REENTRANT TACHYCARDIA

Between 5% and 17% of posteroseptal and left posterior accessory pathways have been reported to be epicardial and ablatable only within a branch of the coronary sinus (most commonly the middle cardiac vein), on the floor of the coronary sinus at the orifice of a venous branch, or within a coronary sinus diverticulum.[69] These pathways may consist of connections between the muscle coat of the coronary sinus and the ventricle. In the presence of a coronary sinus–ventricular accessory pathway, a conventional ablation catheter may completely occlude a branch of the coronary sinus, preventing cooling of the ablation electrode and resulting in high impedance when RF energy is delivered. This markedly reduces the amount of power that can be delivered and may result in adherence of the ablation electrode to the wall of the vein. An externally saline-cooled ablation catheter allows more consistent delivery of RF energy with less heating at the electrode-tissue interface.

A small percentage of left free-wall accessory pathways also may be epicardial, requiring ablation from within the coronary sinus. Other types of unusual accessory pathways that cannot be ablated with a standard endocardial approach at the annulus have been described.[17-19] These include accessory pathways that connect the right atrial appendage to the right ventricle, successfully ablated using a transcutaneous pericardial approach, and accessory pathways closely associated with the ligament of Marshall, ablated by targeting that ligament.[70-72] Several studies[73,74] showed that RF ablation using an irrigated-tip catheter can be useful for the treatment of some right posteroseptal accessory pathways resistant to conventional ablation. The optimal temperature suggested by the authors is no greater than 40°C to 45°C, and the temperature setting should be lower still if cooled-tip RF ablation is applied to the cardiac veins.

Conclusion

Research on cooled-tip catheter ablation has been evolving in the past 10 years. Findings and current applications demonstrate that cooled-tip RF ablation is an important improvement in RF catheter ablation technology, because it allows for creation of larger and deeper lesions. Cooled-tip RF ablation is becoming a safe and feasible treatment in atrial flutter and nonidiopathic VT. With careful setting of power and monitoring of temperature and impedance, cooled-tip RF ablation not only creates larger and deeper lesions but also has a low complication rate compared with standard RF ablation technology. There is also increasing evidence to suggest that cooled-tip RF ablation improves the efficacy of catheter ablation and reduces the procedure time and total radiation time. These potential benefits suggest that ablation systems that incorporate cooled-tip RF ablation technology are likely to become a standard tool for catheter ablation of cardiac arrhythmias in the future.

References

1. Jackman WM, Beckman KJ, McClelland JH, et al.: Treatment of supraventricular tachycardia due to atrioventricular nodal reentry, by radiofrequency catheter ablation of slow-pathway conduction. N Engl J Med 327:313-318, 1992.
2. Haissaguerre M, Gaita F, Fischer B, et al.: Elimination of atrioventricular nodal reentrant tachycardia using discrete slow potentials to guide application of radiofrequency energy. Circulation 85:2162-2175, 1992.
3. Calkins H, Yong P, Miller JM, et al.: Catheter ablation of accessory pathways, atrioventricular nodal reentrant tachycardia, and the atrioventricular junction: Final results of a prospective, multicenter clinical trial. The Atakr Multicenter Investigators Group. Circulation 99:262-270, 1999.
4. Jackman WM, Wang XZ, Friday KJ, et al.: Catheter ablation of accessory atrioventricular pathways (Wolff-Parkinson-White syndrome) by radiofrequency current. N Engl J Med 324:1605-1611, 1991.
5. Kuck KH, Schluterm M, Geiger M, et al.: Radiofrequency current catheter ablation of accessory atrioventricular pathways. Lancet 337:1557-1561, 1991.
6. Chen SA, Chiang CE, Yang CJ, et al.: Sustained atrial tachycardia in adult patients: Electrophysiological characteristics, pharmacological response, possible mechanisms, and effects of radiofrequency ablation. Circulation 90:1262-1278, 1994.
7. Coggins DL, Lee RJ, Sweeney J, et al.: Radiofrequency catheter ablation as a cure for idiopathic tachycardia of both left and right ventricular origin. J Am Coll Cardiol 23:1333-1341, 1994.
8. Nakagawa H, Beckman KJ, McClelland JH, et al.: Radiofrequency catheter ablation of idiopathic left ventricular tachycardia guided by a Purkinje potential. Circulation 88:2607-2617, 1993.
9. Coen TJ, Chien WW, Kurie KG, et al.: Radiofrequency catheter ablation for treatment of bundle branch reentrant ventricular tachycardia: Results and long-term follow-up. J Am Coll Cardiol 18:1767-1773, 1991.
10. Morady F, Harvey M, Kalbfleisch SJ, et al.: Radiofrequency catheter ablation of ventricular tachycardia in patients with coronary artery disease. Circulation 87:363-372, 1993.
11. Stevenson WG, Sager PT, Natterson PD, et al.: Relation of pace mapping QRS configuration and conduction delay to ventricular tachycardia reentry circuits in human infarct scars. J Am Coll Cardiol 26:481-488, 1995.
12. Feld GK, Fleck RP, Chen PS, et al.: Radiofrequency catheter ablation for the treatment of human type 1 atrial flutter: Identification of a critical zone in the reentrant circuit by endocardial mapping techniques. Circulation 86:1233-1240, 1992.
13. Cosio FG, Lopez-Gil M, Goicolea A, et al.: Radiofrequency ablation of the inferior vena cava-tricuspid valve isthmus in common atrial flutter. Am J Cardiol 71:705-709, 1993.
14. Nakagawa H, Lazzara R, Khastgir T, et al.: Role of the tricuspid annulus and the eustachian valve/ridge on atrial flutter: Relevance to catheter ablation of the septal isthmus and a new technique for rapid identification of ablation success. Circulation 94:407-424, 1996.
15. Haissaguerre M, Jais P, Shah DC, et al.: Spontaneous initiation of atrial fibrillation by ectopic beats originating in the pulmonary veins. N Engl J Med 339:659-666, 1998.
16. Tsai CF, Tai CT, Hsieh MH, et al.: Initiation of atrial fibrillation by ectopic beats originating from the superior vena cava: Electrophysiological characteristics and results of radiofrequency ablation. Circulation 102:67-74, 2000.
17. Haissaguerre M, Gaita F, Fischer B, et al.: Radiofrequency catheter ablation of left lateral accessory pathways via the coronary sinus. Circulation 86:1464-1468, 1992.
18. Wang X, McClelland JH, Beckman KJ, et al.: Left free-wall accessory pathways which require ablation from the coronary sinus: Unique coronary sinus electrogram pattern [abstract]. Circulation 86:I-581, 1992.
19. Arruda MS, Beckman KJ, McClelland JH, et al.: Coronary sinus anatomy and anomalies in patients with posteroseptal accessory pathway requiring ablation within a venous branch of the coronary sinus [abstract]. J Am Coll Cardiol 17:224A, 1994.

20. Kim YH, Sosa-Suarez G, Trouton TG, et al.: Treatment of ventricular tachycardia by transcatheter radiofrequency ablation in patients with ischemic heart disease. Circulation 89:1094-1102, 1994.

21. Littmann L, Svenson RH, Gallagher JJ, et al.: Functional role of the epicardium in postinfarction ventricular tachycardia: Observations derived from computerized epicardial activation mapping, entrainment, and epicardial laser photoablation. Circulation 83:1577-1591, 1991.

22. Downar E, Kimber S, Harris L, et al.: Endocardial mapping of ventricular tachycardia in the intact human heart. II: Evidence for multiuse reentry in a functional sheet of surviving myocardium. J Am Coll Cardiol 20:869-878, 1992.

23. Wittkampf FHM, Hauer RN, Robles de Medina EO: Radiofrequency ablation with a cooled porous electrode catheter [abstract]. J Am Coll Cardiol 11:17A, 1988.

24. Huang SKS, Cuenoud H, Tande Guzman W, et al.: Increase in the lesion size and decrease in the impedance rise with saline infusion electrode catheter for radiofrequency catheter ablation [abstract]. Circulation 80:II-324, 1989.

25. Haines DE, Watson DD: Tissue heating during radiofrequency catheter ablation: A thermodynamic model and observation in isolated perfused and superfused canine right ventricular free wall. Pacing Clin Electrophysiol 12:962-976, 1989.

26. Haines DE, Watson DD, Verow AF: Electrode radius predicts lesion radius during radiofrequency energy heating: Validation of a proposed thermodynamic model. Circ Res 67:124-129, 1990.

27. Hoyt RH, Huang SK, Marcus FI, et al.: Factors influencing trans-catheter radiofrequency ablation of the myocardium. J Appl Cardiol 1:469-486, 1986.

28. Wittkampf FHM, Hauer RN, Robles de Medina EO: Control of radiofrequency lesion size by power regulation. Circulation 80:962-968, 1989.

29. Ring ME, Huang SKS, Gorman G, et al.: Determinants of impedance rise during catheter ablation of bovine myocardium with radiofrequency energy. Pacing Clin Electrophysiol 12:170-176, 1989.

30. Haines DE, Verow AF: Observation on electrode-tissue interface temperature and effect on electrical impedance during radiofrequency ablation of ventricular myocardium. Circulation 82:1034-1038, 1990.

31. Langberg JJ, Calkins H, El-Atassi R, et al.: Temperature monitoring during radiofrequency catheter ablation of accessory pathways. Circulation 86:1469-1474, 1992.

32. Haverkamp W, Hindricks G, Gulker H, et al.: Coagulation of ventricular myocardium using radiofrequency alternating current: Biophysical aspects and experimental findings. Pacing Clin Electrophysiol 12:187-195, 1989.

33. Kalbfleisch SJ, Langberg JJ: Catheter ablation with radiofrequency energy: Biophysical aspects and clinical applications. J Cardiovasc Electrophysiol 3:173-186, 1992.

34. Haines DE: The biophysics of radiofrequency catheter ablation in the heart: The importance of temperature monitoring. Pacing Clin Electrophysiol 16:586-591, 1993.

35. Langberg JJ, Gallagher M, Strickberger SA, et al.: Temperature-guided radiofrequency catheter ablation with very large distal electrode. Circulation 88:245-249, 1993.

36. Otomo K, Yamanashi WS, Tondo C, et al.: Why a large tip electrode makes a deeper radiofrequency lesion: Effects of increase in electrode cooling and electrode-tissue interface area. J Cardiovasc Electrophysiol 9:47-54, 1998.

37. Sykes C, Riley R, Pomeranz M, et al.: Cooled tip ablation results in increased radiofrequency power delivery and lesion size. Pacing Clin Electrophysiol 88:782, 1994.

38. Nibley C, Sykes CM, McLaughlin G, et al.: Myocardial lesion size during radiofrequency current catheter ablation is increased by intra-electrode tip chilling [abstract]. J Am Coll Cardiol 25:293A, 1995.

39. Mittleman RS, Huang SKS, De Guzman WT, et al.: Use of the saline infusion electrode catheter for improved energy delivery and increased lesion size in radiofrequency catheter ablation. Pacing Clin Electrophysiol 18:1022-1027, 1995.

40. Ruffy R, Imran MA, Santel DJ, et al.: Radiofrequency delivery through a cooled catheter tip allows the creation of larger endomyocardial lesions in the ovine heart. J Cardiovasc Electrophysiol 6:1089-1096, 1995.

41. Nakagawa H, Yamanashi SW, Pitha JV, et al.: Comparison of in vivo tissue temperature profile and lesion geometry for radiofrequency ablation with a saline-irrigated electrode versus temperature control in a canine thigh muscle preparation. Circulation 91:2264-2273, 1995.

42. Eick OJ, Gerritse B, Schumacher B, et al.: Popping phenomena in temperature controlled radiofrequency ablation: When and why do they occur? Pacing Clin Electrophysiol 23:253-258, 2000.

43. Petersen HH, Chen X, Pietersen A, et al.: Lesion size in relation to ablation site during radiofrequency ablation. Pacing Clin Electrophysiol 21:322-326, 1990.

44. Dorwarth U, Fiek M, Remp T, et al.: Radiofrequency catheter ablation: Different cooled and noncooled electrode systems induce specific lesion geometries and adverse effect profiles. Pacing Clin Electrophysiol 26:1438-1445, 2003.

45. Skrumeda LL, Mehra R: Comparison of standard and irrigated radiofrequency ablation in the canine ventricle. J Cardiovasc Electrophysiol 9:1196-1205, 1998.

46. Petersin HH, Chen X, Pietersen A, et al.: Temperature-controlled irrigated tip radiofrequency catheter ablation: Comparison of in vivo and in vitro lesion dimensions for standard catheter and irrigated tip catheter with minimal infusion rate. J Cardiovasc Electrophysiol 9:409-414, 1998.

47. Petersin HH, Chen X, Pietersen A, et al.: Tissue temperatures and lesion size during irrigated tip catheter radiofrequency ablation: An in vitro comparison of temperature-controlled irrigated tip ablation, power-controlled irrigated tip ablation, and standard temperature-controlled ablation. Pacing Clin Electrophysiol 23:8-17, 2000.

48. Wharton JM, Wilber DJ, Calkins H, et al.: Utility of tip thermometry during radiofrequency ablation in humans using an internally perfused saline cooled catheter [abstract]. Circulation 96(Suppl 1);I-318, 1997.

49. Thiagalingam A, Campbell GR, Boyd A, et al.: Catheter intramural needle radiofrequency ablation creates deeper lesion than irrigated tip catheter ablation. Pacing Clin Electrophysiol 26:2146-2150, 2003.

50. Weiss C, Stewart M, Franzen O, et al.: Transmembraneous irrigation of multipolar radiofrequency ablation catheters: Induction of linear lesions encircling the pulmonary vein ostium without the risk of coagulum formation? J Interv Card Electrophysiol 10:199-209, 2004.

51. Demazumder D, Kallash HL, Schwartzman D: Comparison of different electrodes for radiofrequency ablation of myocardium using saline irrigation [abstract]. Pacing Clin Electrophysiol 20:II-1076, 1997.

52. Nakagawa H, Wittkampf FHM, Yamanashi WS, et al.: Inverse relationship between electrode size and lesion size during radiofrequency with active electrode cooling. Circulation 98:458-465, 1998.

53. Wong WS, VanderBrink BA, Riley RE, et al.: Effect of saline irrigation flow rate on temperature profile during cooled radiofrequency ablation. J Interv Card Electrophysiol 4:321-326, 2000.

54. Weiss C, Antz M, Eick O, et al.: Radiofrequency catheter ablation using cooled electrodes: Impact of irrigation flow rate and

catheter contact pressure on lesion dimensions. Pacing Clin Electrophysiol 25:463-469, 2002.

55. d'Avila A, Houghtaling C, Gutierrez P, et al.: Catheter ablation of ventricular epicardial tissue: A comparison of standard and cooled-tip radiofrequency energy. Circulation 109:2363-2369, 2004.

56. Calkins H, Epstein A, Packer D, et al.: Catheter ablation of ventricular tachycardia in patients with structural heart disease using cooled radiofrequency energy: Results of a prospective multicenter study. Cooled RF Multi Center Investigators Group. J Am Coll Cardiol 35:1905-1914, 2000.

57. Reddy VY, Neuzil P, Taborsky M, et al.: Short-term results of substrate-mapping and radiofrequency ablation of ischemic ventricular tachycardia using a saline-irrigated catheter. J Am Coll Cardiol 41:2228-2236, 2003.

58. Soejima K, Delacretaz E, Suzuki M, et al.: Saline-cooled versus standard radiofrequency catheter ablation for infarct-related ventricular tachycardias. Circulation 103:1858-1862, 2001.

59. Jais P, Shah DC, Haissaguerre M, et al.: Prospective randomized comparison of irrigated-tip versus conventional-tip catheters for ablation of common flutter. Circulation 101:772-776, 2000.

60. Jais P, Haissaguerre M, Shah DC, et al.: Successful irrigated-tip catheter ablation of atrial flutter resistant to conventional radiofrequency ablation. Circulation 98:835-838, 1998.

61. Atiga WL, Worley SJ, Hummel J, et al.: Prospective randomized comparison of cooled radiofrequency versus standard radiofrequency energy for ablation of typical atrial flutter. Pacing Clin Electrophysiol 25:1172-1178, 2002.

62. Scavee C, Jais P, Hsu LF, et al.: Prospective randomized comparison of irrigated-tip and large-tip catheter ablation of cavotricuspid isthmus-dependent atrial flutter. Eur Heart J 25:963-969, 2004.

63. Spitzer SG, Karolyi L, Rammler C, et al.: Primary closed cooled tip ablation of typical atrial flutter in comparison to conventional radiofrequency ablation. Europace 4:265-271, 2002.

64. Schreieck J, Zrenner B, Kumpmann J, et al.: Prospective randomized comparison of closed cooled-tip versus 8-mm-tip catheters for radiofrequency ablation of typical atrial flutter. J Cardiovasc Electrophysiol 13:980-985, 2002.

65. Macle L, Jais P, Weerasooriya R, et al.: Irrigated-tip catheter ablation of pulmonary veins for treatment of atrial fibrillation. J Cardiovasc Electrophysiol 13:1067-1073, 2002.

66. Marrouche NF, Dresing T, Cole C, et al.: Circular mapping and ablation of the pulmonary vein for treatment of atrial fibrillation: Impact of different catheter technologies. J Am Coll Cardiol 40:464-474, 2002.

67. Oral H, Knight BP, Ozaydin M, et al.: Segmental ostial ablation to isolate the pulmonary veins during atrial fibrillation: Feasibility and mechanistic insights. Circulation 106:1256-1262, 2002.

68. Marrouche M, Saad E, Bash D, et al.: Phased-array intracardiac echocardiography monitoring during pulmonary vein isolation in patients with atrial fibrillation: Impact on outcome and complications. Circulation 107:2710-2716, 2003.

69. Sun Y, Arruda M, Otomo K, et al.: Coronary sinus-ventricular accessory connections producing posteroseptal and left posterior accessory pathways: Incidence and electrophysiological identification. Circulation 106:1362-1367, 2002.

70. Lam C, Schweikert R, Kanagaratnam L, Natale A: Radiofrequency ablation of a right atrial appendage – ventricular accessory pathway by transcutaneous epicardial instrumentation. J Cardiovas Electrophysiol 11:1170-1173, 2000.

71. Goya M, Takahashi A, Nakagawa H, Iesaka Y: A case of catheter ablation of accessory atrioventricular connection between the right atrial appendage and right ventricle guided by a three-dimensional electroanatomic mapping system. J Cardiovas Electrophysiol 10:1112-1118, 1999.

72. Hwang C, Peter CT, Chen PS: Radiofrequency ablation of accessory pathways guided by the location of the ligament of Marshall. J Cardiovas Electrophysiol 14:616-620, 2003.

73. Garcia JG, Almendral J, Arenal A, et al.: Irrigated tip catheter ablation in right posteroseptal accessory pathways resistant to conventional ablation. Pacing Clin Electrophysiol 25:799-803, 2002.

74. Yamane T, Jais P, Shah DC, et al.: Efficacy and safety of an irrigated-tip catheter for the ablation of accessory pathways resistant to conventional radiofrequency ablation. Circulation 102:2565-2568, 2000.

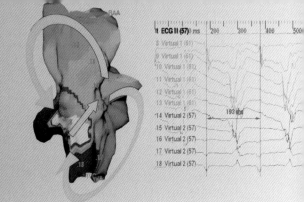

4

Catheter Cryoablation: Biophysics and Applications

Paul G. Novak • *Marc Dubuc*

Key Points

- The biophysics and mechanisms of cryothermal injury comprise three stages: (1) freeze/thaw phase, (2) hemorrhage and inflammation, and (3) replacement fibrosis.

- Advantages of cryoablation include reversibility of cryothermal energy lesions (CryoMapping), decreased thrombus risk, increased cryocatheter stability, and decreased risk of injury to vascular structures.

- Cryoablation has been applied clinically in the following conditions: atrioventricular nodal ablation, atrioventricular nodal reentrant tachycardia (AVNRT), septal and parahisian accessory pathways, atrial flutter (AFL), and atrial fibrillation (AF).

The treatment of cardiac arrhythmias by radiofrequency (RF) lesion creation was first described in experimental animal models in the mid-1980s. Since that time, the clinical subspecialty of cardiac electrophysiology has grown exponentially. RF energy has been investigated and used extensively by invasive cardiac electrophysiologists to create intracardiac lesions for the treatment of cardiac arrhythmias. In fact, currently RF is used as the energy source of choice for the catheter ablation treatment of cardiac arrhythmias. There are, however, limitations to RF as an energy source, which include embolization from charring and thrombus formation, inability to assess electrophysiologic effect before lesion delivery (nonreversibility of lesion effect), and unwanted collateral damage to surrounding vascular and electrical structures.

As a result of such limitations, alternative energy sources for the creation of intracardiac lesions for the treatment of cardiac arrhythmias have been sought. Cryothermal energy is one such source that has numerous advantages as well as an existing track record for safety and efficacy in the arrhythmia surgery forum. The potential advantages of catheter ablation with cryothermal energy sources include decreased thrombogenicity, potential for assessment of lesion effect before delivery of irreversible lesions (Safety and Efficacy CryoMapping), improved catheter stability during ablation procedures, safety within or near vascular structures, and significantly decreased levels of perceived pain by patients.

This chapter attempts to provide the training and practicing electrophysiologist a solid understanding of the field of cryoablation. The history of cryothermal energy use in medicine is reviewed, as is the biophysics of cryoablation and the pathology of cryoablation lesions. A transvenous catheter cryoenergy delivery system is detailed, and the advantages and limitations of cryoablation are reviewed. Finally, current clinical applications of cryothermal energy sources for the treatment of cardiac arrhythmias are discussed.

History of Cryothermal Energy Use in Cardiovascular Medicine

Although cryothermal energy is now commonly used in the treatment of cardiac disorders and particularly cardiac arrhythmias, its initial applications were in noncardiac pathologic conditions, including dermatologic, urologic, gynecologic, ophthalmologic, oncologic, hepatic, and neurosurgical pathologies.[1-4] The earliest descriptions of the use of cryothermal energy, in which carbon dioxide was used for the creation of transmural cardiac lesions, were provided by Hass and Taylor[5] and expanded by Taylor et al.[6] The predecessors of modern cryothermal energy application to specialized conduction tissue were Lister and Hoffman,[7] who described reversible conduction block in the atrioventricular (AV) node after rewarming of a cryothermal energy lesion, currently referred to as *cryomapping*. Since that time, numerous groups of investigators have advanced cryothermal technology, from an experimental energy source for the creation of intracardiac lesions in animals to a modern alternative energy source used by invasive cardiac electrophysiologists for the treatment of a broad range of cardiac arrhythmias (Table 4–1).

TABLE 4–1

Historical Landmarks in Cardiac Cryoablation

Year	Authors (Ref. No.)	Contribution
1948	Hass & Taylor (5)	Cryothermal myocardial lesions
1963	Cooper (8)	Cryosurgical apparatus development
1964	Lister & Hoffman (7)	Cryothermal energy used to retard conductive tissue with evidence of reversibility
1977	Harrison et al. (9)	Surgical application of cryothermal energy by handheld probe
1991	Gillette et al. (10)	Percutaneous application of cryothermal energy by transvenous catheter in animals
1998	Dubuc et al. (11)	Use of steerable cryocatheter system with pacing and recording electrodes
1999	Khairy et al. (12)	Percutaneous transvenous catheter cryoablation in humans

From Khairy P, Dubuc M: Transcatheter cryoablation. In Liem LB, Downar E (eds.): Progress in Catheter Ablation, 2001, p 391, with permission.

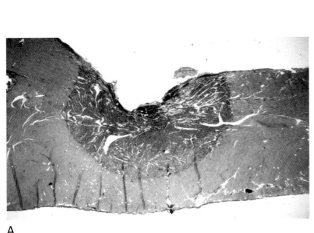
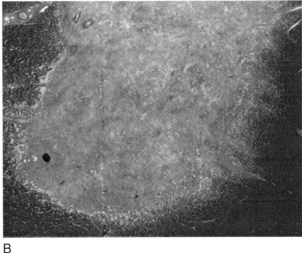

A   B

Figure 4–1. A, Low-power photomicrograph of a subacute cryothermal lesion; note the well-circumscribed borders of the lesion. **B,** Medium-power photomicrograph of a chronic cryothermal lesion with preserved tissue architecture. Both lesions were performed in mongrel dog left ventricular myocardium with a 4-minute cryoapplication to −55°C.

Biophysics and Mechanisms of Cryothermal Energy Tissue Injury

The application of cryothermal energy to cardiac tissue results in the formation of an ice ball, or a hemispherical block of frozen tissue. The tissue goes through a series of stages before forming into a stable lesion. Although these are frequently debated, it is generally accepted that the main stages in the creation of a cryothermal energy lesion include the following: (1) freeze/thaw phase, (2) hemorrhage and inflammation stage, and (3) replacement fibrosis stage.[13-16] Therefore, the lesions created by cryothermal energy sources are morphologically different in the acute and chronic stages (Fig. 4–1).

The freeze/thaw phase results in the initial changes associated with direct cryothermal lesion application that occur within the first hours after delivery. In this phase, freezing results in the formation of intracellular and extracellular ice crystals. The ice crystals do not penetrate cellular membranes; rather, they cause compression and distortion of intracellular organelles. More importantly, extracellular ice crystal formation removes extracellular free water and causes intracellular desiccation. Furthermore, because of the withdrawal of water caused by freezing, the remaining water becomes hyperosmotic, and concentrations of electrolytes become elevated, contributing to cell death. Once thawing begins, first in the extracellular tissues, the hypotonic fluid moves back into the cells,

causing the cells to swell and cell membranes to rupture. The thawing of ice crystals also results in increased membrane permeability in mitochondria and disruption of intracellular transport mechanisms. Once these changes occur, irreversible cell death takes place.

The second stage is termed the hemorrhage and inflammation phase. Within 48 hours after a freeze/thaw cycle, the treated myocardial tissue begins to develop hemorrhage, edema, and inflammation (coagulation necrosis) (see Fig. 4–1A). By 1 week after freezing, the now inflammatory lesions have become sharply demarcated by macrophages, lymphocytes, and fibroblasts and collagen stranding has begun.

The final phase in the evolution of a cryothermal energy lesion is the replacement fibrosis phase. By a number of weeks after ablation, the myocardial tissue within the lesion has become replaced by dense collagen and fat. A short while afterward, the lesion is densely fibrotic, and up to 3 months later has decreased to its final size (see Fig. 4–1B).

The characteristics of lesions created by cryothermal energy tend to differ from those created by RF energy and have been well described by a number of investigators.[11,17,18] Lesions created by a 4-minute cryoablation application at temperatures lower than −50°C grossly appear hemispherical in shape with a sharply defined interface with normal myocardium and well-preserved architecture (Fig. 4–2A, *right panel*). These lesions typically are not associated with any significant endothelial damage and therefore are also typically free of surface thrombosis (see Fig. 4–2B, *right panel*).[19]

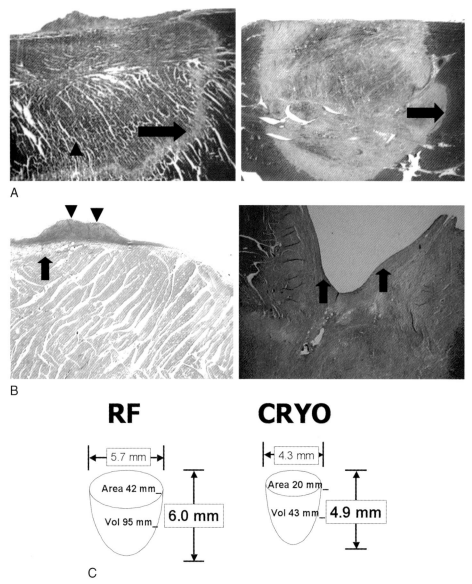

Figure 4–2. A, Photomicrographs of a chronic radiofrequency (RF) lesion (60 seconds at 70° C) *(left)* compared with a chronic cryothermal lesion (4 minutes at −75° C) *(right)*. Note the hemispherical necrosis of the cryothermal lesion, as well as the discrete lesion demarcation *(right, arrow)*, and preserved tissue architecture. In contrast, the RF lesion exhibits less discrete lesion demarcation *(left, arrow)* and less well-preserved architecture *(left, arrowhead)* of the RF lesion. **B,** Photomicrographs of a chronic RF lesion (60 seconds at 70° C) *(left)* compared with a chronic cryothermal lesion (4 minutes at −75° C) *(right)*. Note the well-preserved endothelium free of thrombus in the cryothermal lesion *(right, arrows)*, compared with the disrupted endothelium *(left, arrow)* and associated thrombus *(left, arrowheads)* of the RF lesion. **C,** Schematic diagram comparing lesion geometries between an RF lesion *(left)* and a cryoablation (CRYO) lesion *(right)*. The RF lesion has similar depth but larger lesion volume and area. *(**A,** left panel, reproduced with permission from, and **C** created from data available in, Khairy P, Chauvet P, Lehmann J, et al.: Lower incidence of thrombus formation with cryoenergy versus radiofrequency catheter ablation. Circulation 107:2045-2050, 2003.)*

The average lesion dimensions created by cryothermal lesions have been recently reported[19] to be 20 mm^2 in cross-sectional area and 4.9 mm deep (±1.7 mm) with an average volume of 43.2 mm^3, consistent with earlier reports by others[11,18] (see Fig. 4–2C, *right panel*).

These findings are in contrast to lesions created by RF, which are less sharply demarcated, with less well-preserved architecture (see Fig. 4–2A, *left panel*); they may be associated with surface endothelial disruption and therefore more likely to be associated with surface thrombosis (see Fig. 4–2B, *left panel*).[20,21] However, lesion geometry created by RF energy sources depends on a number of factors, including tissue temperature, power used, duration of ablation, size of ablation electrode, irrigated-tip versus nonirrigated catheter, and electrode-tissue contact.[21-24] The discussion of these factors and their roles in RF lesion size and geometry is beyond the scope of this chapter. However, lesions created by standard 4-mm-tip, temperature-controlled RF application are typically similar in depth but larger in cross-sectional area and volume than lesions created by cryoablation[19] (see Fig. 4–2C, *left panel*).

The difference in lesion cross-sectional area and, consequently, in lesion volume between lesions created by cryothermal versus RF energy sources is most likely due to differences in catheter stability. Because an RF lesion is created with the beating heart moving underneath the catheter, the lesion is delivered over an area slightly larger than the catheter tip as the result of a "brushing" effect. As further discussed later, the ablation catheter is frozen to the tissue during cryoablation, which allows the delivery of a focused lesion without a similar "brushing" effect.[11,18]

Cryoablation Technical Aspects

CONSOLE AND CATHETERS

A number of systems are in commercial use for catheter cryoablation. We describe here our experience with the system (console and catheters) manufactured by CryoCath Technologies, Montreal, Quebec (Fig. 4–3A). The current catheter used is a quadripolar, steerable catheter with a 7 French (F) 4-mm tip (CryoCath Freezor), a 7F 6-mm tip (CryoCath Freezor X-TRA), or a 9F 8-mm tip (CryoCath Freezor MAX) equipped with a thermocouple (see Fig. 4–3B). The current catheters have four electrodes at the distal end: the distal cooling electrode and three proximal electrodes for pacing and recording (see Fig. 4–3C). The distal tip is where the cryothermal

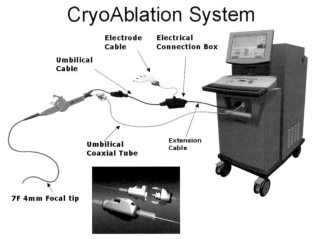

A

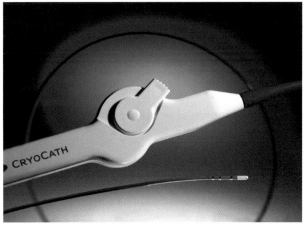

B

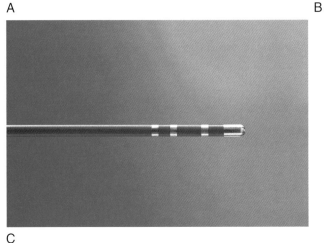

C

Figure 4–3. A, Cryoablation system (CryoCath Freezor) console and connectors. **B,** Cryoablation catheter demonstrating handle design. **C,** Magnification of a 7F catheter tip with 4-mm distal cooling tip and three pacing and sensing electrodes arranged in a 2-5-2 mm array. *(Courtesy of CryoCath Technologies, Montreal, Quebec.)*

lesion is applied and where the temperature is recorded. With respect to cooling, the catheter is composed of two concentric lumens, an inner injection chamber through which liquid nitrous oxide (N_2O) is injected and an outer shaft that is connected to the distal tip and maintained under constant vacuum. The distal tip of the catheter is cooled by the Joule-Thompson effect when the liquid N_2O is injected under pressure from the inner injection chamber into the hollow tip, where its rapid evaporation leads to cooling (Fig. 4–4). The gaseous N_2O is then removed by the vacuum of the outer lumen and vented to the hospital ventilation system. The thermocouple in the tip of the catheter allows for close monitoring of tissue temperatures. The console allows the operator two different modes of operation. The first is the CryoMapping mode, in which the tip is cooled to a temperature not lower than $-30^{\circ}C$ for up to 80 seconds (this is the temperature experimentally demonstrated to be reversible during catheter ablation only, such as during cardiac surgery on a patient under cold cardioplegia; permanent lesions occur at much warmer temperatures). This allows the delivery of an application with reversible effect. The second mode is the CryoAblation mode, which cools the tip to $-75^{\circ}C$ for up to 4 minutes, producing the permanent lesion. The CryoMapping mode can be used an indefinite number of times before the CryoAblation mode is initiated, and the CryoAblation mode may be initiated at any time during a CryoMapping application or without any prior CryoMapping, to allow the operator the greatest degree of versatility for any given ablation case.

CRYOMAPPING AND CRYOABLATION DELIVERY

To perform an ablation procedure with the CryoCath system, the operator advances a 7F quadripolar, steerable cryocatheter (with handling characteristics similar to those of a standard 7F quadripolar, steerable RF catheter) to the region of interest within the heart. The ablation target, such as an accessory pathway (AP) or slow pathway region for ablation of atrioventricular nodal reentrant tachycardia (AVNRT), is then identified with careful mapping techniques, similar to those used to identify targets for RF ablation procedures. Once the target is identified, the operator chooses between the two modes of operation. Typically, a CryoMapping application is performed first, to assess the electrophysiologic effect of the application. As noted earlier, this allows the operator to cool the target tissue to $-30^{\circ}C$. With temperatures of $-20^{\circ}C$ and colder, electrical noise appears on the distal electrode pair, and there is complete loss of local electrogram due to ice ball formation. This electrical noise resolves completely once the temperature warms to greater than $-20^{\circ}C$. During the time that temperatures remain colder than $-20^{\circ}C$, the catheter adheres to the cardiac endocardial tissue and therefore allows the operator to perform programmed stimulation to confirm the desired effect of the lesion (or the absence of unwanted effect) without concern that the catheter will become displaced from the target of interest. Should the operator note an undesired effect of the CryoMapping lesion, such as prolongation or block of the AH interval (i.e., the interval between low right atrial activity and His bundle activity on intracardiac electrograms) or complete AV block, the CryoMapping can be terminated, with recovery of conduction within seconds after rewarming and no permanent effects. Furthermore, because the ice ball melts completely within seconds after cryoapplication is terminated, there is no risk of systemic embolization. The CryoMapping procedure can be terminated and repeated as many times as the operator chooses with no permanent effect on conducting tissue. Once the operator is satisfied with the effect of the CryoMapping lesion (i.e., the arrhythmia substrate is neutralized or the arrhythmia is stopped or is no longer inducible), the CryoAblation mode is started. During CryoAblation mode, the temperature is further decreased to $-75^{\circ}C$, and the catheter is left in contact for up to 4 minutes,

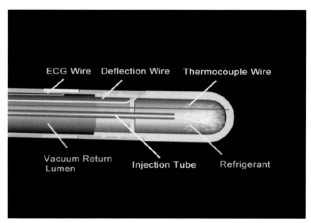

Figure 4–4. Schematic diagram demonstrating the CryoCath Freezor cryocatheter internal design and distal tip cooling by the Joule-Thompson effect. The electrocardiogram (ECG) wire, deflection wire, thermocouple wire, central injection tube, and vacuum return tip and lumen are shown. Refrigerant is injected from the central injection lumen into the distal tip, where it rapidly evaporates. The cooling of the tip causes ice ball formation around the external portion of the distal tip with freezing of adjacent tissue. *(Courtesy of CryoCath Technologies, Montreal, Quebec.)*

resulting in a permanent lesion. A duration of 4 minutes typically is required, because lesion size continues to expand during the cryoablation application, up to a duration of 2 to 3 minutes; therefore applications shorter than 4 minutes may not result in complete lesion delivery (Fig. 4–5A-C). Should the operator note an undesirable electrophysiologic effect during cryoablation, especially when working in a substrate adjacent to the conduction system

(e.g., AH prolongation, AV block), the CryoAblation application can be terminated. If it is terminated immediately upon the appearance of the unwanted effect conduction typically returns to normal on rewarming, with no residual conduction abnormality. Although CryoAblation with one 4-minute application in an optimal position typically is sufficient to result in a permanent effect on conduction, multiple applications may be performed if desired or needed.

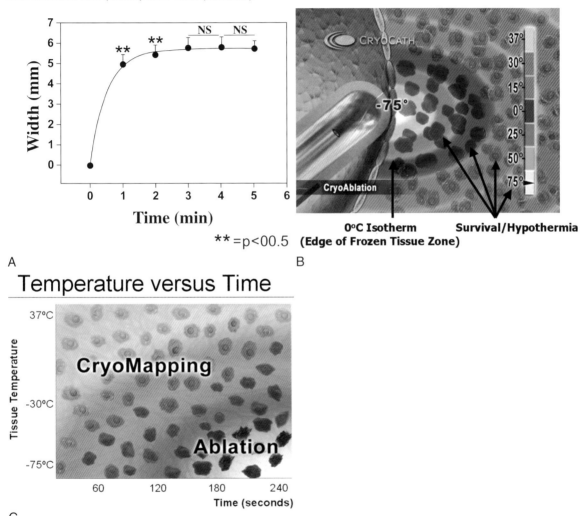

Figure 4–5. A, Plot of lesion width (mm) versus time (min) of lesion application demonstrating continuous and significant increase in lesion size for up to 3 minutes, with no significant further increase with longer application. **, P < .05 versus previous time; NS, not significant. *(From Dubuc M, Roy D, Thibault B, et al. Transvenous catheter ice mapping and cryoablation of the atrioventricular node in dogs. Pacing Clin Electrophysiol 22:1488-1498, 1999, with permission.)* **B,** Schematic diagram demonstrating that as the catheter tip is cooled, the adjacent cardiac tissue is also cooled, with ice ball formation and outward expansion in a concentric fashion from the center of the cooling tip of the catheter. The longer the catheter is cooled, the larger the ice ball formation and the larger the lesion created, with an upper limit at approximately 2 to 3 minutes of application when cooling to −75° C. **C,** Schematic plot of cryothermal energy delivery, demonstrating effect of temperature versus time. In order to create a permanent ablation lesion, the tissue adjacent to the catheter must reach a certain temperature, and this temperature must be applied for a given time. The colder the temperature, the shorter the duration of application necessary to achieve a permanent lesion. *(B and C, Courtesy of Cryo-Cath Technologies, Montreal, Quebec.)*

Clinical Advantages of Cryothermal Energy for Catheter Ablation

Although RF used as an energy source for catheter ablation of cardiac arrhythmias has enjoyed great success and therefore has seen broad applicability, it is associated with some important limitations,[25] most notably the following. The method of tissue destruction caused by RF energy is permanent, and therefore all clinical effects created by RF are essentially irreversible.[22] This translates into an inability to test the clinical effect of a lesion before energy delivery, which has important implications for ablations carried out in close proximity to critical structures such as the AV node. RF energy is also associated with an important risk of tissue charring and thrombus formation with potential for embolization.[26-29] This risk becomes significantly magnified when ablation attempts are made in the left atrium or left ventricle or when large surface areas are ablated, such as in cases of atrial fibrillation (AF) or ventricular tachycardias (VT) of the left ventricle.[26,27] Furthermore, the ability to create successful lesions with RF energy requires adequate catheter tissue contact as well as catheter stability. Finally, the use of RF in or around vascular structures has led to complications such as pulmonary vein stenosis,[30-33] coronary sinus injury or spasm,[34] coronary sinus thrombus and adherence of RF catheter to the coronary sinus wall,[35,36] and coronary artery stenosis and thrombosis.[35,36] The unique biophysical properties associated with cryothermal injury to cardiac tissues have afforded this energy source a number of advantages that overcome these important limitations of RF energy.

REVERSIBILITY OF CRYOTHERMAL LESIONS (CRYOMAPPING)

One of the most exciting and truly remarkable characteristics of cryothermal energy is the ability to create reversible electrophysiologic effects or (CryoMapping). CryoMapping is the ability to deliver a cryothermal application with only temporarily suppressive electrophysiologic effects. Cryothermal energy application has this ability because the temperatures at which reversible tissue effects occur are warmer than -30°C, whereas permanent tissue injury does not occur until the tissue temperatures reach -50°C. (It is of note that these are the temperatures that have been experimentally demonstrated to be reversible and permanent, respectively, in a healthy heart by catheter delivery of cryothermal energy; permanent lesions occur at much warmer

temperatures in patients undergoing cryothermal energy application during cardiac surgery on cold cardioplegia).[11,12,17,37] This broad window between temperatures that suppress electrophysiologic effects of cardiac tissue temporarily and those that cause irreversible tissue damage allows the user of cryothermal energy to perform CryoMapping. Furthermore, CryoMapping can be used for assessment of safety or efficacy. Safety CryoMapping refers to the delivery of a reversible cryothermal energy application that allows the operator to confirm that a CryoAblation at a chosen site will not affect an undesirable target such as the AV node. Efficacy CryoMapping is the delivery of a reversible cryothermal energy application that allows the operator to determine whether a substrate of interest (i.e., slow pathway or AP) will be successfully ablated when a complete irreversible CryoAblation lesion is applied.

Some of the early reports of modern cryothermal mapping were provided by the cardiac surgical experience with cryothermal energy.[38] Camm et al. (1980) described the ability to create reversible partial and complete conduction block in the AV node by placing a cryothermal energy probe in the His bundle position and cooling the tissue to between 0°C and -10°C.[38] They were able to demonstrate AH prolongation followed by complete dissociation, which completely resolved on rewarming.

The feasibility of creating reversible cryothermal energy lesions by a transvenous steerable electrode catheter was first demonstrated by Dubuc et al. in dogs.[11] They were able to demonstrate that complete AV nodal conduction block could be created by cooling tissue to between -20°C and -30°C and then completely recovered after cooling was arrested and tissue was allowed to rewarm. Gross and microscopic examinations of these animals could not identify any evidence of important tissue injury in the AV junction region. These authors further determined that a temperature of approximately -30°C is required to interrupt the tissue electrophysiologic properties, that it takes approximately 10 to 20 seconds of cooling to achieve this temperature, and that rewarming with restoration of AV conduction takes up to 20 seconds.[11]

The feasibility of CryoMapping in humans was also demonstrated by Dubuc et al.[37] They were able to show that reversible AV block could be induced by cooling the tissue of the AV node to no cooler than -30°C, and that further cooling at the site of successful AV block to -60°C would result in permanent AV node ablation (Fig. 4–6). Finally, the large FROSTY trial[39] has validated the concept of CryoMapping on a large clinical scale. This study examined catheter CryoMapping and CryoAblation in more than 160 patients undergoing ablation of the slow pathway region for AVNRT, of AP regions for

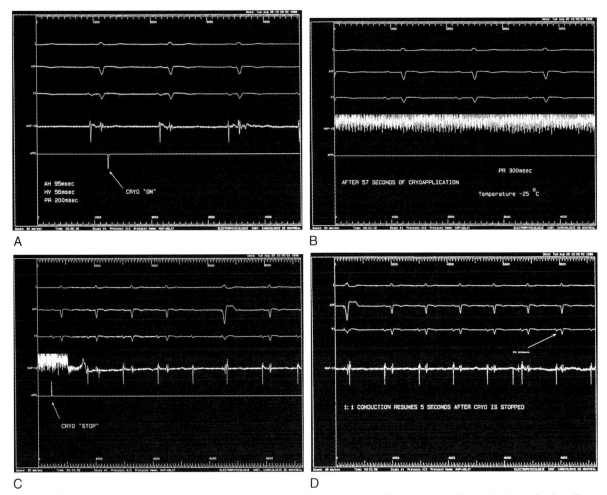

Figure 4–6. Electrograms demonstrating the reversible effect of CryoMapping on the compact atrioventricular node. For all panels, I, AVF, and V1 are surface electrocardiographic (ECG) recordings; MAP 1-2 is the signal from the distal electrode pair of the cryo-catheter; AH is the atrium-to-His activation time; HV is the His-to-ventricle activation time; and PR is the PR interval from the surface ECG. **A,** Normal baseline PR interval of 200 msec and AH interval of 95 msec before cryomapping application (paper speed = 50 mm/sec). **B,** After onset of cryomapping at a temperature of −25° C (evidenced by high-frequency signal on Map 1-2) for 57 seconds, the PR interval has extended to 300 msec (paper speed = 50 mm/sec). **C,** At the end of the cryomapping application, there is evidence of one nonconducted atrial beat with one ventricular backup paced beat. On rewarming, there are no further noncon-ducted atrial beats (paper speed = 25 mm/sec). **D,** After 5 seconds of rewarming, there is normal 1:1 atrioventricular conduction, and the PR interval returns to baseline (paper speed = 25 mm/sec). *(From Dubuc M, Khairy P, Rodriguez-Santiago A, et al. Catheter cryoablation of the atrioventricular node in patients with atrial fibrillation: A novel technology for ablation of cardiac arrhythmias. J Cardiovasc Electrophysiol 12:439-444, 2001, with permission.)*

AV reentry tachycardia, or of the AV junction for AF. The electrophysiologic effects of CryoMapping (Safety CryoMapping) were completely reversible within seconds in 79% of such attempts, and in another 15% of patients complete reversal occurred within 1 to 6 minutes. Six percent of patients had partial reversal of CryoMapping effects at 4 to 21 minutes after rewarming but went on to CryoAbla-tion before complete reversal occurred. Furthermore, CryoMapping successfully identified correct ablation targets in 64% of patients (Efficacy CryoMapping).

This characteristic of reversibility observed with CryoMapping is in stark contrast to the hyperthermal

injury caused by RF energy application.[22] In RF energy delivery, hyperthermal tissue injury leading to reversible loss of excitability occurs at a median tissue temperature of 48° C (range, 42.7° C to 51.3° C), whereas irreversible tissue destruction and irre-versible loss of excitability typically occurs at tissue temperatures greater than 50° C.[22,40] Therefore, when RF energy is used to create lesions to disrupt con-duction in cardiac tissue, there is an extremely narrow window between the temperatures causing reversible and irreversible damage. The window is, in fact, so narrow that it is impractical to attempt to create reversible lesions and study their clinical effects before going on to create permanent lesions. It is for this reason that RF lesions are, for all intents and purposes, irreversible.

The irreversibility of RF lesions becomes a concern when ablations are performed in close proximity to structures critical for normal conduction (e.g., the slow pathway region, parahisian APs). It has resulted in a small but important risk of permanent AV nodal conduction block in conjunction with perinodal ablation for AVNRT (fast pathway ablation, 5.3%; slow pathway ablation, 2.0%),[26,41] with ablation of atrial tachycardia in the triangle of Koch (12.5%),[42] and with AP ablation in the perinodal regions (range, 2.0% to 20%).[43-46] Cryothermal energy, with its ability to produce reversible lesions (CryoMapping), is a very attractive option in these cases. Cryothermal energy allows the operator to "test" the electrophysiologic effects of a lesion before it is made permanent and to abort ablation at a site with potentially harmful effects before these effects become permanent.

MINIMAL THROMBUS RISK

Another extremely appealing characteristic of cryothermal energy for catheter ablation of cardiac arrhythmias is the significantly decreased thrombogenicity associated with lesions created by this energy source, compared with RF.[15,19] Whereas hyperthermic energy results in coagulation and tissue necrosis,[22,47] cryothermal energy preserves tissue architecture with minimal thrombus formation[10,19] (see Fig. 4–2A and B).

Although the true incidence of thromboembolism associated with RF ablation is likely under-reported and perhaps under-recognized, especially in ablations in the right side of the heart, there is good documentation from a number of series and registries, including the large Multicenter European Radiofrequency Survey (MERFS).[26-29] These reports suggest that the overall risk of thromboembolic complications associated with RF ablation procedures ranges from 0.6% to 0.8%. However, this risk increases (to 1.8% to 2.0%) when RF is performed in systemic cardiac chambers and can reach as high as 2.8% when it is performed for left ventricular VT.[26,27] Fortunately, however, the actual risk of cerebral embolization is closer to 0.1%.[26]

Although some investigators have suggested that this thromboembolic risk is simply related to the presence of intracardiac catheters rather than delivery of RF energy, there is evidence to the contrary. This comes, in part, from an elegant study performed by Manolis et al.[48] looking at D-dimer levels in patients undergoing diagnostic electrophysiologic study or RF ablation procedures. D-dimer levels increased by twofold after a diagnostic electrophysiologic study compared with baseline, but after abla-

tion with RF energy they increased an amazing sixfold. Although this study was underpowered to demonstrate a difference in clinical events, there is clearly a thrombogenic effect associated with the delivery of RF energy. Epstein et al.[28] reported an increased thrombus risk associated with prolonged RF duration, further supporting the association of RF with increased thrombogenicity.

There has also been a great deal of effort expended to identify the features of RF ablation that are linked to this increased risk of thrombus formation. It is well known that increased temperatures greater than 100°C during RF ablation results in charring on the ablation electrode and at the tissue-electrode interface, with impedance rise acting as a marker of acute thrombus formation.[22,49,50] The use of intravenous heparin protocols and postprocedure antithrombotic treatment, as well as temperature feedback to control RF current delivery and monitoring for impedance rise, have not been shown to successfully eliminate thromboembolic risk.[27,28,51-53] Therefore, risk of thromboembolism continues to be an important consideration in the use of RF as an energy source for catheter ablation procedures.

Cryothermal energy lesions used for catheter ablation procedures cause tissue destruction in an entirely different manner and have biophysical properties that afford these lesions the benefit of being significantly less thrombogenic, or even clinically nonthrombogenic.[10,19] This was first demonstrated by Dubuc et al.,[11] who investigated the effects of cryothermal energy lesions created by a 9F 4-mm tip electrode. Gross pathologic examinations of dog hearts after ablation failed to reveal any evidence of thrombus formation in a total of 42 lesions. It was only on microscopic examination that occasional thin, flat, white thrombus formation was identified. This finding was further supported by Khairy et al.[19] in a study comparing the risk of thrombus formation in dogs after cryothermal energy lesions (7F or 9F 4-mm tip electrode) versus RF energy lesions (7F 4-mm tip electrode). They found that the incidence of thrombus formation was higher with RF lesions (76% versus 30%) and the median thrombus size was significantly larger ($2.8 \, mm^3$ versus $0.0 \, mm^3$). The result was a 5.6-fold increased risk of thrombus formation with RF energy compared to cryothermal energy (see Fig. 4–2A).

Therefore, cryothermal lesions have been demonstrated to have the distinct advantage over RF lesions of being significantly less thrombogenic. The importance of this fact becomes magnified if ablation procedures are carried out in systemic cardiac chambers or if the lesion set required for successful arrhythmia treatment encompasses a large surface area (e.g., AF, left ventricular VT).

CATHETER STABILITY

Catheter stability is often a technical limitation during attempts to deliver RF for transvenous catheter ablation procedures. With RF energy delivery, the catheter must be held in place by the operator to ensure adequate delivery of power and subsequent tissue heating to the region to obtain the desired electrophysiologic effect. Often, this can prove extremely challenging in the setting of a moving heart. The effect may be significantly magnified during tachycardia, if the tachyarrhythmia abruptly stops during ablation, or if the patient has significant regurgitant valvular lesions. Furthermore, cardiac motion during RF ablation creates a brushing effect of the catheter on the cardiac tissue, which may make the lesion less precise and may augment the risk of undesired damage to adjacent structures. This may become a concern when ablation is performed near critical conduction tissue.

Cryothermal energy used for transvenous catheter ablation of arrhythmias is associated with ice ball formation at the tip of the catheter and adherence of the catheter to the endocardial surface (Fig. 4–7).[11,18] These phenomena were first described by Dubuc et al.[11,18] With the use of intracardiac echocardiography (ICE), they were able to demonstrate ice ball formation approximately 4 seconds after commencement of the freeze cycle, with adherence of the catheter to adjacent tissue after the first 20 seconds of cryothermal energy delivery. This effectively eliminates the possibility of catheter dislodgement from the desired location once ice ball formation occurs and therefore eliminates inadvertent catheter motion away from the desired site of lesion delivery. Furthermore, the increased catheter stability after ice ball formation allows programmed stimulation to be used during the ablation procedure, to confirm the clinical effect of the lesion, without any concern for catheter dislodgement. The increased stability of the cryocatheter may also explain the more focal nature of cryothermal energy lesions.

Therefore, ice ball formation and the consequently augmented catheter stability during lesion creation provide another advantageous characteristic of cryothermal energy compared with RF for use in transvenous catheter ablation procedures.

MINIMAL RISK TO VASCULAR STRUCTURES

Ablation of epicardial left-sided AV APs, posteroseptal AV APs, or atypical AVNRTs occasionally requires ablation within venous structures, such as the coronary sinus. Furthermore, with the advancements in catheter ablation for AF, there is need for ablation at the ostia or adjacent to the pulmonary veins (PV).

There is evidence that delivery of RF lesions within venous structures such as the coronary sinus or PV is associated with a risk of venous stenosis, endoluminal thrombosis, perforation possibly leading to tamponade, or damage to adjacent arterial structures.[30-36,54] Cryothermal energy ablation has proved less harmful to vascular structures.

Catheter ablation within the coronary sinus using cryothermal energy has been investigated by a number of groups. In canine and swine models, cryothermal catheter ablation of APs has been shown to be safe and effective.[55,56] Skanes et al.[55] used a swine model with angiography and pathologic evaluation to investigate the effects of cryothermal lesion production within the distal, middle, and proximal coronary sinus. Yagi et al.[56] performed a similar study using intravascular ultrasound (IVUS), angiography, and pathologic investigation in a canine model. Both groups were able to demonstrate no significant thrombus formation or damage to the coronary sinus and concluded that this technique is safe and feasible.

Gaita et al.[57] were the first to report the clinical use in humans of cryothermal energy deep within the coronary sinus, in a patient with an endocardial left-sided posterolateral AP. They resorted to cryoablation after numerous failed attempts with RF in the left atrium by way of a retrograde aortic approach and also an anterograde fossa ovalis approach, as well as RF within the coronary sinus. They were able to successfully ablate the AP with no evidence of damage to the coronary sinus or circumflex coronary artery, as demonstrated by angiography.

The surgical literature provides evidence as to the safety of cryothermal energy used in close proximity to arterial structures. Misaki et al.[58] performed a study in which epicardial cryothermal energy lesions were applied in close proximity to or directly over large branches of the left coronary artery in sheep models. They reported no evidence of acute blockage or late stenosis despite tissue damage to adjacent myocardium. Other investigators were able to show, in canine or swine models, that catheter cryoablation within the coronary sinus results in minimal or no damage to the adjacent circumflex coronary artery despite ablation within 2 mm of the coronary artery, which is known to be associated with high risk of stenosis when using RF energy.[55,56]

PV ablation procedures require the delivery of cryothermal energy in close proximity to the PVs. Delivery of such lesions is associated with a known risk of PV stenosis.[30-33] There is growing evidence that use of cryothermal energy for ablation within or near the PV is associated with significantly lower rates of PV stenosis, compared with the use of RF energy for ablation.[59] Wong et al.[59] looked at

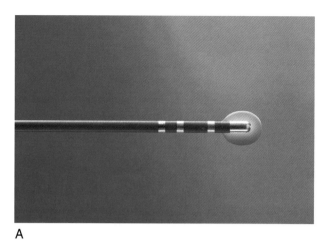

A

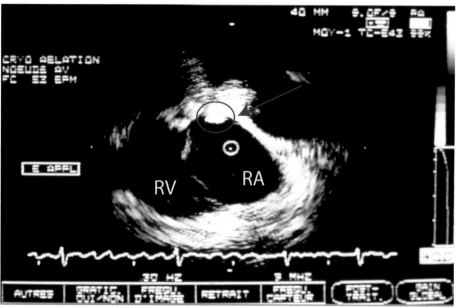

B

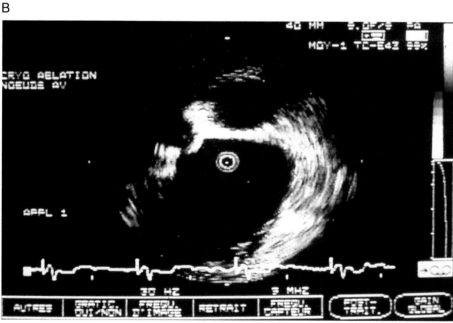

C

Figure 4–7. A, Ice ball formation at tip of cryocatheter during ablation adheres catheter to adjacent cardiac tissue. *(Courtesy of CryoCath Technologies, Montreal, Quebec.)* **B,** Ice ball formation *(oval)* at tip of cryoablation catheter demonstrated by intracardiac echocardiography, showing the right atrium (RA) and right ventricle (RV) with catheter demarcated by the *arrow* before cryoapplication. **C,** After cryoapplication, the ice ball is demonstrated by a hypoechoic zone bordered by a hyperechoic zone with posterior acoustic shadowing. *(From Dubuc M, Khairy P, Rodriguez-Santiago A, et al. Catheter cryoablation of the atrioventricular node in patients with atrial fibrillation: A novel technology for ablation of cardiac arrhythmias. J Cardiovasc Electrophysiol 12: 439-444, 2001, with permission.)*

the use of cryoablation at or near the PV ostia for PV isolation procedures and found no evidence of acute PV stenosis. This finding proved to be robust in a larger study reported by Tse et al.,[60] who reported no cases of PV stenosis in 52 patients at 12-month follow-up with thoracic computed tomographic scan surveillance.

Therefore, if lesion creation is required within or near vascular structures, the use of cryothermal energy to create such lesions is associated with less risk of venous stenosis, perforation, or tamponade, and less injury to adjacent arterial structures. Cryothermal energy offers yet another distinct advantage over RF as an energy source for ablation in specific clinical scenarios.

Clinical Applications

The catheter ablation treatment of cardiac arrhythmias has evolved exponentially since the early 1990s. During this time, RF has become the energy source of choice for the ablation of a broad range of arrhythmias, because of its safety and efficacy.[25] However, because of its many advantages discussed earlier,

cryothermal energy has seen a tremendous amount of interest and investigation for many of the same clinical applications previously reserved for RF. The following sections provide an overview and comparison of the clinical efficacy of cryoablation versus RF and highlight the potential advantages of cryothermal energy. This comparison is summarized in Table 4–2.

ATRIOVENTRICULAR NODAL ABLATION

The first arrhythmia treated by catheter cryoablation in humans was AF; the technique was complete ablation of the AV node. Dubuc et al.[37] were the first to perform and report cryoablation of the AV node in a small feasibility and safety study. They attempted AV node ablation in patients with chronic, drug refractory and poorly rate-controlled ventricular response. They were able to successfully perform complete AV node ablation in 10 of 12 patients. The two other ablations failed because of technical limitations of early versions of the cryoablation catheter system (9F catheter with suboptimal handling characteristics and a console not able to cool to temperatures less than –55°C). Eight of the 10 successfully ablated patients continued to demonstrate complete AV node conduction block at 6 months. These findings were

---

TABLE 4–2

Comparison of Clinical Applications of Cryoablation to Radiofrequency Ablation

Clinical Application	% Success with Cryoablation (Ref. Nos.)	% Success with Radiofrequency Ablation (Ref. Nos.)	Advantages of Cryoablation
AV node ablation for (chronic); drug-refractory AF	67-100 (37,39,61,62)	100 (25)	1. No significant advantage
AVNRT	94 (39,61-63)	97 (25)	1. Ability to perform Safety and Efficacy CryoMapping with decreased risk of AV block
APs	69 (39,61-63)	93 (25)	1. Reversible cryomapping for septal AP's 2. Limitations of cryoablation are related technical limitations of catheterization
Septal and parahisian APs	83-100 (39,64,65)	88-98 (42,43)	1. Ability to perform Safety and Efficacy CryoMapping with decreased risk of AV block
AFL	89-100 (39,62,66,67)	80-100 (68-71)	1. Less pain perception[67]
AF	Acute procedural success: 60-97 (62,72-76) At 1 year: 71 (74)	70-85 (77-79)	1. No pulmonary vein stenosis

AF, atrial fibrillation; AFL, atrial flutter; AP, accessory pathway; AV, atrioventricular; AVNRT, atrioventricular nodal reentrant tachycardia.

validated by other groups looking at the use of cryoablation to perform complete AV node ablation, with the largest study being the recently published FROSTY trial.[39,61,62] Success rates have ranged from 67% of 12 patients in the FROSTY trial to as high as 100% in a smaller trial with only 5 patients.[39,61] These results compare less favorably to the 100% success rate observed with RF for ablation of the AV node.[25] Although efficacious, cryoablation of the AV node for treatment of AF with uncontrolled ventricular response does not offer any significant advantages over traditional ablation techniques using RF as an energy source.

ATRIOVENTRICULAR NODAL REENTRANT TACHYCARDIA

AVNRT is an arrhythmia that is well suited to cryo-mapping and cryoablation because of the potential for procedural complications with inadvertent complete AV node block. As discussed earlier, cryomapping allows the operator to deliver a reversible lesion and to terminate ablation if there is any indication of inadvertent slowing or blockade of AV conduction. For this reason, the use of cryothermal energy for treatment of AVNRT has been studied extensively. Skanes and Dubuc et al.[63] performed some of the earliest investigations of slow pathway elimination by cryoablation for AVNRT; they reported acute procedural success (defined as inability to reinduce AVNRT after slow pathway ablation) in 17 of 18 patients treated. They also reported that cryoablation, unlike RF ablation of slow pathways, did not result in accelerated junctional rhythm identifying successful ablation sites. They described the use of atrial programmed stimulation to search for slow pathway elimination during ablation, to confirm desirable electrophysiologic effect from lesion delivery. This work was further validated by other investigators, who also reported efficacy of cryoablation for slow pathway elimination in patients with AVNRT. Long-term success rates have been as high as 94% in the FROSTY trial.[39,61,62] This success rate is somewhat lower than the 97% success rate reported for ablation of slow pathways for AVNRT with RF.[25] However, this again is offset by the fact that none of the 103 patients with AVNRT treated in the FROSTY trial developed any persistent AV conduction block requiring pacemaker implantation. Therefore, because of the decreased risk of complete AV conduction block, together with the high efficacy, slow pathway ablation of AVNRT by cryothermal energy is an excellent alternative to ablation with RF energy.

SEPTAL AND PARAHISIAN ACCESSORY PATHWAYS

The efficacy of cryothermal energy for ablation of APs has also been investigated extensively.[39,61,62] Unfortunately, unlike the high degrees of efficacy enjoyed for AV node ablation or AVNRT, the efficacy for cryoablation of APs has been lower than the 93% success rate reported for RF ablation.[25] In two smaller trials, including one with 3 patients (all with right-sided AP) and one with 13 patients (right- and left-sided APs), the success rates looked promising at 100% and 77%, respectively.[61,62] However, the largest trial included 49 patients with 50 APs[39] and reported an overall success rate of only 69%. The main reason for lower APS rate for ablation of APs was thought to be problems with the delivery system for cryothermal energy and not with the energy source itself. The high degree of torque often applied to appropriately position ablation catheters on APs can collapse the catheter, impeding adequate delivery of refrigerant to the cooling tip. This leads to suboptimal cooling of the tissue and suboptimal cryothermal lesion delivery and contributes to the failure to successfully eliminate some pathways.

However, there are clinical scenarios in which the augmented safety profile of cryoablation outweighs its lower efficacy. Furthermore, these anatomic locations often are not subjected to the same technical limitations of the cryothermal energy delivery system and therefore are associated with favorable success rates.

Septal APs, including parahisian APs, are arrhythmias well suited to treatment with cryoablation. The risk of AV conduction block with RF ablation of septal APs ranges from 12.5%[42] to 20%,[43] and in many cases this proves to be a significant factor that prohibits offering the patient a chance at successful pathway ablation.

The safety and efficacy of cryoablation for anteroseptal, midseptal, posteroseptal, and parahisian APs has been investigated. Wong et al.[64] reported on their experience with cryoablation in two parahisian pathways. They found the APs to be located at positions recording a significant His signal ($0.18 \pm 0.07\,mV$). However, cryoablation at sites that did not cause prolongation of the AH interval during cryomapping resulted in successful ablation with no AV block. Gaita et al.[65] also looked at cryoablation in 11 anteroseptal and 8 midseptal APs. They observed transient AH interval prolongation in 4 (50%) of 8 patients with midseptal pathways and no AH prolongation in any of the patients with anteroseptal pathways. There were no episodes of complete AV block. The APs rate was 100%, but with 15 months' follow-up there was a 20% recurrence rate (all occurring during the first month after ablation). The FROSTY trial also looked at safety and efficacy of septal pathway ablation and included six right posteroseptal pathways, six right anteroseptal pathways, and one right midseptal pathway.[39] The investigators were able to report acute success rates of 83%, 83%, and 100%, respectively, with no permanent AV conduction block. All acute failures were due to the inability to locate an ablation site that did not result in AV conduction delay or complete block during CryoMapping.

Therefore, because of the superior safety profile afforded to cryothermal energy for ablation of septal APs, resulting from the ability to deliver a reversible CryoMapping lesion, it should be considered the energy source of choice in this high-risk anatomic location despite a possibly lower efficacy.

ATRIAL FLUTTER

The treatment of cavotricuspid isthmus (CTI)-dependent atrial flutter (AFL) by RF catheter ablation has been associated with high success rates and significant improvements in quality of life.[70,71] Although the reported success rates are in the range of 80% to 100%,[68-70] ablation of the CTI with RF has been associated with significant perception of pain during lesion delivery, compared with similar ablations using cryothermal energy.[67] Therefore, numerous investigators have studied the efficacy and safety of cryothermal energy as an alternative energy source for ablation of the CTI.

Rodriguez et al.[62] studied cryoablation of CTI-dependent AFL in 15 patients as part of a larger study of cryoablation in patients with supraventricular tachycardias. They demonstrated a 100% success rate defined by bidirectional CTI block. This result, however, came at a cost of a 4.7-hour mean procedural time. In another study dedicated solely to examination of the efficacy and safety of cryoablation for CTI-dependent AFL, Manusama et al.[66] reported a 97% success rate after application of a median of 10 cryoablation lesions, and an 89% success rate at a mean of 17.6 months' follow-up, which is comparable to CTI ablation with RF. Furthermore, fluoroscopy times were not significantly prolonged by ablation of the CTI with cryothermal energy. However, total procedural time remained long at a mean 3.2 hours.

Therefore, cryothermal energy used as an alternative to RF results in similar rates of efficacy and a similar number of lesions. However, the procedural times are significantly longer with cryoablation. Although the longer procedural times are partially accounted for by a 4-minute application for each lesion, compared with 30 to 60 seconds per RF application, cryoablation is likely to remain the longer procedure. Although the techniques are equally efficacious, RF is likely to remain the energy source of first choice for ablation of the CTI for AFL, with the only real advantage of cryoablation being the significantly decreased level of pain perception during application.

ATRIAL FIBRILLATION

As previously noted, cryothermal energy is being investigated as a possible alternative energy source for the technically demanding PV isolation procedures for AF. This is a procedure in which the PVs are electrically isolated, with guidance by a circumferential mapping catheter, possibly a three-dimensional mapping system, and an RF energy source. Use of RF for a segmental ostial catheter ablation (SOCA) approach is typically associated with 100% immediate postprocedure PV isolation and a 70% to 85% clinical success rate.[77-80]

PV isolation for the SOCA technique has been attempted by groups using either a small-tip single-point lesion cryoablation catheter (Freezor, CryoCath) or a newer, circumferential cryoablation catheter (Arctic Circler, CryoCath). Initial smaller studies identified difficulty achieving complete PV isolation, with immediate postprocedure PV isolation success rates in the 60% to 96% range.[62,72,73] In a larger trial using a small-tip catheter in 52 patients and 152 PVs, an immediate postprocedure PV isolation rate of 97% was reported, as well as a 1-year clinical success rate (no recurrence of symptomatic AF) of 71%.[74] These results did come at a cost of longer procedure time, but that was offset by a 0% PV stenosis rate.

PV isolation by means of a circumferential cryoablation catheter was also investigated with some promising preliminary results.[75,76] This technique involves the use of a circular, expandable catheter (18- to 30-mm diameter) with a 64-mm curvilinear cooling segment (Arctic Circler, CryoCath) (Fig. 4–8). This catheter has reportedly been used to perform rapid and successful complete PV isolation with no evidence of PV stenosis.[75,76] Whether or not this catheter and technique proves to be clinically successful and feasible remains to be proven, with results expected in the next year.

Furthermore, new technologies are currently under development involving a balloon catheter (Arctic Circler Balloon, CryoCath) (Fig. 4–9) for PV isolation. This catheter has a 10F shaft and comes in balloon sizes of 23 and 30 mm. It is used with an over-the-wire technique and is intended to be positioned at the ostium of the PV and inflated to occlude the ostium. Contrast is then injected into the PV through

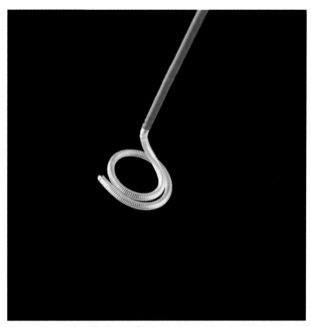

Figure 4–8. CryoCath Arctic Circler cryoablation catheter for pulmonary vein isolation. The distal loop is expandable from an 18 to 30 mm diameter to accommodate the variable pulmonary vein diameters observed clinically. The catheter possesses a 64-mm curvilinear cooling segment for creation of the cryothermal lesion. *(Courtesy of CryoCath Technologies, Montreal, Quebec.)*

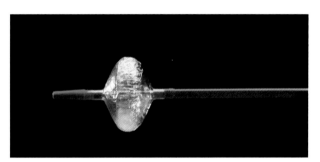

Figure 4–9. CryoCath Arctic Circler balloon cryoablation catheter. This catheter has a 10F shaft with a lumen to aid over-the-wire placement at the ostium of the pulmonary veins and comes in balloon sizes of 23 mm and 30 mm. *(Courtesy of CryoCath Technologies, Montreal, Quebec.)*

the wire lumen to assess completeness of occlusion of the vein. The balloon can then be cooled to create a rapid and complete circumferential cryothermal lesion for rapid PV isolation. The potential advantages for this system include decreased time for PV isolation and the already known decreased risk of PV stenosis observed in other PV isolation cryoablation studies.[74-76]

Overall, cryoablation for PV isolation procedures appears to be a feasible and promising technique. However, it is still undergoing refinement and clinical investigation, and the question of whether a cryothermal energy source will be adapted into routine clinical use for this ablation procedure remains to be answered.

Complications of Cryoablation

The potential complications associated with use of the CryoCath system are similar to those associated with placement of catheters within the heart for diagnostic study or ablation. These theoretically include thrombus formation, cardiac perforation with tamponade, inadvertent AV node ablation, and systemic embolization.[26,27,29] However, as discussed earlier, the characteristics of cryothermal lesions result in significantly lower risk of thrombus formation,[19] and the reversibility of cryothermal lesions during Cryo-Mapping allows the operator to confirm a lesion's effect before delivering it with a permanent effect. The FROSTY trial looked at complications associated with the use of the CryoCath cryoablation system in the largest clinical population ever studied undergoing ablation with a percutaneous cryothermal energy system.[39] Among the 166 patients with many different types of arrhythmias (AVNRT, atrioventricular reciprocating tachycardia, AF), there were no episodes of clinically evident thrombus formation and no episodes of permanent AV block. There was one episode of AV block lasting 10 seconds that occurred during catheter manipulation in the region of the AV node and was thought to be caused by mechanical trauma, one episode of AV block for 25 seconds that occurred during cryomapping, and a few episodes of AV block during cryoablation which all resolved within 1 minute or less. No patient was left with persistent AV block or required permanent pacemaker implantation. These results validate the technology's excellent safety profile in a large-scale clinical trial.

Summary

Cryothermal energy delivery for use in percutaneous catheter ablation procedures is not meant as a technology to replace RF, but rather as a tool in the electrophysiologist's armamentarium to allow further versatility in the ever-diversifying field of invasive clinical electrophysiology. There are clear advantages of cryothermal energy over RF energy in certain clinical scenarios. These may include cases in which the risk of AV block is high (anteroseptal, midseptal, or parahisian APs) or moderate (AVNRT, posteroseptal APs) during ablation with RF energy. They may also include cases in which there is significant catheter instability or the need to ablate within a venous structure or within close proximity to a coronary artery. In these scenarios, ablation with a cryothermal energy source is highly preferable. Conversely, there are clinical scenarios in which RF is the energy source of choice. The well-rounded electrophysiologist, therefore, must be familiar with the advantages and limitations of cryomapping and cryoablation, as well as RF, and use them in a complementary fashion to treat a broad spectrum of clinical arrhythmias with a high level of efficacy and a low level of complications.

References

1. Baust J, Gage AA, Ma H, Zhang C-M: Minimally invasive cryosurgery: Technological advances. Cryobiology 34:373, 1997.

2. Ott DA, Garson AJ, Cooley DA, et al.: Cryoablative techniques in the treatment of cardiac tachyarrhythmias. Ann Thorac Surg 43:138, 1987.

3. Berth-Jones J, Bourke J, Eglitis H, et al.: Value of a second freeze-thaw cycle in cryotherapy of common warts. Br J Dermatol 131:883, 1994.

4. Pease GR, Wong STS, Roos MS, Rubinsky B: MR image-guided control of cryo-surgery. J Magn Reson Imaging 5:753, 1995.

5. Hass GM, Taylor CB: A quantitative hypothermal method for the production of local injury of tissue. Arch Pathol 45:563, 1948.

6. Taylor CB, Davis CB, Vawter GF, Hass GM: Controlled myocardial injury produced by a hypothermal method. Circulation 3:239, 1951.

7. Lister JW, Hoffman BF: Reversible cold block of the specialized conduction tissues of the anaesthetized dog. Science 145:723, 1964.

8. Cooper I: Cryogenic surgery: A new method of destruction or extirpation of benign or malignant tissue. N Engl J Med 268:743, 1963.

9. Harrison L, Gallagher JJ, Kasell J, et al.: Cryosurgical ablation of the A-V node-His bundle: A new method for producing A-V block. Circulation 55:463, 1977.

10. Gillette PC, Swindle MM, Thompson RP, Case CL: Transvenous cryoablation of the bundle of His. Pacing Clin Electrophysiol 14:504, 1991.

11. Dubuc M, Talajic M, Roy D, et al.: Feasibility of cardiac cryoablation using a transvenous steerable electrode catheter. J Interv Card Electrophysiol 2:285, 1998.

12. Khairy P, Rodriguez-Santiago A, Talajic M, et al.: Catheter cryoablation in man: Early clinical experience. Can J Cardiol 15:173D, 1999.

13. Lustgarten DL, Keane D, Ruskin J: Cryothermal ablation: Mechanism of tissue injury and current experience in the treatment of tachyarrhythmias. Prog Cardiovasc Dis 41:481, 1999.

14. Keane D: New catheter ablation techniques for the treatment of cardiac arrhythmias. Cardiac Electrophysiol Rev 6:341, 2002.

15. Ohkawa S, Hackel DB, Mikat EM, et al.: Anatomic effects of cryoablation of the atrioventricular conduction system. Circulation 65:1155, 1982.

16. Gage AA, Baust J: Mechanisms of tissue injury. Cryobiology 37:171, 1998.

17. Rodriguez LM, Leunissen J, Hoekstra A, et al.: Transvenous cold mapping and cryoablation of the AV node in dogs: Observations of chronic lesions and comparison to those obtained using radiofrequency ablation. J Cardiovasc Electrophysiol 9:1055, 1998.

18. Dubuc M, Roy D, Thibault B, et al.: Transvenous catheter ice mapping and cryoablation of the atrioventricular node in dogs. Pacing Clin Electrophysiol 22:1488, 1999.

19. Khairy P, Chauvet P, Lehmann J, et al.: Lower incidence of thrombus formation with cryoenergy versus radiofrequency catheter ablation. Circulation 107:2045, 2003.

20. Huang SK, Bharati S, Lev M, Marcus FI: Electrophysiologic and histologic observations of chronic atrioventricular block induced by closed-chest catheter desiccation with radiofrequency energy. Pacing Clin Electrophysiol 10:805, 1987.

21. Nakagawa H, Yamanashi WS, Pitha JV, et al.: Comparison of in vivo tissue temperature profile and lesion geometry for radiofrequency ablation with a saline-irrigated electrode versus temperature control in a canine thigh muscle preparation. Circulation 91:2264, 1995.

22. Nath S, DiMarco JP, Haines DE: Basic aspects of radiofrequency catheter ablation. J Cardiovasc Electrophysiol 5:863, 1994.

23. Otomo K, Yamanashi WS, Tondo C, et al.: Why a large tip electrode makes a deeper radiofrequency lesion: Effects of increase in electrode cooling and electrode-tissue interface area. J Cardiovasc Electrophysiol 9:47, 1998.

24. Nakagawa H, Wittkampf FHM, Yamanashi WS, et al.: Inverse relationship between electrode size and lesion size during radiofrequency ablation with active electrode cooling. Circulation 8:458, 1998.

25. Calkins H, Yong P, Miller JM, et al., for the Atakr Multicenter Investigators Group: Catheter ablation of accessory pathways, atrioventricular nodal reentrant tachycardia and the atrioventricular junction: Final results of a prospective, multicenter clinical trial. Circulation 99:262, 1999.

26. Hindricks G: The Multicenter European Radiofrequency Survey (MERFS): Complications of radiofrequency catheter ablation of arrhythmias. Eur Heart J 14:1644, 1993.

27. Zhou L, Keane D, Reed G, Ruskin J: Thromboembolic complications of cardiac radiofrequency catheter ablation: A review of the reported incidence, pathogenesis and current research directions. J Cardiovasc Electrophysiol 10:611, 1999.

28. Epstein MR, Knapp LD, Martindill M, et al., for the Atakr Investigator Group: Embolic complications associated with radiofrequency catheter ablation. Am J Cardiol 77:655, 1996.

29. Green TO, Huang SKS, Wagshal AB, et al.: Cardiovascular complications after radiofrequency catheter ablation of supraventricular tachyarrhythmias. Am J Cardiol 74:615, 1994.

30. Scanavacca MI, Kajita LJ, Vieira M, Sosa EA: Pulmonary vein stenosis complicating catheter ablation of focal atrial fibrillation. J Cardiovasc Electrophysiol 11:677, 2000.

31. Yu WC, Hsu TL, Tai CT, et al.: Acquired pulmonary vein stenosis after radiofrequency catheter ablation of paroxysmal atrial fibrillation. J Cardiovasc Electrophysiol 12:887, 2001.

32. Arentz T, Jander N, von Rosenthal J, et al.: Incidence of pulmonary vein stenosis 2 years after radiofrequency catheter ablation of refractory atrial fibrillation. Eur Heart J 24:963, 2003.

33. Saad EB, Marrouche NF, Saad CP, et al.: Pulmonary vein stenosis after catheter ablation of atrial fibrillation: Emergence of a new clinical syndrome. Ann Intern Med 138:634, 2003.

34. Giorgberidze I, Saksena S, Krol RB, Mathew P: Efficacy and safety of radiofrequency catheter ablation of left-sided accessory pathways through the coronary sinus. Am J Cardiol 76:359, 1995.

35. Haissaguerre M, Gaita F, Fischer B, et al.: Radiofrequency catheter ablation of left lateral accessory pathways via the coronary sinus. Circulation 86:1464, 1992.

36. Huang SKS, Graham AR, Bharati S, et al.: Short- and long-term effects of transcatheter ablation of the coronary sinus by radiofrequency energy. Circulation 78:416, 1988.

37. Dubuc M, Khairy P, Rodriguez-Santiago A, et al.: Catheter cryoablation of the atrioventricular node in patients with atrial fibrillation: A novel technology for ablation of cardiac arrhythmias. J Cardiovasc Electrophysiol 12:439, 2001.

38. Camm J, Ward DE, Spurrell RAJ, Rees GM: Cryothermal mapping and cryoablation in the treatment of refractory cardiac arrhythmias. Circulation 62:67, 1980.

39. Friedman PL, Dubuc M, Green MS, et al.: Catheter cryoablation of supraventricular tachycardia: Results of the multicenter prospective "FROSTY" trial. Heart Rhythm 1:129, 2004.

40. Cote J-M, Epstein MR, Triedman JK, et al.: Low-temperature mapping predicts site of successful ablation while minimizing myocardial damage. Circulation 94:253, 1996.

41. Hindricks G: Incidence of complete atrioventricular block following attempted radiofrequency catheter modification of the atrioventricular node in 880 patients: Results of the Multicenter European Radiofrequency Survey (MERFS). Eur Heart J 17:82, 1996.

42. Connors SP, Vora A, Green MS, Tang ASL: Radiofrequency ablation of atrial tachycardia originating from the triangle of Koch. Can J Cardiol 16:39, 2000.

43. Yeh SJ, Wang CC, Wen MS, et al.: Characteristics and radiofrequency ablation therapy of intermediate septal accessory pathway. Am J Cardiol 73:50, 1994.

44. Tai CT Chen S, Chiang CE, et al.: Electrocardiographic and electrophysiologic characteristics of anteroseptal, mid-septal and para-hisian accessory pathways: Implications of radiofrequency catheter ablation. Chest 109:730, 1996.

45. Lin JL, Huang SKS, Lai LP, et al.: Radiofrequency catheter ablation of septal accessory pathways within the triangle of Koch: Importance of energy titration testing other than the local electrogram characteristics for identifying the successful target site. Pacing Clin Electrophysiol 21:1909, 1998.

46. Brugada J, Puigfel M, Mont L, et al.: Radiofrequency ablation of anteroseptal, para-hisian, and mid-septal accessory pathways using a simplified femoral approach. Pacing Clin Electrophysiol 21:735, 1998.

47. Huang SK, Bharati S, Graham AR, et al.: Closed chest catheter desiccation of the atrioventricular junction using radiofrequency energy: A new method of catheter ablation. J Am Coll Cardiol 9:349, 1987.

48. Manolis AS, Melita-Manolis H, Vassilikos V, et al.: Thrombogenicity of radiofrequency lesions: Results with serial D-dimer determinations. J Am Coll Cardiol 28:1257, 1996.

49. Langberg JJ, Calkins H, El-Atassi R, et al.: Temperature monitoring during radiofrequency catheter ablation of accessory pathways. Circulation 86:1469, 1992.

50. Haines DE, Verrow AF: Observations on electrode-tissue interface temperature and effect on electrical impedance during radiofrequency ablation of ventricular myocardium. Circulation 82:1034, 1990.

51. Calkins H, Prystowski E, Carlson M, et al.: for the Atakr Multicenter Investigators Group: Temperature monitoring during radiofrequency catheter ablation procedures using closed loop control. Circulation 90:1279, 1994.

52. Demolin JM, Eick OJ, Munch K, et al.: Soft thrombus formation in radiofrequency catheter ablation. Pacing Clin Electrophysiol 25: 1219, 2002.

53. Matsudaira K, Nakagawa H, Wittkampf FHM, et al.: High incidence of thrombus formation without impedance rise during radiofrequency ablation using electrode temperature control. Pacing Clin Electrophysiol 26:1227, 2003.

54. Sun Y, Po SS, Arruda M, et al.: Risk of coronary artery stenosis with venous ablation for epicardial accessory pathways. Pacing Clin Electrophysiol 24:605, 2001.

55. Skanes A, Jones D, Teefy P, et al.: Cryoablation of accessory pathways via the distal coronary sinus: Safety and feasibility in a swine model. Pacing Clin Electrophysiol 24:660, 2002.

56. Yagi T, Nakagawa H, Chandrasekaran S, et al.: Safety and efficacy of cryo-ablation in the canine coronary sinus. Circulation 104:II-620, 2001.

57. Gaita F, Paperini L, Riccardi R, Ferraro A: Cryothermic ablation within the coronary sinus of an epicardial posterolateral pathway. J Cardiovasc Electrophysiol 13:1160, 2002.

58. Misaki T, Allwork S, Bentall HH: Longterm effects of cryosurgery in the sheep heart. Cardiovasc Res 17:61, 1983.

59. Wong T, Markides V, Chow AWC, et al.: Percutaneous cryoablation pulmonary vein isolation to treat atrial fibrillation. Pacing Clin Electrophysiol 24:552, 2002.

60. Tse HF, Reek S, Timmermans C, et al.: Pulmonary vein isolation using transvenous catheter cryoablation for treatment of atrial fibrillation without risk of pulmonary vein stenosis. J Am Coll Cardiol 42:752, 2003.

61. Lowe MD, Meara M, Mason J, et al.: Catheter cryoablation of supraventricular arrhythmias: A painless alternative to radiofrequency energy. Pacing Clin Electrophysiol 26:500, 2003.

62. Rodriguez LM, Geller JC, Tse HF, et al.: Acute results of transvenous cryoablation of supraventricular tachycardia (atrial fibrillation, atrial flutter, Wolff-Parkinson-White syndrome, atrioventricular nodal reentry tachycardia). J Cardiovasc Electrophysiol 13:1082, 2002.

63. Skanes AC, Dubuc M, Klein GJ, et al.: Cryothermal ablation of the slow pathway for the elimination of atrioventricular nodal reentrant tachycardia. Circulation 102:2856, 2000.

64. Wong T, Markides V, Peters NS, Wyn Davies D: Clinical usefulness of cryomapping for ablation of tachycardias involving perinodal tissue. J Interv Card Electrophysiol 10:153, 2004.

65. Gaita F, Riccardi R, Hocini M, et al.: Safety and efficacy of cryoablation of accessory pathways adjacent to the normal conduction system. J Cardiovasc Electrophysiol 14:825, 2003.

66. Manusama R, Timmermans C, Limon F, et al.: Catheter-based cryoablation permanently cures patients with common atrial flutter. Circulation 109:1636, 2004.

67. Timmermans C, Ayers GM, Crijns HJGM, Rodriguez LM: Randomized study comparing radiofrequency ablation with cryoablation for the treatment of atrial flutter with emphasis on pain perception. Circulation 107:1250, 2003.

68. Rodriguez LM, Nabar A, Timmermans C, et al.: Comparison of results of an 8-mm split-tip versus a 4-mm tip ablation catheter to perform radiofrequency ablation of type I atrial flutter. Am J Cardiol 85:109, 2000.

69. Jais P, Shah D, Haissaguerre M, et al.: Prospective randomized comparison of irrigated-tip versus conventional-tip catheters for ablation of common flutter. Circulation 101:772, 2000.

70. Natale A, Newby KH, Pisano E, et al.: Prospective randomized comparison of antiarrhythmic therapy versus first-line radiofrequency ablation in patients with atrial flutter. J Am Coll Cardiol 35:1898, 2000.

71. Wellens HJJ: Contemporary management of atrial flutter. Circulation 106:649, 2002.

72. Tondo C, Fassini G, De Martino G, et al.: Catheter isolation of the pulmonary veins by cryothermal ablation: Preliminary results. Pacing Clin Electrophysiol 24:612, 2002.

73. Wong T, Markides V, Chow AWC, et al.: Percutaneous cryoablation pulmonary vein isolation to treat atrial fibrillation. Pacing Clin Electrophysiol 24:552, 2002.

74. Tse HF, Reek S, Timmermans C, et al.: Pulmonary vein isolation using transvenous catheter cryoablation for treatment of atrial fibrillation without risk of pulmonary vein stenosis. J Am Coll Cardiol 42:752, 2003.

75. Wong T, Markides V, Peters NS, et al.: Percutaneous isolation of multiple pulmonary veins using an expandable circular cryoablation catheter. Pacing Clin Electrophysiol 27:551, 2004.

76. Rostock T, Weiss C, Ventura R, Willems S: Pulmonary vein isolation during atrial fibrillation using a circumferential cryoablation catheter. Pacing Clin Electrophysiol 27:1024, 2004.

77. Haissaguerre M, Jais P, Shah DC, et al.: Electrophysiological end point for catheter ablation of atrial fibrillation initiated from multiple pulmonary venous foci. Circulation 101:1409, 2000.

78. Macle L, Jais P, Weerasooriya R, et al.: Irrigated-tip catheter ablation of pulmonary veins for treatment of atrial fibrillation. J Cardiovasc Electrophysiol 13:1067, 2002.

79. Oral H, Scharf C, Chugh A, et al.: Catheter ablation for paroxysmal atrial fibrillation: Segmental pulmonary vein ostial ablation versus left atrial ablation. Circulation 108:2355, 2003.

80. From Khairy P, Dubuc M: Transcatheter cryoablation. In Liem LB, Downar E (eds.): Progress in Catheter Ablation, 2001, p 391.

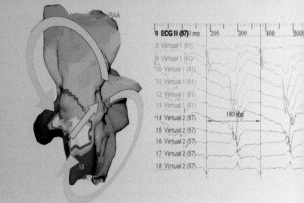

5

Catheter Microwave, Laser, and Ultrasound: Biophysics and Applications

Shephal K. Doshi • David Keane

Key Points

- Alternative energy sources have been explored to overcome the limitations in lesion size and need for tissue contact inherent to radiofrequency (RF) ablation. Microwave (MW), laser, and ultrasound (US) energies have been used in humans.

- Problems with alternative energies have involved their incorporation into a catheter-based platform and titration of energy delivery. MW is particularly suited to penetrating scar tissue. Laser can create large, deep lesions by energy scatter within the tissue. US may be focused to create encircling lesions or focal lesions far from the transducer.

Since the initial descriptions of transcatheter ablation, optimal energy sources for creating myocardial lesions have been sought. Although direct current was initially used, radiofrequency (RF) energy has become the mainstay of transcatheter cardiac ablation.[1,2] RF has provided acceptable results for specific arrhythmias, with success rates in excess of 95% for the treatment of patients with atrioventricular nodal reentrant tachycardia (AVNRT), accessory pathway–mediated tachycardia, and atrioventricular (AV) junction ablation[2-4] with a relatively low complication rate (Fig. 5–1). However, as the targeted substrate for catheter ablation evolves from discrete focal ablation to linear ablation in tissue as thin as the posterior left atrial wall and as deep as the left ventricle, a need for more versatile and effective energy sources arises. This chapter reviews the mechanisms and data behind alternative energy sources for transcatheter ablation, including microwave (MW), laser, and ultrasound (US) energy.

As has been well described, thermal injury to myocardial tissue is a prerequisite for ablation by electromagnetic energy such as RF and MW. When RF voltage is applied, current is induced to flow between a pair of electrodes. RF tissue injury during catheter ablation is a result of resistive (ohmic) heating as electric currents (500 to 750 kHz) flow in radial paths from the ablation catheter electrode tip (high current density) into the tissue to a pad electrode applied to the body surface (low current density).[5,6] With RF, resistive heating decreases to the fourth power as the distance from the ablation electrode increases. Lesions are created beyond the electrode-tissue interface due to passive heat transfer. Lesion volume is primarily determined by conductive heat transfer to adjacent tissue and convective heat loss. Temperatures near 50°C are required to create irreversible tissue injury.[7,8] Once temperatures approach 100°C, coagulum can form at the electrode tip. This desiccation and coagulation of tissue increases the resistance to the flow of current, which hinders tissue heating and limits lesion expansion.[8-10]

Microwave

BASIC PRINCIPLES

Like RF, MW injury is thermally mediated. In contrast to RF-mediated heating by electrical resistance, the mechanism of heating from a high-frequency MW energy source is dielectric.[11] Dielectric heating occurs when electromagnetic radiation stimulates oscillation of dipoles (e.g., water molecules) in the surrounding medium (Fig. 5–2). The electromagnetic energy is converted into kinetic energy (heat).[12] MW frequencies range from 30 to 3000 MHz.[13] These high-frequency electromagnetic waves can propagate in free space or in a conductive medium, through blood or desiccated tissue. Energy can be deposited directly into tissue at a distance regardless of the intervening medium.[14]

It has been described that the propagation of MW in biologic tissue is regulated by tissue composition and dielectric permittivity, source frequency and

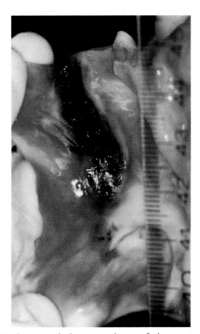

Figure 5–1. Gross pathology specimen of the posterior wall of a caprine right atrium. A radiofrequency (RF) 4-mm electrode catheter was deployed in vivo under electroanatomic guidance to create a linear lesion from the superior vena cava to the inferior cava. The resultant lesion demonstrates some of the limitations of conventional RF ablation, including extensive charring, as well as lack of lesion continuity at its inferior extension. For these reasons, the development of linear ablation approaches to the treatment of atrial fibrillation and ventricular tachycardia have stimulated interest in alternative energy sources for ablation.

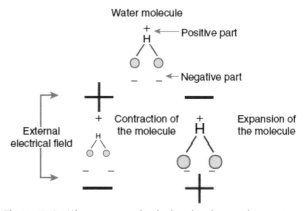

Figure 5–2. Microwave results in heating by causing contraction of expansion and rotation of dipole molecules such as water. The resulting physical motion causes thermal energy.

power, and antenna radiation pattern and polarization.[11,15,16] With regard to biologic tissues of interest such as blood, muscle, and tissues with low water content (i.e., fat, bone, and desiccated tissue), there are differences in conductivity and dielectric constants as a function of frequency.[15,16] These differences can be significant among the three types of tissues. As the MW field propagates in the tissue medium, energy is extracted from the field and absorbed by the medium (converted to heat). This absorption results in a progressive reduction of MW power intensity as the field advances into the tissue.[11]

Because of these differences in dielectric permittivity, tissues with low water content have a depth of penetration four times greater than that of tissues with high water content (e.g., muscle). Lin[15] quantified this reduction of MW power by the depth of penetration at 2450 MHz: 17, 19, and 79 mm for blood, muscle, and fat, respectively. In this way, an MW field can propagate through low-water (desiccated or fat) tissue to deliver energy to deeper tissue. The conductivities for blood and muscle are similar yet almost 300% lower than that of tissue with a low water content.[17] The basic properties of MW that render it favorable for ablation include the following[18]: (1) MW antennas radiate electromagnetic waves into the surrounding cardiac tissue; (2) power deposition follows a second-power law with distance, thereby heating tissue at a greater distance compared with RF; and (3) a dispersive electrode on the skin is not required.

MICROWAVE SYSTEM DESIGN

The first reported use of MW energy for ablation of cardiac arrhythmias in an experimental animal model was by Beckman et al.[19] This report described the application of MW power using a probe applied directly to the His bundle during cardiopulmonary bypass. Langberg et al.[20] first described percutaneous catheter ablation of the AV junction using MW. Multiple reports have described variations in MW antenna design since these landmark studies, but the basic conceptual system design is consistent.

The MW system comprises four primary components: an MW power source, a switch assembly, power monitors, and control circuits.[17] The energy from the power source is transmitted via a coaxial cable to an antenna. MW catheter design is vital for efficient coupling of energy to the tissue. The impedance of the transmission line needs to be matched to the properties of the antenna, to prevent MW energy from being reflected back to its source and thereby minimizing heating of the catheter body (composed of a coaxial cable).[7]

The vital element that determines the efficacy of the MW system is the antenna design. To characterize the MW antenna and its emission properties, the radiation efficiency, radiative field pattern, and power reflection coefficient are studied. The radiative field pattern—the change in temperature from instantaneous heating due to radiation from the MW field emitted from the antenna—is represented by the specific absorption rate (SAR) pattern.[21] The power reflection coefficient represents the amount of return loss of the forward power at a given frequency. This return loss (return of MW current up the transmission cable) should be at a minimum and has been reported to be 1% to 4% with certain antenna designs.[22,23] Multiple studies describing properties of various antenna designs have been published.[9,21,24-37] To date, no one particular antenna design has been universally accepted.

The majority of studies have used MW frequencies of 915 and 2450 MHz. The availability of MW frequencies for noncommunication medical applications is restricted by the U.S. Federal Communications Commission (FCC), which has limited exploration of other frequencies.[38] Because antenna dimensions are based on one-quarter wavelength, 2450 MHz allows use of a significantly smaller antenna, which is more favorable for percutaneous catheter-based systems.[7]

In theory, lower frequencies are associated with deeper lesions and decreased cable heating, however antenna characteristics are highly dependent on MW frequency.[39] The antenna requires a specific design for the selected MW frequency.[38] Large lesions have been reported with both frequencies.[28,30,40,41]

DATA FROM IN VIVO EXPERIMENTS

Atrioventricular Nodal Ablation

MW ablation of the AV node has been studied in open-chest and closed-chest canine models using 2450 MHz frequency and many different MW catheter designs.[20,28,30,31,42] These studies reliably resulted in discrete lesions without evidence of distant damage. Irreversible AV block strongly correlated with temperature rises greater than 55°C.[42] Yang et al.[28] demonstrated that the depth of the ablation lesions increases markedly with increasing power and duration of delivered energy, even beyond 100-second applications. Microscopically, the ablations produced hemorrhagic changes with coagulative necrosis and clearly demarcated borders.[30] There was no evidence of coagulum formation or charring at the catheter tip or antenna.[31]

Ablation of Ventricular Myocardium

Because lesion formation in ventricular myocardium, especially in the presence of scar, limits standard RF

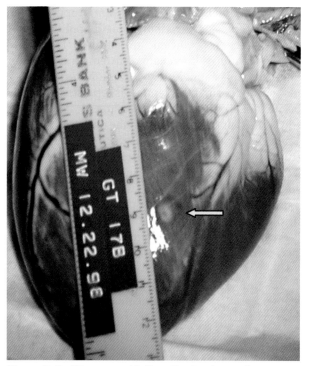

Figure 5–3. Microwave ablation. Caprine heart after percutaneous transvascular endocardial microwave ablation in vivo from an end-firing monopole antenna. The lesion *(arrow)* can be seen to be transmural, with a sharply defined circumferential appearance on the epicardial surface of the left ventricle.

ablation, studies using MW have been performed to assess the efficacy of ablation in the ventricular myocardium.[28,41,43,44] These studies showed the feasibility of creating large lesions in the ventricular myocardium (Fig. 5–3). MW ablation was found to lead to lesion volume expansion through 180 seconds.[28] Using a 4-mm split-tip antenna and 2450 MHz of MW energy, Huang et al.[43] performed closed-chest ablation in mongrel dogs. Each animal received a single pulsed ablation of 30 W for 30 seconds. A total of 40 left ventricular and 18 right ventricular lesions were created. Mean lesion sizes were $10.4 \times 9.1 \times 7.0$ mm (length × width × depth) or 379.0 mm³ (volume) in the left ventricle and $10.4 \times 8.4 \times 5.2$ mm or 249.3 mm³ in the right ventricle. The lesions were discrete and hemielliptical or hemispherical in nature, consisting of a central crater with a thin layer of thrombus, along with a pale necrotic and hemorrhagic peripheral zone. These studies showed that MW energy should be efficacious even when ventricular tachycardia (VT) circuits involve the subepicardium.

Ablation of the Cavotricuspid Isthmus

The efficacy of RF ablation of right atrial cavotricuspid isthmus–dependent flutter has been well docu-

mented.[45-47] Contiguous lesion formation with RF can be difficult due to variable contact and three-dimensionally complex anatomy making contiguous ablation lines difficult. The complexity posed by the ridges and valleys of pectinate muscles and the eustachian ridge may favor the use of MW. A study based on MW energy field measurements was conducted to assess the feasibility of MW ablation without tissue contact at various catheter orientations.[48] Sixty-nine total lesions were created in vitro in bovine hearts with the MW antenna positioned parallel at 0, 1, 2, and 5 mm above the endocardium or perpendicular at 0 mm. Dimensions of lesions created at 0 and 1 mm were significantly greater than those made 2 and 5 mm above the endocardium. The authors concluded that MW lesions were feasible without tissue contact and at different orientations. MW ablation may provide utility especially at sites where there is suboptimal tissue contact.

Iwasa et al.[49] assessed the ability of a linear MW antenna capable of forming lesions up to 4 cm in length to ablate the isthmus from the inferior vena cava to the tricuspid annulus. A steerable 9 French (F) catheter with a 4-cm MW antenna and a 900- to 930-MHz generator were used. Linear MW ablation of the tricuspid valve–inferior vena cava isthmus was successful in producing transmural isthmus ablation with bidirectional block as a treatment for atrial flutter in all 10 dogs studied. Few energy applications were required. The total ablation time ranged from 2 to 10 minutes, and no complications were reported in any of the animals. There was no evidence of charring, coagulum formation, or disruption of the atrial endocardium. Other authors have also concluded that single-application ablation can achieve isthmus block using MW energy delivered through an appropriately sized antenna.[50]

Adragao et al.[51] published the first case of MW ablation of arrhythmia (atrial flutter) in humans. An 8F steerable MW ablation catheter with temperature sensing was used, and the flutter was terminated 50 seconds into the first application. The total application time was 60 seconds and resulted in bidirectional transisthmus conduction block. No coagulum was noted on the ablation catheter tip. No early or late complications occurred. The patient was reported to remain in sinus rhythm 3 months later.

The principal advantages of MW ablation for percutaneous endocardial application include (1) contact forgiveness, (2) depth of penetration and lesion formation, and (3) avoidance of excessive endocardial temperatures in order to achieve adequate tissue temperature in deeper layers of the subepicardium.

In addition to the percutaneous endocardial applications already described, MW energy has been used during the surgical maze procedure both on pump in the arrested heart and, more recently, in a minimally invasive epicardial approach off pump. The ability of MW energy to penetrate through epicardial fat and be absorbed by the atrial myocardium provides another distinct advantage for this latter application.

Laser

BASIC PRINCIPLES

Laser (Light Amplification by Stimulated Emission of Radiation) provides an additional energy source with which tissue ablation can be created. The generation of laser energy involves the basic principles of emission and absorption of electromagnetic radiation that occur when energy states are altered in atoms and molecules.[52] As described by Saksena and Gadhoke,[53] if a large number of identical atoms (or molecules) in a medium undergo a particular change in energy state at the same time, electromagnetic radiation with similar wavelengths, synchronized in time and space, will be emitted. Therefore, laser radiation is of a narrow frequency range (monochromatic), in phase (coherent), and in parallel (collimated). The ability of laser light to be highly focused permits a high power density to be administered to the target tissue.

Laser systems have variable designs but generally consist of a lasing medium of solid, liquid, or gas contained in a chamber of reflecting surfaces. Typically, electricity is used to raise the energy state of the lasing medium, thereby causing a release of photons as the energy level of the medium falls back down to the baseline state. The difference between the two energy states determines the wavelength of the photon. These photons represent laser energy.[54]

Numerous materials are used for laser action. Gaseous mediums used for excimer and argon lasers emit light of wavelengths from 300 to 700 nm in the ultraviolet and visible light bands, respectively. Diode lasers involve the use of semiconductors and emit wavelengths between 700 and 1500 nm (near-infrared). Solid lasers include neodymium-doped yttrium-aluminium-garnet (Nd-YAG) and holmium, which emit energy in the infrared spectrum of 1064 to 2000 nm.[39,55,56] Laser energy can be delivered in either a continuous or a pulsed mode.

Laser energy is thermal in nature, and its effect is a function of laser power density on tissue. During tissue irradiation, light is scattered and absorbed to an extent that depends on beam diameter and the optical properties of the tissue. The laser energy is selectively absorbed by the tissues over a depth of several millimeters and produces heating of a volume of tissue.[57] Tissue heating produces focal myocardial tissue ablation via vaporization and coagulation necrosis. Myocardial tissue coagulation is produced by contraction and dehydration as light energy is absorbed. The volume of coagulated tissue can vary depending on laser energy absorption (transfer ratio) in the irradiated tissue.[58] Tissue temperatures in excess of 100°C typically cause tissue vaporization, whereas those in the range of 42°C to 65°C can cause tissue damage from protein denaturation.[59,60]

The laser beam power decreases within the tissue in an exponential manner. The rate of decay is multifactorial and involves laser beam absorption, scatter, and distance from the laser source.[13] Tissue injury may progress past the target site if the laser exposure time surpasses the thermal relaxation time of the target tissue. The distribution of spread follows a gaussian relationship and is expected to be focal.[61]

In a study by Saksena et al.,[62] argon laser ablation in normal human ventricle was associated with an increase in mean lesion size and depth with increasing mean laser discharge energy dose, with tissue perforation at doses greater than 300 J. The diseased human ventricle had a higher safety margin with respect to perforation. Ultimately, lesion dimensions were determined by the total energy dose, medium used, and tissue characteristics. Isner et al.[63] demonstrated successful ablation of cardiovascular tissues with both infrared and ultraviolet laser radiation.

ARGON LASER

Early work on argon laser radiation produced successful catheter ablation of the specialized AV conduction system in canines using fiberoptics.[64,65] The gross lesions were reported as circular, well-circumscribed areas of thermal injury at the site of discharge. Because the initial use of continuous argon laser discharges was associated with fiberoptic tip damage, the efficacy of pulsed laser ablation was compared with that of continuous laser discharge in the diseased human ventricle.[66] Histologic examination showed crater formation due to tissue vaporization, with the crater lining consisting of charred tissue and a zone of coagulation necrosis. Lesion depth and diameter were comparable in the two approaches.

Evidence has accrued that the mechanical strength of tissue greatly influences the rate of ablation by pulsed lasers. A pulsed or high-energy continuous-wave laser rapidly deposits energy and causes rapid heating of tissue. Because there may not be enough time for expansion of the heated water, there may be a significant pressure increase followed by an explosive abolition of tissue.[67] Argon lasers have been used intraoperatively in clinical settings for patients with refractory sustained VT and for atrial and accessory bypass tract resection.[68,69]

ND-YAG LASER

Initial studies involving the interaction of laser energy with the beating heart in vivo using an Nd-YAG laser created controlled endocardial lesions of 7.9 × 5.4 × 6.6 mm at 40 J.[70] The gross morphologic lesions consisted of a central vaporized crater surrounded by a rim of necrotic tissue. Lesion size increased as a function of total energy delivered. The duration of lasing was a more important determinant of lesion size than the absolute amount of energy delivered. This suggests that short but repetitive laser bursts could create shallow lesions with wider surface area, potentially decreasing the risk of cardiac perforation. Observations have also been made suggesting that, for Nd-YAG and argon lasers, blood enhances laser-induced tissue injury better than saline.[59] Ohtake et al.[58] confirmed that Nd-YAG laser energy was absorbed by blood due to hemoglobin absorption of light, causing more energy to be transferred into the myocardium.

When the Nd-YAG laser is compared with the argon laser, several differences are appreciated. The Nd-YAG laser has much greater forward scatter of energy than absorption at the surface.[58] This scattering effect of the beam on tissue causes coagulation to occur below rather than at the surface.[66] Continuous, percutaneous Nd-YAG laser coagulation was performed by Weber et al.[71,72] in the ventricular and atrial myocardium of canines, producing lesions as large as 7 mm in diameter and 11 mm in depth at 50 J in the ventricle and 5 mm in diameter in the atrium. Focal injuries of homogeneous coagulation or fibrosis were seen to be localized to the target area without vaporizing of tissue or crater formation in the ventricle. Chronic atrial lesions revealed sharply defined, oval-shaped areas of transmural fibrosis.

Initial clinical evaluation of epicardial laser use in patients without left ventriculotomy was performed by Pfeiffer et al.[73] Nine patients with a history of myocardial infarction and monomorphic VT received epicardial laser ablation. The regions of interest where epicardial potentials during VT showed distinct mid-diastolic potentials received epicardial photocoagulation (50 to 80 W) with a continuous wave Nd-YAG laser via a handheld probe. Seven patients remained free of clinical VT for a mean follow-up of 17 ± 11 months. This study elucidated the utility of deep tissue coagulation using the Nd-YAG laser with epicardial application for postinfarction VT caused by midmyocardial or subepicardial reentrant circuits.

Clinical endocardial laser ablation, as described by Weber et al.,[74] involved 10 patients with common AVNRT. Using preshaped guiding catheters and a novel pin-electrode laser catheter, they applied Nd-YAG laser energy (one to five applications per patient) at 20 or 30 W for 10 to 45 seconds in the posteroinferior aspect of the tricuspid annulus. The tachycardia was rendered noninducible after ablation.

DIODE LASER

A large hindrance to acceptance of laser technology has been concern about its size, expense, and complexity. Development of the diode laser, with size and costs analogous to those of an RF generator, has reduced these concerns. Ware et al.[75] used an intramyocardial diode laser operating at 805 nm and low power (2.0 to 4.5 W) in canines to create large, deep, well-circumscribed lesions up to 10 mm in width and depth without disrupting the endocardium or epicardium.

A slow rate of volumetric heating, provided by scattered photons, can enable the creation of deep, large-volume lesions by laser energy. This less intense but strictly intramural heating can permit maximal heat conduction that avoids the endocardium and epicardium.[76] The development of diode laser technology has also created the ability to customize wavelengths for optimal laser ablation, because the optical properties of differing myocardial pathologies vary. An extensive study by d'Avila et al.[77] revealed experimental evidence of the efficacy of near-infrared endocardial and epicardial laser applications for catheter ablation of VT complicating Chagas' disease.

APPLICATIONS FOR LINEAR LESIONS

Interest in contiguous linear ablation lesions, particularly for arrhythmias such as atrial fibrillation (AF), has prompted the study of radial diffusing optical fibers that enable the laser energy to be distributed along the length of the active element. These optical fibers, with a gradient of titanium dioxide particles embedded in the flexible fiber tip, produce scattered radiation with near-uniform 360-degree radial delivery (Fig. 5–4), creating linear thermal lesions.[39] Fried et al.[78] demonstrated linear laser ablation using a Nd-YAG laser source in right ventricular myocardium without evidence of tissue charring and vaporization. Linear laser applications with a diode laser in the trabeculated anterior right atrial wall in a goat model produced transmural conduction block.[79] Use of optical fibers to deliver laser energy also provides a conduit for light transmission and reflectance to provide real-time monitoring of lesion formation (Fig. 5–5A and B). It can also be used to provide endoscopic visualization for direct visual feedback, particularly when a balloon is used.

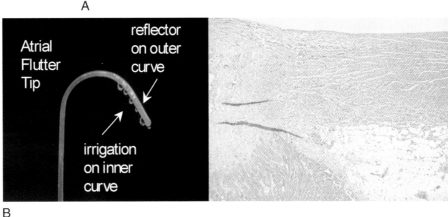

Figure 5–4. A, In vitro analysis of energy distribution of a curvilinear optical light diffuser used for linear lasing in the atrium. Despite the curvature, the uniformity of energy distribution is clear. **B,** Irrigated linear optical diffuser with gold reflector on the outer curve *(left)*. The curvilinear catheter was applied in vivo in the goat atrium and was shown on histology to produce transmural lesions across the isthmus from the inferior vena cava to the tricuspid annulus *(right)*.

LASER BALLOON CATHETER DESIGN

The efficacy of laser energy to create thermocoagulation is influenced by the irradiation angle, the distance between the laser tip and the target tissue, and the properties of the medium.[80] To this end, various catheter designs have been used for laser ablation.[74,75,80,81] The interest in transcatheter ablation of AF by pulmonary vein (PV) isolation and the inherent limitations of RF energy encouraged the design of a laser balloon system capable of projecting forward a circumferential ring of laser energy.[39,82-84] The balloon design has a collapsible profile and is filled with a 3-mL mixture of radiographic contrast agent and deuterium oxide (D_2O). D_2O is intended to eliminate self-heating of the balloon by shifting the absorption of wavelengths to greater than the 980 nm used. The light is transferred from the fiberoptic core with the use of a modified glass fiber tip, through an optically transparent shaft in the balloon, and projected as a ring onto the distal balloon surface (Fig. 5–6). The intensity of the emitted light delivered to the tissue around the ring is uniform and continuous without gaps.[39,83,84]

In an open-thoracotomy caprine model of endocardial access through a left atrial appendage sheath, Reddy et al.[83] demonstrated electrical isolation of 19 of 27 PVs after a single application of photonic energy. With the use of reflectance spectroscopy to ensure adequate orientation and contact of the laser balloon with the left atrial myocardium, complete PV isolation was achieved in 5 of 5 veins. Pathologic examination revealed no PV stenosis, no pericardial damage, minor lung lesions without pleural perforation, minimal endothelium disruption, and, in the presence of adequate heparinization, no endocardial charring or overlying thrombus. Using a percutaneous technique, Lemery et al.[84] delivered photonic energy successfully to 5 of 5 PVs, with gross inspection revealing endocardial lesions at the ostium in 4 of 5 veins.

The use of deflectable delivery systems will facilitate optimal balloon placement. The laser balloon has entered clinical trials in Europe.

Ultrasound

BASIC PRINCIPLES

US is yet another form of energy that can cause thermally mediated tissue injury. A form of vibration energy greater than 18,000 cycles per second (18 kHz), US is propagated as a mechanical wave by the motion of particles within the medium.[85] The motion causes alternating compression and

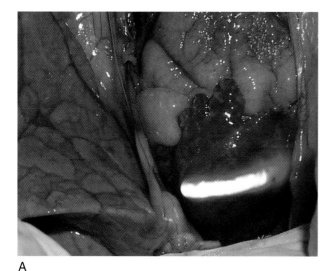

A

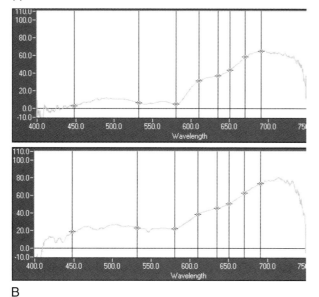

B

Tissue before
coagulation

Tissue after
coagulation

Reflectance
increases overall
but especially at
shorter wavelengths

Figure 5–5. A, Epicardial appearance during endocardial light emission from a linear optical fiber (diffuser) before laser ablation. The reflected light is transmitted back through a second optical fiber and used for reflectance spectroscopy. The linear optical diffuser catheter has been introduced via the right femoral vein of a goat and is seen via an open thoracotomy to be in place for linear ablation of the right atrial free wall. **B,** Reflectance spectroscopy provides a potential means of monitoring lesion progression during ablation. The spectral display of light reflected back through an optical fiber during ablation of caprine atrium is shown. The ratio of green (shorter) to red (longer) wavelengths can provide a metric of lesion formation. If excessive ablation occurs, carbonization of the endocardium results in a reduction of reflected light.

decompression in the medium with the passage of sound waves. Thus, a pressure wave is propagated associated with the mechanical movement of particles. The particulate motion that a US field generates results in mechanical stress and strain. When applied to an absorbing medium, US energy is continuously absorbed and converted to heat within the medium. This thermal effect can cause substantial tissue injury if the temperature elevation is sufficient and is maintained for an adequate period.[86]

Early studies considered high-intensity focused ultrasound (HIFU) energy as a noninvasive technique capable of selectively injuring deep tissues within the body, particularly within the central nervous system.[87,88] Lesions were created in homogeneous tissue without damage to intervening tissue.[88-90] The ablation US transducer contains a piezoelectric element that vibrates at a fixed frequency when elec-

tricity is applied.[39] The lesion is formed within the focal region of the transducer and can be collimated to provide a long depth of penetration.[91]

Using frequencies of 500 kHz to 20 MHz, HIFU can create controlled, localized tissue injury via both mechanical energy (oscillation and collapse of gas bubbles, or microcavitation) and the primary mechanism, thermal energy (tissue absorption of acoustic energy).[92,93] As the incident energy is increased, boiling of tissue water may occur, leading to the formation of vapor cavities (bubbles).[94] The amount of energy transferred from the acoustic wave to the tissue is directly proportional to both the intensity of the wave and the absorption coefficient of the tissue.[95] If the US transducer transmits into a medium with low absorption (e.g., water, blood), then the catheter tip will not need to be in direct contact with the myocardium.[96]

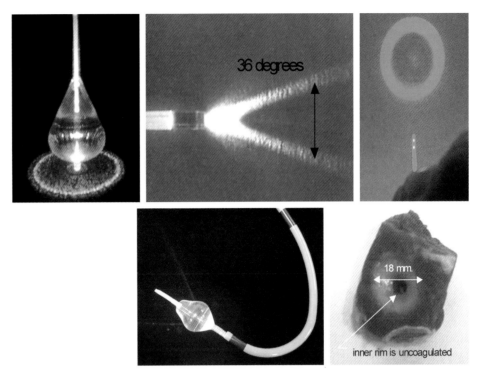

Figure 5–6. Forward-projecting laser balloon. Diode laser energy is emitted circumferentially from the tip of an optical fiber *(top, middle, and right)*. A balloon is used to orient the lasing ring at the pulmonary vein antrum and to eliminate blood from between the diffusing element and the endocardium. Circumferential lasing from the balloon in bovine ventricle in vitro produced a preserved inner circle of myocardium *(bottom right)*.

LESSONS FROM EXPERIMENTAL STUDIES

Zimmer et al.[96] studied the feasibility of using US for cardiac ablation. Frequencies from 10 to 15 MHz produced the deepest lesions at US intensities between 15 and 30 W/cm^2. The results showed the importance of tissue surface temperature monitoring to keep temperatures to less than the boiling threshold of 100°C. When temperatures reached these high levels, the lesions produced by sonication were typically wider and shallower than those created at a lower power level. This was thought to be a result of the scattering of sound by the gas bubbles formed from the boiling of water. Both in vitro and in vivo experiments verified the theoretical calculations that HIFU can ablate cardiac muscle within 60 seconds, creating lesions up to 9 mm deep with large area up to 40 mm^2.

Ohkubo et al.[91] studied the HIFU lesions created with transducers with frequencies in the range of 5 to 10 MHz on a beating heart in canine cardiac tissue and porcine heart specimens. HIFU was delivered through the ablation catheter at a preset temperature of 85°C for 180 seconds. The electrical power input was automatically adjusted to keep the temperature near the preset value, producing sharply demarcated endocardial lesions of varying size. In the in vitro study, when the temperature was maintained stable, lesion depth increased significantly with sonication of longer duration, and when the duration of sonication was kept constant, lesion depth increased significantly with higher temperatures of energy delivery.

Using a 10 MHz HIFU transducer mounted on a 7F catheter in canines, He et al.[86] obtained lesions with sonication for as little as 15 seconds. Myocardial lesions 11 mm in depth were produced with an acoustic power of 1.3 W applied for 60 seconds. Histologically, these lesions were well circumscribed, with a clear border zone between necrosis and intact cell layers. Hemorrhage, inflammation, and fibrin thrombi were consistently absent. Strickberger et al.[97] obtained similar histologic findings when performing extracardiac HIFU in an open-thoracotomy model to create AV block within the canine heart. Parallel two-dimensional US imaging was used to find the AV junction anatomically. Complete AV block was created in each of 10 animals with 30-second applications of HIFU gated to the cardiac cycle at a mean of 6.5 sites. Of interest, the myocardium immediately adjacent to the lesion, including the tissue between the lesion and the ablation US transducer (a distance of up to 6.3 cm), was histologically normal. This study raises the possibility of noninvasive cardiac ablation.

PHASED-ARRAY HIGH-INTENSITY FOCUSED ULTRASOUND SYSTEMS

Phased-array HIFU systems composed of hundreds of US elements may be used to create lesions at specific target depths of up to 15 cm without significant heating of the intervening tissues.[98] Phased-array systems may be better suited to noninvasive cardiac ablation because of the ability to control the position of the target site by switching between different beam patterns at electronic speed, the ability to correct for aberrations that may be present due to complex inhomogeneous intervening tissue such as ribs and lungs, and the ability to change the effective aperture dimensions during treatment by adjusting the driving signals.[97] A novel "combo" catheter with real-time, three-dimensional imaging and a ring transducer for US ablation has been described.[99]

ULTRASOUND BALLOON CATHETERS

Because US remains collimated or focused as it passes through an echolucent fluid medium, it may be advantageous for application through a fluid-filled balloon.[39] US balloon delivery systems are being clinically investigated for ablation around the PVs. Two systems have been evaluated in humans. In the original concept, collimated US was delivered circumferentially around the equator of a balloon perpendicular to the axis of the catheter. Once it was realized that ablation inside the PV orifice may be less efficacious and safe than ablation in the PV antrum, a forward-projecting, focused US balloon was developed by incorporation of a parabolic acoustic reflector at the back of the balloon (Fig. 5–7). The US energy is delivered via a cylindrical transducer mounted on a catheter. The current passes through the transducer at its resonant frequency and causes it to vibrate. The emitted sound waves travel from the transducer through the balloon to the axis of the transducer and are absorbed by the cardiac tissue that is in contact with the balloon surface where the beam is incident with the tissue. This results in tissue heating, which, when applied for a sufficient duration, creates an irreversible thermal lesion of cardiac tissue.[100] Although unfocused collimated US energy has a decremental loss of energy as it emanates from the transducer, it may still penetrate significantly beyond the thin atrial or PV wall.

In animal studies, Lesh et al.[101] reported the creation of uniformly heated lesions with a balloon apparatus for anatomic isolation of the PVs. In a canine study,[102] a single US application targeted at 65° C was placed via a balloon catheter system in the right superior PV. PV stenosis with cartilaginous metaplasia was seen in two animals. All lesions were transmural, but PV branching and shorter applications accounted for incomplete circumferential lesions.

Natale et al.[103] first reported a single-center experience with the use of a through-the-balloon circumferential US ablation system for patients with recurrent AF. Subsequently, these patients were included with patients from other centers who underwent circumferential US ablation.[104] This analysis consisted of 33 patients with a total of 85 veins ablated. The system used consisted of a 0.035-inch-diameter luminal catheter with a distal balloon (maximum diameter, 2.2 cm) that contained a centrally located 8-MHz US transducer. The catheter was advanced over a sheath and guide wire to the ostium of the PV. The balloon was inflated at the ostium, causing total occlusion verified by contrast venography. Activated clotting times were maintained at greater than 250 seconds with heparin. During ablation, the energy was adjusted to maintain target temperatures of at least 60° C. A mean of 6.7 ablations per vein were applied. At 22-month follow-up, a total of 20 patients (60%) experienced recurrence of AF. Variable PV anatomy limiting proper balloon positioning and inability to reach temperatures greater than 60° C were technical limitations thought to be responsible for the high inefficacy rate in this early-generation US balloon catheter. Procedural complications included cerebellar stroke (one patient), phrenic nerve palsy (two patients), severe PV stenosis (one patient), and hematoma (two patients).[104]

A forward-projecting, focused US ablation system for circumferential ablation outside the PV has been developed, and clinical evaluation is in progress.[105] Dispersion of the US energy beyond the highly focused target depth should reduce the risk of deeper extracardiac damage compared with collimated US.

HIFU has also been applied successfully in patients with AF undergoing minimally invasive

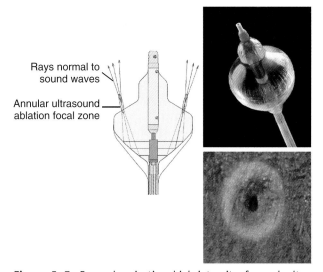

Figure 5–7. Forward-projecting high-intensity focused ultrasound balloon for pulmonary vein isolation. Radially emitted ultrasound is reflected from the back of the balloon, resulting in forward projection of ultrasound energy with a focal point at the balloon-endocardial interface. Application in vitro *(bottom right)* reveals the sharply demarcated edges and preserved inner core.

Rays normal to sound waves

Annular ultrasound ablation focal zone

off-pump epicardial surgical maze procedures. The characteristics of transmission of energy through epicardial fat and contact forgiveness provided by US offer distinct advantages over RF applications (Fig. 5–8).

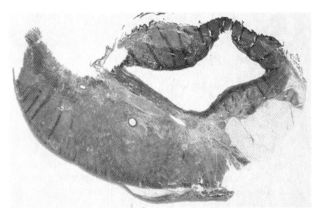

Figure 5–8. Epicardial high-intensity focused ultrasound (HIFU) ablation in a calf heart. Trichrome stain of posterior left atrial wall, including vein of Marshall *(top of image)*. HIFU was delivered in vivo from the epicardium in an open thoracotomy model to demonstrate the ability of HIFU to penetrate epicardial fat and venous tissue. The sharply defined, narrow transmural lesion *(blue)* can be seen to extend through to the endocardium *(bottom of section)*.

Alternative Ablative Techniques

Additional ablative energy sources that have been assessed in preclinical studies include direct heating (heated balloon for PV isolation), infrared radiation (epicardial maze), beta radiation (atrial flutter and PV isolation), and pressure necrosis (PV stenting to produce conduction block). Each of these approaches carries a unique profile of relative merits, potential limitations, and technical challenges. The potential limitations include thermal conductivity properties and temperature monitoring of the heated balloon membrane, predisposition to char formation with infrared ablation, and delayed onset of electrophysiologic end point (conduction block) for beta radiation and pressure necrosis (PV stenting).

Conclusion

The limitations of RF ablation, including dependence on tissue contact, coagulation at the catheter

TABLE 5–1

Energy Sources for Catheter Ablation

Energy Source	Frequency or Wavelength	Mechanism of Heating	Relation of Heating to Distance (r) from Source	Tissue Contact Needed	Advantages	Disadvantages
Radiofrequency	300-700 kHz	Resistive	$1/r^4$	Yes	Easy, inexpensive, vast clinical experience	Limited lesion size, charring
Microwave	915-2450 MHz	Dielectric	$1/r^2$	No	Penetrates scar and fat, large lesions, linear catheters possible	Complex catheter design, energy titration
Laser	300-2000 nm	Photon absorption	Complex exponential decline	No	Large lesions, can spare endocardium, linear catheters possible	Difficulty controlling depth, complex effects with tissue properties and distance from source
Ultrasound	500 kHz to 20 MHz	Mechanical stress and strain	Varies with focal length	No	Can be focused for encircling lesions and focal lesions far from source	Difficulty controlling depth, highly directional

tip–tissue interface that limits power delivery, and difficulty in creating lesions in myocardial scar, have prompted the search for alternative sources of ablative energy (Table 5–1). MW energy has been shown in both in vitro and in vivo studies to be less dependent on tissue contact, to have the ability to transmit energy through desiccated and coagulated tissue, and to create larger lesions that expand with increased application time. The ability to create large, well-circumscribed lesions in myocardial scar is a characteristic favorable to laser energy. Focused ultrasound has the unique property of reaching specific target depths without injuring intervening tissues.

These energy sources, when applied to new catheter designs and delivery techniques, may play an important role in the management of specific arrhythmias, including AF and VT, as the indication for ablation is broadened and the technical requirements shift from conventional focal ablation to linear ablation.

References

1. Scheinman MM, Morady F, Hess DS, et al.: Catheter-induced ablation of the atrioventricular junction to control refractory supraventricular arrhythmias. JAMA 248:851-855, 1982.
2. Olgin JE, Scheinman MM: Comparison of high energy direct current and radiofrequency catheter ablation of the atrioventricular junction. J Am Coll Cardiol 21:557-584, 1993.
3. Jackman WM, Hunzhang W, Friday KJ, et al.: Catheter ablation of accessory atrioventricular pathways (Wolff-Parkinson-White syndrome) by radiofrequency current. N Engl J Med 324:1605-1611, 1991.
4. Jackman WM, Beckman KJ, McClelland JH, et al.: Treatment of supraventricular tachycardia due to atrioventricular nodal entry by radiofrequency catheter ablation of slow-pathway conduction. N Engl J Med 327:313-319, 1992.
5. Organ LW: Electrophysiologic principles of radiofrequency lesion making. Appl Neurophysiol 39:69-76, 1976.
6. Nath S, Lynch C, Whayne JG, et al.: Cellular electrophysiological effects of hyperthermia on isolated guinea pig papillary muscle: Implications for catheter ablation. Circulation 88:1826-1831, 1993.
7. Nath S, Haines DE: Biophysics and pathology of catheter energy delivery systems. Prog Cardiovasc Dis 37:185-204, 1995.
8. Haines DE, Watson DD: Tissue heating during radiofrequency catheter ablation: A thermodynamic model and observations in isolated perfused and superfused canine right ventricular free wall. Pacing Clin Electrophysiol 12:962-971, 1989.
9. Wonnell TL, Stauffer PR, Langberg JJ: Evaluation of microwave and radio frequency catheter ablation in a myocardium-equivalent phantom model. IEEE Trans Biomed Eng 39:1086-1095, 1992.
10. Jumrussirikul P, Chen JT, Jenkins M, et al.: Prospective comparison of temperature guided microwave and radiofrequency catheter ablation in the swine heart. Pacing Clin Electrophysiol 21:1364-1374, 1998.
11. Johnson CC, Guy AW: Nonionizing electromagnetic wave effects in biologic materials and systems. Proc IEEE 60:692-709, 1972.
12. Whayne JG, Nath S, Haines DE: Microwave catheter ablation of myocardium in vitro: Assessment of the characteristics of tissue heating and injury. Circulation 89:2390-2395, 1994.
13. Avitall B, Khan M, Krum D, et al.: Physics and engineering of transcatheter cardiac tissue ablation. J Am Coll Cardiol 22:921-932, 1993.
14. Gadhoke A, Aronovitz M, Zebede J, et al.: Are tissue contact and catheter orientation important variables in microwave ablation? [abstract]. Circulation 86(Suppl 1):I-191, 1992.
15. Lin JC: Microwave propagation in biologic dielectrics with application cardiopulmonary interrogation. In Larson LE, Jacobi JH (eds.): Medical Applications of Microwave Imaging. New York: IEEE Press, 1986, pp 47-58.
16. Lin JC: Engineering and biophysical aspects of microwave and radiofrequency radiation. In Watmough DJ, Ross WM (eds.): Hyperthermia. Glasgow, UK: Blackie and Sons, 1986, pp 42-75.
17. Lin JC: Catheter microwave ablation therapy for cardiac arrhythmias. Bioelectromagnetics 4(Suppl):120-132, 1999.
18. Lin JC: Studies on microwaves in medicine and biology: From snails to humans. Bioelectromagnetics 25:146-159, 2004.
19. Beckman KJ, Lin YC, Wang Y, et al.: Production of reversible and irreversible atrioventricular block by microwave energy. Circulation 76:1612, 1987.
20. Langberg JJ, Wonnell T, Chin MC, et al.: Catheter ablation of the atrioventricular junction using a helical microwave antenna: A novel means of coupling energy to the endocardium. Pacing Clin Electrophysiol 14:2105-2113, 1991.
21. Keane D, Ruskin J, Norris N, et al.: In vitro and in vivo evaluation of the thermal patterns and lesions of catheter ablation with a microwave monopole antenna. J Interv Card Electrophysiol 10:111-119, 2004.
22. Lin JC, Wang YJ: A catheter antenna for percutaneous microwave therapy. Microw Opt Tachnolo Lett 8:70-72, 1995.
23. Lin JC, Wang YJ: The cap-choke catheter antenna for microwave ablation treatment. IEEE Trans Biomed Eng 43:657-660, 1996.
24. Wang PJ, Schoen FJ, Aronovitz M, et al.: Microwave catheter ablation under the mitral annulus: A new method of accessory pathway ablation? Pacing Clin Electrophysiol 16:866, 1993.
25. Huang SKS, Lin JC, Mazzola F, et al.: Percutaneous microwave ablation of the ventricular myocardium using a 4-mm split-tip antenna electrode: A novel method for potential ablation of ventricular tachycardia [abstract]. J Am Coll Cardiol 24A:351, 1994.
26. Mazzola F, Huang SKS, Lin J, et al.: Determinates of lesion size using a 4-mm split-tip antenna electrode for microwave catheter ablation. Pacing Clin Electrophysiol 17:814, 1994.
27. Ruder M, Mead RH, Baron K, et al.: Microwave ablation: In vivo data. Pacing Clin Electrophysiol 17:781, 1994.
28. Yang X, Watanabe I, Kojima T, et al.: Microwave ablation of the atrioventricular junction in vivo and ventricular myocardium in vitro and in vivo: Effects of varying power and duration on lesion volume. Jpn Heart J 35:175-191, 1994.
29. Rho TH, Ito M, Pride HP, et al.: Microwave ablation of canine atrial tachycardia induced by aconitine. Am Heart J 129:1021-1025, 1995.
30. Liem LB, Mead RH, Shenasa M, et al.: In vitro and in vivo results of transcatheter microwave ablation using forward-firing tip antenna design. Pacing Clin Electrophysiol 19:2004-2008, 1996.
31. Liem LB, Mead RH, Shenasa M, et al.: Microwave catheter ablation using a clinical prototype system with a lateral firing antenna design. Pacing Clin Electrophysiol 21:714-721, 1998.
32. Nevels RD, Arndt GD, Raffoul GW, et al.: Microwave catheter design. IEEE Trans Biomed Eng 45:885-890, 1998.

33. Gu Z, Rappaport CM, Wang PJ, et al.: A 2 1/4-turn spiral antenna for catheter cardiac ablation. IEEE Trans Biomed Eng 46:1480-1482, 1999.

34. Thomas SP, Clout R, Deery C, et al.: Microwave ablation of myocardial tissue: The effect of element design, tissue coupling, blood flow, power, and duration of exposure on lesion size. J Cardiovasc Electrophysiol 10:72-78, 1999.

35. Vanderbrink BA, Gu Z, Rodriguez V, et al.: Microwave ablation using a spiral antenna design in a porcine thigh muscle preparation: In vivo assessment of temperature profile and lesion geometry. J Cardiovasc Electrophysiol 11:193-198, 2000.

36. Pisa S, Cavagnaro M, Bernardi P, et al.: A 915-MHz antenna for microwave thermal ablation treatment: Physical design, computer modeling and experimental measurement. IEEE Trans Biomed Eng 48:599-601, 2001.

37. Chiu HM, Mohan AS, Weily AR, et al.: Analysis of a novel expanded tip wire (ETW) antenna for microwave ablation of cardiac arrhythmias. IEEE Trans Biomed Eng 50:890-899, 2003.

38. Wang PJ, Estes NA:. New technologies for catheter ablation. In Saksena S, Luderitz B (eds): Interventional Electrophysiology: A Textbook. New York: Futura, 1996, pp 557-560.

39. Keane D: New catheter ablation techniques for the treatment of cardiac arrhythmias. Card Electrophysiol Rev 6:341-348, 2002.

40. Iwasa A, Storey J, Yao B, et al.: Efficacy of a microwave antenna for ablation of the tricuspid valve–inferior vena cava isthmus in dogs as a treatment for type 1 atrial flutter. J Interv Card Electrophysiol 10:191-198, 2004.

41. VanderBrink BA, Gilbride C, Aronovitz MJ, et al.: Safety and efficacy of a steerable temperature monitoring microwave catheter system for ventricular myocardial ablation. J Cardiovasc Electrophysiol 11:305-310, 2000.

42. Lin JC, Beckman KJ, Hariman RJ, et al.: Microwave ablation of the atrioventricular junction in open-chest dogs. Bioelectromagnetics 16:97-105, 1995.

43. Huang SKS, Lin JC, Mazzola F, et al.: Percutaneous microwave ablation of the ventricular myocardium using a 4-mm split-tip antenna electrode: A novel method for potential ablation of ventricular tachycardia [abstract]. J Am Coll Cardiol 34A, 1994.

44. Pires LA, Huang SKS, Lin JC, et al.: Comparison of radiofrequency (RF) versus microwave (MW) energy catheter ablation of the bovine ventricular myocardium. Pacing Clin Electrophysiol 17:782, 1994.

45. Saoudi N, Atallah G, Kirkorian G, et al.: Catheter ablation of the atrial myocardium in human type I atrial flutter. Circulation 81:762-771, 1990.

46. Feld GK, Fleck P, Chen PS, et al.: Radiofrequency catheter ablation for the treatment of human type 1 atrial flutter: Identification of a critical zone in the reentrant circuit by endocardial mapping techniques. Circulation 86:1233-1240, 1992.

47. Cosio FG, Lopez GM, Goicolea A, et al.: Radiofrequency ablation of the inferior vena cava–tricuspid valve isthmus in common atrial flutter. Am J Cardiol 71:705-709, 1993.

48. Gadhoke A, Aronovitz M, Zebede J, et al.: Are tissue contact and catheter orientation important variables in microwave ablation? [abstract]. Circulation 86(Suppl 1):I-191, 1992.

49. Iwasa A, Storey J, Yao B, et al.: Efficacy of a microwave antenna for ablation of the tricuspid valve–inferior vena cava isthmus in dogs as a treatment for type 1 atrial flutter. J Interv Card Electrophysiol 10:191-198, 2004.

50. Liem LB, Mead RH: Microwave linear ablation of the isthmus between the inferior vena cava and tricuspid annulus. Pacing Clin Electrophysiol 21:2079-2086, 1998.

51. Adragao P, Parreira L, Morgado F, et al.: Microwave ablation of atrial flutter. Pacing Clin Electrophysiol 22:1692-1695, 1999.

52. Einstein A: On the quantum theory of radiation. Physikalische Zeitschrift 18:121, 1917.

53. Saksena S, Gadhoke A: Laser therapy for tachyarrhythmias: A new frontier. Pacing Clin Electrophysiol 9:531-550, 1986.

54. Saksena S: Catheter ablation of tachycardias with laser energy:issues and answers. Pacing Clin Electrophysiol 12:196-203, 1989.

55. Zheng S, Kloner RA, Whittaker P: Ablation and coagulation of myocardial tissue by means of a pulsed holmium:YAG laser. Am Heart J 126:1474-1477, 1993.

56. Tomaru T, Geschwind HJ, Boussignac G, et al.: Comparison of ablation efficacy of excimer, pulsed-dye, and holmium-YAG lasers relevant to shock waves. Am Heart J 123:886-895, 1992.

57. Verdaasdonk RM, Borst C, van Gemert MJC: Explosive onset of continuous wave laser tissue ablation. Phys Med Biol 35:1129-1144, 1990.

58. Ohtake H, Misaki T, Watanabe G, et al.: Myocardial coagulation by intraoperative Nd:YAG laser ablation and its dependence on blood perfusion. Pacing Clin Electrophysiol 17:1627-1631, 1994.

59. Lee BI, Rodriguez ER, Notargiocomo A: Thermal effects of laser and electrical discharge on cardiovascular tissue: Implications for coronary artery recanalization and endocardial ablation. J Am Coll Cardiol 8:193-200, 1986.

60. Splinter R, Semenov SY, Nanney GA, et al.: Myocardial temperature distribution under cw Nd:YAG laser irradiation in "in vitro" and "in vivo" situations: Theory and experiment. Appl Optics 34:391-399, 1995.

61. Levine JH, Merillat JC, Stern M, et al.: The cellular electrophysiologic changes induced by ablation: Comparison between argon laser photo ablation and high-energy electrical ablation. Circulation 76:217-225, 1987.

62. Saksena S, Ciccone JM, Chnadran P, et al.: Laser ablation of normal and diseased human ventricle. Am Heart J 112:52-60, 1986.

63. Isner JM, DeJesus SR, Clarke RH, et al.: Mechanism of laser ablation in an absorbing field. Lasers Surg Med 8:543-554, 1988.

64. Narula OS, Bharati S, Chan MC, et al.: Laser microsection of the His bundle: A pervenous catheter technique. J Am Coll Cardiol 3:537, 1984.

65. Abele GS, Griffin JC, Hill JA, et al.: Transvascular argon laser induced atrioventricular conduction ablation in dogs. Circulation 68:145, 1983.

66. Ciccone J, Saksena S, Pantopoulos D: Comparative efficacy of continuous and pulsed argon laser ablation of human diseased ventricle. Pacing Clin Electrophysiol 9:697-704, 1986.

67. Walsh JT, Deutsch TF: Pulsed CO_2 laser ablation of tissue: Effect of mechanical properties. IEEE Trans Biomed Eng 36:1195-1201, 1989.

68. Saksena S, Hussain SM, Gielchinsky I, et al.: Intraoperative mapping-guided argon laser ablation of malignant ventricular tachycardia. Am J Cardiol 59:78-83, 1987.

69. Saksena S, Hussain SM, Gielchinsky I, et al.: Intraoperative mapping-guided argon laser ablation of supraventricular tachycardia in the Wolff-Parkinson-White syndrome. Am J Cardiol 60:196-199, 1987.

70. Lee BI, Gottdiener JS, Fletcher RD, et al.: Transcatheter ablation: Comparison between laser photoablation and electrode shock ablation in the dog. Circulation 71:579-586, 1985.

71. Weber HP, Enders HS, Keiditisch E: Percutaneous Nd:YAG laser coagulation of ventricular myocardium in dogs using a special electrode laser catheter. Pacing Clin Electrophysiol 12:899-910, 1989.

72. Weber HP, Enders HS, Ruprecht L, et al.: Catheter-directed laser coagulation of atrial myocardium in dogs. Eur Heart J 15:971-980, 1994.

73. Pfeiffer D, Moosdorf R, Svenson RH, et al.: Epicardial neodymium:YAG laser photocoagulation of ventricular tachycardia without ventriculotomy in patients after myocardial infarction. Circulation 94:3221-3225, 1996.

74. Weber HP, Kalternbrunner W, Heinze A, et al.: Laser catheter coagulation of atrial myocardium for ablation of atrioventricular nodal reentrant tachycardia. Eur Heart J 18:487-495, 1997.

75. Ware DL, Boor P, Yang C, et al.: Slow intramural heating with diffused laser light: A unique method for deep myocardial coagulation. Circulation 99:1630-1636, 1999.

76. Pierce J, Thomasen S: Rate process analysis of thermal damage. In Welch AJ, van Gemert MJC (eds.): Optical-Thermal Responses of Laser-Irradiated Tissue. New York: Plenum Press, 1995, pp 561-606.

77. d'Avila A, Splinter R, Svenson RH: New perspectives on catheter-based ablation of ventricular tachycardia complicating Chagas' disease: Experimental evidence of the efficacy of near infrared lasers for catheter ablation of Chagas' VT. J Interv Card Electrophysiol 7:23-38, 2002.

78. Fried NM, Lardo AC, Berger RD, et al.: Linear lesions in myocardium created by Nd:YAG laser using diffusing optical fibers. Lasers Surg Med 27:295-304, 2000.

79. Keane D, Ruskin JN: Linear atrial ablation with a diode laser and fiberoptic catheter. Circulation 100:e59-e60, 1999.

80. Wagshall A, Abela GS, Maheshwari A, et al.: A novel catheter design for laser photocoagulation of the myocardium to ablate ventricular tachycardia. J Interv Card Electrophysiol 7:13-22, 2002.

81. Littmann L, Svenson RH, Chuang CH, et al.: Catheterization technique for laser photoablation of atrioventricular conduction from the aortic root in dogs. Pacing Clin Electrophysiol 16:401-406, 1993.

82. Johnson S, Su W, Da Salva LL, et al.: Power dependance of laser energy in circumferential ablation of pulmonary veins [abstract]. Pacing Clin Electrophysiol 24:552, 2002.

83. Reddy VR, Houghtaling C, Fallon J, et al.: Use of a diode laser balloon catheter to generate circumferential pulmonary venous lesions in an open-thoracotomy caprine model. Pacing Clin Electrophysiol 27:52-57, 2004.

84. Lemery R, Vienot JP, Tang ASL, et al.: Fiberoptic balloon catheter ablation of pulmonary vein ostia in pigs using photonic energy delivery with diode laser. Pacing Clin Electrophysiol 25:32-36, 2002.

85. Stewart HF: Ultrasonic measurement techniques and equipment output levels. In Repacholi MH, Benwell DA (eds.): Essentials of Medical Ultrasound. Clifton, N.J.: Humana, 1982, pp 77-116.

86. He DS, Zimmer JE, Hynynen FI, et al.: Application of ultrasound energy for intracardiac ablation of arrhythmias. Eur Heart J 16:961-966, 1995.

87. Lynn JG, Zwemer RL, Chick AJ, et al.: A new method for the generation and use of focused ultrasound in experimental biology. J Gen Physiol 26:179-193, 1942.

88. Fry W, Mosberg W, Barnard J, et al.: Production of focal destructive lesions in the central nervous system. J Neurosurg 11:471-478, 1954.

89. Ter Haar GR, Robertson D: Tissue destruction with focused ultrasound in vivo. Eur Urol 23:8-11, 1993.

90. Susani M, Madersbacher S, Kratzik C, et al.: Morphology of tissue destruction induced by focused ultrasound. Eur Urol 23:34-38, 1993.

91. Ohkubo T, Okishige K, Goseki Y, et al.: Experimental study of catheter ablation using ultrasound energy in canine and porcine hearts. Japan Heart J 39:399-409, 1998.

92. Repacholi M, Grondolfo M, Rindi A: Ultrasound: Medical Applications, Biological Effects and Hazard Potential. New York: Plenum, 1987.

93. Lee LA, Simon C, Bove EL, et al.: High intensity focused ultrasound effect on cardiac tissues: Potential for clinical application. Echocardiography 17:563-566, 2000.

94. Malcolm AL, Ter Haar GR: Ablation of tissue volumes using high intensity focused ultrasound. Ultrasound Med Biol 22:659-669, 1996.

95. National Council on Radiation Protection: Biological Effects of Ultrasound: Mechanisms and Clinical Implications. NCRP Report No 74. Bethesda, Md.: National Council on Radiation Protection, 1983.

96. Zimmer JE, Hynynen K, He DS, et al.: The feasibility of using ultrasound for cardiac ablation. IEEE Trans Biomed Eng 42:891-897, 1995.

97. Strickberger SA, Tokano T, Kluiwstra JA, et al.: Extracardiac ablation of the canine atrioventricular junction by use of high-intensity focused ultrasound. Circulation 100:203-208, 1999.

98. Wan J, VanBaren P, Ebbini E, et al.: Ultrasound surgery: Comparison of strategies using phased array systems. IEEE Trans UFFC 43:1085-1098, 1996.

99. Gentry KL, Smith SW: Integrated catheter for 3-D intracardiac echocardiography and ultrasound ablation. IEEE Trans UFFC 51:799-807, 2004.

100. Hynynen K, Dennie J, Zimmer JE, et al.: Cylindrical ultrasonic transducers for cardiac catheter ablation. IEEE Trans Biomed Eng 44:144-151, 1997.

101. Lesh MD, Diederich C, Guerra G, et al.: An anatomic approach to prevention of atrial fibrillation: Pulmonary vein isolation with through-the-balloon ultrasound ablation (TTB-USA). Thorac Cardiovasc Surg 47:347-351, 1999.

102. Azegami K, Arruda MS, Anders R: Circumferential ultrasound ablation of pulmonary vein ostia: Relationship between ablation time and lesion formation [abstract]. J Am Coll Cardiol 39:106A, 2002.

103. Natale A, Pisano E, Shewchik J, et al.: First human experience with pulmonary vein isolation using a through-the-balloon circumferential ultrasound ablation system for recurrent atrial fibrillation. Circulation 102:1879-1882, 2000.

104. Saliba W, Wilber D, Packer D, et al.: Circumferential ultrasound ablation for pulmonary vein isolation: Analysis of acute and chronic failures. J Card Electrophysiol 13:957-961, 2002.

105. Meininger GR, Calkins H, Lickfett L, et al.: Initial experience with a novel focused ultrasound ablation system for ring ablation outside the pulmonary vein. J Interv Card Electrophysiol 8:141-148, 2003.

Cardiac Mapping and Imaging

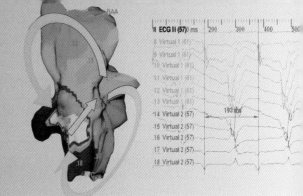

PART II

6

Fluoroscopic and Angiographic Heart Anatomy for Catheter Mapping and Ablation of Arrhythmias

Jerónimo Farré • José A. Cabrera
Damián Sánchez-Quintana • José M. Rubio
Siew Yen Ho • Robert H. Anderson

Key Points

▥ Fluoroscopy remains the primary imaging modality for ablation procedure.

▥ Radiation exposure is reduced by use of collimators, pulsed fluoroscopy, shielding, and avoidance of magnification.

▥ Attitudinally oriented nomenclature should be understood and utilized to standardize anatomic descriptions.

▥ Orthogonal fluoroscopic views are needed to define anatomic positions in the heart.

The adoption of catheter ablation techniques for the treatment of tachyarrhythmias in humans has increased the interest in cardiac anatomy. Interventional arrhythmologists have had to study the gross morphologic and architectural features of the heart. In addition, a new investigational wave has emerged to revisit cardiac anatomic topics for which the information was incomplete or simply wrong. As a result, recent studies have unraveled anatomic features,[1-4] architectural aspects,[5-11] and histologic details of certain components of the heart that are of interest to understanding of the substrates of tachycardias and their ablation.[12-19] Another consequence of catheter ablation techniques is the introduction of a new, fluoroscopically oriented nomenclature that takes into account the correct attitudinal positions of the cardiac structures.[20] In this chapter, as in previous reviews,[21,22] we define the fluoroscopic heart anatomy as observed during an electrophysiologic study and catheter ablation procedure in the light of an attitudinally oriented nomenclature. We discuss some anatomic concepts such as the terminal crest, the sinuatrial region, the triangle of Koch, the pyramidal space, the inferior isthmus, the interatrial groove, the septa, and the sites of ablation of accessory pathways (APs). To facilitate the understanding of the fluoroscopic heart anatomy we have used the Visible Human Slice and Surface Server[23] that uses data sets of the Visible Human Male and Female Project.[24]

Simple Fluoroscopy, Angiography, and Other Techniques

Today there are nonfluoroscopic navigational tools of varying capacity for reconstructing a computer-based surrogate of the endocardial surface of the heart chambers. In spite of these developments, simple fluoroscopy, with or without the aid of angiographic techniques, remains the essential guide for mapping and ablation procedures. With simple fluoroscopy, the only anatomic reference is the heart shadow and its relation to electrode-catheters positioned at certain fixed locations such as the right atrial appendage, the right ventricular apex and/or outflow tract, the region of the His bundle, and the coronary sinus. Recently, attention has been directed to the fluoroscopic identification of a "fat stripe" in the right anterior oblique (RAO) projection that is the landmark of both atrioventricular (AV) grooves.[25]

Angiography is increasingly performed as an aid to catheter-electrode mapping. Right atrial angiography allows definition of the anatomic boundaries of the triangle of Koch and the inferior (cavotricuspid) isthmus.[2,4,26,27] The size and morphology of the inferior isthmus seems to play a crucial role as to the ease of ablation of isthmus-dependent atrial flutter.[27] A coronary sinus venogram has been obtained in patients with inferior paraseptal APs when the presence of a diverticulum was suspected.[28-30] Although pulmonary venous angiography has been used in patients with atrial fibrillation undergoing catheter ablation procedures in and around the pulmonary veins,[31,32] these techniques are not routinely used today. Angiography has also been used to diagnose the development of pulmonary vein stenosis as a complication of applying radiofrequency (RF) pulses inside the pulmonary veins in patients with atrial fibrillation.[33-35]

Magnetic resonance imaging and transesophageal echocardiography are also used to diagnose pulmonary venous stenosis after ablation procedures.[36,37] Magnetic resonance imaging is likely to become the technique of choice not only to diagnose pulmonary venous stenosis but also to obtain, before the ablation procedure, a real view of the anatomy of the pulmonary veins, which have many interindividual variations.[38-40] In the future, computerized systems will superimpose three-dimensional magnetic resonance images acquired before the procedure with an electromagnetically defined catheter-positioning technique, thereby allowing display of the navigating electrode on the real anatomy of the patient.[41]

So-called nonfluoroscopic, electroanatomic mapping technologies enable display of the cardiac chambers and the relative position of ablation spots; they are used to ablate various types of supraventricular and ventricular tachyarrhythmias.[42-53] Intracardiac echocardiography also has been used to identify certain anatomic landmarks and to monitor the effects of ablation.[53-63]

X-ray Protection and Image Quality Recommendations

Catheter ablation procedures require long fluoroscopy times in many instances. To minimize radiation exposure of patients and personnel and to maximize image quality, these rules should be followed[22]:

1. Keep fluoroscopy time as low as possible.
2. Use X-ray beam systems entering the posterior and not the anterior side of the patient, thus attenuating radiation to thyroid, breasts, and eyes of the patient.
3. Use collimation to limit the size of the explored field and to reduce scattered radiation.

4. Use the largest possible field of the image intensifier, because magnification increases the dose.

5. Use pulsed fluoroscopy (with ≤12.5 pulses/second) instead of continuous fluoroscopy.

6. Use digital fluorography (at ≤12.5 images/second) rather than 35-mm filming to store positions of catheters or angiographic information.

7. Use all possible protections such as a leaded acrylic shield between patient and operator, leaded aprons, neck collars and glasses, and filtration of the primary X-ray beam.

8. Maintain all personnel as far as possible from the X-ray beam.

9. Manipulate catheters as little as possible from a subclavian or jugular approach; use preferably the femoral approach, which results in less scattered radiation for the exploring physician.

10. Manipulate catheters as much as possible in the RAO or anteroposterior projections, because the left anterior oblique (LAO) projection is the worst in terms of secondary radiation for the exploring physician.[64-68]

Potential problems associated with radiation exposure during catheter ablation procedures are the development of various forms of malignant tumors, genetic abnormalities, and skin injuries. Failed procedures are associated with significantly longer fluoroscopy times than successful interventions. The experience of the operator and the methods used at each individual laboratory also play an important role.[69] The dose needed to cause radiation skin injury is exceeded in some 20% of procedures.[69] The level of radiation exposure per hour of fluoroscopy during catheter ablation has been estimated to result in an excess of fatal malignancies ranging from 450 to 2600 per million people.[69,70]

Cardiac Fluoroscopic Projections and Nomenclature

Understanding of the attitudinally oriented nomenclature of cardiac anatomy endorsed by the European Society of Cardiology and the North American Society of Pacing and Electrophysiology[20] is facilitated by The Visible Human Slice and Surface Server, a software program developed by Hersch and coworkers from the Geneva Hospitals and WDS Technologies SA[23] from data sets of the Visible Human Male and Female Project of the U.S. National Library of Medicine.[24]

Fluoroscopic examination during catheter-electrode mapping and ablation procedures is performed using the frontal and oblique projections. The frontal view is used to introduce and position catheters in the apex and outflow tract of the right ventricle, in the right atrial appendage or the lateral aspect of the right atrium, and in the region of the His bundle. We also use the frontal projection to enter into the left ventricle from a retrograde aortic approach. Although different laboratories may have their own preferences regarding the rotations selected to obtain the oblique projections, we usually prefer a 45-degree tilt for both of them. The LAO is generally used to catheterize the coronary sinus independently of the type of venous approach. From an attitudinal point of view, the RAO projection defines what is anterior, posterior, superior, and inferior (Fig. 6–1). The LAO defines superior, inferior, anterior, and posterior locations for both the right and left AV grooves, which are almost parallel to the plane of the image intensifier in this projection.

The Right Atrium

TERMINAL CREST AND THE SMOOTH-WALLED RIGHT ATRIUM

The right atrium consists of a flat-walled posterior venous portion and a trabeculated anterolateral sector, the pectinated right atrial appendage. These two areas are separated by the terminal crest (Fig. 6–2). The crest, from its origin at the interatrial groove, anterior to the superior caval vein (superior vena cava), extends laterally and inferiorly as a C-shaped right atrial structure, ramifying to form the pectinate muscles that insert at the smooth vestibule of the tricuspid valve anteriorly (Fig. 6–3). In the RAO projection, the terminal crest is almost perpendicular to the fluoroscopic screen. In the LAO projection, the C-shaped terminal crest is more or less parallel to the plane of the image intensifier.

The terminal crest is important in interventional arrhythmology for three reasons: (1) it is a barrier to conduction, probably more functional than anatomic, in isthmus-dependent atrial flutter[71,72]; (2) it is the origin of many focal right atrial tachycardias in patients without structural heart disease[73]; and (3) catheter ablation of the terminal crest has been used in patients with inappropriate sinus tachycardia.[74,75] It is beyond the scope of this chapter to discuss these issues in detail.[9]

THE REGION OF THE SINUS NODE

The human sinus node is a 13.5 ± 2.5 mm long, crescent-like formation located in the superior part of the terminal groove, close to the junction between the

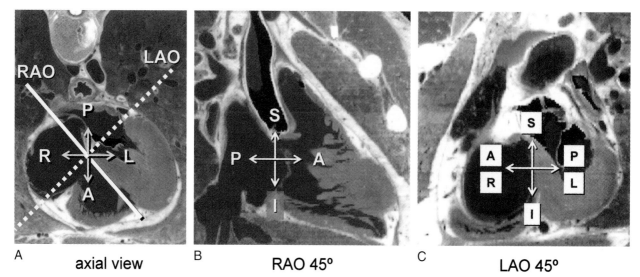

FIGURE 6–1. A, Axial slice obtained with The Visible Human Slice and Surface Server[23] showing the four heart chambers. Two axes have been traced to indicate the planes of the 45-degree right and left anterior oblique projections (RAO and LAO, respectively). Note that the right and left atrioventricular grooves are almost parallel to the plane of the image intensifier in LAO views, whereas the interatrial groove (interatrial septum) is almost perpendicular to it. A, anterior; L, left; P, posterior; R, right. **B,** A 45-degree RAO slice has been obtained at the level indicated in panel A. This projection defines A and P locations, as well as superior (S) and inferior (I) sites. **C,** A 45-degree LAO slice of the heart enables definition of what is R and A, and what is L and P, as well as S and I. Note that the plane of the triangle of Koch (**A** and **B**) is parallel to the input of the image intensifier in the RAO projection.

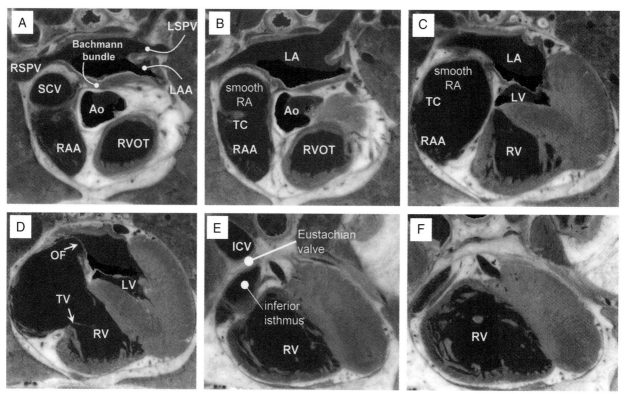

FIGURE 6–2. Right atrial anatomy as depicted on axial slices obtained with The Visible Human Slice and Surface Server.[23] Panel **A** through **F** are successive slides obtained from a cranial to caudal direction. **A,** Slice obtained at the junction between the superior caval vein (SCV) and the right atrium. Anterior to the SCV, the trabeculated right atrium forms the right atrial appendage (RAA). At this very high level, the tip of the appendage is shown; note that it is close to the myocardium of the right ventricular outflow tract (RVOT). Within the left atrium, the left atrial appendage (LAA) is anterior to the left superior pulmonary vein (LSPV). The Bachmann bundle can be traced rightward to the terminal crest at the junction between the right atrium and the SCV. **B,** The terminal crest (TC) separates the posterior smooth right atrium (RA) from the trabeculated RAA. The right superior pulmonary vein (RSPV) is behind the smooth RA. The right and left atrial myocardiums at this level and more caudally (**C**) form a sandwich that contains fibrofatty tissue. Anatomically speaking, this is an interatrial groove more than an interatrial septum. More caudally still (**D**), the oval fossa (OF), a fibrous tissue that is a true interatrial septum, is visible. (See text for details.) The inferior right atrial isthmus is located between the tricuspid valve (TV) and the inferior caval vein (ICV). **E** and **F,** The eustachian valve separates the ICV from the inferior isthmus. Ao, aorta; LA, left atrium; LV, left ventricle; RV, right ventricle.

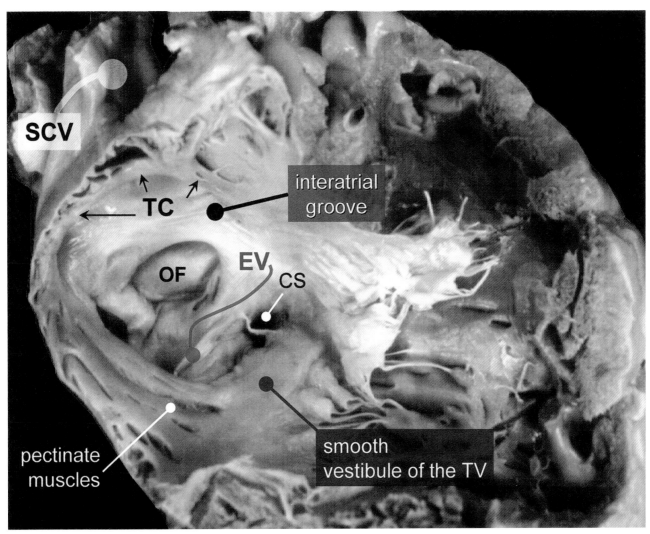

FIGURE 6–3. Gross human necropsy specimen showing the right atrium and its most important anatomic landmarks as viewed in an attitudinal right anterior oblique projection. Note that the so-called muscular interatrial septum is in fact an interatrial groove formed by the apposition of the right and left atrial myocardiums, which are separated by fibrofatty tissue. Anterior to the oval fossa (OF) there is a prominent muscular rim known as the anterior limbus. The terminal crest (TC) is a thick, C-shaped muscular bundle that distally ramifies to form the pectinate muscles. The eustachian valve (EV) separates the inferior caval vein from the inferior right atrial isthmus. Note that at this level and toward the tricuspid valve (TV) insertion, the right atrium forms a smooth vestibule. The thebesian valve guards the entry into the coronary sinus (CS). SCV, superior caval vein.

superior caval vein and the right atrial appendage. The sinus node extends laterally along the terminal groove, gradually penetrating through the thickness of the terminal crest to terminate in a tail that is buried deep in the myocardium of the terminal crest. Despite the lack of a sheath of fibrous tissue insulating the sinus node from the neighboring working myocardium, this structure is relatively protected against RF catheter ablation for several reasons: (1) most of the sinus node is a subepicardial structure, relatively distant from the right atrial endocardium; (2) the constantly present central sinus node artery exerts a cooling effect on the node; (3) a significant mass of the node is separated from the right atrial endocardium by the thick terminal crest; (4) it is an extensive structure not amenable to a focal complete injury; and (5) the nodal cells are packed in a dense matrix of connective tissue. These factors probably explain why endocardial RF catheter ablation is less effective in suppressing inappropriate sinus node tachycardia than it is for other right atrial tachycardias. Epicardial approaches have been attempted with various degrees of permanent success.[76,77,78]

THE RIGHT ATRIAL APPENDAGE

The trabeculated wall of the right atrium anterior to the terminal crest is the right atrial appendage. The trabeculated (or pectinated) right atrium extends all round the smooth vestibule of the tricuspid valve (see

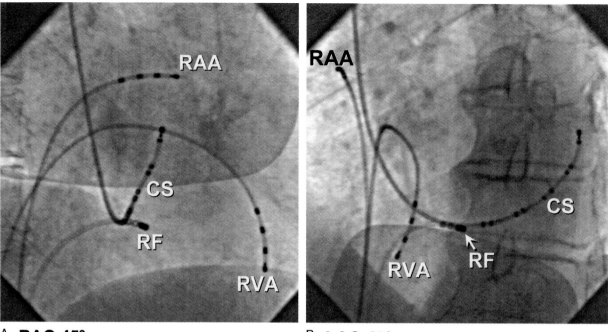

A **RAO 45°**   B **LAO 45°**

FIGURE 6–4. A, A 45-degree right anterior oblique (RAO) projection showing electrode catheters placed at the right atrial appendage (RAA), right ventricular apex (RVA), and coronary sinus (CS). A fourth catheter is used for the ablation of an accessory pathway at the ostium of the coronary sinus (RF). **B,** A 45-degree left anterior oblique (LAO) projection. The CS catheter runs towards the posterior border of the heart. Note that the tip of the RAA points towards the right of the screen in the RAO projection and to the left in the LAO view.

Fig. 6–3). It is an error to consider as the appendage only its triangular tip. To position a catheter-electrode in the triangular tip of the right atrial appendage, we prefer to use the frontal projection. In this fluoroscopic view, the catheter tip, when it is at the apex of the appendage, moves from left to right and from right to left (negation movement). The tip of the right atrial appendage is superior and anterior, and it lies over the anterosuperior aspect of the right AV groove (see Fig. 6–2A and B). When a catheter is placed at the apex of the right atrial appendage, its tip points to the right of the screen in the RAO projection, and to the left in the LAO view (Fig. 6–4). The main arrhythmologic interest of the right atrial appendage is the existence of APs connecting this structure with the right ventricular myocardium (Fig. 6–5). The injection of contrast medium into the right atrium facilitates the correct identification of this very rare type of AV accessory pathway.

EUSTACHIAN VALVE, EUSTACHIAN RIDGE, AND TENDON OF TODARO

In the adult, the eustachian valve separates the inferior caval vein (inferior vena cava) from the smooth vestibular inferior right atrium (see Figs. 6–2E and 6–3). The eustachian valve can be fluoroscopically visualized in the RAO projection only after injection

of contrast material into the inferior caval vein, close to the right atrial junction (Fig. 6–6). The eustachian ridge is a rim between the oval foramen and the coronary sinus that is in continuation with the insertion of the eustachian valve. The eustachian ridge contains the tendon of Todaro, a fibrous structure not constantly present in the adult human heart.[18,79] When the tendon of Todaro is fully developed, it has a superior course under the eustachian ridge toward the central fibrous body, ending at the junction between the AV node and the His bundle, or directly above the bundle.[79] The fluoroscopic equivalent of the tendon of Todaro or, better, of the eustachian ridge, is an imaginary line traced between the upper border of the orifice of the coronary sinus (or the uppermost extreme of the eustachian valve) and the anterosuperior limit of the septal leaflet of the tricuspid valve (see Fig. 6–6). This "fluoroscopic tendon of Todaro" is in fact a sort of imaginary concept, because in reality the superior insertion of the tendon is a few millimeters posteroinferior to the anterosuperior limit of septal leaflet of the tricuspid valve. The anterosuperior limit marks the supraventricular crest and not the central fibrous body. Anterior and inferior to the eustachian valve, there is a pouch-like formation or recess that continues more anteriorly with the smooth-walled vestibule of the tricuspid valve (see Figs. 6–3 and 6–6). This pouch and the vestibule

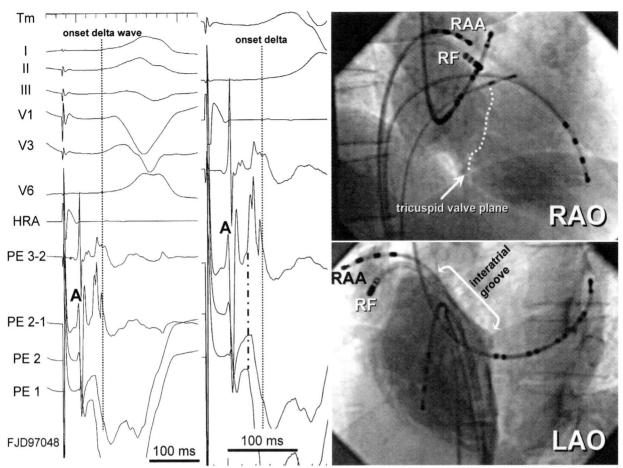

FIGURE 6–5. Accessory pathway connecting the right atrial appendage (RAA) with the right ventricle. The left panel shows the simultaneous display of six surface electrocardiographic (ECG) leads and several intracardiac bipolar and unipolar recordings. HRA, high right atrium; PE, probing electrode. Note that, in the bipolar recording from the two distal electrodes of the ablation catheter (PE 2-1), there is an electrogram between the point of local atrial activation (A) and the onset of the delta wave in the surface ECG leads. This pre-delta local activation is coincidental with the onset of a QS potential in the unfiltered unipolar lead (PE 1), as shown in detail on the magnified recording presented in the middle panel. The right panels show the fluorographic right anterior oblique (RAO) and left anterior oblique (LAO) views of the catheters, with the probing electrode at the site of successful ablation of the accessory pathway (RF). Both fluorographic frames were obtained during the injection of radiographic contrast material into the right atrium. Note that the position of the tip of the ablation catheter is far from the level of the tricuspid valve plane. Also note that the terminal portion of the ablation catheter seems to be "outside" the boundaries of the right atrium as outlined by the contrast agent. This is because the manual injection of contrast did not fill the tip of the RAA, which is where the catheter was located to ablate this very rare type of accessory pathway. Note that the interatrial groove is perpendicular to the plane of the image intensifier in the LAO projection.

of the tricuspid valve are clearly depicted in the RAO projection after contrast is injected into the inferior caval vein (see Fig. 6–6). The degree of development of the pouch and its angiographic demarcation in relation to the tricuspid vestibule vary from patient to patient.[4,26]

THE INFERIOR (CAVOTRICUSPID) ISTHMUS

The inferior right atrial isthmus is the zone of slow conduction of the macroreentrant circuit responsible for the so-called isthmus-dependent atrial flutters (the common anticlockwise flutter, the uncommon clockwise form, and the more exceptional lower-loop reentry atrial flutter).[3,42,61,71,72,80] The inferior isthmus is limited posteriorly by the eustachian valve and anteriorly by the annular insertion of the septal leaflet of the tricuspid valve (see Figs. 6–2E and 6–3). In patients with isthmus-dependent atrial flutter, the relation of the ablation catheter to the inferior isthmus must be explored using both RAO and LAO projections. In the right atrial angiogram obtained in the RAO view, the isthmus consists of three areas: a posterior region that is mainly membranous, an intermediate pouch that is muscular and trabeculated,

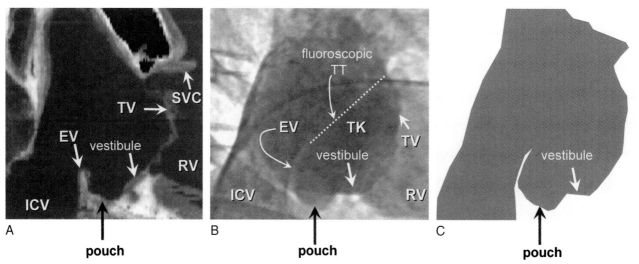

FIGURE 6–6. A, Anatomic slice in 45-degree right anterior oblique (RAO) projection obtained with The Visible Human Slice and Surface Server.[23] **B,** Right atrial angiogram obtained by injecting contrast material into the inferior caval vein (ICV), in a 45-degree RAO projection. **C,** Schematic representation of the angiogram of panel B. The supraventricular crest (SVC) separates the right ventricular outflow and inflow tracts. EV, eustachian valve; RV, right ventricle; TK, triangle of Koch; TT, tendon of Todaro; TV, tricuspid valve.

and an anterior smooth region, also muscular, that is the vestibule of the tricuspid valve (see Figs. 6–3 and 6–6).[5] Fluoroscopically, these three regions of the isthmus cannot be visualized without angiographic techniques. In the LAO projection, three areas must also be distinguished: a medial or paraseptal region (5 o'clock position), a middle or inferior area (6 o'clock position), and a lateral portion which, attitudinally speaking, is anteroinferior (7 o'clock position) (Fig. 6–7; see Fig. 6–3). These three regions can be identified with simple fluoroscopy (see Fig. 6–7C).

Angiographically, the dimensions of the right atrium and the inferior isthmus are larger in patients with isthmus-dependent atrial flutter than in normal controls.[4] This enlarged right atrium including the inferior isthmus region may provide the pathophysiologic basis to sustain atrial flutter within an otherwise universally existing anatomic substrate. The variable angiographic expression of the inferior isthmus may influence the ease of production of a complete line of bidirectional block across this anatomic landmark.[26,27]

THE TRIANGLE OF KOCH

The triangle of Koch is the inferior, paraseptal, right atrial region that contains the AV node and its inferior extensions, as well as the transitional fibers approaching the compact AV nodal area.[1,2,7-9,12,14-18] In addition, the triangle of Koch is the seat of the atrial insertion of many AV APs, usually termed septal and paraseptal.[19-22,81-89] The AV component of the mem-

branous septum forms the anterosuperior apex of the triangle. The eustachian ridge, containing the tendon of Todaro, and the attachment of the septal leaflet of the tricuspid valve are its lateral margins. The base of the triangle is the orifice of the coronary sinus and the vestibular region, from the coronary sinus to the tricuspid valve (see Fig. 6–6). Walter Koch did not describe the landmarks of this area as such, but he produced a celebrated illustration displaying very clearly this anatomic region. The eponym *triangle of Koch* is widely used by morphologists, surgeons, and arrhythmolgists.[15,79]

In the 45-degree RAO projection, the plane of the triangle of Koch is parallel to that of the image intensifier (see Figs. 6–1, 6–3, and 6–6). To establish whether the catheter is on the triangle of Koch, the RAO and LAO views must be combined (Figs. 6–8 and 6–9). The LAO projection differentiates "paraseptal" locations from inferior (formerly posterior), anteroinferior (formerly posterolateral), and anterior (formerly right lateral) positions of the probing electrode. The region of the His bundle is superior, whereas the orifice of the coronary sinus is inferior (Fig. 6–10).

Right atrial angiography obtained in a 45-degree RAO projection allows definition of the size and orientation of the triangle of Koch, as well as the relation between the site of recording of the largest His bundle potential and the plane of the tricuspid valve. The triangle of Koch may have different sizes and configurations. In some patients it is more vertically oriented, and in others it has a more horizontal display. The pre-eustachian pouch and the tricuspid

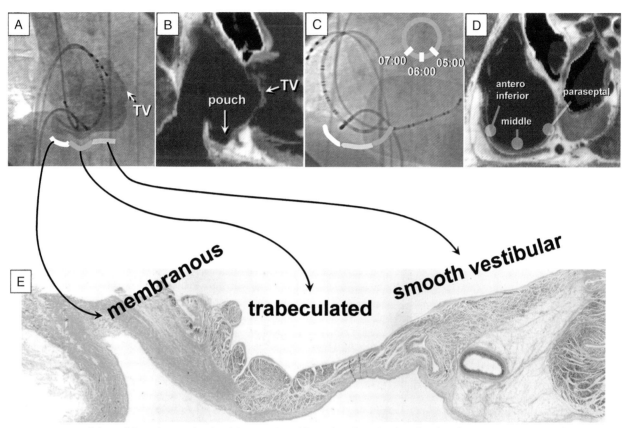

FIGURE 6–7. A, Right atrial angiogram in the right anterior oblique (RAO) projection showing three regions in the inferior isthmus (see text). TV, tricuspid value. **B,** Anatomic slice in RAO projection obtained with The Visible Human Slice and Surface Server.[23] **C,** Fluoroscopic view of the catheters in left anterior oblique (LAO) projection. Note that the ablation catheter is located in the anteroinferior region of the inferior isthmus. The three regions that must be identified in this projection (anteroinferior, middle, and paraseptal) are also shown in white, yellow, and cyan, respectively. **D,** Anatomic slice in LAO projection obtained with The Visible Human Slice and Surface Server.[23] Note the three regions of the inferior isthmus in this projection (see text). **E,** Histologic section of the isthmus obtained between the middle and the paraseptal regions and depicting the architecture of the posterior membranous sector, the inter-mediate trabeculated muscular area, and the smooth anterior vestibular area, which also contains atrial myocardium (see text).

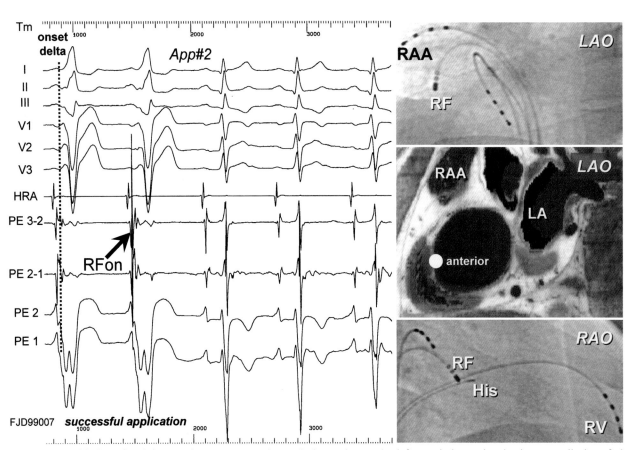

FIGURE 6–8. Ablation of a right anterior accessory atrioventricular pathway. The left panel shows the simultaneous display of six surface electrocardiographic (ECG) leads and several intracardiac bipolar and unipolar recordings. The *arrow* signals the artefact of the onset of the application of radiofrequency current (RF). Preexcitation disappears in the first beat after initiation of the delivery of RF. HRA, high right atrium; PE, probing electrode. The position of the ablation catheter at the site of application of RF is shown in the 45-degree left anterior oblique (LAO) and 45-degree right anterior oblique (RAO) projections. In the right middle panel, the site of RF application is shown on a 45-degree LAO section of the heart obtained with The Visible Human Slice and Surface Server.[23] His, bundle of His; LA, left atrium; RAA, right atrial appendage; RV, right ventricle.

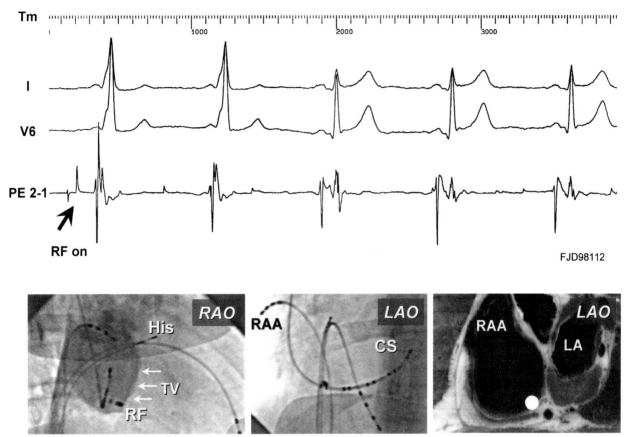

FIGURE 6–9. Ablation of a septal accessory atrioventricular pathway (midseptal, in the traditional nomenclature). The upper panel shows the simultaneous display of two surface electrocardiographic (ECG) leads (I and V6) and the filtered bipolar distal recording from the ablation electrode. The *arrow* signals the onset of the application of radiofrequency current (RF), after which preexcitation disappears within less than 2 seconds. The position of the ablation catheter at the site of application of RF is shown in the 45-degree right anterior oblique (RAO) and 45-degree left anterior oblique (LAO) projections. The lower right panel displays the site of RF application on a 45-degree LAO section of the heart obtained with The Visible Human Slice and Surface Server.[23] CS, coronary sinus; His, bundle of His; LA, left atrium; RAA, right atrial appendage; RF, ablation catheter. The right atrial angiogram (lower right panel) shows that the site of ablation was close to the tricuspid valve (*horizontal arrows*, TV). The LAO projection serves to demonstrate that the ablation catheter has a septal location.

vestibule also vary in size (see Figs. 6–6, 6–7A, and 6–9). The site of recording of the largest His bundle deflection does not always coincide with the anterosuperior vertex of the triangle as judged angiographically (Fig. 6–11). This has implications regarding the position of the compact node that is just proximal to the His bundle. The compact AV node is an unprotected structure, very sensitive to the application of RF current. Mapping in the vicinity of the compact node can induce mechanical AV block. Unless such blockade is intended, delivery of RF current near the AV compact node must be avoided. The node becomes the His bundle as the AV conduction axis enters the membranous septum and is encircled by fibrous tissue. Therefore, the bundle of His is better protected than the compact node against RF current. Parahisian accessory AV pathways are superficial to the collagenous cup of the His bundle and have a subendocardial course; therefore, they are very sen-

sitive to mechanical block during catheter mapping, and their ablation is possible without inducing His bundle block.

Right atrial angiography in the RAO projection not only displays the limits and variable dimensions of the triangle of Koch but also identifies the exact position of the catheter used for ablation in relation to the anterosuperior and posteroinferior limits of the tricuspid valve (see Fig. 6–9). This applies to ablative procedures in patients with AV nodal reentry tachycardia; in patients with inferior paraseptal, truly septal, and superior paraseptal (including parahisian) APs; and in patients with certain forms of atrial tachycardia arising from the triangle of Koch. The dimensions of the triangle of Koch may warn the interventional electrophysiologist about the potential dangers of inducing unwanted damage over the compact node. In ablative procedures aimed at approaching the slow nodal pathway, where the elec-

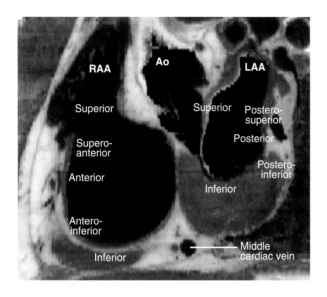

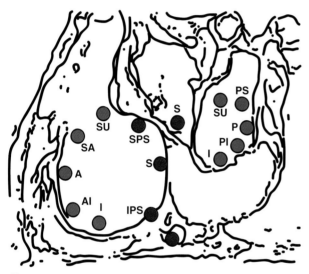

● Attitudinal nomenclature for positions in the right and left

   AV grooves

● Septal and paraseptal locations

FIGURE 6–10. Attitudinal nomenclature for positions in the right and left atrioventricular grooves as well as septal and paraseptal locations in an LAO slice of the heart obtained with The Visible Human Slice and Surface Server.[23] This nomenclature is particularly useful for locations of accessory pathways. A, anterior; AI, anteroinferior; Ao, aorta; I, inferior; IPS, inferior paraseptal; LAA, left atrial appendage; P, posterior; PI, posteroinferior; PS, posterosuperior; RAA, right atrial appendage; S, septal; SA, superoanterior; SPS, superior paraseptal; SU, superior. Note that there are septal accessory pathways at the right but also at the left side of the interventricular septum.

trogram markers for ablation are relatively nonspecific, the LAO fluoroscopic projection enables the operator to determine that the probing electrode is pointing toward the triangle of Koch, rather than toward the inferior isthmus.

Although APs ablated in the region of the triangle of Koch are termed today septal, this area is not a septal structure in the strictest sense, if by that term is understood those cardiac walls that can be excised without exiting from the cardiac cavities.[90] The triangle of Koch is an overlap of the atrial and ventricular musculature previously called AV septum. An extension of the inferior AV groove separates these muscular walls like the content of a sandwich.

THE OVAL FOSSA AND THE INTERATRIAL GROOVE (SEPTUM)

The oval fossa is a depression in the right atrial aspect of the area traditionally considered to be the interatrial septum (see Fig. 6–2D). At the left side of the heart, a membranous valve covers this region; when it fully seals the passage of blood from one atrium to the other, it represents the true interatrial septum in the sense than it can be crossed without exiting the heart.[90] The rest of the so-called muscular interatrial septum is formed by apposition of the right and left atrial myocardiums, which are separated by fibrofatty tissues that extend from the extracardiac fat. This is why we prefer to use the term *interatrial groove* rather than muscular interatrial septum. The interatrial groove has an oblique course from right to left (see Fig. 6–2). In the LAO projection, the interatrial groove is almost perpendicular to the plane of the image intensifier (see Figs. 6–1A and 6–5). Anterior to the oval fossa, there is a prominent muscular border known as the anterior limbus (see Fig. 6–3).

The oval fossa is an interesting anatomic landmark in the electrophysiology laboratory because of the increased need to perform trans-septal punctures, particularly for ablative procedures in patients with atrial fibrillation and left-sided atrial tachyarrhythmias.[31-35,44-47,50,52,53,58,60,62,63,91-94] Electrophysiologists have suggested modifications of the traditional technique for trans-septal catheterization.[93,94] Fluoroscopic angulations used for trans-septal punctures must be individualized because of the variability in the position of the heart in the thorax. Experienced operators may perform very efficiently the puncture of the oval fossa in the posteroanterior (PA) projection; others may prefer a very angulated LAO projection (>45 degrees). In the RAO projection, the oval fossa is posterior and superior or at the same level as the site of recording of the His bundle potential. In this projection, the oval fossa is usually posterior and superior relative to the entry into the coronary sinus.[94]

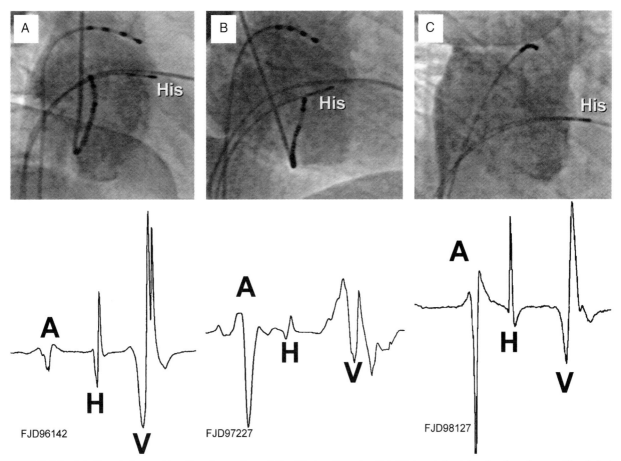

FIGURE 6–11. Relations between the site of recording of the His bundle potential (His) and the triangle of Koch as outlined during right atrial angiography. The His bundle potential was recorded at the level of the tricuspid valve (**A**), at a pretricuspid site (**B**), and beyond the tricuspid valve (**C**). Despite being at a right ventricular location in the right atrioventricular groove, the recording displays not only local His and ventricular deflections (H and V, respectively) of a good voltage, but also a large atrial electrogram (A).

It is important to perform the trans-septal puncture through the oval fossa (Fig. 6–12). A puncture throughout the interatrial groove (muscular interatrial septum) may result in hemopericardium in a highly anticoagulated patient, because blood can dissect the vascular fibrofatty tissue that is sandwiched between the right and left atrial myocardiums at this level.

THE CORONARY SINUS AND THE PYRAMIDAL SPACE

The coronary sinus and the pyramidal space are discussed in the context of the right atrial section because we approach this region from a right atrial entry. The pyramidal space is an area of the heart whose superior vertex is the central fibrous body, whose lateral sides are right and left atria, and whose floor is the muscular ventricular septum and left ventricle. The coronary sinus limits the base of this area, which has a trihedral pyramidal configuration. Tissues that are continuous with the inferior epicar-

dial AV groove occupy the pyramidal space. The term *pyramidal space* was introduced by Sealy and Gallagher[84] during the days of surgical ablation of septal APs.

AV accessory pathways in this region are referred to as septal and paraseptal. This terminology is too broad and simplistic to help the ablationist. Inferior paraseptal APs can be ablated from the right side of the heart, outside or inside the coronary sinus or in the middle cardiac vein, and from the left side of the heart, in the immediate subaortic region (see Fig. 6–10). The middle cardiac vein ends up in the proximal coronary sinus and initially runs an inferior course, as seen in both the LAO and RAO projections (Fig. 6–13), before bending anteriorly along the inferior epicardial surface of the muscular interventricular septum.

Midseptal APs, a terminology introduced by Jackman et al.,[81] are those located between the His bundle region and the orifice of the coronary sinus. These APs are ablated on the triangle of Koch and are termed "septal" in the attitudinally oriented

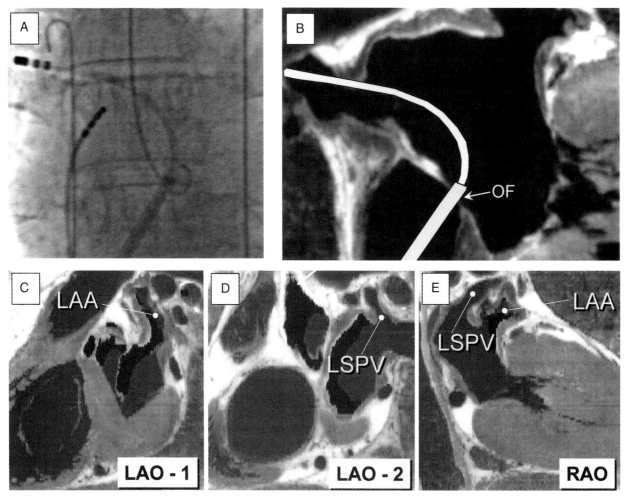

FIGURE 6–12. Panel **A** shows the ablation catheter positioned inside the right superior pulmonary vein through a trans-septal puncture. Panel **B** shows how the oval fossa (OF) has been crossed. **C** through **E**, left anterior oblique (LAO) and right anterior oblique (RAO) sections of the heart depicting the relationship between the left atrial appendage (LAA) and the left superior pulmonary vein (LSPV). In the LAO projection, the LAA and the LSPV project at the same level. The anatomic slice in panel **C** is more anterior than that in panel **D**. The RAO enables the operator to determine whether the catheter is inside the LAA or the LSPV. The LAO is the best projection to explore the left pulmonary veins. Panels B–E from The Visible Human Slice and Surface Server (Ref. 23).

nomenclature, despite the fact that, strictly speaking, the triangle of Koch is not a true septal region. To be certain the ablation catheter is on the triangle of Koch, we must combine the two oblique projections. Figure 6–9 shows an example of an AP whose categorization as septal (midseptal) or right inferior paraseptal (right posteroseptal) could be debated. In our opinion, the important issue here is that this AP was ablated on the triangle of Koch, anterior to and outside the coronary sinus, well below the His bundle, in an inferior position of the triangle.

The right AV groove APs may connect the atrial and ventricular myocardiums across the right AV groove. Most ablative procedures in patients with right-sided APs approach the atrial rather than the ventricular insertion of the bypass tract. Figure 6–8

shows ablation of a right anterior AP. Special sheaths may be used to attain catheter stability during ablation procedures in the right AV groove.

The Right Ventricle

The right ventricle is almost systematically catheterized during an electrophysiologic study and very frequently during an ablation procedure. In some stimulation studies, both the right ventricular apex and its outflow tract are catheterized simultaneously or sequentially. Usually, the frontal fluoroscopic projection is used to position an electrode-catheter at the right ventricular apex. The right ventricular outflow

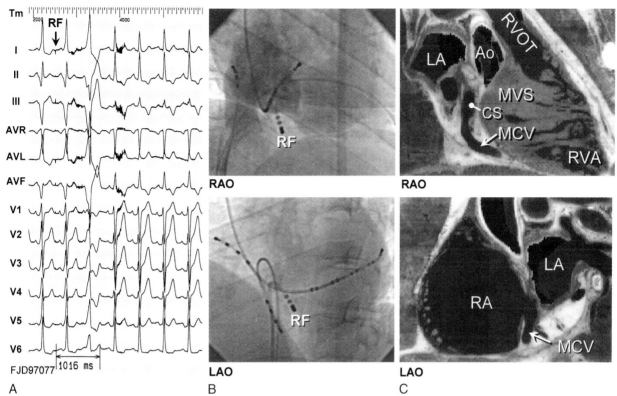

FIGURE 6–13. Ablation of an inferior paraseptal accessory pathway within the midcardiac vein (MCV). The electrocardiographic record (**A**) shows that the accessory pathway is blocked 1016 msec after onset of the application of radiofrequency current (RF). **B,** right anterior oblique (RAO) and left anterior oblique (LAO) fluorographic images displaying the position of the ablation catheter (RF). Note that the injection of contrast material in the RAO projection allows the operator to determine that the ablation catheter is "outside" the outlines of the right atrium as defined by the angiographic contrast. This is indeed true, because the catheter is inside the MCV. **C,** RAO and LAO slices of the heart obtained with The Visible Human Slice and Surface Server.[23] The MCV ends up in the proximal coronary sinus (CS) and runs an inferior course before bending anteriorly along the epicardial surface of the muscular interventricular septum (MVS). Ao, aorta; LA, left atrium; RA, right atrium; RVA, right ventricular apex; RVOT, right ventricular outflow tract.

tract can also be reached via a frontal fluoroscopy view, but it is safer, particularly with the relatively rigid catheters used for ablation, to use an LAO projection, to avoid entering the coronary sinus by mistake. Electrocardiographic (ECG) monitoring can also assist in preventing this error by demonstrating, for example, that atrial and ventricular electrograms are being recorded (typical of the proximal coronary sinus) when it was thought the catheter had entered the right ventricle under the supraventricular crest. The right ventricle is said to be anterior in relation to the left. As seen in Figure 6–2, this relation is true for the right versus the left ventricular cavities, but not for the right and left ventricular myocardial masses. The right ventricular outflow tract is anterior and superior in relation to the supraventricular crest and, therefore, to the bundle of His (see Figs. 6–1 and 6–13C). As far as mapping is concerned, the right ventricular outflow tract becomes important in certain idiopathic ventricular tachycardias that

originate from this region, in some forms of arrhythmogenic right ventricular cardiomyopathy, and in some scar-related ventricular tachycardias developing after complete correction of a tetralogy of Fallot.

The right ventricular outflow tract is separated from the inflow tract of the right ventricle by the supraventricular crest (see Fig. 6–6A). Some APs with a superior paraseptal location (formerly considered as anteroseptal) can have a cristal insertion. If the ventricular insertion of such an AP is in the supraventricular crest, the catheter in the LAO view separates it from the area of the membranous septum fluoroscopically marked by the site of recording of the His bundle potential. The RAO projection cannot differentiate a cristal from a parahisian insertion. Although the cristal ventricular insertion is a safe site at which to apply RF current, slight catheter displacement can damage the normal AV conduction axis, which is very close.

The right bundle branch runs an anterior course. In patients with bundle branch reentry tachycardia, the right bundle branch is the preferred target for RF current. Sites for ablation should be selected as distant as possible from the His bundle. The RAO fluoroscopic projection allows the operator to estimate the distance between the His bundle and the selected target site of the right bundle branch. The LAO projection is helpful in these instances to direct the probing electrode to the superior paraseptal aspect of the right ventricle, where the trunk of the right bundle branch is located, before dividing itself into several fascicles.

ACCESSORY PATHWAYS WITH A MAHAIM PHYSIOLOGY

In 1971, Wellens, in his doctoral thesis, described an 8-year-old boy with a PR interval of 0.12 second, minor "type B" preexcitation during sinus rhythm, and wide QRS-complex tachycardias with left bundle branch block configuration.[95] Although Wellens initially postulated that a nodoventricular Mahaim tract was involved in this form of preexcitation, it was subsequently demonstrated that the bypass tract in most of these patients consists of a right free-wall anomalous node that continues with an accessory His-Purkinje system distally, inserting at the normal right bundle branch or directly at the right ventricular myocardium. The term *Mahaim physiology* has been used for this kind of AP, but such a name is a misnomer, because what Mahaim described were connections between the AV node or left bundle branch and the ventricular myocardium (nodoventricular or fasciculoventricular connections).[96] Several approaches have been suggested for ablation in these APs, including catheter-induced mechanical block of the AP and identification of the AP potential, either the proximal anomalous His or a more distant Purkinje-like potential of the anomalous AV bundle.[97-99] We perform the ablation at sites where a Purkinje-like potential precedes the onset of a maximally preexcited QRS-complex by 20 to 40 msec. More proximal sites may be encased by a shield of connective tissue, making them less susceptible to RF ablation. Approaching the atrial insertion by frequently provoking long-lasting mechanical blockade makes the ablation procedure more difficult. Distal segments close to the ventricular exit probably branch and are inappropriate targets for RF catheter ablation, yielding only temporary success. Although most of these APs have a distal insertion that tends to be close to the right ventricular apex, some of them may end in the neighborhood of the right ventricular outflow tract (Fig. 6–14).

The Left Atrium and the Pulmonary Veins

The left atrial anatomy is more complex than is usually conceived.[6] The left atrial endocardium is smooth except for the left atrial appendage, where the left-sided pectinate muscles are confined. The left atrium is separated from the right atrium by the valve of the oval foramen. In some 25% of adult hearts, this valve can be forced, so that a catheter can access the left atrium from the right atrium without the necessity of puncturing the oval fossa to perforate the valve covering the oval foramen.[6]

The left atrial appendage is anterior in relation to the orifice of the left superior pulmonary vein (see Figs. 6–2A, 6–12C through E). Accessory pathways can connect the left atrial appendage with the left ventricle. Anteriorly, the Bachmann bundle connects the right and left atria (see Fig. 6–2A). The Bachmann bundle can be traced rightward to the terminal crest at the junction between the right atrium and the superior caval vein. The Bachmann bundle that is not well developed in some hearts and is not the only interatrial myocardial bridge.[6] The Bachmann bundle is superior to the His bundle region and oval fossa and posterior relative to the apex of the right atrial appendage (see Fig. 6–2). Axially, it is more or less at the level of the orifice of the right superior and left superior pulmonary veins (see Fig. 6–2). In the frontal fluoroscopic view, the Bachmann bundle also is at the level of the right atrial appendage, provided the catheter located at the latter site is pointing anteriorly or toward the spine. Should we intend to map the Bachmann bundle endocardially, in addition to the aforementioned fluoroscopic references, we must confirm that the probing catheter is pointing anteriorly, using the RAO projection. However, in the RAO view, a catheter exploring the Bachmann bundle must be behind an electrode-catheter positioned inside the apex of the right atrial appendage (see Fig. 6–2).

Defining the venoatrial junction is difficult in the electrophysiology laboratory even with the use of angiographic techniques. A common source of fluoroscopic error is to consider that we are in the pulmonary veins only when the mapping catheter is outside the contour of the heart silhouette in the PA projection. In fact, we can be inside any of the four pulmonary veins without having crossed the projection of the heart on the PA fluoroscopic view. In fact, the initial portion of the right superior pulmonary vein is behind the smooth-walled right atrium at its junction with the posterior side of the superior caval vein (see Fig. 6–2). The best fluoroscopic projection to

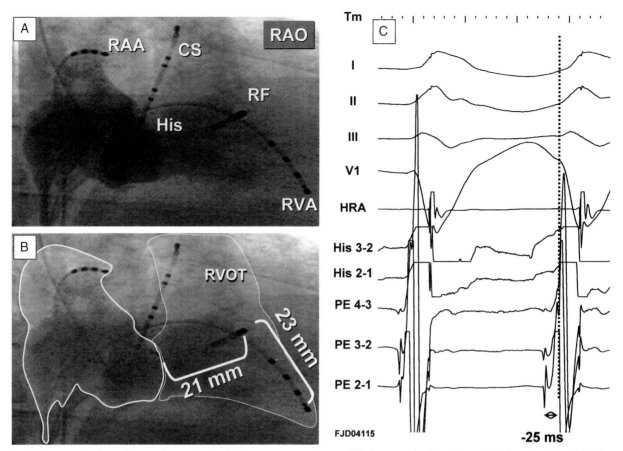

FIGURE 6–14. Ablation of an atrioventricular (AV) accessory pathway with long conduction times (Mahaim physiology) having a ventricular insertion high in right interventricular septum, close to the right ventricular outflow tract (RVOT). **A,** Position of the ablation catheter (RF) in the right anterior oblique (RAO) projection during injection of contrast material into the right atrium. Note that the ablation catheter is far from the tricuspid valve plane. When outlines of the right atrium and right ventricle are superimposed on the fluorographic image (**B**), the tip of the ablation catheter is seen to be 21 mm from the tricuspid plane and 23 mm from the tip of the right ventricular apex (RVA). **C,** Recordings obtained at the site of ablation during pacing from the right atrial appendage. Note the long AV conduction times during atrial pacing. Also note the presence of a Purkinje-like potential, which precedes onset of the maximally preexcited ventricular complexes by 25 msec. CS, coronary sinus; His, bundle of His; HRA, high right atrium; PE, probing electrode; RAA, right atrial appendage.

explore the left-sided pulmonary veins is the LAO (see Fig. 6–12). The best projection to explore the right-sided pulmonary veins is the RAO (Fig. 6–15). Pulmonary venography is best performed by direct catheterization of each individual pulmonary vein. The venous phase of a pulmonary arteriography does not provide sufficient anatomic details.

The Left Ventricle

The left ventricle differs from the right ventricle in four major anatomic details: (1) the musculature of the left ventricular walls is much thicker than that of the right ventricle (see Fig. 6–2); (2) in the left ventricle, there is no muscular separation between inflow

and outflow tracts such as the supraventricular crest in the right ventricle, and there is mitroaortic continuity; (3) the mitral valve has an insertion that is above that of the tricuspid valve; and (4) the right and left AV rings form a divergent angle in the RAO projection, so that they merge anterosuperiorly and separate inferoposteriorly. The latter situation explains why the triangle of Koch consists of supratricuspid right atrial myocardium that overrides the inframitral ventricular myocardium.

Usually, the left ventricle is catheterized to ablate the ventricular insertion of left-sided APs and ventricular tachycardias. Generally, the left ventricle is approached from an aortic retrograde access (Fig. 6–16). A trans-septal approach can also be used. The septal area of the left ventricle is best examined on an LAO fluoroscopic projection. A combination of LAO and RAO projections usually is necessary to locate

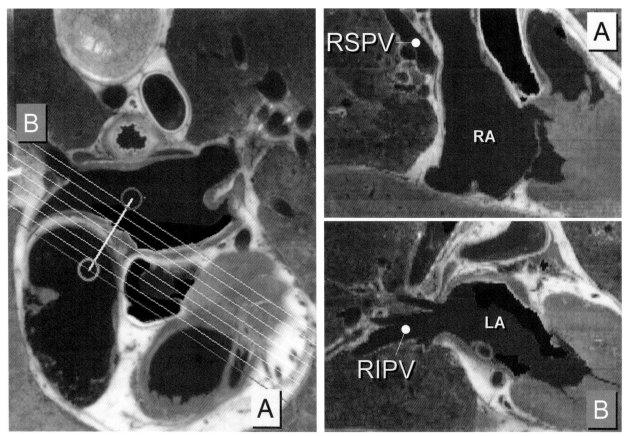

FIGURE 6–15. The right anterior oblique (RAO) view is the best projection for exploring the right pulmonary veins. On the left is an axial slice obtained with The Visible Human Slice and Surface Server.[23] On the right are the respective slices obtained with RAO-oriented cuts through the lines A and B on the left hand image (*top* and *bottom,* respectively). Note that the right superior pulmonary vein (RSPV) has a superiorly oriented course and the right inferior pulmonary vein (RIPV) runs a posteriorly oriented course.

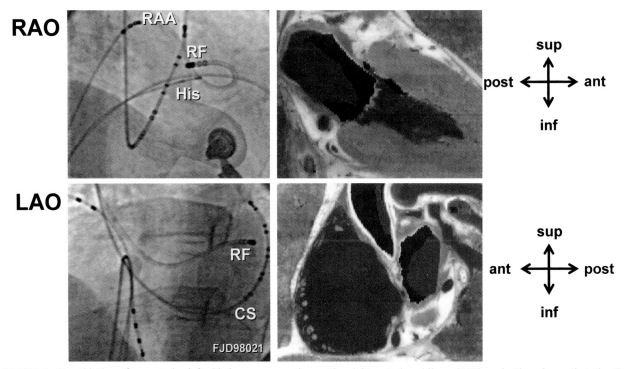

FIGURE 6–16. Ablation of a posterior left-sided accessory pathway. The right anterior oblique (RAO) projection shows that the tip of the ablating electrode (RF) is below the coronary sinus (CS) catheter, indicating that we are approaching the ventricular insertion of the accessory pathway. The left anterior oblique (LAO) view enables us to define the posterior location of the bypass tract. On the right are RAO and LAO slices obtained with The Visible Human Slice and Surface Server.[23] His, bundle of His; RAA, right atrial appendage.

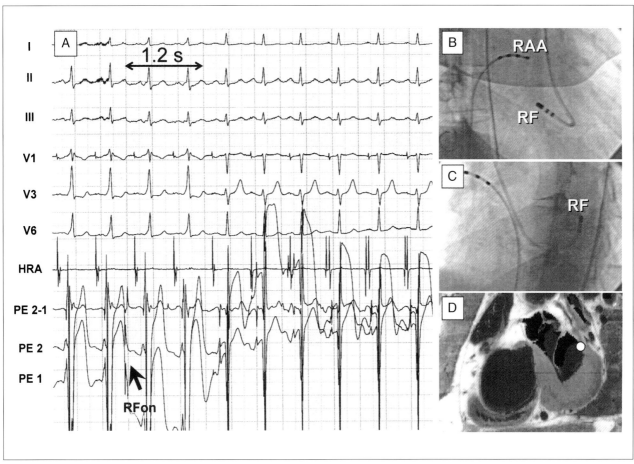

FIGURE 6–17. Ablation of a posterior left-sided accessory pathway with the so-called single-catheter technique. Panel **A** shows the disappearance of preexcitation 1.2 seconds after onset of the radiofrequency (RF) pulse application. Panels **B** and **C** are, respectively, the left and right anterior oblique fluorographic views of the catheters used during this intervention. Note that, apart from the ablation catheter (RF), we used a second catheter that was placed at the right atrial appendage (RAA). In fact, this catheter was used during the procedure for right atrial pacing, to increase the degree of preexcitation, which was not well evident during sinus rhythm. **D,** Left anterior oblique slice obtained with The Visible Human Slice and Surface Server.[23] Note the mitroaortic continuity (see text). HRA, high right atrium; PE, probing electrode.

the site of successful ablation in the three dimensions of the left ventricle. Although many ablationists prefer to have a catheter inside the coronary sinus to guide ablation procedures in patients with left-sided APs, with sufficient fluoroscopic experience it is possible to map the left AV groove without the coronary sinus catheter.[100] The so-called single-catheter technique in practice requires two catheters: the ablation electrode and a right-sided catheter used for subsequent atrial and ventricular pacing after the ablation. Frequently, this pacing catheter is useful during the ablation procedure itself, to increase the contribution of the bypass tract to ventricular activation with atrial pacing in patients with left-sided APs, which may have low levels of preexcitation during sinus rhythm (Fig. 6–17).

Accessory pathways connecting the left atrial appendage with the ventricle must be approached by a trans-septal catheterization. In our experience, this

type of AP cannot be reached with a retrograde aortic approach, because it frequently connects the left atrial myocardium just at or below the mouth of the left atrial appendage with the opposite ventricular myocardium through the epicardial fat. Because the ventricular insertion is rather epicardial, we must approach the atrial insertion of these APs.

References

1. Dean JW, Ho SY, Rowland E, et al.: Clinical anatomy of the atrioventricular junctions. J Am Coll Cardiol 24:1725-1731, 1994.
2. Cabrera JA, Medina A, Suárez-de-Lezo J, et al.: Angiographic anatomy of Koch's triangle, atrioventricular nodal artery, and proximal coronary sinus in patients with and without atrioventricular nodal reentrant tachycardia. In Farre J, Moro C (eds.): Ten Years of Radiofrequency Catheter Ablation. Armonk, N.Y.: Futura, 1998, pp 91-102.

3. Nakagawa H, Lazzara R, Khastgir T, et al.: Role of the tricuspid annulus and the eustachian valve/ridge on atrial flutter: Relevance to catheter ablation of the septal isthmus and a new technique for rapid identification of ablation success. Circulation 94:407-424, 1996.

4. Cabrera JA, Sanchez-Quintana D, Ho SY, et al.: Angiographic anatomy of the inferior right atrial isthmus in patients with and without history of common atrial flutter. Circulation 99:3017-3023, 1999.

5. Cabrera JA, Sanchez-Quintana D, Ho SY, et al.: The architecture of the atrial musculature between the orifice of the inferior caval vein and the tricuspid valve: The anatomy of the isthmus. J Cardiovasc Electrophysiol 9:1186-1195, 1998.

6. Ho SY, Sanchez-Quintana D, Cabrera JA, Anderson RH: Anatomy of the left atrium: Implications for radiofrequency ablation of atrial fibrillation. J Cardiovasc Electrophysiol 10:1525-1533, 1999.

7. Sanchez-Quintana D, Davies DW, Ho SY, et al.: Architecture of the atrial musculature in and around the triangle of Koch: Its potential relevance to atrioventricular nodal reentry. J Cardiovasc Electrophysiol 8:1396-1407, 1997.

8. Sanchez-Quintana D, Ho SY, Cabrera JA, et al.: Topographic anatomy of the inferior pyramidal space: Relevance to radiofrequency catheter ablation. J Cardiovasc Electrophysiol 2:210-217, 2001.

9. Sanchez-Quintana D, Anderson RH, Cabrera JA, et al.: The terminal crest: Morphological features relevant to electrophysiology. Heart 88:406-411, 2002.

10. Ho SY, Cabrera JA, Tran VH, et al.: Architecture of the pulmonary veins: Relevance to radiofrequency ablation. Heart 86:265-270, 2001.

11. Cabrera JA, Sanchez-Quintana D, Farre J, et al.: Ultrasonic characterization of the pulmonary venous wall: Echographic and histological correlation. Circulation 106:968-973, 2002.

12. McGuire MA, de Bakker JM, Vermeulen JT, et al.: Atrioventricular junctional tissue: Discrepancy between histological and electrophysiological characteristics. Circulation 94:571-577, 1996.

13. de Bakker JM, Coronel R, Tasseron S, et al.: Ventricular tachycardia in the infarcted, Langendorff-perfused human heart: Role of the arrangement of surviving cardiac fibers. J Am Coll Cardiol 15:1594-1607, 1990.

14. Ho SY, McComb JM, Scott CD, Anderson RH: Morphology of the cardiac conduction system in patients with electrophysiologically proven dual atrioventricular nodal pathways. J Cardiovasc Electrophysiol 4:504-512, 1993.

15. Ho SY, Kilpatrick L, Kanai T, et al.: The architecture of the atrioventricular conduction axis in dog compared to man: Its significance to ablation of the atrioventricular nodal approaches. J Cardiovasc Electrophysiol 6:26-39, 1995.

16. Inoue S, Becker AE: Posterior extensions of the human compact atrioventricular node: A neglected anatomic feature of potential clinical significance. Circulation 97:188-193, 1998.

17. Medkour D, Becker AE, Khalife K, Billette J: Anatomic and functional characteristics of a slow posterior AV nodal pathway: Role in dual-pathway physiology and reentry. Circulation 98:164-174, 1998.

18. Ho SY, Anderson RH: How constant anatomically is the tendon of Todaro as a marker for the triangle of Koch? J Cardiovasc Electrophysiol 11:83-89, 2000.

19. Becker AE, Anderson RH, Durrer D, Wellens HJ: The anatomical substrates of Wolff-Parkinson-White syndrome: A clinicopathologic correlation in seven patients. Circulation 57:870-879, 1978.

20. Cosio FG, Anderson RH, Kuck KH, et al.: Living anatomy of the atrioventricular junctions: A guide to electrophysiologic mapping. A Consensus Statement from the Cardiac Nomenclature Study Group, Working Group of Arrhythmias, European Society of Cardiology, and the Task Force on Cardiac Nomenclature from NASPE. Circulation 100:e31, 1999.

21. Farre J, Rubio JM, Cabrera JA: Fluoroscopic heart anatomy. In Farre J, Moro C (eds.): Ten Years of Radiofrequency Catheter Ablation. Armonk, N.Y.: Futura, 1998, pp 3-19.

22. Farre J, Anderson RH, Cabrera JA, et al.: Fluoroscopic cardiac anatomy for catheter ablation of tachycardia. Pacing Clin Electrophysiol 25:76-94, 2002.

23. Visible Human Slice and Surface Server. Available at http://visiblehuman.epfl.ch

24. Visible Human Male and Female Project. Available at http://www.nlm.nih.gov/research/visible/visible_human.html

25. Moulton KP: The annular fat stripe as a fluoroscopic guide to anatomic sites during diagnostic and interventional electrophysiology studies. Pacing Clin Electrophysiol 26:2151-2516, 2003.

26. Heidbuchel H, Willems R, van Rensburg H, et al.: Right atrial angiographic evaluation of the posterior isthmus: Relevance for ablation of typical atrial flutter. Circulation 101:2178-2184, 2000.

27. Da Costa A, Faure E, Thevenin J, et al.: Effect of isthmus anatomy and ablation catheter on radiofrequency catheter ablation of the cavotricuspid isthmus. Circulation 110:1030-1035, 2004.

28. Stamato N, Goodwin M, Foy B: Diagnosis of coronary sinus diverticulum in Wolff-Parkinson-White syndrome using coronary angiography. Pacing Clin Electrophysiol 12:1589-1591, 1989.

29. Lesh MD, Van Hare G, Kao AK, Scheinman MM: Radiofrequency catheter ablation for Wolff-Parkinson-White syndrome associated with a coronary sinus diverticulum. Pacing Clin Electrophysiol 14:1479-1484, 1991.

30. Tebbenjohanns J, Pfeiffer D, Schumacher B, et al.: Direct angiography of the coronary sinus: Impact on left posteroseptal accessory pathway ablation. Pacing Clin Electrophysiol 19:1075-1081, 1996.

31. Haissaguerre M, Jais P, Shah DC, et al.: Spontaneous initiation of atrial fibrillation by ectopic beats originating in the pulmonary veins. N Engl J Med 339:659-666, 1998.

32. Lin WS, Prakash VS, Tai CT, et al.: Pulmonary vein morphology in patients with paroxysmal atrial fibrillation initiated by ectopic beats originating from the pulmonary veins: Implications for catheter ablation. Circulation 101:1274-1281, 2000.

33. Robbins IM, Colvin EV, Doyle TP, et al.: Pulmonary vein stenosis after catheter ablation of atrial fibrillation. Circulation 98:1769-1775, 1998.

34. Scanavacca MI, Kajita LJ, Vieira M, Sosa EA: Pulmonary vein stenosis complicating catheter ablation of focal atrial fibrillation. J Cardiovasc Electrophysiol 11:677-681, 2000.

35. Haissaguerre M, Jais P, Shah DC, et al.: Electrophysiological end point for catheter ablation of atrial fibrillation initiated from multiple pulmonary venous foci. Circulation 101:1409-1417, 2000.

36. Yang M, Akbari H, Reddy GP, Higgins CB: Identification of pulmonary vein stenosis after radiofrequency ablation for atrial fibrillation using MRI. J Comput Assist Tomogr 25:34-35, 2001.

37. Sohn RH, Schiller NB: Left upper pulmonary vein stenosis 2 months after radiofrequency catheter ablation of atrial fibrillation. Circulation 101:154-155, 2000.

38. Kato R, Lickfett L, Meininger G, et al.: Pulmonary vein anatomy in patients undergoing catheter ablation of atrial fibrillation: Lessons learned by use of magnetic resonance imaging. Circulation 107:2004-2010, 2003.

39. Vasamreddy CR, Jayam V, Lickfett L, et al.: Technique and results of pulmonary vein angiography in patients undergoing catheter ablation of atrial fibrillation. J Cardiovasc Electrophysiol 15:21-26, 2004.

40. Kluge A, Dill T, Ekinci O, et al.: Decreased pulmonary perfusion in pulmonary vein stenosis after radiofrequency ablation: Assessment with dynamic magnetic resonance perfusion imaging. Chest 126:428-437, 2004.

41. Dickfeld T, Calkins H, Zviman M, et al.: Stereotactic magnetic resonance guidance for anatomically targeted ablations of the fossa ovalis and the left atrium. J Interv Card Electrophysiol 11:105-115, 2004.

42. Shah DC, Jais P, Haissaguerre M, et al.: Three-dimensional mapping of the common atrial flutter circuit in the right atrium. Circulation 96:3904-3912, 1997.

43. Dorostkar PC, Cheng J, Scheinman MM: Electroanatomical mapping and ablation of the substrate supporting intraatrial reentrant tachycardia after palliation for complex congenital heart disease. Pacing Clin Electrophysiol 21:1810-1819, 1998.

44. Pappone C, Oreto G, Lamberti F, et al.: Catheter ablation of paroxysmal atrial fibrillation using a 3D mapping system. Circulation 100:1203-1208, 1999.

45. Pappone C, Rosanio S, Oreto G, et al.: Circumferential radiofrequency ablation of pulmonary vein ostia: A new anatomic approach for curing atrial fibrillation. Circulation 102: 2619-2628, 2000.

46. Leonelli FM, Tomassoni G, Richey M, Natale A: Ablation of incisional atrial tachycardias using a three-dimensional nonfluoroscopic mapping system. Pacing Clin Electrophysiol 24:1653-1659, 2001.

47. Gepstein L, Wolf T, Hayam G, Ben-Haim SA: Accurate linear radiofrequency lesions guided by a nonfluoroscopic electroanatomic mapping method during atrial fibrillation. Pacing Clin Electrophysiol 24:1672-1678, 2001.

48. De Ponti R, Ho SY, Salerno-Uriarte JA, et al.: Electroanatomic analysis of sinus impulse propagation in normal human atria. J Cardiovasc Electrophysiol 13:1-10, 2002.

49. Drago F, Silvetti MS, Di Pino A, et al.: Exclusion of fluoroscopy during ablation treatment of right accessory pathway in children. J Cardiovasc Electrophysiol 13:778-782, 2002.

50. Scavee C, Weerasooriya R, Jais P, et al.: Linear ablation in the left atrium using a nonfluoroscopic mapping system. J Cardiovasc Electrophysiol 14:554, 2003.

51. Soejima K, Stevenson WG, Sapp JL, et al.: Endocardial and epicardial radiofrequency ablation of ventricular tachycardia associated with dilated cardiomyopathy: The importance of low-voltage scars. J Am Coll Cardiol 43:1834-1842, 2004.

52. Nademanee K, McKenzie J, Kosar E, et al.: A new approach for catheter ablation of atrial fibrillation: Mapping of the electrophysiologic substrate. J Am Coll Cardiol 43:2044-2053, 2004.

53. Mesas CE, Pappone C, Lang CC, et al.: Left atrial tachycardia after circumferential pulmonary vein ablation for atrial fibrillation: Electroanatomic characterization and treatment. J Am Coll Cardiol 44:1071-1079, 2004.

54. Ren JF, Schwartzman D, Callans DJ, et al.: Intracardiac echocardiographic imaging in guiding and monitoring radiofrequency catheter ablation at the tricuspid annulus. Echocardiography 15:661-664, 1998.

55. Callans DJ, Ren JF, Schwartzman D, et al.: Narrowing of the superior vena cava-right atrium during radiofrequency catheter ablation for inappropriate sinus tachycardia: Analysis with intracardiac echocardiography. J Am Coll Cardiol 33:1667-1670, 1999.

56. Marchlinski FE, Ren JF, Schwartzman D, et al.: Accuracy of fluoroscopic localization of the crista terminalis documented by intracardiac echocardiography. J Interv Card Electrophysiol 4:415-421, 2000.

57. Schwartzman D, Ren JF, Devine WA, Callans DJ: Cardiac swelling associated with linear radiofrequency ablation in the atrium. J Interv Card Electrophysiol 5:159-166, 2001.

58. Morton JB, Sanders P, Byrne MJ, et al.: Phased-array intracardiac echocardiography to guide radiofrequency ablation in the left atrium and at the pulmonary vein ostium. J Cardiovasc Electrophysiol 12: 343-348, 2001.

59. Ren JF, Callans DJ, Michele JJ, et al.: Intracardiac echocardiographic evaluation of ventricular mural swelling from radiofrequency ablation in chronic myocardial infarction: Irrigated-tip versus standard catheter. J Interv Card Electrophysiol 5:27-32, 2001.

60. Saad EB, Cole CR, Marrouche NF, et al.: Use of intracardiac echocardiography for prediction of chronic pulmonary vein stenosis after ablation of atrial fibrillation. J Cardiovasc Electrophysiol 13:986-989, 2002.

61. Morton JB, Sanders P, Davidson NC, et al.: Phased-array intracardiac echocardiography for defining cavotricuspid isthmus anatomy during radiofrequency ablation of typical atrial flutter. J Cardiovasc Electrophysiol 14:591-597, 2003.

62. Marrouche NF, Martin DO, Wazni O, et al.: Phased-array intracardiac echocardiography monitoring during pulmonary vein isolation in patients with atrial fibrillation: Impact on outcome and complications. Circulation 107:2710-2716, 2003.

63. Ren JF, Marchlinski FE, Callans DJ: Left atrial thrombus associated with ablation for atrial fibrillation: Identification with intracardiac echocardiography. J Am Coll Cardiol 43:1861-1867, 2004.

64. Calkins H, Niklason L, Sousa J, et al.: Radiation exposure during radiofrequency catheter ablation of accessory atrioventricular connections. Circulation 84:2376-2382, 1991.

65. Lindsay BD, Eichling JO, Ambos HD, Cain ME: Radiation exposure to patients and medical personnel during radiofrequency catheter ablation for supraventricular tachycardia. Am J Cardiol 70:218-223, 1992.

66. Scanavacca M, d'Avila A, Velarde JL, et al.: Reduction of radiation exposure time during catheter ablation with the use of pulsed fluoroscopy. Int J Cardiol 63:71-74, 1998.

67. Kovoor P, Ricciardello M, Collins L, et al.: Risk to patients from radiation associated with radiofrequency ablation for supraventricular tachycardia. Circulation 98:1534-1540, 1998.

68. Wittkampf FH, Wever EF, Vos K, et al.: Reduction of radiation exposure in the cardiac electrophysiology laboratory. Pacing Clin Electrophysiol 23:1638-1644, 2000.

69. Rosenthal LS, Mahesh M, Beck TJ, et al.: Predictors of fluoroscopy time and estimated radiation exposure during radiofrequency catheter ablation procedures. Am J Cardiol 82:451-458, 1998.

70. Perisinakis K, Damilakis J, Theocharopoulos N, et al.: Accurate assessment of patient effective radiation dose and associated detriment risk from radiofrequency catheter ablation procedures. Circulation 104:58-62, 2001.

71. Olgin JE, Kalman JM, Fitzpatrick AP, Lesh MD: Role of right atrial endocardial structures as barriers to conduction during human type I atrial flutter: Activation and entrainment mapping guided by intracardiac echocardiography. Circulation 92:1839-1848, 1995.

72. Friedman PA, Luria D, Fenton AM, et al.: Global right atrial mapping of human atrial flutter: The presence of posteromedial (sinus venosa region) functional block and double potentials. A study in biplanefluoroscopy and intracardiac echocardiography. Circulation 101:1568-1577, 2000.

73. Kalman JM, Olgin JE, Karch MR, et al.: "Cristal tachycardias": Origin of right atrial tachycardias from the crista terminalis identified by intracardiac echocardiography. J Am Coll Cardiol 31:451-459, 1998.
74. Lee RJ, Kalman JM, Fitzpatrick AP, et al.: Radiofrequency catheter modification of the sinus node for "inappropriate" sinus tachycardia. Circulation 92:2919-2928, 1995.
75. Boineau JP, Canavan TE, Schuessler RB, et al.: Demonstration of a widely distributed atrial pacemaker complex in the human heart. Circulation 77:1221-1237, 1988.
76. Man KC, Knight B, Tse HF, et al.: Radiofrequency catheter ablation of inappropriate sinus tachycardia guided by activation mapping. J Am Coll Cardiol 35:451-457, 2000.
77. Koplan BA, Parkash R, Couper G, Stevenson WG: Combined epicardial-endocardial approach to ablation of inappropriate sinus tachycardia. J Cardiovasc Electrophysiol 15:237-240, 2004.
78. Schweikert RA, Saliba WI, Tomassoni G, et al.: Percutaneous pericardial instrumentation for endo-epicardial mapping of previously failed ablations. Circulation 108:1329-1335, 2003.
79. James TN: The tendons of Todaro and the "triangle of Koch": Lessons from eponymous hagiolatry. J Cardiovasc Electrophysiol 10:1478-1496, 1999.
80. Cheng J, Cabeen WR, Scheinman M: Right atrial flutter due to lower loop reentry: Mechanism and anatomic substrate. Circulation 99:1700-1705, 1999.
81. Jackman WM, Friday KJ, Fitzgerald DM, et al.: Localization of left free-wall and posteroseptal accessory atrioventricular pathways by direct recording of accessory pathway activation. Pacing Clin Electrophysiol 12:204-214, 1989.
82. Scheinman MM, Wang YS, Van Hare GF, Lesh MD: Electrocardiographic and electrophysiologic characteristics of anterior, midseptal and right anterior free wall accessory pathways. J Am Coll Cardiol 20:1220-1229, 1992.
83. Kuck KH, Schluter M, Gursoy S: Preservation of atrioventricular nodal conduction during radiofrequency current catheter ablation of midseptal accessory pathways. Circulation 86:1743-1752, 1992.
84. Sealy WC, Gallagher JJ: The surgical approach to the septal area of the heart based on experiences with 45 patients with Kent bundles. J Thorac Cardiovasc Surg 79:542-551, 1980.
85. Takahashi A, Shah DC, Jais P, et al.: Specific electrocardiographic features of manifest coronary vein posteroseptal accessory pathways. J Cardiovasc Electrophysiol 9:1015-1025, 1998.
86. Davis LM, Byth K, Ellis P, et al.: Dimensions of the human posterior septal space and coronary sinus. Am J Cardiol 68:621-625, 1991.
87. Sousa J, el-Atassi R, Rosenheck S, et al.: Radiofrequency catheter ablation of the atrioventricular junction from the left ventricle. Circulation 84:567-571, 1991.
88. Schluter M, Kuck KH: Catheter ablation from right atrium of anteroseptal accessory pathways using radiofrequency current. J Am Coll Cardiol 19:663-670, 1992.
89. Haissaguerre M, Marcus F, Poquet F, et al.: Electrocardiographic characteristics and catheter ablation of parahissian accessory pathways. Circulation 90:1124-1128, 1994.
90. Anderson RH, Webb S, Brown NA: Clinical anatomy of the atrial septum with reference to its developmental components. Clin Anat 12:362-374, 1999.
91. Natale A, Breeding L, Tomassoni G, et al.: Ablation of right and left ectopic atrial tachycardias using a three-dimensional nonfluoroscopic mapping system. Am J Cardiol 82:989-992, 1998.
92. Anguera I, Brugada J, Roba M, et al.: Outcomes after radiofrequency catheter ablation of atrial tachycardia. Am J Cardiol 87:886-890, 2001.
93. De Ponti R, Zardini M, Storti C, et al.: Trans-septal catheterization for radiofrequency catheter ablation of cardiac arrhythmias: Results and safety of a simplified method. Eur Heart J 19:943-950, 1998.
94. Gonzalez MD, Otomo K, Shah N, et al.: Transseptal left heart catheterization for cardiac ablation procedures. J Interv Card Electrophysiol 5:89-95, 2001.
95. Wellens HJJ: Electrical Stimulation of the Heart in the Study and Treatment of Tachycardias. Leiden, Germany: Stenfert Kroese, 1971, pp 97-109.
96. Mahaim I: Kent's fibers and the AV paraspecific conduction through the upper connections of the bundle of His-Tawara. Am Heart J 33:651-659, 1947.
97. McClelland JH, Wang X, Beckman KJ, et al.: Radiofrequency catheter ablation of right atriofascicular (Mahaim) accessory pathways guided by accessory pathway activation potentials. Circulation 89:2655-2666, 1994.
98. Cappato R, Schluter M, Weiss C, et al.: Catheter-induced mechanical conduction block of right-sided accessory fibers with Mahaim-type preexcitation to guide radiofrequency ablation. Circulation 90:282-290, 1994.
99. Haissaguerre M, Cauchemez B, Marcus F, et al.: Characteristics of the ventricular insertion sites of accessory pathways with anterograde decremental conduction properties. Circulation 91:1077-1085, 1995
100. Kuck KH, Schluter M: Single-catheter approach to radiofrequency current ablation of left-sided accessory pathways in patients with Wolff-Parkinson-White syndrome. Circulation 84:2366-2375, 1991.

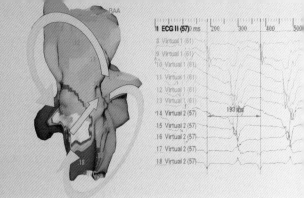

7

Fundamentals of Intracardiac Mapping

Rishi Arora • Alan Kadish

Key Points

- Intracardiac electrograms timing and morphology are used to assess cardiac electrical activation.

- Local tissue activation is best identified by the point of maximal downslope of unipolar electrograms and maximal amplitude of bipolar electrograms.

- Cardiac mapping techniques include activation mapping, electrogram voltage and morphology mapping, pace mapping, entrainment mapping, and computerized mapping.

This chapter discusses the fundamentals of intracardiac mapping, especially as it relates to the mapping and ablation of cardiac arrhythmias. The initial sections are dedicated to the basis and methodology of intracardiac, extracellular recording techniques; this is followed by a description of intracardiac electrograms as recorded in the normal myocardium, and subsequently by a description of intracardiac signals in the abnormal heart. The remainder of the chapter is dedicated to the application of various endocardial mapping techniques (i.e., activation, pace, and entrainment mapping) in the diagnosis and ablation of atrial and ventricular arrhythmias in both normal and diseased hearts. Computerized mapping is discussed in Chapter 8.

Underlying Basis for the Extracellular Electrogram

Cardiac electrical activity originates from ion channel movement across cell membranes. The cardiac action potential is generated within individual cells and reflects cardiac electrical activation. Although some net charge flow occurs in the extracellular space, the majority of cardiac electrical activity is generated within individual myocardial cells. Extracellular electrodes record potentials generated in the extracellular space and therefore differ markedly from action potentials recorded intracellularly. The differences result not only from differences in recording location (extracellular versus intracellular) but also from the inherent summation of electrical activity from multiple cells that occurs when an extracellular potential is generated.

The "field of view" of extracellularly recorded electrograms reflects the relative contributions of individual cells both near to and far from recording electrodes that generate extracellular potentials. Computer modeling studies have created simulated extracellular potentials using various assumptions regarding intracellular action potentials.[1] Factors that affect the field of view of recording electrodes include whether the recordings are unipolar or bipolar, the interelectrode distance (for bipolar recordings), electrode size and composition, and inherent myocardial properties such as tissue resistivity and space constant. In view of the summation of intracellular potentials that occurs to generate extracellular potentials, some fundamental questions regarding cardiac mapping require further investigation.

For example, when one asks what is the "activation time" determined from extracellular potentials,

there may not be a single answer to this question, because different cells within the field of view of an extracellular recording electrode may be activated at different times. Therefore, uniform rules regarding interpretation of extracellular electrograms need to account for differences in underlying physiology, and different "rules" may be appropriate in different circumstances. For example, it has generally been accepted that the His ventricle (HV) interval should be measured from the onset of the His bundle electrogram. The basis for this approach is that, regardless of the location of the recording electrode, one wishes to determine the onset of activation within the His bundle to best evaluate conduction time within the His-Purkinje system. In contrast, mapping of tachycardia origin uses techniques (e.g., baseline crossing in a bipolar electrogram) that seek to determine not the onset of activation but the occurrence of activation at a specific location, in most cases to predict the effects of ablation at that site. Understanding of the physiology that generates extracellular potentials and of the purpose of a particular mapping technique are required to determine the best theoretical as well as practical techniques to use for intracardiac mapping.

Electrogram Recording: Amplification, Filtering, and Digitization of Signals

Physiologic signals acquired via intracardiac electrodes are typically smaller than 10 mV in amplitude and therefore require considerable amplification before they can be digitized, displayed, and stored. In most modern electrophysiology labs, the signal processor (filters and amplifiers), visualization screen, and recording apparatus are incorporated into a computerized laboratory recording system. The amplifiers used for recording intracardiac electrocardiograms (ECGs) must be capable of gain modification as well as alteration of both high- and low-bandpass filters to permit appropriate attenuation of the incoming signals.[2]

After amplification, signals are digitized and filtered by a computerized data acquisition system and are written to a hard disk or optical drive, as well as being displayed in real time on a cathode ray tube or monitor. Digitization is a form of data reduction wherein an analog waveform is "sampled" at a constant rate (sampling rate) by an analog-to-digital (A/D) converter. The amplitude of the analog waveform is translated into a binary number (e.g., 8, 10, or 12-bit conversion, depending on the resolution of the

TABLE 7–1

Typical Filter Settings for Electrophysiology Laboratory Recordings

Recording	High-Pass (Hz)	Low-Pass (Hz)
Surface ECG	0.05-0.1 Hz	100
Bipolar intracardiac	30-50 Hz	300-500
Unipolar intracardiac	Direct current to 0.05	>500

A/D converter), which represents the full dynamic input range of the A/D converter (typically ± 2.5 or ± 10 V). Sampling rates of 600 Hz or greater allow for the recording of most of the data contained in the intracardiac electrogram waveforms, and most modern mapping systems sampling at about 1000 Hz. The ideal system should be able to provide a variety of display configurations with a wide range of sweep speeds (most modern systems can display up to 400 mm/sec) and should allow adjustment of the size/gain and other characteristics of the amplified electrogram.

Filtering is an important aspect of electrogram processing (Table 7–1). High-pass filters eliminate components below a given frequency. In the surface ECG, components such as the T wave are of relatively low frequency, and high-pass filtering of 0.05 to 0.1 Hz is used to preserve these components while eliminating baseline drift. When examining bipolar intracardiac electrograms, high-frequency components are of the most interest, and high-pass filtering of 30 to 50 Hz is used to eliminate the low-frequency components. However, unipolar electrograms usually go through a high-pass filter of 0.05 Hz, because the polarity of the signal (which reflects the direction of myocardial activation) and the signal morphology (and therefore the low-frequency components) must be preserved. To eliminate noise at higher frequencies, low-pass filters are typically set to about 500 Hz for intracardiac signals (because there are essentially no intracardiac signals of interest much above 300 Hz).[3] Figure 7–1 shows the effect of various filter settings on intracardiac atrial, ventricular, and His-Purkinje signals.

Unipolar and Bipolar Signals

The morphology and amplitude of the recorded electrograms depend on (1) the type of normal or abnormal depolarization responsible for the electrical potential and local myocardial characteristics such as ischemia or infarction; (2) the orientation of the activation wavefront in relation to myocardial fiber orientation[4]; (3) the distance between the source of the potential and the recording electrode or electrodes; (4) the size, configuration, and interpolar distance of the recording electrodes[5]; (5) the orientation of the wavefront in relation to the poles of a bipolar electrode; and (6) the conducting medium in which electrograms are recorded,[6] among other factors.

The unipolar electrogram is recorded as the potential difference between a single electrode in direct contact with the heart ("exploring" electrode) and an "indifferent" electrode, which is placed at a distance from the heart[7] or at the Wilson central terminal.[8] The recording is therefore not truly unipolar, because all recordings depend on voltage differences between two poles; the "unipolar" designation signifies that one of the poles is distant from the heart. During cardiac activation, the approach of this dipole toward an exploring electrode results in a small positive deflection, and its passage causes a rapid deflection in the negative direction, with a final return to baseline.[9] The amplitude of the unipolar electrogram is proportional to the area of the dipole layer and the reciprocal value of the square of the distance between the dipole layer and the recording site.[10] Therefore, the unipolar electrogram records a combination of local and distant electrical events, with the contribution of distant electrical events decreasing in proportion to the square of the distance from the exploring electrode.[11] As mentioned previously, extracellular recordings are not synonymous with intracellular microelectrode recordings. Nonetheless, in normal myocardium with relatively homogeneous conduction and repolarization characteristics, several studies (as well as theoretical models) have shown conformity of activation times between an intracellular microelectrode and extracellular recordings (Fig. 7–2), with the maximum downslope of the unipolar electrogram coinciding with the upstroke of the transmembrane potential.[12,13] At least in normal hearts, therefore, there is agreement on using the maximum downslope of the unipolar electrogram for activation detection. However, there is significant controversy as to the optimal value of the slope threshold, with recommended thresholds from different studies ranging from −0.2 to −2.5 mV/msec. The large range can be at least partially attributed to the fact that these studies were performed under a variety of baseline conditions in normal, acutely ischemic, and chronically infracted hearts (animal and human).

The bipolar electrogram is recorded as the potential difference between two closely spaced electrodes

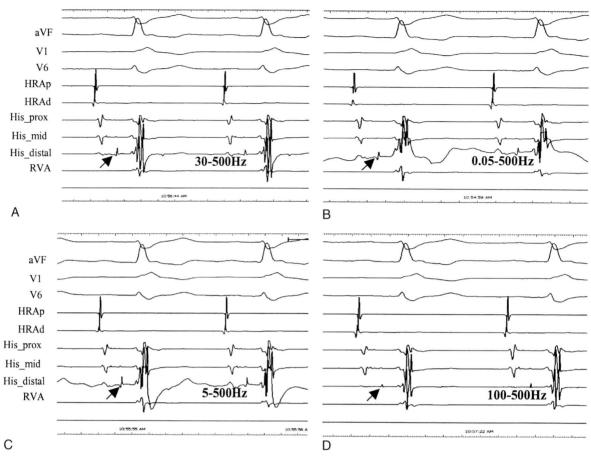

FIGURE 7–1. Effects of various filtering frequencies on the morphologic appearance of intracardiac electrograms. **A** through **D,** The tracings from top to bottom are electrocardiographic leads aVF, V1, V6, right atrial (HRAp, HRAd), three His bundle (His-prox, His-mid, His-distal) electrograms, and right ventricle (RVA). In each panel, both beats are [AA] of sinus origin. The top two His tracings (Prox and mid), RA, and right ventricular (RV) tracings are filtered at 30 to 500 Hz (i.e., the usual filtering frequencies). The bottom His distal tracing shows the effect of various filtering frequencies on the appearance. The low-frequency signals are mostly eliminated at high-bandpass filter frequency settings greater than 10 Hz. It should be pointed out that the high-bandpass setting reduces the overall magnitude of the electrogram, necessitating an increase in amplification. At all frequencies depicted, the His bundle deflection can be clearly identified.

that are in direct contact with the heart; it can be calculated as the difference between two unipolar electrograms at each of the two electrode sites[14] (Fig. 7–3); in the electrophysiology laboratory, this is typically done with analog amplifiers rather than with digital subtraction between unipolar signals. The amplitude of the bipolar electrogram is inversely proportional to the third power of the distance between recording site and dipole.[15]

The major advantage of bipolar recordings lies in the distinction between local and distant activity. A limitation of bipolar electrograms is their directional sensitivity: if the activation wavefront is parallel to the electrode pair, the bipolar spike will be of maximum amplitude, but if it is perpendicular, both

electrodes will record the same waveform at the same time, and no spike will result.[16] In addition, activation at the two poles is not simultaneous, making activation detection more difficult in bipolar electrograms. The following criteria have been suggested for activation detection in bipolar electrograms: (1) the maximum absolute value of the bipolar electrogram; (2) the first elevation of the electrogram of more than 45 degrees from the baseline (45 degrees); (3) the baseline crossing with the steepest slope; and (4) morphologic algorithms that search for symmetry in the bipolar waveform. Of these, the maximum amplitude (and the maximum absolute amplitude) of the bipolar electrogram is most easily measured and has been shown to closely coincide with the

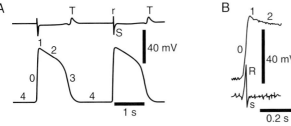

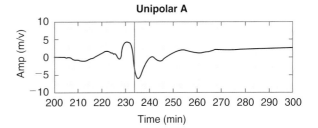

FIGURE 7–2. Concordance between extracellular electrogram and intracellular action potential recordings. **A,** Relationship between unipolar electrogram *(top trace)* and the transmembrane potential *(bottom trace)* recorded simultaneously from bullfrog ventricle. **B,** Display of the initial part of the simultaneously recorded transmembrane action potential *(top trace)* and unipolar electrogram from a different frog *(bottom trace)*, showing concordance between the upstrokes of the two potentials. *(Modified from Yoshida S: Simple techniques suitable for student use to record action potentials from the frog heart. Adv Physiol Edu 25:176-186, 2001, with permission.)*

TABLE 7–2	
Sources of Intracardiac Recording Artifacts	
Cause	**Manifestation**
Electrode polarization	Electrogram drift
Excessive contact pressure	ST elevation
Catheter motion	Fractionation
Poor contact	Low amplitude
Contact with other catheters	High-frequency signals
Repolarization	Late or mid-diastolic potentials
Electromagnetic interference	High-frequency noise
Poor grounding	High-frequency noise

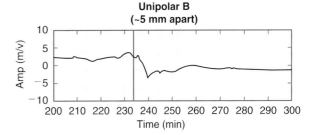

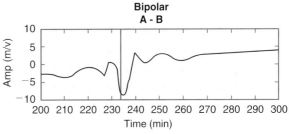

FIGURE 7–3. Relationship between unipolar and bipolar electrograms. The bipolar electrogram represents the difference between two closely spaced unipolar electrodes that have the same reference. The result is that the far-field effects and noise that are present in both unipolar electrograms get canceled out. Amp, amplitude.

RECORDING ARTIFACTS

The correct and timely identification of artifactual electrograms is of crucial importance in any system of cardiac mapping and can have major influence on the final interpretation of an activation sequence (e.g., whether a fractionated electrogram represents a motion artifact or local activation in an assumed zone of slow conduction)[17] (Table 7–2). Typical recording artifacts induced at the myocardium/electrode interface include the following: (1) polarization of electrodes, which can cause slow shifts of the baseline of

maximum downslope of the unipolar electrogram (and the maximum upstroke of the monophasic action potential).[19]

the signals; (2) local myocardial injury resulting from inappropriate pressure by recording electrodes[12]; (3) motion artifacts, which are often rhythmic and repeating, simulating fractionated electrograms, or which can be sudden shifts of potential that may be misinterpreted as activations by computer algorithms; (4) poor contact between electrode and myocardium, which leads to heavier weighing of far-field effects and increased 50- or 60-Hz noise; (5) potential produced by two electrodes from different catheters touching each other; and (6) repolarization signals masquerading as a mid-diastolic potential. Ensuring good contact between the recording electrodes and the underlying myocardium (to remove far-field effects); eliminating all possible sources of noise (including adequate grounding for 50/60 Hz and, if necessary, the use of notch filters); and locating preamplifiers and amplifiers as close as possible to the mapped heart are all key factors that may help eliminate most of the artifacts that are seen in the clinical electrophysiology lab. Undue pressure by the recording catheter on the underlying myocardium can be reflected by the appearance of ST segment elevation on the unipolar electrogram; slight catheter repositioning usually results in resolution of the ST segment to baseline. Motion artifact (from the patient or the surrounding environment) can be minimized by preventing contact of perfusion pumps and other equipment capable of generating cyclic noise with the patient table and mapping equipment.

Characteristics of Intracardiac Signals: Normal Hearts

Unipolar endocardial electrograms obtained from experiments in normal canine hearts, as well as from the human atrium and ventricle, are characterized by a QS morphology with a rapid downstroke in the first part of the QRS complex (intrinsic deflection).[10,18] Bipolar endocardial electrograms in the normal human left ventricle from catheters with 10-mm interelectrode distance have amplitudes of greater than 3 mV and durations of less than 70 msec, and no split, fractionated electrograms are found.[19] Unipolar as well as bipolar electrograms in diseased myocardium are typically characterized by slower upstrokes and fragmentation (see later discussion).

Although slow conduction and fractionated, low-amplitude signals are not as widespread in the normal heart as they are in diseased atrium or ventricle, low-amplitude, high-frequency electrograms have been well described at the thoracic vein–atrial junction, within both the pulmonary veins and the vena cava,[20-22] and at other sites in the normal heart such as the crista terminalis and coronary sinus (the "ring of fire").[23]

ELECTRICAL ABNORMALITIES IN THE ABSENCE OF STRUCTURAL HEART DISEASE

Electrograms need not be entirely "normal" even in the absence of overt fibrosis or fatty replacement. For example, low-amplitude, fractionated bipolar electrograms may be seen at the earliest activation sites of focal tachycardias, even in the presence of a normal-looking unipolar electrogram. Figure 7–4 shows the bipolar electrogram at the successful ablation site of two different focal tachycardias in the absence of any overt structural heart disease (i.e., a focal tachycardia originating from the ostium of the coronary sinus and a focal ventricular tachycardia [VT] arising from the inferolateral left ventricle). At other times, we have noted late potentials during sinus rhythm in hearts that are otherwise morpho-

logically "normal"; Figure 7–5 shows late potentials in the lateral right ventricle of a patient who had exercise-induced left-bundle superior axis VT but no evidence of scar or any other abnormality on an echocardiography or cardiac magnetic resonance imaging (MRI).

The basis for these potentials is not entirely clear. In the absence of overt scar on sensitive imaging modalities such as MRI, it is tempting to speculate that at least some of the delay seen in these electrograms may be functional in nature. In fact, "functional" anisotropic conduction may occur in the normal heart (e.g., at the crista terminalis), and may be responsible for the creation of macroreentrant circuits (e.g., isthmus-dependent atrial flutter). More recently, anisotropic conduction has also been demonstrated within the pulmonary veins[24] and the superior vena cava. Figure 7–6 shows that the conduction times into and out of the pulmonary vein can be very different from each other—an example of anisotropic conduction.[25]

It is conceivable, therefore, that at least some of the focal tachycardias that are described in the normal heart are indeed microreentrant in origin. Other factors that have been postulated include poor intercellular coupling (e.g., due to decreased gap junctions at sites of origin of focal tachycardias) that leads to decreased electronic inhibition of the focus by surrounding tissue.[26] In general, electrograms at successful ablation sites for focal tachycardias occur less than 50 msec before the systolic beat. However, pulmonary vein tachycardias may be more than 50 msec presystolic, at least partially because of the slow conduction noted in this area.

Fractionated, bipolar electrograms (during both tachycardia and sinus rhythm) have also been well described in idiopathic VT arising from the left ventricular septum. In fact, it is the presence of such Purkinje-like potentials some distance away from the septum that has led some to postulate a reentrant circuit of considerable size as the basis for this VT.[27] Split electrograms may sometimes be recorded in the normal heart, such as in the right posteroseptal area from conduction block across the eustachian ridge.

ELECTROGRAM ABNORMALITIES IN THE PRESENCE OF STRUCTURAL HEART DISEASE

The signature of scar in the atrium or ventricle is a low-amplitude, high-frequency electrogram (during sinus rhythm or tachycardia), with the duration and amplitude of the electrogram showing some correlation with the degree of slow conduction in and around the area of fibrosis.[28] Low-amplitude, fractionated electrograms may be recorded during or after the QRS complex and are typically less than

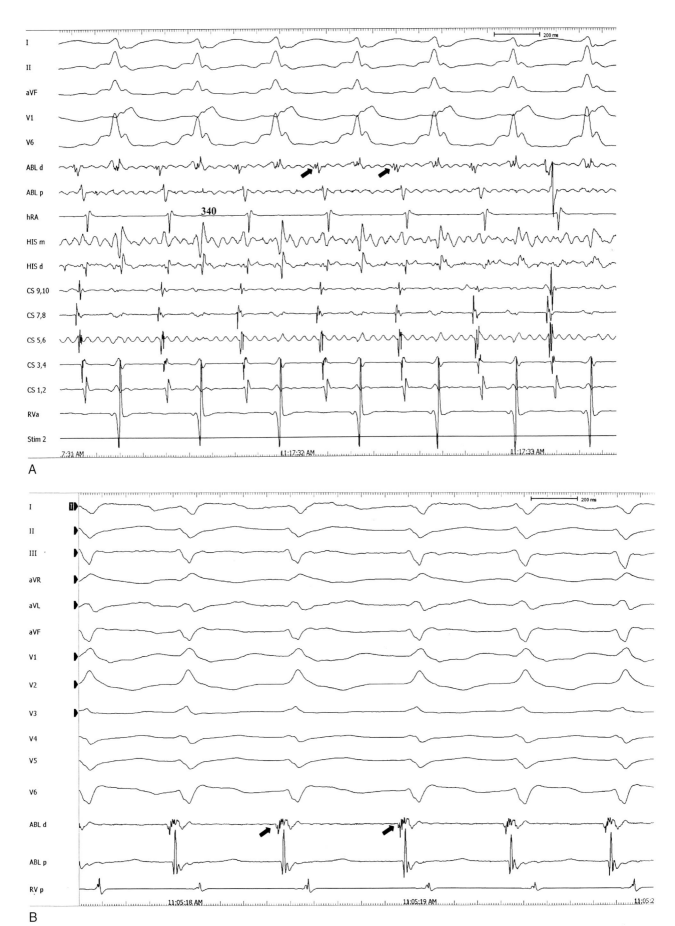

FIGURE 7-4. Low-amplitude bipolar electrogram at successful ablation site of two focal tachycardias: a focal tachycardia originating from the ostium of the coronary sinus (**A**) and a focal ventricular tachycardia arising from the inferolateral left ventricle (**B**). In both instances, notice the lower amplitude and prolonged duration of the electrogram at the site of earliest activation (i.e., the ablation site) *(arrows)*.

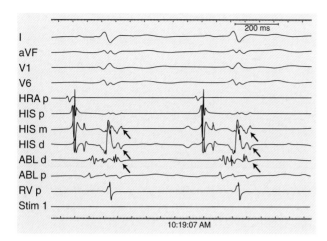

FIGURE 7–5. Late systolic potentials in a heart with no known myocardial disease. The figure demonstrates late potentials that extend beyond the end of the QRS *(arrows)* at the septal right ventricle (base of the right ventricular outflow tract) of a patient who had exercise-induced left-bundle superior axis ventricular tachycardia but no evidence of scar or any other abnormality on echocardiography or cardiac magnetic resonance imaging. HRA, high right atrium; ABL, ablation; RV, right ventricle; p, proximal; m, mid; d, distal; Stim, stimulus.

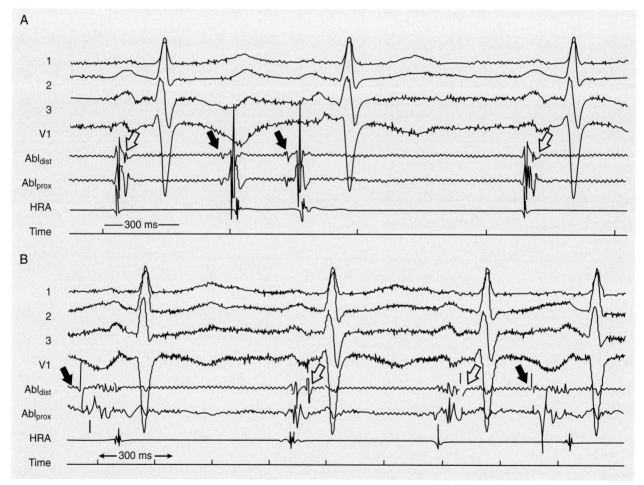

FIGURE 7–6. Anisotropic conduction in the superior vena cava (SVC) and pulmonary vein. In both **A** and **B,** *open arrows* indicate atrial electrograms and *solid arrows* indicate pulmonary vein potentials. **A,** Sinus rhythm with conduction into the posterior superior right atrium (close to its junction with the SVC). **B,** The right superior pulmonary vein. In both **A** and **B,** the bipolar ablation electrogram shows an atrial signal followed by an SVC or a pulmonary vein myocardial signal. Atrial premature contractions (APCs) coming from the SVC or from pulmonary veins show the venous myocardial potential first, followed by the atrial myocardial signal. Note that conduction out of the SVC or pulmonary vein (APCs) is longer than conduction into the SVC or pulmonary vein during sinus rhythm. *(From Figure 9 in Miller JM, Olgin JE, Das MK: Atrial fibrillation: What are the targets for intervention? J Interv Card Electrophysiol 9:249-257, 2003, with permission.)*

1 mV in amplitude; these can be recorded during sinus rhythm or VT. The characteristic unipolar electrogram in the setting of chronic myocardial scar (e.g., after myocardial infarction) may show a single, rapid, biphasic deflection of rs morphology after a wide QS potential, a double rs deflection, or fragmentation with multiple deflections.[29] Continuous, low-amplitude electrical activity (i.e., a fractionated electrogram spanning the entire tachycardia cycle length) can also be seen in the setting of myocardial scar or disease.

Animal studies performed in the setting of chronic experimental myocardial infarction have examined the intracellular basis of the above-mentioned changes on the extracellularly recorded electrogram and have demonstrated that action potential amplitude and upstroke are similar to those of normal myocardium.[30,31] Despite the presence of normal action potentials, slow and discontinuous conduction is present and may provide an electrophysiologic and anatomic basis for arrhythmias. One explanation of the low amplitude, prolonged duration, and notched appearance of extracellular potentials in the infracted areas is that the slow conduction represents activation of normal cells separated by areas of fibrous tissue producing discontinuities in conduction. Kadish et al.[32] used vector mapping, a technique based on summing orthogonally bipolar electrograms, to determine the direction of activation in cardiac tissue. They showed that, although vector loops recorded from normal myocardial tissue were found to be smooth and pointing in a single direction, those recorded from areas of healed myocardial infarction were notched, irregular, and occasionally pointing in more than one direction. Using the vector technique, they demonstrated complex activation patterns in areas where abnormal extracellular electrogram were recorded in which it might be difficult to identify discrete activation times, such as in areas of fractionated electrograms where multiple peaks are present.[33]

Ischemic heart disease is by far the most common cause of scar in the ventricles, although less common conditions (e.g., arrhythmogenic right ventricular dysplasia) may demonstrate similar electrophysiologic characteristics due to fibrofatty replacement in the right (and occasionally the left) ventricle. Fibrosis has also been described in dilated cardiomyopathy, but it is seen far less commonly than in ischemic heart disease. In the atria, scar is commonly the result of surgery for congenital heart disease. Atrial septal defect repair, tricuspid atresia (Fontan repair), tetralogy of Fallot repair, and transposition of great arteries (Mustard/Senning repair) are the most common reasons for scar in the right atrium.[34] Left atrial surgery can create substrate for left or right atrial

reentry,[35] the latter most likely because of cannulation sites during bypass.

As mentioned earlier, the low-amplitude electrograms during sinus rhythm are often noted late in systole; Figure 7–7 shows an example of late systolic potentials in the right ventricle of a patient with arrhythmogenic right ventricular dysplasia. Such low-amplitude, high-frequency electrograms are thought to underlie the late potentials that are seen on a positive signal-averaged ECG.[36] Significantly, even though late potentials are typically seen in and around an area of scar or infarction, late potentials have not been shown to be a clear predictor of ablation success.[37] Although late potentials are frequently noted at or near sites of successful ablation (of reentrant tachycardias), they lack specificity in that they may also be found at sites that are relatively remote from a successful ablation site (indicating diseased myocardium in other areas). A list of abnormal electrogram morphologies and their possible interpretations is given in Table 7–3.

Endocardial Mapping Techniques

"Contact" endocardial mapping can be performed during sinus rhythm or during tachycardia. Mapping techniques can be broadly categorized as follows: (1) activation sequence mapping, (2) fractionated local electrogram and voltage mapping, (3) pace mapping, (4) entrainment mapping, and (5) miscellaneous pacing maneuvers (performed during sinus rhythm or tachycardia). Although these techniques are usually used in combination, the relative utility of each depends on arrhythmia inducibility, stability of the induced arrhythmia, underlying substrate (i.e., normal versus diseased heart), and arrhythmia mechanism, among other factors. For example, entrainment can be used only in the setting of a sustained reentrant arrhythmia. The previous two sections have described the electrogram and voltage characteristics in normal and diseased hearts. The following paragraphs describe the underlying basis for the remainder of the techniques and highlight their use (singly or in combination) in the diagnosis and ablation of atrial and ventricular arrhythmias.

ACTIVATION SEQUENCE MAPPING

The most commonly used method of identifying the site of origin of a tachyarrhythmia is activation mapping to locate the site of "earliest" endocardial

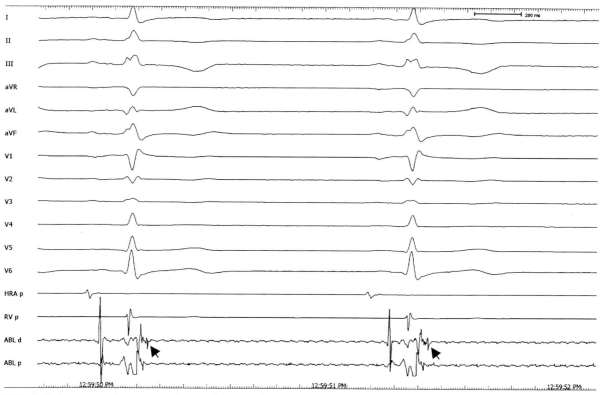

FIGURE 7–7. Late potential mapping in the right ventricle. In a patient with arrhythmogenic right ventricular dysplasia, many of the electrograms were abnormal, especially at the right ventricular (RV) inflow, the RV apex, and the right ventricular outflow tract. The figure shows late potentials during sinus rhythm in the region of the RV apex on the ablation (ABL) catheter *(arrows)*.

TABLE 7–3		
Abnormal Electrogram Morphologies		
Morphology	**Definition**	**Interpretations**
Low amplitude	Atrium: <0.5 mV Ventricle: <1.5 mV	Myocardial infarction, fibrosis, infiltrative process, poor contact, far-field effect
Fractionated	Prolonged (>70 msec), low-amplitude potential with multiple peaks or multiple baseline crossings	Peri-infarction, slow conduction, catheter motion, arborized myocardial connection
Split	Duration >50 msec with two components separated by isoelectric interval	Local conduction block, surgical scar, slow conduction
Late component	Potential occurs after end surface QRS or P wave	Delayed activation, line of block, slow conduction
Continuous	Absence of isoelectric interval throughout diastole	Slow conduction, electromagnetic interference artifact
Mid-diastolic	Potential occurs in mid-diastole, bounded by isoelectric intervals	Protected isthmus, bystander connection, repolarization, or motion artifact
Low frequency	Low dV/dt	Far-field effect, artifact
Monophasic action potential	Injury current pattern	Excessive contact pressure, local tissue injury (unipolar)

dV/dt, maximum negative slope.

activation or determine the activation sequence during the tachycardia. Focal arrhythmias are typically characterized by presystolic timings of less than 50 msec. Reentrant arrhythmias, in both normal and diseased hearts, typically demonstrate diastolic activity that is significantly earlier than 50 msec. In fact, for reentrant arrhythmias, intracardiac activity should be present at some point in the heart throughout the cardiac cycle. In the normal heart (e.g., in the setting of subeustachian isthmus-dependent "typical" atrial flutter), the macroreentrant circuit is of considerable size; it is bounded by two anatomic barriers, the crista terminalis and the tricuspid annulus, and need not demonstrate the low-amplitude, high-frequency electrograms that are typical of scar-related reentrant arrhythmias. In a reentrant arrhythmia in the setting of myocardial scar, a zone of slow conduction over a pathway of possibly quite complex geometry (e.g., nonlinear, nonhomogeneously anisotropic) provides the diastolic limb of the reentrant circuit. After emerging from the zone of slow conduction, the wavefront propagates rapidly throughout the ventricles to generate the QRS complex. Thus, early or presystolic activation occurs in close proximity to the exit region from the zone of slow conduction.

It follows that what is considered early activation and a suitable ablation site in a focal arrhythmia (30 to 50 msec) may not necessarily be "early" activation in a reentrant arrhythmia; reentrant atrial tachycardias (AT) and VTs are characterized by earlier electrogram timing in diastole, and mid-diastolic or even earlier potentials (discussed later) have been correlated with successful ablation sites for these arrhythmias. Figure 7–8 shows an example of AT induced in a patient with no known atrial disease; mapping with the ablation catheter revealed electrograms in and around the tricuspid annulus that were significantly more than 50 msec presystolic, thereby raising suspicion for a reentrant (and not a focal) tachycardia. A halo catheter was subsequently inserted into the left atrium and showed an activation sequence consistent with counterclockwise reentry around the tricuspid annulus. Entrainment maneuvers confirmed the diagnosis and led to successful ablation of the arrhythmia at the subeustachian isthmus.

Mid-diastolic Potentials

If an intervening isoelectric segment exists, the prepotentials are called mid-diastolic potentials (Fig. 7–9); it has been suggested that they identify the region of slow conduction. These prepotentials may precede the major ventricular deflection by tens to hundreds of milliseconds.

It is important to demonstrate that during initiation and resetting of the atrial or ventricular arrhythmia, the mid-diastolic potential always precedes all complexes of the tachycardia in a parallel manner, and that loss of the mid-diastolic potential is associated with termination of the arrhythmia.[27] Although some recent data support the specificity of diastolic potentials during sinus rhythm as successful ablation sites (i.e., critical isthmus sites during VT),[38] most studies have looked at diastolic potentials during sustained ventricular or atrial tachycardia as markers of a protected isthmus.

Mid-diastolic potentials that do not dynamically precede the QRS complex of the VT may represent blind-end alleys of late activation or motion artifact.[27,28] In one study, almost continuous electrical activity spanning the diastolic segment was frequently seen in patients with VT due to ischemic heart disease or arrhythmogenic right ventricular dysplasia; however, in 85% of patients, the episodes of continuous electrical activity could be dissociated from the VT.[23] Such behavior presumably is caused by slow and fractionated conduction into nonessential areas of diseased myocardium.

Unipolar Potential Mapping

Although abnormal endocardial electrograms can be recorded from arrhythmogenic areas, patients with diffuse myocardial abnormalities (e.g., coronary disease, previous infarction) or nonischemic cardiomyopathy can have electrogram abnormalities that are widespread. Therefore, examination of electrogram morphology in sinus rhythm or during tachycardia lacks specificity in mapping tachycardia. However, some electrogram characteristics, particularly of the unipolar electrogram during tachycardia, may have sufficient specificity to be useful in mapping.

The site of origin of an arrhythmia can also perhaps be determined with more precision, at least in the absence of significant myocardial disease, by examination of the unipolar morphology; the absence of a QS pattern is strongly correlated with lack of ablation success. Unipolar electrograms also provide useful adjunctive mapping information to bipolar electrograms during mapping for focal ATs and VTs. Amerendral et al.[39] noted that the presence of a QS complex was highly sensitive in identifying successful ablation sites. However, almost 70% of unsuccessful sites also manifested a QS unipolar complex, with QS complexes being recorded more than 1 cm away in 65% of patients.[40] The unipolar electrogram morphology with standard ablation electrodes is therefore a highly sensitive but nonspecific marker for target sites in patients with idiopathic right ventricular (RV)

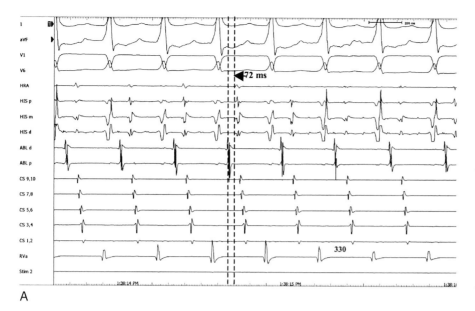

A

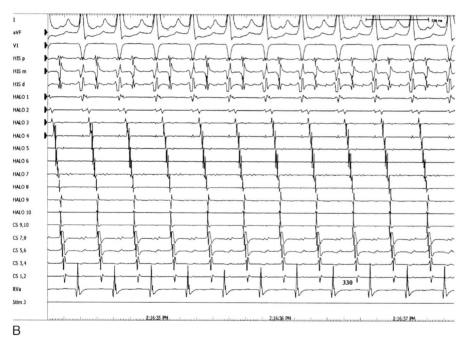

B

FIGURE 7-8. Apparent atrial tachycardia with sites that had greater than 50 msec presystolic activation times in a patient with no known atrial disease. The P wave morphology and cycle length suggested that atrial tachycardia rather than atrial flutter was present. However, the mid-diastolic activation times suggested reentry rather than focal tachycardia. **A,** Mapping with the ablation catheter revealed electrograms in and around the tricuspid annulus that were more than 50 msec presystolic, thereby raising suspicion for a reentrant tachycardia. **B,** A halo catheter inserted subsequently showed an activation sequence consistent with clockwise, isthmus-dependent atrial tachycardia/flutter. Entrainment maneuvers confirmed the diagnosis and led to successful ablation of the arrhythmia.

tachycardia and other VTs as well as ATs. However, unipolar electrograms are of limited utility in the setting of myocardial scar or fibrosis, because the criteria established for unipolar activation (i.e., peak maximum negative slope [dV/dt]), cannot be relied on in the presence of slow, disordered conduction. The initial deflection in unipolar recordings in this setting frequently shows a delayed initial deflection.

Much has been written about the utility of the unipolar electrogram in localizing sites of insertion and successful ablation for accessory pathways (APs),[41] It must be remembered, however, that most of these data are for anterograde mapping in the setting of overt preexcitation, although some investigators have demonstrated the utility of unipolar mapping for retrogradely conducting APs.[42] Electrograms characteristic of the insertion sites of APs are described in Chapter 20.

PACE MAPPING

Pace mapping involves manipulation of the mapping catheter to the region of origin of the tachycardia. Pacing at this site, using the same cycle length as the

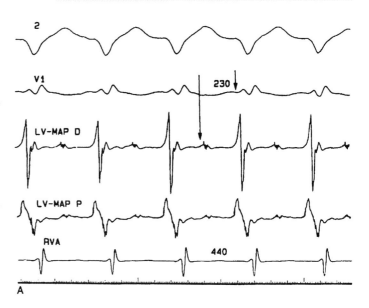

FIGURE 7–9. Activation mapping in a diseased heart. The figure shows mid-diastolic potentials in the setting of infracted-related ventricular tachycardia (VT). Leads 2 and V1 are shown with distal (D) and proximal (P) bipolar signals recorded from a presumed protected isthmus of the VT circuit. An isolated mid-diastolic potential (long arrow) is recorded 230 msec before the QRS during VT (short arrow), with a cycle length of 440 msec. *(From Josephson ME, Clinical Cardiac Electrophysiology: Techniques and Interpretation, 3rd ed. Philadelphia: Lippincott Williams & Wilkins, 2002, with permission.)*

tachycardia, should generate P waves or QRS complexes resembling those observed during tachycardia. The greater the degree of concordance between the P wave or QRS morphology during pacing and the tachycardia, the closer the catheter is to the site of exit of the tachycardia.

Pace mapping has advantages over activation mapping in that induction of arrhythmia is not required; as a result, it allows identification of the site of origin when the induced arrhythmia is poorly tolerated or when VT is not inducible by electrophysiologic techniques but P wave or QRS morphology from a 12-lead ECG is available. However, others have argued that pace mapping is not as sensitive as activation mapping and may be more time-consuming. Pace mapping has been more useful as a means of localizing sites, with a combination of activation and pace-mapping being used to best identify the optimal target site of ablation.

Most investigators report successful ablation at sites with identical or near-identical matches in all 12 surface leads.[43,44] Differences in QRS configuration between pacing and spontaneous tachycardia in a single lead can be critical. An example is shown in Figure 7–10, where ablation success was achieved (in the left coronary cusp) only at the site of a 12/12 or perfect pacemap.

The use of single ECG leads or body surface mapping may improve the precision of pace mapping.[45] Kadish et al.[46] examined the spatial resolution of unipolar pacing with respect to the degree of pacemap matching and found that, under optimal conditions—that is, when minor differences in configuration (e.g., notching, new small component,

change in amplitude of individual component, overall change in QRS shape) in at least one lead were accounted for—the spatial resolution of an exact pacemap match may be less than 5 mm. Bipolar pacing may introduce additional variability in the ventricular-paced ECG, but these changes may be minimized by low pacing outputs and small interelectrode distances (≤ 5 mm) or unipolar pacing.[46] Pace mapping should be performed as close as possible to the cycle length of the spontaneous tachycardia in order to minimize rate-dependent aberration in paced P-wave or QRS configurations caused by increasing degrees of incomplete repolarization and fusion with the preceding T wave during shorter cycle lengths.[47]

Pace mapping during sinus rhythm has been shown to be less sensitive in the setting of scarred myocardium; even if pacing is performed close to the tachycardia circuit, the activation wavefront may take the path of least resistance: instead of mimicking the tachycardia wavefront (through the protected tachycardia isthmus), it may activate normal myocardium first, thereby creating a very different pacemap. In addition, the boundaries of a protected isthmus may be functional in nature, and therefore they may be difficult to replicate with pacing during sinus rhythm. More recently, however, several investigators have shown that pace mapping can be performed at the infarct border[48] with good sensitivity and specificity and can provide successful target sites for ablation based on the closeness of the pacemap to the tachycardia and the stimulus-to-QRS interval (helping outline the critical isthmus from entrance to exit) (Fig. 7–11).

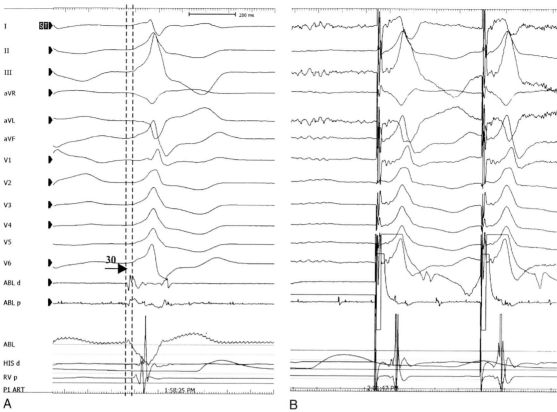

FIGURE 7–10. Excellent pacemap in a patient with right-bundle inferior axis premature ventricular contractions (PVCs). **A,** Right-bundle PVCs mapped to the left coronary cusp. The ablation catheter shows an activation time that was 30 msec presystolic. The distal unipolar electrogram coincides with the earliest bipolar electrogram. Note that the unipolar electrogram (ABL) has a small r wave before the inscription of the QS. **B,** Pace mapping performed at the site shown in **A** revealed a 12/12 match with the PVC in **A.** It was decided to ablate at this site, because activation sites with a QS pattern on the unipolar electrogram (i.e., no r wave) were less than 0.5 cm from the left main artery. Ablation resulted in termination of PVCs.

ENTRAINMENT MAPPING

Entrainment is one of the most powerful tools in the electrophysiologist's arsenal that serves the following purposes: (1) allows confirmation of reentry as the underlying mechanism of a sustained arrhythmia, (2) allows localization of an underlying reentrant circuit (e.g., to the right or left atrium in the setting of a reentrant AT), and (3) allows localization of a portion of myocardium that is critical to the sustenance of a reentrant circuit (i.e., critical isthmus). The critical isthmus may be narrow enough to be amenable to ablation, with resulting interruption of the tachycardia.[49] A full discussion of resetting curves, entrainment criteria, and the pitfalls of entrainment is beyond the scope of this chapter; the reader is referred to other authoritative texts for a more in depth study of the principles of entrainment.[49-52]

The delivery of progressively premature single atrial premature contractions (APCs) during an AT or ventricular premature contractions (VPCs) during a VT (and the resulting return tachycardia cycle length)

allows the construction of a resetting curve: a decreasing curve supports a triggered mechanism, with flat, increasing, and mixed curves being more typical of reentrant tachycardias.[53] Entrainment is continuous resetting of a reentrant circuit with an excitable gap by a series of stimuli. If pacing at a rate faster than the tachycardia cycle length accelerates all P waves or QRS complexes (or intracardiac electrograms) to the pacing rate, and termination of pacing is followed by resumption of the same tachycardia, then the presence of constant surface or intracardiac fusion during pacing (or progressive fusion during pacing at progressively faster cycle lengths) establishes the presence of entrainment. There are four criteria for manifest entrainment:

1. Constant fusion during overdrive pacing except for the last captured beat, which is entrained but not fused.
2. Progressive fusion during overdrive pacing.
3. Localized conduction block to a site (or sites) for one paced beat associated with interruption of the

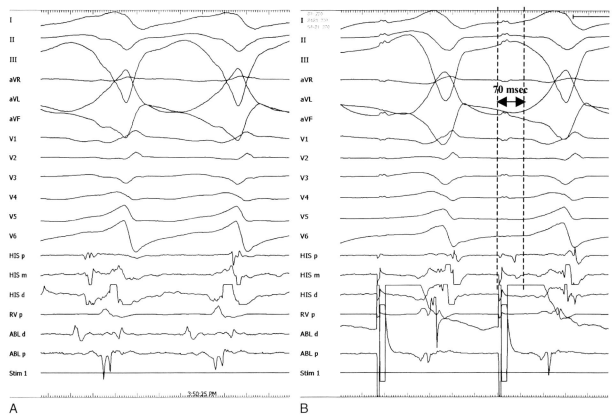

A   **B**

FIGURE 7–11. Pace mapping in the setting of myocardial scar. **A,** Ventricular tachycardia (cycle length, 260 msec). **B,** Pace mapping in a region of scar (low-amplitude potentials) in the right ventricle of a patient with arrhythmogenic right ventricular dysplasia. Note the long 12/12 pacemap and the long, mid-diastolic stimulus-to-QRS interval (70 msec); the stimulus-to-QRS interval was suggestive of a location in the middle of a protected isthmus. Ablation in this region rendered the ventricular tachycardia noninducible.

tachycardia, followed by activation of that site by the next paced beat from a different direction and with a shorter conduction time.

4. During pacing at two different rates during a tachycardia, there is a change in conduction time to and electromyographic morphology at an electrode recording site (this is the intracardiac equivalent of criterion 2, because surface criteria may be difficult to visualize on occasion, as in AT).

Figure 7–12 shows an example of manifest entrainment (based on intracardiac electrograms); activation around the tricuspid annulus is shown during overdrive pacing of what appeared to be typical, counterclockwise atrial flutter in a patient with a normal heart. Pacing at progressively faster rates demonstrates progressive fusion (one of the diagnostic criteria for entrainment) and therefore reentry, which is best demonstrated by a change in activation (as well as timing) of the bipolar electrograms in the distal halo electrodes. Even if changes in timing are subtle, electrogram morphology may provide important clues to a diagnosis.

Once entrainment has been demonstrated (i.e., "manifest" entrainment), it can be used for mapping. Entrainment mapping is centered on obtaining a "match" between the entrained surface P wave or QRS complex and/or intracardiac electrograms and tachycardia morphology ("concealed" entrainment, discussed later), as well as on obtaining a postpacing interval (PPI; described later) that is equal to the tachycardia cycle length. Whereas the demonstration of resetting with fusion (or manifest entrainment) confirms reentry, the presence of concealed entrainment allows the ablationist to "home in" on a protected isthmus—a frequent site of ablation success. Concealed entrainment is characterized by a failure to demonstrate fusion (i.e., criteria 1, 2, and 4) during pacing from a particular site within or outside a circuit. Typically, pacing from a protected isthmus within a tachycardia circuit (Fig. 7–13) is also associated with a PPI that is equal to the tachycardia cycle length. The PPI is the time between the last pacing stimulus that entrained the tachycardia and the next recorded electrogram at the pacing site. The PPI should be equal to the tachycardia cycle length

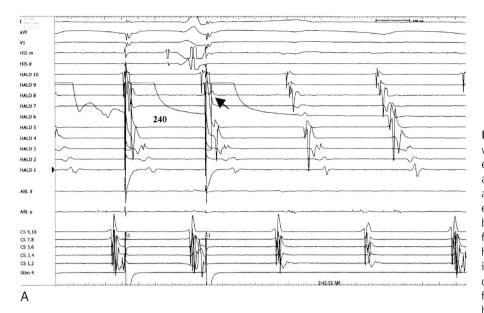

A

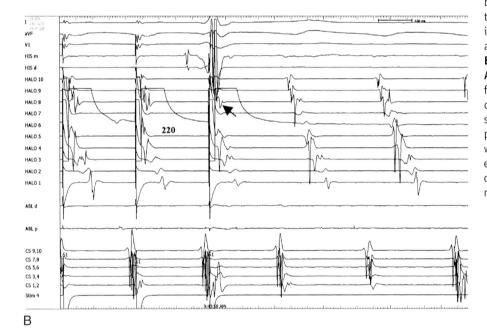

B

FIGURE 7–12. Progression fusion with demonstration of (manifest) entrainment. The figure shows activation around the tricuspid annulus during attempted entrainment of what appeared to be typical, counterclockwise atrial flutter in a patient with a normal heart. **A,** Pacing from halo 6 that is slightly faster than the tachycardia (entrainment) reveals fusion along the halo catheter; halo 7 is captured antidromically, but the rest of the halo is captured orthodromically (no change in activation sequence or polarity along the halo except in halo 7). **B,** Pacing 20 msec faster than in **A** demonstrates progressive fusion: now halo 7 and halo 8 are captured antidromically (*arrows* show clear change in timing and polarity of halo 8 in **B** compared with **A**), thereby confirming entrainment (based on intracardiac fusion, the fourth entrainment criterion).

(within 20 to 30 msec) if the pacing site is within a critical part of the reentrant circuit. If the pacing site is outside the circuit, the PPI should be equal to the tachycardia cycle length plus the time required for the stimulus to propagate from the pacing site to the tachycardia circuit and back.

The protected isthmus may be relatively wide, as in subeustachian isthmus-dependent flutter, which may be seen even in the absence of significant structural heart disease. Most other reentrant atrial flutters or tachycardia are seen in the setting of considerable structural heart disease (e.g., repaired congenital heart defects) and are characterized by low-amplitude, high-frequency, mid-diastolic activity not unlike that seen in scar-related reentrant VT. Of note,

even in the setting of congenital heart disease repair (e.g., Fontan repair, Mustard repair), the most common flutter seen is typical, isthmus-dependent flutter.

Entrainment in the Setting of Myocardial Scar

Chapter 27 describes diastolic potentials in detail (e.g., timing in relation to the entrance or exit site of an isthmus, influence of bystander sites). Important measurements to remember are the electrogram-to-QRS (or P-wave) intervals during tachycardia and the pacing stimulus-to-QRS (or P-wave) and PPIs during entrainment mapping. Although entrainment and pace-mapping criteria are best established for the

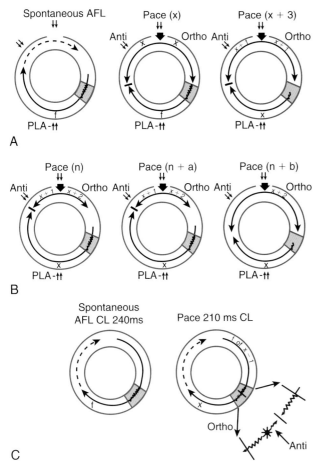

FIGURE 7–13. Manifest and concealed entrainment of atrial flutter. The figure shows schematic diagrams of manifest and concealed entrainment respectively. **A** and **B** demonstrate fixed and progressive fusion, respectively, with overdrive pacing during tachycardia; the contribution of the antidromic wavefront to the tachycardia morphology progressively increases. **C** represents concealed fusion—that is, progressively faster pacing from a protected isthmus does not lead to manifest fusion, because the antidromic wavefront does not contribute significantly to the morphology of the tachycardia beat. Shaded areas = protected isthmus. *(Modified from Waldo AL: Atrial flutter: Entrainment characteristics. J Cardiovasc Electrophysiol 8:337-352, 1997, with permission.)* AFL, atrial flutter; CL, cycle length; x, pacing stimulus in a sequence of stimuli; n, pacing cycle lengths with n > n + a > n + b; anti, antidromic; ortho, orthodromic; PLA, postero-inferior left artium.

surface ECG during VT mapping, multiple intracardiac electrograms should be examined to fulfill the same criteria during macroreentrant AT (because the P-wave is small and is frequently obscured during pace mapping). Standard catheters (quadripolar, decapolar, duodecapolar) allow intracardiac recording from 1 to 20 sites at a time. In the right atrium, we typically use a 20-pole halo catheter and a His catheter; a coronary sinus catheter is helpful to examine activation sequences in the left atrium, although it may be limited in its utility for the study

of activation of the anterior and superior aspects of the left atrium. More detailed pace and entrainment mapping in the right or left atrium can be performed with a 64-electrode "basket" catheter (Boston Scientific, San Jose, Calif.).

MISCELLANEOUS PACING MANEUVERS

Atrial or ventricular pacing during sinus rhythm or during tachycardia is a useful maneuver for determining the mechanism of a tachycardia and may also help in mapping a tachycardia.

Response to Atrial or Ventricular Pacing

We perform overdrive ventricular pacing in an attempt to demonstrate entrainment in the setting of a narrow-complex supraventricular tachycardia (SVT) with a concentric retrograde activation sequence. In this setting, we perform ventricular pacing (entrainment) as a diagnostic maneuver to differentiate among atrioventricular nodal reentrant tachycardia (AVNRT), atrioventricular reentrant tachycardia (AVRT), and AT. We pace 10 to 30 msec faster than the tachycardia cycle length for at least 8 to 10 beats, to allow continuous resetting of the atrial rate to occur. The atrial activation sequence of the tachycardia must remain unchanged during orthodromic capture of an AVRT or reentrant AT circuit as well as during AVNRT; the latter is a microreentrant circuit in which fusion cannot be seen during pacing—only the third entrainment criterion (outlined earlier) has been used to demonstrate entrainment during AVNRT. If the tachycardia resumes after pacing, we look for a ventricle-atrium-ventricle (V-A-V) versus a V-A-A-V response on the return cycle length,[54] with the latter indicating an AT. If a V-A-V response is noted, we proceed to compare the stimulus-to-A interval (and the His-atrium (HA) interval, if a retrograde His signal is visible) during pacing with the ventricle-atrium (VA) (and HA) interval during tachycardia.[54-56] We also measure the PPI and compare it with the tachycardia cycle length,[54] to differentiate between AVRT and AVNRT.[54] Figure 7–14 shows an example each of AVNRT and AVRT in response to ventricular entrainment.

Ventricular pacing can also be performed at the tachycardia cycle length during sinus rhythm, and the diagnostic criteria mentioned earlier (i.e., comparison of VA and HA times during tachycardia and pacing) can be used to differentiate between AVNRT and AVRT.

Another maneuver that may be helpful in deciphering the mechanism of a narrow-complex tachycardia is atrial pacing at the tachycardia cycle length; a comparison of AH times may allow differentiation

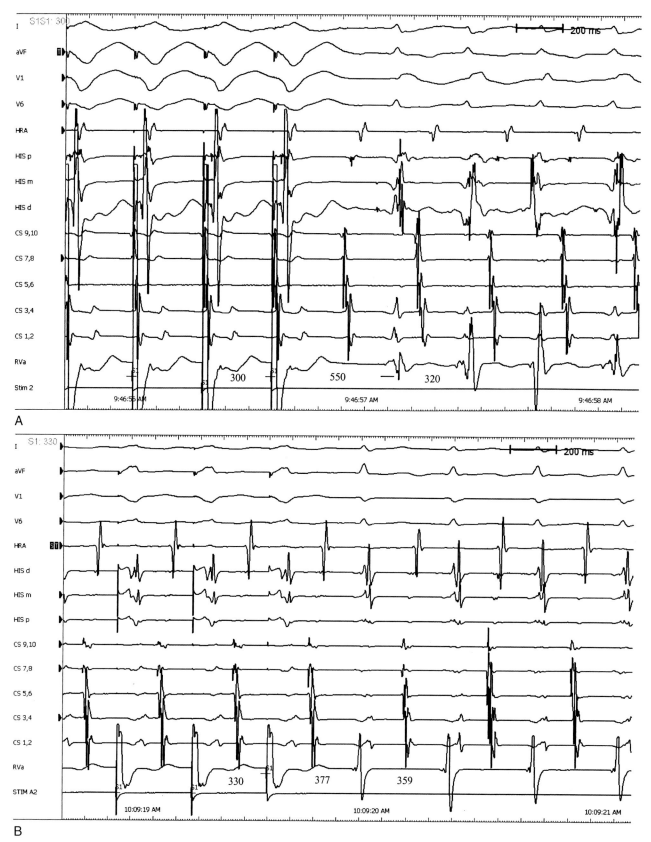

FIGURE 7–14. Entrainment of supraventricular tachycardia. The figure demonstrates the response of atrioventricular nodal reentrant tachycardia (AVNRT) and atrioventricular reentrant tachycardia (AVRT) (with concentric activation sequences) to entrainment from the ventricle. **A,** Entrainment is consistent with AVNRT: the stimulus-to-A interval during ventricular pacing exceeds the VA interval during tachycardia by more than 85 msec. The postpacing interval (PPI) exceeds the tachycardia cycle length by more than 115 msec, also consistent with AVNRT. **B,** Entrainment here is consistent with AVRT, with the difference between the stimulus-to-A interval (during pacing) and the VA interval (during tachycardia) being less than 85 msec and the PPI being approximately equal to the tachycardia cycle length.

between AT, AVNRT, and AVRT. AH intervals during pacing are expected to be similar to those observed during tachycardia (≤ 20 msec), but they are longer during AVRT (difference in AH, 20 to 40 msec) and during AVNRT (difference in AH, ≥40 msec).[57]

PVCs during Narrow-Complex Tachycardia

After determination of the cycle length and the atrial and ventricular sequence of an induced arrhythmia, it is almost standard practice in most laboratories to deliver premature ventricular stimuli at the onset of a sustained, hemodynamically well-tolerated, and regular (i.e., invariable cycle length) tachycardia. Exceptions to this rule include a regular tachycardia with changing VA times, which indicates probable AT, and tachycardias that lack a one-to-one AV association (which exclude AV reentry and making AVNRT unlikely). Single premature ventricular stimuli (PVCs) delivered during His refractoriness are of diagnostic utility if they advance, retard, or terminate the tachycardia—each of these phenomena indicates the presence of a retrogradely conducting AP, and the latter two, if reproducible, confirm the participation of the pathway as the retrograde limb of the tachycardia. Although a PVC on His advancing the atrium with the same retrograde activation

sequence as the tachycardia is highly suggestive of a participating bypass tract, it is by no means diagnostic, and an AT arising from near the insertion of a bypass tract is a remote possibility. Figure 7–15 shows a PVC delivered during His refractoriness. Although no His depolarization is seen, the presence of ECG fusion during the PVC confirms anterograde His depolarization, thereby indicating His refractoriness. More premature PVCs (more than 30 msec before the next expected His bundle depolarization), delivered close to the site of earliest atrial activation, can be considered diagnostic of the absence of an AP if the atrium is not affected.[58] PVCs that reset the A can also help indicate the presence of an AP if they significantly change the VA; for example, during an SVT with an eccentric retrograde atrial activation, a left-bundle PVC (from the RV apex) that advances the A along with an increase in the VA interval is diagnostic of a left-sided AP.

Termination of Tachycardia during Pacing Maneuvers

If a narrow-complex tachycardia terminates during ventricular pacing without any prior change in the atrial cycle length (indicating no depolarization of the atrium by the ventricular stimuli), AT has been

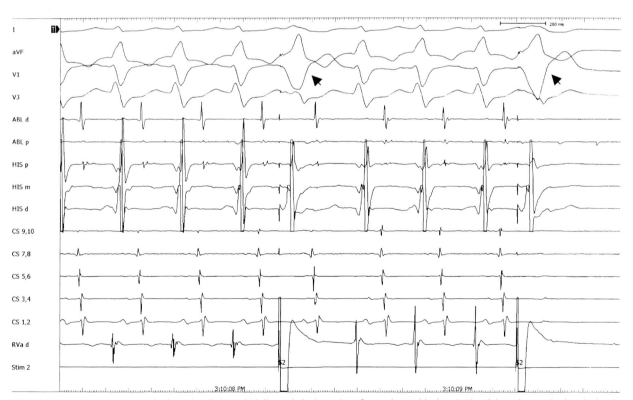

FIGURE 7–15. Premature ventricular stimuli (PVCs) delivered during His refractoriness (during SVT). Although no His depolarization is seen, the presence of electrocardiographic fusion during the first PVC—compared with the second PVC, which closely resembles a fully paced beat during sinus rhythm (not shown here)—confirms anterograde His depolarization, thereby indicating His refractoriness during the first PVC.

excluded as a possible diagnosis (Figue 7–15). (Also see the earlier section on PVCs during narrow-complex tachycardia.)

On occasion, the mode of termination provides valuable information about the location of a protected isthmus in the setting of a scar-related tachycardia. Figure 7–16 shows left ventricular mapping during VT, with mid-diastolic recordings from a site on the anterior wall; pacing at this site showed it to be integral to the VT circuit. A single extrastimulus delivered at this site reproducibly terminated VT without local propagation or depolarization.[59] Moreover, a single extrastimulus delivered at this site during sinus rhythm initiated VT. Radiofrequency energy delivered at this site terminated VT after one beat. This suggests that the ablation catheter tip was positioned in a critical portion of the circuit before tissues in the circuit immediately distal to this site had recovered excitability. The inference is that, because the stimulus did not elicit a QRS complex, it affected cells that were in a protected area, such that (1) a single extrastimulus delivered at that site during sinus rhythm might have only one possible direction of propagation and could initiate VT, and (2) this site would be an excellent ablation target site.

Electrogram Morphology in Response to Pacing

Close observation of electrogram morphology and polarity can also help differentiate between disparate activation pathways during electrophysiologic maneuvers performed in the absence of tachycardia. Bipolar electrogram morphology and polarity during atrial pacing, for example, can be very helpful in targeting successful ablation sites in an otherwise normal, healthy heart in the setting of a reentrant tachycardia (e.g., during typical, isthmus-dependent atrial flutter). Figure 7–17 shows the local bipolar electrogram at a site at which radiofrequency energy was applied with success. Ablation had previously been performed along the isthmus but without resulting in conduction block; the isthmus ablation line was further explored for areas where conduction through the isthmus remained. At one site along the line of block, the electrogram shown in Figure 7–17 was noted; although split, the electrograms were not as far apart as others along the ablation line. A single radiofrequency application at this site (applied during coronary sinus pacing) resulted in further separation of the electrograms (with a change in electrogram polarity for the second component of the

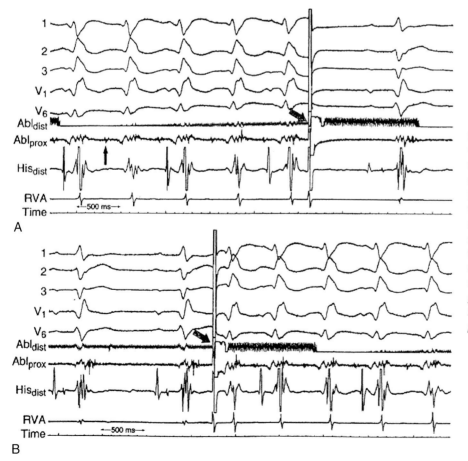

FIGURE 7–16. Termination of ventricular tachycardia (VT) by a nonpropagated extrastimulus. **A,** A single extrastimulus *(arrow)* terminated VT without local propagation. **B,** A single extrastimulus delivered at this site during sinus rhythm initiated VT. See text for discussion. *(From Altemose GT, Miller JM: Termination of ventricular tachycardia by a nonpropagated extrastimulus. J Cardiovasc Electrophysiol 11:125, 2000, with permission.)*

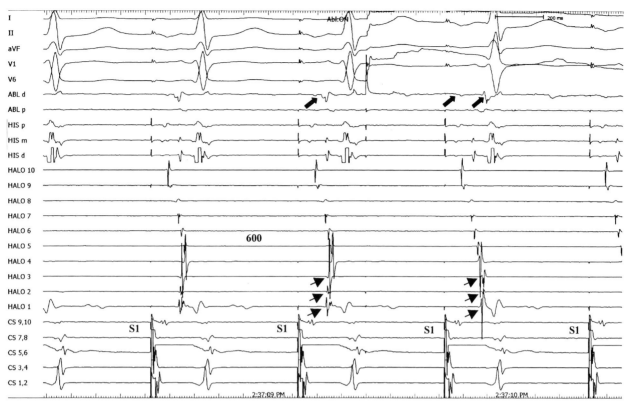

FIGURE 7–17. Reversal of bipolar electrogram polarity with ablation. The figure shows right atrial electrograms from a patient undergoing ablation for typical, isthmus-dependent atrial flutter. Ablation had been performed along the isthmus but without resulting in conduction block. When the isthmus ablation line was further explored for unablated areas, the electrograms shown here were recorded. The *first arrow* highlights the local bipolar electrogram at a 6 o'clock position along the subeustachian isthmus, close to where radiofrequency had been applied previously. Although split, the electrograms were not as far apart here as at other sites along the ablation line. A single radiofrequency application at this site resulted in further separation of the electrograms *(double arrows)*, with a change in electrogram polarity for the second component of the split electrogram, indicating activation from the opposite direction, and evidence of conduction block on the halo catheter.

split electrogram, indicating activation from the opposite direction) and evidence of conduction block on the halo catheter.

More recently, bipolar electrograms have also been found to have utility in mapping the pulmonary veins for ablation of atrial fibrillation. Sites at which the bipolar electrogram changes direction (polarity), thought to indicate breakthroughs from the left atrium into the pulmonary vein, have been found to be predictive for ablation success of a myocardial sleeve (with resulting pulmonary vein isolation from the rest of the atrial myocardium) (Fig. 7–18).[60]

Activation Sequence during Pacing Maneuvers

Close attention to atrial activation sequence and electrogram polarity during ventricular pacing (in sinus rhythm) can also provide important diagnostic clues to underlying AP and AV nodal physiology—clues that may be helpful, for example, in individualizing ablation strategies. Figure 7–19 shows an example in which subtle changes in electrogram morphology occurred during ventricular pacing in the presence of a right lateral AP. A cursory look at the activation sequence suggests that fusion may be present in the first three beats (i.e., retrograde activation may progress up the AP and the AV node), because there is no significant change in timing of the high right atrial electrogram (i.e., the VA time between the first three beats, which have a "concentric" retrograde activation sequence, and the subsequent beats, which have an "eccentric" retrograde sequence). However, the near-reversal of polarity of the distal high right atrial electrogram in the fourth and fifth beats suggests that retrograde activation is solely up the AV node for the first three beats and solely up the AP for the fourth and fifth beats. Detailed assessment of atrial and AV AP activation direction using bipolar mapping was performed by Damle et al.,[61] who showed that vector mapping (performed by summing three orthogonally oriented bipolar electrograms) can help accurately localize AP insertion sites.

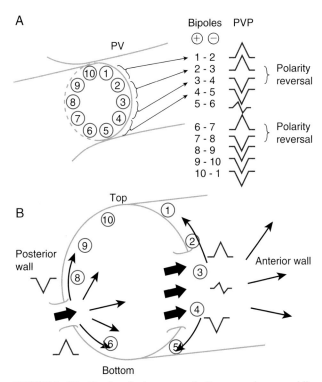

FIGURE 7–18. Bipolar electrogram polarity reversal as an additional indicator of breakthroughs from the left atrium to the pulmonary veins. **A,** Schematic representation of the circular mapping catheter with 10 electrodes. Pulmonary vein (PV) muscle potentials were recorded at the proximal PV in bipolar mode from 10 bipoles. Polarity reversal was defined as a sudden change of the main deflection of pulmonary vein potential (PVP) from positive to negative when analyzing adjacent bipoles in ascending order. **B,** Schematic diagram of radial propagation of activation fronts from two different breakthroughs in the left superior PV. The numbers positioned at the ostium of the vein represent the 10 electrodes of the circular mapping catheter. There are two distinct breakthroughs, at both the anterior and posterior aspect of the vein. Radial propagation of the activation front through one breakthrough (posterior wall) is reflected by an electrogram polarity reversal across the adjacent two bipoles (6 to 7 and 7 to 8). In the case of wider breakthrough (anterior wall), an electrogram polarity reversal is observed across three consecutive bipoles (2 to 3, 3 to 4, and 4 to 5), with the intervening bipole (3 to 4) showing relatively isoelectric initial deflection. *(From Yamane T, Shah DC, Jais P, et al.: Electrogram polarity reversal as an additional indicator of breakthroughs from the left atrium to the pulmonary veins. J Am Coll Cardiol 39:1337-1344, 2002, with permission.)*

Even if directional information is not present on a single bipolar electrogram (e.g., a high-frequency recording such as the His-bundle electrogram, analysis of the electrogram when performed in the presence of its "neighboring" electrograms may indicate the direction of activation. Figure 7–20 provides an example of retrograde His bundle activation, as shown by the distal-to-proximal activation of the His bundle potential with a ventricular extrastimulus

(seen clearly due to retrograde right bundle branch block with a prolonged VH time), as opposed to proximal-to-distal or antegrade activation during sinus rhythm. Knowledge of the direction of activation of the His bundle electrogram may be extremely helpful in the following:

1. To diagnose bundle branch reentry/reentrant beats.
2. To confirm validity of diagnostic maneuvers that rely on anterograde as well as retrograde His activation (e.g., comparison of HA intervals during SVT with those obtained during ventricular pacing or entrainment, in order to differentiate AVNRT from AVRT).[56]
3. To identify disparate pathways of activation during ventricular pacing (e.g., retrograde conduction up an AP versus the normal conduction system). Further analysis of the timing of the retrograde His bundle and atrial recordings (in relation to ventricular capture and to one another) also provides information about delay or blockade in a bundle branch, activation up the fast (versus the slow) AV nodal pathway, and so on (Fig. 7–21).

A caveat to the statements just made is that if the His-bundle catheter lies perpendicular to the underlying His bundle, directional information may be lost. If more sensitive His-bundle mapping is desired, a higher-density mapping electrode (with more closely spaced electrodes) may be required.

Parahisian pacing is of utility in differentiating between a retrogradely conducting septal pathway and the AV node (Fig. 7–22). When direct His-bundle capture is obtained, retrograde conduction can occur rapidly over the AV node if retrograde septal conduction is present.[62] In contrast, if conduction is proceeding only up an AP, His-bundle capture does not alter the VA interval. Therefore, a retrogradely conducting septal pathway can be identified by the presence of a fixed VA interval regardless of capture. Retrograde fusion complicates this finding. Shortening of the VA interval may occur if retrograde conduction is proceeding up both the AV node and an AP. In such a case, examination for closely spaced atrial recording sites can help identify a change in activation sequence that occurs when His-bundle capture shortens the VA interval.

Figure 7–23 shows an instance in which parahisian pacing may be fraught with error, with retrograde activation being different for ventricular versus combined (i.e., ventricular and His-bundle) capture pacing. Ventricular pacing alone causes a longer VA interval, because conduction is over a posteroseptal pathway that conducts more slowly than the AV node, although some AV nodal conduction (i.e., fusion) cannot be ruled out in the His bundle

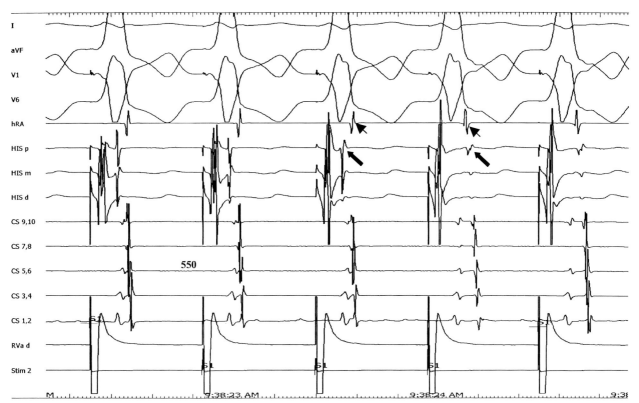

FIGURE 7–19. Reversal of polarity in high right atrial (HRA) bipolar electrogram with a change in retrograde activation sequence during ventricular pacing. Subtle changes in electrogram morphology are noted during ventricular pacing (at 550 msec) in the presence of a right lateral accessory pathway. The first three beats suggest that activation is up the AV node, whereas the fourth and later beats show a change in activation sequence, with the HRA now being earliest, suggesting retrograde activation up a right-sided accessory pathway. Although the stimulus-to-atrium time in the HRA is approximately the same for both activation sequences, suggesting that fusion up the AV node and accessory pathway may be occurring during the first three beats, the polarity of the HRA electrogram changes with the second activation sequence. This suggests that retrograde activation for the first three beats is entirely up the AV node, whereas activation for the fourth and subsequent beats is entirely up the accessory pathway. HRA, high right atrium.

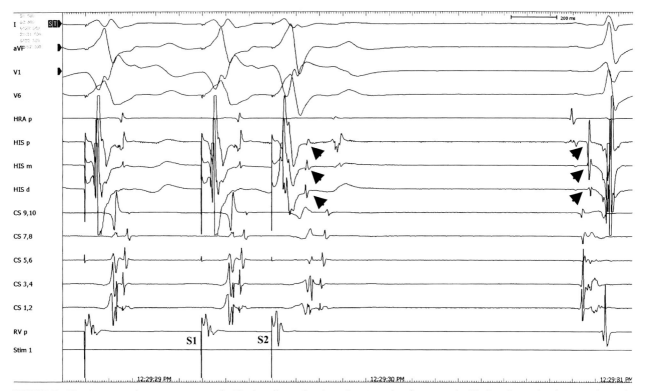

FIGURE 7–20. Anterograde versus retrograde His bundle activation. An example of retrograde His bundle activation, as shown by the distal(d)-to-proximal(p) activation of the His bundle potential *(first set of arrows)* with a ventricular extrastimulus (seen clearly due to retrograde right bundle branch block with a prolonged VH time), as opposed to proximal-to-distal or anterograde activation during sinus rhythm *(second set of arrows)*.

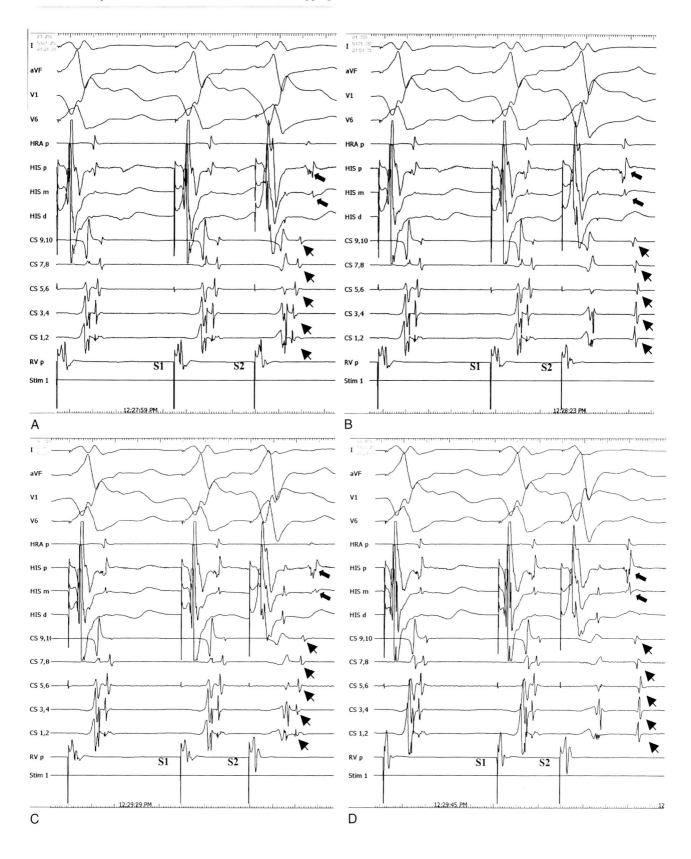

FIGURE 7–21. Changes in retrograde activation sequence with ventricular pacing in a patient with a left lateral accessory pathway. Retrograde activation from the ventricular drive train appears to be fusion up the atrioventricular (AV) node and the accessory pathway. The VA time in the His bundle is shorter, because the His is probably within the early portion of the QRS. Multiple activation sequences are detected by ventricular extrastimulus testing. In the same patient as in Figure 7–12, disparate pathways of activation with single ventricular extrastimulus testing are shown. **A,** Change in atrial activation in the His channel and in coronary sinus (CS) 9, 10 (with a change in polarity in the latter) with the ventricular extrastimulus, with retrograde atrial activation appearing to go entirely up a left-sided accessory pathway. Note that a His deflection can be seen after the ventricular depolarization, suggesting retrograde right bundle branch block (due to the premature extrastimulus) with activation up the left bundle branch. **B,** With a more premature extrastimulus, the VH prolongs further; this is accompanied by a further increase in the VA time in the His recording channels, although the HA time remains unchanged. The atrial activation in the CS has now changed and is more concentric, suggesting activation up the AV node (i.e., block in the accessory pathway). **C,** With a still more premature extrastimulus, there is conduction up the accessory pathway again (with a change in polarity in the CS electrograms); the timing and polarity of the His and HRA electrograms remains unchanged again, with the HA being constant. The retrograde activation represents fusion up the accessory pathway and the AV node. **D,** A further increase in prematurity of the extrastimulus results in block in the accessory pathway once again. There is a further increase in the VH time, with the VA time increasing accordingly (i.e., constant HA), indicating activation up the AV node.

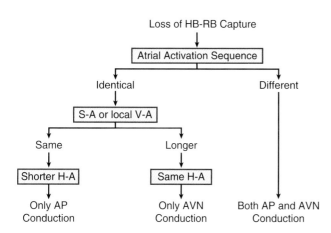

FIGURE 7–22. Schematic for use in parahisian pacing to differentiate retrograde conduction over an accessory pathway from retrograde conduction over the atrioventricular (AV) node. AP, accessory pathway; AVN, atrioventricular node; H-A, interval from His bundle to atrial signal; HB, His bundle; RB, right bundle; S-A, interval from stimulus to atrial signal; V-A, interval from ventricular to atrial signal. *(From Hirao K, Otomo K, Wang X, et al.: Para-hisian pacing: A new method for differentiating retrograde conduction over an accessory AV pathway from conduction over the AV node. Circulation 94:1027-1035, 1996, with permission.)*

recording. Combined His bundle and ventricular capture causes conduction to proceed up the AV node, but with a shorter VA time (and a different activation sequence than when retrograde conduction is over the AP).

Wide-Complex Supraventricular Tachycardia

Once a wide-complex tachycardia with 1:1 AV association has been induced, the surface ECG characteristics as well as the intracardiac intervals and activation sequence should be examined to differentiate VT from SVT. Unless proven otherwise, a typical right or left bundle-branch block appearance represents SVT with aberrancy. Moreover, the HV interval during an aberrant tachycardia is equal to or greater than that observed during non-preexcited sinus rhythm. An obviously preexcited tachycardia (the diagnosis of which is aided by the presence of similar preexcitation during sinus rhythm, a short or negative HV interval) is best approached with single APCs delivered during His refractoriness (i.e., delivered so that the atrial depolarization in the His recording is not affected by the APC). As with PVCs during His refractoriness, an APC that retards the next ventricular activation (or terminates tachycardia without ventricular depolarization) is diagnostic of a participating AP. An APC that advances the ventricle with no change in ventricular/QRS activation and that also resets that tachycardia is also strongly suggestive of a participating pathway. Other maneuvers described earlier for a narrow-complex tachycardia can also be used for a preexcited tachycardia; for example, a comparison of HA intervals can help differentiate between antidromic tachycardia and AVNRT with a bystander AP.[63] The HV interval can be extremely valuable in differentiating the tachycardia mechanism in the presence of an atriofascicular pathway; this is explained in greater detail in related chapters elsewhere in this text.

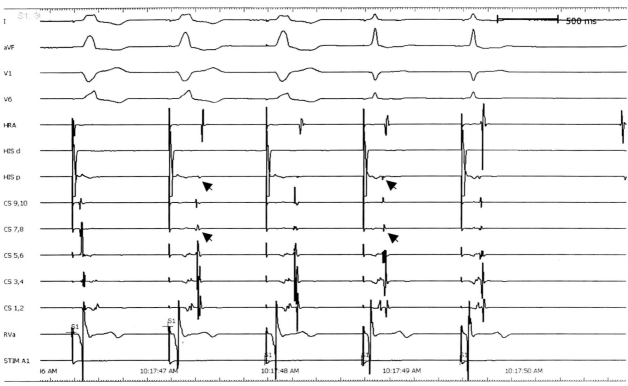

FIGURE 7-23. Parahisian pacing. Parahisian pacing is performed in a patient with a known posteroseptal pathway, with retrograde activation being different with ventricular versus combined (i.e., ventricular and His-bundle capture) pacing. The first arrow shows ventricular pacing (wider QRS) with a longer VA time, whereas the second arrow shows His bundle as well as ventricular capture (narrower QRS) with a shorter VA time. Note, however, that the retrograde activation sequence with the first beat is earliest in the proximal coronary sinus (CS) and with the second beat it is earliest at the AV junction. Conduction in the former instance is up a slowly conducting posteroseptal pathway, although some AV nodal conduction (i.e., fusion) cannot be ruled out in the His bundle recording; in the latter instance, conduction is up the AV node alone. See text for discussion.

References

1. Rudy Y, Luo CH: A dynamic model of the cardiac ventricular action potential. I: Simulations of ionic currents and concentration changes. Circ Res 74:1097-113, 1994.
2. Josephson ME: Clinical Cardiac Electrophysiology: Techniques and Interpretation, 3rd ed. Philadelphia: Lippincott Williams & Wilkins, 2002.
3. Murgatroyd FD, Krahn A: Handbook of Cardiac Electrophysiology: A Practical Guide to Invasive EP Studies and Catheter Ablation. London: ReMedica, 2002.
4. Roberts DE, Hersh LT, Scher AM: Influence of cardiac fiber orientation on wavefront voltage, conduction velocity, and tissue resistivity in the dog. Circ Res 44:701-712, 1979.
5. Witkowski FX, et al.: In Shenasa M, Borggrefe M, Breithardt G (eds.): Cardiac Mapping. Mount Kisco, N.Y.: Futura, 1993, pp 79-84.
6. Green LS, Taccardi B, Ersler PR, Lux RL: Epicardial potential mapping: Effects of conducting media on isopotential and isochrone distributions. Circulation 84:2513-2521,1991.
7. Lewis T, Rothschild MA: The excitatory process in the dog's heart. Part II: The ventricles. Philos Trans R Soc Lond (Biol) 206B:181-226, 1915.
8. Wilson FN, Johnston FD, Maclecd AG, Barker PS: Electrocardiograms that represent the potential variations of a single electrode. Am Heart J 9: 447-458, 1934.
9. Gallagher JJ, Kasell J, Sealy WC, Pritchett EL, Wallace AG: Epicardial mapping in the Wolff-Parkinson-White syndrome. Circulation 57:854-866, 1978.
10. Scher AM, Young AC: Ventricular depolarization and the genesis of the QRS. Ann N Y Acad Sci 65:768-778, 1957.
11. Kupersmith J: Electrophysiologic mapping during open heart surgery. Prog Cardiovasc Dis 19:167-202, 1976.
12. Durrer D, Van der Tweel LH: Excitation of the left ventricular wall of the dog and goat. Ann N Y Acad Sci 65:779-803, 1957.
13. Spach MS, Barr RC, Serwer GA, et al.: Extracellular potentials related to intracellular action potentials in the dog Purkinje system. Circ Res 30:505-519, 1972.
14. Gallagher JJ, Kasell JH, Cox JL, et al.: Techniques of intraoperative electrophysiologic mapping. Am J Cardiol 49:221-240, 1982.
15. Durrer D, Van Der Tweel LH: The spread of the activation in the left ventricular wall of the dog: I. Am Heart J 46:683-691, 1953.
16. Ideker RE, Smith WM, Blanchard SM, et al.: The assumptions of isochronal cardiac mapping. Pacing Clin Electrophysiol 12:456-478, 1989.
17. Biermann M: Precision and reproducibility of Cardiac mapping. In Shenasa M, Borggrefe M, Breithardt G (eds.): Cardiac Mapping, 2nd ed. Elmsford, N.Y.: Futura/Blackwell Publishing, 2003, pp 157-186.

18. Scher AM, Young AC, Malmgren AL, et al.: Spread of electrical activity through the wall of ventricle. Circ Res 1:539-574, 1953.
19. Cassidy DM, Vassallo JA, Marchlinski FE, et al.: Endocardial mapping in humans in sinus rhythm with normal left ventricles: Activation patterns and characteristics of electrograms. Circulation 70:37-42, 1984.
20. Yasuda T, Tojo H, Noguchi H, et al.: Pulmonary vein electrogram characteristics in patients with focal sources of paroxysmal atrial fibrillation. Pacing Clin Electrophysiol 23:1823-1827, 2000.
21. Haissaguerre M, et al.: Role of rapid focal activation in the maintenance of atrial fibrillation originating from the pulmonary veins. Pacing Clin Electrophysiol 23:1828-1831, 2000.
22. Chen PS, Wu TJ, Hwang C, et al.: Thoracic veins and the mechanisms of non-paroxysmal atrial fibrillation. Cardiovasc Res 54:295-301, 2002.
23. Kalman JM, Olgin JE, Karch MR, et al.: "Cristal tachycardias": Origin of right atrial tachycardias from the crista terminalis identified by intracardiac echocardiography. J Am Coll Cardiol 31:451-459, 1998.
24. Arora R, Verheule S, Navarrete A, Vaz DG, Olgin JE: Effects of autonomic stimulation on the electrophysiology of the pulmonary vein and venoatrial junction. Pacing Clin Electrophysiol 24:550, 2001.
25. Miller JM, Olgin JE, Das MK: Atrial fibrillation: What are the targets for intervention? J Interv Card Electrophysiol 9:249-257, 2003.
26. Arora R, Verheule S, Scott L, et al.: Arrhythmogenic substrate of the pulmonary veins assessed by high-resolution optical mapping. Circulation 107:1816-1821, 2003.
27. Wen MS, Yeh SJ, Wang CC, et al.: Successful radiofrequency ablation of idiopathic left ventricular tachycardia at a site away from the tachycardia exit. J Am Coll Cardiol 30:1024-1031,1997.
28. Stevenson WG, Wiss JN, Wiener I, et al.: Fractionated endocardial electrograms are associated with slow conduction in humans: Evidence from pace-mapping. J Am Coll Cardiol 13:369-376, 1989.
29. Lacroix D, Savard P, Shenasa M, et al.: Spatial domain analysis of late ventricular potentials: Intraoperative and thoracic correlations. Circ Res 66:55-68, 1990.
30. Ursell PC, Gardner PI, Albala A, et al.: Structural and electrophysiological changes in the epicardial border zone of canine myocardial infarcts during infarct healing. Circ Res 56:436-451, 1985.
31. Spear JF, Michelson EL, Moore EN: Cellular electrophysiologic characteristics of chronically infarcted myocardium in dogs susceptible to sustained ventricular tachyarrhythmias. J Am Coll Cardiol 1:1099-1110, 1983.
32. Kadish AH, Spear JF, Levine JH, et al.: Vector mapping of myocardial activation. Circulation 74:603-615, 1986.
33. Kadish A, Balke CW, Levine JF, Moore EN, Spear JF: Activation patterns in healed experimental myocardial infarction. Circ Res 65(6):1698-1709, 1989.
34. Van Hare GF, Lesh MD, Ross BA, et al.: Mapping and radiofrequency ablation of intraatrial reentrant tachycardia after the Senning or Mustard procedure for transposition of the great arteries. Am J Cardiol 77:985-991, 1996.
35. Markowitz SM, Brodman RF, Stein KM, et al.: Lesional tachycardias related to mitral valve surgery. J Am Coll Cardiol 39:1973-1983, 2002.
36. Kinoshita O, Fontaine G, Rosas F, et al.: Time- and frequency-domain analyses of the signal-averaged ECG in patients with arrhythmogenic right ventricular dysplasia. Circulation 91:715-721, 1995.
37. Cassidy DM, Vassallo JA, Buxton AE, et al.: The value of catheter mapping during sinus rhythm to localize site of origin of ventricular tachycardia. Circulation 69:1103-1110, 1984.
38. Bogun F, Groenefeld G, et al.: Characteristics of critical reentry sites of postinfarct hemodynamically stable ventricular tachycardia during sinus rhythm. Pacing Clin Electrophysiol 24:726, 2001.
39. Amerandral J, Peinado R: Radiofrequency catheter ablation of idiopathic right ventricular outflow tract tachycardia. In Farre J, Moro C (eds.): Ten Years of Radiofrequency Catheter Ablation. Armonk, N.Y.: Futura, 1998, pp 249-262.
40. Man KC, Daoud EG, Knight BP, et al.: Accuracy of the unipolar electrogram for identification of the site of origin of ventricular activation. J Cardiovasc Electrophysiol 8:974-979, 1997.
41. Barlow MA, Klein GJ, Simpson CS, et al.: Unipolar electrogram characteristics predictive of successful radiofrequency catheter ablation of accessory pathways. J Cardiovasc Electrophysiol 11:146-154, 2000.
42. Farre J, Martinell J, et al.: Atrial unipolar waveform analysis during retrograde conduction over left-sided accessory atrioventricular pathways. In Brugada P, Wellens H (eds.): Cardiac Arrhythmias: Where Do We Go from Here? Mount Kisco, N.Y.: Futura, 1987, p 243.
43. Klein LS, Shih HT, Hackett FK, et al.: Radiofrequency catheter ablation of ventricular tachycardia in patients without structural heart disease. Circulation 85:1666-1674, 1992.
44. Calkins H, Kalbfleisch SJ, el-Atassi R, et al.: Relation between efficacy of radiofrequency catheter ablation and site of origin of idiopathic ventricular tachycardia. Am J Cardiol 71:827-833, 1993.
45. Wilber D: Ablation of idiopathic right ventricular tachycardia. In Huang SKS, Wilber DJ (eds.): Radiofrequency Catheter Ablation of Cardiac Arrhythmias: Basic Concepts and Clinical Applications, 2nd ed. Armonk, N.Y.: Futura/Blackwell Publishing, 2000, pp 621-651.
46. Kadish AH, Childs K, Schmaltz S, Morady F: Differences in QRS configuration during unipolar pacing from adjacent sites: Implications for the spatial resolution of pace-mapping. J Am Coll of Cardiol 17:143-151, 1991.
47. Goyal R, Harvey M, Daoud EG, et al.: Effect of coupling interval and pacing cycle length on morphology of paced ventricular complexes: Implications for pace mapping. Circulation 94:2843-2849, 1996.
48. Brunckhorst CB, Stevenson WG, Soejima K, et al.: Relationship of slow conduction detected by pace-mapping to ventricular tachycardia re-entry circuit sites after infarction. J Am Coll Cardiol 41:802-809, 2003.
49. Stevenson WG, Khan H, Sager P, et al.: Identification of reentry circuit sites during catheter mapping and radiofrequency ablation of ventricular tachycardia late after myocardial infarction. Circulation 88:1647-1670, 1993.
50. Waldo AL: Atrial flutter: Entrainment characteristics. J Cardiovasc Electrophysiol 8:337-352, 1997.
51. Henthorn RW, Okumura K, Olshansky B, et al.: A fourth criterion for transient entrainment: the electrogram equivalent of progressive fusion. Circulation 77:1003-1012, 1988.
52. Waldo AL, Henthorn RW: Use of transient entrainment during ventricular tachycardia to localize a critical area in the reentry circuit for ablation. Pacing Clin Electrophysiol 12:231-244, 1989.
53. Josephson M: Recurrent ventricular tachycardia. In Josephson M (ed.): Clinical Cardiac Electrophysiology: Techniques and Interpretations. Philadelphia: Lippincott Williams & Wilkins, 2002, pp 519-526.
54. Knight BP, Ebinger M, Oral H, et al.: Diagnostic value of tachycardia features and pacing maneuvers during paroxysmal supraventricular tachycardia. J Am Coll Cardiol 36:574-582, 2000.

55. Michaud GF, Tada H, Chough S, et al.: Differentiation of atypical atrioventricular node re-entrant tachycardia from orthodromic reciprocating tachycardia using a septal accessory pathway by the response to ventricular pacing. J Am Coll Cardiol 38:1163-1167, 2001.

56. Miller JM, Rosenthal ME, Gottlieb CD, et al.: Usefulness of the delta HA interval to accurately distinguish atrioventricular nodal reentry from orthodromic septal bypass tract tachycardias. Am J Cardiol 68:1037-1044, 1991.

57. Man KC, Niebauer M, Daoud E, et al.: Comparison of atrial-His intervals during tachycardia and atrial pacing in patients with long RP tachycardia. J Cardiovasc Electrophysiol 6:700-710, 1995.

58. Otomo K, Wang Z, Lazzara R, et al.: Atrioventricular nodal reentrant tachycardia: Electrophysiological characteristics of fours forms and implications for the reentrant circuit. In Zipes DP, Jalife J (eds.): Cardiac Electrophysiology: From Cell to Bedside. Philadelphia: WB Saunders, 2000, pp 504-521.

59. Altemose GT, Miller JM: Termination of ventricular tachycardia by a nonpropagated extrastimulus. J Cardiovasc Electrophysiol 11:125, 2000.

60. Yamane T, Shah DC, Jais P, et al.: Electrogram polarity reversal as an additional indicator of breakthroughs from the left atrium to the pulmonary veins. J Am Coll Cardiol 39:1337-1344, 2002.

61. Damle RS, Choe W, Kanaan NM, et al.: Atrial and accessory pathway activation direction in patients with orthodromic supraventricular tachycardia: Insights from vector mapping. J Am Coll Cardiol 23:684-692, 1994.

62. Hirao K, Otomo K, Wang X, et al.: Para-hisian pacing: A new method for differentiating retrograde conduction over an accessory AV pathway from conduction over the AV node. Circulation 94:1027-1035, 1996.

63. Josephson ME: Preexcitations syndromes. In Josephson M (ed.): Clinical Cardiac Electrophysiology: Techniques and Interpretations. Philadelphia: Lippincott Williams & Wilkins, 2002, pp 338-350.

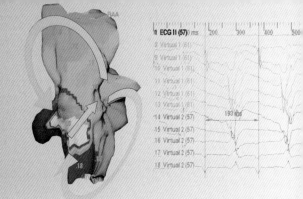

8

Advanced Catheter Mapping and Navigation Systems

Sam Asirvatham • Om Narayan

Key Points

- A variety of mapping and catheter navigation systems are available, each with specific strengths and weaknesses.

- Each system requires familiarity with its principles of operation and serves as an adjunct to basic mapping and diagnostic techniques.

- The "best" system for any patient depends on characteristics of the arrhythmia to be mapped, operator familiarity with the system, and need to use specific mapping/ablation catheters.

- Misinterpretation of the mapping data and improper data acquisition or processing are potential pitfalls.

Ablation procedures have completely changed the way in which cardiac electrophysiology is practiced. For ablation to be successful, two factors need to come together: detailed mapping of the circuit or focus responsible for the arrhythmia, and the ability to navigate catheters that deliver energy to the diagnosed site of arrhythmogenesis. Specific challenges that remain are outlined in Table 8–1 and include the occurrence of multiple arrhythmias, transient arrhythmia, hemodynamically intolerable arrhythmia, and the difficulties in navigation associated with complex anatomy. An ideal mapping system combines several desirable characteristics: (1) accurate and reproducible documentation of both the timing and the amplitude of recorded electrograms; (2) cataloging of the source of the electrogram, be it endocardial, midmyocardial, epicardial, or intracavitary (papillary muscle); (3) a safe method of navigation, with recognition of tissue contact and the prowess to negotiate complex geometry; and (4) the ability to accomplish this within one or a few beats of arrhythmia. Although no present mapping system fulfills all these criteria, the unique features of each of the available major mapping and navigation systems are discussed here. First, an introduction to the principles behind each system is presented. Next, specific uses of each individual system, in particular for cardiac arrhythmias, are discussed. Finally, an approach to the use of these systems in various arrhythmias that includes understanding of the strengths and pitfalls involved is outlined.

Catheter ablation has become first-line therapy for many cardiac arrhythmias, and the number of indi-cations is increasing. In most patients, conventional catheter mapping techniques readily target the arrhythmogenic tissue. However, if patients present with atypical or unstable forms of arrhythmia, conventional mapping becomes more difficult and the success rate is lower. Several new mapping and navigation technologies have emerged in the last 10 years (Table 8–2) that may facilitate mapping and treatment in these complex situations.

Major Mapping and Navigation Systems Available

ELECTROANATOMIC MAPPING

The electroanatomic mapping or CARTO system (Biosense Webster, Baldwin Park, Calif.) has become widely used in ablative procedures, particularly where detailed point-to-point mapping and accurate electroanatomic correlation are required. The system is based on the premise that a metal coil placed in a magnetic field will generate an electric current. The magnitude of this current depends on the field's strength and the orientation of the coil in the field. The catheter used for electroanatomic mapping (Navistar), is a deflectable quadripolar ablation catheter that contains a location sensor embedded in its tip. Three ultra-low magnetic fields are emitted from a unit mounted under the patient table. Data for amplitude, frequency, and phase of the magnetic field are gathered and analyzed by a processing unit to determine the location of the catheter tip and its orientation. A three-dimensional (3-D) map is created by first placing the catheter under fluoroscopic guidance in known anatomic positions that serve as landmarks. Other points can then be identified without the use of fluoroscopy. Computer analysis of these points is used to create a real-time, 3-D model of the mapped chamber. In addition, a local electrogram is produced at each point and gated to a preselected reference electrogram. These electrograms create a voltage, activation, or propagation color-coded map that is superimposed on the anatomic model of the chamber. Specific points of interest, such as the bundle of His, scar tissue, or ablation points, may be tagged by the investigator for later reference. Multiple projections of the model can be viewed on a graphical display unit. In the following section, ventricular tachycardia (VT) is discussed as an introduction to electroanatomic mapping. Other arrhythmias are discussed later.

TABLE 8–1

Potential Difficulty in Ablating Cardiac Arrhythmias

Characteristic	Cause of Difficulty
Hemodynamically intolerable arrhythmia	Adequate time for detailed mapping is not allowed.
Multiple arrhythmias	Detailed mapping is time-consuming and would not allow for mapping of multiple arrhythmia.
Complex cardiac anatomy	The true source of a recognized electrogram has to be assigned. This may be very difficult with overlapping cardiac structures or with fragmented electrograms.
Catheter instability	Catheter moves from ablation site.

TABLE 8–2

Advanced Mapping Systems

System	Principle of Catheter Localization	Activation Mapping	Voltage Mapping	Multiple Catheters Visualized	Special Catheters Required	CT/MRI Image Integration	Advantages	Disadvantages
CARTO (Biosense Webster)	Magnetic field	Yes	Yes	No	Yes	Yes	Activation and voltage mapping, anatomic display	Point-by-point mapping without QuickMap
EnSite (Endocardial Solutions)	Electrical field	Yes	Yes	No	Balloon catheter, any ablation catheter	Yes	Single-beat activation and voltage mapping	Balloon stability, system complexity, loss of accuracy with large chamber sizes
EnSite NavX (Endocardial Solutions)	Electrical field	No	Yes	Yes	No	Yes	Ease of use, 64 electrodes displayed	Available only with EnSite system
LocaLisa (Medtronic)	Electrical field	No	No	Yes	No	No	Inexpensive to use per patient, ease of use	No electrical information, limited to 10 electrodes displayed
RPM (Boston Scientific)	Ultrasound	Yes	No	Yes	Yes	No	Ease of use, multiple catheters, activation displayed	Two references required, proprietary catheters needed

Ventricular Tachycardia

The ability to create the electroanatomic maps in patients with structural heart disease and VT has greatly increased understanding of arrhythmia mechanisms and substrates in these patients.[1] In the simplest construct, postinfarction VT is a reentrant arrhythmia with a critical zone of slow conduction that exists between a dense infarction-related scar and either another scar or an anatomic obstacle such as the mitral valve. In reality, however, the situation is often more complex, with the potential for multiple circuits, circuits traversing through what was considered to be scar, and absence of true normal myocardium making several large areas of slow conduction responsible for the maintenance of macroreentrant circuits. When using electroanatomic mapping for these tachycardias, care must be taken to accurately identify scar versus diseased myocardium, to obtain a sufficiently dense map so as to not miss critical arrhythmogenic zones, and to distinguish near-field electrical activation from that associated with surrounding structures. First, the anatomic reconstruction of the ventricle is created. Onto this, electrophysiologic information, including activation, timing, and bipolar and unipolar voltage information, is recorded (Fig. 8–1).

To eliminate the arrhythmogenic slow zones of present and potential VTs in patients with myocardial infarctions, the central common pathway for these circuits must be mapped and ablated. Conventional mapping methods, including criteria of entrainment mapping and mid-diastolic potentials with pacing maneuvers, have failure rates of 25% to 72% on 5-year follow-up.[1] Further, some VTs are difficult to induce in the electrophysiology laboratory or may be hemodynamically intolerable. A detailed description with scar mapping of the individual patient substrate allows an approach to ablate the arrhythmogenic slow zones in these patients. Marchlinski et al.[2] described the successful ablation of unmappable monomorphic VTs by this method. Patients in this study, in addition to having a remote myocardial infarction, had severely depressed left ventricular function. This is often the case, because generally slow conduction over the entire myocardium facilitates the maintenance and inducibility of multiple VTs. In their study, a 75% success rate was achieved with 8-month follow-up after placement of linear lesions connecting scar to anatomic boundaries guided by voltage mapping and limited pacemaps. Kottkamp[3] described a similar technique but restricted the map to regions near scarred tissue. In this, less time-consuming approach, they did not define a lower voltage limit to address scar tissue but used the combination of a missing electrogram signal and failure to capture by pacing regardless of voltage as a definition of dense scar. Under these criteria, linear ablation was performed in areas with voltages up to 1.5 mV, targeting all potential VT circuits. In their study, 79% of patients had complete noninducibility of VT at the end of the procedure. They reported a 64% success rate at 15-month follow-up in these difficult ablation situations.

Arrhythmogenic Dysplasia

Arrhythmogenic right ventricular dysplasia (ARVD) is a progressive cardiac disease, primarily affecting the right ventricle, in which myocytes are replaced by fibrotic tissue and fat. Because ARVD is an important cause of sudden death in young patients, implantable cardioveter defibrillators (ICD) are often placed. Because of the progressive nature of this disease and difficulty with medical therapy, ablation is often required to decrease the frequency of ICD discharges. In these patients, an approach similar to that employed for patients with scar-related VT (e.g., remote myocardial infarction) can be used.[4,5] Boulos et al.[4] demonstrated that diseased areas defined by electroanatomic mapping correlated well with magnetic resonance imaging (MRI) and echocardiographic findings. The VT can also be mapped using the CARTO system to define the circuit and its relationship to the surrounding fibrofatty substrate, thus allowing individually structured ablation lines.

Ablation of Ventricular Tachycardia of Other Causes

Patients with congenital heart disease (e.g., tetralogy of Fallot with previous surgical repair) or infiltrative disease may have recurrent macroreentrant monomorphic VTs with an underlying mechanism similar to that observed in patients with coronary artery disease or previous myocardial infarction. Voltage maps in association with activation maps using electroanatomic mapping can be similarly employed in these situations.[6,7]

Integration of Cardiac Magnetic Resonance Imaging with Electroanatomic Mapping

Reddy et al., in a series of in vitro and in vivo experiments,[8] evaluated the feasibility of integrating MRI and electroanatomic mapping data to guide real-time left ventricular catheter manipulation. A customized program was employed, initially using a plastic model of the left ventricle and later a porcine infarction model targeting ablation lesions to the scar border. Their in vitro experiments reveal that regis-

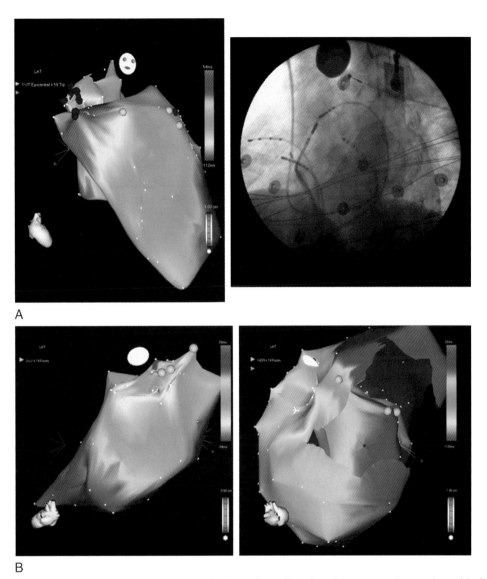

FIGURE 8–1. A, Mapping and ablation of epicardial ventricular tachycardia using electroanatomic mapping. This figure illustrates an important advantage of electroanatomic mapping. Separate maps were created of the endocardial right ventricle and the epicardial right ventricle, particularly the outflow tract, and the maps were superimposed (*left panel*). The right panel shows the pericardial catheter being placed via a subxiphoid approach with fluoroscopic guidance. The ability to compare and catalog endocardial and epicardial points helps to pinpoint the exact location of the focus or, in some cases, the exit of a ventricular tachycardia that can be targeted for ablation. **B,** Another example of electroanatomic mapping. In the left panel, an endocardial activation map of the left ventricle reveals a site (*red area*) about 90 msec prior to the reference electrogram. This site could have been targeted for ablation. However, when the epicardial map/shell was created (*right panel*), the true early site of activation, about 130 msec prior to a standard reference, was found in the epicardium.

tration of the left ventricle alone results in inaccuracies in alignment. Inclusion of the aorta in the registration process rectifies this error. In their in vitro iron oxide injection experiment, ablation lesions were accurately located approximately 1.8 mm from the target. In the porcine infarct model, the catheter could be reliably navigated to the mitral valve annulus, and ablation lesions were uniformly situated at the scar borders. Verma et al.[9] reported the integration of 3-D helical computed tomographic images with elec-

troanatomic mapping (CARTOMERGE; Biosense Webster, and Siemens AG, Munich, Germany).

Although electroanatomic mapping accurately tracks the location of the mapping catheter in 3-D space, an important limitation is that only a single bipolar electrode on the catheter tip can record electroanatomic data. Therefore, construction of high-density electroanatomic maps requires potentially time-consuming, sequential, point-by-point acquisitions throughout the cardiac chambers. Recently introduced is the CARTO XP system (Biosense Webster). Technological advances involve a novel 26-electrode mapping catheter (Qwikstar, Biosense Webster) to acquire multiple distinct electroanatomic points simultaneously from each electrode, thereby potentially reducing the number of point-by-point acquisitions. The electrodes are positioned on the catheter's distal tip and along its shaft. Chauhan et al.[10] evaluated the utility of this system for mapping of arrhythmias in patients with structural heart disease. The electroanatomic map was constructed in two stages: a sculpt map, using the minimum number of tip and shaft electrode data points, that covered more than 70% of tachycardia cycle length and a majority of the chamber volume, and a complete map, using additional tip electrode data points. They found, for large macroreentrant tachycardias or focal arrhythmias in patients with structural heart disease, that the multielectrode catheter can generate a preliminary or sculpt map that accurately guides complete electroanatomic mapping and uses fewer point-by-point acquisitions than with the bipolar catheter alone.

NONCONTACT MAPPING

The noncontact mapping system (EnSite 3000; Endocardial Solutions, St. Paul, Minn.) is made up of a multielectrode array (MEA) probe, an amplifier, and a computer workstation used to display electrical potential maps of the atria in three dimensions (Figs. 8–2 and 8–3). The system uses a mapping catheter that contains 64 filaments with 0.025-inch insulation breaks at specified sites to form an MEA.

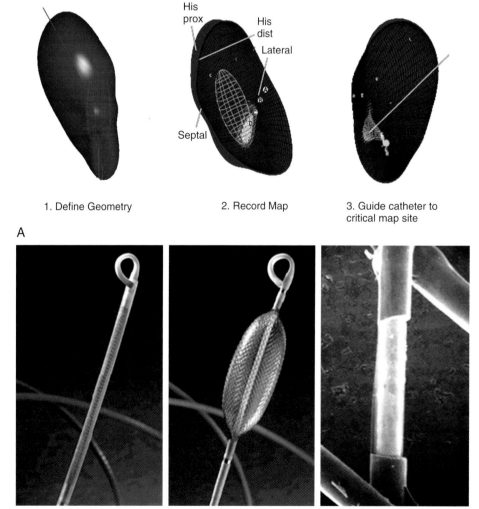

3 Steps to Non Contact Map

His prox   His dist   Lateral   Septal

1. Define Geometry   2. Record Map   3. Guide catheter to critical map site

A

B

FIGURE 8–2. A, This figure illustrates the principles of noncontact mapping. First, the geometry of the chamber of interest is defined. Then, a single beat of tachycardia is mapped by analysis of the color map and the virtual electrogram at different sites in the chamber. The result can be compared with normal rhythm and is best compared with at least one or two other beats of tachycardia. The site of earliest activation or exit from the critical zone of a macroreentrant circuit can be targeted for ablation. B, The multielectrode array probe. Left, multielectrode array (MEA) probe deflated. Middle, MEA balloon inflated. Right, magnification of electrode etched on MEA. See text for details. (A and B, Courtesy of Endocardial Solutions, St. Paul, Minn.)

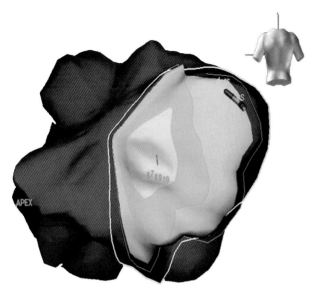

FIGURE 8–3. Procedure similar to scar mapping, explained with electroanatomic mapping, can also be performed with noncontact mapping. This new feature, called dynamic substrate mapping (DSM), can be used to visualize the local voltage amplitude at various sites. Sites of decreased voltage between scarred areas can be targeted for ablation. In addition, hemodynamically unstable ventricular tachycardias can be visualized to be exiting through one or more suspected low-voltage areas.

This array is passed through the vasculature in low profile and expanded when deployed in the chamber of interest to provide 64 noncontact electrodes with a fixed geometry. Any conventional mapping catheter is then swept throughout the cardiac chamber to define the endocardial boundaries. The location of any mapping catheter relative to the MEA is determined by means of a 5.68-kHz low-current locator (signal passed between the mapping catheter and electrodes proximal and distal to the MEA alternately, permitting localization of the signal source). During the definition of the atrial geometry, each passage of the mapping catheter to a new, more distant location in a given direction from the MEA defines the endocardial boundary, thus building a 3-D geometry.

Once the chamber geometry has been determined, the system can create a potential voltage map during a single cardiac cycle. Because the endocardial surface geometry has been defined and the expanded MEA surface is predefined, the inverse solution to the Laplace equation is employed by a computer workstation to process the amplified far-field signals from the noncontact catheter; this creates a 3-D endocardial potential map from a single cardiac cycle, with the potentials changing in time as the computer-generated movie of the cardiac activation is advanced.[11,12] Thus, electrophysiologic and anatomic data are associated in a 3-D "movie" that can be manipulated by the user to facilitate arrhythmia mapping.

Additionally, the user can select "virtual electrodes" at any point on the endocardial surface by selecting the location on the 3-D surface. Local electrograms are reconstructed at the virtual electrode sites; these replicate the signals that a contact catheter would have recorded from those sites, with high fidelity at distances less than 3.5 cm from the MEA.[11,12] Once a potential map has been created, the real-time position of a catheter relative to that map can be displayed (irrespective of arrhythmia termination), permitting targeting of desirable ablation sites during sinus rhythm. Critical locations such as the His bundle can be tagged and appropriately labeled for avoidance of ablation.

Although appropriate changes in the filter settings can be used to detect the site of earliest activation in focal arrhythmias arising from the epicardium, the accuracy of this method with atrial fibrillation is not clearly known. Thiagalingam et al.[13] studied the efficacy of noncontact mapping for recognition of endocardial, midmyocardial, and epicardial sites of activation in a sheep model. They found that noncontact electrograms correlated equally well in morphology and accuracy of timing with endocardial, intramural, and epicardial electrograms, as well as transmurally summated contact electrograms. This was true in sinus rhythm and with pacing from either the endocardium or the epicardium. Investigators also found a nonlinear relationship between noncontact electrogram accuracy, as measured by correlation with a contact electrogram, and distance from the MEA catheter. At distances beyond 40 mm, the accuracy decreased rapidly.[13-15] No data are presently available from the noncontact mapping system for identification of epicardial or midmyocardial sites of activation in diseased hearts.

Normal Activation Patterns

Studies using traditional mapping techniques as well as electroanatomic mapping have shown that electrical pathways in the right and left atria are complex.[16,17] Activation of these structures is clearly not a simple, uniform spread of activation from a point source; instead, it depends on the local myocardial architecture and interfaces with nonconducting obstacles.[18] Noncontact mapping has the advantage that a complete endocardial map can be created from a single sinus beat; therefore, it is suited to analyze normal rhythm propagation. In our analysis of both canine and human left atrial activation patterns in sinus rhythm,[19] we noted fairly predictable patterns of left atrial activation in normal hearts. Markides et al.[20] studied left atrial endocardial activation in 19 patients using noncontact mapping techniques; they importantly showed correlation between these pathways of activation and abrupt changes in subendo-cardial fiber orientation of the myocardial architecture. A knowledge of these normal activation patterns is important for understanding the patterns observed during tachycardia. For example, an automatic tachycardia that arises in the roof of the left atrium and travels around the posterior interpulmonary vein left atrium may give the mistaken impression of reentry around the pulmonary veins. We now introduce the use of noncontact mapping for reentrant flutters; specific arrhythmias are discussed later.

Noncontact Mapping for Atrial Flutter

Tai et al.[21] studied the utility of noncontact mapping (EnSite 3000 with precision software) in 15 patients with atypical right atrial flutter. The right atrial activation time in these patients accounted for 100% of the cycle length. In patients with single-loop reentry, the wavefront was found to circulate around a central obstacle in the anterolateral wall, with conduction through the channel between the central obstacle and the crista terminalis. In patients with double-loop or figure-of-eight reentry, a similar channel was observed. Radiofrequency (RF) ablation of these free-wall channels or gaps within the crista terminalis was effective in eliminating these flutters. These investigators reported complete elimination of the atrial flutters in 13 of 15 patients with follow-up of about 17 months.

Intraatrial Reentry after Fontan Surgery

Betts et al.[22] evaluated the utility of noncontact mapping in patients with complex anatomic and postsurgical substrates. Eleven arrhythmias in six patients who had undergone Fontan surgery were characterized by noncontact mapping. RF linear ablative lesions were placed along recognized critical zones in five patients and cryoablation was performed in one patient. The recurrence rate in this series was high, which the authors suggested might be explained by inadequate lesion creation. However, the known potential for parts of the arrhythmia circuit to be in the excluded portions of the original right atrium also needs consideration.

Role of Filter Settings with Noncontact Mapping

In general, filters are used with electrophysiologic tracings to minimize noise and to remove the unwanted effects of nonpathologic events. The purpose of using filters, therefore, is either to include information that is thought to have electrophysiologic reference or to exclude unwanted information. Understanding of the effect of filter settings is particularly relevant when using noncontact mapping.

An example is the effect of the EnSite high-pass filter. The high-pass filter allows frequencies above the filter setting to remain. That is, if a 2-Hz high-pass filter setting is used, frequencies lower than 2 Hz will be filtered out. Setting a higher number for the high-pass filter allows less of the lower-frequency signals to be included. Far-field electrograms such as those originating within anatomic pouches, adjacent cardiac chambers, or an epicardial site will be excluded from the virtual electrogram isopotential map if a higher high-pass filter setting is used.

The effect of filters alters the wavefront, and this effect is different according to the filter setting and whether the analyzed electrogram is unipolar or bipolar. With noncontact mapping, the high-pass filters may be set from 0.05 to 32 Hz to visualize conduction from other chambers or to include epicardial foci. The higher settings, such as 32 Hz, are used to remove low-frequency influences such as the T-wave diaphragmatic potentials and to specifically exclude contaminating signals from the epicardium or from an adjacent chamber. The highest high-pass filter settings, such as 16 or 32 Hz, are required to clearly define high-frequency signals (e.g., signals from Purkinje fibers, mid-diastolic potentials during reentrant arrhythmias) (see later discussion).

Low-pass filters can be set between 25 and 300 Hz. They are used to control high-frequency interference, usually nonphysiologic environmental noise. It should be recognized that inappropriately set low-pass filters can cause overfiltration of signals and change the baseline; in fact, they can change the timing of the analyzed electrogram in relation to its own neighbors and to surface electrocardiographic deflection.

To summarize, most manipulation with noncontact mapping and filter settings is done with the high-pass filter. The filters are "opened" (i.e., set at a low number) if one wishes to include potential epicardial sites or information from an adjacent chamber, such as the right superior pulmonary vein or left atrium when mapping the right atrium. A higher high-pass filter setting is used if the main interest is high-frequency signals, for example with fascicular tachycardia and the wish to include Purkinje potential signals.

EnSite NavX Methodology

The Endocardial Solutions EnSite system can be used as a pure navigation tool without the use of the noncontact mapping array.[23] A surface-based system is used to define cardiac anatomy and visualize catheter positions. A 5.6-kHz signal is emitted from three pairs of surface electrodes. Each catheter electrode is located 93 times per second. Up to 8 catheters and 64 electrodes can be visualized in 3-D space, and navigation is possible for all cardiac chambers. Navigation of the catheter is also continuously observed during ablation, and the system is compatible with both cryo-ablation and standard RF ablation. Although lesion markers can be tagged to see continuity of ablation lines (e.g., completion of the circumferential ablation for pulmonary vein isolation), simultaneous voltage caliper displays can be used to see the effect on the local electrogram during RF ablation.

LOCALISA

The LocaLisa system (Medtronic, Minneapolis, Minn.) is a catheter positioning system that locates diagnostic and ablation catheters electrods measuring the local field strength at the catheter electrodes during application of three orthogonal currents through the patient's body. An externally applied electrical field is detected via standard catheter electrodes. Regular catheter electrodes are used as sensors for a high-frequency transthoracic electrical field that is applied via standard skin electrodes. The reported localization accuracy is better than 2 mm with an additional scaling area of 8% to 14%.[24] The geometric measurements made using the system sometimes are inaccurate, mainly because of the inhomogeneity of tissues present in the chest.

When an electrical current is externally applied through the thorax, a voltage drop occurs across internal organs such as the heart. The resulting voltage can be recorded via standard catheter electrodes and can be used to determine electrode position. To apply this concept to catheter mapping and ablation procedures, several requirements must be met. First, the method must be applied in three orthogonal directions. Second, the externally applied electrical field must be harmless and must not interfere with standard electrocardiograms or electrograms. Third, cyclic variations due to cardiac contraction and respiration must be offset. Fourth, the localization method must be stable throughout the catheterization procedure. Finally, the system must be calibrated to translate changes in recorded voltages into changes in electrode position.

Analogous to the Frank lead system, three skin electrode pairs were used to send three small, 1-mA currents through the thorax in three orthogonal directions with slightly different frequencies of approximately 30 kHz used for each direction. Standard surface electrocardiographic electrodes are placed at the right and left midaxillary lines at the fourth intercostal space and in the left shoulder and left leg field; 2 × 15 cm skin patches, one anterior above the heart and the other posterior under the heart on the back, are used to create a third orthogo-

nal access. These lateral electrodes are large because their proximity to the heart can create an otherwise too inhomogeneous electrical field. The posterior skin patch simultaneously serves as the return electrode for RF ablation. The 30-kHz signal does not interfere with electrophysiologic signals, and the 1-mA current level is in accordance with international safety standards. The mixture of 30-kHz signals recorded from each catheter electrode is digitally separated to measure the amplitude of each of the three frequency components. The three electrical field strengths are calculated automatically by use of the difference in amplitude measured from neighboring electrode pairs with a known interelectrode distance of at least three different spatial orientations of that bipole. The 3-D position is then calculated for each electrode by dividing each of the three amplitudes by the corresponding electrical field strength. The electrode positions are averaged over 1 or 2 seconds to reduce cyclic cardiac variation. Respiratory variations are too slow to be eliminated by averaging without compromising the real-time nature of the localization method, and their effect on localization accuracy has been shown to be minimal. Examples of the LocaLisa display are presented in Chapter 20.

Kirchhof et al.[25] studied the LocaLisa system for mapping and ablation of supraventricular tachycardias and found that it reduced procedure-related exposure to ionizing radiation by 35% during ablation. In another study, the LocaLisa system was compared in efficacy with a conventional mapping and ablation approach for typical atrial flutter[26]. Total fluoroscopy time was reduced significantly, from approximately 16 minutes to approximately 7 minutes. In 9 of 26 patients studied, the entire ablation procedure could be performed with a fluoroscopy time of 1 minute or less. Macle et al. and others[27-29] described use of the LocaLisa system for pulmonary vein disconnection in the RF ablation of atrial fibrillation. This navigation system was used for real-time 3-D nonfluoroscopic imaging of the circumferential mapping catheter and ablation catheter electrodes in 26 patients. The cumulative duration of RF energy delivery, procedural time, and fluoroscopy time required for isolation of the pulmonary veins were compared in their study. Successful pulmonary vein isolation was achieved in all pulmonary veins without acute complications and the fluoroscopy time required for successful ablation was significantly reduced.

REAL-TIME POSITION MANAGEMENT AND MAPPING SYSTEM

Presently employed mapping systems discussed earlier, such as the CARTO and noncontact mapping systems, have allowed great strides to be made in overcoming the limitations of traditional point-to-point mapping in complex arrhythmia. However, the expense of these systems, the need for stable positioning of reference catheters, and the space occupied by these unique catheters (MEA with noncontact mapping) remain difficulties.

A newly developed 3-D real-time position management system (RPM; Boston Scientific, San Jose, Calif.) attempts to overcome these difficulties (Fig. 8–4). In this system, an ultrasound ranging technique is used to construct a 3-D representation of catheters (including electrodes and transducers), anatomic structures, and ablation sites. The system displays real-time movement of the tips and shafts of the catheters.

The 3-D RPM mapping system uses ultrasound ranging techniques to determine the position of a mapping or ablation catheter relative to two reference catheters. The mapping system consists of an acquisition module and an ultrasound transmitter and receiver unit, both connected to a computer. The system is capable of simultaneously processing 7 position management catheters, 24 bipolar or 48 unipolar electrogram signals, a 12-lead electrocardiogram, and 2 pressure signals. Signals are sampled at 3 kHz per channel with a resolution of 14 bits. The high-pass filters are set at 30 Hz and the low-pass filters at 500 Hz. Electrograms and catheter positions are displayed on a computer monitor. Signals and catheter positions are stored on an optical disk. The original positions can be displayed on a real-time window, allowing repositioning of catheters after

displacement. By measuring the time delay between the departure of the transmitted ultrasound pulse and the reception of this pulse by other transducers, the distance between the individual transducers can be calculated. Once the 3-D reference frame is established, triangulation is used to trace the positions of additional transducers. DeGroot et al. reported on the use of this system in RF ablation. Ten patients with atrial flutter were studied[30]. The proximal His bundle was marked as an electrical landmark to verify reproducibility. After identification of target sites, the position of each lesion created with the ablation catheter was marked. Successful ablation was achieved in all patients. Schreieck et al.[31] used this system in 21 patients with various arrhythmias including atypical atrial flutter and atrial fibrillation. They reported success in 95% of these patients. There were difficulties in steering the real-time position management ablation catheter in 28% of the successfully mapped patients such that ablation at the diagnosed site with another catheter was required. Potential drawbacks of real-time position management include the need for two intracardiac reference catheters and the relation between the distances of the mapping catheter from the reference catheters and the system's location accuracy. The system also assumes a uniform velocity for ultrasound through blood. Interphases with other tissues and the effect of whole blood transmission of ultrasound with ablation may introduce error.

MAGNETIC NAVIGATION WITH REMOTE CATHETER ABLATION

Currently, most catheter ablations are performed with manual catheter ablation guided by fluoroscopy. Catheters are typically deflectable and use a pull-wire mechanism. Recently, a novel magnetic navigation system has been introduced that allows the use of an ablation catheter that can be guided and positioned by magnetic fields to the desired site within a cardiac chamber. The magnetic navigation system (Niobe; Stereotaxis, St. Louis, Mo.) consists of two permanent magnets, the positions of which relative to each other are computer controlled inside a fixed housing. The magnets are positioned on either side of the fluoroscopy table. In the "navigate" position, they create a relatively uniform magnetic field (0.08 Tesla) of approximately 15 cm inside the chest of the patient. The mapping and ablation catheter is equipped with small permanent magnets at its tip that align with the direction of the externally controlled magnetic field so that it can be steered effectively. When the orientation of the outer magnets relative to each other is changed, the orientation of the magnetic field changes, leading to deflection of the catheter (Fig. 8–5). All magnetic field vectors can be stored and, if

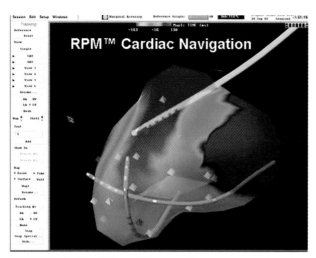

FIGURE 8–4. The RPM real-time position management system uses ultrasonic ranging technology to accurately track the navigation catheter. Advantages include the real-time display synchronized with heart rate, and minimized respiratory effects with the use of intracardiac reference catheters. *(Courtesy of Boston Scientific, San Jose, Calif.)*

necessary, reapplied while the magnetic catheter is navigated automatically. In addition, the computer-controlled catheter advancer system is used to allow truly remote catheter navigation without the need of manual manipulation. A workstation used in conjunction with this unit allows precise orientation of the catheter by 1-degree increments and by 1-mm steps in advancement or retraction. The system is controlled by a joystick or mouse and allows remote control of the ablation catheter from inside the control room. When the external magnet housing is

in navigation position (close to the patient), the angulation of the C arm is limited to 28 degrees for both right anterior oblique and left anterior oblique projections. RF ablation can then be performed using this solid-tip magnetic ablation catheter in the usual temperature-controlled mode with an RF generator.

This technology has evolved fairly rapidly. After an early report in 1991[32] of magnetic navigation of a catheter in a neonate and further evolution of the system in the field of neurosurgery,[33] a novel magnetic navigation system was introduced to interven-

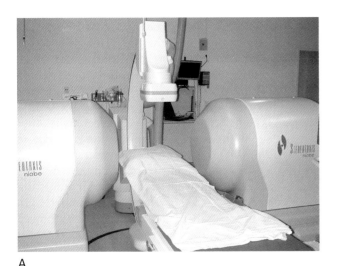

A

FIGURE 8–5. The Niobe Stereotaxis catheter navigation system. **A,** This system comprises a single-plane fluoroscopic arm, two permanent magnets (shown in steering position), the computers and software to control the magnets, and the mapping and ablation catheter with up to three magnets embedded in its distal shaft for steering. **B,** The computer control screen for steering the catheter. Right and left anterior oblique views of the heart are obtained and displayed. Points in these complementary views can be indicated on the screen, and the trajectory for steering the catheter to this location is indicated by the yellow lines displayed. The catheter can also be steered by directing the magnetic vectors in three dimensions.

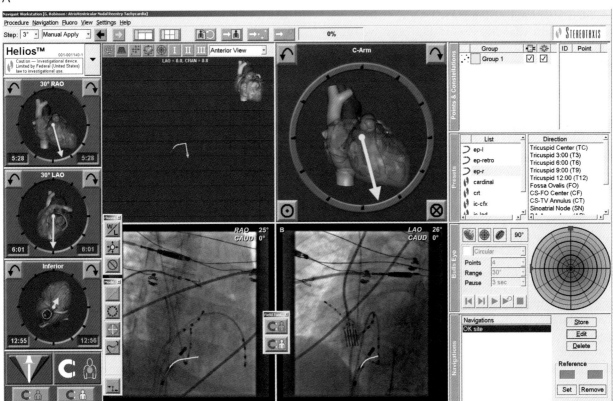

B

tional cardiology.[34] The first generation of these devices (0.15 Tesla, Tellstar; Stereotaxis) consisted of electromagnets and a biplane fluoroscopic imaging system. The present system (Niobe) consists of two permanent magnets (neodymium-boron-iron) and a single-plane fluoroscopic system. Ernst et al.[35] reported the successful use of this system in 42 patients with atrioventricular node reentrant tachycardia (AVNRT). There were no significant procedural complications, perforations, or recurrences with the patients in their study. Fluoroscopy was still used, with a mean fluoroscopy time of 8.9 ± 6.2 minutes, and procedure duration was not significantly shorter than the usual times required for AVNRT (145 ± 43 minutes), but this probably reflects the learning curve with the new system. The obvious major advantages include the ability to perform these procedures free of fluoroscopic exposure for the operator and with minimal fluoroscopic exposure for the patient, the ability to renavigate to a previously ablated site using the stored magnetic field vector without fluoroscopy, and improved stability and maneuverability during ablation.

INTRACARDIAC ULTRASOUND

The use of intracardiac ultrasound is described in detail in Chapter 9. In addition to navigation within the heart, this technology can be used to evaluate "electromechanical mapping" of cardiac arrhythmias associated anatomic anomalies.[36] Other situations in which intracardiac ultrasound has been useful in defining the arrhythmia include the finding of false tendons in patients with fascicular VT and the finding of right atrial pouches and large pectinates traversing the subeustachian isthmus in patients with atrial flutter.

The use of intracardiac ultrasound with a linear phased-array catheter, typically placed in the right atrium involves both facilitation of navigation and electrical mapping of both right and left atrial structures. The use of intracardiac ultrasound as a navigation tool is intuitive. The high-resolution images of the cardiac chambers obtained assist with catheter manipulation within those chambers. When electrophysiologic catheters are navigated in a cardiac chamber, at times no discernible electrical signal is seen. This may occur because there is no viable tissue at the site of catheter contact or because the catheter is free in the cardiac chamber and not making contact. Intracardiac ultrasound allows appropriate interpretation of the lack of electrical signal as either scar or lack of contact. Further, intracardiac echocardiography can visualize akinetic or dyskinetic thinned segments of the ventricular myocardium and allow for an echocardiographically guided ablation

approach, with lines being created between scars or between scars and anatomic obstacles.

In addition to visualization as an aid for navigation, true electrical mapping can also be performed with intracardiac ultrasound. With the technique of Doppler tissue imaging with appropriate filtering for amplitude and velocity, the tissue velocities can be calculated (Fig. 8–6). These velocities can be displayed either as Doppler coded velocity maps or tissue acceleration maps or as M-mode tissue velocity maps. The premise for tissue velocity–related electrical mapping is that an abrupt change in tissue velocity or acceleration is likely to be a result of local electrical activation of that particular myocardial site. The timing for this abrupt change in tissue velocity in relation to onset of the QRS for ventricular mapping, or the onset of the P wave for atrial mapping, can be calculated. Therefore, a site with a long delay from onset of the QRS to the time of abrupt acceleration (local contraction) represents a site that is being activated relatively late. On the other hand, a site with an onset of contraction at or before onset of the QRS deflection may represent the site of earliest activation in a point-source tachycardia or the site of preexcitation in a patient with an antegrade lead conducting accessory pathway. Similarly, in patients with substrate related reentrant arrhythmias, the propagation pattern in the ventricular or atrial myocardium and the anatomic relationships of this circuit to dyskinetic or akinetic segments can be visualized. Tangential tissue velocities (i.e., the velocity of propagation of mechanical contraction) can also be calculated and regions of slow conduction thus identified. One major utility of using intracardiac ultrasound to perform electromechanical mapping is the ability of this technique to visualize tissue velocity changes in the endocardium, epicardium, and midmyocardium. By this means, midmyocardial slow zones of conduction or an epicardial origin for a focal tachycardia can be estimated (Fig. 8–7).

For this method of mapping to be useful, two criteria need to be satisfied. First, the frame rate for the imaging, or the firing rate in the case of M-mode maps, must be sufficiently high to have a useful spatial resolution, particularly in normally conducting tissue. With the knowledge of normal conduction velocities in rapidly conducting regions of the heart, such as in the His-Purkinje system, the frame rate needs to be approximately 1000 frames per second to allow a spatial resolution of 1 mm. Presently existing systems do not allow for such high frame rates. With placement of the intracardiac probe in the chamber of interest and maximum frame rates, a spatial resolution for mapping of approximately 2.5 mm can be obtained. The second criterion for this technique to be useful is that the mechanical events

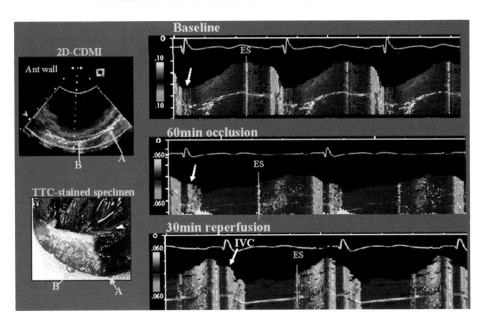

FIGURE 8–6. Use of intracardiac tissue Doppler ultrasound to recognize changes associated with ischemia. A similar principle can be used when noting the timing of the first evidence of contraction with the surface electrocardiogram. This is equivalent to the timing of local electrical activation should a conventional catheter have been placed at this site. *(See text for details.)*

must mirror electrical activity. This is true if there is little or no electromechanical delay. It is also true if the amount of electromechanical delay is uniform throughout the myocardium. However, in diseased myocardium, there can be significant and heterogenous delays between local electrical activation and the onset of mechanical contraction. Therefore, because of these limitations, intracardiac echocardiography is best used as an adjunct to other mapping techniques.

Use of Mapping Systems to Treat Specific Arrhythmias

LIMITATIONS OF MAPPING AND NAVIGATION SYSTEMS

Similar to conventional mapping techniques, noncontact mapping and electroanatomic mapping systems acquire and display data only from the endocardial surface of the heart. Tachycardia circuits are foci that are epicardial or midmyocardial in origin; they may not be accurately represented on these maps, and the visible endocardial breakthrough site may be of limited importance for arrhythmia maintenance. With noncontact mapping using isopotential maps, ventricular repolarization must be distin-

guished from atrial activation, and early diastolic activity may be difficult to map. Judicious use of high-pass filters and virtual electrogram analysis, in addition to existing software enhancements, can help to overcome this difficulty. Automatic tracking of the electrogram at the most depolarized site is an advance in distinguishing local activation from repolarization. Another limitation on noncontact mapping is the degradation of virtual electrograms at distances greater than 4 cm from the center of the MEA. In the rare patient with very large cardiac chambers, the MEA may need to be repositioned to acquire adequate maps. Similarly, when low-amplitude virtual electrograms are recognized, particularly at relatively large distances from the center of the balloon, electrogram degradation must be distinguished from localized scar associated with low-amplitude contact electrograms. The addition of voltage or conduction velocity maps is helpful in making this distinction and accurately identifying scar.

The major limitation of electroanatomic mapping is the need for point-to-point mapping. Creation of these maps is somewhat time-consuming and requires a sustained, hemodynamically stable rhythm. This limitation can be overcome for reentrant arrhythmias if gross substrate abnormalities such as scars and diseased myocardium can be detected using a voltage map. Based on the premise that the arrhythmogenic substrate for reentrant atrial and ventricular arrhythmias involves a zone of slow conduction, typically located between two scarred

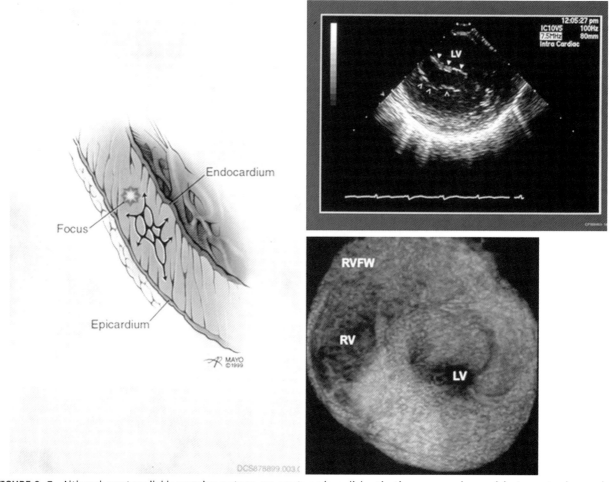

FIGURE 8–7. Although most available mapping systems can create endocardial activation maps, and some (electroanatomic mapping) can be used for epicardial mapping, the myocardial depth creates the possibility of midmyocardial foci or midmyocardial slow zones of reentrant arrhythmia. Doppler tissue imaging can encompass the entire myocardium, and the sites of activation and sequence of activation can be visualized with appropriate reconstruction. LV, left ventricle; RV, right ventricle; RVFW, right ventricle free wall. *(Three-dimensional reconstructed image courtesy of Dr. Douglas L. Packer, Mayo Clinic, Rochester, Minn.)*

regions or between a scarred region and an anatomic obstacle such as the mitral valve, this information can obviate the need for mapping of the tachycardia. Using this premise, ablation lesions are placed between scarred regions or between scars and normal anatomic obstacles. Another limitation of electroanatomic mapping is the need for a specific catheter with a magnetic sensor. Certain catheter features such as bidirectional deflectability and multielectrode mapping or ablation are not available with the presently existing electroanatomic mapping catheters.

FOCAL OR POINT-SOURCE TACHYCARDIAS

Electroanatomic Mapping for Focal Tachycardias

As outlined earlier, the electroanatomic mapping system is set up. Once the tachycardia is induced, the electroanatomic mapping catheter is advanced to the chamber of interest (Fig. 8–8). If the tachycardia is known for certain to be right atrial, then a right atrial map alone is created. If the chamber of origin is in question, separate activation maps of the right atrium, the left atrium, and in some cases the coronary sinus are created. Once the mechanism of the tachycardia is clearly known to be focal, then the site of earliest activation in comparison with a stable reference electrode is targeted for ablation. Care must be taken to exclude reentry as a mechanism of the arrhythmia (Fig. 8–9).

Potential causes of difficulty exist in certain situations. First, with fascicular or junctional tachycardia, the site of earliest activation for a ventricular electrogram can be far removed from the source of the tachycardia. With electroanatomic mapping, it is ideal to set up two maps, using the "remap" feature. The first map is the usual ventricular activation map, used to find the site of earliest local ventricular activation in comparison with a stable reference, usually

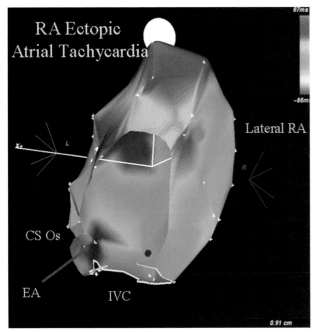

FIGURE 8–8. Use of electroanatomic mapping of the right atrium for a focal tachycardia. A three-dimensional rendering of the activation pattern (posterior view) allows easy visualization and defines a target for ablation (arrow). Conduction velocities also can be estimated with this system. If a large area of early activation is noted, either the true source of the tachycardia is arising from the epicardial surface or an adjacent chamber, causing simultaneous activation of multiple endocardial sites, or conduction velocity is very rapid and more detailed mapping is required to find the actual source of the tachycardia. CS os, ostium of the coronary sinus; EA, ectopic atrial focus; IVC, inferior vena cava; RA, right atrium.

the QRS complex.[37] The second map specifically catalogs the activation pattern of the prepotential or Purkinje sites. Both maps can be analyzed and the site of earliest Purkinje potential activation used to perform a pacing maneuver that compares the local Purkinje potential with the earliest ventricular electrogram, and tachycardia with the stimulus-to-earliest QRS observed with pacing. The advantage of using electroanatomic mapping is that ablation can be performed empirically at these and related sites, should the tachycardia be mechanically traumatized and difficult to induce.

Second, extreme care should be taken in assigning a given electrogram to a particular chamber or location. For example, tachycardias arising near the crista terminalis can be associated with multiple sites with double potentials. If only the site of earliest potential is taken and used for creation of the activation map, an indicated site with earliest activation may be a far-field potential that in fact reflects the true earliest site on the other side of the crista terminalis. Multiple similar early sites may be found with such a mapping technique.[38,39] The best method in this situation is to catalog only the earliest near-field potential sites.

Third, in patients with congenital heart disease, it is vital that all viable tissue relevant to the tachycardia be mapped. This can be difficult if surgery or the patient's inherent anomaly makes catheter access to certain atrial sites challenging.

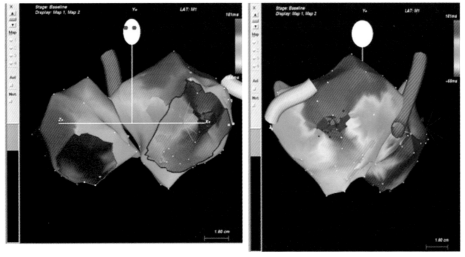

FIGURE 8–9. This figure illustrates a common limitation when using a mapping system in isolation. Left panel: LAO view. Right panel: posterior view. The site of earliest activation (*red area*) is seen in the posterior left atrium. Following the activation sequence, it can be seen that the latest sites of activation (*purple area*) are very close to the early sites. This pattern can be seen with a reentrant arrhythmia having a slow zone in the posterior left atrium, or with an ectopic atrial tachycardia arising from the posterior left atrium and a separate cause of unilateral block just superior to the site of origin, producing much more rapid conduction in an inferior direction. This map needs to be used in conjunction with conventional electrophysiologic maneuvers such as entrainment mapping to ascertain the nature of the arrhythmia and guide ablation.

Noncontact Mapping for Focal Tachycardias

Although catheter ablation for focal tachycardias using point-to-point contact mapping guided by fluoroscopy has been highly successful, some difficulties remain with irregular, transient, and poorly tolerated atrial tachycardias and VTs. Seidl et al.[40] studied the use of noncontact mapping in 18 patients with atrial tachycardia. When the generated isopotential map suggested a discrete origin by displaying a relatively narrow and sharp ring of colors around a discrete white spot (15 out of 18 patients), with simultaneous and rapid spread of activation and virtual electrograms demonstrating a QS morphology, catheter ablation was successful at the endocardial site located by the system. In this series, ablation was not successful when a large area of endocardial breakthrough was found. Hindricks et al.[41] demonstrated successful ablation of nonsustained ectopic atrial tachycardias that arose from a single focus using noncontact mapping.

Technique

Typically, the chamber of origin of the focal tachycardia is identified from the surface electrocardiogram and brief mapping with the use of coronary sinus and other commonly used catheters. The MEA is then advanced to that chamber, and isopotential maps in sinus rhythm are created. Important anatomic landmarks such as the His bundle, the coronary sinus ostium, the fossa ovalis, and the atrioventricular valves are identified on the map. These points are used to facilitate catheter navigation in real time and for orientation during map interpretation. If the automatic tachycardia is sustained, isopotential maps are recorded from 5 to 10 beats of tachycardia, and the virtual electrograms at the site of earliest activation are reviewed. Optimal sites for ablation are characterized by discrete early potentials, which are seen on the isopotential map as a narrow, sharp ring of multiple colors around a focal white center. The unipolar virtual electrograms at optimal sites have an immediately negative QS morphology with a rapid dV/dt in the range of 50 to 200 mV/msec, consistent with an electrical point-source activation. If nonsustained atrial tachycardia is mapped, comparison of at least three episodes is necessary to exclude the presence of multiple foci.

Potential Difficulties

If an ideal site with the characteristics described earlier is not found, or if ablation targeted at such a site is not successful, care must be taken to exclude a nonendocardial focus. With careful analysis of the unipolar virtual electrogram, one often can identify a far-field–type signal preceding the electrogram at the perceived endocardial breakthrough point. Although such a trigger may be truly epicardial, often it represents a far-field detection of an adjacent electrogenic structure, such as the right upper pulmonary vein behind the posterior right atrium or the vein of Marshall adjacent to the lateral left atrium.

Any cul-de-sac such as an atrial pouch, atrial aneurysm, or aneurysmal pulmonary vein that has not been included in the rendering of the atrial geometry will give the appearance of an epicardial trigger, and simultaneous endocardial breakthrough points at the ostium of the vein or at the rim of the cul-de-sac will be seen.

To overcome these difficulties, an accurate knowledge of both the cardiac anatomy at the site of catheter location and the adjacent neighboring anatomy is required. Intracardiac ultrasound, cardiac chamber angiography, or integration with computed tomographic scans or MRI data (NavX technology) is required for appropriate interpretation of the virtual electrogram or actual contact electrogram at the site of contemplated ablation. Sometimes, in cases of congenital cardiac disease and surgical correction, certain cardiac chambers may be completely or partially excluded from the rest of the chambers (e.g., the neo-left atrium in a patient who has undergone certain types of the Fontan procedure). In such instances, the MEA cannot be deployed in the actual chamber of origin of the arrhythmia. In these cases, the role of noncontact mapping is primarily to exclude certain chambers as being involved in the arrhythmogenesis of a particular arrhythmia and then target the anatomically difficult to access chamber of origin of the tachycardia with contact mapping techniques.

REENTRANT TACHYCARDIA

Atrial Flutter

Typical atrial flutter results from a stable macroreentrant circuit for the critical slow zone of conduction bounded by the tricuspid valve annulus and the inferior vena cava (the subeustachian isthmus) (Figs. 8–10 and 8–11). Because of the fixed and accessible anatomic location of the vulnerable zone of this circuit, typical atrial flutter is usually effectively treated with standard mapping and ablation techniques. At times, however, typical isthmus-dependent atrial flutter is difficult to distinguish from atypical non–isthmus-dependent flutters using the 12-lead electrocardiogram. This difficulty is particularly manifest in patients with atriotomy scars from surgery and in those with structural heart disease. The global activation maps generated by noncontact mapping can rapidly identify the arrhythmia mechanism and can be used to target vulnerable circuit components in typical flutters. The use of electroanatomic mapping (CARTO) can be invaluable in cases of persistent conduction and recurrent atrial flutter despite aggressive attempts at ablation in the subeustachian isthmus. Electroanatomic maps can identify the gap in conduction and also correctly diagnose the existence of longitudinal disassociation within the subeustachian isthmus itself (see Fig. 8–11).

Electroanatomic Mapping for Reentrant Arrhythmia

The principles for using electroanatomic mapping with reentrant arrhythmias are as detailed previously. The potential pitfalls and precautions needed are similar to those associated with the use of non-contact mapping for reentrant arrhythmias. To summarize, first, a decision must be made as to whether a pure scar-based approach or tachycardia is going to be induced and mapped. Second, if the tachycardia is going to be mapped, then it must be understood that targeting of the early site (red area) is of little value (Fig. 8–12). Depending on what reference is used, the "early" site can be significantly changed, because there is continuous electrical activity at some point in the myocardium for a given reentrant arrhythmia. Nevertheless, and regardless of what is taken for the arrhythmia window or reference electrogram, the red or early area often approximates the exit site of the tachycardia, probably because a significant portion of the tachycardia cycle length is taken up by the slow zone within or between two scars. Any reproducible electrogram from beat to beat

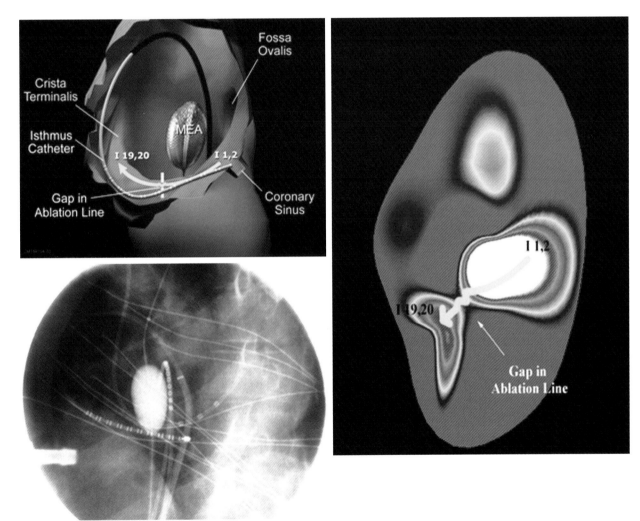

FIGURE 8–10. There are several potential uses of noncontact mapping in cases of atrial flutter. In this example, the activation pattern shows a gap in a previously placed ablation line. This particular site can be targeted for ablation (so-called spot welding). *Top left:* Schematic diagram of catheter positions in the coronary sinus and a multielectrode array (MEA) in the right atrium. *Bottom left:* Fluoroscopic image represented by the schematic. *Right:* Activation map showing conduction through gap in ablation line (arrow). *(Courtesy of Dr. Paul A. Friedman, Mayo Clinic, Rochester, Minn.)*

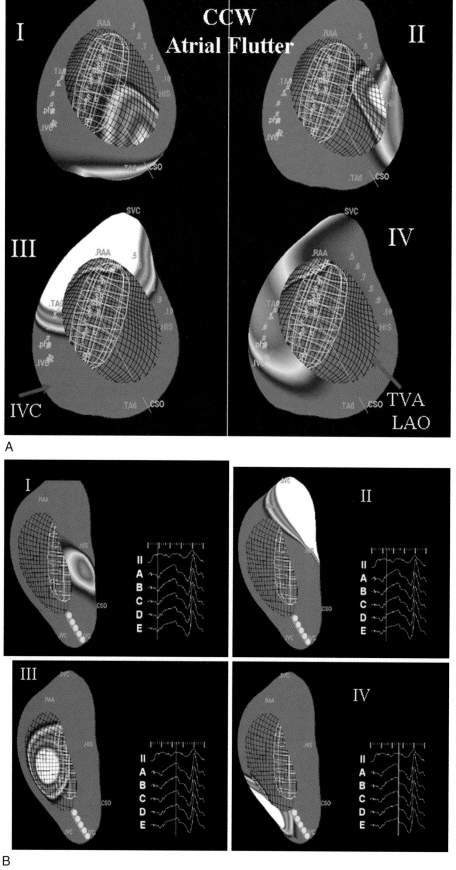

FIGURE 8–11. A, The circuit of counterclockwise (CCW) atrial flutter is shown in sequential still frames obtained with noncontact mapping. Passive activation of the cavotricuspid isthmus from a focal tachycardia cannot be excluded, and analysis of these maps should be done in conjunction with the usual entrainment maneuvers to confirm the nature of the arrhythmia and the participation of the cavotricuspid isthmus tissue in tachycardia. **B,** Once the ablation line has been created for atrial flutter, noncontact mapping can be used to confirm the block across the ablation line. Here, in pacing from the coronary sinus, the wavefront is seen to travel in a CCW direction with no evidence of conduction passing through the ablation line. *(Courtesy of Dr. T. M. Munger.)* CSO, coronary sinusos; SVC, superior vena cava; RAA, right atrial appendage; TVA, tricuspid value annulus.

should be used for the activation map as well as the voltage map, regardless of how low the amplitude is. Only sites with no discernible electrogram activity, and with inability to capture the local myocardium at that site, should be marked as scar. An important cause for failure to eliminate reentrant arrhythmias with this approach (with either a scar-based or an activation map–based approach) is the incorrect tagging of viable myocardial sites as scar. This error may occur because of failure to recognize, or because

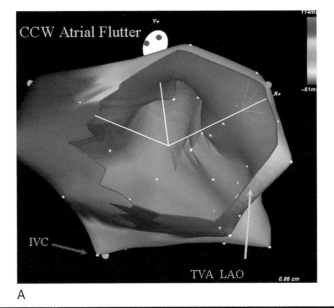

FIGURE 8–12. A, An activation map obtained through electroanatomic mapping in a patient with counterclockwise (CCW) atrial flutter. The entire flutter cycle length should be accounted for when mapping a particular chamber. If it is not, some unmapped structure, either another cardiac chamber or an anatomic anomaly such as a pouch, has not been mapped and included in the circuit. It should be noted that the red area or site of "early" activation is arbitrary in relation to the reentrant circuit and has no specific significance. As noted with noncontact mapping, the activation pattern alone does not prove the existence of a macroreentrant arrhythmia using the circuit. Appropriate pacing maneuvers need to be performed to ascertain the exact nature of the tachycardia and circuit. IVC, inferior vena cava; LAO, left anterior oblique; TVA, tricuspid value annulus. (Courtesy of Dr. T. M. Munger.) **B,** In order to visualize the propagated electrical wavefront, a propagation map can be generated with electroanatomic mapping.

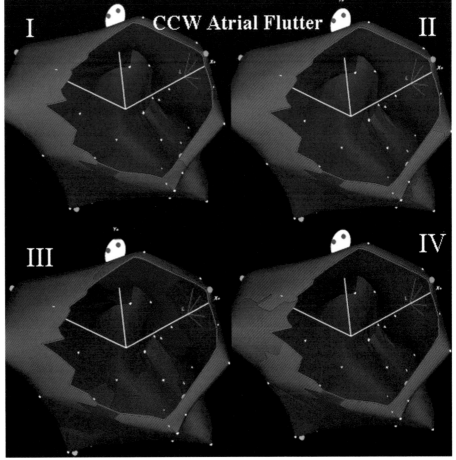

the catheter is not making contact with myocardium and therefore no discernible electrogram is seen. The adjunctive use of intracardiac echocardiography can help eliminate this cause of difficulty. The opposite issue also occurs: if a catheter is wedged between scar and viable papillary muscle tissue, even though that particular site is scarred, the electrogram from the papillary muscle will be seen and tagged as part of the voltage or activation map at that particular site. Again, intracardiac echocardiography can help in anticipating sites where this difficulty may arise.

An important advantage of electroanatomic mapping over noncontact mapping is the specific ability to map the epicardial surface of the myocardium. Although the epicardial location of a slow zone, scar, or exit site can be inferred with careful analysis of the virtual electrograms and noncontact mapping, a direct separate electroanatomic map can be made using the electroanatomic mapping catheter in the pericardial space. Comparison of the epicardial and endocardial maps can sometimes best define the circuit and the best target for ablation.

Regardless of the mapping system used, liberal use should be made of traditional mapping techniques, including entrainment maneuvers and pace mapping, to maximize the chance of success.

Intra-atrial Reentry in Patients with Congenital Heart Disease

Triedman et al.[42] studied the utility of electroanatomic mapping in patients with complex circuits of atrial reentrant tachycardia. A total of 177 procedures were performed in 134 patients. There was a significant increase in clinical status in most patients. However, recurrence rates were high (42%), and there was no decrease in procedure or fluoroscopy time. Improved outcomes were associated with high-saturation electroanatomic mapping, fewer tachycardia circuits, acute procedural success, and improved ablative lesion placement. Nakagawa et al.[39] showed that ablation of relatively narrow channels between large low-voltage areas eliminates tachycardia.

Ablation of Ventricular Tachycardia in Patients with Dilated Cardiomyopathy

Dilated cardiomyopathy involves several disease processes including autoimmune, idiopathic, and certain infiltrative diseases. Because of the lack of fixed or dense scars in these patients, targeting of anatomic sites for ablation is difficult. Some tachycardias in these patient groups are microreentrant or macroreentrant and involve the conduction system

(Purkinje potential–related tachycardia, bundle-branch reentry, interfascicular reentry). Noncontact mapping has the advantage in tachycardias involving microreentry or abnormal automaticity that are nonsustained or hemodynamically stable. However, the critical zone or focus of these tachycardias is often subendocardial in location and can easily be mechanically traumatized by catheters. Therefore, the MEA and even traditional mapping techniques can be challenging. Electroanatomic mapping or real-time position management may allow "tagging" of the site where the mechanical trauma or bump occurred, permitting future energy delivery at this site if the tachycardia cannot be reinduced or mapped. The exit sites or foci may be epicardial, and Doppler ultrasound tissue mapping techniques can be particularly useful in this subset of patients, because the ventricular wall is often thin and endocardial ablation at the recognized early epicardial site may be successful.[43]

Atrial Fibrillation

Clearly, the number of procedures being performed to attempt a cure for atrial fibrillation is growing. Several groups have demonstrated high success rates, with patients being drug free and symptom free after RF ablation for atrial fibrillation.[44-46] Success rates have been reported between 70% and 88%, and complication rates between 2% and 4%. Because of these rates and the attractiveness of a permanent cure for atrial fibrillation (as opposed to continuous drug use), many patients have begun seeking this potentially curative therapy and the electrophysiologists and centers that offer it.

Mapping and navigation systems have an important role to play in the ablation of atrial fibrillation. This section outlines the methods of use and relative merits of the available mapping systems.

Although many methods for ablation of atrial fibrillation exist, the two most accepted premises on which they are based are (1) that the pulmonary and other venous structures represent the arrhythmogenic triggers for atrial fibrillation and need to be electrically isolated from the atria, and (2) that the atrial substrate needs to be modified with ablation, usually in a linear fashion, to decrease or eliminate the ability of this substrate to maintain atrial fibrillation (Fig. 8–13). Mapping and navigation technologies ideally should be flexible, so as to be useful regardless of whether a venous isolation or substrate modification is planned. If substrate modification is planned, then the mapping and navigation system should be able to visualize catheter movement relative to the rendered geometry of the atrium in real time and to catalog ablation points on the atrial geometry. A further utility with a mapping system is the ability to allow documentation of the electrical end point of the ablation, such as entrance block into the pulmonary veins or the completeness and adequacy of linear ablation. Finally, the mapping and navigation system should allow for the diagnosis and ablation of nonvenous atrial triggers initiating atrial fibrillation.

Use of the Noncontact Mapping System for Atrial Fibrillation

Anatomic Ablation. With the use of the EnSite NavX technology described previously, the left atrial geometry is rendered. After transseptal puncture, any catheter that is planned to be used for ablation or mapping can be visualized in real time, and the pulmonary vein and left atrial geometry is outlined. With the use of importing data from computed tomography or MRI, real-time comparison with detailed preimaged anatomy can facilitate catheter movement and understanding of the site of electrograms to be analyzed or targeted for ablation. Once the geometry has been outlined, if a pulmonary isolation approach is planned, real-time cataloging of a mapping catheter position within the pulmonary vein is useful. For example, the use of a circumferential mapping catheter such as a lasso catheter requires exact knowledge of the position of this catheter before and after the ablation process. The nature of the electrograms from the lasso catheter can be quite different when the catheter is deeper into

the vein, is closer to the ostium, or has migrated to a site that has been directly ablated. Mapping catheter shift during the ablation procedure is fairly common. Typically, the ratio of the far-field left atrial electrogram and the near-field pulmonary vein potential, as well as fluoroscopic and intracardiac echocardiographic data, is used to ascertain the mapping catheter location. The advantage of a mapping system such as the EnSite system is that there is continuous documentation of the catheter position, which can quickly be analyzed for distance from the tagged ablation site and pulmonary vein ostia.

When ablation points are cataloged in a circumferential manner, around each pulmonary vein or each set of pulmonary veins, a point may be taken and cataloged as a successful ablation point but there may not have been sufficient contact or sufficient time or power of energy delivery to create a transmural lesion at that site. Therefore, a gap in the conduction line or circle may exist despite a cataloged point. With the EnSite system, the use of voltage calipers, with which a reduction in local electrogram voltage can be visualized during ablation, helps avoid such gaps.

To aid linear ablation, this technology can be used in a similar manner. When the left atrial geometry is created, it is important to accurately identify the pulmonary vein ostia, the mitral valve, the interatrial septum, and the left atrial appendage. When identifying the mitral valve, it is important to take, as the

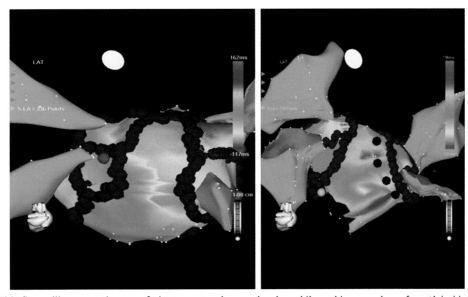

FIGURE 8–13. This figure illustrates the use of electroanatomic mapping in guiding wide-area circumferential ablation for atrial fibrillation (posterior view of left atrium). *Left:* The red dots denote ablation points and the anatomic contiguity of these points. Care must be taken to avoid entering into the geometrically identified pulmonary veins. *Right:* An advantage of electroanatomic mapping is that the mapping catheter can be placed in the esophagus to obtain and catalog areas of posterior left atrium in proximity to the esophagus, thus helping to avoid fatal left atrial-esophageal fistula. The black dots represent the location of the esophagus.

limit of the left atrial geometry, a site where the atrial electrogram on the ventricular side of the annulus is no longer seen. This is because creation of an ablation line from the mitral annulus to the left inferior pulmonary vein, so as to prevent or treat mitral isthmus-dependent atrial flutter, requires ablation from the ventricular portion of the annulus up to the ablation surrounding the left inferior pulmonary vein, avoiding ablation into the vein itself (Fig. 8–14).

Nonanatomic Approach. Although circumferential isolation of the pulmonary vein and substrate modification with linear ablation can often be performed with a purely anatomic approach to ablation, at times further mapping and electrophysiologic analysis is required. The MEA can be used in conjunction with the NavX technology for such mapping.

Electrical end points for complete isolation of the pulmonary veins include entrance block (failure of excitation of the pulmonary vein musculature during sinus rhythm or atrial pacing) and exit block (failure to excite the atrium when pacing and capturing viable pulmonary vein musculature). Noncontact mapping and the virtual electrograms can be used to identify pulmonary vein potentials and compare them before and after ablation to identify entrance block.[48] The wavefront of activation of the left atrium during pacing within the pulmonary vein can also be used to determine whether exit block is present and, if not, to approximate where the activation is exiting to the left atrium.

Nonpulmonary vein foci can trigger atrial fibrillation. These foci may be from the atrial musculature itself or from a nonpulmonary vein such as the coronary sinus or vein of Marshall. Therefore, mapping and ablation is sometimes required even after successful isolation of the pulmonary vein for triggers of atrial fibrillation. The noncontact mapping system, employed in either the left or right atrium after pulmonary vein isolation, can be used to identify and target such sites for ablation. Once the geometry has been rendered using the approach described earlier, the array can be deployed in the left atrium without a need to recreate the geometry. Initiations of atrial fibrillation are then recorded, and the site of earliest activation targeted for ablation.

When the myocardium in an atrial vein such as the Vein of Marshall is triggering atrial fibrillation, the noncontact mapping system can be used to infer such a site of origin. In contrast to the procedure with noncontact mapping for an atrial trigger, the high-pass filter needs to be set at a relatively low level, such as 0.05 or 0.1 Hz. This allows the inclusion of far-field low-frequency potentials. What is sometimes observed in this situation is that the earliest site of activation is a far-field potential, typically filtered out when the high-pass filter is set above 4 Hz, followed by the endocardial breakout point (similar to a focal atrial tachycardia). When this pattern is recognized, ablation can be targeted to the earliest far-field site, or further mapping within the epicardial atrial vein can be done with contact catheters to identify and target the earliest signal within the vein.

Procedure Time and Fluoroscopy Time. It might be expected that newer mapping and navigation systems, by facilitating nonfluoroscopic catheter navigation, would reduce fluoroscopy times. Willems et al.[49] reported a significant reduction in fluoroscopic times, from 29.2 to 7.7 minutes, when electroanatomic

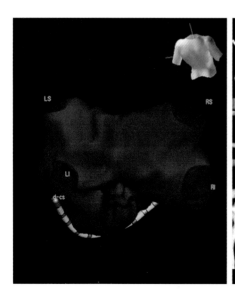
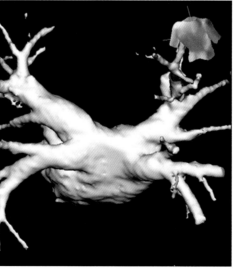

FIGURE 8–14. An advance in the use of the NavX system (*left*) is the ability to use data from other digital imaging—in this example, data from computed tomographic scanning (*right*). This allows better geometric visualization of the pulmonary veins and the ostia (a posterior view of the left atrium is shown in both figures). *(Courtesy of Dr. Douglas L. Packer, Mayo Clinic, Rochester, Minn.)* LS, left superior pulmonary vein; LI, left inferior pulmonary vein; RS, right superior pulmonary vein; RI, right inferior pulmonary vein; CS, coronary sinus catheter.

mapping rather than conventional methods were used to guide ablation of typical atrial flutter. In another published, large series of patients with reentrant atrial tachycardia and congenital heart disease at a single center, the use of electroanatomic mapping was associated, surprisingly, with longer procedural and fluoroscopic times compared with conventional fluoroscopy-based technique.[42] The lack of constant observance of this expected reduction in fluoroscopy time may be related to the complexity of the cases reported as well as the learning curve involved when operators familiar with conventional mapping use the newer systems. Clearly, navigation systems such as the Stereotaxis system, particularly when used in conjunction with accurate electroanatomic mapping and given enough operator experience, should greatly reduce procedural and fluoroscopy times. One challenge in the immediate future of mapping technology is to simplify the user interfaces for the systems, so that these results may be quickly seen even with relatively inexperienced operators.

REENTRANT ARRHYTHMIAS

Noncontact Mapping for Recurrent Flutter

Atrial flutter recurrence after apparently successful ablation results from one or more gaps in the linear ablative lesion between the tricuspid annulus and the inferior vena cava.[50] Noncontact mapping accurately identifies gaps in linear lesions using isopotential maps created during pacing near the ablation line or during arrhythmia. These gaps may be closed with additional ablation lesions. Additionally, noncontact mapping has been used successfully to identify gaps in flutter lesions that were not apparent with traditional mapping because of severe conduction delay. Noncontact mapping can also be used as the initial mapping system for atrial flutter. The MEA is placed in the right atrium so that the equator of the MEA is approximately in the region of the subeustachian isthmus. Maps are obtained during pacing of either the proximal coronary sinus or the lateral right atrium at an annular site. The standard ablation is performed in a pull-back fashion from the tricuspid annulus to the inferior vena cava. Progressive delay in conduction during pacing across the isthmus is noted. When the ablation line has been completed, a reversal of activation on the tricuspid isthmus (e.g., a counterclockwise direction during proximal coronary sinus pacing) is abruptly seen. If such a reversal of activation does not occur, the gap can be identified and the gap site targeted for further ablation. Just as double potentials that are widely spaced (signifying conduction block) are seen with contact catheters, similar widely spaced double potentials can be seen

on the virtual electrograms when measured along the ablation line. A narrowing of the virtual electrogram double potential to a point where a single virtual electrogram is located is another method of identifying the gap in conduction. Similar methods are used for reentrant VT.[15]

Summary

The EnSite and CARTO systems are electroanatomic mapping systems that incorporate a positioning technology. The EnSite mapping system uses a positioning technique that measures the distance of a roving catheter tip from a plurality of electrodes of an intracavitary electrode. The EnSite system uses an intracavitary electrode set as the frame of reference; hence, the repeatability of the positioning information is highly dependent on stable positioning of the intracavitary electrode (Fig. 8–15). The reported accuracy of the EnSite system is $4 \pm 3.2\,\mathrm{mm}$.[51] The CARTO system incorporates a positioning system with six degrees of freedom; it reports catheter position and orientation using an ultra-low-intensity electromagnetic field. The CARTO system enables simultaneous recording of local endocardial electrical activity together with its temporal position.[52] The position of the CARTO system is recorded relative to a fixed extracorporeal reference location sensor that is secured to the patient's back. The reported resolution of the CARTO system is $0.7\,\mathrm{mm}$.

Apart from location resolution, the cardiac pathway positioning system LocaLisa, the EnSite system, and the CARTO system differ significantly in their mapping, intervention planning, and therapy monitoring capabilities. Both the EnSite and CARTO systems offer mapping capability. At present, the EnSite system reports virtual electrograms that are computed using the Infer solution of the recorded intracavitary potential. The benefit of the EnSite system has the capability to map transient and hemodynamically intolerable events. The CARTO system reports the contact electrograms actually measured from the endocardium.

In evaluating the relative merits of positioning systems, one must consider the need for accuracy, reproducibility, the nature of the cardiac arrhythmia, compatibility with various ablation and mapping catheters, and cost issues when choosing a particular system for a given patient. Mapping systems should facilitate the planning and execution of the ablation procedure and, ideally, should decrease the complexity of these procedures, as well as procedure time and fluoroscopic exposure time. True 3-D reconstruc-

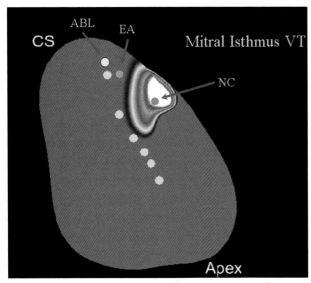

FIGURE 8-15. Example of an exit site in a patient with mitral isthmus ventricular tachycardia demonstrated by noncontact mapping of the left ventricle. It is important that the exit site not be targeted immediately for ablation. Further mapping, entrainment, and knowledge of where the scar and slow zone are located will allow either placement of linear ablation lesions or point ablation after a narrow slow zone is identified. CS, coronary sinus; ABL, ablation site; EA, easly activation; NC, noncontact site of tachycardia origin.

tions of the electroanatomy, including intracavitary electrically active structures and epicardial foci or parts of reentry circuits, need to be easily visualized to allow planning of ablative therapy (Fig. 8–16).

To best use the available mapping systems for a specific patient, several factors should be considered:

1. Familiarity with the specific strengths and pitfalls of each system is an important factor in deciding which system to use for a complex arrhythmia. Dysfamiliarity extends not only to the consulting electrophysiologist but to the local technical staff and support from the manufacturer available on that particular day. If a patient has a transient or nonsustained arrhythmia, even though noncontact mapping is ideally suited for this situation, if local expertise is not available, then mapping of each ectopic beat or nonsustained episode can be undertaken with the available mapping system. Care should be taken in this instance to use ectopic beats of similar coupling intervals.

2. Arrhythmias that are transient in nature or hemodynamically unstable are most expeditiously mapped by noncontact mapping. If a pure anatomic approach to the arrhythmia is being considered, any of the available mapping or navigation systems may be used. However, the highest spatial resolution and the ability to map

individual chambers separately and in combination presently exist with electroanatomic mapping.

3. The flexibility to use any mapping, multielectrode, or ablation catheter should be considered. Presently, electroanatomic mapping can be performed only with the compatible catheter. The use of NavX technology, real-time position management, or the LocaLisa system allows for such flexibility.

4. Finally, the cost of the system, in terms of both initial purchase and use of the required catheters, should be considered. Real-time position management and the LocaLisa system are potentially advantageous in this regard.

Regardless of the mapping system used, the advances in catheter navigation obtained with magnet-aided navigation and the ability to combine electrographic data with intracardiac ultrasound tissue velocity mapping offer great promise in dealing with the most complex situations. For example, if a patient with complex, surgically corrected congenital disease has a nonsustained arrhythmia, noncontact mapping can quickly exclude the accessible portion of the right atrium as a source of the tachycardia. Intracardiac echocardiography may help guide difficult catheter manipulations to obtain separate electroanatomic maps of excluded portions of atrial tissue. Finally, a magnetic navigation system may greatly enhance the ease with which catheters can access these sites to perform linear ablation at targeted sites.

References

1. Wetzel U, Hindricks G, Dorszewski A, et al.: Electroanatomic mapping of the endocardium: Implications for catheter ablation of ventricular tachycardia. Herz 28:583-590, 2003.
2. Marchlinski F, Callans D, Gottlieb C, Zado E: Linear ablation lesions for control of unmappable ventricular tachycardia in patients with ischemic and nonischemic cardiomyopathy. Circulation 101:1288-1296, 2000.
3. Kottkamp H: Catheter ablation of ventricular tachycardia in remote myocardial infarction: Substrate description guiding placement of individual linear lesions targeting noninducibility [see comment]. J Cardiovasc Electrophysiol 14:675-681, 2003.
4. Boulos M, Lashevsky I, Reisner S, Gepstein L: Electroanatomic mapping of arrhythmogenic right ventricular dysplasia. J Am Coll Cardiol 38:2020-2027, 2001.
5. Niroomand F, Carbucicchio C, Tondo C, et al.: Electrophysiological characteristics and outcome in patients with idiopathic right ventricular arrhythmia compared with arrhythmogenic right ventricular dysplasia. Heart 87:41-47, 2002.
6. Fukuhara H, Nakamura Y, Tasato H, et al.: Successful radiofrequency catheter ablation of left ventricular tachycardiology following surgical correction of tetralogy of Fallot. Pacing Clin Electrophysiol 23:1442-1445, 2000.
7. Rodriguez LM, Smeets JL, Timmermans C, et al.: Radiofrequency catheter ablation of sustained monomorphic

RA Activation Map in AFL

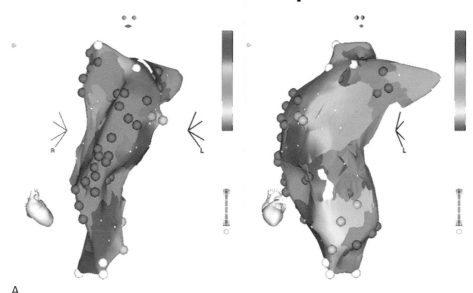

Neo-LA Activation Map in AFL

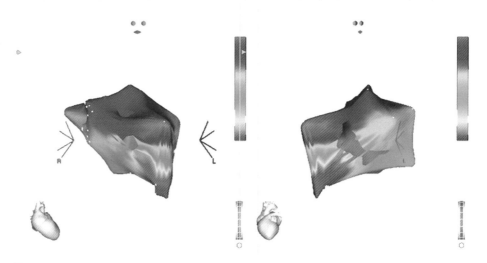

Combined Map - Ablation

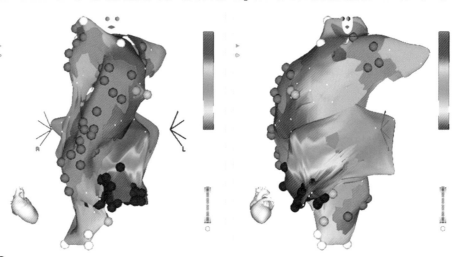

FIGURE 8–16. Mapping the atrium after surgery for congenital heart disease. **A,** When the activation map was created in the right atrium (RA), which was accessible via the superior vena cava or inferior vena cava, a counterclockwise pattern of activation near the annulus was found. However, the entire cycle length map in this chamber was far less than the cycle length of the tachycardia. **B,** When catheter access was obtained to the surgically created neo-left atrium (LA) via a retrograde aortic approach and via the left atrium through an atrial septal defect into the excluded portion of the right atrium (neo-left atrium), the remaining portion of the tachycardia cycle length was seen. **C,** The ablation line, including portions in the neo-left atrium, that successfully eliminated the arrhythmia, are shown. Both the right and left atria are represented in this map. AFL, atrial flutter.

A

B

C

ventricular tachycardia in hypertrophic cardiomyopathy. J Cardiovasc Electrophysiol 8:803-806, 1997.

8. Reddy VY, Malchano ZJ, Holmvang G, et al.: Integration of cardiac magnetic resonance imaging with three-dimensional electroanatomic mapping to guide left ventricular catheter manipulation: Feasibility in a porcine model of healed myocardial infarction. J Am Coll Cardiol 44:2202-2213, 2004.

9. Verma A, Marrouche N, Natale A: Novel method to integrate three-dimensional computed tomographic images of the left atrium with real-time electroanatomic mapping. J Cardiovasc Electrophysiol 15:968, 2004.

10. Chauhan VS, Nair GM, Sevaptisidis E, Downar E: Magneto-electroanatomic mapping of arrhythmias in structural heart disease using a novel multielectrode catheter. Pacing Clin Electrophysiol 27:1077-1084, 2004.

11. Schilling RJ, Davies DW, Peters NS: Characteristics of sinus rhythm electrograms at sites of ablation of ventricular tachycardia relative to all other sites: A noncontact mapping study of the entire left ventricle. J Cardiovasc Electrophysiol 9:921-933, 1998.

12. Schilling RJ, Friedman PA, Stanton MS, et al.: Mathematical Reconstruction of Endocardial Potentials with Non-contact Multi-electrode Array. ESI Press, 1998, pp 1-16.

13. Thiagalingam A, Wallace EM, Boyd AC, et al.: Noncontact mapping of the left ventricle: Insights from validation with transmural contact mapping. Pacing Clin Electrophysiol 27:570-578, 2004.

14. Gornick CC, Adler SW, Pederson B, et al.: Validation of a new noncontact catheter system for electroanatomic mapping of left ventricular endocardium. Circulation 99:829-835, 1999.

15. Friedman PA, Asirvatham SJ, Grice S, et al.: Noncontact mapping to guide ablation of right ventricular outflow tract tachycardia. J Am Coll Cardiol 39:1808-1812, 2002.

16. Scheinman MM, Yang Y: Electroanatomic analysis of sinus impulse propagation in normal human atria. J Cardiovasc Electrophysiol 13:11-12, 2002.

17. Goodman D, van der Steen AB, van Dam RT: Endocardial and epicardial activation pathways of the canine right atrium. Am J Physiol 220:1-11, 1971.

18. Ho SY, Sanchez-Quintana D, Cabrera JA, Anderson RH: Anatomy of the left atrium: Implications for radiofrequency ablation of atrial fibrillation. J Cardiovasc Electrophysiol 10:1525-1533, 1999.

19. Asirvatham S, Packer DL: Evidence of electrical conduction within the coronary sinus musculature by non-contact mapping. Circulation 100:4486, 1999.

20. Markides V, Schilling RJ, Ho SY, et al.: Characterization of left atrial activation in the intact human heart. Circulation 107:733-739, 2003.

21. Tai CT, Chen SA, Chiang CE, et al.: A new electrocardiographic algorithm using retrograde P waves for differentiating atrioventricular node reentrant tachycardia from atrioventricular reciprocating tachycardia mediated by concealed accessory pathway. J Am Coll Cardiol 29:394-402, 1997.

22. Betts TR, Roberts PR, Allen SA, et al.: Electrophysiological mapping and ablation of intra-atrial reentry tachycardia after Fontan surgery with the use of a noncontact mapping system. Circulation 102:2094-2099, 2000.

23. Ventura R, Rostock T, Klemm HU, et al.: Catheter ablation of common-type atrial flutter guided by three-dimensional right atrial geometry reconstruction and catheter tracking using cutaneous patches: A randomized prospective study. J Cardiovasc Electrophysiol 15:1157-1161, 2004.

24. Wittkampf FH, Wever EF, Derksen R, et al.: LocaLisa: New technique for real-time 3-dimensional localization of regular intracardiac electrodes. Circulation 99:1312-1317, 1999.

25. Kirchhof P, Loh P, Eckardt L, et al.: A novel nonfluoroscopic catheter visualization system (LocaLisa) to reduce radiation exposure during catheter ablation of supraventricular tachycardias. Am J Cardiol 90:340-343, 2002.

26. Huang SK, Bharati S, Graham AR,Lev M, Marcus FI, Odell RC. Closed chest catheter desiccation of the atrioventricular junction using radiofrequency energy—a new method of catheter ablation. J Am Coll Cardiol 1987, 9:349-358.

27. Macle L, Jais P, Scavee C, et al.: Pulmonary vein disconnection using the LocaLisa three-dimensional nonfluoroscopic catheter imaging system. J Cardiovasc Electrophysiol 14:693-697, 2003.

28. Simmers TA, Tukkie R: How to perform pulmonary vein isolation for the treatment of atrial fibrillation: Use of the LocaLisa catheter navigation system. Europace 6:92-96, 2004.

29. Weerasooriya R, Macle L, Jais P, et al.: Pulmonary vein ablation using the LocaLisa nonfluoroscopic mapping system. J Cardiovasc Electrophysiol 14:112, 2003.

30. De Groot NMS, Bootsma M, Schalij MJ: Radiofrequency catheter ablation of atrial flutter guided by a new 3-D signal based tracking system: first clinical results [abstract]. PACE 23(II):579, 2000.

31. Schreieck J, Ndrepepa G, Zrenner B, et al.: Radiofrequency ablation of cardiac arrhythmias using a three-dimensional real-time position management and mapping system. Pacing Clin Electrophysiol 25:1699-1707, 2002.

32. Ram W, Meyer H: Heart catheterization in a neonate by interacting magnetic fields: A new and simple method of catheter guidance. Cathet Cardiovasc Diagn 22:317-319, 1991.

33. Grady MS, Howard MA III, Dacey RG Jr, et al.: Experimental study of the magnetic stereotaxis system for catheter manipulation within the brain. J Neurosurg 93:282-288, 2000.

34. Erdogan A, Schulte B, Carlsson J, et al.: Klinische Charakteristika von Patienten mit AV-Knoten-Reentrytachykardie (AVNRT): Beeinflussung durch die Hochfrequenzkatheterablation. Untersuchung an 748 Patienten nach Hochfrequenzkatheterablation. Med Klin 96:708-712, 2001.

35. Ernst S, Ouyang F, Linder C, et al.: Modulation of the slow pathway in the presence of a persistent left superior caval vein using the novel magnetic navigation system Niobe. Europace 6:10-14, 2004.

36. Okumura Y, Watanabe I, Yamada T, et al.: Comparison of coronary sinus morphology in patients with and without atrioventricular nodal reentrant tachycardia by intracardiac echocardiography. J Cardiovasc Electrophysiol 15:274-275, 2004.

37. Ouyang F, Cappato R, Ernst S, et al.: Electroanatomic substrate of idiopathic left ventricular tachycardia: Unidirectional block and macroreentry within the Purkinje network. Circulation 105:462-469, 2002.

38. Nakagawa H, Jackman WM: Use of a three-dimensional, non-fluoroscopic mapping system for catheter ablation of typical atrial flutter. Pacing Clin Electrophysiol 21:1279-1286, 1998.

39. Nakagawa H, Shah N, Matsudaira K, et al.: Characterization of reentrant circuit in macroreentrant right atrial tachycardia after surgical repair of congenital heart disease. Circulation 103:699-709, 2001.

40. Seidl K, Beatty G, Drogemuller A, et al.: Catheter-based right and left atrial compartmentalisation procedure in chronic atrial fibrillation using a novel non-contact mapping system: Feasibility and safety. J Am Coll Cardiol 35:123, 2000.

41. Hindricks G, Mohr FW, Autschbach R, Kottkamp H: Antiarrhythmic surgery for treatment of atrial fibrillation: New concepts. Thorac Cardiovasc Surg 47:365-369, 1999.

42. Triedman JK, Alexander ME, Love BA, et al.: Influence of patient factors and ablative technologies on outcomes of radiofrequency ablation of intra-atrial re-entrant tachycardia

in patients with congenital heart disease. J Am Coll Cardiol 39:1827-1835, 2002.

43. Swarup V, Morton JB, Arruda M, Wilber DJ: Ablation of epicardial macroreentrant ventricular tachycardia associated with idiopathic nonischemic dilated cardiomyopathy by a percutaneous transthoracic approach. J Cardiovasc Electrophysiol 13:1164-1168, 2002.

44. Morady F: Treatment of paroxysmal atrial fibrillation by pulmonary vein isolation. Circulation 67:567-571, 2003.

45. Pappone C, Oreto G, Lamberti F, et al.: Catheter ablation of paroxysmal atrial fibrillation using a 3D mapping system. Circulation 100:1203-1208, 1999.

46. Haïssaguerre M, Shah DC, Jaïs P, Clementy J: Role of catheter ablation for atrial fibrillation. Curr Opin Cardiol 12:18-23, 1997.

47. Asirvatham SA, Friedman PA: Etiology of electrogram "spikes" observed in the pulmonary veins. Circulation 102:II-144, 2000.

48. Shah DC, Jais P, Haissaguerre M, et al.: Three-dimensional mapping of the common atrial flutter circuit in the right atrium. Circulation 96:3904-3912, 1997.

49. Willems S, Weiss C, Ventura R: Catheter ablation of atrial flutter guided by electroanatomic mapping (CARTO): a randomized comparison to the conventional approach. J Cardiovasc Electrophysiol 11(11):1223-1230, 2000.

50. Schilling RJ, Peters NS, Davies DW: Simultaneous endocardial mapping in the human left ventricle using a noncontact catheter: Comparison of contact and reconstructed electrograms during sinus rhythm. Circulation 98:887-898, 1998.

51. Gepstein L, Hayam G, Ben-Haim SA: A novel method for nonfluoroscopic catheter-based electroanatomical mapping of the heart: In vitro and in vivo accuracy results. Circulation 95:1611-1622, 1997.

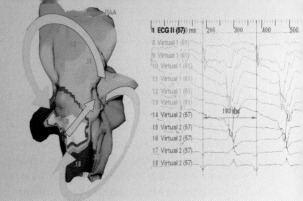

9

Role of Intracardiac Echocardiography in Clinical and Experimental Electrophysiology

Joseph B. Morton • *David J. Wilber* • *Jonathan M. Kalman*

Key Points

- Catheter technology includes mechanical types (single rotating transducer, 360-degree circumferential imaging, 9 to 12 MHz, near-field clarity, poor tissue penetration) and phased-array types (64-element sector scan, 5 to 10 MHz, steerable, full Doppler capability, good depth penetration).

- Intracardiac echocardiography (ICE) is used to help identify atrial endocardial structures, guide radiofrequency (RF) ablation, monitor RF lesions, and perform ablation for atrial fibrillation (AF).

- For identification of atrial endocardial structures, ICE is used to characterize the role of anatomy in arrhythmia mechanisms (e.g., crista terminalis, pulmonary veins [PVs]).

- For guidance of RF ablation, ICE is used to identify the anatomic location of the catheter tip and to ensure tissue contact (distal tip electrode or linear ablation catheter).

- For monitoring of RF lesions, ICE is used for real-time assessment of lesion formation and size (mural swelling and increased tissue echodensity).

- For AF ablation, ICE assists with trans-septal puncture, defines PV anatomy, allows accurate positioning of the lasso catheter at the PV ostium, monitors lesion formation, monitors for complications (e.g., tamponade, thrombus), and identifies and possibly predicts PV stenosis.

- Other uses of ICE include atrial flutter ablation (imaging cavotricuspid isthmus anatomy), ventricular tachycardia (imaging scar border, identifying coronary cusps and left ventricular outflow tract), guidance of trans-septal puncture in difficult cases, assessment of left atrium and appendage mechanical function and thrombus, and guidance of atrial septal defect device closure.

The development of intracardiac echocardiography (ICE) has led to an increasing appreciation of the important relationship between arrhythmia mechanism and anatomy. Uses of ICE in the electrophysiology laboratory have included identification of atrial endocardial structures and manipulation of mapping and ablation catheters in relation to these structures,[1,2] creation and quantification of focal[3-9] and continuous[10-12] radiofrequency ablation (RFA) lesions, guidance in the performance of atrial trans-septal puncture,[13,14] and identification and prevention of procedural complications.

Although ICE has been critical to understanding of the importance of cardiac anatomy in arrhythmia mechanisms, until recently its clinical utility was limited mostly to guidance of difficult transseptal procedures. However, in recent years, ICE has developed a central role in some centers during catheter ablation procedures for atrial fibrillation (AF).

Intracardiac Echocardiography Catheter Design

Technical advances in the construction of compact ultrasound transducers have allowed the development of ICE. Two forms of ICE catheter have been designed which may be described as mechanical ICE and phased-array ICE.

Mechanical ICE catheters have a single ultrasound crystal mounted at the distal end of a 6 to 10 French (F) catheter. The majority of these catheters have been nonsteerable. The transducer is connected to a motor in the handle of the device via a braided drive shaft. Engagement of the mechanism results in rapid rotation of the transducer, providing 360-degree circumferential imaging in a plane perpendicular to the long axis of the catheter. Mechanical ICE uses imaging frequencies of 9 to 12 MHz, which provide near-field clarity but poor tissue penetration and far-field resolution (Fig. 9–1). As a result, these systems have not

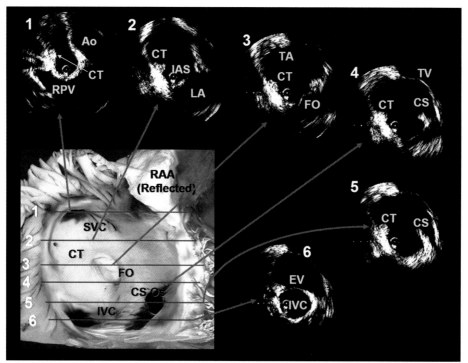

FIGURE 9–1. Serial horizontal slices taken through the right atrium using a conventional 9-MHz mechanical transducer and an intracardiac echocardiography catheter. The inset shows an anatomic cut-away view of the right atrium. The catheter has been withdrawn sequentially from the junction of the superior vena cava (SVC) and right atrium to the inferior vena cava (IVC). The anatomy of the crista terminalis (CT) is highlighted through a series of images. Superiorly, the CT is closely related to the right superior pulmonary vein (RPV). The interatrial septum (IAS) then comes into view with the fossa ovalis (FO). The mouth of the coronary sinus (CS) appears superior to the level of the eustachian valve (EV). The eustachian ridge (continuation of caudal CT) passes septally toward the mouth of the CS (CS Os; posterior rim). Ao, aorta; LA, left atrium; TA, tricuspid annulus; TV, tricuspid valve. *(Inset adapted from Ref. 82.)*

allowed clear imaging of the left atrium and pulmonary veins (PVs) with the catheter located in the right atrium.[2] Imaging with this catheter has been used in experimental and clinical studies to identify endocardial landmarks, guide mapping and ablation catheters in proximity to these landmarks, guide trans-septal puncture, and monitor for procedural complications.[1,4,5,13,15-18]

Ren et al.[19] compared imaging data obtained from transesophageal echocardiography (TEE) and conventional ICE in pigs and concluded that, although the latter provided higher-resolution imaging of individual cardiac chambers and structures, whole heart imaging was limited by ultrasound penetration at 12.5 MHz.

Phased-array ICE is a newer imaging system that incorporates a miniaturized 64-element, phased-array, electronically controlled transducer mounted at the distal end of a 90-cm long, steerable, 8F or 10F catheter. Variable imaging frequencies can be used, ranging from 5 to 10 MHz, and the system permits the full range of two-dimensional, M-mode and Doppler imaging (including pulsed wave, color, continuous wave, and tissue Doppler). The catheter tip can be deflected 160 degrees in two planes (anteroposterior and right-to-left) and then locked in position. Bidirectional steering and locking are performed via three separate controls located in the catheter handle. This catheter produces a wedge-shaped (sector) image, which is displayed on a conventional echocardiographic workstation similar to that used in transthoracic echocardiography or TEE.

Bruce et al.[20] reported the results of a preclinical human trial assessing the feasibility of imaging with this device and concluded that the system provided diagnostic quality, high-resolution, two-dimensional and Doppler imaging.

Phased-array ICE has been shown to provide image quality similar to that obtained with TEE, both for imaging the interatrial septum during device closure of an atrial septal defect (ASD)[21] and for imaging of the left atrial appendage with Doppler assessment of mechanical function in patients with atrial arrhythmias.[22]

Identification of Atrial Endocardial Structures

One of the initial uses of ICE was in the identification of endocardial structures and accurate positioning of diagnostic and ablation electrophysiology catheters in relation to this defined anatomy. This technology facilitated, for the first time, an understanding of the relationship between anatomy and electrophysiology. Kalman et al.[23] and Olgin et al.[1] used conventional ICE to define the tricuspid annulus, crista terminalis, and eustachian ridge as important anatomic barriers to conduction during typical human atrial flutter (AFL). Subsequently, in a study also using ICE guidance of catheter positioning, Friedman et al.[24] suggested that the region of posterior block in typical flutter was actually at the posterior smooth-walled atrium, immediately adjacent to the crista terminalis. This debate revolves around the spatial resolution of a 0.5-cm bipole. Many investigators believe that the area of block is at the medial aspect of the crista terminalis, at the transition between smooth-walled, sinus venosus–derived atrium and the crista terminalis, which marks the beginning of the trabeculated atrium.

Kalman et al.[16] later used ICE to assist in accurate positioning of a multipolar catheter along the crista terminalis, in order to define this structure as a major focus for atrial tachycardia within the right atrium ("cristal tachycardias"). In dogs, ICE allowed accurate ablation and functional modification of the sinus node pacemaker complex located along the long axis of the crista terminalis.[8] In a subsequent clinical study,[15] ICE was used to identify the crista terminalis in patients with inappropriate sinus tachycardia and to guide modification of sinus pacemaker function. Although the anatomic location of the crista terminalis in the right atrium is well known, Marchlinski et al.[25] demonstrated that fluoroscopically guided identification of this structure was frequently inaccurate and was greatly facilitated by the use of ICE.

Guidance of Radiofrequency Ablation Catheter

The creation of lesions during RFA procedures requires stable contact between the ablation catheter electrode and the target tissue. ICE may facilitate this process, leading to more efficient ablation.[4,6,10] RFA catheters can be easily visualized by ICE and have a typical appearance, with a bright tip and a fan-shaped acoustic shadow.[26] Kalman et al.[6] compared traditional criteria for determining tissue contact (stable electrogram signals and fluoroscopic appearance) with conventional ICE–guided ablation in dogs. Without ICE guidance, lateral sliding of the ablation catheter (greater than 5 mm) was frequent (18%), as was poor perpendicular electrode tissue contact (27%) leading to smaller lesion formation and a lower efficiency of heating index (ratio of steady-state temperature to power).[6] Olgin et al.[11] created long linear ablation lesions in the atria of pigs using a multielectrode coil array guided by conventional ICE. ICE allowed accurate positioning of the array between anatomic structures including the tricuspid annulus, fossa ovalis, crista terminalis, and inferior vena cava. In particular, ICE allowed visualization of tissue contact along the length of the multielectrode catheter and demonstrated that, with fluoroscopy alone, frequently more than half of the coil length was not in tissue contact. Similarly, Epstein et al.[10] compared fluoroscopy and ICE for the creation of linear atrial lesions in dogs. ICE led to a higher percentage of successful applications, which were more accurately located and of a larger size as a result of better tissue contact.

Roithinger et al.[12] performed linear left atrial ablation in dogs using a multicoil ablation catheter. Lesions were placed under either fluoroscopic or ICE guidance. In this study, an investigational, nonsteerable, 17F, 9- to 12-MHz phased-array device was used. It provided good imaging of the left atrial free wall, roof, and appendage but poor views of the PVs.[12]

Identification of structures on the left side of the heart may be enhanced if the catheter is introduced into the arterial circulation[18,27]; however, this approach is associated with increased complications. Mangrum et al.[18] introduced a 9F, 9-MHz conventional ICE catheter into the left atrium and PV mouth via a trans-septal sheath. ICE was then used to guide circumferential RFA, ensure good ablation catheter tissue contact, and monitor for PV stenosis. After ablation, the PV wall was observed to be thickened with increased echogenicity. The mean reduction in luminal diameter after RFA was 12%.

Monitoring and Quantification of Radiofrequency Ablation Lesions

In the clinical electrophysiology laboratory, ICE is the only technique available for providing real-time assessment of lesion formation and size. In an excised canine heart model of ablation, Kalman et al.[3] used high-frequency ICE imaging (15 MHz) to measure RFA lesion size and demonstrated a high correlation between ultrasonic and pathologic lesion depth. However, whereas other investigators have used ICE to observe lesion formation in vivo, it is less clear that a correlation exists between the endocardial changes observed in the beating heart and lesion size.

Using conventional ICE (10 MHz), Chu et al.[26] described lesion formation after RFA in the canine right atrium as the development of an endocardial dimple or defect. However, the majority of subsequent studies have described a region of swelling or increased echogenicity (or both) at the ablation site.

In a human study of sinus node modification by RFA techniques, Lee et al.[15] used conventional ICE (10 MHz) to target the sinus node (crista terminalis). In this study, RFA lesion formation was detected by ICE and described as an area of local increase in tissue echogenicity producing an ultrasound shadowing artifact.[15]

In a series of human and porcine studies, Marchlinski et al.[28-30] used conventional ICE to describe the nature of the lesion formed as a result of the application of radiofrequency (RF) energy. They observed the formation of mural swelling and increased tissue echodensity after the application of RF in the right atrium. Furthermore, after transmural linear lesion formation in the posterior right atrium of pigs, the demonstration by ICE of mural swelling correlated with the finding of mural edema on histopathology.[29] In a study of cavotricuspid isthmus ablation by Morton et al.[31] using phased-array ICE and an imaging frequency of up to 10 MHz, it was possible to observe discrete lesion formation after RF applications, manifested predominantly as regions of tissue swelling. Interestingly, without additional RF applications, ICE demonstrated a progression over ensuing minutes to more diffuse swelling and lesion coalescence. The significance of this finding is uncertain, but again it may represent development of tissue edema after the RF application.

This swelling at the region of RF application has in some anatomic locations had important clinical implications. In humans, ICE has allowed the identification of narrowing of the superior vena cava–right atrium junction during RFA of the crista terminalis for inappropriate sinus tachycardia.[30] Indeed, superior vena cava syndrome has been described as a potential complication of circumferential ablation at this junction. This observation predated by several years a similar observation of PV narrowing caused by circumferential ostial ablation (see below).

Role in Atrial Fibrillation Ablation Procedures

Catheter ablation procedures for the treatment of AF have assumed an increasingly important therapeutic role. After initial experience with catheter ablation targeting arrhythmogenic foci within the PV,[32,33] techniques have been evolved to electrically isolate the PV by ablation of left atrial–PV connections. Both circumferential ablation[34] and a segmental approach (targeting sites with early activation[35-37]) have been employed. Current techniques vary in the extent of left atrium ablated with or without linear lesions, in targeting of fractionated electrograms, and in procedural end points.

A key requirement for successful and safe ablation within the left atrium is anatomic characterization of the PVs and accurate localization of the ostia. At the venoatrial junction, the PVs demonstrate considerable anatomic heterogeneity in their ostial diameter, number, location, and pattern of branching[38] (Fig. 9–2). PV imaging can be performed with the use of contrast venography. However this procedure may require separate contrast injections and does not allow real-time monitoring of catheter positioning; nor does it provide physiologic data. Alternatively, electroanatomic and noncontact mapping systems may be used to define anatomy, potentially with a computed tomographic (CT) or magnetic resonance imaging (MRI) template for the three-dimensional chamber reconstruction.

Phased-array ICE has been shown in experimental and clinical studies[20,39] to provide accurate two-dimensional and Doppler imaging of the left atrium and PVs while positioned in the right atrium. Furthermore, ICE has the potential to accurately guide and monitor the positioning of diagnostic and ablation catheters within the left atrium. A negative aspect of existing ICE imaging using a mechanically rotating 9-MHz transducer is that the field of view is limited. As a result, these systems have not allowed clear imaging of the left atrium and PVs[2] except when introduced directly into the left atrium and advanced to the PV ostium.[18]

Wood et al.[40] compared measurements of PV diameter by phased-array ICE with those obtained by CT, contrast venography, and TEE. Ostial PV diameters were significantly correlated between each imaging modality; however, several important observations were made. PV values measured by CT and ICE were similar, whereas venography tended to overestimate and TEE to underestimate the ostial diameter. Furthermore, CT and ICE identified more PV ostia than either venography or TEE.

In general, phased-array ICE is the system of choice for assisting AF catheter ablation.

The main roles of ICE in left atrium ablation procedures are the following:

1. Assisting with trans-septal puncture
2. Defining PV anatomy
3. Allowing accurate positioning of the lasso catheter at the venous ostium
4. Monitoring lesion formation
5. Monitoring for complications
6. Identifying and possibly predicting PV stenosis

ACCURATE POSITIONING OF THE LASSO CATHETER AT THE VENOUS OSTIUM

Recent data indicate that inward migration and misalignment of the lasso catheter are common during

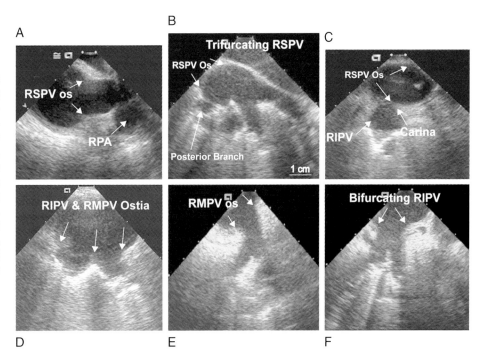

FIGURE 9–2. Intracardiac echocardiographic images demonstrating anatomic variations of the right-sided pulmonary veins (PV): right superior (RSPV), right middle (RMPV), and right inferior (RIPV). **A,** The usual relationship of the RSPV to the right pulmonary artery (RPA). **B,** Posterior RSPV branch. **C,** Carina between RSPV and RIPV. **D** and **E,** RMPV examples. **F,** RIPV early bifurcation. *Small arrows* indicate the pulmonary vein ostia.

AF ablation procedures.[41] ICE allows continuous referencing of the lasso and ablation catheter positions to the PV ostium, permitting frequent readjustment of both before RFA (Figs. 9–3, 9–4, and 9–5).

Early ablation reports suggested that the PV triggers were located deep within the PVs.[32] Although this remains true, later clinical studies have indicated that such triggers may also frequently arise very proximally in the PV and indeed at the PV–left atrium junction.[36] Recent experimental animal data highlight the electrophysiologic importance of the proximal PV and adjacent left atrium as a region of marked anisotropic conduction,[42] spontaneous focal activity,[42] and high-frequency microreentrant sources.[43] Accurate identification of the PV ostium with fluoroscopy alone can be challenging, especially with inexperienced operators. Migration of the lasso catheter into the PV during the course of PV isolation is common and is not readily detectable by fluoroscopy (see Fig. 9–5). In a subset of 30 patients specifically monitored for lasso movement, we found that displacement of the lasso by more than 1 cm inside the ostium occurred at least once during the course of isolation in 32% of PVs (Morton and Wilber, unpublished data). ICE permitted rapid identification of this problem and guided subsequent repositioning to a more ostial location (Fig. 9–6).

MONITORING LESION FORMATION

ICE has been used not only to monitor lesion formation during RFA but also to identify potential com-

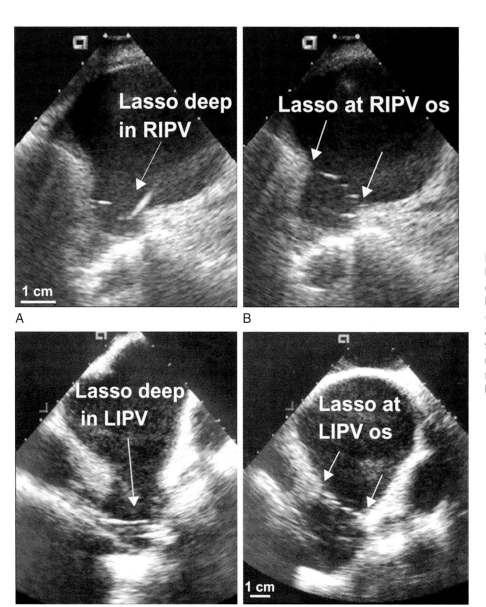

A

B

C

D

FIGURE 9–3. Positioning of lasso catheter. **A** and **C,** Lasso catheter deep within right and left inferior pulmonary vein (RIPV and LIPV, respectively). **B** and **D,** Correction of lasso position to a true ostial location using intracardiac echocardiography. *Small arrows* indicate lasso catheter.

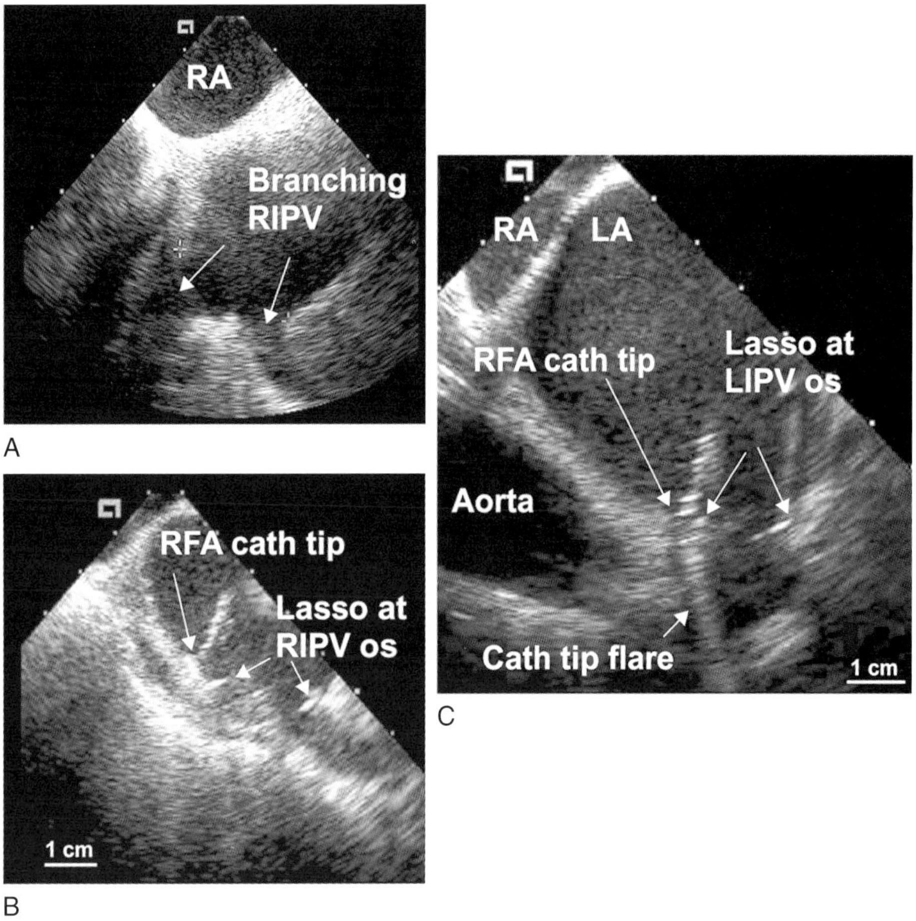

FIGURE 9–4. A and **B,** Complex right inferior pulmonary vein (RIPV) anatomy with two separate branches *(arrows)* opening into a single pulmonary vein (PV) ostium. In **B,** a lasso is positioned at the true ostium of the PV, allowing radiofrequency ablation (RFA) to be delivered to the atrial tissue adjacent to the venoatrial junction. **C,** Lasso catheter and RFA catheter positioned at the true ostium of a left inferior PV (LIPV os). LA, left atrium; RA, right atrium.

plications. In an early study in dogs, Kalman et al.[6] used ICE to observe coagulum formation (shaggy echodensity) on the ablation catheter tip. This occurrence was usually preceded (by 5 to 10 seconds) by local microbubble formation during the ablation.[6] More recently, Marrouche et al.[44] extended these observations and described their clinical utility. These investigators based the titration of power during RF delivery on the real-time observations obtained from ICE during ablation. They defined type 1 and type 2 microbubbles during RF applications. Type 1 are defined as scattered microbubbles. They are presumed to be caused by early tissue overheating and, when observed, lead the operator to reduce the power delivered by 5-W decrements until the microbubbles disappear. Type 2 microbubbles are defined as dense showers of bubbles. They usually herald an imminent impedance rise, and therefore the RF application is immediately interrupted by the operator. Using this approach, this group achieved a greater success rate than when using ICE without bubble monitoring, and with fewer complications. In particular, the incidence of thromboembolic events was significantly reduced. Although these are intriguing and provocative observations, to date they have not been confirmed in prospective and randomized studies. In addition, if externally irrigated catheters are used for AF ablation, type 1 microbubbles cannot be distinguished from the catheter irrigation.

More recently, Bunch et al.[45] demonstrated in an animal model of PV ablation, using an 8-mm-tip catheter, that microbubbles are an inconsistent marker of tissue overheating. Using phased-array ICE and implanted atrial thermocouples, this group showed that type 1 and type 2 microbubbles were not seen during some ablations (13% and 40%, respectively) despite tissue temperatures greater than 80°C. Furthermore, in 40% of ablations, type 1 microbubbles did not precede the development of type 2 microbubbles. Overall, however, microbubble formation was correlated with tissue overheating.

Phased-array ICE has also been used in the left atrium and coronary sinus to achieve novel views during linear lesion formation between the left inferior pulmonary vein and the mitral annulus. In a case report,[46] tissue edema during RF application, together with the appearance of a hypodense region within the atrial musculature, was identified as a prelude to imminent impedance rise and "pop."

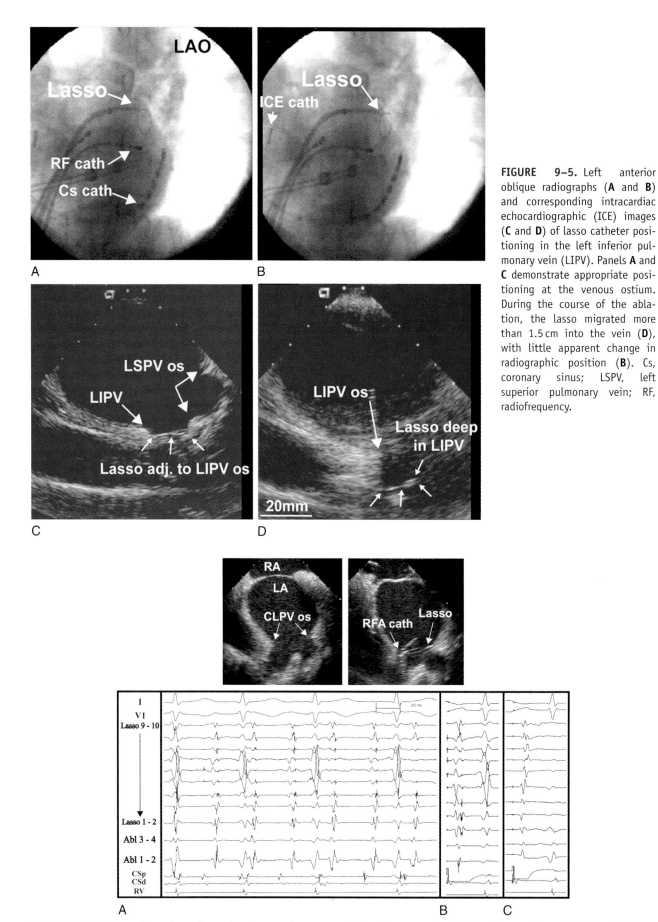

FIGURE 9–5. Left anterior oblique radiographs (**A** and **B**) and corresponding intracardiac echocardiographic (ICE) images (**C** and **D**) of lasso catheter positioning in the left inferior pulmonary vein (LIPV). Panels **A** and **C** demonstrate appropriate positioning at the venous ostium. During the course of the ablation, the lasso migrated more than 1.5 cm into the vein (**D**), with little apparent change in radiographic position (**B**). Cs, coronary sinus; LSPV, left superior pulmonary vein; RF, radiofrequency.

FIGURE 9–6. Intracardiac echocardiographic images of a common left pulmonary vein (CLPV) with superior and inferior divisions. Adjacent image shows lasso and radiofrequency ablation catheter (RFA cath) positioned at the venous ostium. With the lasso in this position, pulmonary vein potentials were recorded from each bipole during spontaneous atrial tachycardia arising from the CLPV (**A**), with the earliest PV potential recorded in lasso 1-2. After several radiofrequency (RF) applications, tachycardia was terminated but sharp PV potentials were still present on the lasso during coronary sinus pacing (panel **B**). Further RF applications targeting the remaining PV potentials were given, and venous isolation was achieved (**C**). LA, left atrium; RA, right atrium.

POSTABLATION IMAGING: CAN PULMONARY VEIN STENOSIS BE PREDICTED?

PV stenosis remains a significant limiting factor to procedures targeting these structures.[47-52] Robbins et al.[47] first reported two cases of symptomatic PV stenosis in individuals who had undergone PV ablation procedures. Both patients presented with dyspnea and pulmonary hypertension and required balloon dilatation of the stenosed veins. Gerstenfeld et al.[48] found evidence of PV stenosis in 8% of those undergoing focal ablation of AF. In a larger series, Yu et al.[49] assessed PV flow by transesophageal pulsed-wave Doppler (PWD) imaging and frequently identified increased flow velocity (suggesting stenosis) after ablation. In their study, most patients remained asymptomatic, and no factors predictive of developing stenosis were identified. However, other groups have suggested that RFA within small PVs increases the risk of stenosis.[51] Taylor et al.[53] performed extensive RFA within canine PVs and observed frequent PV stenosis and occlusion. Histology of the affected veins demonstrated thrombus formation, fibrocellular intimal proliferation, endocardial contraction, and proliferation of the internal elastic lamina.

PV luminal narrowing cannot be detected on fluoroscopic imaging alone; either contrast venography,[47] TEE,[49] CT scanning, or MRI is required.[50] Making the diagnosis of PV stenosis by TEE involves measurement of the PV ostial diameter, color flow Doppler imaging to visualize turbulent flow within the posterior left atrium, and PWD to detect elevated PV inflow velocity.[49,54] A PWD signal of greater than 160 cm/sec with loss of phasic flow has been used to define PV stenosis.[55] In the setting of PV ablation, Yu et al.[49] defined stenosis as an increase in maximal inflow Doppler velocity to greater than two standard deviations above the preablation mean.

Several reports have shown a small but statistically significant decrease in PV dimensions and increase in PV flow velocity after ablation, as measured by ICE for each of the PVs.[18,56-58] Importantly, Saad et al.[58] also demonstrated a lack of relationship between immediate postablation PV measurements and the development of PV stenosis. In a study of 95 patients undergoing PV isolation, the mean preablation and postablation flow velocities were observed to increase, the correlation between flow velocity and PV stenosis was poor. All patients underwent CT scanning of the PVs at 3 months after ablation. Of 380 PVs ablated, the CT scans revealed 2 (1%) with severe stenosis (>70%), 13 (3%) with moderate stenosis (51% to 70%), and 62 (16%) with mild stenosis(≤50%). The authors concluded that "acute changes in PV flow immediately after ostial PV isolation do not appear to be a strong predictor of chronic PV stenosis."

This observation supports the suggestion that the mechanism of PV stenosis is progressive after ablation[59] and may involve thrombus formation or intimal proliferation or both.[53] Nonetheless, it would seem reasonable to closely monitor any patient who has a marked increase (>1.0 m/sec) in PV flow velocity after ablation or a significant acute reduction in luminal diameter for the development of late PV stenosis.

PHASED-ARRAY INTRACARDIAC ECHOCARDIOGRAPHY AND ABLATION OF ATRIAL FLUTTER

RFA for the creation of a bidirectional conduction block across the cavotricuspid isthmus has become first-line therapy in the management of typical cavotricuspid isthmus–dependent atrial flutter[60-65] and has a high success rate. However, the complex and variable anatomy of the cavotricuspid isthmus region may be an impediment to achieving isthmus block. Cabrera et al.[66] reported a wide range of possible anatomic variations within the isthmus, including pouches, recesses, trabeculations, and ridges, that could make successful ablation difficult. Large-tip and irrigated-tip catheters facilitate isthmus ablation, but there is still a potential role for a real-time imaging modality that has the capability to accurately define cavotricuspid isthmus anatomy and guide RFA in difficult cases. The use of ICE for this purpose remains largely experimental. Mechanical ICE has facilitated detailed endocardial mapping of the boundaries to an isthmus-dependent atrial flutter[67,68] but is limited in its discrimination of other cavotricuspid isthmus features.[69] Right atrium angiography may also give a general guide to cavotricuspid isthmus anatomy,[70] but it does not provide detailed endocardial definition or information regarding the thickness of the isthmus.

Recently, Morton et al.[31] used phased-array ICE with a high imaging frequency (7.5 to 10 MHz) in 15 patients who were undergoing ablation of typical atrial flutter. With this modality, they were able to perform detailed analysis of the cavotricuspid isthmus in all patients (Fig. 9–7). The boundaries of the cavotricuspid isthmus (tricuspid annulus, eustachian ridge, coronary sinus, and trabeculated free wall of the right atrium) were well visualized, as was endocardial contour and shape; the presence of pouching, recesses, and trabeculations; and the isthmus thickness along its length before and after ablation. The thickness of the cavotricuspid isthmus measured as follows: anterior cavotricuspid isthmus (at the tricuspid annulus), 4.1 ± 0.8 mm; midcavotricuspid isthmus, 3.3 ± 0.5 mm; and posterior cavotri-

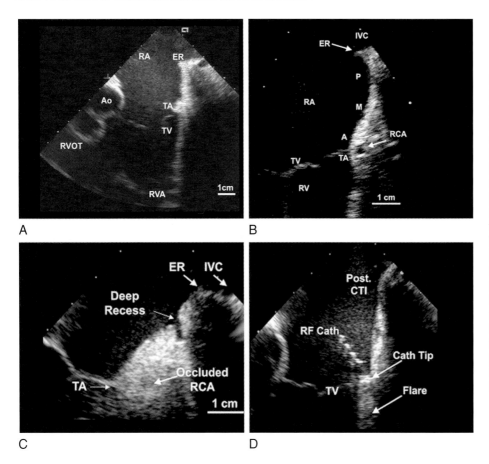

FIGURE 9–7. **A,** Baseline view of the right atrium (RA), ventricle (RVA), and outflow tract (RVOT), tricuspid valve (TV), and annulus (TA). The eustachian ridge (ER) and aortic root (Ao) can also be seen. **B,** View with higher imaging frequency (8.5 MHz) of the central cavotricuspid isthmus (CTI), identifying the RA; right ventricle (RV); TV; TA; right coronary artery (RCA); ER; inferior vena cava (IVC); and anterior (A), middle (M), and posterior (P) isthmus sectors. **C,** Deep recess within the CTI. Note the chronically occluded RCA. **D,** Radiofrequency ablation of the anterior isthmus. Note the prominent flare of the radiofrequency ablation catheter tip. Cath, catheter; Post, posterior.

cuspid isthmus (at the eustachian ridge), 2.7 ± 0.9 mm ($P < .001$ by analysis of variance [ANOVA]).

ICE was used to identify the ablation catheter and guide lesion delivery away from deep recesses and prominent trabeculations. After each RF application, a discrete lesion was usually visible, although this was more prominent when an 8-mm-tip RF catheter was used. Over time (minutes), these lesions lost their definition and were replaced by a diffuse swelling of the cavotricuspid isthmus. Pouching and recesses were commonly seen and usually were deeper in the septal rather than the lateral isthmus. In this study, ICE confirmed a long-held clinical impression, that there may be no single, ideal, anatomically determined location in the cavotricuspid isthmus at which to perform ablation. Although the septal isthmus is narrower in most patients, it is significantly more pouched. The location of thick trabeculae is variable throughout the cavotricuspid isthmus but was more frequently observed in the lateral isthmus.

INTRACARDIAC ECHOCARDIOGRAPHY–GUIDED ABLATION IN THE LEFT VENTRICLE

Experimental studies by Callans et al.[71,72] showed the efficacy of conventional ICE for defining scar in a porcine model of healed anterior infarction when the catheter is introduced directly into the left ventricular cavity via a modified sheath passed from the carotid artery. As in standard non-intracardiac echocardiography, chronically infarcted scarred myocardium was identified as thinned muscle with increased echodensity. ICE was also used to monitor RF lesion formation and again demonstrated tissue thickening after ablation. ICE-defined infarction correlated with that defined by electroanatomic mapping and pathologic analysis.

Clinical experience with ICE and ablation of ventricular tachycardia (VT) is less than with AF ablation. Phased-array ICE can visualize the infarcted area of myocardium when positioned in the right ventricle via the femoral vein approach, and all regions of the left ventricle can be imaged. ICE allows monitoring for the development of either microbubble formation (tissue overheating) or pericardial effusion. Doi et al.[73] used phased-array ICE imaging from the right ventricle to monitor RF lesion formation in a canine model of left ventricular ablation. The ablation catheter was easily visualized by ICE, as were the majority of delivered RF lesions. ICE-detected lesion size tended to overestimate the true pathologic necrotic area, because of the adjacent regions of edema.

Phased-array ICE has also been used to monitor the delivery of RF energy within the left coronary cusp in patients with idiopathic VT arising from this region (Fig. 9–8). Although coronary angiography is the gold standard for identifying the relationship of ablation sites to the left coronary artery, ICE provides real-time visualization of the distance between the RF catheter tip and both the coronary ostium and the proximal left main coronary artery, and it also monitors for microbubble formation.

TRANS-SEPTAL PUNCTURE

ICE has been used to accurately guide trans-septal puncture in both animal and human studies.[5,13,14,74,75] Daoud et al.[13] characterized the variations in the size, thickness, and anatomy of the fossa ovalis. If the fossa is thick and small or very localized, ICE can be effectively used to guide accurate positioning of the trans-septal needle. Needle positioning can be observed by a careful appraisal of the region of maximal "tenting" of the central fossa and can be confirmed by the injection of saline, which appears as bubbles at the needle tip. If the septum in the region of the fossa ovalis is highly mobile, ICE can monitor the distance between the point of maximal tenting and the adjacent lateral left atrium wall, which in the extreme may be impinged upon by the tented fossa. Without ICE, the

trans-septal puncture assembly may slide superiorly during the process of advancing the needle. ICE can monitor for excessive sliding with the potential for puncture of the high septum and atrial roof.

ECHOCARDIOGRAPHIC EVALUATION OF ATRIAL MECHANICAL FUNCTION

At present, TEE remains the clinical gold standard for assessment of left atrial mechanical function and screening for the presence of left atrial appendage thrombus. Phased-array ICE has been evaluated against TEE for measuring atrial mechanical function. In a small prospective study, Morton et al.[22] compared ICE with multiplane TEE for this purpose in patients undergoing RFA for atrial flutter, in whom atrial mechanical stunning occurs after ablation (Fig. 9–9).

Bland and Altman[76] plots were used to measure the limits of agreement between the two techniques. A high correlation and clinically excellent limits of agreement were found to exist between the two imaging modalities for measurement of left atrial appendage emptying velocity, right and left PV flow, mitral E and A wave inflow velocities, severity of left atrial spontaneous echo contrast, and left atrial appendage fractional area change. No patients were identified with left atrial appendage thrombus, and

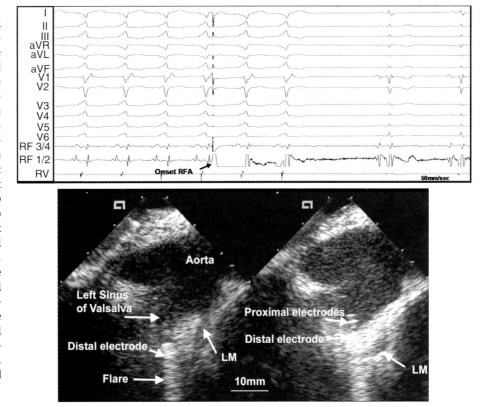

FIGURE 9–8. The top panel shows an inferior-axis ventricular tachycardia mapped to the left coronary cusp, with rapid termination during application of radiofrequency ablation (RFA) using a 4-mm-tip ablation catheter. Radiofrequency (RF) energy application was monitored in real time by an intracardiac echocardiographic catheter positioned in the right side of the heart *(bottom two panels)*, which was able to clearly discern the aortic root and valve, distal and proximal ablation catheter electrodes, catheter tip flare, and both the proximal *(bottom left)* and distal *(bottom right)* left main coronary artery (LM). Note the close relationship of both proximal and distal LM to the distal ablation catheter tip (10 to 13 mm). No arterial injury occurred during RFA.

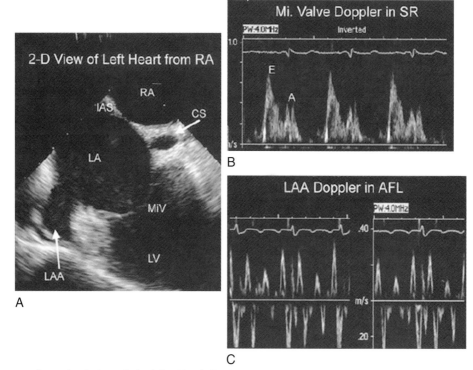

FIGURE 9–9. A, Two-dimensional view of the left side of the heart with the intracardiac echocardiography catheter positioned in the right atrium (RA). The imaging frequency was 7.5 MHz. Visible are the interatrial septum (IAS), left atrium (LA), proximal coronary sinus in cross-section (CS), mitral valve (MiV), left ventricle (LV), and left atrial appendage (LAA). The catheter transducer (which is mounted parallel to the long axis of the catheter shaft) has been directed posterolaterally toward the mitral valve. Note the presence of spontaneous echo contrast within the LA and LAA. **B,** Pulsed-wave (PW). Doppler trace of the mitral valve (Mi. valve) inflow pattern during sinus rhythm (SR), illustrating the E and A wave components to flow. The mean E wave is 0.7 m/sec, and the mean A wave is 0.4 m/sec. **C,** PW. Doppler trace of the LAA emptying velocity recorded during atrial flutter (AFL). *(From Morton JB, Sanders P, Sparks PB, et al.: Usefulness of phased-array intracardiac echocardiography for the assessment of left atrial mechanical "stunning" in atrial flutter and comparison with multiplane transesophageal echocardiography. Am J Cardiol 90:741-746, 2002, with permission of Blackwell Scientific Publishing.)*

this was a limitation of the study. However, previous animal studies have identified left atrial thrombus with ICE (Morton et al.[39]), and small, highly mobile strands of thrombus attached to long vascular sheaths deployed in the left atrium are occasionally seen using ICE.

Therefore, ICE may be an alternative to TEE for the measurement of left atrium mechanical function and surveillance for left atrial thrombus formation in selected patients undergoing atrial catheter ablation procedures.

SUGGESTED IMAGING PROTOCOL FOR PHASED-ARRAY INTRACARDIAC ECHOCARDIOGRAPHY

Under fluoroscopic guidance, the catheter is advanced into the body of the right atrium. For inexperienced operators, it is helpful to obtain a view of the tricuspid valve, right ventricle, and right ventricular infundibulum and use this as a reference point for the examination. An imaging frequency of either 5.0 or 7.5 MHz is used. To achieve this view, the catheter is positioned vertically in the mid-right atrium and then simply rotated without either left-right or anterior-posterior steering. Next, clockwise rotation of the catheter brings septal structures into view, and the fossa ovalis is easily visualized. Further clockwise rotation brings important left atrial structures into view. The mitral annulus and left atrial appendage are imaged with clockwise rotation on a level at or just inferior to the fossa ovalis. To image the mitral valve in a long-axis, two-chamber view (left atrium, mitral valve, and left ventricle), a mild degree of apically directed ICE catheter tip deflection may be required. At the level of the left atrial appendage, the catheter shaft is rotated and the tip is deflected, using the steering mechanism, until the mouth and body of the appendage are clearly visualized. PWD imaging of the left atrial appendage can be performed and an assessment made for spontaneous echo contrast or thrombus.[22]

The PVs are visualized with further clockwise rotation on a level at or immediately superior to the fossa. The left sided PVs are visualized first, and a common left PV ostium is seen in up to 25% of patients. A common left PV may be defined by the ICE appearance of a single left-sided PV ostium with a common segment (neck) of at least 5 mm between the left atrium–PV junction and first-order branching. The mean common left PV ostial diameter is approximately 26 ± 4 mm (range, 20 to 40 mm) with a common venous segment (neck) of variable length $(12 \pm 4$ mm; range, 6 to 23 mm).[77]

If the ostia are separate, it usually is not possible to clearly discern the left atrium–PV junction of both PVs in the same view, and small amounts of adjustment in steering and rotation are required to distinguish each vein. Occasionally, a third left PV is identified.

After imaging of the left-sided PVs is complete, further clockwise rotation of the catheter at the same level brings the right inferior PV into view. If the ICE catheter is advanced and rotated to direct the transducer more posteriorly, the right superior PV (RSPV) can be seen; the right pulmonary artery passes superiorly to it. Variations in right PV anatomy detected by ICE are common. A right middle PV occurs in 5% to 15% of patients, although a posterior branch of the RSPV may be mistaken for a right middle PV if it does actually enter the RSPV just proximal to the PV–left atrium junction. A common right PV may be observed, or, alternatively, there may be very closely related right superior and inferior PVs with a discrete carina or ridge between them.

The left and right inferior PVs are easily visualized in their longitudinal axis. Some degree of catheter manipulation is almost always required to visualize the left and right superior PVs in their long axis.

For each PV, the vein diameter at the left atrium–PV junction and the maximal PV inflow velocity by PWD are acquired before and after ablation (see later discussion). For the PV inflow velocity measurement using PWD, the sample volume is placed approximately 5 mm inside the PV ostium.

To visualize the left ventricle, the ICE catheter is advanced with apically directed tip deflection into the right ventricle and rotated clockwise against the interventricular septum. Excellent images of the left ventricle and mitral valve are obtained, and this view also permits easy and rapid identification of any pericardial effusion. If the catheter is further advanced and rotated, the apex of the right ventricle can be inspected and false tendons identified.

Withdrawing the catheter back to the base of the right ventricular outflow tract and rotating the shaft allows the tract to be seen in its long axis, with a cross-sectional view of the pulmonic valve.

Alternatively the right and left outflow tracts and aortic root with coronary artery ostia can be imaged by advancing the catheter in the right atrium to the level of the outflow tracts. The aortic valve can also be imaged in its cross-section from this region.

OTHER AND NOVEL USES OF INTRACARDIAC ECHOCARDIOGRAPHY

Hijazi et al.[21] compared the efficacy of TEE and ICE in guiding the performance of percutaneous ASD device closure. There was a high correlation between TEE and ICE for measuring the defect size, and it was concluded that ICE could potentially replace TEE as a guiding imaging tool for this procedure. More recently, Bartel et al.[78] demonstrated shorter fluoroscopy and procedural times when using ICE rather than conventional monitoring (TEE) for ASD and PFO device closure.

More varied uses of this catheter have been reported and include the assessment of left ventricular function[79] as well as peripheral vascular anatomy and atherosclerotic burden.[79,80]

ICE may also be used to facilitate the performance of complex pacemaker procedures, pacemaker lead extraction, and the identification of endocarditis if TEE is nondiagnostic.[81]

Summary

The development of ICE provided the initial and perhaps critical insights into the role of cardiac anatomy in electrophysiology and helped define the mechanism of a variety of different arrhythmias. Since that time, an array of sophisticated three-dimensional mapping tools that superimpose electrical activation on cardiac anatomy have been developed. They are now in everyday use in cardiac electrophysiology laboratories. In contrast, the true role of ICE in electrophysiology remains both limited and uncertain. Although it remains an exceedingly useful tool in clinical research and experimental models, its clearly defined and accepted clinical application may be limited to the guidance of difficult trans-septal punctures. Beyond that, however, its role is more controversial, and despite extensive experience and literature in RF ablation, no randomized studies as yet have clearly delineated its efficacy. In AF ablation, some centers advocate routine use of ICE to identify anatomy, guide ablation, and monitor for complications. However, many other centers achieve similar outcomes without its use. Similarly, ICE may play a helpful role in monitoring RF lesion formation and in ablation of atrial flutter, atrial tachycardia, and certain VTs, but its clinical utility in these circumstances remains uncertain. There is no doubt that phased-array ICE has represented a quantum advance in the field over mechanical ICE, and, as image quality continues to improve with further development, the true utility of ICE in day-to-day electrophysiology may be become clearer.

References

1. Olgin JE, Kalman JM, Fitzpatrick AP, Lesh MD: Role of right atrial endocardial structures as barriers to conduction during human type I atrial flutter: Activation and entrainment mapping guided by intracardiac echocardiography. Circulation 92:1839-1848, 1995.
2. Kalman JM, Olgin JE, Karch MR, Lesh MD: Use of intracardiac echocardiography in interventional electrophysiology. Pacing Clin Electrophysiol 20:2248-2262, 1997.
3. Kalman JM, Jue J, Sudhir K, et al.: In vitro quantification of radiofrequency ablation lesion size using intracardiac echocardiography in dogs. Am J Cardiol 77:217-219, 1996.
4. Chu E, Kalman JM, Kwasman MA, et al.: Intracardiac echocardiography during radiofrequency catheter ablation of cardiac arrhythmias in humans. J Am Coll Cardiol 24:1351-1357, 1994.
5. Ren JF, Schwartzman D, Callans D, et al.: Imaging technique and clinical utility for electrophysiologic procedures of lower frequency (9 MHz) intracardiac echocardiography. Am J Cardiol 82:1557-1560, 1998.
6. Kalman JM, Fitzpatrick AP, Olgin JE, et al.: Biophysical characteristics of radiofrequency lesion formation in vivo: Dynamics of catheter tip-tissue contact evaluated by intracardiac echocardiography. Am Heart J 133:8-18, 1997.
7. Chugh SS, Chan RC, Johnson SB, Packer DL: Catheter tip orientation affects radiofrequency ablation lesion size in the canine left ventricle. Pacing Clin Electrophysiol 22:413-420, 1999.
8. Kalman JM, Lee RJ, Fisher WG, et al.: Radiofrequency catheter modification of sinus pacemaker function guided by intracardiac echocardiography. Circulation 92:3070-3081, 1995.
9. Asirvatham S, Johnson SB, Wahl MR, Packer DL: Superiority of ultrasound over fluoroscopic assessment of electrode tissue contact for optimal lesion formation [abstract]. Circulation 100(Suppl 1):I-374, 1999.
10. Epstein LM, Mitchell MA, Smith TW, Haines DE: Comparative study of fluoroscopy and intracardiac echocardiographic guidance for the creation of linear atrial lesions. Circulation 98:1796-1801, 1998.
11. Olgin JE, Kalman JM, Chin M, et al.: Electrophysiological effects of long, linear atrial lesions placed under intracardiac ultrasound guidance. Circulation 96:2715-2721, 1997.
12. Roithinger FX, Steiner PR, Goseki Y, et al.: Low-power radiofrequency application and intracardiac echocardiography for creation of continuous left atrial linear lesions. J Cardiovasc Electrophysiol 10:680-691, 1999.
13. Daoud EG, Kalbfleisch SJ, Hummel JD: Intracardiac echocardiography to guide transseptal left heart catheterization for radiofrequency catheter ablation. J Cardiovasc Electrophysiol 10:358-363, 1999.
14. Epstein LM, Smith T, TenHoff H: Nonfluoroscopic transseptal catheterization: Safety and efficacy of intracardiac echocardiographic guidance. J Cardiovasc Electrophysiol 9:625-630, 1998.
15. Lee RJ, Kalman JM, Fitzpatrick AP, et al.: Radiofrequency catheter modification of the sinus node for "inappropriate" sinus tachycardia. Circulation 92:2919-2928, 1995.
16. Kalman JM, Olgin JE, Karch MR, et al.: "Cristal tachycardias": Origin of right atrial tachycardias from the crista terminalis identified by intracardiac echocardiography. J Am Coll Cardiol 31:451-459, 1998.
17. Fisher WG, Pelini MA, Bacon ME: Adjunctive intracardiac echocardiography to guide slow pathway ablation in human atrioventricular nodal reentrant tachycardia: Anatomic insights. Circulation 96:3021-3029, 1997.
18. Mangrum JM, Mounsey JP, Kok LC, et al.: Intracardiac echocardiography-guided, anatomically based radiofrequency ablation of focal atrial fibrillation originating from pulmonary veins [abstract]. J Am Coll Cardiol 39:1964-1972, 2002.
19. Ren JF, Schwartzman D, Lighty GWJ, et al.: Multiplane transesophageal and intracardiac echocardiography in large swine: Imaging technique, normal values, and research applications. Echocardiography 14:135-148, 1997.
20. Bruce CJ, Packer DL, Seward JB: Intracardiac doppler hemodynamics and flow: New vector, phased-array ultrasound-tipped catheter. Am J Cardiol 83:1509-1512, 1999.
21. Hijazi Z, Wang Z, Cao Q, et al.: Transcatheter closure of atrial septal defects and patent foramen ovale under intracardiac echocardiographic guidance: Feasibility and comparison with transesophageal echocardiography. Catheter Cardiovasc Interv 52:194-199, 2001.
22. Morton JB, Sanders P, Sparks PB, et al.: Usefulness of phased-array intracardiac echocardiography for the assessment of left atrial mechanical "stunning" in atrial flutter and comparison with multiplane transesophageal echocardiography. Am J Cardiol 90:741-746, 2002.
23. Kalman JM, Olgin JE, Saxon LA, et al.: Activation and entrainment mapping defines the tricuspid annulus as the anterior barrier in typical atrial flutter. Circulation 94:398-406, 1996.
24. Friedman PA, Luria D, Fenton AM, et al.: Global right atrial mapping of human atrial flutter: The presence of postero-medial (sinus venosa region) functional block and double potentials. A study in biplane fluoroscopy and intracardiac echocardiography. Circulation 101:1568-1577, 2000.
25. Marchlinski FE, Ren JF, Schwartzman D, et al.: Accuracy of fluoroscopic localization of the Crista terminalis documented by intracardiac echocardiography. J Interv Card Electrophysiol 4:415-421, 2000.
26. Chu E, Fitzpatrick AP, Chin MC, et al.: Radiofrequency catheter ablation guided by intracardiac echocardiography. Circulation 89:1301-1305, 1994.
27. Schwartz SL, Gillam LD, Weintraub AR, et al.: Intracardiac echocardiography in humans using a small-sized (6F), low frequency (12.5 MHz) ultrasound catheter: Methods, imaging planes and clinical experience. J Am Coll Cardiol 21:189-198, 1993.
28. Ren JF, Marchlinski FE, Callans DJ, Zado ES: Echocardiographic lesion characteristics associated with successful ablation of inappropriate sinus tachycardia. J Cardiovasc Electrophysiol 12:814-818, 2001.
29. Schwartzman D, Ren JF, Devine WA, Callans DJ: Cardiac swelling associated with linear radiofrequency ablation in the atrium. J Interv Card Electrophysiol 5:159-166, 2001.
30. Callans DJ, Ren JF, Schwartzman D, et al.: Narrowing of the superior vena cava-right atrium junction during radiofrequency catheter ablation for inappropriate sinus tachycardia: Analysis with intracardiac echocardiography. J Am Coll Cardiol 33:1667-1670, 1999.
31. Morton JB, Sanders P, Davidson NC, Sparks PB, Vohra JK, Kalman JM: Phased array intracardiac echocardiography for defining cavotricuspid isthmus anatomy during radio-

frequency ablation of typical atrial flutter. J Cardiovasc Electrophysiol 14:591-597, 2003.

32. Haissaguerre M, Jais P, Shah DC, et al.: Spontaneous initiation of atrial fibrillation by ectopic beats originating in the pulmonary veins. N Engl J Med 339:659-666, 1998.

33. Chen SA, Hsieh MH, Tai CT, et al.: Initiation of atrial fibrillation by ectopic beats originating from the pulmonary veins: Electrophysiological characteristics, pharmacological responses, and effects of radiofrequency ablation. Circulation 100:1879-1886, 1999.

34. Natale A, Pisano E, Shewchik J, et al.: First human experience with pulmonary vein isolation using a through-the-balloon circumferential ultrasound ablation system for recurrent atrial fibrillation. Circulation 2000;102:1879-1882.

35. Haissaguerre M, Jais P, Shah DC, et al.: Electrophysiological end point for catheter ablation of atrial fibrillation initiated from multiple pulmonary venous foci. Circulation 101:1409-1417, 2000.

36. Marrouche NF, Dresing T, Cole C, et al.: Circular mapping and ablation of the pulmonary vein for treatment of atrial fibrillation: impact of different catheter technologies. J Am Coll Cardiol 40:464-474, 2002.

37. Oral H, Knight BP, Tada H, et al.: Pulmonary vein isolation for paroxysmal and persistent atrial fibrillation. Circulation 105:1077-1081, 2002.

38. Ho SY, Sanchez-Quintana D, Cabrera JA, Anderson RH: Anatomy of the left atrium: Implications for radiofrequency ablation of atrial fibrillation. J Cardiovasc Electrophysiol 10:1525-1533, 1999.

39. Morton JB, Sanders P, Byrne MJ, et al.: Phased-array intracardiac echocardiography to guide radiofrequency ablation in the left atrium and at the pulmonary vein ostium. J Cardiovasc Electrophysiol 12:343-348, 2001.

40. Wood MA, Wittkamp M, Henry D, et al.: A comparison of pulmonary vein ostial anatomy by computerized tomography, echocardiography, and venography in patients with atrial fibrillation having radiofrequency catheter ablation. Am J Cardiol 93:49-53, 2004.

41. Packer DL, Darbar D, Bhulm CM, et al.: Utility of phased array intracardiac ultrasound for guiding the positioning of the lasso mapping catheter in pulmonary veins undergoing AF ablation [abstract]. Circulation 104:620, 2001.

42. Arora R, Verheule S, Scott L, et al.: Arrhythmogenic substrate of the pulmonary veins assessed by high-resolution optical mapping. Circulation 107:1816-1821, 2003.

43. Mandapati R, Skanes A, Chen J, et al.: Stable microreentrant sources as a mechanism of atrial fibrillation in the isolated sheep heart. Circulation 101:194-199, 2000.

44. Marrouche NF, Martin DO, Wazni O, et al.: Phased-array intracardiac echocardiography monitoring during pulmonary vein isolation in patients with atrial fibrillation: Impact on outcome and complications. Circulation 107:2716, 2003.

45. Bunch TJ, Bruce GK, Johnson SB, et al.: Analysis of catheter-tip (8-mm) and actual tissue temperatures achieved during radiofrequency ablation at the orifice of the pulmonary vein [abstract]. Circulation 110:2988-2995, 2004.

46. Weerasooriya R, Jais P, Sanders P, et al.: Images in cardiovascular medicine: Early appearance of an edematous tissue reaction during left atrial linear ablation using intracardiac echo imaging. Circulation 108:e80, 2005.

47. Robbins IM, Colvin EV, Doyle TP, et al.: Pulmonary vein stenosis after catheter ablation of atrial fibrillation. Circulation 98:1769-1775, 1998.

48. Gerstenfeld EP, Guerra P, Sparks PB, et al.: Clinical outcome after radiofrequency catheter ablation of focal atrial fibrillation triggers. J Cardiovasc Electrophysiol 12:900-908, 2001.

49. Yu WC, Hsu TL, Tai CT, et al.: Acquired pulmonary vein stenosis after radiofrequency catheter ablation of paroxysmal atrial fibrillation. J Cardiovasc Electrophysiol 12:887-892, 2001.

50. Yang M, Akbari H, Reddy GP, Higgins CB: Identification of pulmonary vein stenosis after radiofrequency ablation for atrial fibrillation using MRI. J Comput Assist Tomogr 25:34-35, 2001.

51. Moak JP, Moore HJ, Lee SW, et al.: Case report. Pulmonary vein stenosis following RF ablation of paroxysmal atrial fibrillation: Successful treatment with balloon dilation. J Interv Card Electrophysiol 4:621-631, 2000.

52. Scanavacca MI, Kajita LJ, Vieira M, Sosa EA: Pulmonary vein stenosis complicating catheter ablation of focal atrial fibrillation. J Cardiovasc Electrophysiol 11:677-681, 2000.

53. Taylor GW, Kay GN, Zheng X, et al.: Pathological effects of extensive radiofrequency energy applications in the pulmonary veins in dogs. Circulation 101:1736-1742, 2000.

54. Feigenbaum H: Echocardiography. Philadelphia: Lea & Febiger, 1993.

55. Minich LL, Tani LY, Breinholt JP, et al.: Complete follow-up echocardiograms are needed to detect stenosis of normally connecting pulmonary veins. Echocardiography 18:589-592, 2001.

56. Swarup V, Azegami K, Arruda MS, et al.: Four vessel pulmonary vein isolation guided by intracardiac echocardiography without contrast venography in patients with drug refractory paroxysmal atrial fibrillation [abstract]. J Am Coll Cardiol 39:114A, 2002.

57. Martin RE, Ellenbogen KA, Lau YR, et al.: Phased-array intracardiac echocardiography during pulmonary vein isolation and linear ablation for atrial fibrillation. J Cardiovasc Electrophysiol 13:873-879, 2002.

58. Saad EB, Cole CR, Marrouche NF, et al.: Use of intracardiac echocardiography for prediction of chronic pulmonary vein stenosis after ablation of atrial fibrillation. J Cardiovasc Electrophysiol 13:986-989, 2002.

59. Dill T, Neumann T, Ekinci O, et al.: Pulmonary vein diameter reduction after radiofrequency catheter ablation for paroxysmal atrial fibrillation evaluated by contrast-enhanced three-dimensional magnetic resonance imaging. Circulation 107:845-850, 2003.

60. Nakagawa H, Lazzara R, Khastgir T, et al.: Role of the tricuspid annulus and the eustachian valve/ridge on atrial flutter: Relevance to catheter ablation of the septal isthmus and a new technique for rapid identification of ablation success. Circulation 94:407-424, 1996.

61. Poty H, Saoudi N, Nair M, et al.: Radiofrequency catheter ablation of atrial flutter: Further insights into the various types of isthmus block. Application to ablation during sinus rhythm. Circulation 94:3204-3213, 1996.

62. Shah DC, Haissaguerre M, Jais P, et al.: Simplified electrophysiologically directed catheter ablation of recurrent common atrial flutter. Circulation 96:2505-2508, 1997.

63. Lesh MD, Kalman JM, Olgin JE: New approaches to treatment of atrial flutter and tachycardia. J Cardiovasc Electrophysiol 7:368-381, 1996.

64. Cosio FG, Arribas F, Lopez-Gil M, Gonzalez HD: Radiofrequency ablation of atrial flutter. J Cardiovasc Electrophysiol 7:60-70, 1996.

65. Schwartzman D, Callans DJ, Gottlieb CD, et al.: Conduction block in the inferior vena caval-tricuspid valve isthmus: Association with outcome of radiofrequency ablation of type I atrial flutter. J Am Coll Cardiol 28:1519-1531, 1996.

66. Cabrera JA, Sanchez-Quintana D, Ho SY, et al.: The architecture of the atrial musculature between the orifice of the inferior caval vein and the tricuspid valve: The anatomy of the isthmus. J Cardiovasc Electrophysiol 9:1186-1195, 1998.

67. Olgin JE, Kalman JM, Fitzpatrick AP, Lesh MD: Role of right atrial endocardial structures as barriers to conduction during human type I atrial flutter: Activation and entrainment mapping guided by intracardiac echocardiography. Circulation 92:1839-1848, 1995.

68. Kalman JM, Olgin JE, Saxon LA, et al.: Activation and entrainment mapping defines the tricuspid annulus as the anterior barrier in typical atrial flutter. Circulation 94:398-406, 1996.

69. Darbar D, Olgin JE, Miller J, Friedman PA: Localization of the origin of arrhythmias for ablation: From electrocardiography to advanced endocardial mapping systems. J Cardiovasc Electrophysiol 12:1309-1325, 2001.

70. Heidbuchel H, Willems R, van Rensburg H, et al.: Right atrial angiographic evaluation of the posterior isthmus: Relevance for ablation of typical atrial flutter. Circulation 101:2178-2184, 2000.

71. Callans DJ, Ren JF, Michele J, et al.: Electroanatomic left ventricular mapping in the porcine model of healed anterior myocardial infarction: Correlation with intracardiac echocardiography and pathological analysis. Circulation 100:1744-1750, 1999.

72. Callans D, Ren JF, Narula N, et al.: Effects of linear, irrigated-tip radiofrequency ablation in porcine healed anterior infarction. J Cardiovasc Electrophysiol 12:1037-1042, 2001.

73. Doi A, Takagi M, Toda I, et al.: Real time quantification of low temperature radiofrequency ablation lesion size using phased array intracardiac echocardiography in the canine model: Comparison of two dimensional images with pathological lesion characteristics. Heart 89:923-927, 2003.

74. Mitchel JF, Gillam LD, Sanzobrino BW, et al.: Intracardiac ultrasound imaging during transseptal catheterization. Chest 108:104-108, 1995.

75. Cafri C, de la Guardia B, Barasch E, et al.: Transseptal puncture guided by intracardiac echocardiography during percutaneous transvenous mitral commissurotomy in patients with distorted anatomy of the fossa ovalis. Cathet Cardiovasc Interv 50:463-467, 2000.

76. Bland JM, Altman DG: Statistical methods for assessing agreement between two methods of clinical measurement. Lancet 1:307-310, 1986.

77. Morton JB, Swarup V, Stobie P, et al.: The common left pulmonary vein: Intracardiac ultrasound characteristics and impact upon pulmonary vein isolation [abstract 846-2]. J Am Coll Cardiol 41:124A, 2003.

78. Bartel T, Konorza T, Arjumand J, et al.: Intracardiac echocardiography is superior to conventional monitoring for guiding device closure of interatrial communications. Circulation 107:795-797, 2004.

79. Premawardhana U, Hoskins M, Celermajer DS: Transvenous echo Doppler in baboons: A new window to the cardiovascular system. Clin Sci (Colch) 99:141-147, 2000.

80. Premawardhana U, Adams MR, Birrell A, et al.: Cardiovascular structure and function in baboons with Type 1 diabetes: A transvenous ultrasound study. J Diabetes Complications 15:174-180, 2001.

81. Dalal A, Asirvatham S, Chandrasekaran K, et al.: Intracardiac echocardiography in the detection of pacemaker endocarditis. J Am Soc Echocardiogr 15:1027-1028, 2002.

82. Anderson RH and Becker AE: The Heart: Structure in health and disease. London: Gower Medical, 1992.

Catheter Ablation of Atrial Tachycardia and Flutter

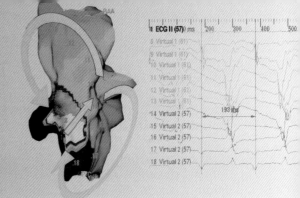

PART III

10

Ablation of Focal Atrial Tachycardias

Byron K. Lee • Jeffrey E. Olgin

Key Points

- The mechanism of focal atrial tachycardia (AT) can be automatic, triggered, or reentry.

- Mapping of the P-wave morphology on a 12-lead electrocardiogram gives a general idea of the origin of the focal AT. Other techniques include determining the earliest atrial activation during tachycardia and pace mapping of the P-wave morphology.

- Ablation targets comprise abnormal atrial tissue from which the tachycardia originates as identified by the site of earliest atrial activation.

- Three-dimensional mapping systems are often useful, and intracardiac echocardiography (ICE) can be helpful, especially for crista terminalis tachycardias.

- Difficulty arises when the tachycardia is not inducible or is not sustained.

Atrial tachycardia (AT) is a tachycardia that originates from and is confined to one or both atria. By definition, AT does not use the atrioventricular (AV) junction or an accessory pathway as an essential portion of its circuit and can continue indefinitely and independently of them.[1] More specifically, *focal atrial tachycardias* are defined as ATs that originate from a single site in either atrium, in contrast to *macroreentrant atrial tachycardias (or flutters)*, which are discussed in Chapters 11 through 13.

Anatomy

Focal ATs usually occur along the crista terminalis in the right atrium and near the pulmonary veins in the left atrium.[2-10] Less frequently, they arise from the coronary sinus, the coronary sinus os, the parahisian region, the appendages, or, rarely, along the tricuspid or mitral annulus.

Pathophysiology

Chen et al.[11] showed that focal AT can occur in any age group, with a greater incidence in the adult middle-aged population and no gender preference. It more commonly arises from the right atrium, and a second focus of AT may be found in up to 13% of the patients.

Focal ATs may have an automatic, triggered, or microreentrant mechanism. Although it can be difficult to precisely define the basic mechanism of a particular AT, understanding the basic principles of focal ATs may help with certain therapeutic decisions.[3,12] The arrhythmogenic mechanisms should not be used with stringency, and flexibility should be used in the judgment of apparent inconsistencies in a particular tachycardia mechanism.

Abnormal automaticity, most likely caused by a positive ionic influx during phase 4 depolarization, is thought to be the most common underlying mechanism for focal ATs. Clinically, automatic tachycardias are characterized by sudden onset with a "warm-up" period and facilitation by adrenergic surge or exogenous catecholamines. Vagal stimulation, beta-blockers, and calcium channel blockers may suppress these types of ATs, and adenosine may provoke an ambiguous response.[13] In the electrophysiology laboratory, these tachycardias are not inducible by programmed stimulation and may be suppressed by overdrive pacing.

Triggered activity is the mechanism by which the cardiac cell depolarizes due to afterpotentials. Delayed afterpotentials occur after the repolarization of the cell action potential and are able to depolarize the cell membrane to the depolarization threshold. This triggers activation of the inward ionic currents, causing an action potential. The role of afterdepolarizations in ATs appears to be limited and is inferential from single-cell recordings; however, evidence suggests that this mechanism may play a role in AT during digitalis toxicity.[14] Triggered tachycardias usually are inducible by programmed stimulation—commonly, constant-rate pacing. They may have a warm-up period and are facilitated by catecholamines. They may also be accelerated by overdrive pacing. Vagal maneuvers, beta-blockers, calcium channel blockers, and adenosine may terminate this type of AT.

Reentry is another mechanism of focal ATs. In reentry, the arrhythmia is maintained by a self-perpetuating circuit that travels around an area of scar or slow conduction. If the reentry circuit is discrete (microreentrant), the AT is still classified as focal. However, if the reentry circuit is larger, it is classified as a macroreentrant AT. Focal reentrant tachycardias can be ablated with a single ablation lesion, whereas macroreentrant ATs typically require a series of ablation lesions. Macroreentrant ATs are discussed in detail in Chapters 11 through 13. Focal reentrant AT is characterized by initiation and termination with atrial pacing. Because of the small circuit size, criteria for entrainment of these tachycardias can be difficult to demonstrate. Focal reentrant ATs are also frequently terminated by verapamil or adenosine.[15]

Although there are no large-scale trials in the medical treatment of focal ATs, it appears, based on the reported data, that beta-blockers[16] and calcium channel blockers are at least partially effective, particularly if the underlying mechanism of the tachycardia is abnormal automaticity or triggered activity.[13,15] Because of their safety profile, these drugs are usually first-line medical therapy.

Other (membrane-active) antiarrhythmic drugs may be effective in treating some patients with AT. However, there are no large-scale trials comparing the drugs or even trials comparing drugs to placebo. Therefore, drug therapy is largely empiric, and drug choice is determined more by the side effect profile and risk of proarrhythmia than by suspected efficacy. The use of class IC antiarrhythmic drugs may be somewhat successful.[17-19] Flecainide and propafenone are often well tolerated in patients without structural heart disease and can be considered a reasonable first-line antiarrhythmic therapy. Quinidine and procainamide are less well tolerated. Class IB agents are generally not effective for AT; however, there may be a small subset of lidocaine-sensitive ATs for which mexiletine is effective.[20] Sotalol may also be effective, in part because of its inherent beta-blocking properties. It typically is better tolerated than quinidine and may provide rate control during recurrences.[21] Nevertheless, because sotalol is also a class III drug, it prolongs the QT interval and may predispose to torsades de pointes, similar to quinidine and procainamide. Amiodarone may be effective, especially in resistant tachycardias such as multifocal ATs. In addition, it is the least proarrhythmic choice and is generally used as first-line drug therapy in patients with depressed left ventricular function. Newer class III drugs such as dofetilide and azimilide may be effective for AT, but there is currently a lack of reported data on their use in atrial arrhythmias, except for atrial fibrillation and atrial flutter.[22]

Clinically, patients with AT may present with varying degrees of symptoms, from being only mildly symptomatic to having overt congestive heart failure due to tachycardia-induced cardiomyopathy. The latter scenario warrants emphasis because patients with incessant ATs and tachycardia-induced cardiomyopathy can be misdiagnosed as having a compensatory sinus tachycardia in the setting of an idiopathic dilated cardiomyopathy. Often this distinction is difficult to make, but curing the AT with ablation can save a patient from eventual cardiac transplantation.

Diagnosis and Differential Diagnosis

Analysis of the 12-lead scalar electrocardiogram P-wave morphology can be very helpful in determining the origin of the tachycardia (Fig. 10–1). Leads aVL and V1 are the most useful to distinguish between left and right origin.[9] A positive or biphasic P wave in aVL predicts a right atrial origin of the tachycardia with a sensitivity of 88% and a specificity of 79%. A positive P wave in V1 has a sensitivity of 93% and a specificity of 88% in predicting a left atrial origin. In addition, leads II, III, and aVF may help differentiate a superior focus (positive P wave) from an inferior one (negative P wave).[9] Furthermore, a negative P wave in lead aVR suggests a right lateral location, specifically the crista terminalis, with 100% sensitivity and 93% specificity, whereas a negative P wave in leads V5 and V6 suggests an inferomedial location.[23] The presence of an isoelectric segment between P waves in all leads is more consistent with a focal AT than an atrial flutter. A P-wave morphology identical to that in sinus rhythm may be present in sinus node reentry or inappropriate sinus tachycardia.

Although these rules generally hold true, there are some limitations to using P-wave vectors for diagnosis. For example, the presence of 1:1 AV conduction can cause distortion of the P waves by the QRS

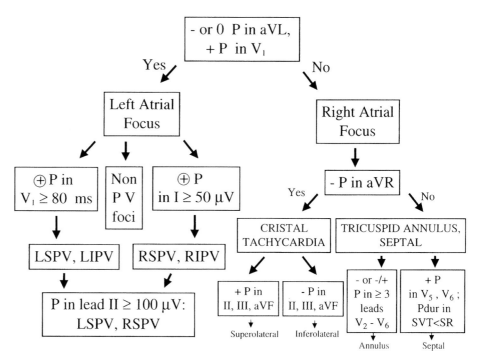

FIGURE 10–1. Algorithm for localization of atrial tachycardia origin based on surface electrocardiogram. +, upright P-wave morphology; −, inverted P-wave morphology; I, inferior; L, left; R, right; PV, pulmonary vein; S, superior. *(From Ellenbogen KA, Wood MA: Atrial tachycardia. In Zipes DP, Jalife J [eds.]: Cardiac Electrophysiology: From Cell to Bedside, 4th ed. Philadelphia: WB Saunders, 2004, pp 500-511.)*

complex or T wave. In such cases, pharmacologic or vagal-induced AV block or induced PVCs may be useful to analyze the P wave. Even so, analysis of the origin of the AT based on P-wave morphology alone can be misleading. There is a spatial limitation of morphology that makes P waves indistinguishable if they originate from paced sites 17 mm apart or less.[24] Another frequent problem encountered is the differentiation of left ATs originating in the right pulmonary veins, which anatomically are located behind the right atrium, from those originating in the right atrium. An intracardiac echocardiography (ICE) image can illustrate the close anatomic relationship between these structures (Fig. 10-2).

The R-P relationship is often useful in the differential diagnosis.[25] AT is typically a long R-P supraventricular tachycardia, whereas atrioventricular nodal reentrant tachycardia (AVNRT) and atrioventricular reentrant tachycardia (AVRT) are usually short R-P supraventricular tachycardias. However, in rare circumstances, these expected R-P relationships do not hold. For example, an AT with prolonged AV nodal conduction would be a short R-P tachycardia, whereas atypical AVNRT or AVRT using a slowly conducting accessory pathway would be a long R-P tachycardia. Distinguishing AT from

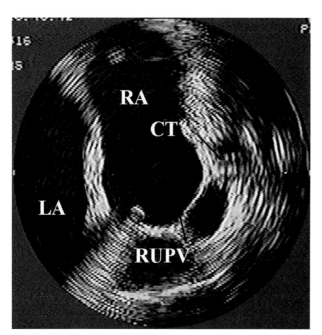

FIGURE 10-2. Intracardiac echocardiogram shows the relationship of the right upper pulmonary vein (RUPV) to the right atrium (RA) and crista terminalis (CT). Atrial tachycardias (ATs) arising from the RUPV may have very similar activation sequence as those arising from the superior CT. Both areas are common sites for focal ATs. Intracardiac echocardiography may be used to precisely position a mapping catheter in relationship to these structures.

AVNRT or AVRT requires analysis of conventional intracardiac electrogram recordings during tachycardia and the response of the arrhythmia to stimulation maneuvers and pharmacologic manipulation. Spontaneous termination of the tachycardia with an atrial depolarization not followed by a ventricular depolarization makes AT unlikely. Variable AV conduction with more atrial than ventricular signals strongly suggests AT and excludes a reciprocating tachycardia (Fig. 10-3). Conditions such as AV node reentry with block in the lower common pathway are rarely seen.[26] In addition, for ATs originating away from the AV valve annuli or coronary sinus ostium, atrial activation is usually inconsistent with AVRT using an accessory pathway or with AVNRT. However, if there is 1:1 AV conduction and the atrial activation sequence suggests an annular location, differentiation from AVNRT and AVRT can be more difficult, and standard electrophysiologic maneuvers to determine the necessity of the AV node for the arrhythmia are used.

Ventricular pacing maneuvers can be very helpful in differentiating AT from AVNRT and AVRT. If burst pacing in the right ventricle at a rate slightly faster than the tachycardia rate dissociates the ventricle from the tachycardia, AVRT is excluded. If ventricular pacing reproducibly terminates the tachycardia without conduction to the atrium (Fig. 10-4), AT is excluded. If burst pacing in the ventricle entrains the atrium and there is a V-A-A-V response after the last paced beat (Fig. 10-5A), AT is the most likely diagnosis. In contrast, a V-A-V response (see Fig. 10-5B) is more consistent with AVNRT or AVRT.[27]

Atrial pacing maneuvers can also be helpful. One can pace in the atrium at a rate faster than the tachycardia rate. If the VA interval of the return cycle length is within 10 msec of the VA interval during the tachycardia, there is "VA linking" and AVNRT or AVRT is the most likely diagnosis. If the VA interval is variable, AT is most likely. The difference between the A-H interval during right atrial pacing at the tachycardia cycle length and the A-H interval during tachycardia can be used to differentiate among long R-P tachycardias. If the A-H interval with atrial pacing is less than 20 msec longer than in tachycardia, an AT is most likely. If the difference is between 20 and 40 msec, a reciprocating tachycardia is likely. Differences greater than 40 msec are consistent with AV nodal reentry.

Finally, the response to pharmacologic termination with adenosine also may be helpful. Although adenosine can be useful to dissociate the tachycardia from the AV node and ventricle, some ATs are adenosine sensitive.[28] Termination of the tachycardia in the atrium (last electrogram seen), if reproducible, makes the diagnosis of AT unlikely.

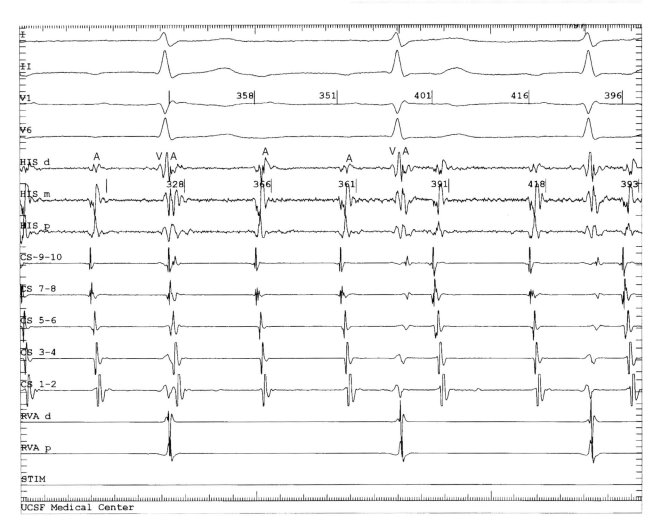

FIGURE 10–3. Variable atrioventricular conduction with more atrial (A) than ventricular (V) signals strongly suggests atrial tachycardia. I, II, V₁, V₆, surface ECG leads; CS, coronary sinus; RVA, right ventricular apex; d, distal; m, mid; p, proximal.

TABLE 10–1
Diagnostic Criteria

- Ventricular pacing during tachycardia results in a V-A-A-V response before tachycardia resumes.

- A-H interval during atrial pacing at tachycardia cycle length minus A-H interval during tachycardia is less than 20 msec.

- Spontaneous termination of tachycardia with an atrial activation makes AT unlikely.

- Ventricle can be dissociated from tachycardia.

- Ventricular pacing that reproducibly terminates the tachycardia without conduction to the atrium excludes AT.

- Variable VA intervals during sustained tachycardia or with ventricular pacing suggests AT.

- Macroreentrant AT has been excluded.

Mapping

Regardless of the tachycardia mechanism, successful ablation of a focal AT requires precise mapping of the tachycardia focus. Activation mapping, in which the earliest local activation is compared with onset of the tachycardia P wave, is the most common technique for mapping. With this technique, sites with local activation ranging from 15 to 60 msec before P-wave onset are targeted for ablation. The unipolar atrial electrogram should show a QS complex (Fig 10–6B). Often, the electrogram at the earliest site is fractionated (Fig. 10–6). Activation mapping is most effective when there is sustained tachycardia to map. Multielectrode catheters (such as a 20-pole catheter placed along the crista terminalis and a multipolar coronary sinus catheter) can be useful to guide initial mapping.[2] Because the majority of focal ATs originate

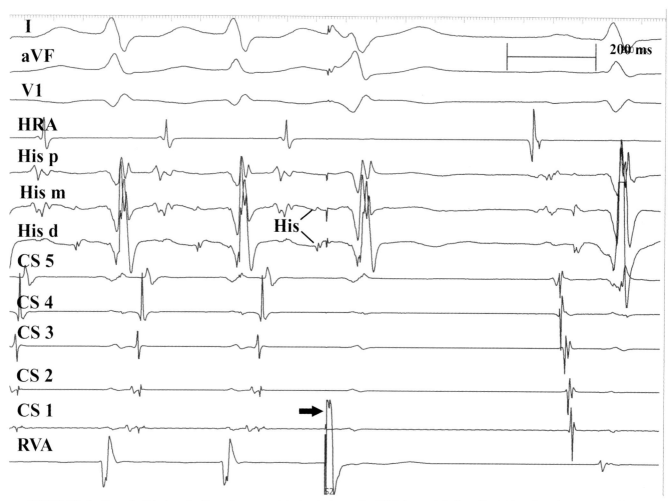

FIGURE 10–4. Reproducible termination of supraventricular tachycardia (SVT) by ventricular stimulation that does not conduct to the atrium excludes an atrial tachycardia. In this figure SVT occurs with earliest atrial activation in the distal coronary sinus (CS1). A premature ventricular stimulus (arrowhead) is delivered approximately 30 msec after activation of the His (labeled) followed by termination of the tachycardia. This finding was reproducible and the patient underwent successful ablation of a left lateral accessory pathway. CS 5, proximal coronary sinus; CS 1, distal coronary sinus. Other abbreviations per Figure 10-3.

from the right atrium, a crista terminalis catheter can rapidly identify the best region in which to start mapping (Fig. 10–7). Furthermore, the activation sequence in the multielectrode catheters, in combination with the His atrial signal, can also suggest the location of foci.[29,30] The inability to record early atrial activation should suggest the possibility of AT arising from the coronary sinus musculature. These tachycardias are rare, and atrial activation may be confusing because of the pattern of electrical attachment between the coronary sinus and atrial musculatures. Also rare are atrial tachycardias that arise from the ligament of Marshall. This epicardial atrial structure is positioned between the left atrial appendage and the left superior pulmonary vein and may be mapped from the distal coronary sinus.

For instances in which tachycardia is not sustained or is difficult to induce, pace mapping can be useful. It is also useful as an adjunct to activation mapping. Pace mapping is performed by pacing at the lowest capture output; the paced P-wave morphology is then compared with the P wave recorded during tachycardia. This technique has the limitation of requiring a "pure" P wave on the 12-surface-lead electrocardiogram, undisturbed by the QRS or T wave. However, use of surrogate markers such as multiple intracardiac recordings has been proposed.[31]

Three-dimensional (3-D) mapping systems offer many advantages in the ablation of focal ATs. In general, these systems allow construction of a 3-D image of the heart chamber that is suspected to be the source of the tachycardia. If mapping is done during sustained AT, these systems can produce an activation map that identifies the earliest site of atrial activation, which can then be targeted for ablation. The 3-D mapping systems can also show the tip of the ablation catheter moving in the generated 3-D image. Use of this image to guide mapping and ablation minimizes fluoroscopy exposure. Finally, 3-D systems allow

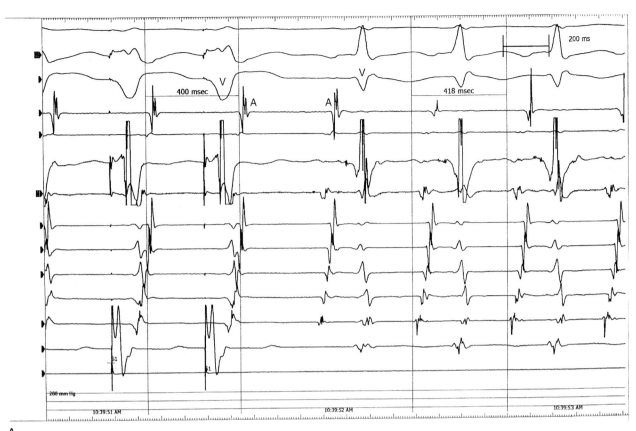

A

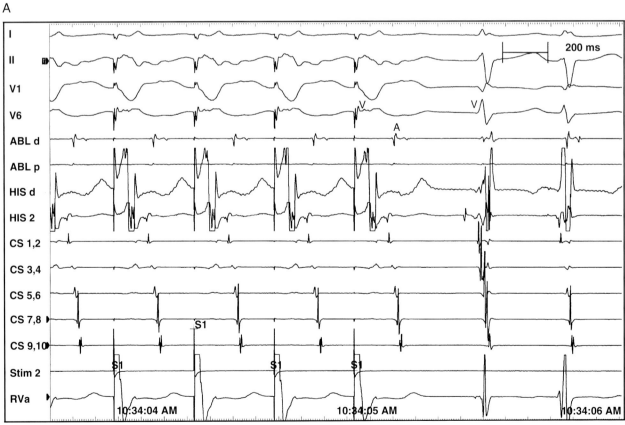

B

FIGURE 10–5. A, V-A-A-V response after the last right ventricular-paced beat (S1 on stim channel) suggests atrial tachycardia acceleration of the atrial rate to the ventricular pacing rate of 400 msec indicates entrainment of the atrium. **B,** V-A-V response after the last right ventricular-paced beat (S1 on stim channel) suggests atrioventricular nodal reentrant tachycardia or atrioventricular reentrant tachycardia.

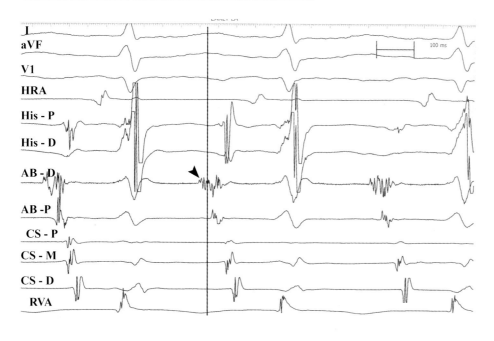

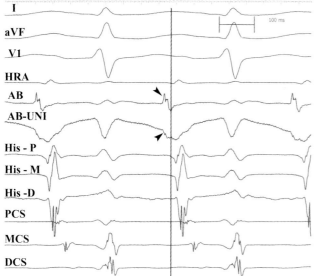

FIGURE 10–6. Electrogram targets for ablation of atrial tachycardias. A. The distal ablation electrogram (AB-D) shows electrical activity beginning 30 msec (arrow) before the surface P wave onset that is indicated by the vertical line. Note the marked fractionation of the electrogram at this site. Ablation at this site terminated an atrial tachycardia in the lateral left atrium. B. In this patient with a right atrial tachycardia, the ablation catheter distal bipolar recording (AB) shows local activation 35 msec (arrowhead) before surface P wave onset (vertical line). The distal ablation unipolar electrogram (AB-UNI) shows a QS morphology with the point of maximal negative dv/dt also 30 msec before P wave onset (arrowhead). Ablation at this site terminated the tachycardia and rendered it non-inducible. For both figures the time scale (upper left) indicates 100 msec. Other abbreviations per Figure 10-3.

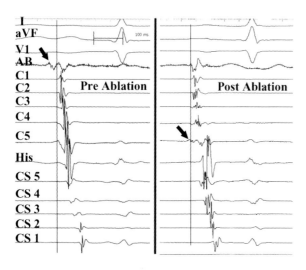

FIGURE 10–7. Ablation of inappropriate sinus tachycardia arising from the crista terminalis using a multipolar crista mapping catheter. Left panel—A 10 pole mapping "crista" catheter is positioned along the crista terminalis with the distal bipole (C1) cranial and the proximal bipole (C5) caudal. The activation is cranial to caudal with the ablation electrogram (AB) preceding all other atrial activity (arrow) and the surface P wave onset (vertical line). Ablation delivered to this site reduced the atrial rate from 120 to 100 bpm. Right Panel—After ablation, the activation of the crista is changed with the caudal bipole recording the earliest activity. Additional ablation was then performed about this site of early activation to further reduce the atrial rate. The time scale represents 100 msec.

marking of interesting sites noted during mapping. Marking of the His "cloud" to show areas to avoid during ablation can be helpful, particularly in cases of parahisian AT. If the ablation catheter is unstable during tachycardia, marking of the earliest site during tachycardia facilitates returning to that same site for ablation during sinus rhythm.

The generated 3-D activation map can also be very helpful in distinguishing a focal AT from a macroreentrant tachycardia. In macroreentrant AT, the activation map spans the entire tachycardia cycle length, and the earliest site meets the latest site. In focal ATs, the activation map typically spans less than 60% of the tachycardia cycle length, and the latest site usually does not meet the earliest site.

Some of the 3-D mapping systems have unique features that make them particularly useful. The CARTO (Biosense Webster; Baldwin Park, Calif.) 3-D mapping system can create voltage maps that accurately identify areas of scar with no electrical signal. Voltage maps are more useful for marcroreentrant ATs, in which the circuit often revolves around a scar. The CARTO system has been successfully used for ablation of focal ATs with a relatively short mapping time (Fig. 10–8).[32] One of its major limitations is its inability to map transient nonsustained tachycardias and sustained tachycardias that are hemodynamically unstable. The EnSite (Endocardial Solutions; St. Paul, Minn.) 3-D mapping system uses a 64-wire array mounted to a 10-mL balloon-catheter. Once the anatomy has been obtained by tracing of the chamber

with a standard catheter, the system superimposes over it the data from 3200 electrograms obtained by mathematical reconstruction simultaneously, to create an isopotential map.[33] The biggest advantage of this system is its ability to map nonsustained tachycardias, and even single beats. The spatial resolution, however, is lost if the system is used in a very large atrium (Fig. 10–9). The LocaLisa (Medtronic; Minneapolis, Minn.) 3-D catheter navigation system uses standard catheter electrodes as sensors for a high-frequency transthoracic electrical field, which is applied via standard skin electrodes.[34] Unlike the CARTO and EnSite systems, which require specialized expensive mapping catheters, LocaLisa uses all catheters and also multiple mapping catheters, allowing for a combination of sequential and simultaneous

TABLE 10–2
Target Sites
• Atrial electrogram precedes P-wave onset by at least 15 to 60 msec.
• Early fractionated electrograms are present.
• Pacing from site produces a surface P wave identical to the P wave of tachycardia.
• Earliest site identified by 3-D mapping.

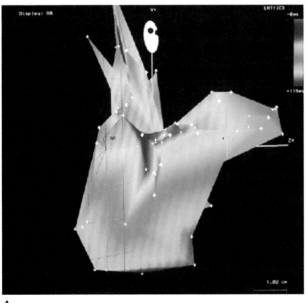
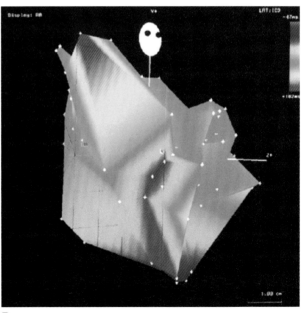

A   B

FIGURE 10–8. A, Right atrial electroanatomic (CARTO) map of a focal atrial tachycardia originating on the posterolateral right atrium in right anterior oblique view. **B,** Right atrial CARTO map of sinus rhythm after successful ablation. Note sinus rhythm origin on the superior portion of the sinus node complex on the crista terminalis.

mapping (Fig. 10–10). The RPM system (Boston Scientific; San Jose, Calif.) functions similarly to the CARTO system in that special catheters are required and mapping is performed sequentially (Fig. 10–11).

Ablation

Although focal ATs may result from automatic, triggered, or microreentry mechanisms, their precise mechanism does not affect the mapping technique or the success rate of ablation therapy.

Once mapping identifies the optimal site, 25 to 50 W of radiofrequency energy is delivered for 30 to 60 seconds. Standard ablation catheters with 4-mm tips are usually satisfactory. Large-tip catheters, high-energy generators, or irrigated ablation systems are rarely necessary. Acceleration of the tachycardia before termination suggests that ablation will be successful, as does termination within 10 seconds. A suc-

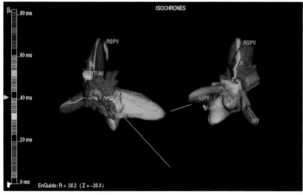

FIGURE 10–9. ESI (St. Paul, MN) noncontact activation map of a focal atrial tachycardia originating from the ostium of the right superior pulmonary vein (RSPV). LIPV, left inferior pulmonary vein.

cessful ablation is verified by the inability to reinduce the tachycardia after ablation. If isoproterenol was necessary for induction before ablation, it should be used again during attempts at reinduction to confirm success.

Some ATs originate from the coronary sinus or pulmonary veins. Lower energy and temperature settings are used in these vascular structures to minimize the risk of perforation and thrombosis. Before ablation in the coronary sinus, angiography of the arterial system can be helpful to rule out proximity to the coronary arteries. The use of irrigated radiofrequency catheters (50°C at 20 to 30 W) may reduce the risk of impedance rises within the coronary sinus. Cryoablation may be a safe alternative to radiofrequency ablation in these cases. Aggressive ablation near the coronary arteries can lead to myocardial infarction.

ICE (see Fig. 10–2) can also help with ablation by localizing anatomic structures, aiding with catheter positioning and catheter tip contact, and confirming and identifying lesion size and location.[2,35-37] It is particularly useful in helping to guide fine catheter movement between the upper crista terminalis and the right atrial posterior wall opposing the right upper pulmonary vein; in this context, ICE can quickly differentiate a crista terminalis AT from a right upper pulmonary vein AT before a decision for or against trans-septal puncture is made. ICE also can help with trans-septal puncture in terms of recognizing early complications, such as perforations and clot formation, and with reducing fluoroscopy time.

Catheter ablation for focal ATs has been proven safe and effective,[2,4,5,8,9,11,31,38,39] with reported success rates between 77% to 100%. It also has been shown to improve patient quality-of-life scores.[40] Complications are rare and usually reflect the risks of vascular access and intracardiac catheter manipulation. Abla-

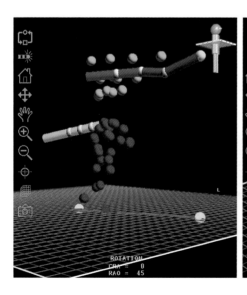
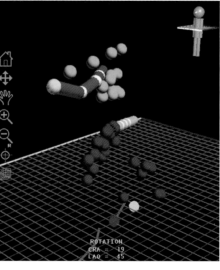

FIGURE 10–10. LocaLisa image showing the His cloud *(blue dots)* and ablation sites *(red dots)* for a parahisian atrial tachycardia in the right anterior oblique *(left image)* and left anterior oblique *(right image)* projections.

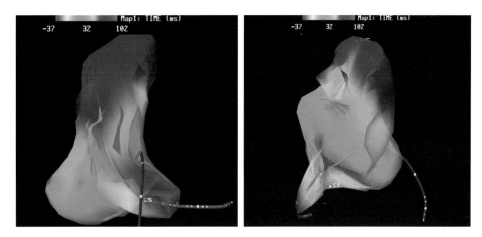

FIGURE 10–11. RPM image showing a focal atrial tachycardia arising from the coronary sinus in the right anterior oblique *(right image)* and left anterior oblique *(left image)* projections. *(Courtesy of N. Badhwar.)*

tion near the AV node or conduction system may risk heart block. Ablation along the lateral right atrium may damage the phrenic nerve. Before ablation in the area of the phrenic nerve, it is recommended to pace at high output (10 mA) from the ablation catheter. If phrenic nerve stimulation is noted on fluoroscopy, the risk of phrenic nerve injury may be substantial. Therefore, ablation should be indicated for all symptomatic patients who have persistent symptoms despite medical therapy or intolerable side effects from medicines. Patients who are not willing to undergo medical therapy should also be considered.

Troubleshooting the Difficult Case

One of the common problems with ablation of focal ATs is the inability to induce the tachycardia once the patient is in the electrophysiology laboratory. Although the patient may have frequent bouts of tachycardia outside the laboratory, the artificial environment of the laboratory, combined with sedation, may change the milieu enough to make the tachycardia noninducible. Occasionally, the use of high doses of isoproterenol (up to 8 μg/min) is necessary to induce the tachycardia. Additionally, some ATs are observed during the "washout" phase of isoproterenol. Other adrenergic stimuli, such as norepinephrine or aminophylline, are rarely useful. Minimizing or eliminating sedation may be helpful. For a female patient, scheduling a procedure at a different point in the menstrual cycle may also help.

Sometimes focal ATs are inducible but not sustained. Occasionally only one or two beats of the tachycardia can be induced at a time. A nonsustained AT can usually be successfully mapped and ablated with repeated inductions of the nonsustained tachycardia. However, this makes mapping much more time-consuming and painstaking. Pace mapping can be a useful technique in this situation. The EnSite 3-D mapping system can also be particularly helpful in this situation, because, with even a single beat of tachycardia, it can grossly map and localize the AT origin. If ablation is unsuccessful because the AT was noninducible or nonsustained, it may be necessary to bring the patient back for a repeat procedure at times of frequent tachycardia.

Inappropriate sinus tachycardia is one type of focal AT that deserves special consideration. It is a syndrome characterized by an increased sinus rate, either at rest or with minimal exertion. The P-wave morphology is generally identical to that of normal sinus rhythm. The resting heart rate often is in excess of 100 beats per minute, with an exaggerated response to minimal exertion or postural changes. It is a rare clinical syndrome and usually affects young women. The clinical presentation is palpitations, easy fatigability, dizziness, lightheadedness, shortness of breath, and sometimes presyncope or syncope.

The mechanism of inappropriate sinus tachycardia is poorly understood. Possible mechanisms have been postulated, among them a depressed cardiovagal reflex with an elevated intrinsic heart rate and beta-adrenergic sensitivity,[41] abnormal autonomic control of the sinus node,[42] and a primary abnormality of the sinus node.[43] Although inappropriate sinus tachycardia is often difficult to differentiate from a focal AT, it appears that the mechanism is different.[44,45]

The treatment of inappropriate sinus tachycardia has not been tested in any large-scale trial and currently it is largely empiric. The use of beta-blockers or calcium channel blockers is the first line of treatment, because these drugs are usually well tolerated and do not cause serious side effects. Other drugs are generally ineffective.

If medical therapy has failed and the patient's symptoms are related to a fast heart rate, catheter ablation of a portion of the sinus node (so-called sinus node modification) can be offered.[44,46] This technique entails mapping and ablation of a portion of the crista terminalis during isoproterenol infusion. A thorough diagnostic electrophysiologic study must be performed before sinus node modification to rule out another type of tachycardia. Once the diagnosis has been established, a multipole (20-pole) diagnostic crista terminalis catheter is positioned along the crista terminalis, if possible with echocardiographic guidance to ensure its precise position. The sinus rhythm activation sequence is then analyzed in the crista catheter at baseline and after isoproterenol infusion. A shift of the earliest crista terminalis activation sequence is gradually noted with increased sinus rate. The ablation catheter is then positioned at the more cranial portion of the crista terminalis, and radiofrequency energy is applied in a craniocaudal fashion, again preferably guided by intracardiac ultrasound, along the crista terminalis, shifting the sinus node function and causing a reduction in the sinus rate. This technique has a high acute success rate,[44,46] defined as an increase in the sinus rate cycle length of at least 10%. Others have reported using CARTO or EnSite technology to help guide ablation

or modification of the sinus node. Although sinus node modification is effective at lowering the sinus rate, the long-term results of symptomatic relief have been at most modest.[47]

Ablation of parahisian ATs, which originate from near the AV node or His region is often difficult and requires careful mapping to avoid ablation-induced complete heart block. Starting ablation with lower energy and temperature settings, and stopping immediately if A-H prolongation or heart block occurs, may avert permanent damage to the conduction system. Use of a 3-D mapping system to create a His cloud can also help delineate areas to avoid ablating (see Fig. 10–10). Finally, the CryoTherapy system (CryoCath, Montreal, Quebec), which uses cooling to ablate tissue, has been employed successfully to ablate parahisian ATs.[48,49] CryoTherapy allows testing of potential ablation sites by adhering the catheter tip to the target tissue and chilling it to create a reversible electrical effect. If there is no heart block, the catheter tip can be cooled further to create a permanent lesion.

Troubleshooting difficulties are summarized in Table 10–3.

TABLE 10-3

Troubleshooting the Difficult Case

Problem	Causes	Solution
Unable to induce tachycardia	Residual drug effects	Stop antiarrhythmic medicine at least 5 half-lives before the procedure
	Catecholamine dependence	Use isoproterenol, epinephrine use
	Sedation	Minimize sedation, hand grip exercise
Tachycardia not sustained long enough for mapping	Characteristic of the tachycardia	Use EnSite 3-D mapping system
	Catecholamine dependence	High-dose isoproterenol
Poor catheter stability	Excessive heart motion	Pace during RF ablation
		Ablate in sinus rhythm
	Poor catheter characteristics	Try alternative catheters or cryoablation
		Use a preformed sheath
Failure despite precise mapping	Poor catheter contact	Adjust catheter
		Try alternative catheters
		Use preformed sheath
	Low temperature or current	High-output or irrigated RF system
Origin of right-sided focal AT changing with each ablation	Inappropriate sinus tachycardia	Ablate along crista until sinus cycle length increases >10%
AT origin near the AV node or His region	Parahisian AT	Map His "cloud" before ablation
		Ablate initially with lower energy and temperature settings
		Use CryoTherapy
No early atrial sites	Coronary sinus origin	Map/ablate in coronary sinus

AT, atrial tachycardia; AV, atrioventricular; RF, radiofrequency

Conclusion

Advances in the past several years have improved the ability to ablate focal ATs. 3-D mapping systems provide a straightforward approach that can identify the origin of focal ATs even if these arrhythmias are unstable or nonsustained. ICE can facilitate mapping and ablation. Finally, 3-D mapping of the His cloud and the use of CryoTherapy has improved the ability to safely ablate parahisian focal ATs. Although ablation of focal ATs can still be complex and challenging, these advances have allowed safe and successful expansion of the use of curative catheter ablation for these arrhythmias.

References

1. Scheinman MM, Basu D, Hollenberg M: Electrophysiologic studies in patients with persistent atrial tachycardia. Circulation 50:266-273, 1974.
2. Kalman JM, Olgin JE, Karch MR, et al.: "Cristal tachycardias": Origin of right atrial tachycardias from the crista terminalis identified by intracardiac echocardiography. J Am Coll Cardiol 31:451-459, 1998.
3. Callans DJ, Schwartzman D, Gottlieb CD, Marchlinski FE: Insights into the electrophysiology of atrial arrhythmias gained by the catheter ablation experience: "Learning while burning, Part II." J Cardiovasc Electrophysiol 6:229-243, 1995.
4. Lesh MD, Van Hare GF, Epstein LM, et al.: Radiofrequency catheter ablation of atrial arrhythmias: Results and mechanisms. Circulation 89:1074-1089, 1994.
5. Pappone C, Stabile G, De Simone A, et al.: Role of catheter-induced mechanical trauma in localization of target sites of radiofrequency ablation in automatic atrial tachycardia. J Am Coll Cardiol 27:1090-1097, 1996.
6. Chen SA, Chiang CE, Yang CJ, et al.: Radiofrequency catheter ablation of sustained intra-atrial reentrant tachycardia in adult patients: Identification of electrophysiological characteristics and endocardial mapping techniques. Circulation 88:578-587, 1993.
7. Walsh EP, Saul JP, Hulse JE, et al.: Transcatheter ablation of ectopic atrial tachycardia in young patients using radiofrequency current [see comments]. Circulation 86:1138-1146, 1992.
8. Kay GN, Chong F, Epstein AE, et al.: Radiofrequency ablation for treatment of primary atrial tachycardias [see comments]. J Am Coll Cardiol 21:901-909, 1993.
9. Tang CW, Scheinman MM, Van Hare GF, et al.: Use of P wave configuration during atrial tachycardia to predict site of origin. J Am Coll Cardiol 26:1315-1324, 1995.
10. Jais P, Shah DC, Haissaguerre M, et al.: Atrial fibrillation: role of arrhythmogenic foci. J Interv Card Electrophysiol 4(Suppl 1):29-37, 2000.
11. Chen SA, Tai CT, Chiang CE, et al.: Focal atrial tachycardia: Reanalysis of the clinical and electrophysiologic characteristics and prediction of successful radiofrequency ablation. J Cardiovasc Electrophysiol 9:355-365, 1998.
12. Steinbeck G, Hoffmann E: 'True' atrial tachycardia. Eur Heart J 19(Suppl E):E10-E12, E48-E49, 1998.
13. Engelstein ED, Lippman N, Stein KM, Lerman BB: Mechanism-specific effects of adenosine on atrial tachycardia. Circulation 89:2645-2654, 1994.
14. Rosen MR: Cellular electrophysiology of digitalis toxicity. J Am Coll Cardiol 5:22A-34A, 1995.
15. Chen SA, Chiang CE, Yang CJ, et al.: Sustained atrial tachycardia in adult patients: Electrophysiological characteristics, pharmacological response, possible mechanisms, and effects of radiofrequency ablation [see comments]. Circulation 90:1262-1278, 1994.
16. Coumel P, Escoubet B, Attuel P: Beta-blocking therapy in atrial and ventricular tachyarrhythmias: Experience with nadolol. Am Heart J 108:1098-1108, 1984.
17. Coumel P, Leclercq JF, Assayag P: European experience with the antiarrhythmic efficacy of propafenone for supraventricular and ventricular arrhythmias. Am J Cardiol 54:60D-66D, 1984.
18. Pool PE, Quart BD: Treatment of ectopic atrial arrhythmias and premature atrial complexes in adults with encainide. Am J Cardiol 62:60L-62L, 1988.
19. Brugada P, Abdollah H, Wellens HJ: Suppression of incessant supraventricular tachycardia by intravenous and oral encainide. J Am Coll Cardiol 4:1255-1260, 1984.
20. Chiale PA, Franco DA, Selva HO, et al.: Lidocaine-sensitive atrial tachycardia: Lidocaine-sensitive, rate-related, repetitive atrial tachycardia: a new arrhythmogenic syndrome. J Am Coll Cardiol 36:1637-1645, 2000.
21. Anderson JL, Prystowsky EN: Sotalol: An important new antiarrhythmic. Am Heart J 137:388-409, 1999.
22. Torp-Pedersen C, Moller M, Bloch-Thomsen PE, et al.: Dofetilide in patients with congestive heart failure and left ventricular dysfunction: Danish Investigations of Arrhythmia and Mortality on Dofetilide Study Group. N Engl J Med 341:857-865, 1999.
23. Tada H, Nogami A, Naito S, et al.: Simple electrocardiographic criteria for identifying the site of origin of focal right atrial tachycardia. Pacing Clin Electrophysiol 21:2431-2439, 1998.
24. Man KC, Chan KK, Kovack P, et al.: Spatial resolution of atrial pace mapping as determined by unipolar atrial pacing at adjacent sites. Circulation 94:1357-1363, 1996.
25. Kalbfleisch SJ, el-Atassi R, Calkins H, et al.: Differentiation of paroxysmal narrow QRS complex tachycardias using the 12-lead electrocardiogram. J Am Coll Cardiol 21:85-89, 1993.
26. Miller JM, Rosenthal ME, Vassallo JA, Josephson ME: Atrioventricular nodal reentrant tachycardia: Studies on upper and lower "common pathways." Circulation 75:930-940, 1987.
27. Knight BP, Ebinger M, Oral H, et al.: Diagnostic value of tachycardia features and pacing maneuvers during paroxysmal supraventricular tachycardia. J Am Coll Cardiol 36:574-582, 2000.
28. Glatter KA, Cheng J, Dorostkar P, et al.: Electrophysiologic effects of adenosine in patients with supraventricular tachycardia. Circulation 99:1034-1040, 1999.
29. Kistler PM, Sanders P, Fynn SP, et al.: Electrophysiological and electrocardiographic characteristics of focal atrial tachycardia originating from the pulmonary veins: Acute and long-term outcomes of radiofrequency ablation. Circulation 108:1968-1975, 2003.
30. Ashar MS, Pennington J, Callans DJ, Marchlinski FE: Localization of arrhythmogenic triggers of atrial fibrillation. J Cardiovasc Electrophysiol 11:1300-1305, 2000.
31. Tracy CM, Swartz JF, Fletcher RD, et al.: Radiofrequency catheter ablation of ectopic atrial tachycardia using paced activation sequence mapping [see comments]. J Am Coll Cardiol 21:910-917, 1993.
32. Hoffmann E, Nimmermann P, Reithmann C, et al.: New mapping technology for atrial tachycardias. J Interv Card Electrophysiol 4(Suppl 1):117-120, 2000.

33. Kadish A, Hauck J, Pederson B, et al.: Mapping of atrial activation with a noncontact, multielectrode catheter in dogs. Circulation 99:1906-1913, 1999.

34. Wittkampf FH, Wever EF, Derksen R, et al.: Accuracy of the LocaLisa system in catheter ablation procedures. J Electrocardiol 32:7-12, 1999.

35. Lesh MD, Kalman JM, Karch MR: Use of intracardiac echocardiography during electrophysiologic evaluation and therapy of atrial arrhythmias. J Cardiovasc Electrophysiol 9:S40-S47, 1998.

36. Kalman JM, Olgin JE, Karch MR, Lesh MD: Use of intracardiac echocardiography in interventional electrophysiology. Pacing Clin Electrophysiol 20:2248-2262, 1997.

37. Chu E, Kalman JM, Kwasman MA, et al.: Intracardiac echocardiography during radiofrequency catheter ablation of cardiac arrhythmias in humans. J Am Coll Cardiol 24:1351-1357, 1994.

38. Feld GK: Catheter ablation for the treatment of atrial tachycardia. Prog Cardiovasc Dis 37:205-224, 1995.

39. Poty H, Saoudi N, Haissaguerre M, et al.: Radiofrequency catheter ablation of atrial tachycardias. Am Heart J 131:481-489, 1996.

40. Bubien RS, Knotts-Dolson SM, Plumb VJ, Kay GN: Effect of radiofrequency catheter ablation on health-related quality of life and activities of daily living in patients with recurrent arrhythmias [see comments]. Circulation 94:1585-1591, 1996.

41. Morillo CA, Klein GJ, Thakur RK, et al.: Mechanism of "inappropriate" sinus tachycardia: Role of sympathovagal balance. Circulation 90:873-877, 1994.

42. Bauernfeind RA, Amat YLF, Dhingra RC, et al.: Chronic non-paroxysmal sinus tachycardia in otherwise healthy persons. Ann Intern Med 91:702-710, 1979.

43. Lowe JE, Hartwich T, Takla M, Schaper J: Ultrastructure of electrophysiologically identified human sinoatrial nodes. Basic Res Cardiol 83:401-409, 1988.

44. Lee RJ, Kalman JM, Fitzpatrick AP, et al.: Radiofrequency catheter modification of the sinus node for "inappropriate" sinus tachycardia. Circulation 92:2919-2928, 1995.

45. Krahn AD, Yee R, Klein GJ, Morillo C: Inappropriate sinus tachycardia: Evaluation and therapy. J Cardiovasc Electrophysiol 6:1124-1128, 1995.

46. Kalman JM, Lee RJ, Fisher WG, et al.: Radiofrequency catheter modification of sinus pacemaker function guided by intracardiac echocardiography. Circulation 92:3070-3081, 1995.

47. Man KC, Knight B, Tse HF, et al.: Radiofrequency catheter ablation of inappropriate sinus tachycardia guided by activation mapping. J Am Coll Cardiol 35:451-457, 2000.

48. Wong T, Markides V, Peters NS, Davies DW: Clinical usefulness of cryomapping for ablation of tachycardias involving perinodal tissue. J Interv Card Electrophysiol 10:153-158, 2004.

49. Ellenbogen KA, Wood MA: Atrial tachycardia. In Zipes DP, Jalife J (eds.): Cardiac Electrophysiology: From Cell to Bedside, 4th ed. Philadelphia: WB Saunders, 2004, pp 500-511.

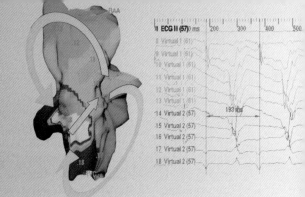

11

Ablation of Isthmus-Dependent Atrial Flutters

Gregory K. Feld • *Uma Srivatsa* • *Bobbi Hoppe*

Key Points

- The mechanism of isthmus-dependent atrial flutter is a macroreentrant circuit around the tricuspid valve (TV) annulus.

- The diagnosis is confirmed by demonstration of concealed entrainment from the cavotricuspid isthmus (CTI) or by multielectrode catheter or computerized activation mapping.

- The ablation target is the CTI between the TV annulus and the inferior vena cava (IVC).

- Special equipment that may be used includes a large-tip catheter with a high-power radiofrequency generator or a cooled-tip ablation catheter, a large-curve catheter with or without preformed sheaths, an electroanatomic or noncontact three-dimensional mapping system, and a multielectrode "Halo" catheter.

- Sources of difficulty may include complex anatomy/topography of the CTI area and failure to achieve isthmus block despite extensive ablation.

- Acute success rates range from 95% to 100%, and chronic success rates from 95% to 97%, with large-tip or cooled-tip catheters.

Type 1 (or typical) atrial flutter (AFL) is a common atrial arrhythmia, often occurring in association with atrial fibrillation, that can cause significant symptoms and serious adverse effects including embolic stroke, myocardial ischemia and infarction, and, rarely, a tachycardia-induced cardiomyopathy resulting from rapid atrioventricular (AV) conduction. The electrophysiologic substrate underlying type 1 AFL has been shown to be a combination of slow conduction velocity in the cavotricuspid isthmus (CTI) and anatomic and/or functional conduction block along the crista terminalis and eustachian ridge. This electrophysiologic milieu produces a long enough reentrant path length, relative to the average tissue wavelength around the tricuspid valve (TV) annulus, to allow for sustained reentry. The triggers of AFL may include premature atrial contractions or nonsustained episodes of atrial fibrillation, which originate most commonly in the left atrium and pulmonary veins, respectively, and most likely account for the fact that counterclockwise AFL occurs most frequently clinically. Type 1 AFL is also relatively resistant to pharmacologic suppression.

As a result of the well-defined anatomic substrate and the pharmacologic resistance of type 1 AFL, radiofrequency (RF) catheter ablation has emerged in the last decade as a safe and effective first-line treatment. Although several procedures have been described for ablating type 1 AFL, the most widely accepted and successful technique is an anatomically guided approach targeting the CTI. Recent technological developments, including three-dimensional (3-D) electroanatomic contact and noncontact mapping and the use of large-tip ablation electrode catheters with high-power generators, have produced almost uniform efficacy without increased risk. This chapter reviews the electrophysiology of human type 1 AFL and techniques currently employed for its diagnosis, mapping, and ablation.

Atrial Flutter Terminology

Because of the variety of terms used to describe AFL in humans—including type 1 and type 2 AFL, typical and atypical AFL, counterclockwise (CCW) and clockwise (CW) AFL, and isthmus-dependent and non–isthmus-dependent AFL—the Working Group of Arrhythmias of the European Society of Cardiology and the North American Society of Pacing and Electrophysiology convened and published a consensus document in 2001 in an attempt to develop a generally accepted standardized terminology for AFL.[1] The consensus was that the widely accepted

terms "typical" and "type 1" AFL were most commonly used to describe macroreentrant right atrial tachycardia, involving the CTI, in either a CCW or a CW direction as visualized from a left anterior oblique perspective. Therefore, the consensus terminology derived from this working group to describe CTI-dependent, right atrial macroreentry tachycardia in the CCW direction is "typical" AFL, and a similar tachycardia in the CW direction is called "reverse typical" AFL.[1] For the purposes of this book, these two arrhythmias are referred to specifically as typical and reverse typical AFL when being individually described, but as type 1 AFL when being referred to jointly. Other isthmus-dependent flutters, including lower loop reentry and partial isthmus-dependent flutter, are also discussed in this chapter.

Anatomy and Pathophysiology

The development of successful RF catheter ablation techniques for human type 1 AFL was dependent in part on the delineation of its electrophysiologic mechanism. Through the use of advanced electrophysiologic techniques, including intraoperative and transcatheter activation mapping,[2-7] type 1 AFL was determined to be caused by a macroreentrant circuit rotating in either a CCW (typical) or a CW (reverse typical) direction in the right atrium around the TV annulus, with an area of relatively slow conduction velocity in the low posterior right atrium (Fig. 11–1). The predominant area of slow conduction in the AFL reentry circuit has been shown to be in the CTI, through which conduction times may reach 80 to 100 msec, accounting for one third to one half of the AFL cycle length.[8-10]

The CTI is anatomically bounded by the inferior vena cava (IVC) and eustachian ridge posteriorly and by the TV annulus anteriorly (see Fig. 11–1); these boundaries form lines of conduction block or barriers delineating a protected zone of slow conduction in the reentry circuit.[11-14] The presence of conduction block along the eustachian ridge[11-14] has been confirmed by the demonstration of double potentials along its length during AFL (Fig. 11–2A). Double potentials have also been recorded along the crista terminalis,[11-14] suggesting that it too forms a line of block separating the smooth septal right atrium from the trabeculated right atrial free wall (see Fig. 11–2B). Such lines of block, which may be either functional or anatomic, are necessary to create an adequate path length for reentry to be sustained, even in the

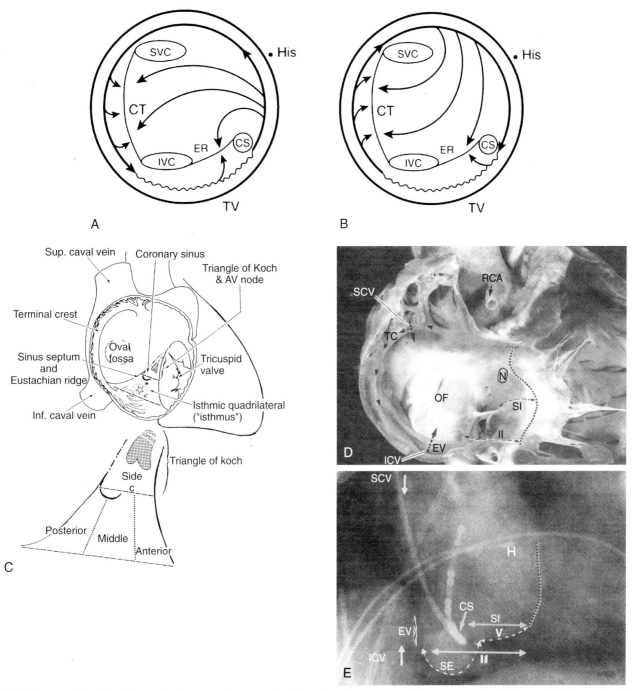

FIGURE 11–1. **A** and **B,** Schematic diagrams demonstrating the activation patterns of human type 1 atrial flutter (AFL), as viewed from below the tricuspid valve (TV) annulus, looking up into the right atrium. In the typical form of AFL (**A**) the reentrant wavefront rotates counterclockwise in the right atrium, whereas in the reverse typical form (**B**) reentry is clockwise. Note that the eustachian ridge (ER) and crista terminalis (CT) form lines of block, and that an area of slow conduction (wavy line) is present in the isthmus between the inferior vena cava (IVC) and ER and the TV annulus. CS, coronary sinus ostium; His, His bundle; SVC, superior vena cava. **C** through **E,** Anatomy of the isthmus area. The schematic diagram of the right atrium (**C**) shows the cavotricuspid isthmus *(expanded insert),* which is posterior and inferior to the triangle of Koch. **D,** Pathologic specimen showing the heart in right anterior oblique (RAO) view. The hinge of the TV is shown by the *dotted line.* Note the complex anatomy along the inferior isthmus line, with a fenestrated thebesian valve present. SI, septal isthmus line; II, inferior isthmus; EV, eustachian valve; OF, foramen ovale; N, AV nodal area; SVC, superior vena cava. **E,** RAO angiogram of the isthmus. A pouchlike subeustachian sinus (SE) is clearly seen adjacent to the vestibule region (V). H, His catheter. *(From Cabrera JA, Sanchez-Quintana D, Ho SY, et al.: The architecture of the atrial musculature between the orifice of the inferior caval vein and the tricuspid valve: The anatomy of the isthmus. J Cardiaovasc Electrophysiol 9:1186-1195, 1998, with permission.)*

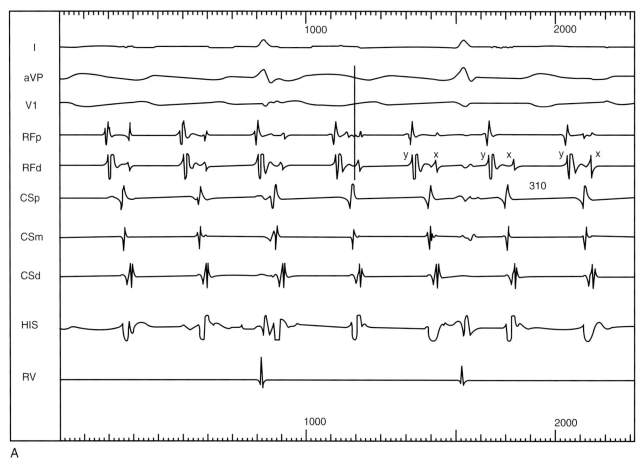

A

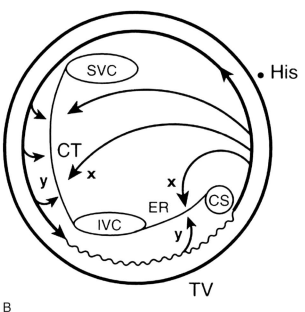

B

FIGURE 11–2. A, Surface electrocardiographic leads I, aVF, and V1 and endocardial electrograms in a patient with typical atrial flutter (AFL) demonstrating double potentials (XY) recorded along the eustachian ridge (ER) by the ablation catheter (RFd). Note that the X and Y potentials straddle the onset of the initial downstroke of the F wave in lead aVF *(vertical line),* indicating that the X potential is recorded immediately after the activation wavefront exits the subeustachian isthmus and circulates around the coronary sinus above the ER. The Y potential is recorded after the activation wavefront has rotated entirely around the atrium and is proceeding through the subeustachian isthmus below the ER. Double potentials may similarly be recorded along the crista terminalis (CT). **B,** A schematic diagram of the right atrium indicates where such double potentials (XY) may be recorded along the ER and CT during typical AFL. CSp, CSm, and CSd are electrograms recorded, respectively, from the proximal, middle, and distal electrode pairs on a quadripolar catheter in the coronary sinus (CS) with the proximal pair at the ostium. His, electrogram from the His bundle catheter; IVC, inferior vena cava; RFp and RFd, electrograms from the proximal and distal electrode pairs of the mapping/ablation catheter with the distal pair positioned on the ER, RV, right ventricle electrogram; SVC, superior vena cava; TV, tricuspid valve.

presence of an area of slow conduction, and to prevent short-circuiting of the reentrant wavefront.[12-15]

The medial and lateral CTI, which are contiguous, respectively, with the interatrial septum near the coronary sinus (CS) ostium and with the low lateral right atrium near the IVC (see Fig. 11–1), correspond electrophysiologically to the exit and entrance to the zone of slow conduction, depending on whether the direction of reentry is CCW or CW in the right atrium.[2-15] The path of the reentrant circuit outside the confines of the CTI (see Fig. 11–1) consists of a broad activation wavefront in the interatrial septum and right atrial free wall around the crista terminalis and the TV annulus.[12-15]

The slower conduction velocity in the CTI, relative to the interatrial septum and right atrial free wall, may be caused by anisotropic fiber orientation in the CTI.[7-10,16,17] This may also predispose to the develop-

ment of unidirectional block during rapid atrial pacing, accounting for the observation that typical (CCW) AFL is more likely to be induced when pacing is performed from the CS ostium, and reverse typical (CW) AFL when pacing is from the low lateral right atrium.[18-21]

Lower loop reentry is an isthmus-dependent flutter in which the caudal-to-cranial limb of the wavefront crosses over gaps in the crista terminalis in the low to middle right atrium (Fig. 11–3).[22,23] The circuit is essentially around the ostium of the inferior vena cava in the right atrium. The direction of rotation may be CW or CCW. This variant activation sequence may be sustained, or it may interconvert with other forms of AFL.

Partial isthmus flutter is another variant in which the CCW reentrant wavefront "short-circuits" through the eustachian ridge barrier to pass between

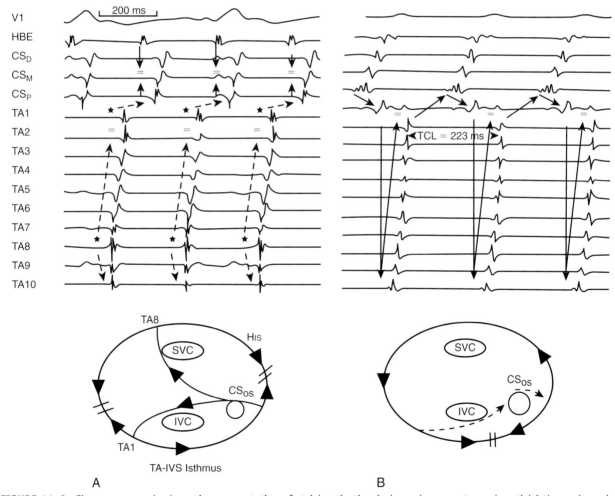

FIGURE 11–3. Electrograms and schematic representation of atrial activation in lower loop reentry and partial isthmus-dependent flutter. **A,** In lower loop reentry, the posterior right atrium is part of the reentry circuit and wavefronts collide in the lateral right atrium. The electrograms show multiple collisions at TA1 and TA8 *(stars)*. **B,** In partial isthmus-dependent flutter, the wavefront bypasses the cavotricuspid isthmus (CTI) through the eustachian ridge to enter it laterally and medially. The coronary sinus ostium (CS_os) is activated prematurely, and the tachycardia is not entrained from the CTI itself. IVC, inferior vena cava; SVC, superior vena cava; TA10, proximal recording electrodes on Halo catheter near upper septum; TA1, distal recording electrodes on Halo catheter near lateral aspect of the CTI. *(From Yang Y, Cheng J, Bochoeyer A, et al.: Atypical right atrial flutter patterns. Circulation 103:3092-3098, 2001, with permission.)*

the IVC and the CS ostium (see Fig. 11–3).[22] The wavefront then propagates in a CW direction through the medial end of the CTI to collide with the wavefront that is also conducting through the isthmus from its lateral aspect.

Diagnosis

SURFACE ELECTROCARDIOGRAPHY

The surface 12-lead electrocardiogram (ECG) is helpful in establishing a diagnosis of type 1 AFL, particularly the typical form (Table 11–1). In typical AFL, an inverted sawtooth F-wave pattern is observed in the inferior ECG leads II, III, and aVF, with low-amplitude biphasic F waves in leads I and aVL, an upright F wave in precordial lead V1, and an inverted F wave in lead V6 (Fig. 11–4A). In contrast, in reverse typical AFL, the F-wave pattern on the 12-lead ECG is less specific and variable, often with a sine wave pattern in the inferior ECG leads (see Fig. 11–4B). The

determinants of F-wave pattern on ECG are largely dependent on the activation pattern of the left atrium resulting from reentry in the right atrium. Inverted F waves are inscribed in the inferior ECG leads in typical AFL as a result of activation of the left atrium initially posterior, near the CS, and upright F waves are inscribed in the inferior ECG leads in reverse typical AFL as a result of activation of the left atrium initially anterior, near Bachman's bundle.[24,25] However, because the typical and reverse typical forms of type 1 AFL utilize the same reentry circuit, but in opposite directions, their rates are usually similar.

Recently developed algorithms using signal processing software to assess stability of the F wave on the surface ECG may allow the clinician to determine whether the CTI is a critical zone in the reentry circuit of any AFL observed on ECG, regardless of the F-wave pattern.[26] Data from these studies suggest that CTI-dependent AFL, both typical and reverse typical forms, has a significantly more stable cycle length and activation pattern than does atypical AFL. A potential explanation for this observation is that CTI-dependent AFL has a more stable macroreentrant

TABLE 11–1	
Diagnostic Criteria for Isthmus-Dependent Flutters	
Type of Flutter	**Criteria**
Surface ECG	
Typical flutter	Sawtooth upright F-wave pattern in the inferior ECG leads and in V1
Reverse typical flutter	Sine wave or upright F-wave pattern in the inferior ECG leads
Lower loop reentry	Variable; often resembles typical flutter if counterclockwise; clockwise rotation usually yields upright F waves inferiorly and inverted in V1
Partial isthmus-dependent flutter	Poorly described; probably similar to typical flutter
Electrophysiologic testing	
All isthmus-dependent flutters	Demonstration of entrainment criteria during pacing from the CTI, including the following: First postpacing interval ≤30 msec longer than tachycardia cycle length Stimulus-to-F-wave interval equal to electrogram-to-F-wave interval on pacing catheter Identical paced F-wave morphology and atrial activation sequence Macroreentrant RA activation by standard activation or electroanatomic mapping
Typical flutter	Concealed entrainment from CTI and counterclockwise macroreentrant RA activation
Reverse typical flutter	Concealed entrainment from CTI and clockwise macroreentrant RA activation
Lower loop reentry	Concealed entrainment from both CTI *and* low posterior right atrium with clockwise or counterclockwise macroreentrant RA activation
Partial isthmus-dependent flutter	Concealed entrainment from lateral but *not* medial margin of CTI; early coronary sinus ostium activation; wavefront collision in CTI; counterclockwise macroreentrant RA activation

CTI, cavotricuspid isthmus; ECG, electrocardiogram; RA, right atrial.

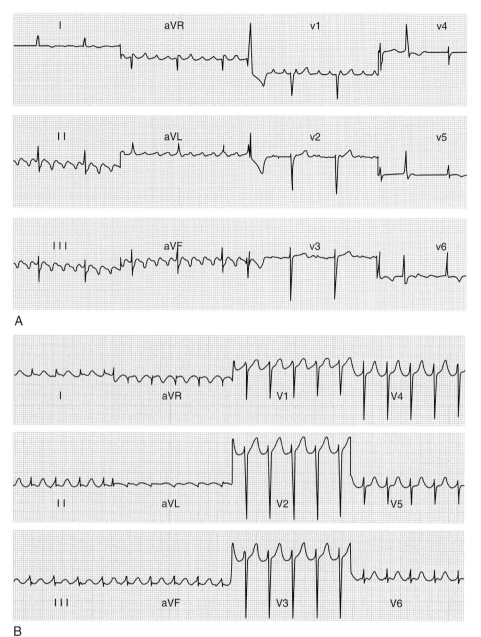

FIGURE 11–4. A, A 12-lead electrocardiogram recorded from a patient with typical atrial flutter (AFL). Note the typical sawtoothed pattern of inverted F waves in the inferior leads II, III, and aVF. Typical AFL is also characterized by flat to biphasic F waves in I and aVL, respectively; an upright F wave in V_1; and an inverted F wave in V_6. **B,** A 12-lead electrocardiogram from a patient with the reverse typical AFL. The F wave in the reverse typical form of AFL has a less distinct sine wave pattern in the inferior leads. In this case, the F waves are upright in the inferior leads II, III, and aVF; biphasic in leads I, aVL, and V_1; and upright in V_6.

activation pattern than atypical AFL does, most likely because of its anatomically restricted boundaries. This is important mechanistically and may have clinical implications in planning approaches to mapping and ablation.

The ECG presentation of lower loop reentry is highly variable, depending on the caudal-to-cranial level of wavefront breakthrough across the crista terminalis.[23] CCW lower loop reentry may resemble typical AFL because of similar patterns of activation of the atrial septum and left atrium. A decrease in the late inferior forces may be evident in lower loop reentry due to wavefront collision in the lateral right atrium. With multiple or variable wavefront breaks in the lateral atrium, unusual and changing ECG patterns may be observed. Alternation of P-wave polarity from positive to negative in V1 may occur.[23] CW lower loop reentry typically demonstrates positive flutter waves in the inferior leads and negative flutter waves in V1.

The ECG description of partial isthmus-dependent flutter is incomplete but may be expected to resemble typical AFL, given the similar patterns of atrial activation.[22]

ELECTROPHYSIOLOGIC DIAGNOSIS

Despite the utility of the 12-lead ECG in making a presumptive diagnosis of typical AFL, an electrophysiologic study with mapping and entrainment must be performed to confirm the underlying mechanism if RF catheter ablation is to be successfully performed (see Table 11–1). This is particularly true in the case of reverse typical AFL, which is much more difficult to diagnose on 12-lead ECG.

For the electrophysiologic study of AFL, activation mapping may be performed using standard multielectrode catheters or one of the currently available 3-D computerized activation mapping systems. For standard multielectrode catheter mapping, catheters are positioned in the right atrium, His bundle region, and CS. To most precisely elucidate the endocardial activation sequence, a Halo 20-electrode mapping catheter (Cordis-Webster, Diamond Bar, Calif.) is most commonly used in the right atrium, positioned around the TV annulus (Fig. 11–5). Recordings obtained during AFL from all electrodes are then analyzed to determine the right atrial activation sequence.

For patients who present to the laboratory in sinus rhythm, it is necessary to induce AFL to confirm its mechanism. Induction of AFL is accomplished by atrial programmed stimulation or burst pacing. Preferred pacing sites are the CS ostium and low lateral right atrium; the type of AFL induced may depend in part on the pacing site (CCW and CW, respectively). Burst pacing is the preferred method to induce AFL. Pacing cycle lengths between 180 and 240 msec are typically effective in producing unidirectional CTI block and inducing AFL. Induction of AFL typically occurs immediately after the onset of unidirectional CTI isthmus block, which can be directly observed during standard electrode catheter mapping, or after a brief period of rapid atrial tachycardia or atrial fibrillation.[18,19] During electrophysiologic study, a diagnosis of either typical or reverse typical AFL is

suggested by observing, respectively, a CCW or CW activation pattern in the right atrium and around the TV annulus. For example, as seen in Figure 11–6A in a patient with typical AFL, the atrial electrogram recorded at the CS ostium is timed with the initial downstroke of the F wave in the inferior surface ECG leads, followed by caudal-to-cranial activation in the interatrial septum-to-His bundle atrial electrogram, then cranial-to-caudal activation in the right atrial free wall from proximal to distal on the Halo catheter, and finally signal to the ablation catheter in the CTI, indicating that the underlying mechanism is a CCW macroreentry circuit with electrical activity encompassing the entire tachycardia cycle length. In a patient with reverse typical AFL, the mirror image of this activation pattern is seen (see Fig. 11–6B).

In addition, confirmation that the reentry circuit utilizes the CTI requires demonstration of the classic criteria for entrainment—specifically, concealed entrainment during pacing from the CTI.[5] Criteria for demonstrating concealed entrainment of AFL include acceleration of the tachycardia to the pacing cycle length without a change in the F-wave pattern on surface ECG or in the endocardial atrial activation pattern and electrogram morphology, as well as immediate resumption of the tachycardia at the original cycle length on termination of pacing, including the first postpacing interval (Fig. 11–7). Concealed entrainment is further confirmed, during pacing performed within the CTI, if the stimulus-to-F wave or stimulus-to-reference electrogram interval during pacing and the pacing electrode electrogram-to-F wave or electrogram-to-reference electrogram interval during AFL are the same (see Fig. 11–7). Furthermore, during typical AFL the stimulus-to-F wave or stimulus-to-proximal CS electrogram is shorter when

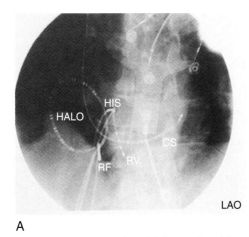
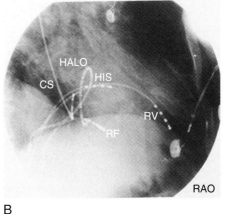

A   B

FIGURE 11–5. Right anterior oblique (**A**) and left anterior oblique (**B**) fluoroscopic projections showing the intracardiac positions of the right ventricular (RV), His bundle (HIS), coronary sinus (CS), Halo (HALO), and mapping/ablation catheter (RF). Note that the Halo catheter is positioned around the tricuspid valve annulus, with the proximal electrode pair at 1 o'clock and the distal electrode pair at 7 o'clock in the LAO view. The mapping/ablation catheter is positioned in the subeustachian isthmus, midway between the interatrial septum and the low lateral right atrium, with the distal 8-mm ablation electrode near the tricuspid valve annulus.

FIGURE 11–6. Endocardial electrograms from the mapping/ablation, Halo, coronary sinus (CS), and His bundle catheters and surface electrocardiogram leads I, aVF, and V1, demonstrating a counterclockwise (CCW) rotation of activation in the right atrium in a patient with typical atrial flutter (AFL) (**A**) and a clockwise (CW) rotation of activation in the right atrium in a patient with reverse typical AFL (**B**). The AFL cycle length was 256 msec for both CCW and CW forms. Arrows demonstrate activation sequence. The HALOD through HALOP tracings are 10 bipolar electrograms recorded from the distal (low lateral right atrium) to the proximal (high right atrium) poles of the 20-pole Halo catheter positioned around the tricuspid valve annulus with the proximal electrode pair at 1 o'clock and the distal electrode pair at 7 o'clock. CSP electrograms were recorded from the CS catheter proximal electrode pair positioned at the ostium, HISP electrograms from the proximal electrode pair of the His bundle catheter, and RF electrograms from the mapping/ablation catheter positioned with the distal electrode pair in the cavotricuspid isthmus. ms, microseconds.

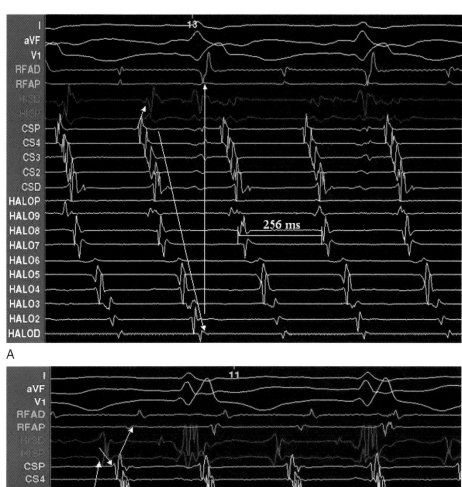

A

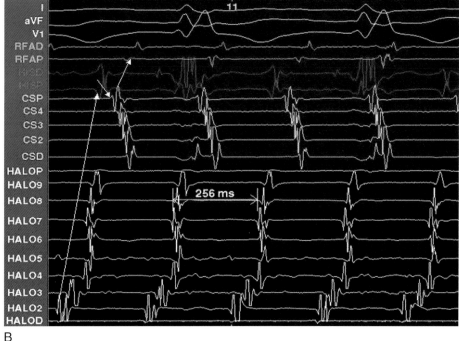

B

the pacing site is medial, near the exit from the CTI (e.g., 30 to 50 msec), and longer when the pacing site is lateral, near the entrance to the CTI (e.g., 80 to 100 msec); the converse is true during reverse typical AFL. In contrast, pacing at sites outside the CTI results in overt entrainment of AFL, with variable degrees of constant fusion of the F-wave pattern and endocardial atrial electrograms.

The diagnosis of lower loop reentrant AFL is confirmed by the demonstration of concealed entrainment of the tachycardia from not only the CTI but also the posterior right atrium.[22] Partial isthmus-dependent flutter is confirmed by the demonstration of concealed entrainment from the lateral margin of the CTI but not from the medial portion. In addition, there is early activation of the CS ostium and evidence of collision within the CTI. Concealed entrainment should be demonstrable from the area of short circuit through the eustachian ridge.

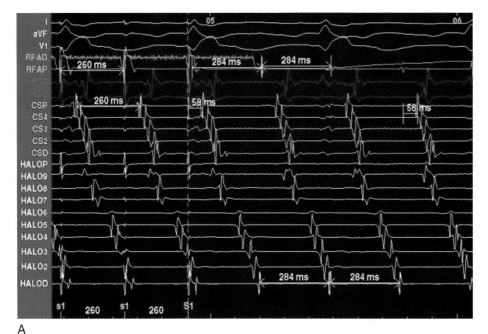

A

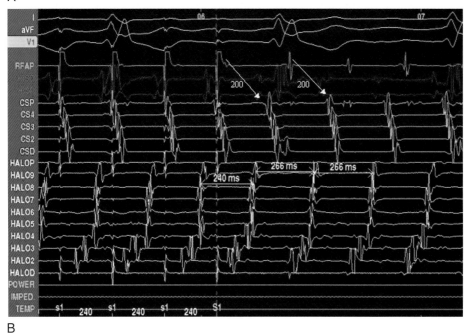

B

FIGURE 11-7. A 12-lead electrocardiogram (ECG) and endocardial electrogram recordings during pacing entrainment from the cavotricuspid isthmus in patients with typical atrial flutter (AFL) (**A**) and reverse typical AFL (**B**). Note in both examples that the tachycardia is accelerated to the pacing cycle length, and that the F-wave morphology on surface ECG and endocardial waveforms and the activation pattern are unchanged during pacing compared with AFL, indicating concealed entrainment. Furthermore, the stimulus-to-F wave or local electrogram intervals are comparable to the electrogram-to-F wave or local electrogram intervals recorded on the mapping/ablation catheter (RFAP) during entrainment and AFL in both examples, indicating concealed entrainment. Halo catheter tracings are as described in Figure 11-6. ms, microseconds; S1, pacing stimulus artifact. (Abbreviations per Fig. 11-6).

The differential diagnosis of AFL from other supraventricular arrhythmias is usually apparent given typical ECG manifestations and variable ventricular-atrial relationships. The most likely differential to be made is the exclusion of a focal atrial tachycardia. Rarely, atrial tachycardia in the low posteroseptal right atrium may be confused with AFL if unidirectional CTI block is present. Otherwise, the atrial tachycardia can be recognized by failure to entrain from the CTI and by a radial activation pattern.

Ablation

RF catheter ablation of typical AFL and other isthmus-dependent flutters is performed with a steerable mapping/ablation catheter with a large distal ablation electrode, ranging in available length from 4 to 5 mm, that is positioned in the right atrium via a femoral vein.[2-4,6,27-30] The typical RF generator used by most laboratories is capable of automatically adjusting applied power (i.e., up to 50W) to achieve an operator-programmable tissue-electrode interface temperature. Tissue temperature is monitored via a thermistor or thermocouple embedded in the distal ablation electrode. Programmable temperature with automatic power control is important, because successful ablation requires a stable temperature of at least 50°C to 60°C, and occasionally 70°C, whereas temperatures in excess of 70°C can cause tissue vaporization (steam pops), tissue charring, and formation of blood coagulum on the ablation electrode, resulting in a rise in impedance that limits energy delivery and lesion formation, possibly leading to complications such as cardiac perforation or embolization.

A variety of mapping/ablation catheters, with different shapes and curve lengths, as well as RF generators, are currently available from several commercial manufacturers. We prefer to use a larger-curve catheter (K2 or mid-distal large curve; EP Technologies, San Jose, Calif.), with or without a preshaped guiding sheath such as an SR0, SL1, or ramp sheath (Daig, Minnetonka, Minn.), to ensure that the ablation electrode will reach the TV annulus, especially in patients with an enlarged right atrium.

Recently, RF ablation catheters with either saline-cooled ablation electrodes or large distal ablation electrodes (i.e., 8 to 10mm) have been approved by the U.S. Food and Drug Administration for ablation of type 1 AFL; these are available from EP Technologies, Biosense Webster, and Medtronic, (Minneapolis, MN). During ablation with saline-cooled catheters, the use of lower power and temperature settings is recommended to avoid steam pops, because higher intramyocardial tissue temperatures are produced than those measured at the tissue-electrode interface, due to the electrode cooling effect of saline perfusion.[31-34] Typically, a maximum power of 35 to 40W and a temperature of 40°C to 45°C should be used initially, although studies have reported use of up to 50W and 60°C for ablation of AFL without higher than expected complication rates.[31-34] In contrast, the large-tip (8 to 10mm) ablation catheters require a higher power, up to 100W, to achieve target temperatures of 50°C to 70°C, because of the greater energy-dispersive effects of the larger ablation electrode, which also requires the use of two grounding pads applied to the patient's skin to avoid skin burns.[34-39] The target for type 1 AFL ablation is the CTI (Table 11–2), which, when standard multipolar electrode catheters are used for mapping and ablation, is localized with a combined fluoroscopically and electrophysiologically guided approach.[2-4,6,27-39] Typically, a steerable mapping/ablation catheter is initially positioned fluoroscopically (see Fig. 11–5) in

TABLE 11–2
Targets for Ablation of Isthmus-Dependent Flutters

Type of Flutter	Targets
CTI-dependent	CTI from tricuspid valve annulus to IVC
	Tricuspid valve annulus–eustachian ridge isthmus
	Tricuspid valve annulus–CS ostium–eustachian ridge isthmus
Partial isthmus-dependent	CS ostium to IVC

CS, coronary sinus; CTI, cavotricuspid isthmus; IVC, inferior vena cava.

the CTI, with the distal ablation electrode on or near the TV annulus in the right anterior oblique view, and midway between the septum and low right atrial free wall (6 or 7 o'clock position) in the left anterior oblique view. The distal ablation electrode position is then adjusted toward or away from the TV annulus, based on the ratio of atrial and ventricular electrogram amplitudes (A/V ratio) recorded by the bipolar ablation electrode. An optimal ratio is 1:2 or 1:4 at the TV annulus, as seen in Figure 11–6A on the ablation electrode. After the ablation catheter is positioned on or near the TV annulus, it is very slowly withdrawn during ablation toward the IVC while RF energy is applied continuously; alternatively, it can be withdrawn in a stepwise manner, a few millimeters at a time (usually the length of the distal ablation electrode), with 30- to 60-second pauses at each location, during a continuous or interrupted energy application. Electrogram recordings may be employed in addition to fluoroscopy to ensure that the ablation electrode is in contact with viable tissue in the CTI throughout each energy application. Ablation across the entire CTI (Fig. 11–8) may require several sequential 30- to 60-second energy applications during a stepwise catheter pullback, or a prolonged energy application of up to 120 seconds or longer during a continuous catheter pullback. The catheter should be gradually withdrawn until the distal ablation electrode records no atrial electrogram, indicating that it has reached the IVC, or until the ablation electrode is noted to abruptly slip off the eustachian ridge fluoroscopically. RF energy application should be immediately interrupted when the catheter has reached the IVC, because ablation in venous structures is known to cause significant pain to patients.

Alternatively, ablation of the TV-CS and CS-IVC isthmuses (see Fig. 11–8) may be performed using an approach similar to that used to ablate the CTI.[40] However, for this approach to be successful, it may be necessary to ablate within the CS ostium as well,

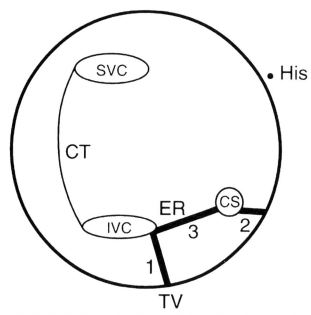

FIGURE 11–8. Schematic diagram of the right atrium, showing the typical locations for linear ablation of the cavotricuspid isthmus *(line 1)*, the tricuspid valve (TV)–coronary sinus (CS) isthmus *(line 2)*, and the CS–inferior vena cava (IVC) isthmus *(line 3)*. CT, crista terminalis; ER, eustachian ridge; His, His bundle; SVC, superior vena cava.

which may be associated with a higher risk of complications such as AV node block. It has also been reported that type 1 AFL may be cured by ablating between the TV annulus and eustachian ridge only, which is a narrower isthmus than the CTI.[41] During repeat ablation, it may be necessary to rotate the ablation catheter away from the initial line of energy application, either medially or laterally in the CTI, to create new or additional lines of block, or to use a slightly higher power and/or ablation temperature. In addition, if ablation is initially attempted using a standard 4- to 5-mm-tip electrode and fails, repeat ablation with a large-tip electrode catheter or a cooled-tip ablation catheter may be successful.[31-39] Ablation of partial isthmus-dependent flutter requires creation of a block from the CS ostium to the IVC, eliminating conduction across the eustachian ridge. Completion of this line may convert the tachycardia to typical isthmus-dependent flutter, which then requires full ablation of the CTI.[22]

PROCEDURAL END POINTS FOR RADIOFREQUENCY CATHETER ABLATION OF TYPE 1 ATRIAL FLUTTER

Ablation may be performed during sustained AFL or during sinus rhythm. If it is performed during AFL, the first end point is its termination during energy application (Fig. 11–9). However, even if AFL termi-

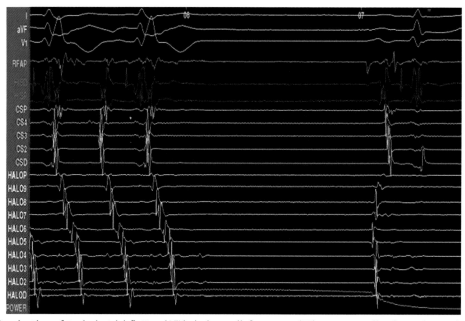

FIGURE 11–9. Termination of typical atrial flutter (AFL) during radiofrequency (RF) energy application using a slow drag technique across the cavotricuspid isthmus (CTI). AFL usually terminates just as the distal ablation electrode on the mapping/ablation catheter (RFAP) approaches the inferior vena cava. Conduction fails at the CTI, as indicated by block developing between the low lateral right atrium and coronary sinus in the typical form, or between the coronary sinus and the low lateral right atrium in the reverse typical form (not shown). The power readout from the RF energy generator is shown in the bottom tracing. Halo catheter and other tracings are as described in Figure 11–6.

nates, it is common to find that CTI conduction persists. Therefore, the entire CTI ablation should first be completed, after which electrophysiologic testing can be performed. After completion of CTI ablation as determined by fluoroscopic and electrophysiologic criteria described previously, programmed stimulation and burst pacing should be performed immediately and repeated over the course of at least 30 minutes to ensure that bidirectional CTI block has been achieved and that neither typical nor reverse typical AFL can be reinduced.[2-4,6,27-39] If AFL is not terminated during the first attempt at CTI ablation, the activation sequence and isthmus dependence of the AFL should be reconfirmed, and ablation should be repeated.

If AFL is terminated during ablation, pacing should then be done at a cycle length of 600 msec or less, depending on the sinus cycle length, to determine whether there is a bidirectional conduction block in the CTI (Figs. 11–10 through 11–13). If ablation is done during sinus rhythm, pacing can also be done during energy application to monitor for the development of conduction block in the CTI (Fig. 11–14). The use of this end point for ablation may be associated with a significantly lower recurrence rate of type 1 AFL during long-term follow-up.[42-45] Conduction in the CTI is commonly evaluated by comparing activation patterns in the right atrial free wall and interatrial septum or around the TV annulus, while pacing during sinus rhythm at slow rates (i.e., cycle lengths ≥600 msec) from the low lateral right atrium and CS ostium, before and after ablation. It is important to pace at relatively slow rates during assessment for CTI block, because conduction block

across the CTI may be functional and rate dependent in some patients after ablation. In addition, conduction block across the crista terminalis may be functional in some patients, and at slow pacing rates conduction across the midcrista region can result in uncertainty regarding the presence or absence of bidirectional CTI block after ablation.[46-48] Therefore, it may be necessary to pace not only from the proximal CS but also adjacent to the ablation line in the CTI, or in the posterior-inferior right atrial septum, to confirm the presence of CTI isthmus block.[48] Bidirectional conduction block in the CTI is confirmed by demonstration of a change, from a bidirectional wavefront with collision in the right atrial free wall or interatrial septum before ablation, to a strictly cranial-to-caudal activation sequence after ablation during pacing from the CS ostium or low lateral right atrium, respectively[42-45] (see Figs. 11–10 through 11-13). The presence of bidirectional conduction block in the CTI is also strongly supported by recording widely spaced (>90 to 110 msec) double potentials along the entire ablation line, during pacing from the low lateral right atrium or CS ostium (see Fig. 11–14).[49,50] In order to expedite the assessment of bidirectional conduction block after CTI ablation, and to obviate the need for multipolar electrode catheter recordings, several algorithms based on transisthmus conduction times, changes in P-wave polarity, reversal of electrogram polarity at the ablation line, and use of unipolar electrograms have been employed, with varying degrees of accuracy.[51-54] These methods are summarized in Figure 11–15. However, in most electrophysiology laboratories, these methods alone are not relied on to confirm the presence or absence

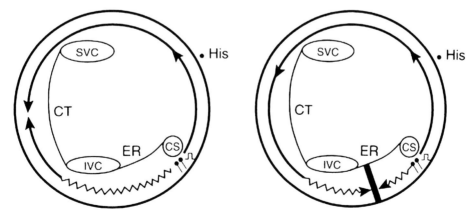

FIGURE 11–10. Schematic diagrams of the expected right atrial activation sequence during pacing in sinus rhythm from the coronary sinus (CS) ostium before *(left panel)* and after *(right panel)* ablation of the cavotricuspid isthmus (CTI). Before ablation, the activation pattern during CS pacing is caudal to cranial in the interatrial septum and low right atrium, with collision of the septal and right atrial wavefronts in the midlateral right atrium. After ablation, the activation pattern during CS pacing is still caudal to cranial in the interatrial septum, but the lateral right atrium is now activated in a strictly cranial-to-caudal pattern (i.e., counterclockwise), indicating complete clockwise conduction block in the CTI. CT, crista terminalis; ER, eustachian ridge; His, His bundle; IVC, inferior vena cava; SVC, superior vena cava.

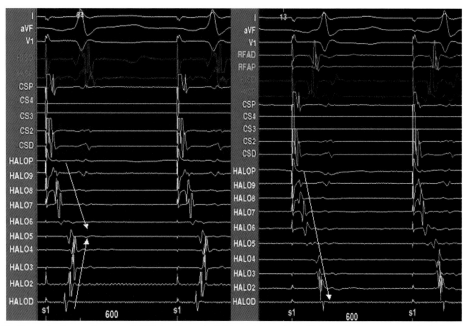

FIGURE 11–11. Surface electrocardiogram (ECG) leads and right atrial endocardial electrograms recorded during pacing in sinus rhythm from the coronary sinus (CS) ostium before *(left panel)* and after *(right panel)* ablation of the cavotricuspid isthmus (CTI). Tracings include surface ECG leads I, aVF, and V1 and endocardial electrograms from the proximal coronary sinus (CSP), His bundle (HIS), tricuspid valve annulus at 1 o'clock (HALOP) to 7 o'clock (HALOD), and high right atrium (HRA or RFA). Before ablation during CS pacing there is collision of the cranial and caudal right atrial wavefronts in the midlateral right atrium (HALO5). After ablation, the lateral right atrium is activated in a strictly cranial-to-caudal pattern (i.e., counterclockwise), indicating complete medial-to-lateral conduction block in the CTI.

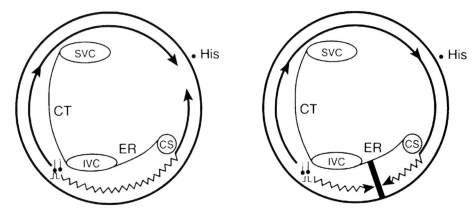

FIGURE 11–12. Schematic diagrams of the expected right atrial activation sequence during pacing in sinus rhythm from the low lateral right atrium before *(left panel)* and after *(right panel)* ablation of the cavotricuspid isthmus (CTI). Before ablation, the activation pattern during coronary sinus (CS) pacing is caudal to cranial in the right atrial free wall, with collision of the cranial and caudal wavefronts (i.e., through the CTI) in the midseptum; there is simultaneous activation at the His bundle (HISP) and proximal coronary sinus (CSP). After ablation, the activation pattern during low lateral right atrial sinus pacing is still caudal to cranial in the right atrial free wall, but the septum is now activated in a strictly cranial-to-caudal pattern (i.e., clockwise), indicating complete counterclockwise conduction block in the CTI. CT, crista terminalis; ER, eustachian ridge; His, His bundle; SVC, superior vena cava.

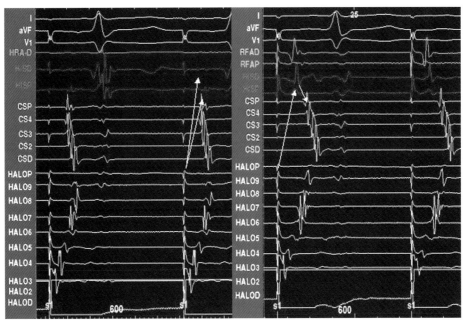

FIGURE 11–13. Surface electrocardiogram (ECG) and right atrial endocardial electrograms during pacing in sinus rhythm from the low lateral right atrium before *(left panel)* and after *(right panel)* ablation of the cavotricuspid isthmus (CTI). Tracings include surface ECG leads I, aVF, and V1 and endocardial electrograms from the proximal coronary sinus (CSP), His bundle (HIS), tricuspid valve annulus at 1 o'clock (HALOP) to 7 o'clock (HALOD), and high right atrium (HRA or RFA). Before ablation, during low lateral right atrial pacing there is collision of the cranial and caudal right atrial wavefronts in the midseptum (HIS and CSP). After ablation, the septum is activated in a strictly cranial-to-caudal pattern (i.e., clockwise), indicating complete lateral-to-medial conduction block in the CTI.

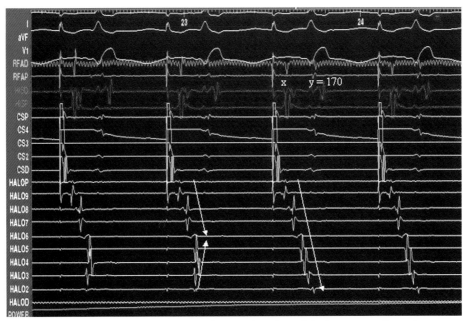

FIGURE 11–14. Surface electrocardiogram leads I, aVF and V1, and endocardial electrograms from the coronary sinus (CS), His bundle, Halo, mapping/ablation (RF), and right ventricular catheters during radiofrequency catheter ablation of the cavotricuspid isthmus (CTI), while pacing from the CS ostium. Note the change in activation of the lateral right atrium on the Halo catheter from a bidirectional to a unidirectional pattern, indicating the development of clockwise block in the CTI. This was associated with the development of widely spaced (170 msec) double potentials (x and y) on the ablation catheter in the CTI, further confirming medial-to-lateral conduction block. Halo catheter and other tracings are as described in Figure 11–6.

Methods: Point to point activation mapping along ablation line during PCS pacing post ablation
Measure: Interval between split components of isthmus electrogram (DP1-2) on ablation (Abl) catheter
Definition of Complete Isthmus Block: DP1-2 $\geq$ 110 or $\geq$ 90 ms with $\leq$ 15 ms variation along line
Reference: Tada. JACC 2001;38:750-755

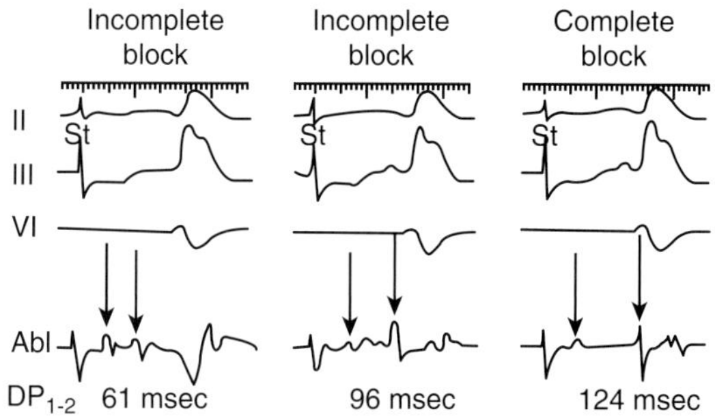

Methods: Pacing at sites (A, B, C, and D) on both sides of ablation line and record bipolar EGM activation times at points A, B, C, and D pre- and post-ablation
Measure: Conduction times among sites A, B, C, and D
Definition of Complete Isthmus Block: Conduction times AD > BD and DA > CA after ablation
Reference: Chen. Circulation 1999;100:2507-2513

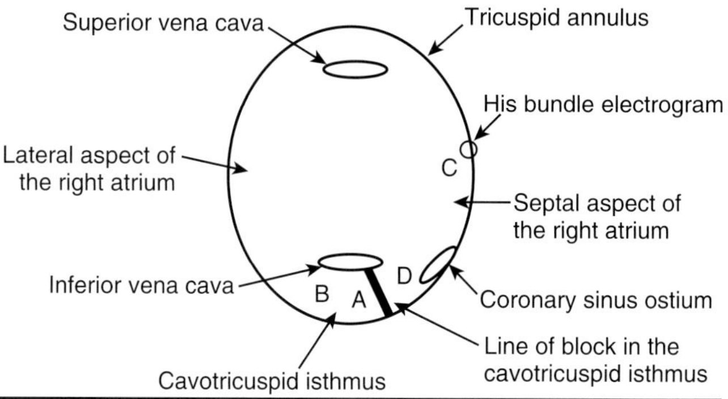

Methods: Pacing PCS and record 2 bipolar EGM (E1 and E2, 2mm spacing each) 2mm apart just lateral to ablation line
Measure: Polarity of E1 and E2 during PCS pacing pre- and post-ablation
Definition of Complete Isthmus Block: Transition of EGM polarity from positive to negative at both E1 and E2
Reference: Tada H. JCE 2001;12:393-399

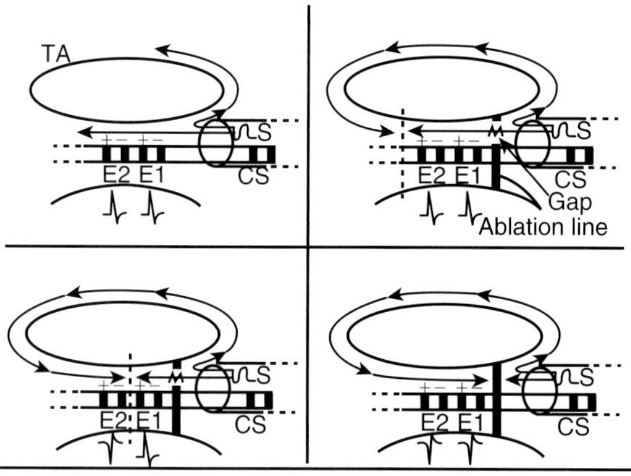

Methods: Unipolar EGM recording during PCS pacing pre- and post-ablation
Measure: Unipolar EGM polarity immediately lateral to ablation line
Definition of Complete Isthmus Block: Loss of negative components and development of R or Rs pattern in unipolar EGM
Reference: Villacastin J. Circulation 2000; 102:3080-3085

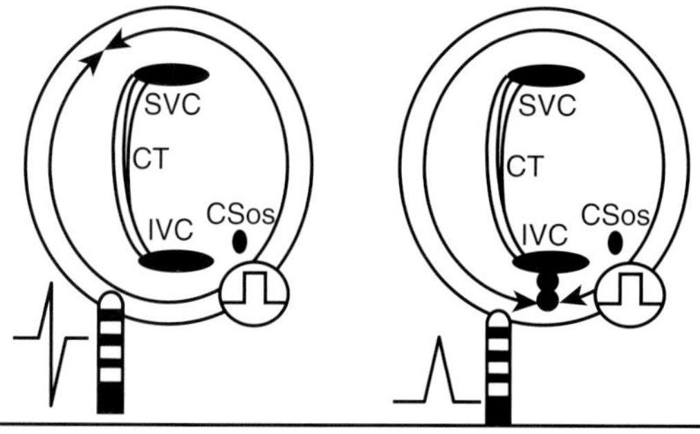

Methods: Pacing PCS and low lateral right atrium and recording bipolar EGM for conduction time across isthmus
Measure: $\triangle = CT_1 + CT_2 - TCL$. CT_1 – conduction time low lateral atrium (LLRA) in flutter and CT_2 – conduction time from PCS to LLRA with PCS pacing. TCL – flutter cycle length
Definition of Isthmus Block: $\triangle \geq 0$ ms
Reference: Johna R. AJC 1999;83:1666-1668

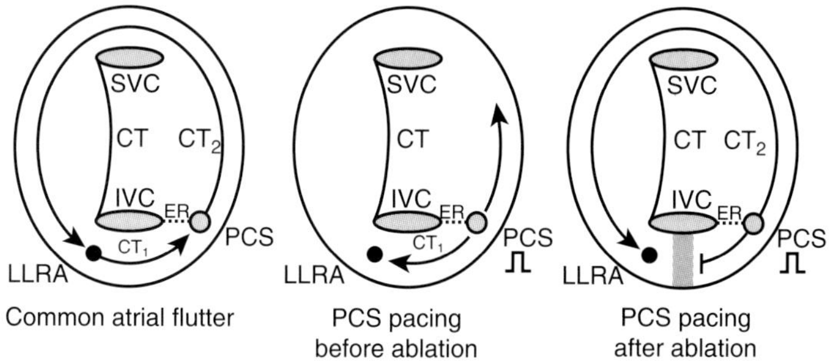

FIGURE 11-15. Methods of determining bidirectional isthmus block after ablation. AJC, *American Journal of Cardiology*; EGM, electrogram; JACC, *Journal of the American College of Cardiology*; JCE, *Journal of Cardiovascular Electrophysiology*.

of bidirectional CTI conduction block, and they are unlikely to replace the gold standard of multielectrode recordings or 3-D activation mapping.[2-4,6,27-39]

OUTCOMES AND COMPLICATIONS OF RADIOFREQUENCY CATHETER ABLATION OF TYPE 1 ATRIAL FLUTTER

Early reports[1-6] of RF catheter ablation of AFL revealed high initial success rates but with recurrence rates as high as 20% to 45% (Table 11–3). However, as experience with RF catheter ablation of AFL has increased,[27-39] both acute success rates (defined as termination of AFL and bidirectional isthmus block) and chronic success rates (defined as no recurrence of type 1 AFL) have risen to 85% to 95%. Contributing in large degree to these improved results has been the introduction of bidirectional conduction block in the CTI as an end point for successful RF catheter ablation of AFL.[27-39] In the most recent studies using either large-tip electrode ablation catheters with high-power RF generators or cooled-tip electrode ablation catheters with standard RF generators, acute success rates as high as 100% and chronic success rates as high as 98% have been reported.[36-39] Randomized comparisons of internally cooled, externally cooled, and large-tip ablation catheters suggest a slightly better acute and chronic success rate with the externally cooled ablation catheters (which are available in Europe but not in the United States).[31-34,39] In addition, in one recent, very large study (169 patients) of the safety and efficacy of large-tip catheters for ablation of type 1 AFL,[35-37] it was demonstrated that acute success (defined as bidirectional CTI block) was achieved with fewer RF energy applications (10 ± 8 versus 14 ± 8 applications, $P = .002$) and shorter ablation time (0.5 ± 0.4 versus 0.8 ± 0.6 hours, $P = .0002$) with a 10-mm-tip catheter, compared with an 8-mm-tip catheter.

In almost all of the large-scale studies in which CTI ablation has successfully eliminated recurrence of type 1 AFL and quality-of-life scores (QOL) have been assessed, there has been statistically significant improvement, primarily resulting from reduced symptoms and antiarrhythmic medication use.[36-38]

Despite the excellent acute results and long-term outcome after RF catheter ablation for freedom from type 1 AFL, the development of atrial fibrillation and/or atypical AFL occurs at a high rate in this population of patients (up to 67% over 5 years), especially if there is a history of atrial fibrillation or underlying heart disease.[55,56] Nonetheless, ablation of

---

TABLE 11–3

Success Rates for Radiofrequency Catheter Ablation of Typical Atrial Flutter*

Author	Year (Ref. No.)	No. Patients	Electrode Length (mm)	% Acute Success	Follow-up (Months)	% Chronic Success
Feld et al.	1992 (2)	16	4	100	4 ± 2	83
Cosio et al.	1993 (3)	9	4	100	2-18	56
Kirkorian et al.	1994 (28)	22	4	86	8 ± 13	84
Fischer et al.	1995 (27)	80	4	7	20 ± 8	81
Poty et al.	1995 (42)	12	6/8	100	9 ± 3	92
Schwartzman et al.	1996 (43)	35	8	100	1-21	92
Chauchemez et al.	1996 (44)	20	4	100	8 ± 2	80
Tsai et al.	1995 (35)	50	8	92	10 ± 5	100
Chen et al.	1996 (30)	65	8	93	20 ± 11	92
Atiga et al.	2002 (32)	59	4 vs cooled	88	13 ± 4	93
Scavee et al.	2004 (33)	80	8 vs cooled	80	15	98
Feld et al.	2004 (37)	169	8 or 10	93	6	97
Calkins et al.	2004 (38)	150	8	88	6	87
Ventura et al.	2004 (39)	130	8 vs cooled	100	14 ± 2	98

*Acute success is defined as termination of atrial flutter during ablation and/or demonstration of isthmus block after ablation. Chronic success is defined as no recurrence of type 1 atrial flutter during follow-up. Acute and chronic success rates are reported as overall results in randomized or comparison studies.

the CTI may also reduce or, in rare cases, eliminate recurrences of atrial fibrillation,[56,57] and it is especially effective in patients undergoing pharmacologic treatment for atrial fibrillation who have antiarrhythmic drug–induced type 1 AFL (i.e., the so-called hybrid approach). Ablation of the CTI may be required as well in patients undergoing ablation for atrial fibrillation who also have a history of type 1 AFL.[58]

RF catheter ablation of the CTI for type 1 AFL is relatively safe, but serious complications can rarely occur, including heart block, cardiac perforation and tamponade, myocardial infarction from right coronary artery injury, and thromboembolic events including pulmonary embolism and stroke. In recent large-scale studies, even with cooled-tip and large-tip ablation catheters, major complications were observed in 2.5% to 3.5% of patients.[37-39] In addition, in the studies of large-tip ablation electrode catheters, there did not appear to be any relation between complication rates and the use of higher power (i.e., >50 W) for ablation of the CTI.

Although conversion of AFL to sinus rhythm is less likely to cause thromboembolic complications (e.g., stroke) than atrial fibrillation is, there is still a significant risk, and anticoagulation with warfarin before ablation must be considered in patients who have chronic type 1 AFL.[59-61] This may be particularly important in those patients with depressed ventricular function, mitral valve disease, or left atrial enlargement with left atrial thrombus or spontaneous contrast (i.e., smoke) on echocardiography. As an alternative, the use of transesophageal echocardiography to rule out left atrial clot or smoke before ablation may be acceptable, but subsequent anticoagulation with warfarin is still recommended, because atrial stunning may occur after conversion of AFL, as it does with atrial fibrillation.[59-61]

ROLE OF COMPUTERIZED THREE-DIMENSIONAL MAPPING IN DIAGNOSIS AND ABLATION OF TYPE 1 ATRIAL FLUTTER

The 3-D electroanatomic CARTO (Biosense Webster, Baldwin Park, Calif.) or noncontact EnSite (Endocardial Solutions, St. Paul, Minn.) activation mapping systems and the LocaLisa tracking system (EP Systems/Medtronic), although certainly not required for successful ablation of type 1 AFL, have specific advantages that have made them widely used and accepted technologies.[62,63] These systems are described in Chapter 8. There are unique characteristics of each system that make them more or less suitable for mapping and ablation of AFL.

The EnSite system uses a saline-inflated balloon catheter, on which is mounted a wire mesh containing electrodes that are capable of sensing the voltage

potential of surrounding atrial endocardium without actual electrode-tissue contact; from this catheter, the computerized mapping system can generate up to 3000 virtual endocardial electrograms and create a propagation map of the AFL (Fig. 11–16). In addition, a low-amplitude, high-frequency electrical current emitted from the ablation catheter can be sensed and tracked in 3-D space by the mapping balloon. The 3-D anatomy is delineated by roving the mapping catheter around the right atrial endocardium, and the propagation map is superimposed upon it. The appropriate ablation target, in this case the CTI, can then be localized, and the ablation catheter can be positioned appropriately and tracked while ablation is performed. After ablation, the mapping system can be used to assess for bidirectional CTI conduction block during pacing from the low lateral right atrium and CS ostium.

The advantages of the EnSite system include the ability to map the entire AFL activation sequence in one beat, precise anatomic representation of the right atrium including the CTI and adjacent structures, precise localization of the ablation catheter within the right atrium, and propagation maps of endocardial activation during AFL and during pacing after abla-

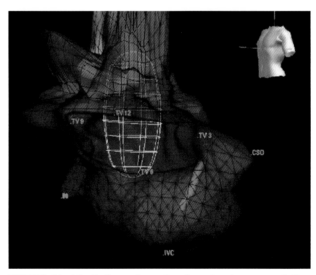

FIGURE 11–16. A three-dimensional anatomic representation of the right atrium in a patient with typical atrial flutter (AFL), using the EnSite balloon (Endocardial Solutions). This system uses an inflatable, wire mesh–coated balloon mounted on a pigtail catheter to record up to 3000 virtual electrograms simultaneously, allowing reconstruction of a virtual anatomy and virtual activation sequence. Virtual electrograms are reconstructed from voltage potentials recorded by the balloon mapping catheter from the endocardial surface. The location of the ablation catheter can also be tracked in three-dimensional space by the system. CSO, coronary sinus ostium; IVC, inferior vena cava; TV, tricuspid valve.

tion, to assess for CTI conduction block. In addition, any ablation catheter system can be used with the EnSite system. The major disadvantage of the EnSite system is the need to use the balloon mapping catheter, with its large (10 French) introducer sheath, and the need for full anticoagulation during the mapping procedure.

The CARTO system uses a magnetic sensor in the ablation catheter and a magnetic field (generated by a grid placed under the patient and a reference pad on the skin) to track the ablation catheter in 3-D space; a computer system sequentially records anatomic locations and electrograms for on-line analysis of activation time and computation of isochronal patterns, which are then superimposed on the endocardial geometry (Fig. 11–17A). A live propagation map can also be produced. The advantages of the CARTO system include precise anatomic representation of the right atrium including the CTI and adjacent structures, precise localization of the ablation catheter within the right atrium, and static activation and propagation maps of endocardial activation during AFL and during pacing after ablation, to assess for CTI conduction block[64] (see Fig. 11–17B). The disadvantages of the CARTO system

include the need to use a magnet, as well as the proprietary catheters and ablation generator, and the inability to map the entire endocardial activation sequence in one beat.

The 3-D computerized mapping systems, again while not required to map and ablate AFL, may be particularly useful in difficult cases such as in patients for whom prior ablation has failed, those with complex anatomy including idiopathic or postoperative scarring, and those with unoperated or surgically corrected congenital heart disease. For example, in Figure 11–18, a CARTO map of the right atrium shows an area of extensive scar in the CTI. However, near the TV annulus, a rim of viable myocardium persists and allows propagation of the macroreentrant wavefront through the CTI, perpetuating CCW type 1 AFL. Ablation in this case required a large-curve ablation catheter to reach the TV annulus and successfully ablate AFL.

Finally, 3-D activation mapping systems may be useful in ablation of type 1 AFL because they can mark the location of each ablation as it is done, thereby allowing the operator to reposition the ablation catheter precisely along the ablation line in the event the catheter moves inadvertently during abla-

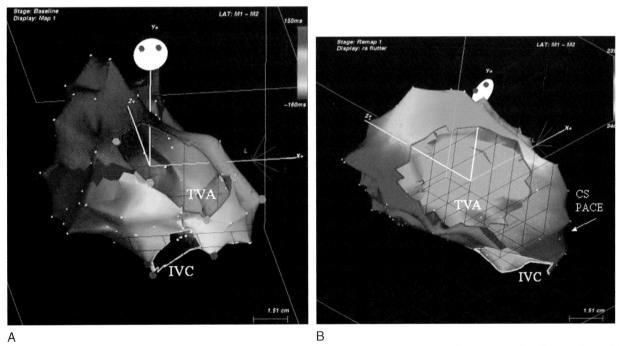

A   B

FIGURE 11–17. A three-dimensional electroanatomic (CARTO system, Biosense Webster) map of the right atrium in a patient with typical atrial flutter (AFL), before (**A**) and after (**B**) cavotricuspid isthmus (CTI) ablation. Note the counterclockwise activation pattern around the tricuspid valve during AFL (**A**), which is based on a color scheme indicating activation time from orange (early) to purple (late). After ablation of the CTI (**B**), during pacing from the coronary sinus (CS) ostium, there is evidence of medial-to-lateral isthmus block, as indicated by juxtaposition of orange and purple color in the CTI. A three-dimensional propagation map can also be produced using the CARTO system; in some cases, this allows better visualization of the atrial activation sequence during AFL. IVC, inferior vena cava; ms, microseconds; TVA, tricuspid valve annulus.

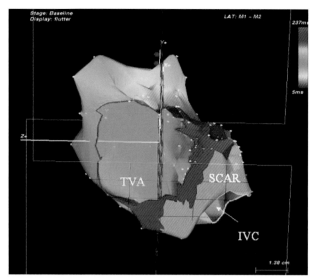

FIGURE 11–18. A three-dimensional electroanatomic (CARTO system, Biosense Webster) map of the right atrium is shown in a patient who underwent a previous failed ablation attempt for typical atrial flutter (AFL). An area of extensive scar *(gray)* is present in the cavotricuspid isthmus (CTI) due to previous ablation, but a surviving rim of tissue is observed along the tricuspid valve annulus (TVA), through which an activation wavefront propagates slowly, perpetuating AFL. This narrow rim of surviving tissue was easily ablated, curing the AFL. IVC, inferior vena cava; ms, microseconds.

tion, or to create a new ablation line adjacent to the previous one if ablation is initially unsuccessful.

ALTERNATIVE ENERGY SOURCES FOR ABLATION OF TYPE 1 ATRIAL FLUTTER

The development of new energy sources for ablation of cardiac arrhythmias is an ongoing effort, largely in response to the disadvantages of the use of RF energy for ablation, which include but are not limited to risk of coagulum formation, tissue charring, subendocardial steam pops, embolization, failure to achieve transmural ablation, and long procedure and fluoroscopy times required to ablate large areas of myocardium. Many of these disadvantages have been overcome in the case of ablation of type 1 AFL in the past decade of RF ablation catheter use. Nonetheless, several clinical and preclinical studies have been published on the use of catheter cryoablation and microwave ablation of AFL and other arrhythmias.[65-69] Two recent studies demonstrated that catheter cryoablation of type 1 AFL can be achieved with results similar to those observed with RF ablation.[65,66] The potential advantages of cryoablation include the lack of pain associated with ablation, the ability to produce a large transmural ablation lesion, and the lack of tissue charring or coagulum formation.[65-67] Further clinical research is

ongoing with respect to the safety and efficacy of catheter cryoablation for AFL and atrial fibrillation in the United States and Europe (CryoCor, San Diego, Calif.). In addition, preclinical and early work has begun on the use of a linear microwave ablation catheter system (Medwaves, San Diego, Calif.) with antenna lengths up to 4 cm.[67-69] These studies have shown the feasibility of linear microwave ablation, which has the advantage of very rapid ablation of the CTI with a single energy application over the entire length of the ablation electrode.[67-69] Clinical studies of this system are planned in Europe and Asia beginning in 2005.

Troubleshooting Difficult Cases of Atrial Flutter Ablation

With the high acute ablation success rates for AFL reported in most recent series, difficult cases may be encountered only occasionally, but with a large enough caseload this will eventually happen to most electrophysiologists, and those with a smaller clinical experience may encounter seemingly difficult cases more often. When this happens, several measures can be employed to increase the likelihood of successful ablation (Table 11–4). First and most important, it is critical to ensure that the mechanism of the spontaneous or induced arrhythmia is CTI dependent. If multielectrode catheter mapping with pacing entrainment is not sufficient to confirm this mechanism, 3-D computerized activation may be helpful to rule out other mechanisms of AFL.

Once the CTI dependence of the AFL has been reconfirmed, if initial ablation attempts are unsuccessful, it is essential to ensure that the ablation catheter has reached the extreme borders of the CTI isthmus, including the TV annulus and eustachian ridge or IVC. This again may require the use of large-curve catheters or the use of preformed guiding sheaths, such as the Daig SL1, SRO, or ramp sheaths, to ensure catheter contact across the entire CTI. Careful mapping of the CTI with the appropriate catheter may also help identify a gap in the ablation line, by demonstrating an area of narrowly spaced double potentials or continuous fragmented electrical activity, which when ablated may terminate AFL and produce bidirectional CTI conduction block (Fig. 11–19). Persistent CTI conduction after initial failed ablation may also sometimes be identified by 3-D computerized activation mapping, if use of standard multielectrode catheters has been unsuccessful.

TABLE 11–4

Troubleshooting Difficult Cases

Problem	Cause	Solution
Lack of termination of AFL during ablation	Non–isthmus-dependent AFL as initial rhythm or change during ablation	Repeat activation map and pacing entrainment to confirm AFL mechanism
	Incomplete CTI ablation line	Use large-curve catheter or preformed sheath to reach TV annulus (1:2 or 1:4 AV ratio)
		Use large-tip (8-10 mm) or cooled-tip ablation catheter
		Map gap in line with standard electrograms or 3-D computerized mapping system
		Deliver a more medial or lateral ablation line
Termination of AFL without bidirectional CTI conduction block	Incomplete CTI ablation line	Use large-curve catheter or shaped sheath to reach TV annulus (1:2 or 1:4 AV ratio)
		Increase ablation temperature (to 70° C)
		Use large-tip (8-10 mm) or cooled-tip ablation catheter
		Use 3-D computerized mapping system to guide ablation
		Map gap in ablation line by standard electrograms or 3-D mapping system
AFL reinducible 30 min after ablation	Recovery of CTI conduction	Repeat CTI ablation with higher power and temperature
		Use large-curve catheter or shaped sheath to reach TV annulus (1:2 or 1:4 AV ratio)
		Drag new ablation line lateral or medial to first line
		Repeat ablation with large-tip or cooled-tip ablation catheter
Changing pattern of atrial activation with or without ablation	Changing activation of left or right atrium (e.g., variable breakthrough of CT in lower loop reentry) or conversion to non–isthmus-dependent flutter	Confirm mechanism of sustained arrhythmias
		Use noncontact mapping for nonsustained arrhythmias
		Re-evaluate after creating bidirectional CTI block
Painful RF delivery	Electrical/thermal stimulation of cardiac nerves	Deep sedation
		Use cryoablation

3-D, three-dimensional; AFL, atrial flutter; AV, atrioventricular; CT, crista terminalis; CTI, cavotricuspid isthmus; RF, radiofrequency energy; TV, tricuspid valve.

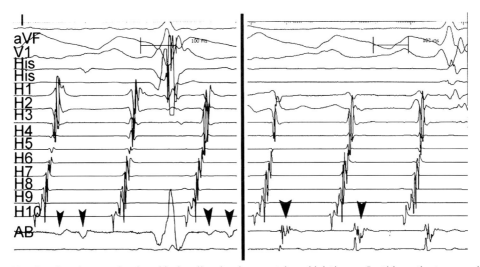

FIGURE 11–19. Mapping for the gap in the ablation line in the cavotricuspid isthmus. In this patient, a previous attempt to terminate typical atrial flutter had failed. *Left panel:* In this procedure, the ablation catheter (AB) recorded low-amplitude but split electrograms *(arrowheads)* along the prior ablation line. The interval between electrogram components was 70 msec during flutter. *Right panel:* With further interrogation of the ablation line, a site with a single-component but fractionated electrogram *(arrowheads)* was identified. Ablation at this site terminated the flutter in less than 2 seconds and created bidirectional block. Surface electrocardiogram leads I, aVF, and V1 are shown. His, His channels; H1 through H10, Halo catheter channels from distal to proximal.

We recommend that ablation be performed in the 6 o'clock position on the TV annulus initially; if this is unsuccessful, a new ablation line should be created more laterally, at the 7 or 8 o'clock position on the TV annulus. Large right atrial trabeculae may enter the lateral CTI tangentially and require ablation to achieve a bidirectional conduction block. If this also is ineffective, an ablation line may be created more medially, at the 5 o'clock position, but care must be taken in this position to monitor AV conduction, because the risk of AV block is increased. Typically, an ablation temperature of 60°C is initially targeted for CTI ablation, but occasionally successful ablation requires a temperature as high as 70°C. If standard ablation electrodes of 4 or 5 mm are used initially and ablation fails, the use of either a large-tip (8- to 10-mm) ablation catheter with a high-power generator or a cooled-tip catheter is recommended. We prefer large-tip or cooled-tip catheters as the first-line approach for CTI ablation, because they have been shown to have greater efficacy than standard catheters in most studies, or at least to produce CTI block with fewer energy applications and shorter procedure times. The use of temperatures in excess of 70°C with standard or large-tip ablation catheters, or in excess of 50°C with cooled-tip catheters, in an attempt to improve success rates, is not recommended due to the increased risk of steam pops, which can in rare instances cause cardiac rupture.

Summary

RF catheter ablation has become a first-line treatment for type 1 AFL, with almost uniform acute and chronic success and a low complication rate. The most effective approach, preferred by most laboratories, is combined anatomically and electrophysiologically guided ablation of the CTI, with procedural end points of arrhythmia noninducibility and bidirectional CTI conduction block. Currently, the use of a large-tip (8 to 10 mm) ablation catheter with a high-output RF generator (i.e., up to 100 W), or a cooled-tip ablation catheter with a standard RF generator, is recommended for optimal success rates. Computerized 3-D activation mapping is an adjunctive method that is not mandatory to cure AFL but may have significant advantages in some cases, resulting in overall improved success rates. New, alternative energy sources, including cryoablation and microwave ablation, are under investigation with the hope of further improving procedure times and success rates and potentially reducing the risk of complications during AFL ablation.

References

1. Saoudi N, Cosio F, Waldo A, et al.: Classification of atrial flutter and regular atrial tachycardia according to electrophysiologic mechanism and anatomic bases: A statement from a joint expert group from the Working Group of Arrhythmias of the European Society of Cardiology and the North American Society of Pacing and Electrophysiology. J Cardiovasc Electrophysiol 12:852-866, 2001.
2. Feld GK, Fleck RP, Chen PS, et al.: Radiofrequency catheter ablation for the treatment of human type 1 atrial flutter: Identification of a critical zone in the re-entrant circuit by endocardial mapping techniques. Circulation 86:1233-1240, 1992.
3. Cosio FG, Lopez-Gil M, Goicolea A, et al.: Radiofrequency ablation of the inferior vena cava-tricuspid valve isthmus in common atrial flutter. Am J Cardiol 71:705-709, 1993.
4. Lesh MD, Van Hare GF, Epstein LM, et al.: Radiofrequency catheter ablation of atrial arrhythmias: Results and mechanisms. Circulation 89:1074-1089, 1994.
5. Cosio FG, Goicolea A, Lopez-Gil M, et al.: Atrial endocardial mapping in the rare form of atrial flutter. Am J Cardiol 66:715-720, 1990.
6. Tai CT, Chen SA, Chiang CE, et al.: Electrophysiologic characteristics and radiofrequency catheter ablation in patients with clockwise atrial flutter. J Cardiovasc Electrophysiol 8:24-34, 1997.
7. Olshansky B, Okumura K, Gess PG, et al.: Demonstration of an area of slow conduction in human atrial flutter. J Am Coll Cardiol 16:1639-1648, 1990.
8. Feld GK, Mollerus M, Birgersdotter-Green U, et al.: Conduction velocity in the tricuspid valve-inferior vena cava isthmus is slower in patients with a history of atrial flutter compared to those without atrial flutter. J Cardiovasc Electrophysiol 8:1338-1348, 1997.
9. Kinder C, Kall J, Kopp D, et al.: Conduction properties of the inferior vena cava-tricuspid annular isthmus in patients with typical atrial flutter. J Cardiovasc Electrophysiol 8:727-737, 1997.
10. Da Costa A, Mourot S, Romeyer-Bouchard C, et al.: Anatomic and electrophysiological differences between chronic and paroxysmal forms of common atrial flutter and comparison with controls. Pacing Clin Electrophysiol 27:1202-1211, 2004.
11. Feld GK, Shahandeh-Rad F: Mechanism of double potentials recorded during sustained atrial flutter in the canine right atrial crush-injury model. Circulation 86:628-641, 1992.
12. Olgin JE, Kalman JM, Fizpatrick AP, et al.: Role of right atrial endocardial structures as barriers to conduction during human type 1 atrial flutter: Activation and entrainment mapping guided by intracardiac echocardiography. Circulation 92:1839-1848, 1995.
13. Olgin JE, Kalman JM, Lesh MD: Conduction barriers in human atrial flutter: Correlation of electrophysiology and anatomy. J Cardiovasc Electrophysiol 7:1112-1126, 1996.
14. Kalman JM, Olgin JE, Saxon LA, et al.: Activation and entrainment mapping defines the tricuspid annulus as the anterior barrier in typical atrial flutter. Circulation 94:398-406, 1996.
15. Tai CT, Huang JL, Lee PC, et al.: High-resolution mapping around the crista terminalis during typical atrial flutter: New insights into mechanisms. J Cardiovasc Electrophysiol 15:406-414, 2004.
16. Spach MS, Miller WT III, Dolber PC, et al.: The functional role of structural complexities in the propagation of depolarization in the atrium of the dog: Cardiac conduction disturbances due to discontinuities of effective axial resistivity. Circ Res 50:175-191, 1982.
17. Spach MS, Dolber PS, Heidlage JF: Influence of the passive anisotropic properties on directional differences in propaga-

tion following modification of sodium conductance in human atrial muscle: A model of reentry based on anisotropic discontinuous propagation. Circ Res 62:811-832, 1988.

18. Olgin JE, Kalman JM, Saxon LA, et al.: Mechanisms of initiation of atrial flutter in humans: Site of unidirectional block and direction of rotation. J Am Coll Cardiol 29:376-384, 1997.

19. Suzuki F, Toshida N, Nawata H, et al.: Coronary sinus pacing initiates counterclockwise atrial flutter while pacing from the low lateral right atrium initiates clockwise atrial flutter: Analysis of episodes of direct initiation of atrial flutter. J Electrocardiol 31:345-361, 1998.

20. Feld GK, Shahandeh-Rad F: Activation patterns in experimental canine atrial flutter produced by right atrial crush-injury. J Am Coll Cardiol 20:441-451, 1992.

21. Haissaguerre M, Sanders P, Hocini M, et al.: Pulmonary veins in the substrate for atrial fibrillation: The "venous wave" hypothesis. J Am Coll Cardiol 43:2290-2292, 2004.

22. Yang Y, Cheng J, Bochoeyer A, et al.: Atypical right atrial flutter patterns. Circulation 103:3092-3098, 2001.

23. Bochoeyer A, Yang Y, Cheng J, et al.: Surface electrocardiographic characteristics of right and left atrial flutter. Circulation 108;60-66, 2003.

24. Oshikawa N, Watanabe I, Masaki R, et al.: Relationship between polarity of the flutter wave in the surface ECG and endocardial atrial activation sequence in patients with typical counterclockwise and clockwise atrial flutter. J Interv Card Electrophysiol 7:215-223, 2002.

25. Okumura K, Plumb VJ, Page PL, et al.: Atrial activation sequence during atrial flutter in the canine pericarditis model and its effects on the polarity of the flutter wave in the electrocardiogram. J Am Coll Cardiol 17:509-518, 1991.

26. Narayan SM, Feld GK, Hassankhani A, et al.: Quantifying intracardiac organization of atrial arrhythmias using temporospatial phase of the electrocardiogram. J Cardiovasc Electrophysiol 14:971-981, 2003.

27. Fischer B, Haissaguerre M, Garrigues S, et al.: Radiofrequency catheter ablation of atrial flutter in 80 patients. J Am Coll Cardiol 25:1365-1372, 1995.

28. Kirkorian G, Moncada E, Chevalier P, et al.: Radiofrequency ablation of atrial flutter: Efficacy of an anatomically guided approach. Circulation 90:2804-2814, 1994.

29. Calkins H, Leon AR, Deam G, et al.: Catheter ablation of atrial flutter using radiofrequency energy. Am J Cardiol 73:353-356, 1994.

30. Chen SA, Chiang CE, Wu TJ, et al.: Radiofrequency catheter ablation of common atrial flutter: Comparison of electrophysiologically guided focal ablation technique and linear ablation technique. J Am Coll Cardiol 27:860-868, 1996.

31. Jais P, Haissaguerre M, Shah DC, et al.: Successful irrigated-tip catheter ablation of atrial flutter resistant to conventional radiofrequency ablation. Circulation 98:835-838, 1998.

32. Atiga WL, Worley SJ, Hummel J, et al.: Prospective randomized comparison of cooled radiofrequency versus standard radiofrequency energy for ablation of typical atrial flutter. Pacing Clin Electrophysiol 25:1172-1178, 2002.

33. Scavee C, Jais P, Hsu LF, et al.: Prospective randomized comparison of irrigated-tip and large-tip catheter ablation of cavotricuspid isthmus-dependent atrial flutter. Eur Heart J 25:963-969, 2004.

34. Calkins H: Catheter ablation of atrial flutter: Do outcomes of catheter ablation with "large-tip" versus "cooled-tip" catheters really differ? J Cardiovasc Electrophysiol 15:1131-1132, 2004.

35. Tsai CF, Tai CT, Yu WC, et al.: Is 8-mm more effective than 4-mm tip electrode catheter for ablation of typical atrial flutter? Circulation 100:768-771, 1999.

36. Feld GK: Radiofrequency ablation of atrial flutter using large-tip electrode catheters. J Cardiovasc Electrophysiol 15:S18-S23, 2004.

37. Feld G, Wharton M, Plumb V, et al., and EPT-1000 XP Cardiac Ablation System Investigators: Radiofrequency catheter ablation of type 1 atrial flutter using large-tip 8- or 10-mm electrode catheters and a high-output radiofrequency energy generator: Results of a multicenter safety and efficacy study. J Am Coll Cardiol 43:1466-1472, 2004.

38. Calkins H, Canby R, Weiss R, et al., and 100W Atakr II Investigator Group: Results of catheter ablation of typical atrial flutter. Am J Cardiol 94:437-442, 2004.

39. Ventura R, Klemm H, Lutomsky B, et al.: Pattern of isthmus conduction recovery using open cooled and solid large-tip catheters for radiofrequency ablation of typical atrial flutter. J Cardiovasc Electrophysiol 15:1126-1130, 2004.

40. Nakagawa H, Lazzara R, Khastgir T, et al.: Role of the tricuspid annulus and the eustachian valve/ridge on atrial flutter: Relevance to catheter ablation of the septal isthmus and a new technique for rapid identification of ablation success. Circulation 94:407-424, 1996.

41. Nakagawa H, Imai S, Schleinkofer M, et al.: Linear ablation from tricuspid annulus to eustachian valve and ridge is adequate for patients with atrial flutter: Extending ablation line to the inferior vena cava is not necessary. J Am Coll Cardiol 29:199A, 1997.

42. Poty H, Saoudi N, Aziz AA, et al.: Radiofrequency catheter ablation of type 1 atrial flutter: Prediction of late success by electrophysiologic criteria. Circulation 92:1389-1392, 1995.

43. Schwartzman D, Callans D, Gottlieb CD, et al.: Conduction block in the inferior caval-tricuspid valve isthmus: Association with outcome of radiofrequency ablation of type 1 atrial flutter. J Am Coll Cardiol 28:1519-1531, 1996.

44. Cuachemez B, Haissaguerre M, Fischer B, et al.: Electrophysiologic effects of catheter ablation of the inferior vena cava-tricuspid annulus isthmus in common atrial flutter. Circulation 93:284-294, 1996.

45. Mangat I, Tschopp DR Jr, Yang Y, et al.: Optimizing the detection of bidirectional block across the flutter isthmus for patients with typical isthmus-dependent atrial flutter. Am J Cardiol 91:559-564, 2003.

46. Arenal A, Almendral J, Alday JM, et al.: Rate-dependent conduction block of the crista terminalis in patients with typical atrial flutter: Influence on evaluation of cavotricuspid isthmus conduction block. Circulation 99:2771-2778, 1999.

47. Liu TY, Tai CT, Huang BH, et al.: Functional characterization of the crista terminalis in patients with atrial flutter: Implications for radiofrequency ablation. J Am Coll Cardiol 43:1639-1645, 2004.

48. Anselme F, Savoure A, Ouali S, et al.: Transcristal conduction during isthmus ablation of typical atrial flutter: Influence on success criteria. J Cardiovasc Electrophysiol 15:184-189, 2004.

49. Tai CT, Haque A, Lin YK, et al.: Double potential interval and transisthmus conduction time for prediction of cavotricuspid isthmus block after ablation of typical atrial flutter. J Interv Card Electrophysiol 7:77-82, 2002.

50. Tada H, Oral H, Sticherling C, et al.: Double potentials along the ablation line as a guide to radiofrequency ablation of typical atrial flutter. J Am Coll Cardiol 38:750-755, 2001.

51. Johna R, Eckardt L, Fetsch T, et al.: A new algorithm to determine complete isthmus conduction block after radiofrequency catheter ablation for typical atrial flutter. Am J Cardiol 83:1666-1668, 1999.

52. Hamdan MH, Kalman JM, Barron HV, et al.: P-wave morphology during right atrial pacing before and after atrial flutter ablation: A new marker for success. Am J Cardiol 79:1417-1420, 1997.

53. Tada H, Oral H, Sticherling C, et al.: Electrogram polarity and cavotricuspid isthmus block during ablation of typical atrial flutter. J Cardiovasc Electrophysiol 12:393-399, 2001.

54. Villacastin J, Almendral J, Arenal A, et al.: Usefulness of unipolar electrograms to detect isthmus block after radiofrequency ablation of typical atrial flutter. Circulation 102:3080-3085, 2000.

55. Gilligan DM, Zakaib JS, Fuller I, et al.: Long-term outcome of patients after successful radiofrequency ablation for typical atrial flutter. Pacing Clin Electrophysiol 26:53-58, 2003.

56. Tai CT, Chen SA, Chiang CE, et al.: Long-term outcome of radiofrequency catheter ablation for typical atrial flutter: risk prediction of recurrent arrhythmias. J Cardiovasc Electrophysiol 9:115-121, 1998.

57. Feld GK: New approaches for the management of atrial fibrillation: Role of ablation of atrial flutter. J Cardiovasc Electrophysiol 10:1188-1191, 1999.

58. Scharf C, Veerareddy S, Ozaydin M, et al.: Clinical significance of inducible atrial flutter during pulmonary vein isolation in patients with atrial fibrillation. J Am Coll Cardiol 43:2057-2062, 2004.

59. Welch PJ, Afridi I, Joglar JA, et al.: Effect of radiofrequency ablation on atrial mechanical function in patients with atrial flutter. Am J Cardiol 84:420-425, 1999.

60. Prater S, Wades M, Reynerston S, et al.: Incidence of atrial thrombus in patients with type 1 atrial flutter undergoing catheter ablation. Circulation 94:I-728, 1996.

61. Gronefeld GC, Wegener F, Israel CW, et al.: Thromboembolic risk of patients referred for radiofrequency catheter ablation of typical atrial flutter without prior appropriate anticoagulation therapy. Pacing Clin Electrophysiol 26:323-327, 2003.

62. Ventura R, Rostock T, Klemm HU, et al.: Catheter ablation of common-type atrial flutter guided by three-dimensional right atrial geometry reconstruction and catheter tracking using cutaneous patches: A randomized prospective study. J Cardiovasc Electrophysiol 15:1157-1161, 2004.

63. Sporton SC, Earley MJ, Nathan AW, et al.: Electroanatomic versus fluoroscopic mapping for catheter ablation procedures: A prospective randomized study. J Cardiovasc Electrophysiol 15:310-315, 2004.

64. Shah D, Haissaguerre M, Jais P, et al.: High-density mapping of activation through an incomplete isthmus ablation line. Circulation 99;211-215, 1999.

65. Manusama R, Timmermans C, Limon F, et al.: Catheter-based cryoablation permanently cures patients with common atrial flutter. Circulation 109:1636-1639, 2004.

66. Timmermans C, Ayers GM, Crijns HJ, et al.: Randomized study comparing radiofrequency ablation with cryoablation for the treatment of atrial flutter with emphasis on pain perception. Circulation 107:1250-1252, 2003.

67. Adragao P, Parreira L, Morgado F, et al.: Microwave ablation of atrial flutter. Pacing Clin Electrophysiol 22:1692-1695, 1999.

68. Liem LB, Mead RH: Microwave linear ablation of the isthmus between the inferior vena cava and tricuspid annulus. Pacing Clin Electrophysiol 11:2079-2086, 1998.

69. Iwasa A, Storey J, Yao B, et al.: Efficacy of a microwave antenna for ablation of the tricuspid valve-inferior vena cava isthmus in dogs as a treatment for type 1 atrial flutter. J Int Card Electrophysiol 10:191-198, 2004.

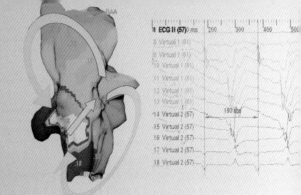

12

Ablation of Non–Isthmus-Dependent Atrial Flutters and Atrial Macroreentry

Steven M. Markowitz • Bruce B. Lerman

Key Points

- Atypical atrial flutter (AFL) requires fixed and/or functional barriers and regions of slow conduction.

- Activation mapping is performed to demonstrate early or mid-diastolic potentials, fractionated potentials, and double potentials. Concealed entrainment demonstrates participation in the tachycardia circuit. Electroanatomic mapping is used to visualize the reentrant circuit.

- Special equipment includes the multipolar electrode ("Halo") catheter for mapping of the right atrial free wall and tricuspid valve annulus. Electroanatomic mapping systems (contact or noncontact) are essential for many cases. Large-tip (8-mm) or irrigated ablation systems may be needed.

- Sources of difficulty include defining complex reentrant circuits, ablation in the mitral isthmus, and spontaneous conversion of AFL to atrial fibrillation (AF) or other arrhythmias.

Atypical atrial flutter (AFL) comprises a heterogeneous group of arrhythmias that arise from both the right and left atria. In many cases, these arrhythmias coexist with atrial fibrillation (AF) and may play transitional roles in the initiation or termination of AF or in transformation to typical AFL. Studies defining atypical AFL and its treatment invariably have involved small numbers of patients, and it is expected that understanding of these arrhythmias will continue to evolve.

Historically, there has been confusion over the use of the terms *atrial flutter* and *atrial tachycardia*.[1] It has been proposed that these terms be applied based on rate or on the presence of isoelectric intervals on the electrocardiogram (ECG). But this classification has little clinical relevance, because it does not correlate with mechanisms of arrhythmia. In this text, the term "atypical AFL" is used preferentially to refer to macroreentrant atrial tachycardias other than right atrial isthmus-dependent flutters.

Atypical AFLs may be classified based on their chamber of origin (Table 12–1). Subclassification of these arrhythmias is based on their pathophysiology (e.g., single or dual loop reentry), location of the circuit, and the clinical substrate. For reporting purposes, an atypical AFL should be described with regard to the type of circuit and anatomic location.

Anatomy

The specific configuration of an AFL circuit is highly dependent on the anatomy of the atrium, as well as its conduction and refractory properties. As a general rule, reentry requires the presence of two limbs that are anatomically and/or functionally dissociated. These limbs are dependent on the presence of a central barrier (atrioventricular annulus, venous ostium, or scar) or a functional line of block. In the right atrium (RA), natural barriers to conduction include the tricuspid valve, inferior vena cava (IVC), superior vena cava (SVC), crista terminalis, and fossa ovale. In the left atrium (LA), the mitral annulus, pulmonary venous ostia, and coronary sinus (CS) serve as critical conduction barriers, in addition to electrically silent areas that may be found in myopathic atria.

Pathophysiology

The risk factors for atypical AFL are those of AF. Although atypical AFL may uncommonly arise in a structurally normal heart, it predominantly occurs in patients with hypertension or organic heart disease or after cardiac surgery. The pathogenesis is thought to involve atrial hypertension, which causes interstitial fibrosis resulting in slowing of conduction and block. Left atrial macroreentry that arises de novo frequently involves regions of patchy scar, which presumably occur as the result of an atrial myopathy. Other important features include shortening of atrial refractoriness and a role for initiating or triggering foci.

In response to premature stimuli, arcs of functional block develop and—if of sufficient length—initiate and support reentry. Functional lines of block develop in other structures, such as the crista terminalis or the eustachian ridge, both of which play a critical role in the formation of typical isthmus-dependent AFL.[2] Gaps in these functional lines of block, as in the crista terminalis, permit atypical circuits to form. Functional lines of block develop in many other locations, including variable sites in the LA. A combination of fixed and functional block has been demonstrated in animal models of lesional tachycardia, in which a line of functional block develops as an extension to a fixed anatomic lesion.[3] In this case, the anatomic lesion might not be large enough to support reentry, but the combined fixed and functional barrier provides the critical length needed to maintain reentry. Formation and breakdown of these

TABLE 12–1
Types of Non–Isthmus-Dependent Atrial Flutter

Right Atrium

Upper loop reentry
Right atrial free wall reentry
Dual loop reentry (combined lower loop, upper loop, free wall, and/or tricuspid valve)
Double-wave reentry (observed with programmed stimulation)

Left Atrium

Circuits	Examples	Clinical scenarios
Single loop reentry	Perimitral annular reentry	De novo
Dual loop reentry	Peripulmonary vein reentry	s/p mitral valve surgery
Complex reentrant	Periseptal tachycardia	s/p AF catheter ablation
	Lesional tachycardia	s/p Maze surgery

Miscellaneous

Coronary sinus–mediated reentry

AF, atrial fibrillation; s/p, status post.

arcs of block are responsible for interconversion of AFL circuits with each other and for the transition to AF.

Diagnosis

MACROREENTRANT VERSUS FOCAL ATRIAL TACHYCARDIA

A fundamental consideration in evaluating an atrial tachyarrhythmia is to establish whether the arrhythmia is macroreentrant or focal in origin (Table 12–2). ECG criteria are not sufficiently sensitive or specific to establish the mechanism of an atrial tachycardia. For example, an isoelectric baseline does not reliably distinguish a focal from a macroreentrant atrial arrhythmia. For localization of atypical reentrant circuits, the AFL wave morphology similarly has limited utility. Although "typical" AFL waves (the so-called sawtooth AFL wave pattern, with deep negative deflections in the inferior leads and a positive deflection in V_1) are usually associated with counterclockwise typical right AFL, other atypical right AFLs or even left AFLs may demonstrate a similar AFL wave morphology. In the LA, in particular, there is a large overlap in AFL morphologies among different circuits.

Proof of a macroreentrant mechanism can be obtained through manifest entrainment, entrainment with concealed fusion ("concealed entrainment"), or electroanatomic mapping (see later discussion). The demonstration of manifest entrainment provides strong proof against a focal mechanism, but it does not provide information on the location of the reentrant circuit. Manifest entrainment is recognized as fixed but progressive fusion with progressively rapid overdrive pacing.[4] Because the surface P-wave morphology may not be visible or may be obscured by ventricular depolarization or repolarization, intracardiac electrograms provide the surrogate for orthodromic and antidromic capture and the degree of fusion. During entrainment, the last beat of overdrive pacing is entrained at the paced cycle length but is not fused.

Manifest entrainment may also give indirect information about the distance of a recording site from the elements of the reentrant circuit.[5] Return cycle lengths equal to the tachycardia cycle length indicate that the recording site is orthodromically captured (and may be within the circuit or outside it). A return cycle length longer than the tachycardia cycle length (TCL) indicates that the site is outside the circuit, with more distant sites having longer return cycle lengths. A short return cycle length is consistent with antidromic capture of a site within the circuit. These general rules may break down if there are separate entrance and exit sites to the reentrant circuit.

Adenosine may be useful in distinguishing macroreentrant from focal atrial tachycardias in that it exerts mechanistic-specific effects on atrial arrhythmias.[6,7] Adenosine does not affect most macroreentrant atrial arrhythmias, but it either terminates or transiently suppresses focal atrial tachycardias. In a review of 74 atrial tachycardias, we found that the sensitivity and specificity of adenosine for identifying a macroreentrant mechanism were 100% and 98%, respectively. This simple tool provides a reliable means to establish a tachycardia mechanism before mapping.

LOCALIZATION OF REENTRY TO THE RIGHT OR LEFT ATRIUM

Left atrial tachycardias typically manifest as positive deflections in lead V_1. The limb leads are highly variable and depend on the particular circuit and conduction characteristics. They may show inferior or superior axes or low-amplitude oscillating deflections. Some cases of left atrial tachycardia can give rise to typical AFL morphologies.

It is possible to establish a diagnosis of left atrial tachycardia during mapping in the RA and thus identify the need for transseptal catheterization and LA mapping.[8,9] Left atrial tachycardias often exhibit distal-to-proximal CS activation. However, a proximal-to-distal sequence does not necessarily

TABLE 12–2
Diagnostic Criteria
Macroreentrant tachycardias
Entrainment with fusion (with last beat entrained but not fused)
Electroanatomic mapping of >90% of tachycardia cycle length with adjacent early and late areas of activation
Insensitivity to adenosine (in dose sufficient to cause AV block)
Left atrial tachycardias
Passive conduction in the RA, with early septal activation and fusion of wave fronts in the right atrial lateral wall
Absence of right atrial activation during long segments of the cycle length (mapping of <50% of tachycardia cycle length in the RA)
Large variations in right atrial cycle length with a relatively fixed cycle length in the LA
Entrainment pacing at multiple sites in the RA yielding postpacing intervals >30 msec

AV, atrioventricular; LA, left atrium; RA, right atrium.

locate the arrhythmia to the RA; such a pattern may be seen with forms of perimitral annular reentry or periseptal reentry. Other unusual activation sequences in the CS can be explained by complex wavefront interactions at the mitral annulus (Fig. 12–1). It should be recognized that activation of the CS can be dissociated from the left atrial endocardium because of a muscular sleeve that envelops the CS and is attached to the LA through discrete connections. A case of macroreentry involving the CS musculature as a critical part of the circuit has been reported.[10]

Criteria for identifying a left atrial origin through intracardiac mapping include the following (see Table 12–2):

1. Passive conduction into the RA, which may be demonstrated as fused wavefronts in the lateral wall of the RA (Fig. 12–2).
2. Early septal activation in the RA, typically in the region of Bachmann's bundle or the CS ostium.
3. Absence of right atrial activation during long segments of the cycle length. In the case of a macroreentrant rhythm, if more than 50% of the

TCL cannot be mapped in the RA, it is highly likely that the origin arises in the LA.
4. Large variations in right atrial cycle length with a relatively fixed cycle length in the LA, implying left atrial/right atrial dissociation or conduction block.
5. Entrainment pacing at multiple sites in the RA, including the cavotricuspid isthmus (CTI) and the right atrial free wall, yielding postpacing intervals longer than 30 msec.

Although fusion of wavefronts in the lateral wall of the RA is common during left atrial tachycardias, it is possible to record a single wavefront mimicking counterclockwise or clockwise AFL. This situation depends on (1) the location of the multipolar catheter in the lateral wall, (2) the location of conduction breakthrough from the LA (i.e., preferential conduction over Bachmann's bundle or the CS), and (3) the presence of conduction block in the CTI. Typically, activation time for the RA is substantially less than the TCL. Exceptions occur if the TCL is short or if conduction is substantially slowed in the RA, thus falsely implying the presence of a right atrial tachycardia.

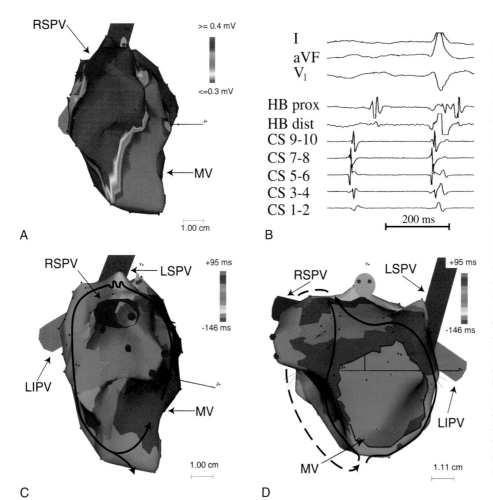

FIGURE 12–1. Left atrial reentrant tachycardia occurring after a left atriotomy for mitral valve surgery. **A,** Voltage map in the right lateral projection. An extensive region of low voltage (in red) is present in the posteroseptal wall adjacent to the right pulmonary veins. **B,** Coronary sinus recording reveals earliest activation at the posterior mitral annulus (CS pole 5 to 6). **C** and **D,** Isochronal maps in the right lateral and anteroposterior projections. Reentry occurs around the posteroseptal lesion and right pulmonary veins, with a zone of slow conduction and low amplitude electrograms in the roof of the left atrium. The wavefront bifurcates at the posterior aspect of the mitral annulus, which explains early CS activation in CS pole 5 to 6. *(From Markowitz SM, Brodman RF, Stein KM, et al.: Lesional tachycardias related to mitral valve surgery. J Am Coll Cardiol 39:1973-1983, 2002, with permission.)*

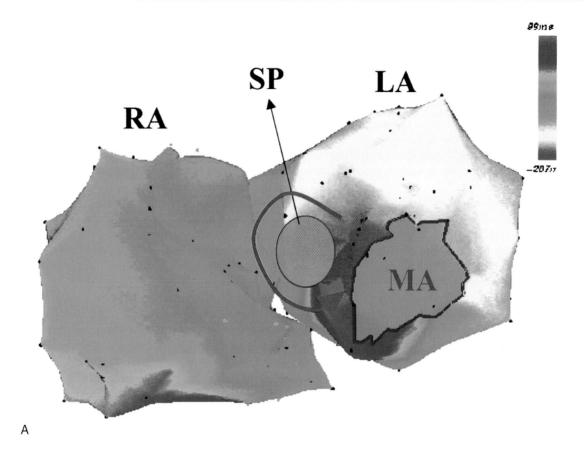

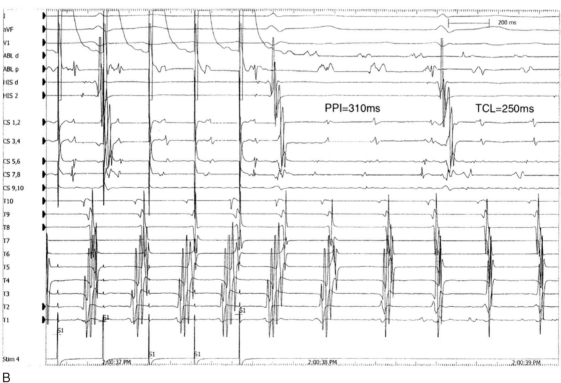

FIGURE 12–2. Left atrial septal flutter. **A,** Left anterior oblique view of the activation map of both atria. Note that the right atrium (RA) is activated from the septum to the lateral wall. **B,** Entrainment pacing around the mitral annulus excluded a periannular circuit. *(From Marrouche NF, Natale A, Wazni OM, et al.: Left septal atrial flutter: Electrophysiology, anatomy, and results of ablation. Circulation 109:2440-2447, 2004, with permission.)*

Mapping

ACTIVATION MAPPING

Conventional activation mapping with multielectrode catheters may be the chief means to define some mechanisms of atypical AFL.

Double potentials, which usually signify lines of block, may be identified through conventional activation mapping. If reentry proceeds around a line of block, double potentials are widely split in the middle of the line and progressively narrow toward the end of the line, where the wavefront pivots.[12] An example of this may be found in right atrial free wall macroreentry (Fig. 12–3A). Mid-diastolic and fragmented potentials are consistent with sites within critical zones of slow conduction, but verification of participation in the tachycardia circuit is required through other means.

ENTRAINMENT MAPPING

Concealed entrainment is an essential tool for identifying sites that participate in a reentrant arrhythmia.[13] Criteria for identifying sites within a circuit are (1) concealed entrainment (with P-wave and intracardiac activation sequences resembling those in tachycardia), (2) a postpacing interval within 20 msec of the tachycardia cycle recorded at the pacing site, and (3) a stimulus-to-P wave interval during pacing equal to the electrogram-to-P wave interval during tachycardia. Because the P wave may not be visible in the case of atypical AFL, identification of the initial inscription of the P wave may be arbitrary, and an intracardiac reference is often used as a surrogate.

Limitations or pitfalls in using concealed entrainment must be recognized. (1) Rate-related conduction slowing may be present, and therefore the postpacing interval might not equal the TCL. This can be minimized by pacing for 10 to 30 msec less than the TCL. (2) Failure to capture might occur in some critical regions of a reentrant circuit. (3) Acceleration or termination of atrial tachycardia with pacing occurs commonly. (4) Concealed entrainment can be confused with resetting of a focal tachycardia if the stimulus-to-P wave interval is short. If pacing is performed in a protected zone of slow conduction within a reentrant circuit, there is a long stimulus-to-P wave interval, depending on the proximity of the pacing site to the isthmus "exit site"; on the other hand, pacing near the exit site results in a short stimulus-to-P wave interval. However, pace-mapping at the origin of a focal arrhythmia also gives rise to a short stimulus-to-P wave interval, which makes differentiation from a reentrant tachycardia difficult.

ELECTROANATOMIC MAPPING

Electroanatomic mapping provides direct visualization of a reentrant circuit, which is defined as the shortest distance of continuous activation comprising the TCL. A hallmark of macroreentrant arrhythmias is the presence of areas of early activation adjacent to late regions, with intermediate values connecting these two regions. In practice, it is necessary to account for 90% or more of the TCL to visualize a reentrant circuit. Both contact and noncontact electroanatomic mapping systems have proved invaluable in defining atypical AFL circuits.

Contact electroanatomic mapping (CARTO, Biosense Webster, Baldwin Park, Calif.; RPM, Boston Scientific, San Jose, Calif.) involves the sequential recording of contact bipolar or unipolar electrograms and their display on a three-dimensional navigation system. When mapping a reentrant atrial tachycardia, the user defines a window that approximates the TCL, and activation times are assigned as "early" or "late" relative to a reference. Designation of activation times in a macroreentrant circuit as "early" or "late" is arbitrary. In theory, a change in the window or reference would not change the circuit but would result only in a "phase shift" of the map. Display of activation information as an isochronal map may clearly demonstrate the direction of wavefront propagation, which is perpendicular to the isochronal steps.

Entrainment mapping may be combined with electroanatomic mapping to define critical components of a reentrant circuit. This combined technique is especially useful if the electroanatomic map is ambiguous and it is difficult to distinguish critical components from bystander regions.

Misinterpretation of electroanatomic maps may occur unless care is taken to avoid the following pitfalls:

1. *Incomplete mapping and low resolution:* If a map is incomplete, bystander sites may be mistakenly identified as part of the reentrant circuit. Depending on the arrhythmia, 80 to 100 points or more may be required to obtain adequate resolution to define the circuit, as is often the case in left atrial macroreentry.
2. *Mapping a single chamber:* If mapping is limited to the RA, left atrial macroreentrant tachycardias may be mistaken for focal arrhythmias with an origin in the region of Bachmann's bundle, the intra-atrial septum, or the CS.

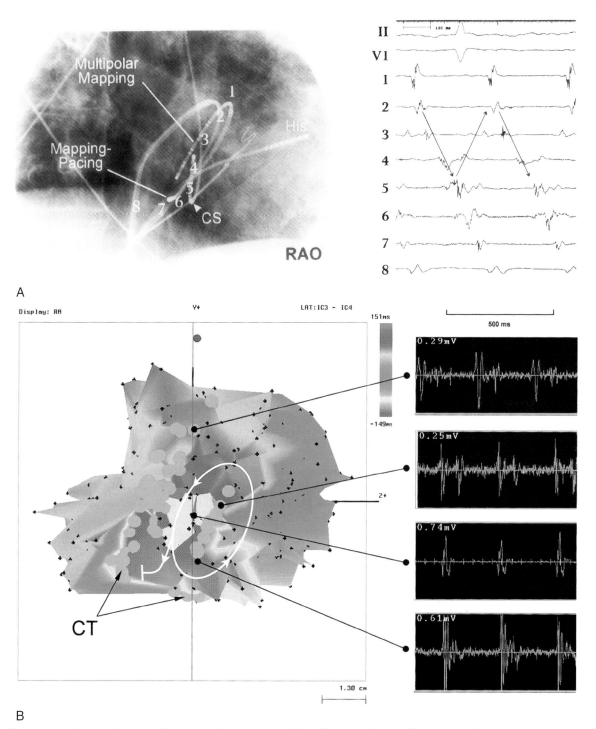

FIGURE 12–3. Right atrial free wall flutter. **A,** Right anterior oblique fluoroscopic view illustrates positions of multipolar mapping and mapping/pacing catheters in lateral right atrial free wall. Numeric designations signify free wall recording sites. Double potentials were recorded from sites 3 and 4 and fractionated electrograms from sites 5 and 8. Analysis indicated that sites 2 through 5 were within and site 8 was outside the atrial flutter circuit. **B,** Electroanatomic activation map depicting sites with double potentials *(olive tags)*. The inferoposterior line of double potentials corresponds to the location of the crista terminalis (CT). In this patient, counterclockwise activation around a vertical line of double potentials 1.5 cm anterior to the CT was observed. Fractionated electrograms were recorded at sites near turnaround points. *(From Kall JG, Rubenstein DS, Kopp DE, et al.: Atypical atrial flutter originating in the right atrial free wall. Circulation 101:270-279, 2000, with permission.)*

3. *Fractionated electrograms:* If highly fractionated and wide potentials are present, it might be difficult to assign an activation time. In this case, reentrant arrhythmias may be confused with focal arrhythmias.

4. *Central obstacles or conduction block:* Failure to identify areas of scar or central obstacles to conduction may confuse an electroanatomic map, because interpolation of activation times through areas of conduction block may give the appearance of wavefront propagation and obscure the reentrant circuit. If this occurs, it is impossible to identify a critical isthmus to target for ablation. A line of conduction block can be inferred if there are adjacent regions with wavefront propagation in opposite directions, separated either by a line of double potentials or by dense isochrones (typically >100 msec difference in activation over <2 cm distance).[14]

5. *Inappropriate activation window:* Focal arrhythmias may give rise to confusing electroanatomical maps if the window overlaps two sequential beats, falsely assigning electrograms from the first beat as "early" and electrograms from the second beat as "late". This may give the inaccurate appearance of adjacent regions of early and late activation.

6. *Conduction delay in either atrium:* Slow conduction or local block may prolong activation in either the RA or LA, and conduction time in the passively activated chamber may approach the TCL. For example, if conduction block is present in the CTI, a left atrial tachycardia can give rise to a counterclockwise activation pattern of the lateral RA. If there is substantial conduction delay in the RA, it may appear that early sites are adjacent to late sites. Even if conduction is present in the CTI, right atrial activation in the lateral wall may be craniocaudal if conduction occurs over Bachmann's bundle; if the isthmus and septum are not mapped in sufficient detail, this activation pattern may mimic typical counterclockwise AFL. In these situations, entrainment is an important adjunctive tool to define the RA as a bystander and clarify the electroanatomic map.

If an atrial voltage map is displayed, areas of scar can be identified to permit the localization of channels that form potential reentrant circuits. Areas with no detectable voltage (defined as the noise limit of recording systems, usually 0.05 mV) represent a dense scar and therefore a region of fixed conduction block.

Noncontact electroanatomic mapping (EnSite, Endocardial Solutions, St. Paul, Minn.) uses a multielectrode array that records intracavitary potentials and software to construct virtual unipolar electrograms on a three-dimensional representation of a chamber. This technique is useful in delineating transitory arrhythmias and has been used to visualize upper loop reentry. Care must be taken to analyze atrial beats without ventricular depolarization or repolarization, which can obscure the atrial unipolar electrograms. The presence of lines of block can be inferred based on activation sequence rather than direct imaging of scar.

Ablation

The guiding principle in ablating macroreentrant atrial tachycardias is to target a critical isthmus that participates in the tachycardia circuit (Table 12–3). For successful ablation, it is often not necessary to delineate the complete reentrant circuit, because interruption of the circuit at any one site terminates the tachycardia and prevents its initiation. The critical isthmus may be a narrow channel or a relatively broad region, and boundaries may include scar or anatomic structures. Fixed anatomic boundaries are most amenable to this strategy of ablation. In the case of dual-loop tachycardias, it is important to identify the common isthmus or corridor. Ablation can be performed by targeting the common isthmus or each loop separately. The technique of ablation involves the creation of a linear lesion between two boundaries to transect the isthmus. Less commonly, a single lesion suffices to interrupt a narrow isthmus.

Standard radiofrequency ablation with a 4-mm-tip catheter is often sufficient, but creation of large linear lesions may be necessary through the use of catheters with larger tips (6 or 8 mm) or irrigated radiofrequency ablation, especially with a relatively broad isthmus. It is common to see electrogram reduction at sites of effective ablation. Ideally, conduction block should be verified after ablation by pacing on one side of the ablation line and recording from the other side. Double potentials, as well as the absence of atrial electrograms, along the ablation line provide supporting evidence for conduction block after ablation.

Noninducibility may be applied as another end point. However, atypical AFLs are frequently associated with other inducible atrial arrhythmias, and judgment is required to decide whether to target other inducible arrhythmias. Strategies that involve ablation of all inducible atrial arrhythmias and channels for potential reentrant circuits have been successful in preventing recurrences, particularly in patients with prior surgery for congenital heart disease.[15]

In several clinical series, short-term follow-up reveals that most patients are free of symptomatic arrhythmias, including AF. For example, in two series of left AFL, 73% and 71% of patients were free of symptomatic recurrences with average follow-up of 16 and 14 months, respectively. This degree of success may require up to three staged procedures.

The long-term recurrence rates of atrial arrhythmias after ablation are unknown, and this issue is of particular importance because atypical AFLs are associated with other atrial arrhythmias and AF. Furthermore, some forms of atypical AFL described in this chapter were induced with rapid pacing during programmed stimulation and were not necessarily observed clinically. Their prognostic significance is uncertain, and it is unknown whether ablation changes the patient's natural history.

Specific Forms of Atypical Flutter

UPPER LOOP REENTRY

The upper loop reentry macroreentrant circuit involves reentry around the SVC and conduction along the crista terminalis but not the CTI.[11,16] This arrhythmia occurs in patients who also have isthmus-dependent AFL, but it also can occur in isolation. Upper loop reentry may be observed in the electrophysiology laboratory as a result of pacing maneuvers in patients undergoing ablation of typical isthmus-dependent AFL, or it may occur during spontaneous transitions of isthmus-dependent AFL. Upper loop reentry typically occurs in patients with underlying heart disease or hypertension, and it can coexist with AF.

Most examples of upper loop reentry circuits reported in the literature are clockwise in direction. The ECG demonstrates either positive or negative deflections in inferior leads, which correlate with the direction of wavefront propagation recorded in the CS. Electrograms show clockwise activation of the high lateral RA (with early breakthrough in the lateral RA). Collision of wavefronts may occur in the CTI or in the low lateral RA. Concealed entrainment may be demonstrated in the septum between the fossa ovale and the SVC.

Most experience with upper loop reentry has used noncontact electroanatomic mapping to define the circuit. Using this technology, the reentrant circuit has been identified as circuit movement around a central obstacle, consisting of the crista terminalis, an area of functional block, and the SVC (Fig. 12–4).

TABLE 12–3
Target Sites for Ablation
General principles
Critical isthmus identified by electroanatomic mapping bounded by two conduction barriers
Entrainment demonstrates orthodromic capture of most of atrium ("concealed entrainment" is present) and postpacing interval ≤30 msec longer than tachycardia cycle length
Anatomic considerations and ablation strategies for specific arrhythmias
Upper loop reentry   Gap in crista terminalis
Right atrial free wall reentry   Linear lesion from conduction barrier to inferior vena cava   Linear lesion from conduction barrier to crista terminalis
Left septal reentry   Linear lesion from septum primum to mitral annulus
Perimitral reentry   Linear lesion from left pulmonary vein to mitral annulus   Linear lesion from right pulmonary vein to mitral annulus

Although the published literature on upper loop reentry is limited and follow-up is relatively short (between 3 and 17 months), small clinical series reveal that ablation can be accomplished with a low recurrence rate of AF or other AFLs (23% in one clinical series).[17] When guided by noncontact electroanatomic mapping, an effective strategy is to create a linear lesion through a gap in the crista terminalis.

RIGHT ATRIAL FREE WALL FLUTTER

Macroreentry may occur in the free wall of the RA in patients without an atriotomy (see Figs. 12–3 and 12–5).[12,17,18] Approximately 50% of patients have no apparent structural heart disease. Right atrial free wall reentry occurs spontaneously or is induced with rapid atrial pacing. It may manifest as a stable rhythm, although it also interconverts with typical AFL. AFL waves are typically negative in the inferior leads, even if the direction of rotation is clockwise or counterclockwise around the line of block, but spontaneous transitions to positive AFL waves occur if there are changes in septal and left atrial activation.

The pathophysiology of this arrhythmia is reentry around a line of block in the lateral RA, which is thought to be distinct from the crista terminalis, thus creating a corridor between this central obstacle and

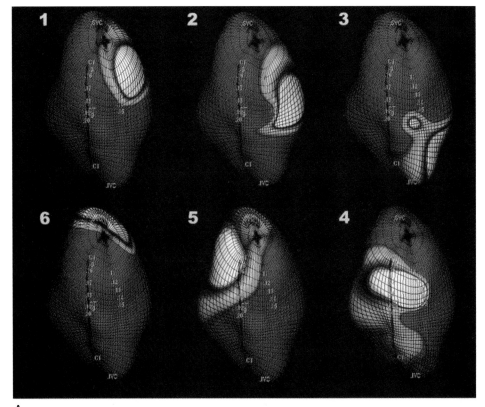

A

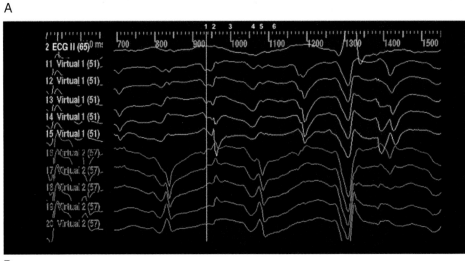

B

FIGURE 12–4. Upper loop reentry demonstrated by noncontact electroanatomic mapping. **A,** Isopotential maps show the activation sequence of counterclockwise upper loop reentry in the right posterior oblique view. The color scale for each isopotential map has been set so that white indicates the most negative potential and blue indicates the least negative potential. The activation wavefront propagates down the anterolateral right atrium (RA) near the superior vena cava (SVC) (frame 1) to the middle and inferior anterolateral RA (frame 2), then splits into two wavefronts (frame 3); one passes around the area of functional block, and the other passes through the cavotricuspid isthmus. The wavefront in the lateral RA continues through the gap (g) in the crista terminalis (CT) (frame 4) to the superior posterior RA (frame 5) and activates the atrial wall surrounding the SVC before reactivation of the anterolateral RA once again. **B,** The virtual electrograms from the area of functional block (virtual 11 to 15) and the CT (virtual 16 to 20) including the conduction gap (virtual 16 to 18) demonstrate double potentials. *(From Tai CT, Huang JL, Lin YK, et al.: Non-contact three-dimensional mapping and ablation of upper loop re-entry originating in the right atrium. J Am Coll Cardiol 40:746-753, 2002, with permission.)*

the crista terminalis. The line of block is functional and appears to be rate related.

Mapping with conventional multipolar catheters reveals a line of double potentials in the lateral wall with single fractionated potentials at the inferior end of the line, reflecting the lower pivot point (see Fig. 12–3A). Entrainment from both sides of the central line of block results in postpacing intervals within 30 msec of the TCL, but pacing from the CTI or the posterior RA results in longer return cycle lengths. The location of the upper pivot point is different in series that use different mapping modalities. One series identified the upper pivot point in the free wall of the RA (see Fig. 12–3),[12] and another series described involvement of the SVC (Fig. 12–5).[17]

Electroanatomic mapping demonstrates clockwise or counterclockwise rotation around the line of block anterior to the crista terminalis (see Figs. 12–3 and 12–5). Catheter ablation may be performed by creating linear lesions from the lateral RA (the area of double potentials) to the IVC. Alternatively, ablation may be performed in the corridor between the line of block in the lateral wall and the crista terminalis. With follow-up periods of approximately 17 to 18 months, no recurrences of free wall reentry were reported, but all patients also had ablation of the CTI.

DUAL LOOP RIGHT ATRIAL REENTRY

Dual loop reentry may occur in the RA if two atypical circuits described earlier coexist or combine with rotation around the tricuspid annulus. Noncontact mapping has permitted the identification of upper loop reentry combined with lower loop reentry or free wall reentry (Fig. 12–6).[17] Entrainment and contact electroanatomic mapping have been used to identify combined lower loop reentry (around the IVC) and simultaneous activation around the tricuspid annulus.[19] Ablation of one component usually transforms the tachycardia to another arrhythmia. For example, when upper loop reentry coexists with lower loop reentry, ablation in the CTI transforms the arrhythmia to upper loop reentry alone, and complete ablation requires additional treatment in the crista terminalis gap.

LEFT ATRIAL MACROREENTRY

A variety of reentrant circuits have been described in the LAs of patients with structural heart disease and those who have undergone surgery for acquired heart disease.[8,9,14] Anatomic obstacles to conduction include the mitral valve orifice, the pulmonary vein ostia, and electrically silent patches. In patients with prior left atrial surgery, low-voltage areas may be found in the vicinity of atrial incisions, or they may be remote from these sites, reflecting an underlying atrial myopathy in this population. Functional block, which can occur adjacent to areas of fixed block, may also play a role in facilitating reentry. Examples of left atrial reentrant circuits include circus movement around the mitral valve, around the pulmonary veins (see Fig. 12–1), around electrically silent areas, or involving a variety of these barriers. Dual-loop circuits are common.

Electroanatomic mapping is essential to define left atrial circuits. After a right atrial origin is excluded, the LA should be mapped in sufficient detail. Recognizing lines of block or central obstacles through the use of electroanatomic mapping is crucial in defining the circuit. Double-loop reentry (or multiple-loop reentry) should be recognized as a common variant of left atrial tachycardias, and a common segment should be identified.

Because the configurations of left atrial AFL are highly variable, there is no single anatomic approach to ablation that is universally successful. Typical sites of ablation include the following: (1) from the left pulmonary veins to the mitral annulus (the "mitral isthmus"), (2) from the right pulmonary veins to the mitral annulus, (3) from a pulmonary vein to an electrically silent area in the posterior wall, and (4) between two electrically silent areas in the posterior wall or roof of the LA.

Completion of the ablation line in the "mitral isthmus" may be difficult to achieve and may require ablation within the CS with an irrigated-tip catheter.[20] Verification of a line of block along the mitral isthmus can be demonstrated by pacing distal and proximal to the ablation line, using one catheter in the CS and one in the LA. In addition, the presence of double potentials along the line supports the existence of conduction block. To distinguish slow conduction from complete block, the technique of differential pacing may be used. This involves comparing conduction times during pacing from distal and proximal poles of a CS catheter. If complete conduction block is present, clockwise conduction time around the mitral annulus is longer with distal pacing than with proximal pacing. A risk of ablation in the mitral isthmus, as in other locations in the LA, is cardiac tamponade. This can be avoided by limiting power to 42 W or less.[20] Interestingly, this complication was observed with endocardial ablation but not with ablation within the CS.

LEFT SEPTAL FLUTTER

Reentry around the septum primum has been recognized as a mechanism of left atrial AFL in the absence

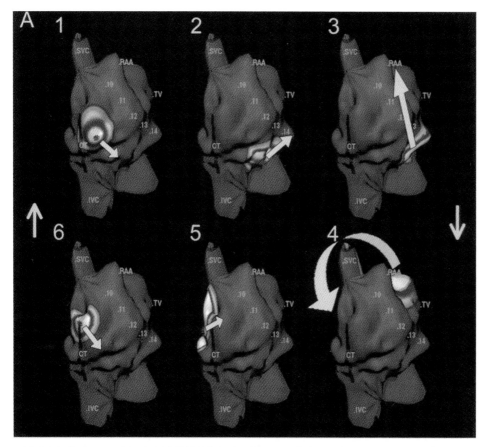

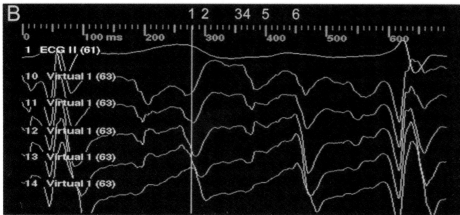

FIGURE 12–5. Right atrial free wall reentry as demonstrated by noncontact electroanatomic mapping. **A,** Isopotential maps show the activation sequence (frames 1 to 6) in the right lateral view. The activation wavefront proceeds through the channel between the crista terminalis (CT) and the central obstacle (frame 1), activates the low anterior wall (frame 2), and turns around the line of block (frame 3). Then the wavefront propagates upward to the roof in front of the right atrial appendage (frame 4), turns around the superior vena cava (SVC) to activate the posterior wall (frame 5), and spreads over the top of the CT to complete the reentrant circuit (frame 6). **B,** The virtual electrograms (virtual 10 to 14) on the line of block showed double potentials. *(From Tai CT, Liu TY, Lee PC, et al.: Non-contact mapping to guide radiofrequency ablation of atypical right atrial flutter. J Am Coll Cardiol 44:1080-1086, 2004, with permission.)*

of previous cardiac surgery, in most cases in patients with AF that has been treated with antiarrhythmic drugs.[21] The reentrant circuit is bounded by the right pulmonary veins posteriorly (which demonstrate a line of double potentials) and the mitral annulus anteriorly. The ECG shows positive or negative AFL waves in V_1 and low-amplitude AFL waves in the other leads.

The ablation strategy involves creation of a linear lesion between the septum primum and the right pulmonary veins, or between the septum primum and the mitral annulus. The anterior approach appears to

have a higher success rate. After a follow-up of 13 months, 76% of patients were in sinus rhythm.[21]

ATRIAL MACROREENTRY AFTER MITRAL VALVE SURGERY

Atypical AFL occurs in both the RA and the LA after mitral valve surgery.[8,9,14] The substrate for these arrhythmias involves atriotomy incisions, as well as intrinsically diseased myocardium, which give rise to anatomic and functional regions of block as well as slowed conduction. Reentry in the RA may be attrib-

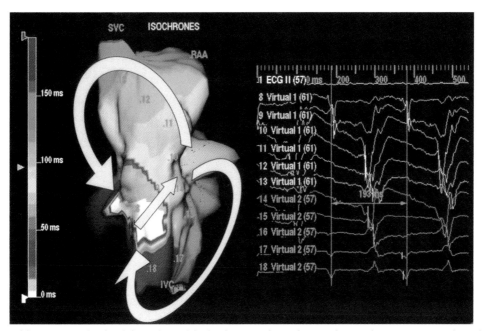

FIGURE 12–6. Dual loop reentry in the right atrium with simultaneous lower loop and upper loop reentry. Isochronal map from non-contact mapping (right posterior oblique view) shows that the activation wavefront propagated through the conduction gap in the crista terminalis and separated into two wavefronts. The counterclockwise wavefront (virtual 8 to 13) rotated around the superior vena cava (SVC) and upper crista, and the clockwise wavefront (virtual 14 to 18) rotated around the inferior vena cava (IVC) and lower crista. The virtual electrogram 9 at the crista gap showed low-amplitude potential between double potentials, representing slow conduction. *(From Tai CT, Liu TY, Lee PC, et al.: Non-contact mapping to guide radiofrequency ablation of atypical right atrial flutter. J Am Coll Cardiol 44:1080-1086, 2004, with permission.)*

uted to several factors, including surgical approaches to the mitral valve that involve right atrial incisions (such as the superior septal approach), cannula insertion in the RA, and underlying myocardial disease. Tachycardias in the RA include single- and dual-loop circuits that involve the right atrial free wall (Fig. 12–7). In the LA, areas of low voltage are often identified, anterior to the right pulmonary veins, that correspond to left atrial incisions (see Fig. 12–1). Reentry around the right pulmonary veins (involving this zone of low voltage) may be present as a single circuit or in a dual-loop configuration (one loop round the right pulmonary veins and a second around the left pulmonary veins, a posterior scar, or the mitral annulus). Other variations in this population include single-loop reentry around the mitral annulus and around a posterior scar.

ATRIAL MACROREENTRY AFTER CATHETER ABLATION FOR ATRIAL FIBRILLATION

With the growing application of linear left atrial ablation for treatment of AF, it has become apparent that left AFL may manifest as a late complication in up to 10% of patients.[22-24] These forms of atypical AFL present as persistent or paroxysmal arrhythmias approximately 1 to 6 months after AF ablation, often in patients who are still taking antiarrhythmic drugs after the procedure. Both focal and macroreentrant tachycardias occur late after ablation, and high-density electroanatomic mapping is required to delineate the mechanism of arrhythmia and guide ablation. The macroreentrant arrhythmias consist of single- or dual-loop tachycardias that use gaps in previous ablation lines or newly created protected isthmuses. Electrograms at these gap sites may demonstrate single fragmented signals, as opposed to double electrograms, which usually indicate barriers to conduction. Gaps may occur in any ablation line, including lesions encircling the pulmonary veins, along the posterior or superior wall, and in the mitral isthmus (Fig. 12–8). In one series, there was a tendency for proarrhythmic gaps to form in the septal aspect of the right pulmonary veins and anterior/superior to the left pulmonary veins.[23] Reentry around the mitral annulus may occur despite a linear ablation in the mitral isthmus because of difficulty achieving conduction block near the mitral annulus.[20] These iatrogenic atrial tachycardias can be treated effectively with catheter ablation, targeting the mitral isthmus or other critical components of the circuits, with initial success rates greater than 90%.

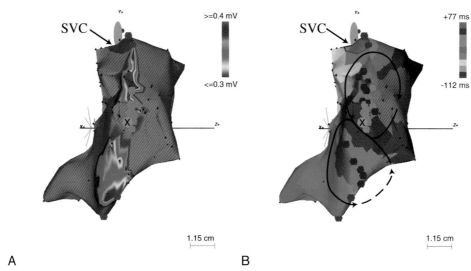

A   B

FIGURE 12–7. Dual loop right atrial tachycardia in a patient who had undergone mitral valve surgery, with a separate left atriotomy and reoperation with the superior trans-septal approach. **A,** Bipolar electroanatomic voltage map of the right artium (RA) in a right posterolateral projection. A zone of low voltage is present in the lateral wall of the RA, extending to the superior vena cava (SVC) and the inferior vena cava. Blue tags indicated double potentials. The green tag (×) is a site of concealed entrainment where ablation terminated atrial tachycardia. At this site, the stimulus-to-P wave interval during pacing was identical to the electrogram-to-P wave interval during tachycardia (125 msec). **B,** Isochronal activation map. Dual loop reentry is present, with a common isthmus between two lesions in the lateral wall. *(From Markowitz SM, Brodman RF, Stein KM, et al.: Lesional tachycardias related to mitral valve surgery. J Am Coll Cardiol 39:1973-1983, 2002, with permission.)*

MACROREENTRANT ATRIAL TACHYCARDIA AFTER MAZE SURGERY

It is generally recognized that atypical AFL may occur later after Maze surgery for AF, but there is little published information with regard to frequency and mechanism of these arrhythmias. Preliminary observations suggest that reentrant arrhythmias may occur due to gaps in the operative lesions, similar to the situation described for arrhythmias after catheter ablation.[25] If lesions are limited to the LA, typical right AFL occurs in up to 10% of patients late after surgery. Even if lesions are placed in the CTI, reentrant circuits can occur in the RA, possibly related to cannula locations or gaps in the right atrial ablation lines. An example of a dual-loop tachycardia in the RA after Maze surgery is given in Figure 12–9. In the LA, gaps in the posterior wall lesions have been described, resulting in reentrant circuits around the right pulmonary veins.[25] It is not clear whether these gap-related AFLs occur more commonly with any particular surgical modality (i.e., conventional incisions, radiofrequency, cryoablation, or microwave energy). Catheter ablation of gap-related AFL after Maze surgery is feasible, using the same mapping techniques as for other complex atrial reentrant circuits.

Troubleshooting the Difficult Case

Cases involving non–isthmus-dependent AFLs are typically complex, and the sources of difficulty are many. Perhaps the most critical difficult aspect of these cases is accurate mapping and understanding of the reentrant circuit. For most cases, electroanatomic mapping capabilities are invaluable. Even with this capability, problems may arise from interpretation of low-voltage electrograms, frequent termination of the tachycardia of interest, or spontaneous oscillation between different tachycardia circuits. Incomplete maps, resulting from an inadequate number of sampled sites, can also be confusing. Meticulous attention to the generation of maps is necessary to minimize confusion. Reassessment of the maps using different system control settings or different threshold levels for voltage mapping can clarify channels not previously evident. Once identified, the targets for ablation may be broad channels requiring creation of linear lesions. Ablation to complete lines to the mitral annulus can require extensive endocardial ablation or ablation within the CS itself. A list of common problems and potential solutions is given in Table 12–4.

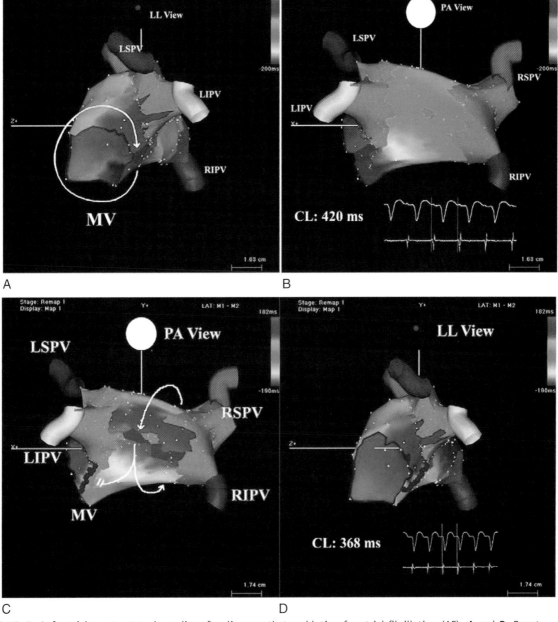

FIGURE 12–8. Left atrial reentrant tachycardias after linear catheter ablation for atrial fibrillation (AF). **A** and **B,** Reentry uses the mitral isthmus. The tachycardia cycle length was 420 msec. **C** and **D,** After ablation and block at the mitral isthmus *(dark red line),* a new single loop tachycardia, now with a cycle length of 368 msec, was induced. The critical isthmus was identified at the posterior wall, between two previously ablated areas. Ablation at this site eliminated the tachycardia. *(From Mesas CE, Pappone C, Lang CC, et al.: Left atrial tachycardia after circumferential pulmonary vein ablation for atrial fibrillation: Electroanatomic characterization and treatment. J Am Coll Cardiol 44:1071-1079, 2004, with permission.)*

TABLE 12–4

Troubleshooting the Difficult Case

Problem	Cause	Solution
Unstable rhythm interconverting with AF or other forms of atypical AFL	Instability of lines of block	Consider noncontact electroanatomic mapping Consider long linear lesions or ablation of AF or both
Uninterpretable electroanatomic map	Incomplete map Failure to identify lines of block and areas of scar	Map 80-100 points during tachycardia Review voltage map to identify areas of scar (<0.1 mV)
Failure to achieve conduction block in mitral isthmus	Persistent epicardial conduction	Use irrigated RF ablation catheter Ablate within coronary sinus

AF, atrial fibrillation; AFL, atrial flutter; RF, radiofrequency.

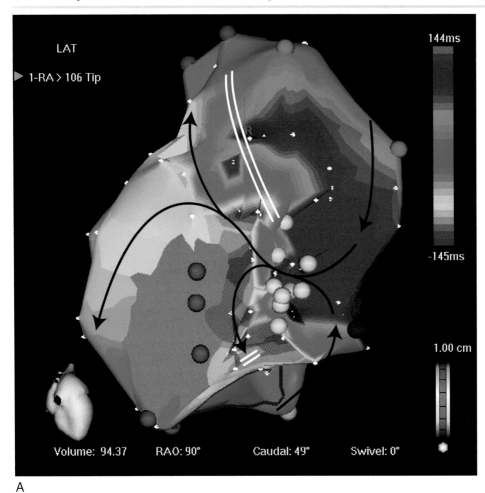

A

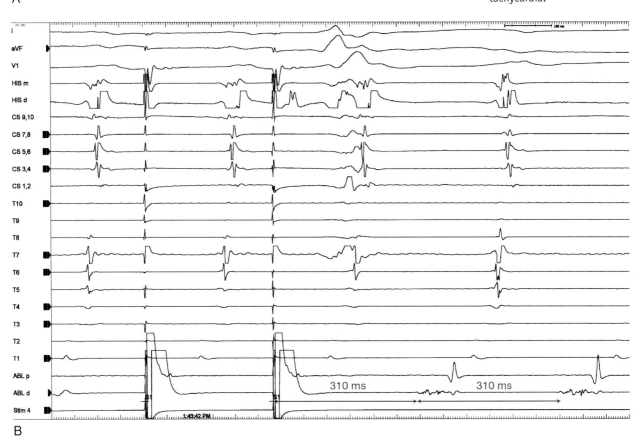

B

FIGURE 12–9. Reentrant atrial tachycardia after Maze surgery. This patient had surgical cryoablation in the cavotricuspid isthmus, an intercaval line, and a line between the right atrial appendage and the lateral right atrium, in addition to left atrial lesions. **A,** Right atrial electroanatomic activation map in right lateral, caudal view, which demonstrates a line of block in the lateral wall with double potentials *(pink tags)*. A gap in this line served as the critical isthmus for the reentrant tachycardia. **B,** The electrogram at this site *(green tag)* was of low amplitude and fractionated. Concealed entrainment from this site indicated participation in the tachycardia circuit (postpacing interval, 310 msec, identical to the tachycardia cycle length). The lower line of block was thought to correspond to the position of the inferior vena cava cannula. Note block in the cavotricuspid isthmus caused by prior surgical ablation, which prevented dual loop tachycardia.

References

1. Saoudi N, Cosio F, Waldo A, et al.: Classification of atrial flutter and regular atrial tachycardia according to electrophysiologic mechanism and anatomic bases: A statement from a joint expert group from the Working Group of Arrhythmias of the European Society of Cardiology and the North American Society of Pacing and Electrophysiology. J Cardiovasc Electrophysiol 12:852-866, 2001.

2. Olgin JE, Kalman JM, Lesh MD: Conduction barriers in human atrial flutter: Correlation of electrophysiology and anatomy. J Cardiovasc Electrophysiol 7:1112-1126, 1996.

3. Tomita Y, Matsuo K, Sahadevan J, et al.: Role of functional block extension in lesion-related atrial flutter. Circulation 103:1025-1030, 2001.

4. Waldo AL: Atrial flutter: Entrainment characteristics. J Cardiovasc Electrophysiol 8:337-352, 1997.

5. Cosio FG, Martin-Penato A, Pastor A, et al.: Atypical flutter: A review. Pacing Clin Electrophysiol 26:2157-2169, 2003.

6. Markowitz SM, Stein KM, Mittal S, et al.: Differential effects of adenosine on focal and macroreentrant atrial tachycardia. J Cardiovasc Electrophysiol 10:489-502, 1999.

7. Iwai S, Markowitz SM, Stein KM, et al.: Response to adenosine differentiates focal from macroreentrant atrial tachycardia: Validation using three-dimensional electroanatomic mapping. Circulation 106:2793-2799, 2002.

8. Jais P, Shah DC, Haissaguerre M, et al.: Mapping and ablation of left atrial flutters. Circulation 101:2928-2934, 2000.

9. Ouyang F, Ernst S, Vogtmann T, et al.: Characterization of reentrant circuits in left atrial macroreentrant tachycardia: Critical isthmus block can prevent atrial tachycardia recurrence. Circulation 105:1934-1942, 2002.

10. Olgin JE, Jayachandran JV, Engesstein E, et al.: Atrial macroreentry involving the myocardium of the coronary sinus: A unique mechanism for atypical flutter. J Cardiovasc Electrophysiol 9:1094-1099, 1998.

11. Yang Y, Cheng J, Bochoeyer A, et al.: Atypical right atrial flutter patterns. Circulation 103:3092-3098, 2001.

12. Kall JG, Rubenstein DS, Kopp DE, et al.: Atypical atrial flutter originating in the right atrial free wall. Circulation 101:270-279, 2000.

13. Stevenson WG, Sager PT, Friedman PL. Entrainment techniques for mapping atrial and ventricular tachycardias. J Cardiovasc Electrophysiol 6:201-216, 1995.

14. Markowitz SM, Brodman RF, Stein KM, et al.: Lesional tachycardias related to mitral valve surgery. J Am Coll Cardiol 39:1973-1983, 2002.

15. Nakagawa H, Shah N, Matsudaira K, et al.: Characterization of reentrant circuit in macroreentrant right atrial tachycardia after surgical repair of congenital heart disease: Isolated channels between scars allow "focal" ablation. Circulation 103:699-709, 2001.

16. Tai CT, Huang JL, Lin YK, et al.: Noncontact three-dimensional mapping and ablation of upper loop re-entry originating in the right atrium. J Am Coll Cardiol 40:746-753, 2002.

17. Tai CT, Liu TY, Lee PC, et al.: Non-contact mapping to guide radiofrequency ablation of atypical right atrial flutter. J Am Coll Cardiol 44:1080-1086, 2004.

18. Iesaka Y, Takahashi A, Goya M, et al.: Nonlinear ablation targeting an isthmus of critically slow conduction detected by high-density electroanatomical mapping for atypical atrial flutter. Pacing Clin Electrophysiol 23:1911-1915, 2000.

19. Zhang S, Younis G, Hariharan R, et al.: Lower loop reentry as a mechanism of clockwise right atrial flutter. Circulation 109:1630-1635, 2004.

20. Jais P, Hocini M, Hsu LF, et al.: Technique and results of linear ablation at the mitral isthmus. Circulation 110:2996-3002, 2004.

21. Marrouche NF, Natale A, Wazni OM, et al.: Left septal atrial flutter: Electrophysiology, anatomy, and results of ablation. Circulation 109:2440-2447, 2004.

22. Gerstenfeld EP, Callans DJ, Dixit S, et al.: Mechanisms of organized left atrial tachycardias occurring after pulmonary vein isolation. Circulation 110:1351-1357, 2004.

23. Mesas CE, Pappone C, Lang CC, et al.: Left atrial tachycardia after circumferential pulmonary vein ablation for atrial fibrillation: Electroanatomic characterization and treatment. J Am Coll Cardiol 44:1071-1079, 2004.

24. Pappone C, Manguso F, Vicedomini G, et al.: Prevention of iatrogenic atrial tachycardia after ablation of atrial fibrillation: A prospective randomized study comparing circumferential pulmonary vein ablation with a modified approach. Circulation 110:3036-3042, 2004.

25. Thomas SP, Nunn GR, Nicholson IA, et al.: Mechanism, localization and cure of atrial arrhythmias occurring after a new intraoperative endocardial radiofrequency ablation procedure for atrial fibrillation. J Am Coll Cardiol 35:442-450, 2000.

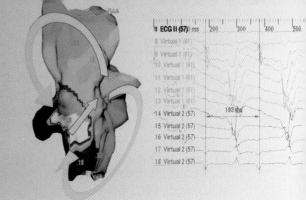

13

Ablation of Postoperative Atrial Tachycardia in Patients with Congenital Heart Disease

Edward P. Walsh

Key Points

■ Activation and entrainment mapping are used to identify macroreentrant circuits.

■ Ablation is targeted at critical points or channels in reentrant circuits.

■ Electroanatomic mapping systems are often helpful. Cooled ablation systems and long preformed sheaths may be needed. Intracardiac or transesophageal echocardiography may be helpful, and angiographic catheters may be needed to delineate anatomy.

■ Sources of difficulty include complex cardiac anatomy, complex or multiple reentrant circuits, and thick or scarred tissue that is resistant to ablation.

It is hard to imagine a more fertile environment for tachyarrhythmias than the postoperative atria of patients with congenital heart disease (CHD). The pathology begins with chambers that are dilated and thickened due to variable volume or pressure loads of long duration, which then suffer the additional insults of an atriotomy incision, caval cannulation scars, and septal patches with running suture lines. This substrate may be further compromised by sinus node dysfunction and suboptimal hemodynamics, all of which ultimately contribute to a high probability of tachycardia events. It should come as no surprise that recurrent atrial arrhythmias are a major source of morbidity and mortality among the rapidly growing population of adolescent and young adult survivors of CHD.[1-3] Some follow-up studies have placed the risk of long-term sudden death as high as 6% to 10% in association with these tachycardias, due to either acute hemodynamic collapse or thromboembolic complications.[4]

Atrial tachycardias can occur after almost any form of CHD surgery, including uncomplicated closure of a simple atrial septal defect. However, the incidence is clearly highest for patients who have undergone extensive atrial manipulation as part of the Mustard or Senning operations for transposition of the great arteries, or the Fontan operation for single ventricle. The most common tachycardia mechanism is macroreentry within the right atrial muscle. Unlike typical atrial flutter in an anatomically normal heart, which traverses a very predictable counterclockwise course through the cavotricuspid isthmus (CTI) at a cycle length of approximately 200 msec, the reentrant circuits in CHD patients tend toward much longer cycle lengths and can follow novel routes related to a wide variety of natural and surgical conduction barriers. It has become customary to distinguish this type of atrial circuit from typical flutter by the label *intra-atrial reentrant tachycardia (IART)*, or *incisional tachycardia*. Less commonly, CHD patients demonstrate *focal atrial tachycardia (FAT)* with gross electrophysiologic behavior consistent with microreentry or triggered activity. Atrial fibrillation can also occur in a subset of CHD patients, especially those with left-sided heart defects such as congenital aortic stenosis or mitral valve disease.[5]

The treatment options available for CHD patients with recurrent atrial tachycardias include catheter ablation,[6] pharmacologic therapy,[4,7] atrial antitachycardia pacemakers,[8,9] and arrhythmia surgery.[10,11] Although therapeutic decisions still are largely made on a case-by-case basis, catheter ablation has become a preferred intervention at many centers. It is the purpose of this chapter to review the current techniques and outcome data for radiofrequency (RF) ablation of IART and FAT in the CHD population. Ablation has not yet been extended to atrial fibrillation in any systematic way for these patients but is likely to be considered in the near future.

TABLE 13–1

*Diagnostic Features of Intra-atrial Reentry Observed on Electrophysiologic Study**

Fixed atrial cycle length (very wide range: 270-450 msec)
Adenosine resistance

Features of macroreentry
    Inducible with programmed stimulation
    Excitable gap
    Entrainment
    Reentrant circuit defined by electroanatomic mapping

*The surface electrocardiogram often is not diagnostic because classic "flutter waves" are uncommon and discrete P waves with isoelectric intervals possible.

Anatomic Considerations

With only rare exceptions, atrial tachycardias arise from right atrial tissue in the CHD group. This is easily visualized in patients with relatively straightforward anatomy, such as those who have undergone atrial or ventricular septal defect closures or tetralogy of Fallot repair (Fig. 13–1), in whom caval return to the right atrium (RA) is normal and an obvious CTI can be identified. Most IART circuits found in such patients do not differ fundamentally from typical atrial flutter, and they can usually be ablated by the standard maneuver of blocking conduction through the CTI.[12] Although IART may occasionally involve a circuit around an atriotomy scar along the lateral RA wall, it is more common for these scars to function as modulators of isthmus flutter by simply channeling conduction along the lateral edge of the tricuspid ring. Therefore, IART circuits in CHD patients with simple anatomy can be understood reasonably well by applying the same mapping and ablation principles used for typical flutter.

The situation becomes less intuitive when complex atrial anatomy is considered. Even though embryologic right atrial tissue is still the source of most tachycardias, the exact orientation of the RA can be grossly distorted by abnormalities of atrial situs,

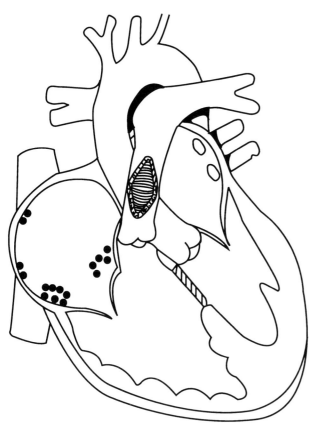

FIGURE 13–1. Diagrammatic view of "simple" congenital heart disease, in this case repaired tetralogy of Fallot. The black dots represent sites of successful ablation for intra-atrial reentrant tachycardia. The cavotricuspid isthmus is typically the most productive ablation site in this group of patients.

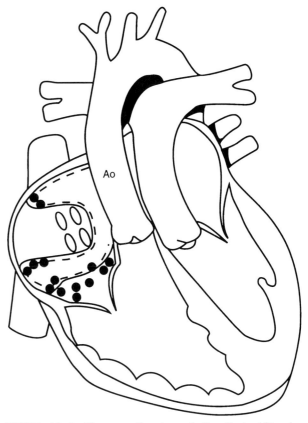

FIGURE 13–2. Diagrammatic view of the Mustard/Senning operation for transposition of the great arteries. The black dots represent sites of successful ablation for intra-atrial reentrant tachycardia. The cavotricuspid isthmus is typically the most productive ablation site in this group, although it is located within the left side of the heart and must be approached with a retrograde or transbaffle technique. Ao, aorta.

atresia of an atrioventricular (AV) valve and ventricle, and surgical septation or baffling, which segregates portions of the RA into the pulmonary venous atrium. A classic example is the patient who has undergone the Mustard or Senning operation, where vena caval flow is baffled toward the mitral valve by a large atrial patch (Fig. 13–2). As a result of this arrangement, the critical right atrial segment containing the CTI is now on the systemic side of the circulation. The isthmus remains the most likely region for an IART circuit to develop,[12-14] but in order to reach this site for mapping and ablation, the catheter must be delivered to the left side of the heart by a retrograde arterial approach or a transbaffle puncture.[15]

By far the most difficult atrial anatomy and least predictable IART circuitry occurs in patients with a single ventricle. Surgery for these cases typically involves one of the many modifications of the Fontan operation, in which the RA is connected directly to the pulmonary arteries (Fig. 13–3). Because there is usually no AV valve associated with the RA, there is no actual CTI. Instead, reentrant circuits tend to

propagate through regions of fibrotic right atrial muscle around lateral wall atriotomy scars, atrial septal patches, or the region of anastomosis with the pulmonary artery. Natural conduction barriers, such as the crista terminalis and the superior and inferior caval orifices, also influence these circuits.[12] Often, multiple IART circuits are present in the same patient, making mapping and ablation a challenging exercise in the Fontan population.

Atrial anatomy for CHD patients can be further complicated by abnormal wall thickness, chamber dilation, and diffuse fibrosis. The RA in some cases can become hypertrophied almost to the thickness of ventricular muscle, and it may exhibit layered myocytes sandwiched between thick sheets of scar (Fig. 13–4). This adds yet another dimension to the already disordered process of atrial conduction, and it almost certainly increases the potential for reentry. The dramatic wall thickness also confounds the effectiveness of RF ablation, because it can be difficult to achieve full transmural tissue destruction with conventional RF techniques.

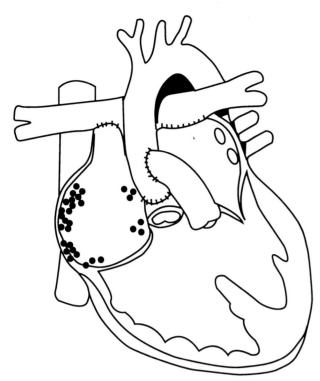

FIGURE 13–3. Diagrammatic view of a single-ventricle heart repaired with an older modification of the Fontan operation, in which the right atrium (RA) is connected directly to the pulmonary arteries. The RA in such cases tends to be very thickened and dilated. The black dots represent sites of successful ablation for intra-atrial reentrant tachycardia, which are widely scattered throughout the chamber.

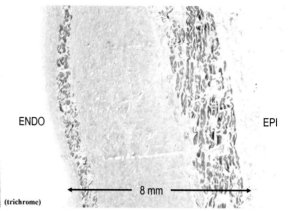

FIGURE 13–4. Microscopic section of the lateral right atrial wall from a patient who had undergone the Fontan operation. A trichrome stain accentuates the diffuse scarring in the atrium. Wall thickness approaches 8 mm. ENDO, endocardial surface; EPI, epicardial surface.

Pathophysiology

As mentioned, macroreentry is by far the most common mechanism for atrial tachycardia in the CHD population. These circuits have an excitable gap and tend to rotate around a central obstacle that has either a fixed or a rate-related conduction block.[16] The conduction velocity through atrial muscle can vary from point to point within the circuit, typically including at least one region of slow conduction. However, slow conduction zones are not absolutely required for IART to develop. Animal models of incisional reentry have demonstrated that circuits can be sustained with a uniform velocity[17] if the total conduction time is prolonged by diffusely abnormal tissue or a physically long path for the circuit.

In general, the atrial rate in IART tends to be much slower than that in typical atrial flutter, with cycle lengths on the order of 270 to 450 msec. Furthermore, the morphology of the P wave on the surface electrocardiogram rarely takes on the classic sawtooth appearance of atrial flutter. Instead, more discrete P waves tend to be seen, with long isoelectric periods

between them (Fig. 13–5). The initial deflection of the P wave usually corresponds to the moment of breakout for atrial activation from a zone of slow conduction, whereas atrial activation during the isoelectric period usually corresponds to conduction within the slow zone itself. These timing features can be of strategic importance during IART mapping, because they help localize regions that might be the most productive sites for ablation.

Figure-of-eight reentry circuits using a common narrow corridor with inner and outer loops have been well demonstrated in patients with IART, especially among the Fontan population of patients with massively dilated right atrial chambers and unconventional circuits. Likewise, it is common for a given IART circuit to be capable of supporting both clockwise and counterclockwise patterns of conduction. During ablation, abrupt slowing of IART without interruption can indicate a shift to a slower outer loop of conduction; similarly, an abrupt change in atrial activation pattern and P-wave morphology could represent reversal in direction of propagation through the same tissue rather than a completely novel IART circuit.

The presence of an excitable gap allows IART circuits to be entrained with pacing maneuvers.[18-20] This assists with accurate circuit localization using the principles of postpacing interval analysis and concealed entrainment (Fig. 13–6). Although these techniques have become somewhat less critical in the era of three-dimensional (3-D) mapping, they nevertheless represented the mainstay of IART mapping for many years and are still used on a regular basis to help decipher complex circuits.

The focal variety of atrial tachycardia is far less common than IART in the CHD population,

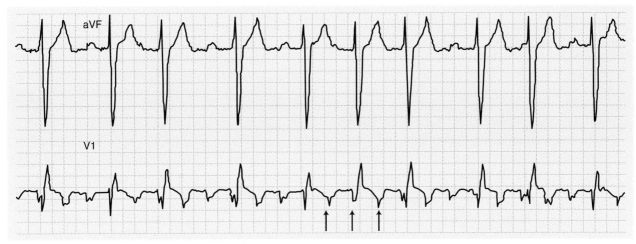

FIGURE 13-5. Rhythm strip (simultaneous electrocardiographic leads aVF and V₁) showing intra-atrial reentrant tachycardia at cycle length of 355 msec. The P waves in this case are discrete, with a high-frequency onset and clear isoelectric times.

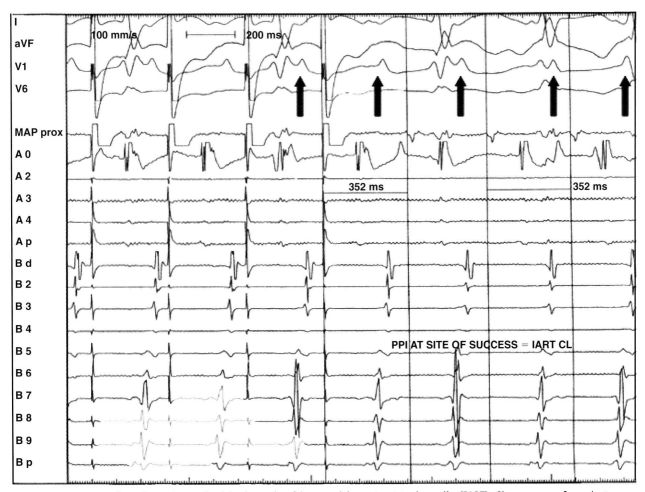

FIGURE 13-6. Recordings from electrophysiologic study of intra-atrial reentrant tachycardia (IART). Shown are surface electrocardiographic leads (I, aVF, V₁, and V₆) along with intracardiac signals from a mapping catheter (MAP) and two multipolar reference catheters (A and B). The tachycardia has a cycle length of 352 msec. Entrainment pacing at cycle length 320 msec is performed from the mapping catheter at a site that is a critical component of the reentrant circuit. The postpacing interval (PPI) is identical to the tachycardia cycle length (CL), and both the electrogram and P-wave morphologies *(arrows)* are perfectly reproduced by atrial pacing. These two findings prove that the pacing site is involved in the circuit, most likely as part of the zone for slow conduction.

representing fewer than 10% of cases in our institutional experience. This paucity of clinical material makes it difficult to characterize the mechanism of FAT exactly, and no doubt different mechanisms could be operative in individual patients.[21] However, there are some fairly consistent clinical features that might best be explained by microreentry or triggered activity. First, these tachycardias can usually be initiated by programmed atrial stimulation and can be terminated with overdrive pacing and direct-current cardioversion. Secondly, mapping strongly suggests a point source for tachycardia origin, with atrial activation on 3-D maps emanating in all directions from the site. Finally, effective ablation can usually be accomplished by targeting the epicenter of atrial activation with a single RF application. Nothing conclusive can be said beyond these observations, except that FAT frequently maps to atrial tissue that is immediately adjacent to suture lines and sometimes can be terminated with adenosine administration. Although FAT is uncommon in CHD patients, failure to consider its possibility could result in a long and frustrating search for missing segments of a traditional macroreentry circuit when none really exists.

Why some CHD patients develop atrial tachycardias, and others with the same lesion do not, is a difficult question. Certainly the position of surgical scars is important,[17] but there is more to this issue than unfortunate placement of an atriotomy incision or septal patch, because otherwise the problem would be ubiquitous and immediate. In fact, these arrhythmias occur only in a subset of CHD patients, and they usually do not surface until a decade or longer after the operation. Clinical series seeking risk factors for IART have identified sinus node dysfunction and older age at time of surgery as two important predictive variables.[22] Sinus bradycardia can result from direct surgical injury to the node or its arterial supply at the time of surgery and may contribute indirectly to the incidence of IART by promoting wider dispersion in atrial muscle refractoriness. The importance of this tachycardia-bradycardia link is underscored by the observation that simple correction of the atrial rate (back to a physiologic range) with a standard pacemaker reduces or even eliminates IART events in many patients.[8] The association of IART with late age at repair may relate to the more advanced degrees of atrial hypertrophy or fibrosis that result from delayed correction of cyanosis and other hemodynamic burdens. Observations such as these have contributed in large measure to revisions in the technical approach and timing for CHD surgery. Nowadays, corrective operations are performed at much younger ages, using techniques that minimize the insult to atrial muscle and the sinus node, including substitution of the arterial switch procedure for the Mustard and Senning operations and new modifications in the Fontan operation that bypass the RA by channeling caval blood flow directly to the pulmonary arteries.[23,24] The incidence of atrial arrhythmias for the current generation of CHD patients has been reduced dramatically by these innovations, but the large population who were repaired with older techniques will continue to require rhythm interventions.

Diagnosis

Making a clinical diagnosis of IART or FAT in CHD patients is not difficult (Table 13–1). The electrocardiographic picture of atrial tachycardia at an unvarying rate is confusing only if there is a 1:1 or 2:1 ratio of atrial and ventricular electrogram amplitudes (A/V ratio) that results in the P waves being obscured by the QRS complex (Fig. 13–7). This is easily clarified whenever necessary by modifying AV conduction with vagal maneuvers or adenosine administration and proving that rapid atrial activity is truly independent of the ventricle. As already implied, P-wave morphology should not be expected to resemble classic flutter waves (Fig. 13–8) and may take on a broad range of appearances. The index of suspicion is usually high enough among physicians caring for CHD patients that these tachycardias are rarely misinterpreted.

The relatively long cycle lengths for atrial tachycardias in the CHD population frequently result in rapid patterns for AV conduction in the absence of

TABLE 13–2
Target Sites for Ablation of Intra-atrial Reentry
Sites generally with low-amplitude, fractionated electrograms
If P wave is discrete, local timing precedes P by about 50-80 msec
Sites with entrainment features 　Electrogram-to-P-wave time = stimulus-to-P-wave time 　Postpacing interval − atrial cycle length ≤30 msec 　Perfect concealed entrainment
Physically narrow corridor based on identification of conduction barriers
Common anatomic targets 　Cavotricuspid isthmus (if present) 　Lateral right atrial wall atriotomy area (Fontan patients)

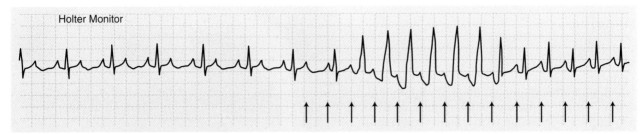

FIGURE 13–7. Holter monitor recording from a patient with intra-atrial reentrant tachycardia at an atrial cycle length of 290 msec. Initially the ventricle responds in a 2:1 fashion, but then shifts to 1:1 conduction with an initial period of rate-related aberration.

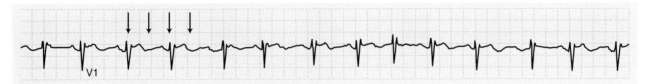

FIGURE 13–8. Rhythm strip (electrocardiographic lead V₁) showing intra-atrial reentrant tachycardia at a cycle length of 360 msec. The P waves do not resemble classic flutter waves. During periods of predominantly 2:1 conduction in this case, the rhythm can be hard to differentiate from mild sinus tachycardia unless the clinical index of suspicion is high.

medications. This, in conjunction with the fact that many of these patients have suboptimal hemodynamics, accounts for the severe symptomatology these arrhythmias tend to produce. Hypotension and syncope are common, and there are well-documented cases of rapid 1:1 conduction degenerating into ventricular fibrillation.[8] Such concerns cannot be underestimated in the electrophysiology laboratory during a long mapping procedure. Diltiazem should always be readily available to titrate the ventricular response back to a tolerable range should rapid conduction occur in the course of a procedure.

The diagnosis of IART is usually straightforward in the electrophysiology laboratory. These tachycardias can be reliably initiated with pacing maneuvers during electrophysiology study. In our institutional experience, burst pacing seems more productive for inducing IART than conventional extrastimulus testing. Our standard protocol now usually begins with S₂ atrial and ventricular stimulation to assess functional characteristics and rule out alternative tachycardia mechanisms, but then shifts directly to 8-beat atrial bursts at a cycle length that is shortened in 10-msec decrements down to a 2:1 pattern of atrial capture. If this fails to induce the tachycardia of interest, an alternative atrial pacing site is chosen. This entire process is then repeated with an isoproterenol infusion if necessary. Nonspecific atrial fibrillation is rarely induced in CHD patients despite such aggressive atrial stimulation, but in the rare case when it does occur, cardioversion is performed and stimulation is reattempted after a loading dose of intravenous procainamide. The diagnosis rests on the

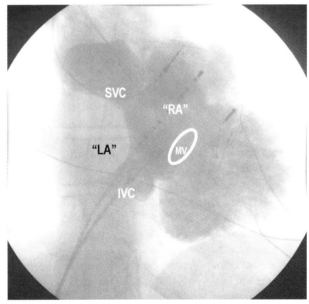

FIGURE 13–9. Angiogram in the modified right atrium ("RA") of a patient who has undergone a Mustard operation, in which blood flow from the inferior vena cava (IVC) and superior vena cava (SVC) is redirected to the mitral valve (MV). "LA," modified left atrium.

demonstration of macroreentrant atrial arrhythmias by dissociation from the ventricles and AV node and the ability to demonstrate features of entrainment that are consistent with the reentrant nature of the arrhythmia (see Table 13–1). The differential diagnosis is also straightforward, in most cases requiring exclusion of AV nodal reentry and reciprocating tachycardias.

Mapping

ANATOMIC DETAIL

The underlying anatomy must be extremely well defined before mapping IART or FAT in the CHD population, beginning with careful analysis of all recent echocardiograms, angiograms, or magnetic resonance images. In addition, prior catheterization reports should be reviewed to anticipate potential difficulties with vascular access or redirected vasculature that could thwart catheter positioning at a potential ablation target site. This is particularly true for patients with complicated intra-atrial baffles of the type used for the Mustard, Senning, and Fontan operations. Operative notes should also be reviewed to ascertain the potential location of all patches and suture lines that might serve as a substrate for the tachycardia.

The specific cardiac lesion and surgical details must be understood, not just for anatomic orientation but also as a guide to the position of the specialized conduction tissues. The AV node and His bundle can be displaced far outside Koch's triangle in some cardiac malformations,[25,26] especially among patients with AV discordance (e.g., "corrected" transposition) and in those with AV canal defects. In order to minimize the chance of inadvertent damage to the AV node or His bundle during ablation of atrial tachycardias, it is essential to have a good working knowledge of conduction system embryology and anatomy in CHD and to spend time carefully locating a high-quality His potential.[27]

Biplane fluoroscopy and angiography are indispensable for mapping and ablation in CHD patients with complex anatomy. As an initial maneuver during these procedures, an angiogram should be performed in the RA to outline gross anatomic landmarks that can serve as a roadmap throughout the mapping process (Figs. 13–9 and 13–10). Such imaging is mandatory whenever conventional electrogram analysis is used as the principal mapping tool,[28] but it is valuable even during sophisticated 3-D mapping, because it helps ensure that the tip of the mapping catheter has truly sampled the entire endocardial surface of a chamber of interest. Additional imaging with transesophageal echocardiography can be used if specific anatomic questions arise or to help guide difficult Brockenbrough procedures or other forms of transbaffle puncture if necessary. We have not had occasion to use intracardiac ultrasound imaging in our own laboratory during ablation in CHD patients, but we acknowledge its potential utility in experienced hands.

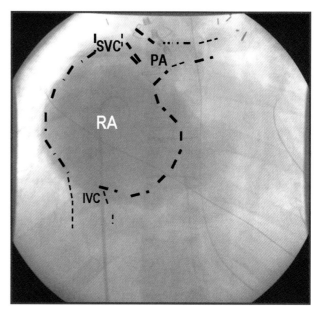

FIGURE 13–10. Angiogram in a patient with tricuspid atresia who underwent a Fontan operation with an old-style connection of the right atrium (RA) directly into the pulmonary artery (PA). The right atrium is severely dilated. IVC, inferior vena cava; SVC, superior vena cava.

CONVENTIONAL ELECTROGRAM MAPPING

The elegant 3-D displays that are available with electroanatomic and noncontact mapping technology sometimes seem to overshadow the value of conventional recordings. However, failure to appreciate the importance of standard electrogram analysis and entrainment pacing techniques is likely to result in a high failure rate for ablation in CHD patients. These techniques are all synergistic in localizing circuits and pinpointing potential ablation targets.

Once the anatomy has been clearly delineated and sustained atrial tachycardia has been induced, the electrogram pattern in the RA (or at least those portions of the RA that can be reached) is sampled to generate an activation sequence map.[29,30] Whether this is accomplished with linear catheters, basket catheters, inflatable balloons, or point-by-point mapping is irrelevant. The more critical issue is compulsive sampling of all possible areas of right atrial endocardium and correct synthesis of this information in the context of the known anatomy.

The electrogram from each sample site is indexed in time against the onset of the surface P wave or, if this is indistinct or uncertain, against some stable atrial reference signal (Fig. 13–11). Electrograms must be collected until sites have been identified to account for the entire duration of the tachycardia cycle length. That is to say, it must be possible to trace out the full

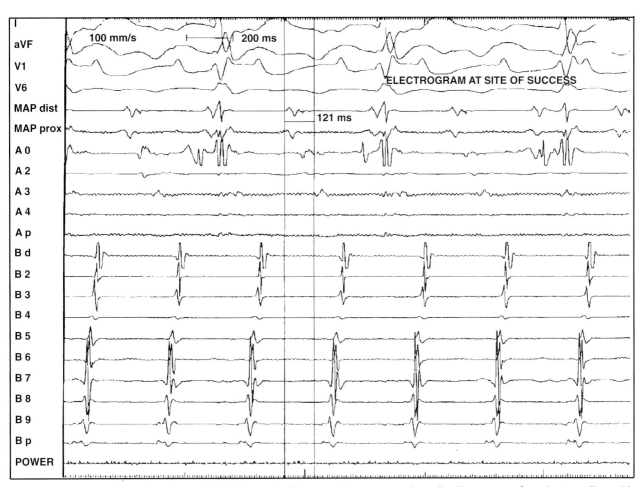

FIGURE 13–11. Recordings from electrophysiologic study of intra-atrial reentrant tachycardia. Shown are surface electrocardiographic leads (I, aVF, V_1, and V_6) along with intracardiac signals from a mapping catheter (MAP) and two multipolar reference catheters (A and B). The atrial cycle length is 365 msec. The mapping catheter is located at a site of successful ablation, where the local electrogram has a fractionated signal that occurs during the isoelectric period between P waves, covering an interval of 60 to 120 msec before P-wave onset. dist, distal; prox, proximal.

path of activation, from the beginning of one P wave to the next, without big gaps in timing.[31] If all electrogram times within the RA cluster toward one end of the tachycardia cycle length, there are only three possible explanations. Most likely, the remaining portion of the circuit is located on the opposite side of the atrial septum or on a surgical baffle, and the other atrial chamber must be entered by trans-septal puncture or via a retrograde approach to find the missing conduction times. This is a common issue in Mustard or Senning patients, as well as many patients with "lateral tunnel" modifications of the Fontan operation. A second possibility is that a small region of the RA with very slow conduction was inadequately sampled. This option should be considered strongly if the missing portion of the cycle length is confined to the isoelectric or diastolic period between P waves and all other activation times have been clearly accounted for within the RA. A third

possibility is that the mechanism of atrial tachycardia is actually FAT, in which activation propagates from a single point rather than involving a large reentry circuit. It usually does not take long to rule in or dismiss this option by brief supplemental mapping in the vicinity of the earliest atrial activation site.

Beyond timing, each electrogram must also be examined for special traits that might indicate an important conduction feature.[32,33] For example, registration of a very-low-amplitude signal from a site where the operator is sure of good endocardial contact strongly suggests a region of scar or a surgical patch. Similarly, a distinctly split electrogram is consistent with recording along the crista terminalis, an old ablation site, an atriotomy incision, or some other suture line (Fig. 13–12). Fractionated electrograms of long duration (Fig. 13–13) can suggest a zone of slow conduction (although not necessarily one that is critical to the circuit). Finally,

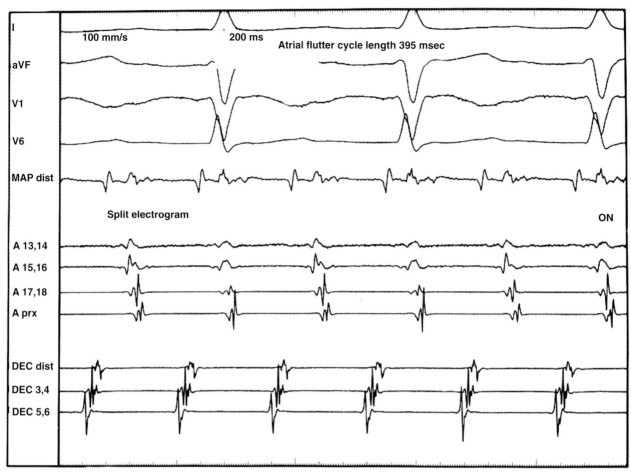

FIGURE 13–12. Recordings from electrophysiologic study of intra-atrial reentrant tachycardia. Shown are surface electrocardiographic leads (I, aVF, V$_1$, and V$_6$) along with intracardiac signals from a mapping catheter (MAP) and two multipolar reference catheters (A and DEC). The atrial cycle length is 395 msec. The mapping catheter is located along a presumptive atriotomy scar, showing a split electrogram pattern.

a discrete island of entrance block can sometimes be found at which the atrial rate is clearly slower than the underlying tachycardia, and the edges of such an island often correspond to important conduction barriers.

All data regarding atrial anatomy, activation patterns, and conduction features must be combined to generate one or more potential models for IART circuit location. The validity of the model can then be tested by entrainment pacing techniques.[18,34] Although there is always a small risk of interrupting or changing the tachycardia while pacing into an IART circuit, this risk is small as long as the pacing rate is just marginally faster than the tachycardia rate. If circuit localization seems quite firm on the basis of activation sequence and the model makes good anatomic sense, then perhaps entrainment pacing might be deferred. However, if there is any ambiguity at all about the circuit, this exercise can be extremely helpful in confirming or refuting the model.

In our electrophysiology laboratory, entrainment is performed with bipolar pacing from the distal electrode pair of the mapping catheter. Some centers perform unipolar pacing from the distal electrode, but we have not found this to be a major advantage for the CHD population. We prefer the reduced pacing artifact that accompanies bipolar pacing over any incremental precision that unipolar pacing might provide. The return atrial signal can usually be measured directly from the pacing electrode pair with modern recording systems (Fig. 13–14), unless the amplitude of the electrogram at the pacing site was exceptionally low to begin with. If the return electrogram from the distal electrode pair is too indistinct for accurate measurement, it is usually sufficient to rely on the proximal electrode pair on the mapping catheter as a proxy, while simply adjusting for the difference in timing between the pacing and recording sites during tachycardia.[35,36] Similar to the experience reported with mapping of reentrant ventricular tachycardia,[18] sites at which the postpacing interval

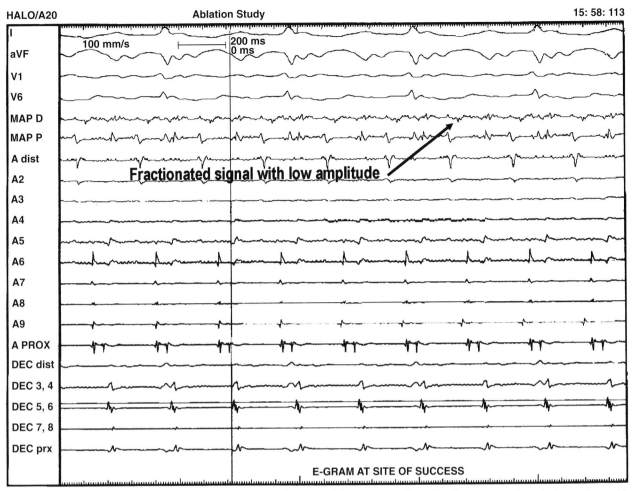

FIGURE 13–13. Recordings from electrophysiologic study of intra-atrial reentrant tachycardia. Shown are surface electrocardiographic leads (I, aVF, V₁, and V₆) along with intracardiac signals from a mapping catheter (MAP) and two multipolar reference catheters (A and DEC). The atrial cycle length is 270 msec. The mapping catheter is located at a site of successful ablation, where the local electrogram has a highly fractionated signal that spans almost the entire duration of atrial diastole. D, distal; dist, distal; prox, proximal.

does not exceed the IART cycle length by more than 30 msec tend to indicate tissue within the path of the circuit, and the smaller this difference, the better the localization.

Accurately identifying the full path of an IART circuit does not necessarily imply that one has pinpointed the correct spot to ablate. In order for RF ablation to succeed, the target area must be as small as possible, so that permanent transmural block can be achieved. Therefore, the atrium must be examined for anatomic and electrogram features[37,38] that are most likely to funnel the circuit into a narrow corridor between two conduction barriers (see Table 13–2). As it turns out, the narrowest corridor usually translates to the zone of slowest conduction, and this further translates to electrogram timings that occur just before the rapid deflection of the P wave on the surface electrocardiogram. Whenever clear and discrete P-wave activity can be identified during

IART, the most optimistic ablation targets usually register electrogram times toward the end of the isoelectric period, approximately 50 to 80 msec before P-wave onset.[6] Electrograms at such a site are quite often fractionated and relatively low in amplitude. Obviously, if the P-wave onset is indistinct on the surface electrocardiogram, slow conduction zones cannot be identified with these simple methods. Instead, one can search for locations within the circuit that generate perfectly concealed entrainment, consisting of a paced P-wave morphology and electrogram patterns that are identical to those observed in spontaneous tachycardia. Such sites should be located in or near a narrow protected conduction corridor. If all else fails, likely corridors of vulnerability can be identified by simply considering the anatomy and picking a region with the narrowest linear dimensions between two well-defined conduction barriers.

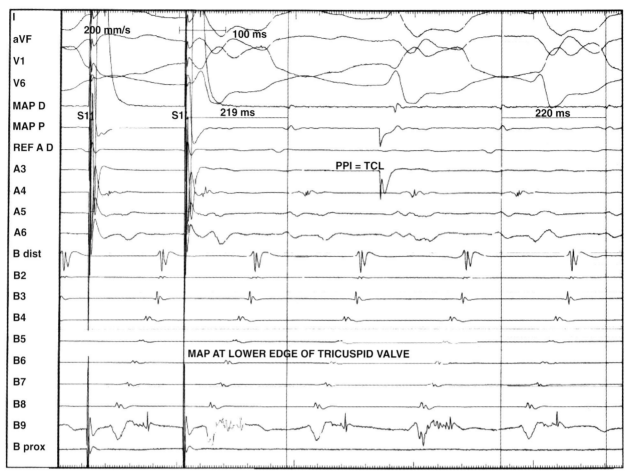

FIGURE 13-14. Recordings from electrophysiologic study of intra-atrial reentrant tachycardia. Shown are surface electrocardiographic leads (I, aVF, V_1, and V_6) along with intracardiac signals from a mapping catheter (MAP) and two multipolar reference catheters (A and B). The tachycardia has a cycle length of 220 msec. Entrainment pacing (S_1) at cycle length of 205 msec is performed from the mapping catheter at a site that is a critical component of the reentrant circuit. The postpacing interval (PPI) measured on the distal MAP electrogram is identical to the tachycardia cycle length (TCL), indicating that the pacing site is involved in the circuit.

THREE-DIMENSIONAL MAPPING

Electroanatomic and noncontact mapping have simplified and improved ablation of atrial tachycardia in CHD patients.[39,40] This is not to say that 3-D technologies have revolutionized understanding of the pathophysiology of IART or FAT in any substantial way. Rather, the major benefit has been that electrogram data are presented in a user-friendly format that enhances catheter positioning and keeps track of subtle conduction features that might go unnoticed or become forgotten during the tedious process of mapping with older recording systems. Moreover, these sophisticated mapping tools have greatly improved the ability to confirm complete conduction block across an ablated region in 3-D space, a process that formerly was highly prone to error for any site other than the CTI. Once these technologies began to

be applied to tachycardia in CHD patients, acute ablation success rates rose and recurrence rates declined.[41]

Most CHD patients have sustained IART circuits with stable cycle lengths, so that high-quality electroanatomic maps can be achieved reliably with point-by-point sampling of the right atrial endocardial surface and, if necessary, of the left atrium as well (Figs. 13–15 and 13–16). The ability to tag this 3-D display with markers indicating scar regions, split potentials, caval orifices, and valve rings assists greatly in fashioning a rational model for IART propagation.[42] In addition, the ability to project maps of both atrial chambers simultaneously (Fig. 13–17) allows prompt identification of circuits that may have to be ablated from the left side of the heart. Electroanatomic displays also remove most confusion about the differential diagnosis between IART and

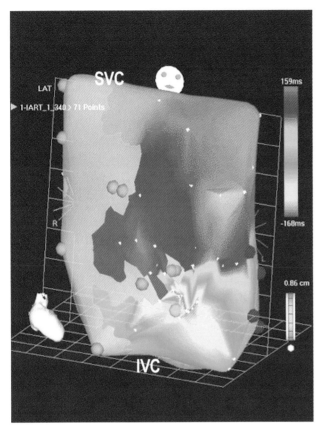

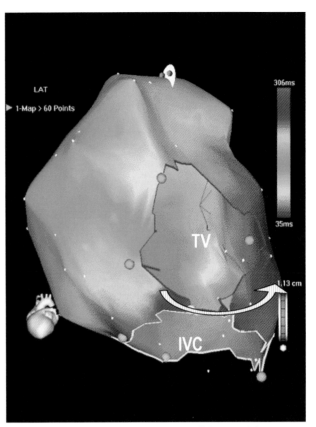

FIGURE 13–15. Electroanatomic map of intra-atrial reentrant tachycardia (cycle length, 330 msec) in a patient with a Fontan operation for tricuspid atresia. This projection shows the lateral wall of the right atrium, with a large area of scar *(gray)* that extends all the way from the superior vena cava (SVC) to the inferior vena cava (IVC), including a small extension that juts forward along the lower half of the right atrial free wall. There was a very narrow conduction channel through this scar extension, and it proved to be a critical part of the tachycardia circuit. Activation proceeds through this channel according to the following color code: blue → purple → red → yellow → green.

FIGURE 13–16. Electroanatomic map of intra-atrial reentrant tachycardia (cycle length, 340 msec) in the right atrium of a patient with repaired tetralogy of Fallot. This LAO caudal projection highlights the isthmus between the inferior vena cava (IVC) and the tricuspid valve (TV), which proved to be a critical part of the tachycardia circuit. Activation proceeds through this isthmus *(arrow)* according to the following color code: blue → purple → red.

FAT, because radial propagation of the latter usually is readily apparent (Fig. 13–18). With experienced staff, full acquisition of a detailed IART or FAT map in the RA can usually be accomplished in less than 15 minutes.

One important caveat with electroanatomic mapping is that the catheter tip must be in good contact with the endocardial surface for each electrogram collected. In CHD patients with very dilated atria, this can be difficult to ensure. Failure to recognize poor contact could result in collection of phantom data points suggesting a low-amplitude scar region, when in fact the catheter tip was simply floating in the atrial cavity. Using the baseline right atrial angiogram as a guide, the catheter operator must periodically check to ensure that the tip of the mapping electrode has reached the true edge of the atrial silhouette. This sometimes requires the use of a long guiding sheath to extend the reach of the catheter curve.

The major limitation of electroanatomic mapping is that tachycardia must remain stable for the duration of data acquisition. Occasionally, CHD patients, particularly in the Fontan group, have multiple IART circuits, and tachycardias can shift or terminate during the mapping process in response to the mechanical ectopy that accompanies catheter manipulation. If this problem repeatedly stymies mapping efforts, it is often useful to revert to a more simple map of sinus rhythm and create a basic anatomic shell of the RA that is focused primarily on the major conduction barriers.[43] This sinus rhythm map can then be examined to identify the most likely narrow conduction corridors, and repeat mapping during any subsequent episodes of tachycardia can concentrate on these regions of interest.

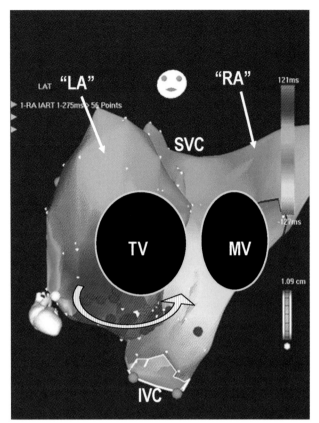

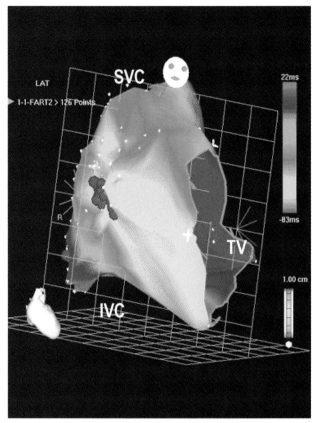

FIGURE 13–17. Electroanatomic map of intra-atrial reentrant tachycardia (cycle length, 255 msec) in a patient who underwent the Mustard operation for transposition of the great arteries. This AP display combines activation times from both the modified right atrium ("RA") and the modified left atrium ("LA") and highlights the isthmus between the inferior vena cava (IVC) and the tricuspid valve (TV), which proved to be a critical part of the tachycardia circuit. Activation proceeds through this isthmus *(arrow)* according to the following color code: blue → purple → red → yellow. MV, mitral valve; SVC, superior vena cava.

FIGURE 13–18. Electroanatomic map of focal atrial tachycardia in the right atrium of a patient who had undergone closure of atrial and ventricular septal defects. Earliest atrial activation was mapped to the lateral right atrial wall, where electrogram features suggested a nearby atriotomy scar. Activation spread in a radial fashion from this site. The red dots mark the site of successful ablation. IVC, inferior vena cava; SVC, superior vena cava; TV, tricuspid valve.

Noncontact mapping[44] may also be used for IART or FAT mapping, and it seems to be particularly well suited to patients with poor hemodynamics, who might not tolerate long episodes of tachycardia, and for those with multiple unstable IART circuits that are too fleeting to map by other techniques (Fig. 13–19). However, this technology has some limitations in CHD patients with very dilated atrial chambers, because data quality can suffer to some degree whenever the inflated recording balloon is too far away from the atrial endocardial surface.

Propagation maps of IART generated by either of these 3-D techniques must still be viewed critically before deciding exactly where to place ablation lesions. Just because an atrial region displays suspicious conduction features on a 3-D map does not prove that it is part of a circuit. It may still be helpful to perform entrainment pacing maneuvers

to confirm the model before embarking on RF applications.[34]

Ablation

Accurate mapping is only half the battle in IART ablation. Even if the tachycardia location is firm, it can still be difficult to create effective ablation lesions in CHD patients using standard RF technology (Table 13–3). The target tissue selected in these cases can be heavily trabeculated and thickened due to hypertrophy or surgical scar, and it almost always has a width greater than that achieved by a single RF application. Multiple overlapping lesions may need to be placed when attempting a line of conduction block, leaving open the possibility of gaps in the line or varying depths of RF penetration that fail to produce full

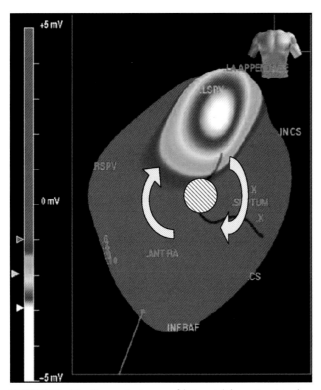

FIGURE 13-19. Noncontact map of intra-atrial reentrant tachycardia in a patient who had undergone a Fontan operation. This projection highlights the atrial septal surface as recorded by the balloon catheter within the left atrium. The activation pattern *(arrows)* indicates a circuit around an atrial septal patch (nashed area). CS, coronary sinus; LA appendage, left atrial appendage; LSPV, left superior pulmonary vein; RSPV, right superior pulmonary vein.

transmural tissue injury. In addition, the biophysics of RF lesion creation may be compromised in some CHD patients, particularly those who have undergone the Fontan operation and have massively enlarged RAs. These patients can have remarkably low atrial blood flow velocity,[45] as evidenced by the common echocardiographic observation of spontaneous cavitation or "smoke" within the body of the RA. As a consequence, there is low convective cooling of the ablation catheter tip by circulating blood, so that RF power delivery becomes severely limited by high catheter-tip temperatures. This limitation has been dealt with fairly effectively by the widespread adoption of alternative catheter designs for RF delivery in CHD patients, including both large-tip and irrigated-tip catheters.

Ablation efforts can usually begin with a standard 4-mm-tip catheter and a temperature-controlled 50-W RF generator set to a maximum of 70°C. As RF applications are made in a region of interest, careful attention should be given to the biophysical parameters measured from the generator. If maximum tip temperatures are achieved quickly but peak RF powers register much less than 25 W, it usually predicts inadequate tissue injury. Even if there is an acute tachycardia termination, true conduction block is unlikely to be achieved, and IART will almost always be reinducible (or recur during later follow-up) when these feeble amounts of RF power are applied. It is probably advisable in these cases to

TABLE 13-3		
Troubleshooting the Difficult Case		
Problem	**Cause**	**Solution**
Complex anatomy and cardiac access	Congenital malformations, prior surgery with patches, baffles, and so on	Extensive review of prior surgical procedures and all imaging modalities Contrast angiography, intracardiac or transesophageal echocardiography during case
Incomplete reentrant circuit mapped	Small zone of slow conduction missed, portions of atria not mapped, inaccessible Circuit involves "the other" atrium True focal mechanism	High-density mapping and pace-mapping for areas of slow conduction thorough mapping of baffles, pouches, and so on Map contralateral atrium Verify with electroanatomic and/or entrainment mapping
Failure of radiofrequency (RF) ablation at favorable site	Thick tissue from scar, hypertrophy, trabeculae Broad reentry circuit Low-flow area yielding high temperatures/low power	Cooled RF ablation Linear lesions, large-tip ablation catheter Cooled ablation
Multiple reentry circuits and arrhythmias	Extensive scarring and surgical procedures (Fontan)	Noncontact mapping for nonsustained arrhythmias Extensive use of electroanatomic and entrainment mapping

switch promptly to either a 6- to 8-mm-tip catheter or an irrigated-tip ablation catheter. We have had experience with various large-tip designs and several irrigation systems, and so long as improved RF power delivery is accomplished, there does not appear to be any obvious advantage of one technique over the other. However, it is abundantly clear that these alternative catheter techniques can succeed in IART cases after standard ablation with a 4-mm-tip catheter has failed.

The acute response of IART to accurately positioned RF applications varies according to the dimensions and conduction properties of the corridor being targeted. Abrupt termination early into a single RF application may be seen if the corridor is narrow and discrete (Fig. 13–20), but this is actually a fairly rare occurrence in CHD patients. It is far more common to observe a pattern of gradual and progressive cycle length prolongation as cumulative RF applications slowly close off conduction through the critical corridor (Fig. 13–21).

It is important to emphasize that the isolated observation of IART termination is not a sufficient end point for ablation. Granted, interruption of tachycardia is an optimistic sign that the map was correct, but it does not prove that complete conduction block has been achieved. Pacing from both sides of the target zone must be performed, and follow-up propagation maps should be constructed to investigate the possibility of residual gaps through the corridor. If there is any hint of residual conduction, additional RF applications should be delivered at the site (using large-tip or irrigation-tip catheters, if necessary) until unequivocal block has been established.[38,41,46] As mentioned, 3-D mapping has greatly improved the accuracy of these follow-up maps for the CHD population (Fig. 13–22).

For the rare CHD patient with FAT, ablation of the focal abnormality with RF current is relatively uncomplicated. The epicenter of early atrial activation can often be ablated with a single application, but, once again, if thermodynamics during RF deliv-

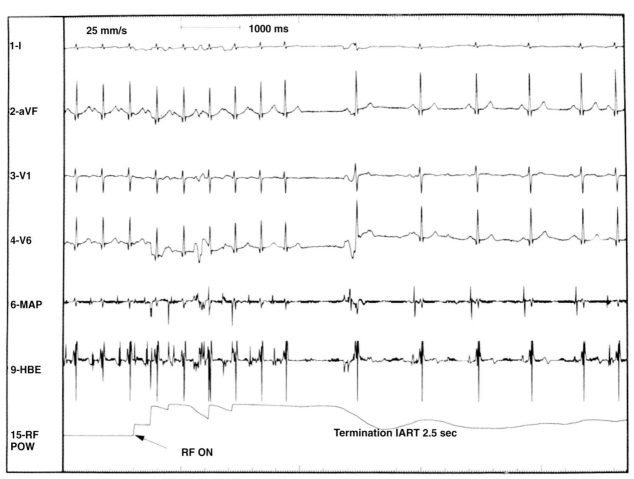

FIGURE 13–20. Recordings from ablation of intra-atrial reentrant tachycardia. Shown are surface electrocardiographic leads (I, aVF, V₁, and V₆) along with intracardiac signals from a mapping catheter (MAP) and a His bundle recording. In this case, tachycardia terminated promptly on initial radiofrequency application. RF Pow, radiofrequency power.

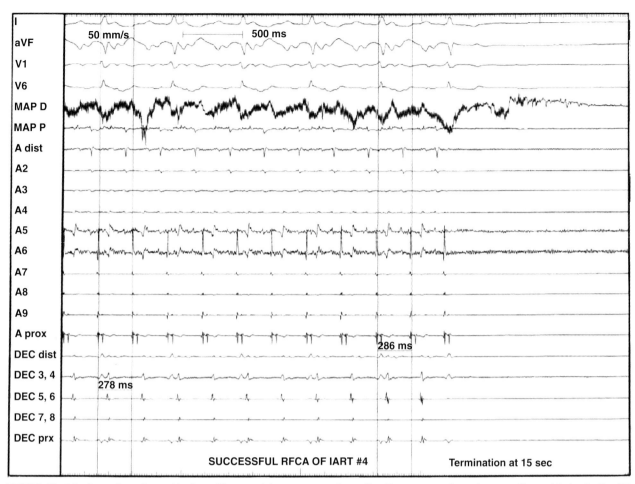

FIGURE 13–21. Recordings from ablation of intra-atrial reentrant tachycardia. Shown are surface electrocardiographic leads (I, aVF, V_1, and V_6) along with intracardiac signals from a mapping catheter (MAP) and two atrial reference catheters (A and DEC). The starting tachycardia cycle length was 260 msec. In this case, tachycardia slowed in a gradual and progressive fashion to 286 msec but did not terminate until 15 seconds into the radiofrequency application. (Abbreviations as in figure 13-13).

ery indicate low wattage because of high tip temperatures, a large-tip or irrigated-tip catheter should be used.

After successful ablation of an IART circuit or FAT focus, repeat atrial stimulation should be performed to rule out additional sources of atrial tachycardia. Among Fontan patients in particular, multiple tachycardias are very common. If the patient has a true CTI that did not participate in the original target arrhythmia, it is probably still wise to close off isthmus conduction as a precaution in the electrophysiology laboratory, even if no tachycardia was identified as involving this site.

Clinical Outcomes

Long-term results for ablation of atrial tachycardias in patients with CHD have been improving steadily as new mapping and ablation technologies have been introduced, but there is still room for improvement. Acute ablation success, defined according to rigorous conduction block criteria, can now be achieved in as many as 90% of cases in the modern era of 3-D mapping and aggressive RF lesion creation. This compares with acute success rates of only about 60% that were seen with older mapping technology and standard 4-mm-tip ablation catheters. However, despite generally excellent acute outcomes, recurrence of some form of atrial tachycardia during longer-term follow-up is still disappointingly common. These recurrences can involve return of the original target arrhythmia, but quite often they represent appearance of a totally new atrial substrate. Recurrence is particularly problematic in Fontan patients with multiple IART circuits, as many as 40% of whom achieve acute success but experience at least one episode of atrial tachycardia within 2 years after the procedure. Recurrence is less common in patients with two ventricles and routine anatomy, in whom

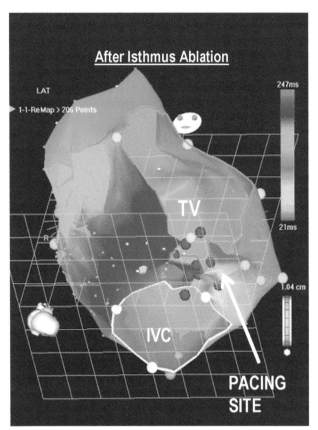

FIGURE 13–22. Electroanatomic map of atrial activation while pacing near the mouth of the coronary sinus in a patient who had just undergone successful interruption of conduction through the cavotricuspid isthmus. The red dots mark the sites of radiofrequency applications. The late electrogram times *(blue and purple)* recorded just on the other side of the ablation line suggest that propagation of atrial activation away from the pacing site had to occur in a counterclockwise manner all the way around the tricuspid valve ring, rather than across the isthmus. IVC, inferior vena cava; TV, tricuspid valve.

ablation can usually be focused on the familiar territory of the CTI. The recurrence risk in this setting is now reasonably low, on the order of 20%.

Contemporary outcome data for atrial tachycardia ablation in CHD patients, although not perfect, may still be viewed as encouraging when compared with the option of pharmacologic therapy,[7] which is associated with a recurrence risk at 2 years as high as 70%. Moreover, even among patients who have a recurrent tachycardia after ablation, global rhythm status is still likely to be improved compared with their preablation condition. This improvement was quantified in a large clinical study from our center using a scoring system that incorporated such items as severity of symptoms, antiarrhythmic drug dependency, the need for cardioversion, and observations on whether tachycardia episodes were sustained or self-termi-

nating.[41] When scored in this fashion, almost all CHD patients (regardless of anatomy) had a substantial improvement in quality of life after ablation for atrial tachycardia.

Conclusion

RF ablation of atrial tachycardia in postoperative CHD patients presents many unique challenges in terms of anatomic complexity, atypical tachycardia substrates, and abnormally thick atrial muscle that can be difficult to ablate. Technological advances in 3-D mapping and the broader availability of ablation catheters designed to make more effective RF lesions have significantly improved outcomes.

Looking forward, it is reasonable to expect a continued reduction in tachycardia recurrence rates with more liberal use of large-tip or irrigated-tip RF ablation catheters, or perhaps the application of novel ablation modalities such as microwave energy or cryoablation.[47] It is anticipated that improved lesion creation, in conjunction with adherence to stringent conduction block criteria for success, may reduce recurrence rates to the range currently seen with ablation of typical atrial flutter in normal hearts.[48] As a spinoff benefit, the clinical experience with catheter ablation of these tachycardias will continue to influence the surgical approach to various forms of CHD. By illustrating the exact spatial relations between scar regions and macroreentry circuits, certain arrhythmogenic locations for atriotomy incisions and patch placement can now be anticipated and avoided for future generations of CHD patients.[49]

References

1. Flinn CJ, Wolff GS, Dick M, et al.: Cardiac rhythm after the Mustard operation for complete transposition of the great arteries. N Engl J Med 3310:1635-1638, 1984.
2. Fishberger SB, Wernovsky G, Gentles TL, et al.: Factors that influence the development of atrial flutter after the Fontan operation. J Thorac Cadiovas Surg 113:80-86, 1997.
3. Walsh EP: Arrhythmias in patients with congenital heart disease. Card Electrophysiol Rev 4:422-430, 2002.
4. Garson A, Bink-Boelkens MTE, Hesslein PS, et al.: Atrial flutter in the young: A collaborative study of 380 cases. J Am Coll Cardiol 6:871-878, 1985.
5. Kirsh JA, Walsh EP, Triedman JK: Prevalence of and risk factors for atrial fibrillation and intraatrial reentrant tachycardia among patients with congenital heart disease. Am J Cardiol 90:338-340, 2002.
6. Triedman JK, Saul JP, Weindling SN, Walsh EP: Radiofrequency ablation of intraatrial reentrant tachycardia following surgical palliation of congenital heart disease. Circulation 91:707-714, 1995.

7. Triedman JK: Atrial reentrant tachycardias. In Walsh EP, Saul JP, Triedman JK (eds.): Cardiac Arrhythmias in Children and Young Adults with Congenital Heart Disease. Philadelphia: Lippincott Williams & Wilkins, 2001, pp 137-160.

8. Rhodes LA, Walsh EP, Gamble WJ, et al: Benefits and potential risks of atrial antitachycardia pacing after repair of congenital heart disease. Pacing Clin Electrophysiol 18:1005-1016, 1995.

9. Stevenson EA, Casavant D, Tuzi J, et al.: Efficacy of atrial anti-tachycardia pacing using the Medtronic AT500 pacemaker in patients with congenital heart disease. Am J Cardiol 92:871-876, 2003.

10. Mavroudis C, Backer CL, Deal BJ, et al.: Total cavopulmonary conversion and maze procedure for patients with failure of the Fontan operation. J Thorac Cardiovasc Surg 122:863-871, 2001.

11. Kreutzer J, Keane JF, Lock JE, et al.: Conversion of modified Fontan procedure to lateral atrial tunnel cavopulmonary anastomosis. J Thorac Cardiovas Surg 111:1169-1176, 1996.

12. Collins KK, Love BA, Walsh EP, et al.: Location of acutely successful radiofrequency catheter ablation of intraatrial reentrant tachycardia in patients with congenital heart disease. Am J Cardiol 86:969-974, 2000.

13. Kanter RJ, Papagiannis J, Carboni MP, et al.: Radiofrequency catheter ablation of supraventricular tachycardia substrates after Mustard and Senning operations for d-transposition of the great arteries. J Am Coll Cardiol 35:428-441, 2000.

14. Van Hare GF, Lesh MD, Ross BA, et al.: Mapping and radiofrequency ablation of intraatrial reentrant tachycardia after the Senning or Mustard procedure for transposition of the great arteries. Am J Cardiol 77:985-991, 1996.

15. Perry JC, Boramanand NK, Ing FF: "Transseptal" technique through atrial baffles for 3-dimensional mapping and ablation of atrial tachycardia in patients with d-transposition of the great arteries. J Interv Card Electrophysiol 9:365-369, 2003.

16. Waldo AL, MacLean WAH, Karp RB, et al.: Entrainment and interruption of atrial flutter with atrial pacing: Studies in man following open-heart surgery. Circulation 56:737-745, 1977.

17. Bromberg BI, Schuessler RB, Gandhi SK, et al.: A canine model of atrial flutter following the intra-atrial lateral tunnel Fontan operation. J Electrocardiol 30:85-93, 1998.

18. Khan HH, Stevenson WG: Activation times in and adjacent to reentry circuits during entrainment: Implications for mapping ventricular tachycardia. Am Heart J 127:833-842, 1994.

19. El-Shalakany A, Hadjis T, Papageorgiou P, et al.: Entrainment/mapping criteria for the prediction of termination of ventricular tachycardia by single radiofrequency lesion in patients with coronary artery disease. Circulation 99:2283-2289, 1999.

20. Kalman JM, Olgin JE, Saxon LA, et al.: Activation and entrainment mapping defines the tricuspid annulus as the anterior barrier in typical atrial flutter. Circulation 94:398-406, 1996.

21. Walsh EP: Ablation of ectopic atrial tachycardia in young patients. In Huang SKS, Wilber DJ (eds.): Radiofrequency Catheter Ablation of Cardiac Arrhythmias, 2nd ed. Armonk, N.Y.: Futura, 2000, pp 115-138.

22. Fishberger SB, Wernovsky G, Gentles TL, et al.: Factors that influence the development of atrial flutter after the Fontan operation. J Thorac Cardiovas Surg 113:80-86, 1997.

23. Rhodes LA, Wernovsky G, Keane JF, et al.: Arrhythmias and intracardiac conduction after the arterial switch operation. J Thorac Cardiovasc Surg 109:303-310, 1995.

24. Stamm C, Friehs I, Mayer JE, et al.: Long-term results of the lateral tunnel Fontan operation. J Thorac Cardiovasc Surg 121:28-41, 2001.

25. Levine J, Walsh EP, Saul JP: Catheter ablation of accessory pathways in patients with congenital heart disease including heterotaxy syndrome. Am J Cardiol 72:689-694, 1993.

26. Epstein MR, Saul JP, Weindling SN, et al.: Atrioventricular reciprocating tachycardia involving twin atrioventricular nodes in patients with complex congenital heart disease. J Cardiovasc Electrophysiol 12:671-679, 2001.

27. Mullen MP, VanPraagh R, Walsh EP: Development and anatomy of the cardiac conduction system. In Walsh EP, Saul JP, Triedman JK (eds.): Cardiac Arrhythmias in Children and Young Adults with Congenital Heart Disease. Philadelphia: Lippincott Williams & Wilkins, 2001, pp 93-111.

28. Walsh EP: Catheter ablation of ectopic atrial tachycardia. In Walsh EP, Saul JP, Triedman JK (eds.): Cardiac Arrhythmias in Children and Young Adults with Congenital Heart Disease. Philadelphia: Lippincott Williams & Wilkins, 2001, pp 93-111.

29. Jenkins JK, Walsh EP, Colan SD, et al.: Multipolar endocardial mapping of the right atrium during cardiac catheterization: Description of a new technique. J Am Coll Cardiol 22:1105-1110, 1993.

30. Triedman JK, Jenkins KJ, Colan SD, et al.: Intra-atrial reentrant tachycardia after palliation of congenital heart disease: Characterization of multiple macroreentrant circuits using fluoroscopically based three-dimensional endocardial mapping. J Cardiovasc Electrophysiol 8:259-270, 1997.

31. Triedman JK, Bergau DM, Saul JP, et al.: Efficacy of radiofrequency ablation for control of intraatrial reentrant tachycardia in patients with congenital heart disease. J Am Coll Cardiol 30:1032-1038, 1997.

32. De Groot NM, Kuijper AF, Blom NA, et al.: Three-dimensional distribution of bipolar atrial electrogram voltages in patients with congenital heart disease. Pacing Clin Electrophysiol 24:1334-1342, 2001.

33. Kalman JK, Van Hare GF, Olgin JE, et al.: Ablation of "incisional" reentrant atrial tachycardia complication surgery for congenital heart disease. Circulation 93:502-512, 1996.

34. Delacretaz E, Ganz LI, Friedman PL, et al.: Multiple atrial macroreentry circuits in adults with repaired congenital heart disease: Entrainment mapping combined with three-dimensional electroanatomic mapping. J Am Coll Cardiol 37:1665-1676, 2001.

35. Triedman JK, Alexander ME, Berul CI, et al.: Estimation of atrial response to entrainment pacing using electrograms recorded from remote sites. J Cardiovasc Electrophysiol 11:1215-1222, 2000.

36. Hadjis TA, Harada T, Stevenson WG, Friedman PL: Effect of recording site on postpacing interval measurement during catheter mapping and entrainment of postinfarction ventricular tachycardia. J Cardiovasc Electrophysiol 8:398-404, 1997.

37. Baker BM, Lindsay BD, Bromberg B, et al.: Catheter ablation of intraatrial reentrant tachycardias resulting from previous atrial surgery: Locating and transecting the critical isthmus. J Am Coll Cardiol 28:411-417, 1996.

38. Poty H, Saoudi N, Nair M, et al.: Radio frequency catheter ablation of atrial flutter—Further insights into the various types of isthmus block: Application to ablation during sinus rhythm. Circulation 94:3204-3213, 1996.

39. Triedman JK, Alexander ME, Berul CI, et al.: Electroanatomic mapping of entrained and exit zones in patients with repaired congenital heart disease and intra-atrial reentrant tachycardia. Circulation 103:2060-2065, 2001.

40. Nakagawa H, Jackman WM: Use of a three-dimensional, non-fluoroscopic mapping system for catheter ablation of typical atrial flutter. Pacing Clin Electrophysiol 21:1279-1286, 1998.

41. Triedman JK, Alexander MA, Love BA, et al.: Influence of patient factors and ablative technologies on outcomes of radiofrequency ablation of intra-atrial tachycardia in patients with congenital heart disease. J Am Coll Cardiol 39:1827-1835, 2002.

42. Mandapati R, Walsh EP, Triedman JK: Pericaval and periannular intra-atrial reentrant tachycardias in patients with congenital heart disease. J Cardiovasc Electrophysiol 14:119-125, 2003.

43. Love BA, Collins KK, Walsh EP, Triedman JK: Electroanatomic characterization of conduction barriers in sinus/atrial paced rhythm and association with intra-atrial reentrant tachycardia circuits following congenital heart disease surgery. J Cardiovasc Electrophysiol 12:17-25, 2001.

44. Schumacher B, Jung W, Lewalter T, et al.: Verification of linear lesions using a noncontact multielectrode array catheter versus conventional contact mapping techniques. J Cardiovasc Electrophysiol 10:791-798, 1999.

45. Be'eri E, Maier SE, Landzberg MJ, et al.: In vivo evaluation of Fontan pathway flow dynamics by multidimensional phase-velocity magnetic resonance imaging. Circulation 98:2873-2882, 1998.

46. Willems S, Weiss C, Hoffmann M, Meinertz T: Atrial flutter ablation using a technique for detection of conduction block within the posterior isthmus. Pacing Clin Electrophysiol 22:750-758, 1999.

47. Lustgarten DL, Keane D, Ruskin J: Cryothermal ablation: Mechanism of tissue injury and current experience in the treatment of tachyarrhythmias. Prog Cardiovasc Dis 41:481-498, 1999.

48. Tai CT, Chen SA, Chiang CE, et al.: Long-term outcome of radiofrequency catheter ablation for typical atrial flutter: Risk prediction of recurrent arrhythmias. J Cardiovasc Electrophysiol 9:115-121, 1998.

49. Collins KK, Rhee EK, Delucca JM, et al.: Modification to the Fontan procedure for the prophylaxis of intra-atrial reentrant tachycardia: Short-term results of a prospective randomized blinded trial. J Thorac Cardiovasc Surg 127:721-729, 2004.

Catheter Ablation for Atrial Fibrillation

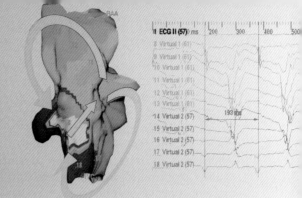

PART IV

14

Atrioventricular Junction Ablation and Modification for Heart Rate Control of Atrial Fibrillation

Ling-Ping Lai • Jiunn-Lee Lin • Shoei K. Stephen Huang

Key Points

- The mechanism of atrial fibrillation is multiple wavelets or rotors in the atria with rapid ventricular response through the atrioventricular (AV) junction.

- Diagnosis is based on the 12-lead electrocardiogram (ECG), which shows a fibrillating baseline or P waves with irregularly irregular QRS complexes at a rate greater than 120 per minute.

- Mapping uses a combined anatomy- and electrogram-guided approach.

- The right-sided approach target is just proximal to or below the His bundle electrode position or at the proximal His position. The left-sided approach target is just below the aortic valve at the septal site where a His potential can be recorded.

- Use of preformed sheaths may be helpful, and cooled ablation is sometimes necessary.

- Sources of difficulties include inability to record the His potential and failure of the right-sided approach.

Atrial fibrillation (AF) is a very common tachyarrhythmia in humans.[1,2] It is responsible for low cardiac output, symptoms of palpitations, and systemic thromboembolic events. For the treatment of AF, rhythm control and rate control strategies are both widely used. Restoration and maintenance of sinus rhythm are sometimes difficult, however, and recent trials have demonstrated no benefit to rhythm control over rate control strategies.[3,4] The traditional way of achieving ventricular rate control is the use of atrioventricular (AV) nodal blocking agents including β-blockers, calcium channel blockers, and digitalis. With the advent of catheter ablation techniques, AV junction ablation has evolved as an important and effective means to achieve ventricular rate control. This chapter describes the techniques of radiofrequency (RF) catheter ablation for ventricular rate control in patients with AF.

Complete Atrioventricular Junction Ablation

Complete AV junction ablation provides a very effective way to control the ventricular rate during AF. However, a permanent pacemaker must be implanted to provide adequate heart rate, because the junctional escape rhythm after ablation is typically slow and unreliable.[5] Initially, this technique was used in patients with tachycardia-bradycardia syndrome, who also need a pacemaker. Its indication was later extended to those with drug-refractory, poorly controlled, rapid ventricular rates. This technique has also been used in patients with AF and a normal ventricular rate.[6] Early works on AV junction ablation were achieved by direct current (DC) shock.[5,6] Today, RF energy has completely replaced DC shock as the energy source for catheter ablation of the AV junction.[7-30] Cryoablation of the AV node has also been reported.[31] However, it has not gained popularity, because RF energy is widely available and highly effective and there has been no demonstrable advantage to cryoablation for this application.

Before AV junction ablation is performed, appropriate ventricular backup pacing must be ensured. This can be achieved by placing a temporary electrode catheter at the right ventricular apex or, more typically, by implanting a permanent pacemaker before the ablation procedure. By implanting the device weeks before the ablation procedure, the problems associated with postimplantation pacemaker system malfunction are avoided. For those with a permanent pacemaker implanted before ablation, care should be taken to ensure effective pacing during ablation, because interaction between RF energy and the pacemaker may occur. The skin patch should be placed as far away as possible from the pacemaker. The pacemaker should be set to VVI or VOO mode at 40 to 50 beats per minute before ablation. Ventricular asystole or extreme bradycardia may occur during RF energy application because of destruction of the AV junction and inhibition of the permanent pacemaker by RF energy. Turning off the ablation power supply restores pacemaker activity. Further ablation can be performed with the pacemaker in the VOO mode. After ablation, permanent pacemakers should be interrogated to assess for alterations in pacemaker programming or changes in pacing or sensing thresholds.

Mapping and Ablation

For the ablation procedure, an approach from the right side is usually tried first.[10] The anatomy of the AV node and conduction system is reviewed in Chapters 18 and 19. The procedure can be performed under the guidance of fluoroscopy and electrograms. Ideally, the ablation catheter is positioned at the compact node region, which is located at the atrial midseptal region, just proximal and inferior to the His bundle catheter position, under fluoroscopy (Fig. 14–1A). Ablation of the AV conduction system as proximally as possible increases the chance that an escape rhythm will emerge. Typically, the electrograms here show an atrial-to-ventricular electrogram ratio (A/V ratio) greater than 1:2.

More typically, the ablation is guided by mapping very proximal His bundle recordings. The ablation catheter is positioned to record the maximal His potential. Although it is often tempting to ablate at the site of maximal His recording, this site often produces right bundle branch block only. The catheter is then withdrawn toward the atrium to record an A/V ratio of 1:1 or 1:2 and a small His electrogram, usually less than 0.15 mV in amplitude (Fig. 14–2). The catheter tip may need to be deflected slightly inferiorly to follow the course of the AV conduction system. During AF, mapping may be complicated by variable atrial electrogram amplitudes and obfuscation of the His electrogram by the continuous atrial activity (Fig. 14–3). With standard 4-mm-tip ablation electrodes, RF is delivered for 60 seconds at 50 to 60 W with target temperatures of 55°C to 65°C. The use of preformed sheaths with a slight septal angulation and large-curve catheters may improve the

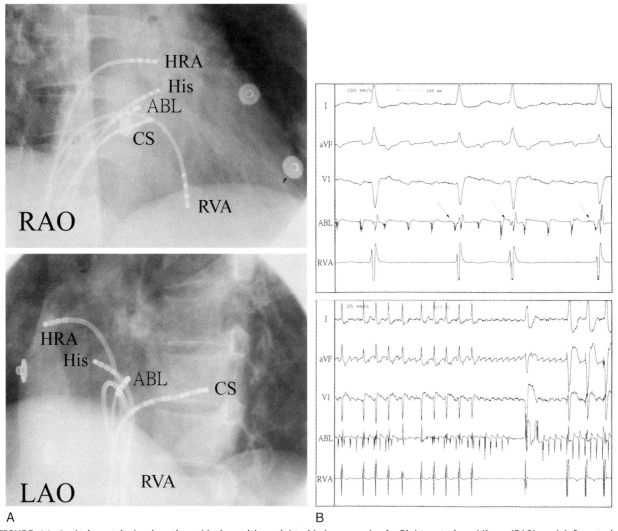

FIGURE 14–1. Atrioventricular junction ablation with a right-sided approach. **A,** Right anterior oblique (RAO) and left anterior oblique (LAO) fluoroscopic images of catheter position during ablation. The ablation catheter (ABL) was positioned just below the His catheter (His). CS, coronary sinus; HRA, high right atrium; RVA, right ventricular apex. **B,** Surface electrocardiogram leads (I, aVF, and V₁) and local electrograms. A His-like potential *(arrows)* is present at the ablation (ABL) site in the top tracing. The bottom tracing shows the onset of complete heart block and ventricular pacing. RVA, right ventricular apex.

stability of the catheter at the desired position. It is highly advisable to carefully map and ensure catheter stability, to avoid delivering ineffective lesions. Multiple ineffective deliveries may produce tissue edema and swelling that then obscure the His recording and distance the ablation catheter from the target tissue. During energy application, effective AV junction ablation is usually marked by accelerated junctional rhythm followed by slowing of the ventricular response and emergence of a paced ventricular rhythm.

A left-sided approach is used as an alternative if the approach from the right side of the heart is undesirable or unsuccessful,[10,11] which occurs in approximately 5% of patients. The ablation catheter enters the left ventricle from the retrograde transaortic

approach. The left-sided portion of the His bundle emerges on the septum just below the aortic valve (Fig. 14–4). It is helpful to maintain a catheter in the His position in the right side of the heart as an anatomic reference while mapping the left side of the septum. After the aortic valve is crossed with a tight curve on the ablation catheter, the curve can be maintained on the catheter while it is rotated toward the septum and withdrawn to the aortic valve. Alternatively, the ablation catheter can be directed toward the inferior apical septum, then withdrawn toward the His bundle until the His potential is recorded beneath the noncoronary aortic cusp. A His electrogram is recorded at the site of ablation. The His potential must be differentiated from the left bundle branch recording.

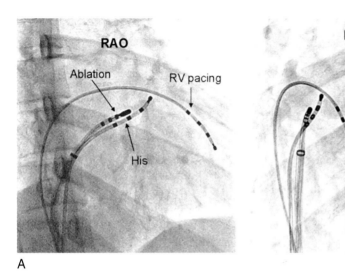

A

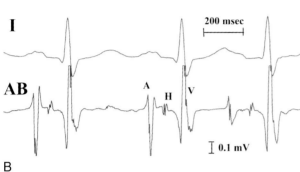

B

FIGURE 14–2. Standard right-sided approach for ablation of the atrioventricular junction. **A,** Right anterior oblique (RAO) and left anterior oblique (LAO) fluoroscopic views showing the ablation catheter aligned with the proximal His catheter (His) along the septum. RV, right ventricle. **B,** Surface electrocardiographic lead I and electrograms from the distal ablation catheter (AB) showing an atrial (A)-to-ventricular (V) electrogram ratio of 1:1.5 and a small His potential (H) with amplitude of 0.12 mV.

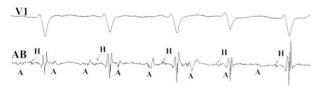

FIGURE 14–3. Mapping of the His bundle in atrial fibrillation. Electrocardiographic lead V_1 and the distal ablation (AB) electrograms are shown. The irregular atrial electrograms (A) may obscure the His recording (H). In addition, variation in the amplitude of A complicates estimation of the atrial to ventricular electrogram ratio.

The left-sided His activation should occur essentially at the same time as the right-sided His. The left bundle branch is typically recorded 1 to 1.5 cm inferior to the optimal His bundle recording site. The left bundle branch recording is identified by a potential-to-ventricular electrogram interval of 20 msec or less and an A/V ratio of 1:10 or less. Electrogram recordings and catheter positions for the left conduction system are discussed in Chapter 28. In rare circumstances in which standard right-sided and left-sided approaches are both unsuccessful, energy delivery to the region of the noncoronary aortic cusp where the His bundle potential is recorded may lead to complete AV block.[12]

In patients with preexisting complete bundle branch block, ablation of the contralateral bundle branch results in complete heart block. Mapping and ablation of the bundle branches are described in Chapter 28. Complete heart block may also result from ablation of both fast and slow pathway inputs to the AV node (Fig. 14–5). The targets for ablation are listed in Table 14–1.

For patients with chronically elevated ventricular rates, abrupt normalization of the heart rate by ablation and pacing may produce repolarization abnormalities and fatal polymorphic ventricular tachycardia.[27-30] This phenomenon resulted in a significant incidence of sudden death after AV junctional ablation before it was appreciated in the early experience. Currently, the risk of postprocedure polymorphic ventricular arrhythmias has been essentially eliminated by programming the permanent pacemaker lower rate limit to 80 to 90 bpm immediately after ablation. The lower rate limit is then reduced by 10 bpm each month until the desired lower rate limit is achieved.

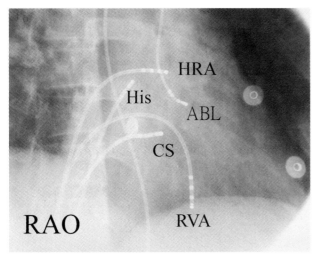

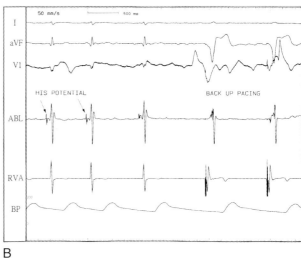

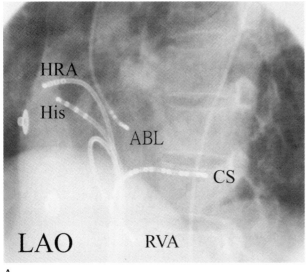

B

A

FIGURE 14–4. Atrioventricular junction ablation with a left-sided approach. **A,** Right anterior oblique (RAO) and left anterior oblique (LAO) fluoroscopic images of catheter position during ablation. The ablation catheter (ABL) was just below the aortic valve. CS, coronary sinus; His, His catheter; HRA, high right atrium; RVA, right ventricular apex. **B,** Surface electrocardiographic leads (I, aVF, and V_1) and local electrograms. A His potential *(arrows)* was present at the ablation site. BP, blood pressure.

Outcomes

The overall success rate for AV junction ablation is essentially 100% in recent reports.[13-20] A recurrence of AV conduction occurs in about 5% of patients. Brignole et al.[13] performed a multicenter, randomized study in 43 patients to compare AV junction versus pharmacologic treatment in patients with symptomatic AF. The report showed that AV junction ablation with pacemaker implantation was superior in controlling symptoms related to palpitations, dyspnea, and exercise intolerance in a 6-month follow-up period. The improvement of quality of life was also greater in the ablation group. Similar results were shown in another, noncontrolled but larger series of 107 patients.[14] In the latter series, not only did the

quality of life improve, but the number of doctor visits, hospital admissions, and episodes of heart failure were all significantly decreased. Therefore, the medical costs were substantially reduced. With regular R-R intervals, the cardiac output and overall cardiac performance as well as exercise capacity can be improved.[15,16] A reduction of left ventricular dimension and increased contractility have also been shown 6 months after ablation.[17] For those with tachycardia-related cardiomyopathy, a recovery of left ventricular size and function has been reported.[18,19]

A meta-analysis of clinical outcomes after AV junctional ablation and pacing in 1181 patients reported in 21 studies demonstrated improvements in quality of life, ejection fraction, and exercise time.[20] Symptoms and health care utilization were decreased. Total mortality in this study was 6% at 1 year, and in long-

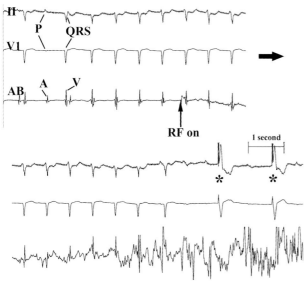

FIGURE 14–5. Induction of complete heart block by ablation of the fast and slow pathway atrioventricular (AV) nodal inputs. Electrocardiographic leads II and V₁ and the ablation (AB) electrograms are shown in this continuous tracing. A clear His recording could not be obtained in this patient. This recording was made after attempts at ablation of the proximal His bundle by anatomic guidance resulted only in fast pathway ablation and a very long PR interval of 600 msec. At the start of the tracing, there is a blocked P wave in sinus rhythm, revealing the very long PR interval. With radiofrequency energy delivery to the slow pathway region (RF on), there is the development of complete AV block and a ventricular paced rhythm (*). A, atrial electrogram; P, P wave; QRS, QRS interval; RF, radiofrequency energy; V, ventricular electrogram.

TABLE 14-1
Targets for Ablation

Distal AV Node–Proximal His Junction (Right-sided Approach)
Small His electrogram (≤0.15 mV)
A/V ratio 1:1 or 1:2

Left-sided His bundle
H-V interval >30-40 msec
A/V ratio approximately 1:10
Site <1-1.5 cm below aortic valve

Compact AV Node
Site proximal and slightly inferior to His catheter in Koch's triangle
A/V ratio 1:1 or 1:2

Bundle Branches
Right Bundle Branch Absent or minimal atrial electrogram BB-V interval <30-35 msec
Left Bundle Branch A/V ratio ≤1:10 BB-V interval ≤20 msec Site approximately 1-1.5 cm below aortic valve

AV, atrioventricular; A/V ratio, atrial-to-ventricular electrogram ratio; BB, bundle branch.

term follow-up it was similar to that in the general population with AF.[21]

Complications directly related to the ablation procedure are rare, especially with right-sided procedures. The risk of postablation polymorphic ventricular arrhythmias has largely been eliminated by programming the pacemaker lower rate limit to 80 to 90 bpm after the procedure (see earlier discussion). Alterations in pacemaker function are common during RF delivery and include inhibition, asynchronous pacing, and induction of pacemaker-mediated tachycardia.[25,29] Interference may be enhanced in unipolar pacing systems. Problems persisting after termination of RF delivery are uncommon but include persistent reset mode requiring reprogramming, elevation of pacing or sensing thresholds, and direct damage to pacemaker leads.[25] For these reasons, permanent pacemakers should be thoroughly evaluated both before and after ablation.

Troubleshooting the Difficult Case

AV junctional ablation is usually a simple and straightforward procedure. It is perhaps this fact that compounds the operator's frustration when a case becomes difficult. The most common problem encountered is the inability to record a clear His potential. This may result from an intramyocardial course of the His bundle or from obfuscation of the His by scar or fibrosis (e.g., from prior surgery). In this instance, localization of the His bundle may be facilitated by use of a separate multipolar mapping catheter. A systematic search of the septum inferiorly and superiorly at variable extents into the ventricle often reveals its location. Pacing from the distal ablation electrodes at high output may identify areas of QRS narrowing, identifying His capture. The continuous atrial activity of AF may obscure the proximal His recording. By cardioversion, even if brief, the His may become apparent. The inability to record the His is a frequent problem after delivery of multiple ineffective lesions to the target area. The resulting edema and tissue swelling may physically distance the ablation catheter from the target tissue. This problem is best avoided by careful mapping and selective RF delivery only to favorable sites with stable catheter positions. If the His can not be identified by any means, anatomically based lesions may be attempted from the right side of the heart before left-sided ablation is attempted. In this instance, the use of irrigated-tip or large-tip catheters may compensate for the absence of precise mapping. A line of lesions on the septum perpendicular to the course of the His bundle may be effective (Fig. 14–6).

Despite clear His recordings, RF lesions may fail to induce heart block. This typically results from unstable catheter positions or poor tissue contact. The use of long preformed sheaths with septal angulation can be very helpful, especially in the setting of enlarged cardiac chambers. The use of irrigated-tip or large-tip catheters coupled with high-output genera-

tors is sometimes necessary. If heart block cannot be achieved from the right ventricle, the left ventricular approach should be tried. If this also fails to target the compact AV node, individual bundle branches or AV nodal inputs are possible.

Loss of ventricular pacing may interrupt an otherwise successful lesion delivery. For patients with permanent pacemakers, reprogramming to VOO mode is usually corrective. Pacemakers should be interrogated fully before ablation, to assess thresholds and battery status. If near elective replacement indicators, reversion to magnet noise or reset mode may result in loss of capture. Rarely, damage to pacing leads or to the electrode-tissue interface can result in more lasting problems. Loss of pacing from temporary pacing leads is usually the result of lead dislodgement. If the ablation catheter is preset for pacing from the distal electrodes, the catheter can readily be advanced into the ventricle for pacing if the other systems fail. Common problems to AV junctional ablation and their solutions are listed in Table 14–2.

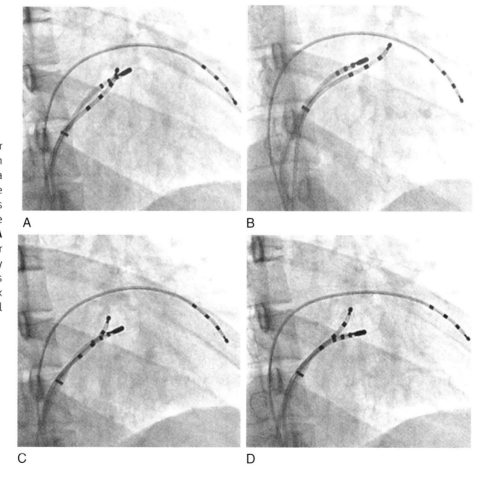

FIGURE 14–6. Right anterior oblique views of ablation catheter positions to create a linear lesion perpendicular to the estimated course of the His bundle when the His bundle cannot be recorded. From **A** through **D,** the ablation catheter is moved superiorly to inferiorly with the His catheter as reference. Complete heart block was achieved at the site in panel D.

A

B

C

D

TABLE 14–2

Troubleshooting the Difficult Case

Problem	Cause	Solution
Inability to record His potential	Intramyocardial course or His obscured by scar or fibrosis	Map with multipolar catheter Pace-map from ablation catheter for His capture (QRS narrowing) Create anatomically based linear lesion perpendicular to His Ablate from left ventricle Target compact AV node or AV nodal inputs
	Acute tissue edema from ineffective RF lesions	Careful initial mapping and catheter stability to limit ineffective lesions As above
	His obscured by atrial activity in AF	Cardiovert and reinitiate AF after ablation
Ineffective RF delivery	Poor tissue contact	Use preformed sheath; change catheter reach, curve, or stiffness Overdrive ventricular pacing to reduce cardiac motion Ablate from left ventricle
	Intramyocardial course, insufficient lesion size	Use irrigated RF or large-tip catheter with high-output generator Ablate from left ventricle Ablate right and left bundle branches separately
Loss of pacing during ablation	Pacemaker inhibition from EMI Pacemaker reset mode Displacement of temporary pacemaker wire	Program VOO or asynchronous pacing Check battery status before ablation Careful catheter manipulation; use screw in temporary pacemaker wire, temporary pacing from ablation catheter advanced into right ventricle

AF, atrial fibrillation; AV, atrioventricular; EMI, electromagnetic interference; RF, radiofrequency energy.

Atrioventricular Junction Modification

AV junction modification without causing complete AV block can also be achieved by catheter ablation. It has been reported that selective ablation of the slow pathway of the AV node results in an increase in AV refractoriness and therefore decreases the ventricular rate.[32-39] In practice, the technique is similar to that used for treating AV nodal reentrant tachycardia. Ablation is begun in the slow pathway region of the low posteroseptal right atrium during AF. It is delivered at sites with A/V ratios of 1:2 to 1:4. While the ventricular response is monitored, lesions are delivered in incremental steps superiorly toward the mid-septal area. Ablation is not given at sites in which a His potential is recorded or that exceed 0.02 mV.[38] The end point is reduction of the ventricular response to less than 100 bpm, and ideally to between 60 and 80 bpm. At this point, an isoproterenol or atropine challenge may be administered and ablation contin-

ued until the heart rate is less than 120 bpm during the pharmacologic stress.[36] The patient should be monitored for 24 to 72 hours after the procedure for recurrences of rapid ventricular rates (which are not uncommon), excessively slow rates, and AV block or polymorphic ventricular arrhythmias. AV junction modification leads to satisfactory ventricular rate control in 25% to 85% of patients.[32-41]

Complications of the procedure include AV block necessitating permanent pacing in as many as 21% of patients.[41] The onset of complete AV block may be delayed for days after the procedure.[38] The occurrence of transient high-grade AV block during the ablation procedure may identify those at risk for late heart block.[38] The occurrence of repolarization abnormalities with polymorphic ventricular tachycardia has also been documented after AV nodal modification without pacemaker implantation.[38]

This technique has been largely abandoned because of the high incidence of AV block and polymorphic ventricular arrhythmias, both of which may occur days after the procedure.[38] These problems are overcome by the presence of a permanent pacemaker, the avoidance of which is the primary benefit of AV junctional modification. In addition, there have been consistent benefits to complete AV junctional ablation and pacing in the literature, with no reported superiority of the AV nodal modification approach.[20,40]

References

1. Kannel WB, Abbott RD, Savage DD, et al.: Epidemiologic features of atrial fibrillation. N Engl J Med 306:1018-1022, 1982.

2. Alpert JS, Petersen P, Godtfredsen J: Atrial fibrillation: Natural history, complications and management. Ann Rev Med 39:41-52, 1988.

3. Van Gelder IC, Hagens VE, Bosker HA, et al., and Rate Control versus Electrical Cardioversion for Persistent Atrial Fibrillation Study Group: A comparison of rate control and rhythm control in patients with recurrent persistent atrial fibrillation. N Engl J Med 347:1834-1840, 2002.

4. Wyse DG, Waldo AL, DiMarco JP, et al.: Atrial Fibrillation Follow-up Investigation of Rhythm Management (AFFIRM) Investigators. A comparison of rate control and rhythm control in patients with atrial fibrillation. N Engl J Med 347:1825-1833, 2002.

5. Curtis AB, Kutalek SP, Prior M, et al.: Prevalence and characteristics of escape rhythms after radiofrequency ablation of the atrioventricular junction: Results from the registry for AV junction ablation and pacing in atrial fibrillation. Ablate and Pace Trial Investigators. Am Heart J 139:122-125, 2000.

6. Natale A, Zimerman L, Tomassoni G, et al.: Impact on ventricular function and quality of life of transcatheter ablation of the atrioventricular junction in chronic atrial fibrillation with a normal ventricular response. Am J Cardiol 78:1431-1433, 1996.

7. Evans T, Scheinman M, Zipes D, et al.: The percutaneous cardiac mapping and ablation registry: Final summary of results. Pacing Clin Electrophysiol 11:1621-1626, 1988.

8. Evans T, Scheinman M, Bardy G, et al.: Predictors of in-hospital mortality after direct current catheter ablation of atrioventricular junction: Results of a prospective, international, multicenter study. Circulation 84:1924-1937, 1991.

9. Simantirakis EN, Vardakis KE, Kochiadakis GE, et al.: Left ventricular mechanics during right ventricular apical or left ventricular-based pacing in patients with chronic atrial fibrillation after atrioventricular junction ablation. J Am Coll Cardiol 43:1013-1018, 2004.

10. Sousa O, Gursoy S, Simonis F, et al.: Right-sided versus left-sided radiofrequency ablation of the His bundle. Pacing Clin Electrophysiol 15:1454-1459, 1992.

11. Sousa J, El-Atassi R, Rosenheck S, et al.: Radiofrequency catheter ablation of the atrioventricular junction from the left ventricle. Circulation 84:567-571, 1991.

12. Cuello C, Huang SKS, Wagshal AB, et al.: Radiofrequency catheter ablation of the atrioventricular junction by a supravalvular non-coronary aortic cusp approach. Pacing Clin Electrophysiol 17:1182-1185, 1994.

13. Brignole M, Gianfranchi L, Menozzi C, et al.: Assessment of atrioventricular junction ablation and DDDR mode-switching pacemaker versus pharmacological treatment in patients with severely symptomatic paroxysmal atrial fibrillation a randomized controlled study. Circulation 96:2617-2624, 1997.

14. Fitzpatrick AP, Kourouyan HD, Siu A, et al.: Quality of life and outcomes after radiofrequency His-bundle catheter ablation and permanent pacemaker implantation: Impact of treatment in paroxysmal and established atrial fibrillation. Am Heart J 131:499-507, 1996.

15. Buys EM, Hemel NM, Kelder JC, et al.: Exercise capacity after his bundle ablation and rate response ventricular pacing for drug refractory chronic atrial fibrillation. Heart 77:238-241, 1997.

16. Rodriguez LM, Smeets JL, Xie B, et al.: Improvement in left ventricular function by ablation of atrioventricular nodal conduction in selected patients with lone atrial fibrillation. Am J Cardiol 72:1137-1141, 1993.

17. Brignole M, Menozzi C, Gianfranchi L, et al.: Assessment of atrioventricular junction ablation and VVIR pacemaker versus pharmacological treatment in patients with heart failure and chronic atrial fibrillation: A randomized, controlled study. Circulation 98:953-960, 1998.

18. Redfield MM, Kay GN, Jenkins LS, et al.: Tachycardia-related cardiomyopathy: A common cause of ventricular dysfunction in patients with atrial fibrillation referred for atrioventricular ablation. Mayo Clin Proc 75:790-795, 2000.

19. Lemery R, Brugada P, Cheriex E, Wellens HJ: Reversibility of tachycardia-induced left ventricular dysfunction after closed-chest catheter ablation of the atrioventricular junction for intractable atrial fibrillation. Am J Cardiol 60:1406-1408, 1987.

20. Wood MA, Brown-Mahoney C, Kay GN, Ellenbogen KA: Clinical outcomes after ablation and pacing therapy for atrial fibrillation: A meta-analysis. Circulation 101:1138-1144, 2000.

21. Ozcan C, Jahangir A, Friedman PA, et al.: Long-term survival after ablation of the atrioventricular node and implantation of a permanent pacemaker in patients with atrial fibrillation. N Engl J Med 344:1043-1051, 2001.

22. Willems R, Wyse DG, Gillis AM, and Atrial Pacing Periablation for Paroxysmal Atrial Fibrillation (PA3) Study Investigators. Total atrioventricular nodal ablation increases atrial fibrillation burden in patients with paroxysmal atrial fibrillation despite continuation of antiarrhythmic drug therapy. J Cardiovasc Electrophysiol 14:1296-1301, 2003.

23. Gianfranchi L, Brignole M, Menozzi C, et al.: Progression of permanent atrial fibrillation after atrioventricular junction ablation and dual-chamber pacemaker implantation in patients with paroxysmal atrial tachyarrhythmias. Am J Cardiol 81:351-354, 1998.

24. Wood MA, Curtis AB, Takle-Newhouse TA, et al.: Survival of DDD pacing mode after atrioventricular junction ablation and pacing for refractory atrial fibrillation. Am Heart J 137:682-685, 1999.

25. Buurke MC, Kopp DE, Alberts M, et al.: Effects of radiofrequency current on previously implanted pacemaker and defibrillator lead systems. J Electrocardiol 34(Suppl):143-148, 2001.

26. Gillis AM, Connolly SJ, Lacombe P, et al.: Randomized crossover comparison of DDDR versus VDD pacing after atrioventricular junction ablation for prevention of atrial fibrillation: The Atrial Pacing Periablation for Paroxysmal Atrial Fibrillation (PA3) Study Investigators. Circulation 102:736-741, 2000.

27. Darpo B, Walfridsson H, Aunes M, et al.: Incidence of sudden death after radiofrequency ablation of the atrioventricular junction for atrial fibrillation. Am J Cardiol 80:1174-1177, 1997.

28. Ozcan C, Jahangir A, Friedman PA, et al.: Sudden death after radiofrequency ablation of the atrioventricular node in patients with atrial fibrillation. J Am Coll Cardiol 40:105-110, 2002.

29. Sadoul N, Blankoff I, de Chillou C, et al.: Effects of radiofrequency catheter ablation on patients with permanent pacemakers. J Interv Card Electrophysiol 1:227-233,1997.

30. Geelen P, Brugada J, Andries E, et al.: Ventricular fibrillation and sudden death after radiofrequency ablation of the atrioventricular junction for atrial fibrillation. Pacing Clin Electrophysiol 20:343-348, 1997.

31. Dubuc M, Khairy P, Rodriguez-Santiago A, et al.: Catheter cryoablation of the atrioventricular node in patients with atrial fibrillation: A novel technology for ablation of cardiac arrhythmias. J Cardiovasc Electrophysiol 12:439-444, 2001.
32. Tebbenjohanns J, Schumacher B, Korte T, et al.: Bimodal RR interval distribution in chronic atrial fibrillation: Impact of dual atrioventricular nodal physiology on long-term rate control after catheter ablation of the posterior atrionodal input. J Cardiovasc Electrophysiol 11:497-503, 2000.
33. Blanck Z, Dhala AA, Sra J, et al.: Characterization of atrioventricular nodal behavior and ventricular response during atrial fibrillation before and after a selective slow-pathway ablation. Circulation 91:1086-1094, 1995.
34. Della Bella P, Carbucicchio C, Tondo C, et al.: Modulation of atrioventricular conduction by ablation of the "slow" atrioventricular node pathway in patients with drug-refractory atrial fibrillation or flutter. J Am Coll Cardiol 25:39-46, 1995.
35. Menozzi C, Brignole M, Gianfranchi L, et al.: Radiofrequency catheter ablation and modulation of atrioventricular conduction in patients with atrial fibrillation. Pacing Clin Electrophysiol 17:2143-2149, 1994.
36. Feld G: Radiofrequency catheter ablation versus modification of the AV node for control of rapid ventricular response in atrial fibrillation. J Cardiovasc Electrophysiol 6:217-228, 1995.
37. Canby RC, Roman CA, Kessler DJ, et al.: Selective radiofrequency ablation of the "slow" atrioventricular nodal pathway for control of the ventricular response to atrial fibrillation. Am J Cardiol 77:1358-1361, 1996.
38. Morady F, Hasse C, Strickberger A, et al.: Long-term follow-up after radiofrequency modification of the atrioventricular node in patients with atrial fibrillation. J Am Coll Cardiol 27:113-121, 1997.
39. Fleck RP, Chen PS, Boyce K, et al.: Radiofrequency modification of atrioventricular conduction by selective ablation of the low posterior septal right atrium in a patient with atrial fibrillation and a rapid ventricular response. Pacing Clin Electrophysiol 16:377-381, 1993.
40. Proclemer A, Della Bella P, Tondo C, et al.: Radiofrequency ablation of atrioventricular junction and pacemaker implantation versus modulation of atrioventricular conduction in drug refractory atrial fibrillation. Am J Cardiol 83:1437-1442, 1999.
41. Williamson BD, Ching Man K, Daoud E, et al.: Radiofrequency catheter modification of atrioventricular conduction to control the ventricular rate during atrial fibrillation. N Engl J Med 331:910-917, 1993.

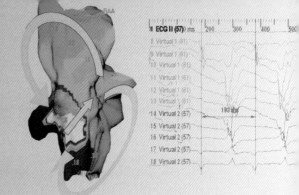

15

Pulmonary Vein Isolation for Atrial Fibrillation

Prashanthan Sanders • *Mélèze Hocini* • *Pierre Jaïs*
Chrishan J. Nalliah • *Yoshihide Takahashi*
Li-Fern Hsu Thomas Rostock • *Martin Rotter*
Fréderic Sacher Jacques Clémenty • *Michel Haïssaguerre*

Key Points

- The mechanism of pulmonary vein (PV) related atrial fibrillation (AF) is uncertain; possible causes are automaticity, triggered activity, and/or reentry.

- Diagnosis is made from the basic criteria for AF and by identifying the arrhythmogenic vein.

- Ablation targets include sites of ectopic activity triggering AF, PV potentials for PV isolation, and atrial myocardium for substrate modification.

- Special equipment that may be used includes circumferential PV mapping catheters, irrigated ablation catheters (to provide reliable achievement of desired power delivery), computerized catheter navigational and mapping systems (optional but can be useful), and echocardiography to exclude preprocedural thrombus (which has also been proposed to be useful for monitoring ablation and catheter positions).

- In general, 60% to 75% of patients with paroxysmal AF will be arrhythmia free without antiarrhythmic drugs after PV ablation.

- The success rate is significantly less for patients with persistent or permanent AF.

Atrial fibrillation (AF) is the most frequent sustained cardiac arrhythmia affecting humans. It has a prevalence of 2% in the unselected adult population and increases with each decade of life. The clinically apparent manifestations of this condition result from thromboembolic complications, loss of atrial systole, and tachycardia-mediated atrial and ventricular cardiomyopathy.[1,2] In addition, AF is associated with an increased mortality rate in both men and women.[3] Although antiarrhythmic drugs have been the mainstay of treatment for AF, their limited efficacy and potential for significant adverse effects have led to a renewed interest in rate control measures, stimulated by publication of the Atrial Fibrillation Follow-Up Investigation of Rhythm Management (AFFIRM),[4] the Rate Control versus Electrical Cardioversion (RACE),[5] and the Pharmacological Intervention in Atrial Fibrillation (PIAF)[6] trials, which suggested an equivalent outcome for pharmacologic rhythm and rate control strategies. However, these findings have highlighted the fact that the benefits of sinus rhythm can be negated by the deleterious effects of antiarrhythmic drugs. A further analysis of the AFFIRM results demonstrated that sinus rhythm was associated with a 47% lower risk of death, whereas the use of antiarrhythmic drugs significantly increased mortality risk by 49%.[7] Therefore, restoration and maintenance of sinus rhythm is of potential benefit if it can be achieved without the use of antiarrhythmic drugs, and this fact underscores the need to strive for the development of nonpharmacologic treatments to achieve and maintain sinus rhythm.

Pulmonary Vein as a Source of Triggers Initiating Atrial Fibrillation

Clinical AF results from the complex interaction of triggers with the perpetuators and substrate predisposing to AF.[8] Although a number of potential sources of triggers exist, the pulmonary veins (PVs) initiate up to 94% of AF.[9] Ectopic beats from these structures may arise from multiple sites within a given PV or from multiple PVs in the one individual.[10,11] These triggers interact with the atrial substrate by conduction, using discrete or wide fascicles connecting the PV and left atrium (LA); ablation at these connections electrically isolates the PVs (Fig. 15–1). However, even after electrical isolation, up to 33% of PVs have spontaneous dissociated slow rhythms and can sustain spontaneous or induced tachycardia within the PV (Fig. 15–2), further highlighting their arrhythmogenic potential.[12-14]

Pulmonary Veins in the Maintenance of Atrial Fibrillation

PVs have also been implicated in the maintenance of AF in some patients. Jais et al.[15] reported a small series of patients who had irregular rapid focal discharges, which persisted sometimes for hours, days or even longer, driving sustained AF; this represents the true "focally driven AF." These patients were cured of their arrhythmia by focal application of radiofrequency (RF) energy. In these cases, the PVs formed not only the trigger but also the substrate maintaining AF.

More recently, investigators have observed paroxysmal short cycle length activity within the PV during AF and have suggested that this may represent a continual fueling of the fibrillatory process from the PV.[16-18] Such paroxysmal bursts of activity demonstrate a distal-to-proximal activation sequence, implicating the distal PV in their origin.[19] Others have demonstrated a gradient of high-frequency activity emanating from the PVs during paroxysmal AF and have suggested that activity from these structures may maintain AF.[20,21] We have provided further evidence to demonstrate the direct participation of PV activity in the maintenance of paroxysmal AF.[22] PV isolation performed during AF in patients with paroxysmal AF produced progressive slowing of the AF process (prolongation of the AF cycle length measured within the coronary sinus), which varied in extent from vein to vein and from individual to individual, culminating in the termination of AF in 75% of patients.[22] Remarkably, PV isolation in these patients rendered AF noninducible in 57%, providing evidence that the PVs or the PV-LA junction formed the perpetuators and substrate of AF in this significant proportion of patients with paroxysmal AF.[23] In concert, these observations have led us to posit a much greater role of the PVs in the maintenance of AF, which we have termed "the venous wave hypothesis" (Fig. 15–3).[23]

Mechanisms of Pulmonary Vein Arrhythmogenicity

The substrate implicated in the arrhythmogenicity of the PVs is the striated myocardial sleeves that extend a variable distance from the LA into the PVs.[24,25] The mechanisms (automaticity or reentry) by which these

FIGURE 15-1. Gross appearance of myocardial sleeves around the pulmonary veins (PVs). *Dotted lines* indicate the presumed junction between the PV and the left atrium (LA); however, the conical nature of the proximal vein in **A** makes this distinction difficult. In **A,** there is a non-uniform arrangement of the fibers, with terminal finger-like extensions over the vein *(arrows)*. In **B,** the myocardial sleeve is smooth and uniform, with a distinct peripheral termination over the vein. **C,** Histologic section of the muscular extension onto the pulmonary vein. The section highlighted by the box is shown at increased magnification on the right. The tip of the extension contains atrophic myocardial cells embedded in fibrous tissue. *(From Saito T, Waki K, Becker AE: Left atrial myocardial extensions onto pulmonary veins in humans: Anatomic observations relevant for atrial arrhythmias. J Cardiovasc Electrophysiol 11:888-894, 2000, with permission.)*

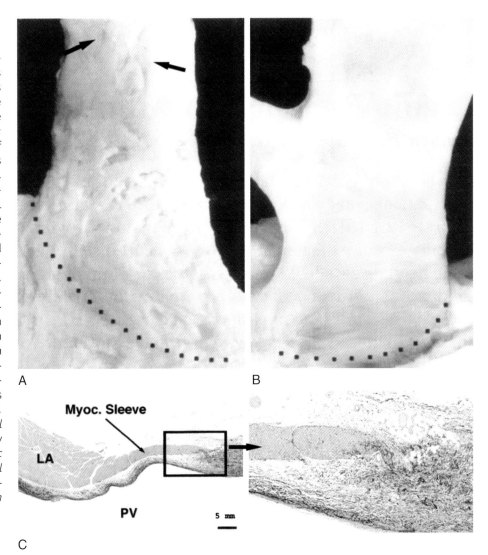

FIGURE 15-2. Persistent rapid, high-frequency bursts of activity in the isolated pulmonary vein (PV), indicating its role in maintaining this patient's atrial fibrillation. Note that the atria are in sinus rhythm, as shown on the surface electrocardiographic leads (I, II, III, and V1).

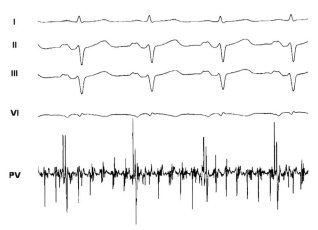

structures are arrhythmogenic are still the subject of intense research.

Studies have suggested that larger or dilated PVs may be a marker of arrhythmogenicity at the time of ablation.[26] This hypothesis is further corroborated by evidence suggesting that patients with AF have significantly larger PV diameters than do those without AF.[27,28] These findings have been extended by the demonstration of structural changes within the PVs of patients with AF, with greater degrees of discontinuous myocardium, hypertrophic myocytes, and fibrosis,[29] suggesting that dilatation may in fact be a marker of such structural changes that are capable of promoting PV arrhythmogenesis.

Several experimental studies have demonstrated that the PV musculature is capable of generating electrical impulses independently due to abnormal automaticity (either early or delayed afterdepolariza-

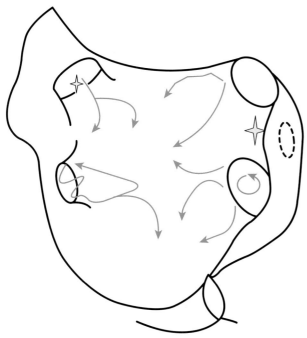

FIGURE 15–3. Schematic diagram demonstrating the "venous wave hypothesis," highlighting the role of focal activity or reentry within the pulmonary vein or at the pulmonary vein–left atrium junction in the initiation and maintenance of atrial fibrillation.

tion) under certain conditions.[30-32] In addition, the complex muscle fibers that interdigitate with fibrous tissue create areas of non-uniform anisotropy that have implicated this region in supporting reentry.[30,33,34]

Clinical studies have shown that the PVs and the PV-LA region have distinctive electrophysiologic properties. Chen et al.[35] demonstrated that the distal PV has significantly shorter refractory periods than the adjacent LA. Jais et al.[36] demonstrated significantly shorter effective refractory periods of the PV (as short as 80 msec in some) in patients with paroxysmal AF compared with patients without a history of AF. In addition, those patients with AF had, more frequently and to a greater degree, decremental conduction to the LA with a tendency for PV extrastimuli to initiate AF. In a clinical study of patients with known AF, Kumagai et al.[37] extended these observations by demonstrating preferential conduction, unidirectional conduction block, and reentry within the PVs. These clinical studies have implicated reentry as the predominant mechanism of PV arrhythmogenesis.

Catheter Ablation of the Pulmonary Veins

An accumulating body of evidence has demonstrated the value of ablation targeting the PVs for cure of AF. Ablation of these structures forms the central theme in all strategies currently used for AF ablation. Current indications for curative ablation of AF are limited to patients who remain symptomatic despite the use of antiarrhythmic agents (Table 15–1). The group in whom PV isolation alone achieves the greatest benefit consists of those patients with short episodes (<24 hours) of paroxysmal AF who have no evidence of structural heart disease and have normal LA size.[14] Accumulating evidence suggests that patients with structural heart disease have diffuse atrial abnormalities that could maintain AF.[38-40] In addition, as the fibrillatory process becomes more established (persistent or permanent AF), the ability of PV ablation alone to clinically suppress arrhythmia is reduced.[41-44] Nevertheless, there is emerging evidence for the wider use of a primary ablation strategy to maintain sinus rhythm in patients.[45]

FOCAL ABLATION OF PULMONARY VEIN TRIGGERS OF ATRIAL FIBRILLATION

Initially, catheter ablation was performed by identifying the arrhythmogenic PV, so as to target ablation at the site of earliest activation during spontaneous ectopy.[9] To identify the culprit vein, several strategies were employed. Studies characterizing the morphology of the ectopic P wave have facilitated recognition of the arrhythmogenic PV.[50,51] These features have been extended to recognize the characteristic endocardial activation sequence, in a bid to guide mapping.[51,52] Other researchers have positioned

TABLE 15–1
Selection of Patients for Ablation of Atrial Fibrillation
Established indication
Symptomatic AF refractory to antiarrhythmic treatment[46]
Evolving indications
AF complicating congestive heart failure[47,48]
Prolonged pauses after termination of AF and the bradycardia-tachycardia syndrome[45,49]
Possibly patients with complications related to AF

AF, atrial fibrillation.

multiple catheters within several of the PVs and mapped the earliest activity during spontaneous ectopy or during the use of pacing maneuvers and isoproterenol.[35,53]

Our initial experience using this strategy was in patients with frequent spontaneous ectopy, bursts of atrial tachycardia, and paroxysmal AF (Fig. 15–4). Of 45 patients, spontaneous ectopy was mapped in 94% to the distal PV, with depolarization marked by a spike (PV potential) preceding the onset of atrial activation.[9] RF ablation at this earliest site resulted in acute abolition of atrial ectopy, and, after 8 ± 6 months, 62% of these patients remained free of AF without the use of antiarrhythmic agents. However, although this technique was a useful strategy in this highly selected group of patients, its applicability has been limited by the infrequency or complete lack of spontaneous ectopy during the procedure in many patients. It also became evident that, in many patients with AF, multiple PVs and multiple sites within a given PV could give rise to spontaneous triggers,[10] necessitating further procedures.[54,55] Improved understanding of the mechanisms of PV arrhythmogenicity and the limited outcomes of focal ablation in the broader population has led to curative AF ablation techniques that have progressively evolved to ostial and even atrial ablation aimed at electrical isolation of all PVs.

PULMONARY VEIN ISOLATION

Circumferential mapping has enabled determination of the perimetric distribution and activation sequence of PV activity, with PV potentials signifying the location and extent of the local striated muscle that electrically connects the PV to the LA.[56] The electrophysiologic features of PV potentials are listed in Table 15–2.

In general, these potentials are sharp, of high frequency, and of short duration (<50 msec). The recog-

TABLE 15–2
Electrophysiologic Features of Pulmonary Vein Potentials
Rapid, high-frequency initial deflection
Short duration (<50 msec)
Follows far-field atrial electrogram during atrial pacing
Precedes far-field atrial electrogram during pulmonary vein pacing

From Tada H, Oral H, Greenstein R, et al. Differentiation of atrial and pulmonary vein potentials recorded circumferentially within pulmonary veins. J Cardiovasc Electrophysiol 13:118-123, 2002, with permission.

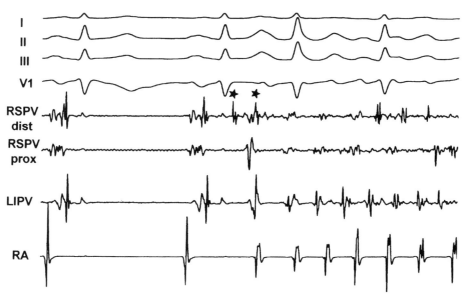

FIGURE 15–4. Initiation of atrial fibrillation by a premature atrial contraction (PAC) originating from the right superior pulmonary vein (RSPV). After the second sinus beat, there is a high-frequency pulmonary vein (PV) potential *(first star)* in the RSPV that precedes the onset of the ectopic P wave. The low-frequency atrial potential follows the PV potential associated with the PAC but precedes the PV potential associated with the sinus beats, indicating a reversal of the activation sequence. A second high-frequency PV potential *(second star)* follows the first by 160 msec. I, II, III, and V1 are surface electrocardiographic leads. dist, distal; prox, proximal; LIPV, left inferior pulmonary vein; RA, right atrium. *(From Haissaguerre M, Jais P, Shah DC, et al.: Catheter ablation of chronic atrial fibrillation targeting the reinitiating triggers. J Cardiovasc Electrophysiol 11:2-10, 2000, with permission.)*

nition of PV potentials as separate from local and far-field atrial potentials is facilitated by comparing the activation timing relative to adjacent structures and by pacing from these structures.[57] During pacing from a site generating a far-field electrogram on the circumferential mapping catheter, the potential is anticipated. Far-field potentials may contribute to the potentials recorded on the circumferential mapping catheter from the left atrial appendage or the adjacent atria, and pacing to differentiate these potentials may be performed from the atrium, the coronary sinus, or the left atrial appendage. During pacing within the PV itself, the PV potentials follow closely after the pacing artifact and are followed by the atrial electrograms after delayed conduction out of the vein.

By sequential ablation at sites of earliest activity, the PVs can be electrically isolated from the LA. The technique involves gravitating circumferentially around the PV, applying longer RF energy at sites that change PV activation; these sites represent critical connections between the PV and LA. Ablation can be started in either right or left PVs and can be performed individually or en bloc, particularly if two or three ostia are coalescent.[14,56,58] It is started at the posterior wall and then continued around the venous perimeter. When ablation is performed along the anterior and inferior aspects of the left PVs, infringement of the PV is frequently required to achieve catheter stability, because the ridge separating the left PV from the appendage is relatively narrow and prohibits stability during ablation in the beating heart. In this latter situation, we use reduced power (25 to 30 W) and perform ablation at critical PV-LA connections by mapping the earliest PV activity.

LOCALIZATION OF ABLATION

Although there has been debate as to the extent of the ostium that is incorporated by various ablation strategies, defining the PV-LA junction is relatively semantic, because, even anatomically, this junction is funnel shaped and a continuum (Fig. 15–5). Nevertheless, identifying the most proximal part of the PV (the ostium) is useful to minimize the risk of PV stenosis and to eliminate a larger portion of the PV-LA ostia that may participate in the fibrillatory process. Identification of the ostia can be achieved in a number of ways (see later discussion). However, although increasingly wider atrial ablation with longer RF application is being advocated, this approach needs to be balanced with the potential for creating an isthmus along the posterior wall that can then support reentry.[59]

NAVIGATION DURING RADIOFREQUENCY ABLATION

Proximal ablation is facilitated with the use of selective PV angiography, intracardiac echocardiography, and three-dimensional mapping systems (Fig. 15–6). Although the use of circumferential mapping provides not only electrophysiologic guidance but also an anatomic framework for PV ablation, navigational tools may further assist this process. Any combination of these tools may be used to ensure the comfort of the operator during PV isolation, which in most experienced centers is being performed within 1 to 2 hours.

Knowledge of the PV anatomy provided by computed tomography or magnetic resonance imaging is useful, particularly in the presence of anatomic variation. Catheter tracking systems such as CARTO (Biosense Webster, Baldwin Park, Calif.), NavX (Endocardial Solutions, St. Paul, Minn.), LocaLisa (Medtronic, Minneapolis, Minn.), or RPM (Boston Scientific, San Jose, Calif.) are useful for nonfluoroscopic monitoring of the catheter position and to tag regions being ablated[60,61] (Table 15–3). Intracardiac

TABLE 15–3
Tools Used during Pulmonary Vein Isolation for Atrial Fibrillation
Mapping
Point-by-point mapping using a rove catheter[11]
Circumferential catheter mapping (Lasso)[56]
Basket catheter mapping[63]
Navigation
Fluoroscopic guidance
LocaLisa catheter tracking (Medtronic)[60]
NavX (Endocardial Solutions)[61]
Electroanatomic mapping (CARTO, Biosense Webster)[64]
Intracardiac echocardiography (AcuNav, Siemens Medical, Malvern, Pa.)[58]
Other
Ablation
Conventional 4-mm-tip ablation
8-mm-tip ablation[58]
Internally irrigated ablation
Externally irrigated ablation[65]
Cryoablation
Other investigational modalities

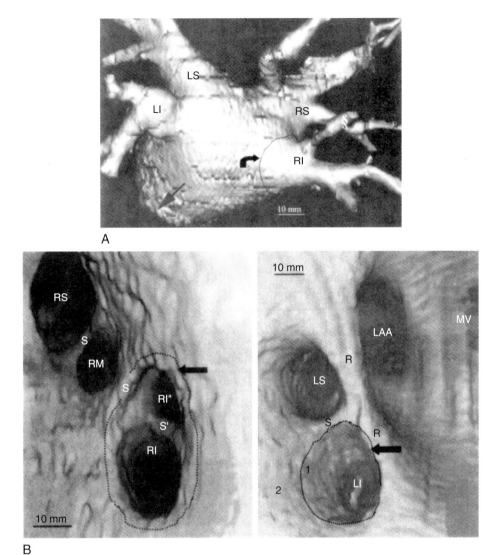

FIGURE 15–5. Computerized tomographic imaging reconstruction of the atrial and pulmonary vein anatomy. **A,** Three-dimensional reconstruction of the left atrium (LA) and pulmonary veins (PVs) viewed from a posterior perspective. LI, left inferior PV; LS, left superior PV; RI, right inferior PV; RS, right superior PV. Note the conical nature of the junctions of the veins with the body of the atrium, which makes definition of a true ostium difficult. **B,** Intra-atrial reconstructed views of the posterior LA. Note the "saddles" (S) between adjacent PVs. The complex, funnel-shaped approaches to the veins are apparent. The position of the inferior venous ostia is denoted by the dotted lines. In this case, it would be preferable to ablate the right PVs together, because they are contiguous. Also demonstrated on the right panel is the narrow ridge that separates the left PVs from the left atrial appendage (LAA). Ablation along this ridge in the beating heart frequently is not possible and necessitates infringing the first component of the PV to achieve stability for ablation. MV, mitral valve; R, ridge between LAA and PVs; RI and RI″, ostia of a complex right inferior PV; RM, right middle PV. The dotted line and arrows indicate the inferior PVs, but note that particularly on the right the superior and inferior PVs are contiguous and require isolation as a pair. Similarly, the antrum of these PVs is more proximal than indicated by the dotted lines. Also note the variation in pulmonary venous anatomy. The asterisk indicates the superior early branching of the RSPV. *(From Schwartzman D, Lacomis J, Wigginton WG: Characterization of left atrium and distal pulmonary vein morphology using multidimensional computed tomography. J Am Coll Cardiol 41:1349-1357, 2003, with permission.)*

echocardiography has been advocated for monitoring the power delivered during these procedures using microbubble formation[58]; however, we have not found this technology to be useful for monitoring power delivery with the externally irrigated catheter. However, it has been useful for performing trans-septal puncture, localizing the PVs, and positioning catheters. In our laboratory, the PV ostia are identified by advancing the catheter into the PV, applying downward deflection of the tip, and then dragging the catheter tip back while monitoring fluoroscopically the fall off the ostial edge. Angiography is performed if further delineation is required.

Another fluoroscopic landmark that is helpful during ablation to localize the PV-LA junction is the right and left border of the spine (in the anteroposte-

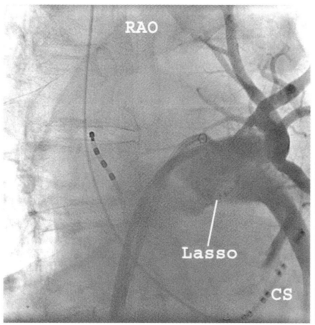

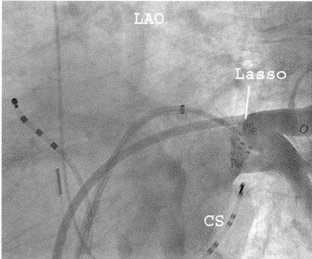

A

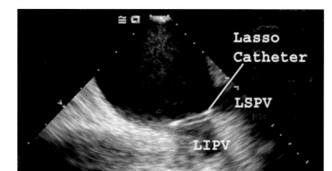

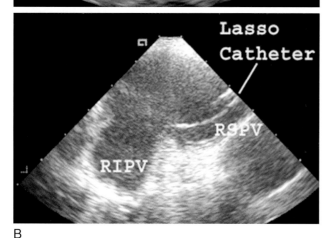

B

FIGURE 15–6. Methods of maintaining the circular mapping catheter at a pulmonary vein (PV) ostium. **A,** Venography. Injection of the left inferior pulmonary vein (LIPV) shows the circular lasso mapping catheter at the ostium of the vein in the right anterior oblique (RAO) and left anterior oblique (LAO) views. CS, coronary sinus catheter. **B,** Intracardiac echocardiography (ICE). Lasso catheter is seen at the ostium of the LIPV in the top panel and at the ostium of the right superior pulmonary vein (RSPV) in the bottom panel. LSPV, left superior pulmonary vein; RIPV, right inferior pulmonary vein. **C,** LocaLisa catheter tracking system (Medtronic). The image shows a representation of the quadripolar ablation catheter in proximity to the representation of the circular mapping catheter in the LSPV. At top left, the ablation catheter tip *(red electrode)* is near electrode 2 of the mapping catheter, which records the earliest PV potentials on bipole 2-3 electrograms *(top right)*. The contact between the ablation catheter and electrodes 2-3 is confirmed by the contact artifact on the electrogram recordings *(asterisk)*. After ablation at this site, the earliest PV activity is shifted to electrodes 4-5 on the mapping catheter electrograms *(bottom right)*. In the bottom left panel, the ablation catheter is shown in approximation with this bipole. *(From Macle L, Jais P, Scavee C, et al.: Pulmonary vein disconnection using the LocaLisa three-dimensional nonfluoroscopic catheter imaging system. J Cardiovasc Electrophysiol 14:693-697, 2003, with permission.)*

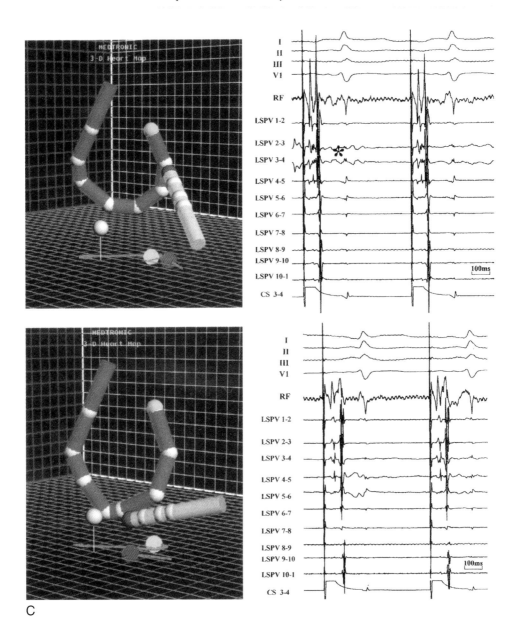

FIGURE 15–6, cont'd

C

rior projection); staying along this border in general ensures that ablation is atrial (1 cm away from both right and left PVs) and thereby minimizes the risk of PV stenosis. The posterior wall of the right PV is reached by turning the catheter counterclockwise; on the left, clockwise rotation is required. If ablation is required at the anterior portions of the left PVs, energy must be delivered within the first few millimeters of the vein (rather than at the posterior wall of the appendage or attempting to balance on the narrow rim of tissue that usually separates these structures) to achieve effective disconnection. A misconception, however, is that the use of these navigation systems prevents or replaces the need for circumferential mapping after ablation and an electrophysiologic end point to the procedure and prevents PV stenosis. In our experience and that of others, anatomically guided coalescent RF lesions are associated with persistent PV potentials in almost half of the patients.[59,62] More importantly, none of these systems is able to exclude the risk of RF delivery within the PVs and the consequent risk of PV stenosis.

At our institution, circumferential mapping is performed with the Lasso catheter (Biosense Webster, Diamond Bar, Calif.) under variable guidance using a combination of fluoroscopy, LocaLisa, NavX, and CARTO systems. Ablation is performed exclusively with an externally irrigated ablation catheter to ensure delivery of the desired power. Ablation is usually performed circumferentially, with longer application at critical sites of the PV-to-LA connection. These sites may be identified as those sites with the earliest PV activity during antegrade conduction

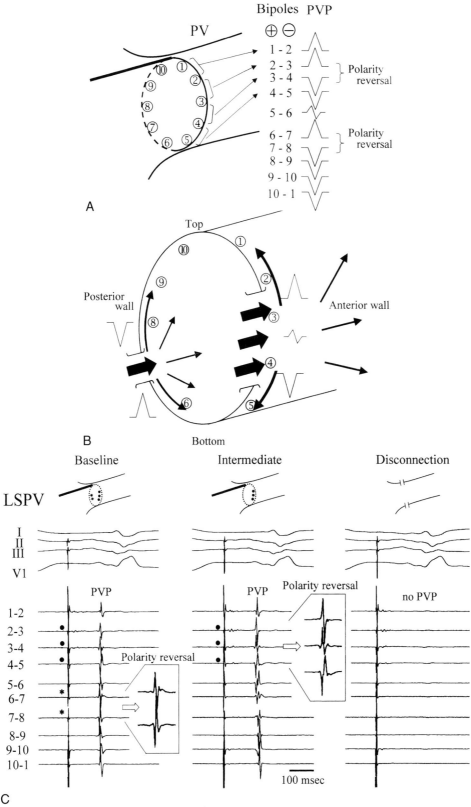

FIGURE 15–7. Electrogram polarity reversal indicating breakthrough from left atrium to pulmonary vein (PV). **A.** A 10-pole circular mapping catheter is represented in the ostium of a PV *(top)*. Polarity reversal is defined as a sudden change in the main deflection of the pulmonary vein potential (PVP). The reversal occurs as the wavefront of activation propagates radially in the PV from its connection with the left atrium *(bottom)*, thus reaching contiguous bipolar recording electrodes in opposing directions. **B and C.** Demonstration of use of electrogram reversal to isolate a left superior pulmonary vein (LSPV) with a wide synchronous breakthrough front. At baseline (left panel), electrogram reversal is identified over lasso bipoles 2-3 to 4-5 *(filled circles)* and between 6-7 and 7-8 *(asterisks)*, consistent with two connection sites to the PV. In the middle panel, RF ablation to bipoles 6-7 and 7-8 has delayed activation of these PVPs, leaving the reversal site between bipoles 2-3 to 4-5. Ablation at this site eliminated all PV potentials (right panel). *(From Yamane T, Shah DC, Jais P, et al.: Electrogram polarity reversal as an additional indicator of breakthroughs from the left atrium to the pulmonary veins. J Am Coll Cardiol 39:1337-1344, 2002, with permission.)*

into the vein, as sites showing electrogram reversal (Fig. 15–7), or as sites at which a change in PV activation occurs during ablation. Targeting of these sites with longer durations of RF application reduces the recurrence of PV conduction, the most common cause of recurrent AF after successful ablation. Other target sites include sites producing atrial ectopy, especially those producing AF, and possibly sites of very-high-frequency atrial activation that are acting as drivers to maintain AF (Fig. 15–8). The potential target sites for AF ablation are listed in Table 15–4.

RADIOFREQUENCY ABLATION

RF energy is the modality most frequently used for ablation. In our institution, the externally irrigated

ablation catheter is routinely used for ablation of AF.[65] Irrigated ablation offers important advantages, allowing higher power delivery, if needed, with a lower risk of char or coagulum formation on both the electrode and the endocardium, and consequently reducing the risk of embolic events during ablation in the LA. This has been particularly useful for delivering adequate power in patients with reduced atrial flow, such as may be encountered in patients with chronic AF.

Ablation is performed with the use of continuous temperature-feedback control of power output to achieve a target temperature of $50°C$. The rate of irrigation is adjusted to between 5 and $20 mL/minute$ to achieve the desired power for ablation. For ablation within the atria, a power of 30 to $35 W$ is delivered; this is reduced to 25 to $30 W$ during ablation within the PV (for the anterior aspect of the left PV). For PV ablation, we deliver RF energy for 30 to 60 seconds at each point, depending on the local effect, and this application is prolonged for 1 to 2 minutes if a change occurs in activation or morphology of the PV potentials, as determined by circumferential mapping recorded downstream (Fig. 15–9). Additional ostial applications targeting fragmented electrograms (more than two deflections) are performed after PV isolation to eliminate any ostial PV potentials and thereby reduce the risk of recurrence due to ostial foci.

TABLE 15–4
Targets for Ablation
Ectopic activity triggering AF
Earliest PV potential activation in PV
All ostial PV potentials
Sites of PV polarity reversal
Possible sites of dominant frequency or rapid activity during AF

AF, atrial fibrillation; PV, pulmonary vein.

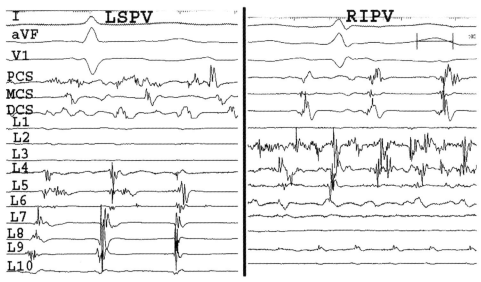

FIGURE 15–8. High-frequency source of electrical activity acting as a driver for atrial fibrillation (AF). During AF, pulmonary vein (PV) potentials in the left superior pulmonary vein (LSPV) were discrete and of low frequency, as seen on lasso (L) bipoles 4-9 with the catheter at the PV os. Electrical isolation of the left PV failed to prevent recurrent AF in the laboratory. In the right inferior pulmonary vein (RIPV), very-high-frequency activity was observed at bipoles 2-4, with almost continuous activity on bipole L2. Ablation of these PV potentials eliminated recurrent AF, suggesting that these sites were drivers for the arrhythmia. I, aVF, and V1, surface electrocardiographic leads. The time scale indicates 100 msec. PCS, proximal coronary sinus; MCS, mid coronary sinus; DCS, distal coronary sinus.

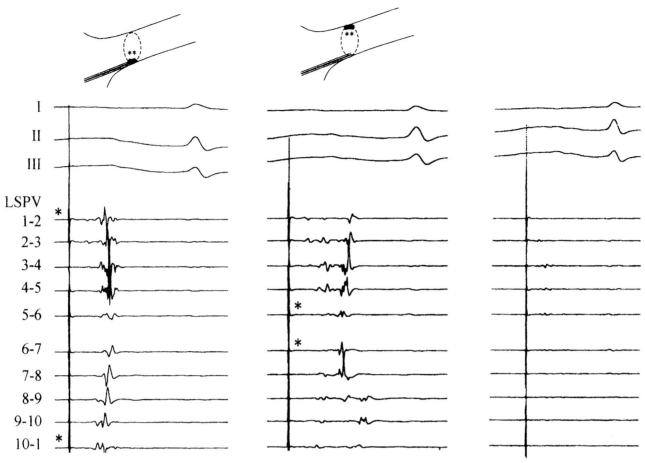

FIGURE 15–9. Change in activation of left superior pulmonary vein (LSPV) potentials with ablation. Bipoles recorded electrograms from the circular mapping catheter at the venous ostium. In the left panel, the earliest pulmonary vein (PV) potentials are recorded at the inferior aspect of the vein, from bipoles 10-1 and 1-2 *(asterisks)*. In the middle panel, after ablation to the inferior aspect of the vein, the PV activation is delayed by 90 msec, and the sequence is changed so that the earliest activation is now at the superior portion of the vein covered by bipoles 5-6 and 6-7 *(asterisks)*. Ablation to these sites eliminated all PV electrical activity (right panel). *(From Haissaguerre M, Shah DC, Jais P, et al.: Electrophysiologic breakthroughs from the left atrium to the pulmonary veins. Circulation 102:2463-2465, 2000, with permission.)*

END POINT AND RESULTS OF ABLATION

Although most groups now agree that lesions around PVs are sufficient to cure a significant proportion of patients with paroxysmal AF, there remains controversy as to whether complete electrical disconnection is superior to incomplete disconnection (Table 15–5).

A purely anatomic approach has been advocated, whereby circumferential lesions are deployed without evaluation of the distal PV potentials.[64,67] With this technique, up to 45% of PVs are not isolated with persistent PV-LA conduction; these PVs remain potentially arrhythmogenic.[59] Although incomplete PV isolation may annihilate the arrhythmogenic potential of PVs at a given percentage of PV-LA conduction delay, the parameters defining this percentage are unknown. Experimental and clinical studies have demonstrated that the PV-LA region is able to

TABLE 15–5
End Points for Ablation of Atrial Fibrillation
Entrance block electrical isolation of all PVs
Exit block electrical isolation of all PVs
Elimination of all atrial ectopic activity
*AF noninducible/nonsustainable
*Elimination of high-frequency "drivers" during AF
Elimination of fractionated electrograms[66]
PV isolation plus completion of linear lesion (e.g., left atrial isthmus line, roof line, anterior line)[43,44]

*Evolving end point.
AF, atrial fibrillation; PV, pulmonary vein.

sustain a variety of potential arrhythmogenic mechanisms, and experience has shown that discrete residual fascicles or prolonged conduction times can still induce AF. In addition, even after isolation, this region is able to produce active rhythm in up to 97% of cases.[12-14] Any interaction between such activity from the PV-LA region and the atria could potentially initiate and maintain AF. Whereas isolation of the PV ensures elimination of this possibility, incomplete isolation provides a spectrum of potential interactions, as reflected in the wide-ranging results observed with a purely anatomic strategy. Pappone et al.,[46] who developed the purely anatomic strategy, reported arrhythmia suppression in 78% of their patients without the use of antiarrhythmic drugs. More recently, however, the experience from their laboratory has supported the conclusion that complete lesions are likely to be superior to incomplete ones.[68] Oral et al.[69] achieved "absence of AF" without the use of antiarrhythmic drugs in 88% of their patients. In contrast, Stabile et al.[70] and Karch et al.[62] reported success rates of 38% and 42%, respectively (i.e., patients in sinus rhythm not treated with antiarrhythmic drugs).

Further evidence corroborating the need for electrical isolation of the PVs has been provided by studies evaluating patients with recurrent AF after PV isolation; these have found that, in almost all patients, recurrence of paroxysmal AF is caused by recovery of PV-LA conduction (Fig. 15–10).[14,22,71]

Despite the insurmountable evidence demonstrating the arrhythmogenicity of the PVs and the potential consequences of PV-LA interactions in the generation and maintenance of arrhythmias, in the absence of studies comparing the outcomes of complete versus incomplete PV isolation, no definitive statement can be made arguing the need for complete PV isolation at this stage. Nevertheless, one could argue theoretically that, whereas incomplete lesions may result in a spectrum of possible PV-LA interactions, complete isolation results in elimination of all such interactions, and, therefore, complete PV isolation should provide at least a similar if not superior efficacy compared with incomplete isolation.

Finally, electrical isolation of the PVs (elimination or dissociation of PV potentials) provides a defined procedural end point that can be achieved in 100% of patients with the use of a cooled-tip catheter. Data

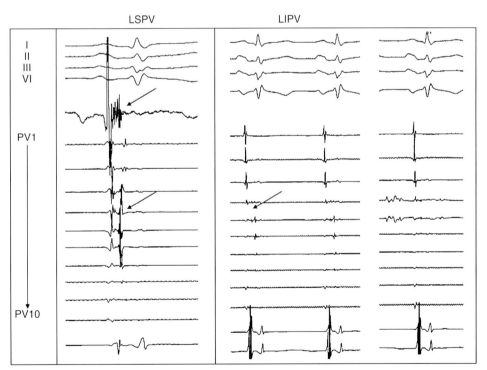

FIGURE 15–10. Mapping of pulmonary veins (PV) in a patient with recurrence of atrial fibrillation (AF) 2 months after PV isolation. In this patient, both the left superior pulmonary vein (LSPV) and the left inferior pulmonary vein (LIPV) demonstrate recovery. The tracing of the LSPV demonstrates the typical appearance of PV conduction slowing, separating the far-field atrial component from the PV potential without the need for pacing the left atrial appendage. Note the continuous slowed activity detected on the ablation catheter at the site of the conduction gap *(arrows)*. A similar finding is observed in the LIPV. The panel on the far right demonstrates ablation at the site of gap (noise on electrograms) and the loss of PV potentials with isolation of the LIPV. Since isolation of both PVs, this patient has not had further AF. Abl, ablation catheter; I, II, III, and V1, electrocardiographic surface leads.

from our institution demonstrate that PV isolation can be achieved with 35 ± 15 minutes of RF energy application and takes 70 ± 21 minutes to perform.[72] Reports of immediate procedural success have ranged from 82% to 100%[14,58,65,71]; however, 27% to 48% of patients develop early recurrence of AF within days after ablation. Patients with early recurrence of AF after PV isolation have been observed to have a significantly lower long-term success rate. In our institution, mapping has demonstrated that 30% of recurrences are caused by recovery of the previously isolated PV, and 70% by non-PV foci. Half of the latter are located chiefly within the LA (posterior wall), in close proximity to the PV ostia, and the remainder are distant from the ablation site (e.g., coronary sinus, superior vena cava, and right atrium). The success of ablation when PV isolation is used as an end point has been remarkably similar in reports from a number of groups.[14,22,58,62,65,73] In our experience, at 10 ± 5 months of follow-up, 69% of patients with paroxysmal AF remained in sinus rhythm without antiarrhythmic drugs.[44] Up to 30% of failed cases have led to additional ablation using lines.[43,44,74,75] Most authors use them during a second procedure for recurrent AF if PV isolation is still complete. In addition, in a selected subset of patients with permanent AF, mapping and ablation of the reinitiating foci after cardioversion has been reported to be successful in up to 60% of cases.[76] However, in most patients with persistent or permanent AF, ablation of the PVs has a limited effect, and these patients require additional substrate modification.[41-44]

COMPLICATIONS OF ABLATION

One of the most concerning complications of these procedures is PV stenosis.[77] The current incidence of angiographic PV stenosis (>50% reduction in PV diameter) is less than 2%, with most patients being asymptomatic. This incidence is reduced significantly with lower-power ostial ablation and operator experience. Of more than 2400 patients having PV ablation in our experience so far, we have observed severe symptomatic PV stenosis (>70%) in only 4 patients, who required PV dilatation and stenting. In addition, 5 of these 2400 patients developed right phrenic nerve injury during ablation of right superior PV, with complete recovery within 8 months.

Ablation anywhere within the atria can result in the creation of conduction abnormalities that then may be able to anchor reentry. After PV isolation alone, we have observed that 12% of patients have inducible macroreentry, and 5% present with spontaneous macroreentry.[78] Mapping and ablation have demonstrated that most of these pathways use the ablated zone as a central obstacle, resulting in either

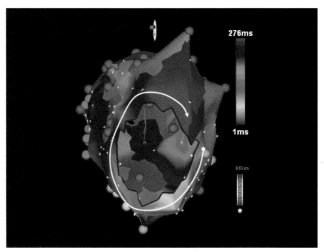

FIGURE 15–11. Perimitral flutter after pulmonary vein (PV) isolation. In this patient, ablation of the mitral isthmus (left inferior PV to lateral mitral annulus) terminated flutter. The image is from an electroanatomic activation map (CARTO, Biosense Webster). ms, microseconds.

perimitral or peri-PV reentry (Fig. 15–11), the latter being more prevalent in patients with larger atria.[78,79] However, there is a subset of these arrhythmias that use the previous ablation lesion or other abnormally conducting zones within the atria to support reentry.[68,80-83] When an anatomic approach to PV encircling has been used, including additional lines, the reported incidence of reentrant arrhythmias has been higher; some groups have reported spontaneous arrhythmias in up to 27% of their patients.[46,59,62,74]

More recently, a rapidly accumulating number of cases of atrial-esophageal fistula are being reported, often associated with a fatal outcome.[84,85] To date, this complication has been observed in patients undergoing an anatomic ablation strategy, with high power (up to 100 W) delivered along the posterior LA via an 8-mm-tip catheter. Although this complication has focused much interest on the position and motility of the esophagus in relation to the LA, it seems likely that this complication is a direct result of the power used during ablation at the posterior LA. We strongly advocate that power be limited to 30 to 35 W during ablation along the posterior LA.

An Individual Rationalized Approach to Ablation

Between 20% and 40% of patients with paroxysmal AF and almost all patients with persistent or permanent AF require additional substrate modification to improve clinical outcome (in terms of eliminating all episodes of AF). However, substrate modification is technically challenging, is associated with increased risk, and can be proarrhythmic in the setting of incomplete lesions.[43,44,86] Although it has been proposed that empiric linear ablation should be used to improve the outcome of AF ablation, we strongly advocate a rationalized approach that targets the individual rather than a "one size fits all" approach to substrate modification in paroxysmal AF.

The ideal modality to individualize our approach is still evolving. It may be based on the cycle length of activation, on the change in cycle length with ablation, on inducibility of the AF, or on clinical outcome.[22] To identify patients who would benefit from PV isolation alone, we have been evaluating the role of the inducibility of AF. We use a standardized protocol of AF induction that consists of burst atrial pacing at maximum output (20 mA) for 5 to 10 seconds, commencing at a cycle length of approximately 250 msec and decreasing to refractoriness. This is performed three times from three sites (left atrial appendage, right atrial appendage, or coronary sinus). Sustained AF, thought to indicate the presence of potential atrial substrate capable of maintaining AF, is defined as AF lasting 10 minutes or longer. Induction of AF is performed before ablation and again after each step of the ablation process (PV isolation and substrate modification). We have found that a significant proportion of patients with paroxysmal AF (up to 57%) have no inducible AF after PV isolation alone. This subset represents a group that will benefit from PV isolation alone and do not require additional substrate modification.

Troubleshooting the Difficult Case

Common difficulties with PV isolation procedures are listed in Table 15–6.

Identification of PV potentials and their differentiation from LA potentials can be accomplished by pacing maneuvers described previously. Unstable ablation or mapping catheter positions may be resolved by changing to mapping catheters with different (or variable) lasso diameters or by the use of preformed sheaths to restrict catheter movement. The use of venography or intracardiac echocardiography may aid in stabilizing the catheter. For patients in whom AF recurs in the laboratory despite complete PV isolation, consideration may be given to substrate modification with linear lesions or targeting of areas of fractionated, high-frequency activity or non-PV foci of ectopic activity.

The elimination PV potentials with ablation at times is difficult. It is important to confirm the nature of the persistent potentials as arising from the PV and not from atrial or far-field sources. Broad or thick muscular connections with the PVs may be difficult to eliminate with focal RF applications. Segmental

---

TABLE 15–6

Troubleshooting the Difficult Case

Problem	Causes	Solutions
Difficult to identify PV potentials	Fusion with atrial electrogram	Determine the activation timing of adjacent structures
	Prominent far-field electrogram	Pacing from adjacent structures (coronary sinus, atrium, or appendage)
PV potentials persist after ablation	Broad/thick PV connection	Prolonged RF delivery; use cooled/irrigated catheter, segmental ablation at ostium
	Connection inserts into contiguous PV	Map/ablate contiguous PV
	Far-field electrogram	Activation timing and pacing from adjacent structures to identify true PV potentials
Unstable catheter positions	Unfavorable PV anatomy	Visualize catheters with ICE or mapping system
Recurrent AF after PV isolation	Non-PV triggers	Map and ablate all triggers
	Arrhythmogenic atrial substrate	Substrate modification with linear lesions or target dominant frequency sources

AF, atrial fibrillation; ICE, intracardiac echocardiography; PV, pulmonary vein; RF, radiofrequency energy.

isolation may be required. The use of cooled or irrigated ablation systems has been helpful to ensure adequate power delivery for ablation of the PVs. Finally, interconnection of muscular fascicles between contiguous PVs may result in inability to ablate the potentials in the vein removed from the fascicles connection with the atrium (Fig. 15–12). By ablating the true atrial connection in an adjacent vein, the refractory potentials may also be eliminated.

in approximately 70% of patients with paroxysmal AF, as well as 20% to 60% of those with persistent or permanent AF. The clinical outcome of ablation can be further improved with the use of additional substrate modification. However, an individually tailored approach to substrate modification based on clinical recurrence or persistent inducibility is advocated.

Conclusion

In patients with paroxysmal AF, PV electrical isolation remains a pivotal strategy. It can technically be achieved in 100% of cases with the use of circumferential mapping, and it is associated with arrhythmia suppression without the use of antiarrhythmic agents

ACKNOWLEDGMENTS

Dr. Sanders is supported by the Neil Hamilton Fairley Fellowship from the National Health and Medical Research Council of Australia and the Ralph Reader Fellowship from the National Heart Foundation of Australia. Mr. Nalliah is supported by the National Heart Foundation of Australia. Dr. Rostock

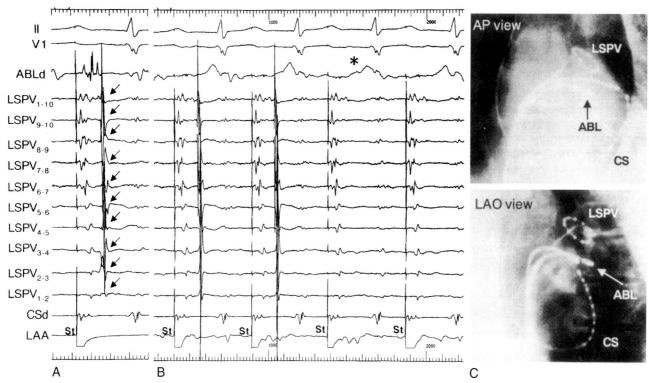

FIGURE 15–12. An example of ablation-induced conduction block between the left atrium (LA) and the left superior pulmonary vein (LSPV) in a patient with electrical connections between the LSPV and the left inferior pulmonary vein (LIPV). **A.** A fractionated potential was recorded from the LIPV ostium during left atrial appendage (LAA) pacing after inability to eliminate the pulmonary vein (PV) potential *(arrows)* with a 1-minute delivery of radiofrequency (RF) energy to the LSPV ostium. 1-2, 2-3, and so on are the circular mapping catheter bipoles. II and V1, electrocardiographic surface leads; ABL, ablation catheter; CS, coronary sinus; d, distal; LAA, left atrial appendage; St, LAA stimulation artifact. **B.** LSPV potentials were eliminated during RF delivery to the anterior aspect of the LIPV ostium. **C.** Radiograms show anteroposterior (AP) and left anterior oblique (LAO) projections of ABL placed at the LIPV ostium and circular catheter placed in the LSPV. *(From Takahashi A, Iesaka Y, Takahashi Y, et al.: Electrical connections between pulmonary veins. Implications for ostial ablation of pulmonary veins in patients with paroxysmal atrial fibrillation. Circulation 105:2998-3003, 2002, with permission.)*

is supported by the German Cardiac Society. Dr. Rotter is supported by the Swiss National Foundation for Scientific Research, Bern, Switzerland.

References

1. Grogan M, Smith HC, Gersh BJ, Wood DL: Left ventricular dysfunction due to atrial fibrillation in patients initially believed to have idiopathic dilated cardiomyopathy. Am J Cardiol 69:1570-1573, 1992.

2. Zipes DP: Atrial fibrillation: A tachycardia-induced atrial cardiomyopathy. Circulation 95:562-564, 1997.

3. Benjamin EJ, Wolf PA, D'Agostino RB, et al.: Impact of atrial fibrillation on the risk of death: The Framingham Heart Study. Circulation 98:946-952, 1998.

4. The Atrial Fibrillation Follow-up Investigation of Rhythm Management (AFFIRM) Investigators: A comparison of rate control and rhythm control in patients with atrial fibrillation. N Engl J Med 347:1825-1833, 2002.

5. Van Gelder IC, Hagens VE, Bosker HA, et al., for the Rate Control Versus Electrical Cardioversion for Persistent Atrial Fibrillation Study Group: A comparison of rate control and rhythm control in patients with recurrent persistent atrial fibrillation. N Engl J Med 347:1834-1840, 2002.

6. Hohnloser SH, Kuck KH, Lilienthal J, for the PIAF Investigators: Rhythm or rate control in atrial fibrillation. Pharmacological Intervention in Atrial Fibrillation (PIAF): A randomised trial. Lancet 356:1789-1794, 2000.

7. The AFFIRM Investigators: Relationships between sinus rhythm, treatment, and survival in the Atrial Fibrillation Follow-up Investigation of Rhythm Management (AFFIRM) study. Circulation 109:1509-1513, 2004.

8. Allessie MA, Boyden PA, Camm AJ, et al.: Pathophysiology and prevention of atrial fibrillation. Circulation 103:769-777, 2001.

9. Haissaguerre M, Jais P, Shah DC, et al.: Spontaneous initiation of atrial fibrillation by ectopic beats originating in the pulmonary veins. N Engl J Med 339:659-666, 1998.

10. Hocini M, Haissaguerre M, Shah D, et al.: Multiple sources initiating atrial fibrillation from a single pulmonary vein identified by a circumferential catheter. Pacing Clin Electrophysiol 23:1828-1831, 2000.

11. Haissaguerre M, Jais P, Shah DC, et al.: Electrophysiological end point for catheter ablation of atrial fibrillation initiated from multiple pulmonary venous foci. Circulation 101:1409-1417, 2000.

12. Weerasooriya R, Jais P, Scavee C, et al.: Dissociated pulmonary vein arrhythmia: Incidence and characteristics. J Cardiovasc Electrophysiol 14:1173-1179, 2003.

13. Takahashi Y, Iesaka Y, Takahashi A, et al.: Reentrant tachycardia in pulmonary veins of patients with paroxysmal atrial fibrillation. J Cardiovasc Electrophysiol 14:927-932, 2003.

14. Ouyang F, Bansch D, Ernst S, et al.: Complete isolation of left atrium surrounding the pulmonary veins: New insights from the double-lasso technique in paroxysmal atrial fibrillation. Circulation 110:2090-2096, 2004.

15. Jais P, Haissaguerre M, Shah DC, et al.: A focal source of atrial fibrillation treated by discrete radiofrequency ablation. Circulation 95:572-576, 1997.

16. Kumagai K, Yasuda T, Tojo H, et al.: Role of rapid focal activation in the maintenance of atrial fibrillation originating from the pulmonary veins. Pacing Clin Electrophysiol 11:1823-1827, 2000.

17. O'Donnell D, Furniss SS, Bourke JP: Paroxysmal cycle length shortening in the pulmonary veins during atrial fibrillation correlates with arrhythmogenic triggering foci in sinus rhythm. J Cardiovasc Electrophysiol 13:124-128, 2002.

18. Oral H, Ozaydin M, Tada H, et al.: Mechanistic significance of intermittent pulmonary vein tachycardia in patients with atrial fibrillation. J Cardiovasc Electrophysiol 13:645-650, 2002.

19. Haissaguerre M, Shah DC, Jais P, et al.: Mapping-guided ablation of pulmonary veins to cure atrial fibrillation. Am J Cardiol 86:K9-K19, 2000.

20. Lazar S, Dixit S, Marchlinski FE, et al.: Presence of left-to-right atrial frequency gradient in paroxysmal but not persistent atrial fibrillation in humans. Circulation 110:3181-3186, 2004.

21. Sanders P, Berenfeld O, Hocini M, et al. Spectral analysis identifies sites of high frequency activity maintaining atrial fibrillation in humans. Circulation 112:789-797, 2005.

22. Haissaguerre M, Sanders P, Hocini M, et al.: Changes in atrial fibrillation cycle length and inducibility during catheter ablation and their relation to outcome. Circulation 109:3007-3013, 2004.

23. Haissaguerre M, Sanders P, Hocini M, et al.: Pulmonary veins in the substrate for atrial fibrillation: The "venous wave" hypothesis. J Am Coll Cardiol 43:2290-2292, 2004.

24. Nathan H, Eliakim M: The junction between the left atrium and the pulmonary veins: An anatomic study of human hearts. Circulation 34:412-422, 1966.

25. Ho SY, Cabrera JA, Tran VH, et al.: Architecture of the pulmonary veins: Relevance to radiofrequency ablation. Heart 86:265-270, 2001.

26. Yamane T, Shah DC, Jais P, et al.: Dilatation as a marker of pulmonary veins initiating atrial fibrillation. J Interv Card Electrophysiol 6:245-249, 2002.

27. Lin WS, Prakash VS, Tai CT, et al.: Pulmonary vein morphology in patients with paroxysmal atrial fibrillation initiated by ectopic beats originating from the pulmonary veins: Implications for catheter ablation. Circulation 101:1274-1281, 2000.

28. Tsao HM, Yu WC, Cheng HC, et al.: Pulmonary vein dilation in patients with atrial fibrillation: Detection by magnetic resonance imaging. J Cardiovasc Electrophysiol 12:809-813, 2001.

29. Hassink RJ, Aretz HT, Ruskin J, Keane D: Morphology of atrial myocardium in human pulmonary veins: A postmortem analysis in patients with and without atrial fibrillation. J Am Coll Cardiol 42:1108-1114, 2003.

30. Hamabe A, Okuyama Y, Miyauchi Y, et al.: Correlation between anatomy and electrical activation in canine pulmonary veins. Circulation 107:1550-1555, 2003.

31. Chen YJ, Chen SA, Chang MS, Lin CI: Arrhythmogenic activity of cardiac muscle in pulmonary veins of the dog: Implication for the genesis of atrial fibrillation. Cardiovasc Res 48:265-273, 2000.

32. Chen YJ, Chen SA, Chen YC, et al.: Effects of rapid atrial pacing on the arrhythmogenic activity of single cardiomyocytes from pulmonary veins: Implication in initiation of atrial fibrillation. Circulation 104:2849-2854, 2001.

33. Hocini M, Ho SY, Kawara T, et al.: Electrical conduction in canine pulmonary veins: Electrophysiological and anatomic correlation. Circulation 105:2442-2448, 2002.

34. Arora R, Verheule S, Scott L, et al.: Arrhythmogenic substrate of the pulmonary veins assessed by high-resolution optical mapping. Circulation 107:1816-1821, 2003.

35. Chen SA, Hsieh MH, Tai CT, et al.: Initiation of atrial fibrillation by ectopic beats originating from the pulmonary veins: Electrophysiological characteristics, pharmacological responses, and effects of radiofrequency ablation. Circulation 100:1879-1886, 1999.

36. Jais P, Hocini M, Macle L, et al.: Distinctive electrophysiological properties of pulmonary veins in patients with atrial fibrillation. Circulation 106:2479-2485, 2002.

37. Kumagai K, Ogawa M, Noguchi H, et al.: Electrophysiologic properties of pulmonary veins assessed using a multielectrode basket catheter. J Am Coll Cardiol 43:2281-2289, 2004.

38. Morton JB, Sanders P, Vohra JK, et al.: The effect of chronic atrial stretch on atrial electrical remodeling in patients with an atrial septal defect. Circulation 107:1775-1782, 2003.

39. Sanders P, Morton JB, Davidson NC, et al.: Electrical remodeling of the atria in congestive heart failure: Electrophysiological and electroanatomic mapping in humans. Circulation 108:1461-1469, 2003.

40. Sanders P, Morton JB, Kistler PM, et al.: Electrophysiological and electroanatomic characterization of the atria in sinus node disease: Evidence of diffuse atrial remodeling. Circulation 109:1514-1522, 2004.

41. Kanagaratnam L, Tomassoni G, Schweikert R, et al.: Empirical pulmonary vein isolation in patients with chronic atrial fibrillation using a three-dimensional nonfluoroscopic mapping system: Long-term follow-up. Pacing Clin Electrophysiol 24:1774-1779, 2001.

42. Oral H, Knight BP, Tada H, et al.: Pulmonary vein isolation for paroxysmal and persistent atrial fibrillation. Circulation 105:1077-1081, 2002.

43. Sanders P, Jais P, Hocini M, et al.: Electrophysiologic and clinical consequence of linear catheter ablation to transect the anterior left atrium in patients with atrial fibrillation. Heart Rhythm 1:176-184, 2004.

44. Jais P, Hocini M, Hsu LF, et al.: Technique and results of linear ablation at the mitral isthmus. Circulation 110:2996-3002, 2004.

45. Hocini M, Sanders P, Deisenhofer I, et al.: Reverse remodeling of sinus node function after catheter ablation of atrial fibrillation in patients with prolonged sinus pauses. Circulation 108:1172-1175, 2003.

46. Pappone C, Rosanio S, Augello G, et al.: Mortality, morbidity, and quality of life after circumferential pulmonary vein ablation for atrial fibrillation: Outcomes from a controlled nonrandomized long-term study. J Am Coll Cardiol 42:185-197, 2003.

47. Chen MS, Marrouche NF, Khaykin Y, et al.: Pulmonary vein isolation for the treatment of atrial fibrillation in patients with impaired systolic function. J Am Coll Cardiol 43:1004-1009, 2004.

48. Hsu LF, Jais P, Sanders P, et al.: Catheter ablation of atrial fibrillation in congestive heart failure. N Engl J Med 351:2373-2383, 2004.

49. Khaykin Y, Marrouche NF, Martin DO, et al.: Pulmonary vein isolation for atrial fibrillation in patients with symptomatic sinus bradycardia or pauses. J Cardiovasc Electrophysiol 15:784-789, 2004.

50. Yamane T, Shah DC, Peng JT, et al.: Morphological characteristics of P waves during selective pulmonary vein pacing. J Am Coll Cardiol 38:1505-1510, 2001.

51. Kistler PM, Sanders P, Fynn SP, et al.: Electrophysiological and electrcardiographic characteristics of focal atrial tachycardia originating from the pulmonary veins: Acute and long-term outcomes of radiofrequency ablation. Circulation 108:1968-1975, 2003.

52. Fynn SP, Morton JB, Deen VR, et al.: Conduction characteristics at the crista terminalis during onset of pulmonary vein atrial fibrillation. J Cardiovasc Electrophysiol 15:855-861, 2004.

53. Hsieh MH, Chen SA, Tai CT, et al.: Double multielectrode mapping catheters facilitate radiofrequency catheter ablation of focal atrial fibrillation originating from pulmonary veins. J Cardiovasc Electrophysiol 10:136-144, 1999.

54. Gerstenfeld EP, Guerra P, Sparks PB, et al.: Clinical outcome after radiofrequency catheter ablation of focal atrial fibrillation triggers. J Cardiovasc Electrophysiol 12:900-908, 2001.

55. Sanders P, Morton JB, Deen VR, et al.: Immediate and long-term results of radiofrequency ablation of pulmonary vein ectopy for cure of paroxysmal atrial fibrillation using a focal approach. Intern Med J 32:202-207, 2002.

56. Haissaguerre M, Shah DC, Jais P, et al.: Electrophysiological breakthroughs from the left atrium to the pulmonary veins. Circulation 102:2463-2465, 2000.

57. Shah D, Haissaguerre M, Jais P, et al.: Left atrial appendage activity masquerading as pulmonary vein potentials. Circulation 105:2821-2825, 2002.

58. Marrouche NF, Martin DO, Wazni O, et al.: Phased-array intracardiac echocardiography monitoring during pulmonary vein isolation in patients with atrial fibrillation: Impact on outcome and complications. Circulation 107:2710-2716, 2003.

59. Hocini M, Sanders P, Jais P, et al.: Prevalence of pulmonary vein disconnection after anatomical encircling ablation for atrial fibrillation. Eur Heart J 26:696-704, 2005.

60. Macle L, Jais P, Scavee C, et al.: Pulmonary vein disconnection using the LocaLisa three-dimensional nonfluoroscopic catheter imaging system. J Cardiovasc Electrophysiol 14:693-697, 2003.

61. Rotter M, Takahashi Y, Sanders P, et al.: Reduction of fluoroscopy exposure and procedure duration during ablation of atrial fibrillation using a novel anatomical navigation system. Eur Heart J 26:1415-1421, 2005.

62. Karch MR, Zrenner B, Deisenhofer I, et al. Freedom from atrial tachyarrhythmias after catheter ablation of atrial fibrillation. A randomized comparison between 2 current ablation strategies. Circulation 111:2875-2880, 2005.

63. Arentz T, von Rosenthal J, Blum T, et al.: Feasibility and safety of pulmonary vein isolation using a new mapping and navigation system in patients with refractory atrial fibrillation. Circulation 108:2484-2490, 2003.

64. Pappone C, Rosanio S, Oreto G, et al.: Circumferential radiofrequency ablation of pulmonary vein ostia: A new anatomic approach for curing atrial fibrillation. Circulation 102:2619-2628, 2000.

65. Macle L, Jais P, Weerasooriya R, et al.: Irrigated-tip catheter ablation of pulmonary veins for treatment of atrial fibrillation. J Cardiovasc Electrophysiol 13:1067-1073, 2002.

66. Nademanee K, McKenzie J, Kosar E, et al.: A new approach for catheter ablation of atrial fibrillation: Mapping of the electrophysiological substrate. J Am Coll Cardiol 43:2044-2053, 2004.

67. Pappone C, Oreto G, Rosanio S, et al.: Atrial electroanatomic remodeling after circumferential radiofrequency pulmonary vein ablation: Efficacy of an anatomic approach in a large cohort of patients with atrial fibrillation. Circulation 104:2539-2544, 2001.

68. Pappone C, Manguso F, Vicedomini G, et al.: Prevention of iatrogenic atrial tachycardia after ablation of atrial fibrillation: A prospective randomized study comparing circumferential pulmonary vein ablation with a modified approach. Circulation 110:3036-3042, 2004.

69. Oral H, Scharf C, Chugh A, et al.: Catheter ablation for paroxysmal atrial fibrillation: Segmental pulmonary vein ostial ablation versus left atrial ablation. Circulation 108:2355-2360, 2003.

70. Stabile G, Turco P, La Rocca V, et al.: Is pulmonary vein isolation necessary for curing atrial fibrillation? Circulation 108:657-660, 2003.

71. Cappato R, Negroni S, Pecora D, et al.: Prospective assessment of late conduction recurrence across radiofrequency lesions producing electrical disconnection at the pulmonary vein ostium in patients with atrial fibrillation. Circulation 108:1599-1604, 2003.

72. Hocini M, Sanders P, Jais P, et al.: Techniques for curative treatment of atrial fibrillation. J Cardiovasc Electrophysiol 15:1467-1471, 2004.

73. Oral H, Knight BP, Ozaydin M, et al.: Segmental ostial ablation to isolate the pulmonary veins during atrial fibrillation:

Feasibility and mechanistic insights. Circulation 106:1256-1262, 2002.

74. Oral H, Chugh A, Lemola K, et al.: Noninducibility of atrial fibrillation as an end point of left atrial circumferential ablation for paroxysmal atrial fibrillation: A randomized study. Circulation 110:2797-2801, 2004.

75. Pappone C, Santinelli V, Manguso F, et al.: Pulmonary vein denervation enhances long-term benefit after circumferential ablation for paroxysmal atrial fibrillation. Circulation 109:327-334, 2004.

76. Haissaguerre M, Jais P, Shah DC, et al.: Catheter ablation of chronic atrial fibrillation targeting the reinitiating triggers. J Cardiovasc Electrophysiol 11:2-10, 2000.

77. Robbins IM, Colvin EV, Doyle TP, et al.: Pulmonary vein stenosis after catheter ablation of atrial fibrillation. Circulation 98:1769-1775, 1998.

78. Jais P, Hocini M, Weerasooriya R, et al.: Left atrial macroreentry after pulmonary vein isolation for atrial fibrillation: Incidence and mechanism. Pacing Clin Electrophysiol 25:363, 2002.

79. Gerstenfeld EP, Callans DJ, Dixit S, et al.: Mechanisms of organized left atrial tachycardias occurring after pulmonary vein isolation. Circulation 110:1351-1357, 2004.

80. Villacastin J, Perez-Castellano N, Moreno J, Gonzalez R: Left atrial flutter after radiofrequency catheter ablation of focal atrial fibrillation. J Cardiovasc Electrophysiol 14:417-421, 2003.

81. Oral H, Knight BP, Morady F: Left atrial flutter after segmental ostial radiofrequency catheter ablation for pulmonary vein isolation. Pacing Clin Electrophysiol 26:1417-1419, 2003.

82. Nakagawa H, Aoyama H, Beckman KJ, et al.: Incidence and location of the reentrant circuit in macroreentrant left atrial tachycardia following pulmonary vein isolation. Pacing Clin Electrophysiol 26:970, 2003.

83. Jais P, Sanders P, Hsu LF, et al.: Tachycardias from the Bachmann region observed in the course of atrial fibrillation ablation. Heart Rhythm 1:S18, 2004.

84. Pappone C, Oral H, Santinelli V, et al.: Atrio-esophageal fistula as a complication of percutaneous transcatheter ablation of atrial fibrillation. Circulation 109:2724-2726, 2004.

85. Scanavacca MI, Avila AD, Parga J, Sosa E: Left atrial-esophageal fistula following radiofrequency catheter ablation of atrial fibrillation. J Cardiovasc Electrophysiol 15:960-962, 2004.

86. Ernst S, Ouyang F, Lober F, et al.: Catheter-induced linear lesions in the left atrium in patients with atrial fibrillation: An electroanatomic study. J Am Coll Cardiol 42:1271-1282, 2003.

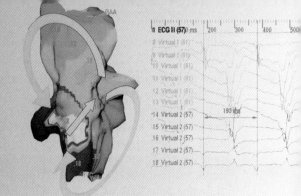

16

Catheter Ablation of Paroxysmal Atrial Fibrillation Originating from the Non–Pulmonary Vein Areas

Satoshi Higa • Ching-Tai Tai • Shih-Ann Chen

Key Points

- The mechanisms of paroxysmal atrial fibrillation (AF) originating from the non–pulmonary vein areas are automaticity, triggered activity, and microreentry.

- Diagnosis is made on the basis of spontaneous onset of ectopic beats initiating AF during baseline or after provocative maneuvers.

- Ablation targets are the earliest activation sites for focal ablation and the myocardial sleeve surrounding the ostium of vena cava for isolation.

- Special equipment includes the circular catheter, basket catheter, noncontact balloon catheter, and electroanatomic mapping is useful.

- The success rates are greater than 95% for vena cava, 95% for the crista terminalis, 50% for the left atrial posterior wall, and 50% for the ligament of Marshall.

The pulmonary veins (PVs) are a major source of ectopies initiating atrial fibrillation (AF), and isolation of PVs from the left atrium (LA) can cure paroxysmal AF.[1-3] On the other hand, several laboratories have demonstrated that ectopies originating from non-PV areas can also be AF initiators.[1-17] Shah et al. reported that non-PV ectopies caused AF recurrence in more than 24% of patients after isolation of four PVs.[15] Several institutions have reported a lower recurrence rate and a higher cure rate of AF in patients for whom non-PV ablation was added after multiple AF ablation procedures.[18,19] Those findings support the important role of non-PV ectopies in AF initiation and recurrence, as was previously proposed by our laboratory.[2,4,5,7,14] Based on these reports and our recent study, non-PV ectopy can play an important role in AF initiation.

The aim of this chapter is to review the current state of knowledge about the electrophysiologic features, mapping and ablation strategy, safety, and efficacy associated with catheter ablation of AF initiated by ectopic foci originating from non-PV areas.

Characteristics of Atrial Fibrillation Originating from Non–Pulmonary Vein Areas

INCIDENCE OF NON–PULMONARY VEIN ATRIAL FIBRILLATION INITIATORS

We have proposed several important concepts regarding the role of non-PV ectopy in initiating AF.[4,5,7,14] Other investigators also have demonstrated ectopies initiating AF that originated from non-PV areas, with an incidence as great as 47%.[3,15-17,20-23] The most recent data, from the Heart Rhythm Society's 25th Annual Scientific Sessions in 2004, showed that 14% to 28% of patients have non-PV AF initiators. In addition, the majority of non-PV ectopic beats initiating AF have a characteristic anatomic distribution, with the preferential distribution in the superior vena cava (SVC) and left posterior free wall, followed by crista terminalis, coronary sinus ostium, ligament of Marshall, and interatrial septum (Table 16–1).[14,16,17]

PATHOPHYSIOLOGY OF NON–PULMONARY VEIN ATRIAL FIBRILLATION INITIATORS

Embryonic sinus venosus has been found in the musculature of the SVC, coronary sinus, and crista terminalis of the mammalian heart.[24] The possible mechanisms of the ectopic beats initiating AF include abnormal automaticity and triggered activity. Several investigators have demonstrated that the SVC is one of the major foci for causing AF.[5,15,25-28] We also found that heterogeneity in the myocardial sleeve is present in the SVC and that cardiomyocytes isolated from the SVC show spontaneous depolarization.[29,30] The myocardial fiber of the SVC sleeve are connected to the right atrium (RA), and atrial excitation can conduct to the SVC.[31-33] Previous reports showed that sustained tachyarrhythmias are induced by abnormal automaticity or triggered activity in human atrial fibers.[34-36] The human diseased atria show hypopolarized activities compared with normal atria.[35,36] Therefore, the posterior free wall of the LA might have abnormal electrical activity. The crista terminalis, which is an area with abnormal automaticity, anisotropy, and slow conduction, may serve as an arrhythmogenic substrate for developing microreentry.[37,38] We have demonstrated catecholamine-sensitive ectopies from the crista terminalis that showed very fast depolarization with fibrillatory conduction in the atrium.[14] The ligament of Marshall is an embryologic remnant of the left SVC, and the myocardial fibers of this structure may connect with the LA and coronary sinus musculatures. Recently, several investigators have reported the presence of catecholamine-sensitive tissue within the ligament of Marshall that have abnormal automaticity and therefore could be a potential source of AF.[6,14,39,40] Myocardial fibers within the coronary sinus also have been reported to have the capability of spontaneous depolarization associated with catecholamine.[41,42]

Diagnosis of Non–Pulmonary Vein Atrial Fibrillation Initiators

PROVOCATIVE MANEUVERS

In our laboratory, we first tried to record the spontaneous onset of ectopic beats initiating AF during baseline monitoring or after isoproterenol infusion (up to 4 to 8 μg/minute). If ectopy did not occur, a short duration of atrial pacing with intermittent pause (8 to 12 beats at a cycle length of 200 to 300 msec) was applied to induce the ectopy with AF initiation. If AF still did not appear, burst atrial pacing was used to induce AF. If pacing-induced AF was sustained for longer than 5 minutes, external cardioversion was performed to terminate the AF, and spontaneous reinitiation of AF would be recorded. If a consistent location of ectopy and onset pattern of

TABLE 16-1

Incidence of Atrial Fibrillation Originating from Non–Pulmonary Vein Areas

| Authors, Year (Ref. No.) | No. of Patients | | Age (Mean ± SD) and Gender | No. of Ectopic Foci | | Mapping Tool | Location of Ectopy (No. of Foci) | | | | | | | |
	Total	Non-PV Ectopy		Total	Non-PV		RA	SVC	CS	IAS	LA	LOM	SVT	Other
Lin et al., 2003[14]	240	68 (28%)	61 ± 13, 43M/25F	358	73 (20%)	C, Basket, ICE	CT (10)	27	1	1	PW (28)	6	—	—
Shah et al., 2003[15]	160[†]	36 (24%)	53 ± 11, 130M/30F	NA	85	C	5	3[‡]	4	—	PW (30), PV os (39), Other (5)	—	—	—
Beldner et al., 2004[16]	401	68 (17%)	NA NA	NA	83	C, ICE, CARTO	CT (11), TA (4), ER (13)	4	3	FO (4)	PW (15), MA (7)	—	20*	2
Suzuki et al., 2004[17]	127[§]	18 (14%)	53 ± 11, 106M/21F	NA	20	C	CT (4)	5	1	7	2	1	—	—
Total	928	190 (20.5%)	—	—	261	—	47 (17.9%)	39 (14.9%)	9 (3.4%)	12 (4.6%)	126 (48.1%)	7 (2.7%)	20 (7.6%)	2 (0.8%)

*Atrioventricular nodal reentrant tachycardia (19) and atrioventricular reentrant tachycardia (1) triggered atrial fibrillation.
[†]After isolation of one to four PVs, non-PV triggers were identified, but at least 16 foci were of unknown origin.
[‡]Includes persistent left superior caval vein.
[§]After isolation of four PVs, non-PV triggers were identified in the first and second sessions.

Basket, basket catheter; C, conventional mapping; CARTO, electroanatomic mapping; CS, coronary sinus; CT, crista terminalis; ER, Eustachian ridge; F, female; FO, fossa ovalis; IAS, interatrial septum; ICE, intracardiac echocardiography; LA, left atrium; LOM, ligament of Marshall; M, male; MA, mitral annulus; NA, data not available; PV, pulmonary vein; PVos, ostia of ablated pulmonary vein including the zone between ipsilateral veins; PW, left atrial posterior wall; RA, right atrium; SVC, superior vena cava; SVT, supraventricular tachycardia; TA, tricuspid annulus.

spontaneous AF were confirmed, the earliest activation site during ectopy would be defined as the AF initiator.[2,4,5,7,14]

MAPPING TECHNIQUES

An ectopic focus can be localized by detailed endocardial mapping using several multipole catheters, especially during frequent atrial ectopies initiating burst AF. We have demonstrated that the use of endocardial activation sequences in the high RA, His bundle, and coronary sinus ostium can predict the location of AF ectopic foci.[2,4,5,7,14]

Predicting the Location of Atrial Fibrillation Initiators

With the difference in time interval between high RA and His bundle atrial activation during sinus rhythm and ectopy being less than 0 msec, the accuracy for discriminating ectopy in the SVC or upper portion of the crista terminalis from PV ectopy is 100%.[43] Because of the close spatial opposition, potentials from the right superior pulmonary vein (RSPV) can be recorded from a contiguous area of the RA, and ectopies from both areas show similar P-wave morphologies. Therefore, if the ectopy originates from the upper portion of the crista terminalis or from the RA-SVC junction, ectopy from the RSPV should be excluded.[37,44,45] If far-field potentials from the right PV are recorded at the high posteromedial right atrial wall, the true origin of ectopy can be clarified by simultaneous mapping of the SVC and the RSPV using two multipolar catheters.[5]

Another concern to be raised is ectopy from the left side of the interatrial septum. Atrial ectopy may originate from either side of the interatrial septum.[46] If the earliest atrial activation site is considered to be from the interatrial septum, left atrial mapping should be considered before ablation of the right-sided septum in cases with a shorter activation time (≤15 msec) preceding the P-wave onset or a monophasic positive P wave in lead V_1 during ectopy, or if the earliest site is near the area of Bachmann's bundle.[46,47] If the earliest endocardial activation site is around the posterolateral mitral annulus or the left PV ostium, a ligament of Marshall potential may be identified by differential pacing or by detailed epicardial mapping through the distal coronary sinus, or both (Table 16–2).[7,48]

TABLE 16–2

Diagnostic Criteria for Non–Pulmonary Vein Ectopy Initiating Atrial Fibrillation

Location	Criteria
AF initiators from RA	Difference in time interval between atrial activation at high RA and His bundle area during sinus rhythm and ectopy <0 msec
IVC, SVC	Positive (SVC) and negative (IVC) P waves in the inferior leads, positive or biphasic P wave in V1 (SVC) Earliest ectopic activity in the VC during simultaneous mapping of VC and right PV Reversal of the double-potential sequence during ectopy (VC potentials with a rapid deflection–far-field atrial potential sequence; distal-to-proximal venous activation sequence)
Crista terminalis (CT)	Polarity of P waves in the inferior leads: upper portion of CT, positive; middle portion, biphasic; lower portion, negative Earliest ectopic activity along the CT during simultaneous mapping of CT, VC, and right PV
Coronary sinus (CS) ostium	Negative P waves in the inferior leads Earliest ectopic activity in the CS ostium
AF initiators from LA	Difference in time interval between atrial activation at high RA and His bundle area during sinus rhythm and ectopy >0 msec
Left atrial free wall or left artial appendage	Atrial potentials with a rapid deflection–PV potential found after the earliest atrial activation
Ligament of Marshall (LOM)	Earliest activation site along the vein of Marshall, posterolateral portion of mitral annulus, or left PV ostium Reversal of the triple-potential sequence; LOM potential is earlier than LA or left PV potential (LOM–LA–PV potentials sequence)

AF, atrial fibrillation; IVC, inferior vena cava; LA, left atrium; PV, pulmonary vein; RA, right atrium; SVC, superior vena cava; VC, vena cava.

Atrial Fibrillation Initiators from the Right Atrium

Analysis of P-wave polarity of the AF ectopy has been a useful method to predict the approximate location of the AF ectopy.[49] Ectopy originating from the SVC or upper portion of the crista terminalis exhibits upright P waves in the inferior leads; ectopy from the coronary sinus ostium produces a negative P-wave polarity in the inferior leads; and ectopy from the middle portion of crista terminalis causes biphasic P waves. If RA ectopy is being considered, we place a duodecapolar catheter (1-mm electrode length and 2-mm interelectrode spacing) from the crista terminalis to the SVC with the most distally recorded electrogram amplitude larger than 0.05 mV.[2,4,5,7,14] The intracardiac recordings from the proximal portion of the SVC usually show a blunted atrial potential followed by a discrete SVC potential (Fig. 16–1). The activation sequence of these double potentials is reversed during SVC ectopy. Intracardiac recordings from the distal portion of the SVC usually show double potentials: the first one represents the SVC potential, and the second one, the RSPV far-field potential. During SVC ectopy, the activation sequence of these double potentials remains unchanged. Simultaneous recordings from the SVC and RSPV demonstrate double potentials.

Intracardiac recordings along the crista terminalis also show double potentials during sinus rhythm, with a high-to-low activation sequence, and the activation sequence of the double potentials reverses during crista terminalis ectopy (Fig. 16–2). To identify the ectopic foci and the mechanism of AF, three-dimensional mapping is also useful (Fig. 16–3).[50]

Atrial Fibrillation Initiators from the Left Atrium

After right atrial ectopy is excluded by the surface P-wave polarity and endocardial activation sequence, we start to map the left atrial free wall ectopy by using two multipolar catheters introduced through the interatrial septum. The major sites of the ectopies are distributed in the area between the four PVs or near the PV ostial edge. The interval between atrial activation of the decapolar catheter in the proximal coronary sinus and distal coronary sinus during ectopy is useful to predict ectopic foci located near the right PV ostium (>0 msec) or near the left PV ostium (<0 msec).[43] During sinus rhythm, the left posterior free wall atrial potential with a rapid deflection is recognized; it may be fused with the local PV potential around the edge of PV ostium. An atrial-PV fusion potential can be found in the earliest activation site during the ectopy preceding AF. An alter-

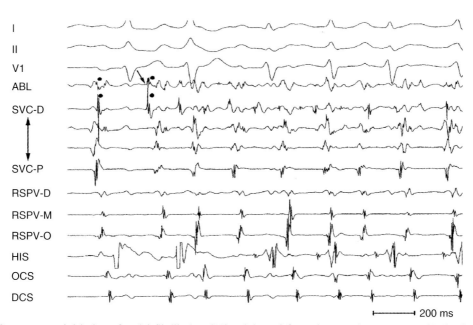

FIGURE 16–1. Spontaneous initiation of atrial fibrillation (AF) originated from the superior vena cava (SVC) after the first sinus beat *(arrow)*. It was marked by the rapid deflection potential preceding the lower-amplitude, slower, far-field atrial activities *(black dots)*. Note that the SVC potential follows the atrial potential during sinus rhythm, in contrast to the onset of AF. Black dots represent local SVC potentials. I, II, and V1, surface electrocardiographic leads; ABL, ablation catheter; -D, distal; DCS, distal coronary sinus; HIS, His bundle; -M, middle portion; ms, microseconds; -O, ostial portion; OCS, coronary sinus ostium; -P, proximal; RSPV, right superior pulmonary vein. *(Adapted from Tsai CF, Tai CT, Hsieh MH, et al.: Initiation of atrial fibrillation by ectopic beats originating from the superior vena cava: Electrophysiological characteristics and results of radiofrequency ablation. Circulation 102:72, 2000.)*

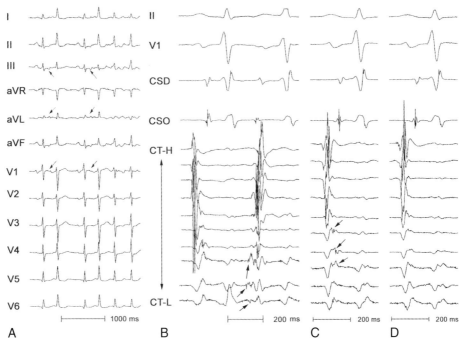

FIGURE 16–2. The tracings on the left show ectopic beats *(arrows)* followed by initiation of atrial fibrillation (AF) in the 12-lead electrocardiogram (ECG) (**A**). Intracardiac recordings on the right show crista terminalis potentials *(arrows)* during ectopic beat originating from the lower portion of the crista terminalis (**B**) and during sinus rhythm before ablation (**C**). The final tracing on the right shows the disappearance of crista terminalis potentials after ablation (**D**). CSD, distal coronary sinus; CSO, coronary sinus ostium; CT-H, high crista terminalis; and CT-L, low crista terminalis; ms, microseconds. *(Adapted from Lin WS, Tai CT, Hsieh MH, et al.: Catheter ablation of paroxysmal atrial fibrillation initiated by non-pulmonary vein ectopy. Circulation 107:3180, 2003.)*

nating pattern of atrial and PV potentials can also be recognized during ectopy (Fig.16–4A).[14]

For ectopy from the ligament of Marshall, the earliest Marshall potential preceding AF is the ablation target site (see Fig. 16–4B).[7,51,52] It has been suggested that this ligament has multiple electrical connections with the left atrial posterior free wall, near or inside the PV ostium. Therefore, it is necessary to differentiate a Marshall potential from a PV or left atrial posterior free wall potential. Differential pacing or direct recording of the ligament of Marshall potential using the microelectrode catheter cannulated in the vein of Marshall can distinguish a Marshall potential from a PV potential to avoid misdiagnosis and inappropriate radiofrequency energy application (Tables 16–3 and 16–4).[6,7]

Assessing the Geometry around the Atrial-Venous Junctions

Selective PV angiography, venous phase imaging after pulmonary artery angiography, and intracardiac echocardiography help to identify the PV ostium, to locate mapping catheters at the PV ostium, and to map ectopy from the left atrial posterior free wall.[2,4,5,7,14] SVC angiography using a pigtail catheter injection of 40 mL of a contrast medium and intra-

cardiac echocardiography help to determine the SVC orifice and the RA-SVC junction. Balloon-occluded coronary sinus angiography using appropriate fluoroscopic views also helps to visualize the vein of Marshall.[8] Integration of three-dimensional computed tomography or magnetic resonance imaging with the LA-PV geometry is the best way to identify the true locations of ectopies and ablation sites.

Ablation Techniques

We have performed mapping-guided ablation techniques for the elimination and electrical isolation of non-PV AF initiators. In general, the ablation target site of non-PV ectopy is the site that shows the earliest bipolar deflection or a unipolar QS pattern recorded from the ectopic foci preceding AF.[2,4,5,7,14] However, specific mapping and ablation techniques can be applied to different non-PV foci. Radiofrequency energy with temperature control (50°C to 55°C) is delivered for 20 to 40 seconds per pulse but should be discontinued immediately if the ablation catheter moves or the patient complains of chest pain, coughs, or shows a Bezold-Jarisch–like reflex.[2,4,5,7,14]

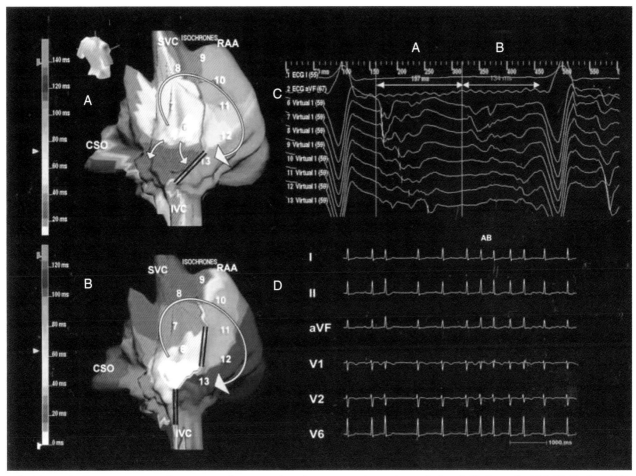

FIGURE 16–3. Noncontact mapping system demonstrating the propagation pattern during initiation of atrial fibrillation (AF). Isochronal maps on the left show the first *(top)* and second *(bottom)* beats initiating reentry in the modified right posterior oblique view. At the upper right is the unipolar virtual electrogram along the activation followed by the ectopy. At the lower right is the surface electrocardiogram recorded during initiation of AF. On the isochronal maps, the color scale ranges from white for the earliest activation to purple for the latest activation site. At first, the wavefront propagated centrifugally from the earliest site of the middle portion of crista terminalis *(top, yellow long arrow)*. Then, unidirectional block occurred in the lower portion of crista terminalis *(yellow short arrows)* and the activation wavefront spread around the upper portion of crista terminalis to initiate reentry into the second cycle of AF *(bottom, yellow long arrow)*. Note that the unipolar virtual signal from the ectopic foci (virtual 6) demonstrates a "QS" morphology in the first cycle, and "rS" morphology in the second cycle. CSO, coronary sinus ostium; IVC, inferior vena cava; ms, microseconds; RAA, right atrial appendage; SVC, superior vena cava. *(Adapted from Lin YJ, Tai CT, Liu TY, et al.: Electrophysiological mechanisms and catheter ablation of complex atrial arrhythmias from crista terminalis: Insight from three-dimensional noncontact mapping. Pacing Clin Electrophysiol 27:1239, 2004.)*

The protocols for facilitating AF initiation before ablation are repeated afterward to assess the effects of ablation.

SUPERIOR VENA CAVA

For patients with SVC AF, isolation of the SVC from the RA (below the level of the SVC-RA junction) is a preferable approach to avoid recurrence and SVC stenosis. High output pacing from the distal ablation catheter should be performed before each ablation in the lateral SVC to exclude catheter proximity to the phrenic nerve. The end point is electrical conduction block between the RA and the SVC. Exit block of the focal repetitive activity inside the SVC may be observed before and/or after ablation (Fig. 16–5).[5,25] Circular catheter, basket catheter, and three-dimensional mapping including the CARTO system (Biosense Webster, Baldwin Park, Calif.) and the EnSite and NavX mapping systems (both from Endocardial Solutions, St. Paul, Minn.) can guide the electrical isolation of the SVC.[14,18,27,28,53-56]

Noncontact mapping can localize the electrical breakthroughs at the RA-SVC junction and guide ablation of SVC AF (Fig. 16–6).[53,55,56] When the noncontact balloon catheter is deployed, only 3 mL of

TABLE 16–3

Targets for Ablation of Atrial Fibrillation Originating from Non–Pulmonary Vein Areas

AF Initiators	Target Sites	Mapping Tools
Right Side		
IVC, SVC	Breakthrough sites around RA-VC junction for isolation	Circular, Basket, EnSite, CARTO
Crista terminalis (CT)	Earliest CT activation site for focal ablation	Unipolar recording with multipolar catheter, Basket, EnSite
Coronary sinus (CS)	Connection sites between CS and atrial musculature for isolation	EnSite, CARTO
Left Side		
Left atrial free wall, septum, appendage, mitral annulus	Earliest activation site for focal ablation	Unipolar recording with multipolar catheter, Basket, EnSite
Ligament of Marshall (LOM)	Earliest LOM potential for focal ablation	Multipolar recording of triple potentials during ectopy, direct mapping of LOM potentials by microelectrode catheter, Basket, EnSite
	Connection sites between LA and LOM for isolation	Multipolar recording of triple potentials during ectopy, direct mapping of LOM potentials by microelectrode catheter, Basket, EnSite, CARTO

AF, atrial fibrillation; Basket, basket catheter; CARTO, electroanatomic contact mapping system; Circular, circular catheter; EnSite, noncontact mapping system; IVC, inferior vena cava; LA, left atrium; RA, right atrium; SVC, superior vena cava; VC, vena cava.

TABLE 16–4

Troubleshooting for the Difficult Cases of Atrial Fibrillation Originating from the Non–Pulmonary Vein Areas

Problem	Causes	Solutions
Unable to induce ectopy initiating AF	Inconsistent ectopic activation or mechanical trauma of ectopy	Repeat the provocative maneuvers Isolation of SVC without provocation of ectopy Ablation of the left atrial wall with Marshall potential
Unable to localize ectopy initiating AF	Misinterpretation of ectopic beat electrogram	Exclude far-field potentials by simultaneous mapping of SVC, CT, and RSPV Exclude far-field potentials by simultaneous mapping of LSPV, LIPV, LA, and LOM, and apply differential pacing method to identify PV or atrial potential
	Immediate degeneration to AF	Use 3-D noncontact mapping system Perform atrial substrate ablation (the ectopic activation will become stable atrial tachycardia, without degeneration to AF, and mapping will become easier)
	Outside the mapping area	Use 3-D noncontact mapping system
Refractory to focal ablation	Epicardial foci	Use 8-mm-tip catheter or irrigated-tip catheter, or use the epicardial approach

3-D, three-dimensional; AF, atrial fibrillation; CT, crista terminalis; LA, left atrium; LIPV, left inferior pulmonary vein; LOM, ligament of Marshall; LSPV, left superior pulmonary vein; PV, pulmonary vein; RSPV, right superior pulmonary vein; SVC, superior vena cava.

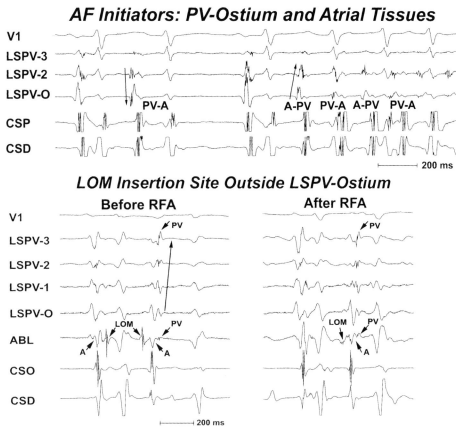

FIGURE 16–4. *Top panel,* Initiation of atrial fibrillation (AF) from the pulmonary vein (PV) and left atrial posterior free wall. The first beat is a sinus beat. The second beat is an ectopic beat originating from the left superior pulmonary vein (LSPV), recorded at the second pair of electrodes in the LSPV (LSPV-2), with conduction to the atrial tissue. The third beat is a sinus beat, and the fourth beat is an ectopic beat originating from A with conduction to the PV. Alternating activation from the PV ostium and the atrial wall was noted. *Bottom left,* Ectopic beat originating from the ligament of Marshall (LOM) before radiofrequency ablation (RFA). The LOM potential can be found in the ablation catheter (ABL), which is outside the ostium of the LSPV (LSPV-O). The typical triple potentials (LOM-A-PV) were noted. *Bottom right,* Diminished LOM potential amplitude after RFA. ABL, ablation catheter; and CSO, coronary sinus ostium; CSD, distal coronary sinus; ms, microseconds; V1, electrocardiographic surface lead. *(Adapted from Lin WS, Tai CT, Hsieh MH, et al.: Catheter ablation of paroxysmal atrial fibrillation initiated by non-pulmonary vein ectopy. Circulation 107:3178, 2003.)*

saline–contrast medium solution is infused, to reduce balloon size and allow positioning closer to the SVC surface. The atriocaval junction can be confirmed by an SVC venogram, intracardiac echocardiography, and electrical signals. In our previous study, we used these three tools simultaneously to identify the SVC-RA junction.[5,14] Recently, we also divided the SVC into three parts. The first part extends from the junction of the right and left brachiocephalic veins to the upper end of the right pulmonary artery. The second part is the part of the SVC that is crossed posteriorly by the right pulmonary artery (i.e., from the upper border of the right pulmonary artery to the lower border of the right pulmonary artery). The third part begins from the lower end of the second part and extends to the site of the SVC-RA junction. The SVC-RA junction is defined as the point below which the cylindrical SVC flares into the RA.[54,55]

CRISTA TERMINALIS

For ectopy from the crista terminalis, we perform focal ablation of the earliest activation site of the ectopy until there is total elimination of the ectopy initiating AF or greater than 50% reduction in the initial electrogram amplitude of the ectopic focus.[14] The crista terminalis ectopy is usually located around the transverse gap conduction region in the crista terminalis. For patients who have accompanying right atrial atypical flutter involving the transverse gap conduction region in the crista terminalis, we perform linear ablation around the gap to eliminate the ectopy and to block transverse conduction through this gap (see Fig. 16–3).[50] Intracardiac echocardiography is helpful to clarify the anatomic relation between the crista terminalis and the catheter position during ablation.

AF: Multiple Migrating Foci with Conduction Block within SVC

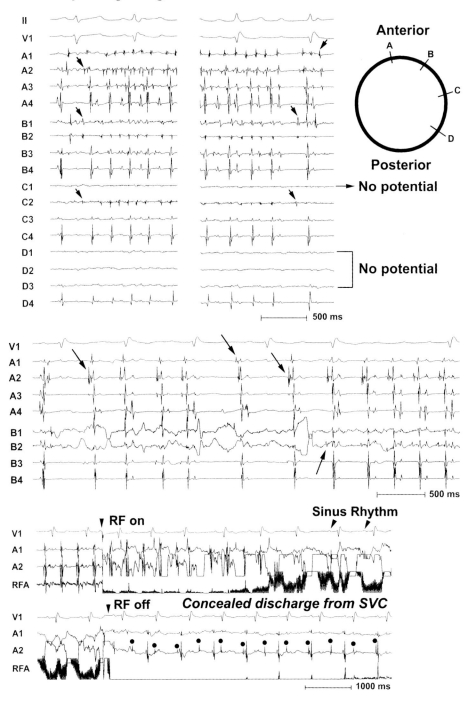

FIGURE 16–5. Multiple migrating foci with conduction block during superior vena cava (SVC) atrial fibrillation (AF) recorded by a basket catheter (*upper panels*). *Left panel,* The first beat is a sinus beat, and the second beat is an ectopic beat from spline B1 and C2, followed by A2 (*arrowheads*). *Right panel,* Spontaneous early reinitiation of ectopic beats from spline B1, C2, and A1 (*arrowheads*). As shown in the diagram on the far right, A through D indicate the wall of the SVC from anterior to posterolateral; 1, 2, 3, and 4 are the bipolar recordings from each spline located along the distal to proximal SVC. *Middle panel,* Ectopies from the SVC recorded by a basket catheter in a different patient. *Top panel,* The earliest activation sites during ectopic beats changed from spline A2, A1, and A2 to B2 (*arrows*). *Bottom panels,* AF termination during segmental isolation of the SVC sleeve by radiofrequency ablation (RFA). After termination, concealed discharge from the SVC is still present (*black dots*). (Adapted from Lin WS, Tai CT, Hsieh MH, et al.: Catheter ablation of paroxysmal atrial fibrillation initiated by non-pulmonary vein ectopy. Circulation 107:3179, 2003.)

CORONARY SINUS

For patients with coronary sinus AF, electrical disconnection of the coronary sinus from the atrium by endocardial or epicardial ablation (or both) is a preferable approach to avoid recurrence. A circular catheter or three-dimensional mapping system is useful for the ablation procedure. The disappearance or isolation of the coronary sinus potential is the end point.[11]

LEFT ATRIAL WALL

For ectopy from the left atrial posterior free wall, we perform focal ablation of the earliest activation site

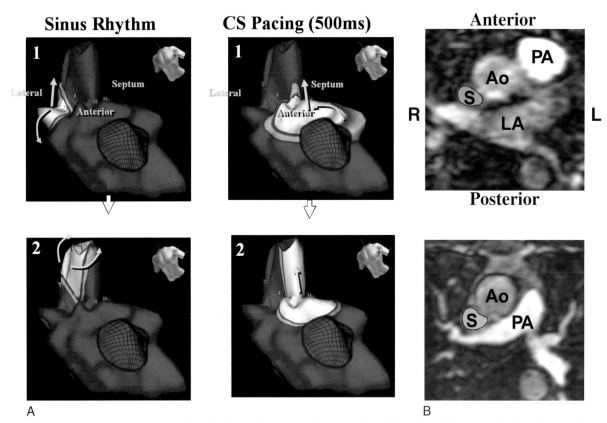

FIGURE 16–6. A, Noncontact mapping showed the activation wavefront conducted from the right atrium (RA) to the superior vena cava (SVC) along the lateral wall of the RA-SVC junction during the sinus beat, and along the septal side of the RA-SVC junction during coronary sinus pacing. In the color scale for each isopotential map, white indicates the most negative potential and purple indicates least negative potential. **B,** Upper panel shows lower portion of SVC near the level of pulmonary artery main trunk. Lower panel shows the higher portion of SVC near the level of right pulmonary artery. AO, ascending aorta; PA, pulmonary artery; S, superior vena cava; L, left; R, right. *(Adapted from Chen SA, Tai CT: Catheter ablation of atrial fibrillation originating from the non-pulmonary vein foci. J Cardiovasc Electrophysiol 16:229-232, 2005.)*

during ectopy. If ectopy still remains, a box-shaped linear ablation (1.5 × 1.5-cm square area) is added around the ectopy.[14] The end point is total elimination of the ectopy initiating AF or a reduction in electrogram amplitude of the ectopic focus to less than 50% of the initial amplitude.

LIGAMENT OF MARSHALL

For patients with ligament of Marshall AF, the earliest ligament of Marshall potential preceding onset of AF is targeted for ablation by an endocardial and/or epicardial approach. Both the ligament of Marshall and the left PVs can be isolated from the LA with guidance by simultaneous mapping of ligament of Marshall and left PV ostia.[6,51]

Efficacy and Safety

ABLATION RESULTS AND RECURRENCES

Recently, we demonstrated that catheter ablation of non-PV ectopy is feasible, but the success rate depends on the origin of the ectopy.[14] Right atrial non-PV ectopy was eliminated with a higher success rate and a lower recurrence rate than left atrial non-PV ectopy. Rates of success, recurrences, and complications reported in journals have been 98.3%, 6.9%, and 0%, respectively, for AF originating from the vena cava, and 76.3%, 17.2%, and 2.6% for ligament of Marshall AF (Tables 16–5, 16–6, and 16–7). In our study, a higher success rate was demonstrated for AF initiated from the RA, including the SVC and crista terminalis.[14] On the other hand, AF initiated from the LA had a higher recurrence rate.

TABLE 16–5

Results of Radiofrequency Catheter Ablation of Atrial Fibrillation Originating from the Vena Cava

Authors, Year (Ref. No.)	No. of Patients	Mean Age by Gender	Mapping Tool	Location of Ectopies	Ablation Method (No. of Patients)	Multiple Foci	Success	Complications	Recurrence	Follow-up (mo)
Chang et al., 2001[26]	2	57 (F), 50 (M)	C	SVC	Focal	NA	Yes	NA	No	6, 3
Ooie et al., 2002[27]	1	42 (F)	Circular	SVC	Isolation	NA	Yes	No	No	7
Goya et al., 2002[18]	16	59 ± 5 (NA)	CARTO, Circular	SVC*	Isolation	NA	100 (100%)	0 (0%)	NA†	13 ± 1
Shah et al., 2002[15]	1	50 (M)	Basket	SVC	Isolation	NA	Yes	NA	No	12
Mansour et al., 2002[10]	2	60 (F), 22 (M)	EnSite, C	IVC-os PL	Focal	No	Yes	No	No	9, 2
Liu et al., 2003[56]	2	57 (F), 73 (M)	EnSite	SVC	Isolation	NA	Yes	No	No	2, 2
Weiss et al., 2003[53]	1	54 (M)	EnSite	SVC	Isolation	NA	Yes	NA	No	4
Lin et al., 2003[14]	27	57 ± 12 (NA)	Basket, C	SVC	Focal (20), Isolation (7)	12 (44%)	100 (100%)	0 (0%)	3 (11%)	NA
Scavee et al., 2003[9]	1	44 (NA)	Circular	IVC-os PM	Isolation	No	Yes	No	No	14
Jayam et al., 2004[28]	1	39 (M)	Basket	SVC	Isolation	NA	Yes	NA	NA	NA
Hsu et al., 2004[13]	5	46 ± 11 (total for 1F and 4M)	CARTO, Circular	PLSVC	Isolation	NA	4 (75%)‡	No	1 (25%)	15 ± 10
Total	59	—	—	—	—	—	58 (98.3%)	0 (0%)	4 (6.9%)	—

*This study included patients with or without SVC ectopy.

†Sinus rhythm was maintained in 13 of 16 patients, but authors did not specify the true recurrence rate of SVC atrial fibrillation.

‡Successful isolation of PLSVC in 4 patients.

Basket, basket catheter; C, conventional mapping; CARTO, electroanatomic mapping system; Circular, circular catheter; EnSite, noncontact mapping system; F, female; Focal, focal ablation of ectopic focus; Isolation, electrical isolation of caval vein; IVC-os PL, posterolateral wall of ostial portion of inferior vena cava; IVC-os PM, posteromedial wall of ostial portion of inferior vena cava; M, male; NA, data not available; PLSVC, persistent left superior vena cava; SVC, superior vena cava.

TABLE 16-6

Results of Radiofrequency Catheter Ablation of Atrial Fibrillation Originating from the Ligament of Marshall

Authors, Year (Ref. No.)	No. of Patients	Mean Age by Gender	Mapping Tool	Mapping Sites	Ablation Sites (No. of Patients)	Ablation Method	Multiple Foci	Success	Complications	Recurrence	Follow-up (mo)
Katritsis et al., 2001[51]	10*	54.2 ± 9.4 (NA)	C	LA, CS	LA (4), CS (1), LA/CS (5)	Focal	Yes	7 (70%)[†]	1 (10%)[‡]	NA	11 ± 5
Hwang et al., 2004[6]	21	43.2 ± 8.7 (total for 5 F and 16 M)	Microelectrode	VOM	VOM insertion sites	Focal	Yes	18 (85.7%)	No	2 (11.1%)	19 ± 10
Polymeropoulos et al., 2002[52]	1	66 (F)	CARTO	LA, CS	LA	Focal	Yes	Yes	No	No	3
Lin et al., 2003[14]	6	66 ± 13 (NA)	C	LA, CS	LSPV-os (5), LSPV-inside (1)	Focal	5 (83%)	3 (50%)	No	3 (50%)	NA
Total	38	—	—	—	—	—	—	29 (76.3%)	1 (2.6%)	5 (17.2%)	—

*Ten of 18 patients received catheter ablation.

[†]Seven patients showed symptomatic improvement after LOM ablation.

[‡]One patient showed pericardial effusion requiring pericardiocentesis.

C, conventional mapping-guided radiofrequency ablation; CARTO, electroanatomic mapping; CS, coronary sinus; F, female; Focal, focal ablation of ectopic focus; LA, left atrium; LSPV-os, left superior pulmonary vein ostium; LSPV-inside, inside the left superior pulmonary vein; M, male; NA, data not available; VOM, vein of Marshall.

TABLE 16–7

Results of Radiofrequency Catheter Ablation of Atrial Fibrillation Originating from the Coronary Sinus

Authors, Year (Ref. No.)	No. of Patients	Mean Age by Gender	Mapping Tool	Location of Ectopies	Ablation Method	Multiple Foci	Success	Complications	Recurrence	Follow-up (mo)
Lin et al., 2003[14]	1	67 (M)	C	CS-os	Focal	No	Yes	No	No	NA
Rotter et al., 2004[12]	1	59 (M)	C	CS-mid to os	Isolation	Yes	Yes	NA	NA	NA
Sanders et al., 2004[11]	1	53 (M)	C	CS-dis to os	Focal, Isolation	Yes	Yes	No	No	2

C, conventional mapping-guided radiofrequency ablation; CS-dis, distal portion of coronary sinus; CS-mid, middle portion of coronary sinus; CS-os, ostial portion of coronary sinus; Focal, focal ablation of ectopic focus; Isolation, electrical isolation of coronary sinus; M, male; NA, data not available.

AVOIDING COMPLICATIONS

Several issues are discussed here on the efficacy and safety of ablation procedures. Radiofrequency energy application around the atrial-venous junction and the left atrial posterior wall can cause sick sinus syndrome, SVC and PV stenosis, phrenic nerve injury, and atrioesophageal fistulas.[57-60] Use of a lower power level of radiofrequency energy, with a temperature of 50°C to 55°C, can avoid these acute or late complications. Pacing to capture the phrenic nerve before ablation can predict phrenic nerve injury. Acceleration of the sinus rate during ablation around the RA-SVC junction is a sign predicting sinus node injury. Avoiding the application of high radiofrequency energy on the left atrial posterior wall close to the esophagus line is also essential to avoid the fatal complication of LA-esophageal fistula.

Conclusions

In most cases, AF is initiated by ectopic beats originating from the PV; however, it can be initiated from non-PV areas. Considering the high incidence (approximately 20%) of non-PV AF before and after isolation of four PVs, provocation of non-PV ectopy initiating AF should be considered in both the primary procedure and repeat procedures. Catheter ablation in non-PV areas is safe and effective in eliminating non-PV ectopy initiating AF.[55]

References

1. Haissaguerre M, Jais P, Shah DC, et al.: Spontaneous initiation of atrial fibrillation by ectopic beats originating in the pulmonary veins. N Engl J Med 339:659-666, 1998.
2. Chen SA, Hsieh MH, Tai CT, et al.: Initiation of atrial fibrillation by ectopic beats originating from the pulmonary veins: Electrophysiological characteristics, pharmacological responses, and effects of radiofrequency ablation. Circulation 100:1879-1886, 1999.
3. Oral H, Knight BP, Tada H, et al.: Pulmonary vein isolation for paroxysmal and persistent atrial fibrillation. Circulation 105: 1077-1081, 2002.
4. Chen SA, Tai CT, Yu WC, et al.: Right atrial focal atrial fibrillation: Electrophysiologic characteristics and radiofrequency catheter ablation. J Cardiovasc Electrophysiol 10:328-335, 1999.
5. Tsai CF, Tai CT, Hsieh MH, et al.: Initiation of atrial fibrillation by ectopic beats originating from the superior vena cava: Electrophysiological characteristics and results of radiofrequency ablation. Circulation 102:67-74, 2000.
6. Hwang C, Chen PS: Clinical electrophysiology and catheter ablation of atrial fibrillation from the ligamnet of Marshall. In Chen SA, Haissaguerre M, Zipes DP (eds): Thoracic Vein Arrhythmias: Mechanisms and Treatment. Malden, Mass.: Blackwell Futura 2004, pp 226-284.
7. Tai CT, Hsieh MH, Tsai CF, et al.: Differentiating the ligament of Marshall from the pulmonary vein musculature potentials in patients with paroxysmal atrial fibrillation: Electrophysiological characteristics and results of radiofrequency ablation. Pacing Clin Electrophysiol 23:1493-1501, 2000.
8. Tuan TC, Tai CT, Lin YK, et al.: Use of fluoroscopic views for detecting Marshall's vein in patients with cardiac arrhythmias. J Interv Card Electrophysiol 9:327-331, 2003.
9. Scavee C, Jais P, Weerasooriya R, Haissaguerre M: The inferior vena cava: An exceptional source of atrial fibrillation. J Cardiovasc Electrophysiol 14:659-662, 2003.
10. Mansour M, Ruskin J, Keane D: Initiation of atrial fibrillation by ectopic beats originating from the ostium of the inferior vena cava. J Cardiovasc Electrophysiol 13:1292-1295, 2002.

11. Sanders P, Jais P, Hocini M, Haissaguerre M: Electrical disconnection of the coronary sinus by radiofrequency catheter ablation to isolate a trigger of atrial fibrillation. J Cardiovasc Electrophysiol 15:364-368, 2004.

12. Rotter M, Sanders P, Takahashi Y, et al.: Images in cardiovascular medicine: Coronary sinus tachycardia driving atrial fibrillation. Circulation 110:e59-e60, 2004.

13. Hsu LF, Jais P, Keane D, et al.: Atrial fibrillation originating from persistent left superior vena cava. Circulation 24;109:828-832, 2004.

14. Lin WS, Tai CT, Hsieh MH, et al.: Catheter ablation of paroxysmal atrial fibrillation initiated by non-pulmonary vein ectopy. Circulation 107:3176-3183, 2003.

15. Shah DC, Haissaguerre M, Jais P, Hocini M: Nonpulmonary vein foci: Do they exist? Pacing Clin Electrophysiol 26:1631-1635, 2003.

16. Beldner SJ, Zado ES, Lin D, et al.: Anatomic targets for non-pulmonary triggers: Identification with intracardiac echo and magnetic mapping. Heart Rhythm 1(Suppl):S237, 2004.

17. Suzuki K, Nagata Y, Goya M, et al.: Impact of non-pulmonary vein focus on early recurrence of atrial fibrillation after pulmonary vein isolation. Heart Rhythm 1(Suppl):S203-S204, 2004.

18. Goya M, Ouyang F, Ernst S, et al.: Electroanatomic mapping and catheter ablation of breakthroughs from the right atrium to the superior vena cava in patients with atrial fibrillation. Circulation 106:1317-1320, 2002.

19. Cappato R, Negroni S, Pecora D, et al.: Prospective assessment of late conduction recurrence across radiofrequency lesions producing electrical disconnection at the pulmonary vein ostium in patients with atrial fibrillation. Circulation 108:1599-1604, 2003.

20. Mangrum JM, Mounsey JP, Kok LC, et al.: Intracardiac echocardiography-guided, anatomically based radiofrequency ablation of focal atrial fibrillation originating from pulmonary veins. J Am Coll Cardiol 39:1964-1972, 2002.

21. Natale A, Pisano E, Beheiry S, et al.: Ablation of right and left atrial premature beats following cardioversion in patients with chronic atrial fibrillation refractory to antiarrhythmic drugs. Am J Cardiol 85:1372-1375, 2000.

22. Jais P, Weerasooriya R, Shah DC, et al.: Ablation therapy for atrial fibrillation (AF): Past, present and future. Cardiovasc Res 54:337-346, 2002.

23. Schmitt C, Ndrepepa G, Weber S, et al.: Biatrial multisite mapping of atrial premature complexes triggering onset of atrial fibrillation. Am J Cardiol 89:1381-1387, 2002.

24. Keith A, Flack M: The form and nature of the primary divisions of the vertebrate heart. J Anat 41:189, 1907.

25. Ino T, Miyamoto S, Ohno T, Tadera T: Exit block of focal repetitive activity in the superior vena cava masquerading as a high right atrial tachycardia. J Cardiovasc Electrophysiol 11:480-483, 2000.

26. Chang KC, Lin YC, Chen JY, et al.: Electrophysiological characteristics and radiofrequency ablation of focal atrial tachycardia originating from the superior vena cava. Jpn Circ J 65:1034-1040, 2001.

27. Ooie T, Tsuchiya T, Ashikaga K, Takahashi N: Electrical connection between the right atrium and the superior vena cava, and the extent of myocardial sleeve in a patient with atrial fibrillation originating from the superior vena cava. J Cardiovasc Electrophysiol 13:482-485, 2002.

28. Jayam VK, Vasamreddy C, Berger R, Calkins H: Electrical disconnection of the superior vena cava from the right atrium. J Cardiovasc Electrophysiol 15:614, 2004.

29. Chen YJ, Chen YC, Yeh HI, et al.: Electrophysiology and arrhythmogenic activity of single cardiomyocytes from canine superior vena cava. Circulation 105:2679-2685, 2002.

30. Yeh HI, Lai YJ, Lee SH, et al.: Heterogeneity of myocardial sleeve morphology and gap junctions in canine superior vena cava. Circulation 104:3152-3157, 2001.

31. Spach MS, Barr RC, Jewett PH: Spread of excitation from the atrium into thoracic veins in human beings and dogs. Am J Cardiol 30:844-854, 1972.

32. Zipes DP, Knope RF: Electrical properties of the thoracic veins. Am J Cardiol 29:372-376, 1972.

33. Hashizume H, Ushiki T, Abe K: A histological study of the cardiac muscle of the human superior and inferior venae cavae. Arch Histol Cytol 58:457-464, 1995.

34. Mary-Rabine L, Hordof AJ, Danilo P Jr, et al.: Mechanisms for impulse initiation in isolated human atrial fibers. Circ Res 47:267-277, 1980.

35. Gelband H, Bush HL, Rosen MR, et al.: Electrophysiologic properties of isolated preparations of human atrial myocardium. Circ Res 30:293-300, 1972.

36. Ten Eick RE, Singer DH: Electrophysiological properties of diseased human atrium. Circ Res 44:545-557, 1979.

37. Kalman JM, Olgin JE, Karch MR, et al.: "Cristal tachycardias": Origin of right atrial tachycardias from the crista terminalis identified by intracardiac echocardiography. J Am Coll Cardiol 31:451-459, 1998.

38. Boineau JP, Canavan TE, Schuessler RB, et al.: Demonstration of a widely distributed atrial pacemaker complex in the human heart. Circulation 77:1221-1237, 1988.

39. Scherlag BJ, Yeh BK, Robinson MJ: Inferior interatrial pathway in the dog. Circ Res 31:18-35, 1972.

40. Doshi RN, Wu TJ, Yashima M, et al.: Relation between ligament of Marshall and adrenergic atrial tachyarrhythmia. Circulation 100:876-883, 1999.

41. Erlanger J, Blackman JR: A study of relative rhythmicity and conductivity in various regions of the auricles of the mammalian heart. Am J Physiol 19:125-174, 1907.

42. Andrew LW, Paul FC: Triggered and automatic activity in the canine coronary sinus. Circ Res 41:435-445, 1977.

43. Lee SH, Tai CT, Lin WS, et al.: Predicting the arrhythmogenic foci of atrial fibrillation before atrial transseptal procedure: Implication for catheter ablation. J Cardiovasc Electrophysiol 11:750-757, 2000.

44. Belhassen B, Viskin S: Atrial tachycardia and "kissing catheters." J Cardiovasc Electrophysiol 11:233, 2000.

45. Soejima K, Stevenson WG, Delacretaz E, et al.: Identification of left atrial origin of ectopic tachycardia during right atrial mapping: Analysis of double potentials at the posteromedial right atrium. J Cardiovasc Electrophysiol 11:975-980, 2000.

46. Frey B, Kreiner G, Gwechenberger M, Gossinger HD: Ablation of atrial tachycardia originating from the vicinity of the atrioventricular node: Significance of mapping both sides of the interatrial septum. J Am Coll Cardiol 38:394-400, 2001.

47. Marrouche NF, Sippens-Groenewegen A, Yang Y, et al.: Clinical and electrophysiologic characteristics of left septal atrial tachycardia. J Am Coll Cardiol 40:1133-1139, 2002.

48. Katritsis D, Giazitzoglou E, Korovesis S, et al.: Epicardial foci of atrial arrhythmias apparently originating in the left pulmonary veins. J Cardiovasc Electrophysiol 13:319-323, 2002.

49. Kuo JY, Tai CT, Tsao HM, et al.: P wave polarities of an arrhythmogenic focus in patients with paroxysmal atrial fibrillation originating from superior vena cava or right superior pulmonary vein. J Cardiovasc Electrophysiol 14:350-357, 2003.

50. Lin YJ, Tai CT, Liu TY, et al.: Electrophysiological mechanisms and catheter ablation of complex atrial arrhythmias from crista terminalis: Insight from three-dimensional noncontact mapping. Pacing Clin Electrophysiol 27:1232-1239, 2004.

51. Katritsis D, Ioannidis JP, Anagnostopoulos CE, et al.: Identification and catheter ablation of extracardiac and intracardiac components of ligament of Marshall tissue for treatment of

paroxysmal atrial fibrillation. J Cardiovasc Electrophysiol 12:750-758, 2001.

52. Polymeropoulos KP, Rodriguez LM, Timmermans C, Wellens HJ: Images in cardiovascular medicine: Radiofrequency ablation of a focal atrial tachycardia originating from the Marshall ligament as a trigger for atrial fibrillation. Circulation 105:2112-2113, 2002.

53. Weiss C, Willems S, Rostock T, et al.: Electrical disconnection of an arrhythmogenic superior vena cava with discrete radiofrequency current lesions guided by noncontact mapping. Pacing Clin Electrophysiol 26:1758-1761, 2003.

54. Huang BH, Wu MH, Tsao HM, et al.: Morphology of the thoracic veins and left atrium in paroxysmal atrial fibrillation initiated by superior caval vein ectopy. J Cardiovasc Electrophysiol 16:411-417, 2005.

55. Chen SA, Tai CT: Catheter ablation of atrial fibrillation originating from the non-pulmonary vein foci. J Cardiovasc Electrophysiol 16:229-232, 2005.

56. Liu TY, Tai CT, Lee PC, et al.: Novel concept of atrial tachyarrhythmias originating from the superior vena cava: Insight from noncontact mapping. J Cardiovasc Electrophysiol 14:533-539, 2003.

57. Lee RJ, Kalman JM, Fitzpatrick AP, et al.: Radiofrequency catheter modification of the sinus node for "inappropriate" sinus tachycardia. Circulation 92:2919-2928, 1995.

58. Callans DJ, Ren JF, Schwartzman D, et al.: Narrowing of the superior vena cava-right atrium junction during radiofrequency catheter ablation for inappropriate sinus tachycardia: Analysis with intracardiac echocardiography. J Am Coll Cardiol 33:1667-1670, 1999.

59. Man KC, Knight B, Tse HF, et al.: Radiofrequency catheter ablation of inappropriate sinus tachycardia guided by activation mapping. J Am Coll Cardiol 35:451-457, 2000.

60. Pappone C, Oral H, Santinelli V, et al.: Atrio-esophageal fistula as a complication of percutaneous transcatheter ablation of atrial fibrillation. Circulation 109:2724-2726, 2004.

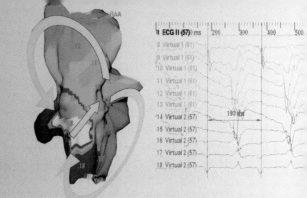

17

Linear Ablation for Atrial Fibrillation

Carlo Pappone • *Kenneth A. Ellenbogen*
Vincenzo Santinelli

Key Points

- Mapping for linear ablation of atrial fibrillation is anatomically based.

- Ablation targets include atrial myocardium around pulmonary venous ostia and sites eliciting vagal reflexes.

- Special equipment used includes an electroanatomic mapping system with a large-tip (8-mm) ablation catheter and a high-output generator, which are essential, as well as preformed sheaths and apparatus for trans-septal access.

- Sources of difficulty include incomplete ablation lines and the potential for postablation macroreentrant atrial tachyarrhythmias.

The poor success of pharmacologic therapy for the treatment of atrial fibrillation[1] (AF) has encouraged clinical investigators to explore alternative therapeutic strategies including multisite atrial pacing, atrial antitachycardia pacing, and atrial defibrillation, but these therapies still remain largely unsatisfactory. A palliative therapy for "drug-refractory" AF is ventricular pacing after atrioventricular junction ablation, but this approach still requires anticoagulation.

Surgical treatment of AF (e.g., the Maze approach) was described by Cox et al. in 1991.[2] Its high long-term success rate has encouraged clinical electrophysiologists to develop a variety of different strategies for ablation of this arrhythmia.[3,4] Percutaneous transcatheter ablation to cure AF currently is an evolving therapy, and different groups have advocated different techniques. At present, ablation approaches for AF can be divided into two major strategies: anatomic ablation[5-13] and electrically guided ablation[14-25] (Fig. 17–1). The relative merits and potential limitations of each approach are currently debated, although the anatomic approach appears to be highly effective and safe in patients with either paroxysmal or chronic AF.[9,13] Although segmental ostial isolation may cure about two thirds of patients with paroxysmal AF,[16,23-25] this approach does not address non–pulmonary venous triggers of AF or the importance of the left atrium (LA) itself. Conversely, the circumferential approach, as developed by Pappone, can not only eliminate the triggers of AF but also modify the left atrial substrate; furthermore, it can be performed in a relatively short period compared with the pulmonary vein (PV) isolation approach.[5-13]

The high success rates after left atrial circumferential ablation in patients with paroxysmal and chronic AF, first reported by Pappone et al.[5-12] and subsequently confirmed by other investigators,[13] have led to increased interest in an ablation approach to AF (Fig. 17–2). This chapter reviews the clinical trials on linear ablation in the right atrium (RA) and LA and discusses the practical aspects of performing left atrial linear ablation. The efficacy and safety of the anatomic approach are described, and practical aspects of management in these patients are detailed. The defined end points of the circumferential approach are discussed, and the extensive experience of Pappone's group with this approach (in more than 4000 patients with paroxysmal or chronic AF, many with structural heart disease) is reported.

Right Atrial Linear Ablation

The initial catheter ablation approaches to AF were focused in the RA.[4,26-28] Right atrial linear ablation was developed to alter atrial substrate that perpetuated AF. Initial enthusiasm was engendered by the belief that the creation of linear right atrial lesions would be simple, quick, safe, and effective. Two major strategies were employed. The first consisted of the "drag and burn" technique, with stepwise movement of a catheter with a 4- to 5-mm tip from spot to spot in the RA. The second strategy consisted of placing a multipolar catheter in the RA and delivering radiofrequency (RF) energy simultaneously or sequentially from each electrode. The objective was to create one or more linear lesions in the RA, usually between one or more anatomic structures, such as the right atrial appendage, superior vena cava, inferior vena cava, crista terminalis, or fossa ovalis. Rarely was conduction block from a linear lesion confirmed electrophysiologically.

The results from these approaches have been disappointing. The number of patients studied in these trials was relatively small, with study sizes ranging from 12 to 91 patients.[4,26-28] All studies included a "typical" atrial flutter ablation line across the right atrial isthmus. Most groups also included a posterior ablation line between the superior vena cava and the inferior vena cava. Other groups included additional lines, such as a septal ablation line, an anterior ablation line between the right atrial appendage and the tricuspid annulus, or a line from the superior vena cava to the tricuspid annulus or the fossa ovalis.

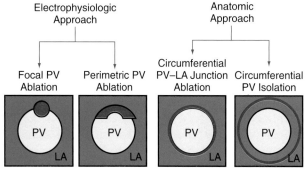

FIGURE 17–1. Summary of the two major strategies for pulmonary vein (PV) ablation therapy: anatomic guided ablation versus electrically guided ablation. Focal ablation refers to localized elimination of atrial fibrillation (AF) triggers, perimetric ablation is segmental ablation at the PV ostium to isolate the vein, Circumferential PV-LA junction ablation is complete encircling of the PV at the ostium, and circumferential PV isolation is isolation of the vein by ablation in the atrium away from the os. The schematics represent the relation of ablation lesions (*red circles or lines*) to the PV ostium and left atrium. LA, left atrium.

Ablative Studies in Atrial Fibrillation

Author	Year	Patients	AF Type	Guidance	Ablative Approach	Overall Freedom from AF (%)	Follow-up (months)
Haissaguerre et al.	1996	45	PAF	Fluoro	Linear Ablation RA **Biatrial**	33 60	11 ± 4
Maloney et al.	1998	15	CAF	Fluoro	Linear Ablation RA	81	23 ± 10
Haissaguerre et al.[18]	1998	45	PAF	Fluoro	Focal PV Ablation	62	8 ± 6
Pappone et al.[17]	1999	27	PAF	CARTO	Linear Ablation RA LA **Biatrial**	50 60 85	11 ± 3
Ernst et al.	1999	45	PAF	CARTO	Linear Ablation LA **Biatrial**	0 0	1 ± 1
Haissaguerre et al.[19]	2000	70	PAF	Fluoro	Segmental PV Isolation	73	4 ± 5
Pappone et al.[24]	2000	26	PAF, CAF	CARTO	Circumferential PV Ablation	85	9 ± 3
Pappone et al.[25]	2001	251	PAF, CAF	CARTO	Circumferential PV Ablation	80	10 ± 5
Oral et al.[20,21]	2002	110	PAF, CAF	Fluoro	Segmental PV Isolation	65	7 ± 4
Pappone et al.[11]	2003	589	PAF, CAF	CARTO	Circumferential PV Ablation	80	29 ± 7
Stabile et al.	2003	51	PAF, CAF	CARTO	Circumferential PV Ablation	80	17 ± 4
Oral et al.[26]	2003	80	PAF	CARTO **vs** Fluoro	Circumferential PV Ablation **vs** Segmental PV Ablation	88 67	6
Pappone et al.[27]	2004	297	PAF	CARTO	Circumferential PV Ablation	85	12

FIGURE 17–2. Summary of results of studies on pulmonary vein (PV) ablation for atrial fibrillation. Anatomic approaches are in red, and electrically guided approaches are shown in blue.

Most of the patients studied had no structural heart disease (lone AF) or hypertension only. The incidence of AF recurrence was high, ranging from 48% to 86%. Most patients were taking antiarrhythmic drugs after the ablation procedure was finished. The patient population studied in these clinical trials was generally young, with a mean age ranging from 51 to 61 years. The mean follow-up ranged from 11 to 22 months.

A major disappointment with right atrial ablation was the lengthy mean procedure times (range, 248 to 474 minutes). In one study, the mean procedure time was 211 ± 111 minutes, but the range in individual patients was great (100 to 755 minutes). The mean fluoroscopy times ranged from 40 to 155 minutes, also with a great deal of variability among different patients and with different study protocols. There was not a great deal of difference with respect to procedural success rate related to technique (i.e., drag and burn versus multipolar catheter) or to the use of two versus three or four ablation lines. Another disappointment was the unexpectedly high incidence of complications. Complication rates varied, and were usually less than 5%. Complications reported included damage to the sinus node requiring pacemaker placement, phrenic nerve injury, pericarditis, atrioventricular (AV) fistula, and cardiac tamponade.

Several lessons were learned from our experience with right atrial linear ablation. First and foremost, right atrial linear ablation rarely results in a successful long-term cure of AF. Second, the procedure is not simple, and it can be lengthy and difficult, exposing the patient to a considerable duration of radiation exposure. Review of a variety of studies indicates that no specific series of lesions or technique has been shown to be superior. Finally, the risk of complications is not inconsequential, although stroke has not yet been reported to occur during right-sided atrial ablation.

Linear Left Atrial Ablation

The feasibility of left atrial linear ablation was demonstrated by John Swartz,[3] who performed drag and burn, point by point catheter ablation with a 4-mm-tip ablation catheter, creating lines from the right superior pulmonary vein (RSPV) to the left superior pulmonary vein (LSPV); from the left inferior pulmonary vein (LIPV) to the mitral annulus; from the RSPV to the right inferior pulmonary vein (RIPV) and toward the mitral annulus; and from the LSPV to the roof of the LA and then across Bachmann's bundle, to a point immediately posterior to the transverse sinus, between the anterior LA and the aortic root.[3] He placed a variety of additional lesions, including a line midway between the LSPV and the LIPV extended parallel to the mitral annulus, and a line between the membranous fossa and the RSPV. Additional right atrial ablation lines included an isthmus line and an intercaval line. Haissaguerre et al.[4] also developed a series of similar but simpler left atrial lines which passed near the PVs and joined the PV lines to the mitral annulus. These approaches were associated with a fair success rate (>50%) for maintenance of sinus rhythm without drugs. The importance of these studies is the proof of concept that the LA should be the central focus for successful cure of AF.

LEFT ATRIAL PULMONARY VEIN ANATOMIC VARIABILITY: IMPLICATIONS FOR CATHETER ABLATION TECHNIQUES

Structural anatomic variability may have potential implications regarding the choice of an ablation approach (Fig. 17–3).[29,30] Among patients undergoing left atrial circumferential ablation, anatomic PV variability does not appear to affect success and complication rates, because RF energy application is delivered away from the PV ostia. Therefore, ipsilateral PVs or veins with adjacent ostia can be safely encircled with a single ablation line. Conversely, several anatomic variations make a segmental ostial

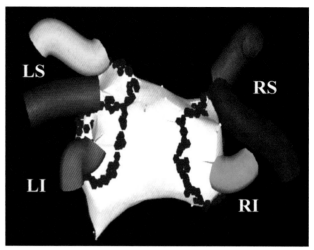

FIGURE 17–3. Anatomic variability of the pulmonary vein (PV)–left atrial junction. Multiple branches with a common ostium are detected in up to 6% of patients, whereas separately branching PVs can be observed in 3% of patients undergoing ablation. This patient has multiple ostia or very early branching of both the right superior (RS) and the left superior (LS) pulmonary vein. LI, left inferior pulmonary vein; RI, right inferior pulmonary vein.

approach for PV isolation challenging. These include a small PV ostium, an early branching PV, PVs arising with a vertical takeoff from the LA, and the presence of a middle PV. A small diameter increases the risk of PV stenosis after ostial ablation, and many electrophysiologists avoid or limit RF applications at the ostia of small veins. A large (>25 mm) PV ostium or a funnel-shaped PV can result in an unstable position and/or inadequate contact of the circumferential mapping catheter (Lasso catheter; Biosense Webster, Baldwin Park, Calif.). Conversely, a PV ostium smaller than 10 mm may not accommodate the Lasso catheter. In addition, large variations in PV ostia in a single patient often result in the need to use multiple Lasso catheters to achieve adequate contact in the smallest and largest PVs. Such anatomic variations imply a significant degree of versatility in the design of any new technology, especially in the dimension of the device, whether it is a balloon, a coil, or a loop catheter. More sophisticated technologies are needed for true guidance of percutaneous, endocardial-based left atrial interventions such as PV ablation, to permit fine interaction between the interventional tool and the anatomic target.

ATRIAL FIBRILLATION PATHOPHYSIOLOGY: IMPLICATIONS FOR CATHETER ABLATION TECHNIQUES

The mechanisms of AF are complex and not yet well defined (Fig. 17–4). The presence of triggers from the

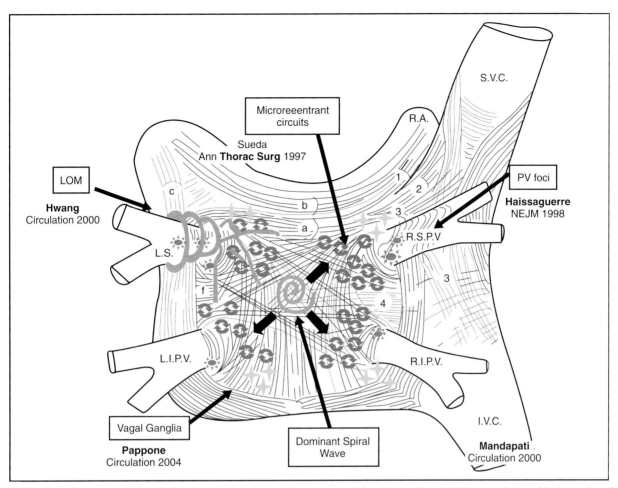

FIGURE 17-4. Summary of the electrophysiologic substrate in posterior left atrial wall amenable to catheter ablation using the linear approach described in this chapter. IVC, inferior vena cava; LI, left inferior; LOM, ligament of Marshall; LS, left superior; PV, pulmonary vein; RI, right inferior; RS, right superior; SVC, superior vena cava.

PVs as initiators of AF in humans has been confirmed,[31-33] but other triggering regions exist.[34-40] The findings of both multiple triggers and organized tachycardias lend credence to the view that the substrate is much more dominant in patients with chronic AF and structural heart disease, and any solution will have to deal with this pathophysiologic reality. Chronic AF is a highly heterogeneous and complex disease, and different mechanisms may operate in different patients, particularly at different stages of the disease. Further insight into all of these factors is needed to effectively devise more rational therapeutic approaches, but it has become increasingly evident that AF is a disease of the LA, and specifically of the posterior wall, which represents a critical zone to restore sinus rhythm, housing critical targets including vagal ganglia.[11,41-43]

The spatial distribution of AF foci coincides markedly with the distribution of pressure-sensitive receptors (eliciting a Bezold-Jarish–like reflex) observed in some patients during PV ablation. Our experience demonstrated the presence of abundant vagal fibers and ganglia at the atrial-venous junction.[11] Postablation heart rate variability analysis also showed a shift of sympathovagal balance toward parasympathetic withdrawal after circumferential left atrial ablation (Fig. 17–5), suggesting that destruction of local vagal innervation also prevents AF recurrences in almost all patients in whom it is possible to elicit and ablate vagal reflexes (overall, 30% of patients in our approach). Based on multiple AF mechanisms, ablation strategies would target either the drivers—whether they originate within a PV,[31-33] in the LA,[34-37] or elsewhere[38]—or the left atrial substrate, such that AF can no longer occur even in the presence of a driver. Therefore, ablation of AF also requires modification of the atrial substrate, including rotors, autonomic tone, and mother wavelets[11,42,43] (see Fig. 17–4), to prevent the critical number of circulating wavelets from developing. Left circumfer-

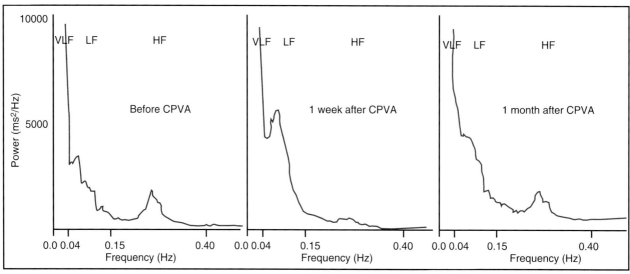

FIGURE 17–5. Empiric observations that suggest an autonomic component to linear atrial fibrillation (AF) ablation in patients with paroxysmal AF. This graphic representation of heart rate variability shows a shift toward the lower frequency spectrum after pulmonary vein isolation. (CPVA). VLF, very low frequency; LF, low frequency; HF, high frequency.

ential PV ablation eliminates both triggers and substrate, and also includes local vagal denervation, whereas ostial PV isolation affects only triggers. Consequently, it is not surprising that left circumferential atrial ablation may be more effective than ostial ablation alone, especially in patients with chronic AF.[5-13]

Circumferential Pulmonary Vein Ablation Procedure

PATIENT SELECTION

Patients with AF and clear contraindications to anticoagulation (heparin and/or warfarin) therapy are not considered potential candidates for the procedure (Figs. 17–6 and 17–8). Patients with esophageal varices and those in whom transesophageal echocardiography (TEE) cannot be safely performed also are not suitable candidates to undergo left atrial ablation. We also recommend that patients adopt a soft diet for 2 to 3 days before and after the ablation procedure, to avoid subclinical injury to the esophagus, in view of the small risk of atrioesophageal fistula that recently has come to light.[12] The procedure is indicated in (1) patients who experience at least one monthly episode of AF despite antiarrhythmic therapy with one or more drugs and who require electrical cardioversion to restore sinus rhythm; (2) patients who have one or more weekly episodes of spontaneously terminating AF but for whom

therapy with one or more antiarrhythmic drugs has failed to control symptoms; and (3) patients who wish an opportunity to have a long-term cure of their arrhythmia and thus avoid lifelong anticoagulation. Circumferential LA ablation can also be performed in elderly patients (up to 80 years of age) who have chronic AF and/or an LA diameter up to 65 mm, and even in patients with mitral and/or aortic metallic prosthetic valves, although longer fluoroscopic exposure times are usually required. In general, a low left ventricular ejection fraction does not represent an absolute contraindication to circumferential left atrial ablation. Patients who, before the procedure, are taking calcium or β-adrenoceptor blocking agents and/or angiotensin II receptor (ATR) blockers may continue therapy after the procedure, particularly in the presence of left ventricular enlargement and/or heart failure. Antiarrhythmic drugs (except amiodarone) and digoxin are discontinued for more than five half-lives. *To prevent stroke or other embolic events in patients not already receiving chronic anticoagulation therapy, a TEE is performed with short-term anticoagulation therapy instead of a 3-week course.*

PREPROCEDURE PREPARATION

One month before the procedure, transthoracic echocardiography (TTE), 24-hour electrocardiogram (ECG) monitoring, and daily transtelephonic random or symptom-triggered recordings are usually scheduled. Among patients with chronic AF, three or more consecutive international normalized ratio (INR) values ranging between 2.5 and 3.5 are required

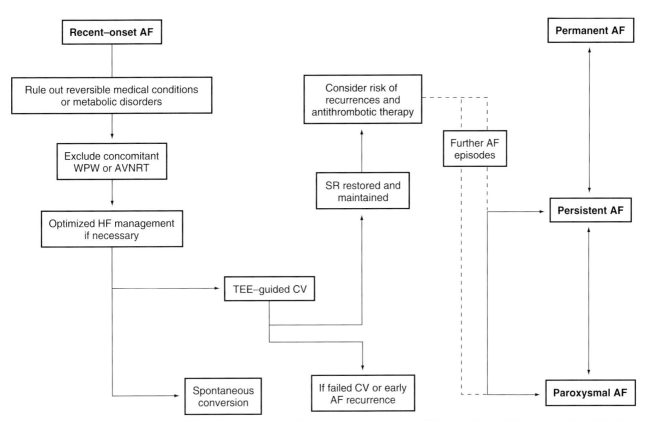

FIGURE 17–6. Algorithm used to guide atrial fibrillation (AF) ablation based on the Milan experience. CV, cardioversion; SR, sinus rhythm; TEE, transesophageal eletrocardiography.

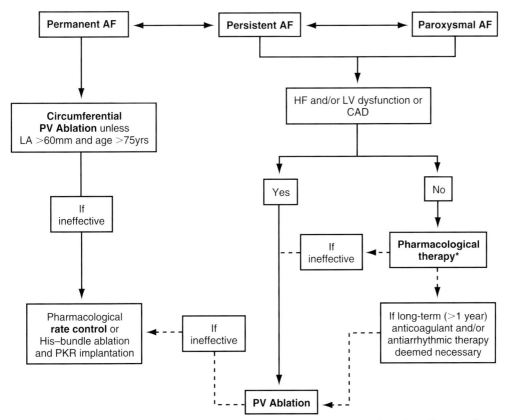

FIGURE 17–7. Algorithm used to guide atrial fibrillation (AF) ablation based on the Milan experience. LA, left atrium; PKR, pacemaker; HF, heart failure; LV, left ventricule; CAD, coronary artery disease.

before the procedure; in some laboratories, INRs between 2.0 and 3.0 are satisfactory. A chest radiograph and laboratory tests are also required to exclude lung and liver disease, which can preclude anticoagulant therapy and/or use of iodine contrast media.

At admission, we perform TEE routinely, but in patients with failed prior focal or segmental ablation of PVs we usually schedule a nuclear magnetic resonance imaging (MRI) examination to exclude significant PV stenosis caused by the prior procedure. Conversely, some laboratories perform spiral computed tomography (CT) with slices of 1 mm or thinner before the procedure, in place of MRI scanning.

PERIPROCEDURAL MANAGEMENT

Three days before the procedure, patients taking anticoagulants (usually those with persistent or chronic AF) stop oral anticoagulant therapy. The night before the procedure, heparin infusion is started to achieve activated clotting time (ACT) values between 200 and 250 seconds. Heparin is usually stopped 2 hours before the procedure, to obtain vascular access and to safely perform the trans-septal puncture. Some laboratories in the United States treat patients with low-molecular-weight (LMW) heparin from the time oral anticoagulation is stopped, discontinuing it 12 to 24 hours before the procedure. In the absence of echocardiographic abnormalities correlated with high thromboembolic risk (left atrial thrombus, spontaneous echocardiographic contrast, or abnormal left atrial appendage peak velocities), heparin is restarted to maintain an ACT between 250 and 300 seconds. In the presence of smoke and/or decreased velocity without left atrial thrombus, the ACT is maintained between 300 and 350 seconds. The presence of a left atrial thrombus is an absolute contraindication to the procedure. Patients with left atrial thrombi receive conventional anticoagulation therapy and have their ablation postponed until intracardiac thrombi can be excluded by a repeat TEE. An initial heparin bolus (1000 U per 10 kg body weight) is injected intravenously, after which heparin is titrated to maintain appropriate ACT values, which are usually checked every 15 to 20 minutes.

Because ablation in the LA, particularly around the LIPV and the posterior wall, may be uncomfortable or painful, we use a weight-adjusted infusion of an intravenous narcotic such as remifentanil (0.025 to 0.05 μg/kg/minute). A number of medications may be given if a patient experiences pain during left atrial ablation, including propofol and midazolam.

Mapping

Three catheters are typically used: a standard bipolar or quadripolar catheter in the RV apex to provide backup pacing; a quadripolar or decapolar catheter in the coronary sinus to allow pacing of the LA; and the ablation catheter, which is passed into the LA after trans-septal puncture with a standard Mullins sheath. A pigtail catheter is temporarily positioned above the aortic valve to act as a landmark at the time of trans-septal puncture. It is then removed, but arterial vascular access is maintained throughout the procedure for continuous arterial pressure monitoring. Particular attention should be paid to avoid aortic puncture while performing trans-septal puncture. Other laboratories use intracardiac echocardiography to aid the trans-septal puncture. A reference patch (Ref-Star; Cordis-Webster, Diamond Bar, Calif.) is also placed on the back of the patient. After the trans-septal puncture, the Mullins sheath is withdrawn into the RA, leaving only the 8-mm F- or D-curve ablation catheter (Navistar, Biosense Webster) in the LA. During the procedure the Mullins sheath is flushed every 10 minutes with heparinized solution. During navigation and ablation, both power and impedance, as well as electrical activity, are continuously and accurately monitored.

Real-time three-dimensional (3-D) maps of the LA and PV profiles are carried out with a nonfluoroscopic electroanatomic mapping system (CARTO, Biosense Webster) (Fig. 17–8), paying particular attention to the PV ostia. This system allows the electrophysiologist to accurately reconstruct the anatomy of the venous-atrial junction and to tailor the number and size of lesions to the complex morphology of the PV-LA junction in an individual patient (see Fig. 17–8). We normally start by acquiring all four PVs and the mitral annulus as anatomic landmarks for the CARTO navigation, and we create the map by entering each PV in turn. Three locations are recorded along the mitral annulus to tag the valve orifice. To acquire PVs, we use three criteria, based on fluoroscopy, impedance, and electrical activity (Table 17–1). Entry into the vein is clearly identified as the catheter leaves the cardiac shadow on fluoroscopy. As the catheter moves further into the vein, the impedance usually rises to greater than 140 to 150 ohms (Ω), and electrograms are no longer recorded. Because of the orientation of some veins and the limitations of catheter shape, it can be difficult to deeply enter some veins, but the impedance still rises when the ablation catheter passes into the vein. To better differentiate between PVs and the LA, we use voltage criteria (fractionation of the local bipolar electrogram) and

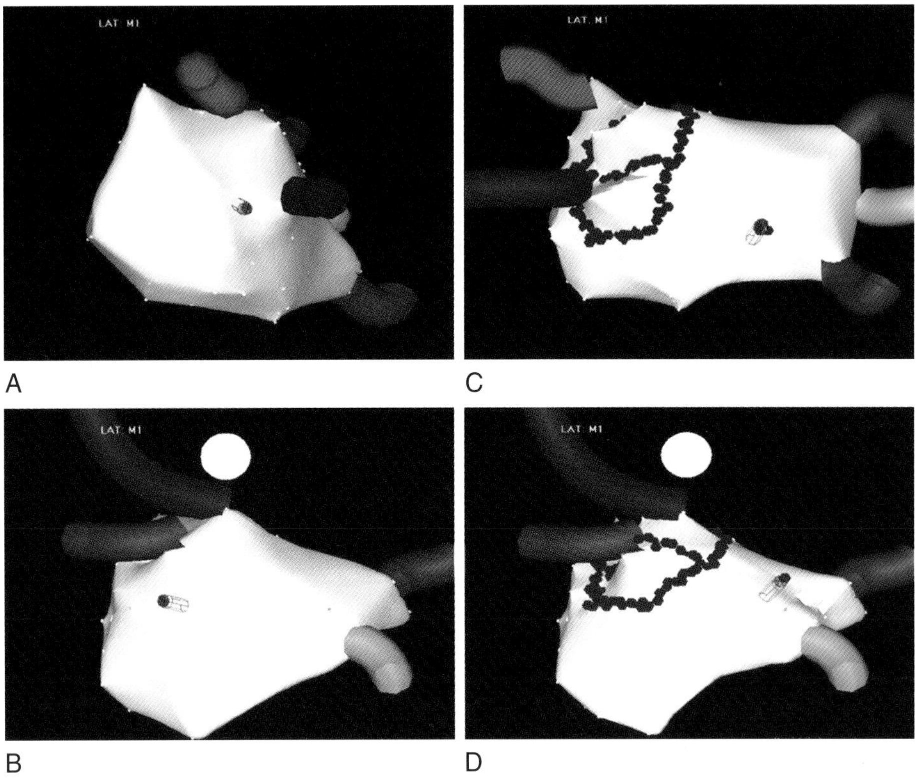

FIGURE 17–8. Monochromatic maps showing left atrial anatomy for ablation of all four pulmonary veins. **A,** Left lateral view. Note the location of the ablation catheter tip in the center of the image. **B,** Posteroanterior view. **C,** Inferior view. **D,** Posteroanterior view after isolation of the left veins. The catheter is positioned to begin circumferential ablation of the right pulmonary veins.

TABLE 17–1
Defining Pulmonary Venous Ostia
Fluoroscopy
Venography
Catheter outside cardiac shadow
Impedance rise >4 Ω above left atrial impedance
Fractionation of bipolar electrograms

impedance (a rise of $>4\,\Omega$ above mean left atrial impedance) to define the PV ostium. The anatomic appearance on CARTO acts as added confirmation of catheter entry into the PV ostium, and an 8-mm-tip deflectable catheter (Navi-Star, Cordis-Webster) is used for mapping and ablation.

The mapping and ablation procedures are performed by using the coronary sinus atrial signal if the patient is in sinus rhythm, or the right ventricular signal if the patient is in AF, as the synchronization trigger for CARTO. Each endocardial location is recorded while a stable catheter position is maintained, as assessed by both end-diastolic stability (a distance of 2 mm between two successive locations) and local activation time (LAT) stability (an interval

of 2 msec between two successive LATs). If spontaneous ventricular rates during AF are too low, we usually pace the right ventricle at higher rates to increase the CARTO system sampling rates. If sinus rhythm is present, we map during continuous coronary sinus pacing to increase the refresh rate. Atrial volumes are calculated by the CARTO system at the end of diastole, independently of the underlying rhythm (AF or sinus rhythm). The mapping catheter is introduced into the LA under fluoroscopic guidance, and its location is recorded relative to the location of the fixed reference. A minimum of 100 points are required to create adequate LA maps.

MAPPING SYSTEM

The anatomic reconstruction of the LA obtained with the CARTO system is reliable, as compared with MRI (Fig. 17–9). As the catheter is moved inside the heart, the mapping system continuously analyzes its location and orientation and presents these data to the user on the monitor of a graphic workstation, thereby allowing navigation without the use of fluoroscopy. The mapping procedure is performed by moving the catheter to numerous and sequential points within the LA and PVs and acquiring the location in 3-D space together, with the local unipolar and bipolar voltages and the LAT relative to the chosen reference interval. The system continuously monitors the

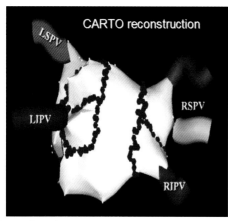
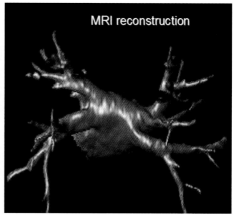

FIGURE 17–9. Comparison between reconstruction of the pulmonary vein–left atrial junction using an electroanatomic guidance system (CARTO, Biosense Webster) and reconstruction based on magnetic resonance imaging (MRI) with contrast. Note the high correlation between the two imaging techniques with respect to identification of the antrum and ostium. LIPV, left inferior pulmonary vein; LSPV, left superior pulmonary vein; RIPV, right inferior pulmonary vein; RSPV, right superior pulmonary vein.

quality of catheter-tissue contact and LAT stability to ensure the validity and reproducibility of each local measurement. The acquired information is then color-coded and displayed. As each new site is acquired, the reconstruction is updated in real time to progressively create a 3-D chamber geometry color-encoded with activation time. Additionally, the collected data can be displayed as voltage maps depicting the magnitude of the local peak voltage in a 3-D model. The chamber geometry is reconstructed in real time by interpolation of the acquired points. LATs can be used to create activation maps, which are of enormous importance when attempting to map and ablate focal or macroreentrant atrial tachycardias (ATs) but are not used during ablation of AF.

Ablation

Once the main PVs and the LA have been adequately reconstructed, RF energy is delivered to the atrial endocardium at a distance greater than or equal to 5 mm from the PV ostia, with RF generator settings of 55° C to 65° C and a power limit of 100 W, to create circumferential lines of conduction block (Table 17–2). This energy is reduced in the posterior wall to 50 W and 55° C to reduce the risk of injury to the surrounding structures.[12] If there is an impedance rise or if the patient has a cough or burning pain, RF delivery is stopped immediately. The monochromatic location map is used for the ablation procedure, because it avoids presentation of unnecessary information to the operator (see Fig. 17–8). Usually, circumferential ablation lines are created, starting at the lateral mitral

TABLE 17–2
Targets for Ablation
Atrial myocardium circumferentially ≥5 mm from pulmonary venous ostia
Sites of vagal reflex activation during ablation

annulus and withdrawing posteriorly, then anterior to the left-sided PVs, passing between the LSPV and the left atrial appendage before completing the circumferential line on the posterior wall of the LA. The "channel" between the LSPV and the left atrial appendage can be identified by fragmented electrograms caused by collision of activity from the left atrial appendage and LSPV/LA. The appendage is identifiable by a significantly higher impedance (>4 Ω greater than the left atrial mean), a high-voltage local bipolar electrogram, and also, frequently, a large ventricular electrogram, with characteristically organized activity in fibrillating patients (Table 17–3). The right PVs are isolated in a similar fashion, and then a posterior line connecting the two circumferential lines is performed to reduce the risk of macroreentrant ATs (Fig. 17–10). Usually, four discrete orifices are identified, permitting separate ablation lines to be created around each vein. However, a single circular line around two ipsilateral veins is created in the presence of (1) ostia less than 20 mm apart from each other, (2) a common ostium with early branching, or (3) a separately branching PV. As a result, we can easily tailor the lesion set based on the individual PV-LA junction morphology.

A number of other centers have adapted this technique with modification. For example, some centers

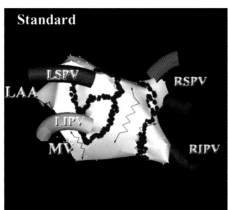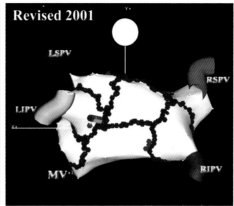

FIGURE 17-10. Standard and modified approach to avoid postablation left atrial tachycardia. The revised approach includes additional ablation lines on the posterior left atrial wall that connect contralateral pulmonary veins (PV) with each other and the left inferior pulmonary vein (LIPV) with the mitral annulus (MV). LAA, left atrial appendage; LSPV, left superior pulmonary vein; RIPV, right inferior pulmonary vein; RSPV, right superior pulmonary vein.

TABLE 17-3
Defining the Left Atrial Appendage

Fluoroscopy
  Venography
  Catheter outside cardiac shadow

Impedance rise 4 Ω above left atrial impedance
High-amplitude atrial electrogram
Large ventricular electrogram
Organized electrical activity in atrial fibrillation

have performed linear left atrial ablation using alternative mapping systems (Endocardial Solutions, St. Paul, Minn.). The Mayo Clinic group has modified this technique by combining left atrial linear ablation with PV isolation; they have termed their variation "wide area circumferential ablation."

ASSESSMENT OF PULMONARY VEIN INNERVATION

Potential vagal target sites are identified during the procedure in at least one third of patients.[11] Vagal reflexes are considered to include sinus bradycardia (<40 beats per minute), asystole, AV block, and hypotension that occurs within a few seconds after the onset of RF application. If a reflex is elicited, RF energy is delivered until such reflexes are abolished, or for up to 30 seconds. The end point for ablation at these sites is termination of the reflex, followed by sinus tachycardia or AF. Failure to reproduce the reflexes with repeat RF is considered confirmation of denervation. Complete local vagal denervation is defined by the abolition of all vagal reflexes. The

most common sites are tagged on electroanatomic maps (Fig. 17-11).

POTENTIAL THROMBUS FORMATION DURING RADIOFREQUENCY APPLICATIONS

We typically use 8-mm-tip catheters to avoid thrombus formation, particularly because we use power up to 100 W and temperature settings up to 65°C. If thrombus forms on the catheter tip, the impedance suddenly increases, although in our experience a much more useful indicator of such complication is a reduction of 40% to 50% in the power being delivered to reach target temperature. If there is reason to suspect thrombus formation, we strongly recommend withdrawing the catheter from the LA without advancing the trans-septal sheath, to preserve trans-septal access. This is to avoid stripping away any potential thrombus present on the catheter tip as the catheter is withdrawn into the sheath, which might result in systemic embolization. Unfortunately, this means that access to the LA will need to be achieved by trying to find the previous trans-septal puncture using the CARTO map. A smart trick is to acquire multiple location points on the electroanatomic map as the catheter is being withdrawn across the atrial septum. When the catheter tip enters the RA, it will suddenly fall, indicating the right aspect of the septum. These points can then act as markers for repeat passage of the catheter into the LA, which can be achieved without repuncture in about 80% of cases.

END POINTS FOR ABLATION

Among patients in sinus rhythm, postablation remapping of the LA is performed using the preab-

Preablation voltage map   Postablation voltage map

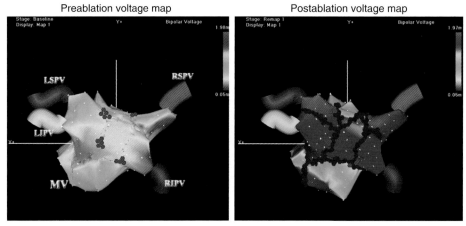

FIGURE 17–11. Preablation and postablation voltage maps depicting "hot spots" *(blue circles)* at which radiofrequency energy (RF) ablation evoked vagal reflexes with subsequent vagal denervation. LIPV, left inferior pulmonary vein; LSPV, left superior pulmonary vein; MV, mitral valve; RIPV, right inferior pulmonary vein; RSPV, right superior pulmonary vein. A posterior view is shown. Note also the marked reduction in the atrial voltages (red) within the ablation lines arter ablation.

lation map for the acquisition of new points to permit accurate comparison of preablation and postablation bipolar voltage maps (see Fig. 17–12). Among patients in AF, after restoration of sinus rhythm, postablation remapping is done using the anatomic map acquired during AF, so as to have the same landmarks and lesion tags for accurate lesion validation. There are no significant intrapatient differences between the anatomic map of a fibrillating atrium and the map obtained during pacing, because location points are recorded at end-diastole. Usually, we do not validate circumferential lesions around PVs by pacing maneuvers, but we validate the bipolar voltage abatement within the encircled areas, by simply performing a voltage remap (i.e., acquiring new points on the existing geometry to provide voltage measurements) (Table 17–4). The end point for circumferential left atrial ablation is a reduction of greater than 90% in voltage within the isolated regions. Therefore, to validate circumferential lesions around each PV, only one postablation voltage map is usually required, without the need for time-consuming mapping studies. In addition, all points inside and around the lesions (e.g., inside the circumferential lesions or lines) with an amplitude of less than 0.1 mV can be selected and tagged, and the software can calculate the surface area in square millimeters of the 3-D reconstruction inside the marked region of interest. Conversely, completeness of lesion lines, particularly at the mitral isthmus, is critical to prevent postablation macroreentrant left atrial tachycardias, which in most cases are mitral isthmus–dependent and incessant.[44] Gaps are defined as breakthroughs in an ablated area, and they are identified by sites with single potentials and by early

TABLE 17–4
End Points for Ablation

>90% reduction electrogram amplitude within isolated regions

Electrogram amplitude <0.1 mV within isolated region

Elimination of vagal reflexes at innervation sites

Complete mitral isthmus line
  Absence conduction across line on activation map
  Double potentials along line with >150 msec separation during coronary sinus pacing

local activation. The completeness of the mitral isthmus line is demonstrated during coronary sinus pacing by endocardial and coronary sinus mapping, looking for widely spaced double potentials across the line of block, and are confirmed by differential pacing. In our experience, the minimum double-potential interval at the mitral isthmus during coronary sinus pacing after block is achieved is 150 msec, depending on the atrial dimensions and the extent of scarring and lesion creation.

After the planned lines of block have been created, the LA is remapped, and the preablation and postablation activation maps are compared. Incomplete block is revealed by impulse propagation across the line; in such a case, further RF applications are given to complete the line of block. Patients with a history of common atrial flutter also undergo ablation of the cavotricuspid isthmus line.

MECHANISMS OF SUCCESSFUL ABLATION

Pappone and colleagues have proposed multiple mechanisms for the high success rate of anatomically guided circumferential ablation. As already discussed, these include ablation of PV triggers, modification of left atrial substrate for maintenance of AF, ablation of non-PV triggers, and ablation of parasympathetic inputs to the posterior left atrial wall.[5-11] Other possible mechanisms can also be envisaged. Several points of continued debate include the importance of complete linear lesions and the importance of PV isolation.

Ernst et al.[44,45] showed that complete left atrial lesions are difficult to achieve using conventional RF energy delivery. Specifically, relatively few patients had complete lines of block attained by trying to create a variety of proposed left atrial linear lesions in a series of patients using the CARTO electroanatomic mapping system and 4-mm-tip catheters with ablation energy limited to 50 W. This study was severely limited in that many patients achieved successful results despite the lack of complete lines of block with the linear lesions, and because the RF delivery was limited to 50 W. A follow-up study from Kuck's group[45] argued for the primacy of PV isolation as being necessary for a high success rate. The authors placed simultaneous Lasso catheters inside both left or both right PVs and used the them to guide ablation. The end point of the procedure was (1) absence of all PV potentials within both Lasso catheters of the ipsilateral veins and (2) no recurrence of PV potentials after adenosine infusion. In contrast, Morady's group[46] was able to show that PV isolation is not necessary for a successful long-term result. A number of other clinical and surgical studies have shown good AF cure rates despite lesions that do not target the PVs.[47] Further prospective studies are needed to better define the mechanisms that explain the high success rate achieved with the circumferential anatomic technique.[5-11]

POSTPROCEDURE MANAGEMENT

At the end of procedure, protamine sulphate is intravenously administered to permit removal of sheaths. Other laboratories allow the ACT to drift down before the sheaths are removed, and some laboratories use closure devices to close the vein and artery. Thirty to 60 minutes after removal of the sheaths, heparin infusion is restarted for 12 to 18 hours, to maintain an ACT between 200 and 250 seconds. In North America, many laboratories start LMW heparin 4 hours after sheath removal. The dose of LMW heparin varies from 0.5 to 1.0 mg/kg, assuming normal renal function. Thereafter, oral anticoag-

ulant therapy is started while subcutaneous calcium heparin (12,500 U two times daily) or LMW heparin is jointly administered for the first few days, until the INR values range between 2.5 and 3.5. After the procedure, patients are anticoagulated for at least 30 days in the presence of a stable sinus rhythm and managed according to the LA size and characteristics of AF before ablation (discussed later). Oral anticoagulation is continued for 3 months after the procedure and is then stopped in case of restoration of sinus rhythm associated with improved or normal left atrial transport and left atrial appendage peak velocities.

Patients with Left Atrial Diameter Greater Than 55 mm and Chronic Atrial Fibrillation

In this patient group, we prescribe oral amiodarone, with a total dose of 1200 mg/week for 30 days and 600 mg/week for the next 30 days. If TTE, performed before the 60th day, shows a reduction in left atrial diameter of greater than 3.5 mm, associated with an improvement of atrial transport function and persistent sinus rhythm documented by daily transtelephonic recordings, amiodarone is replaced by oral sotalol (120 mg daily for 30 days). Usually, sotalol is discontinued after 30 days if sinus rhythm persists.

Patients with Left Atrial Diameter between 40 mm and 55 mm and Paroxysmal Atrial Fibrillation

In this patient category we prescribe sotalol, 40 mg twice daily, and flecainide, 50 mg twice daily, for 30 days. If, after this period, the left atrial diameter decreases, sotalol is continued for 30 days longer.

Patients with Left Atrial Diameter Less Than 40 mm and Paroxysmal Atrial Fibrillation

Among patients with paroxysmal AF and small atria, we prescribe sotalol, 40 mg daily, for 30 days. Because it is not uncommon for patients to have early recurrence of AF after ablation, we discharge many patients on antiarrhythmic medication (as detailed earlier). However, recurrence during the first 4 weeks is not necessarily associated with a poor outcome, and long-term success may still be achieved after restoration of sinus rhythm. Incessant atrial tachyarrhythmias (AT) usually occurs within the first few months as a complication of the procedure in 10% of patients, and in some patients AT may drive AF, but a redo procedure is required in only about 5% of patients.[44,50]

All patients are given a daily transtelephonic event recorder for at least 1 year after the procedure and are requested to send recordings weekly, regardless of the presence or absence of symptoms. We usually arrange for clinical assessment, TTE, and 24-hour ambulatory recordings at 1, 3, 6, and 12 months after the procedure. Because recurrences of AF and/or AT occurring within the first 4 weeks after ablation may be transient phenomena, they are not considered true recurrences if limited to the first 4 weeks. Other laboratories use continuous transtelephonic monitoring for 1 week to 1 month at 3 to 6 months after ablation.[45]

Clinical Outcomes

EFFICACY

Since we first started performing this procedure in 1998, the procedure duration has dropped substantially; it now stands at less than 90 minutes from the time of femoral sheath insertion. Overall, long-term success rates (at 2 years) are approximately 90% for patients with paroxysmal AF, and 80% for those with chronic AF (Fig. 17–13). In patients with paroxysmal AF in whom vagal reflexes are elicited and abolished by RF applications, the long-term success rate is almost 100%.[11] The high success rates achieved by

this procedure in the large experience of Pappone and colleagues have been reported for an extremely diverse group of patients (Figure 17-12). The low complication rates are notable in this context. For example, in the series of 589 consecutive ablations performed between January 1998 and March 2001, with a median follow-up of 900 days, the risk of complications was only 0.7%, and no patients suffered stroke, transient ischemic attack, or pulmonary steno-

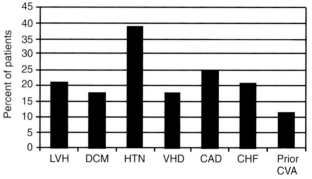

FIGURE 17–12. Clinical characteristics of patients who underwent linear atrial fibrillation ablation in the Milan program from 1998 to 2004. A total of 4177 patients were treated. CHF, congestive heart failure; CAD, coronary artery disease; HTN, hypertension; DCM, dilated cardiomyopathy; LVH, left ventricular hypertrophy; CVA, cerebrovascular accident.

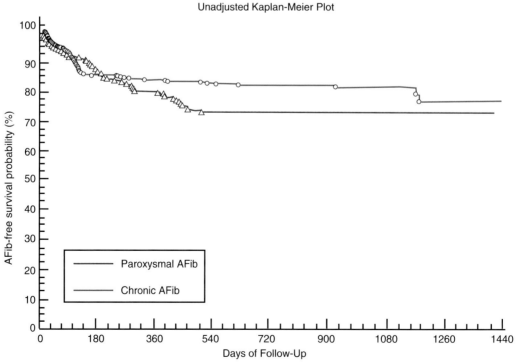

FIGURE 17–13. Timing and pattern of atrial fibrillation (AF) recurrences after ablation for both chronic and paroxysmal AF. For patients with paroxysmal AF, the majority of recurrences occurred in the first weeks after ablation; while for patients with chronic AF a more gradual pattern of recurrence during the first 6 months was noted.

TABLE 17–5

Troubleshooting the Difficult Case

Problem	Causes	Possible Solution
Difficult catheter navigation	Incomplete or inaccurate electroanatomic map	Confirm accuracy of map especially in relation to vein ostia
	Unusual cardiac anatomy	Review preprocedure cardiac imaging
Catheters repeatedly enter pulmonary veins or appendage	Inaccurate electroanatomic map	Confirm accuracy of map, especially in relation to vein ostia
	Unusual cardiac anatomy	Review preprocedure cardiac imaging
	Unstable catheter positions	Try different catheter curve or preformed sheath
Residual high voltage in isolated segments	Incomplete lines	Review continuity of lines, repeat ablation

sis.[9] In this series, the mean age of patients undergoing circumferential ablation was 65 ± 9 years; 66% of patients had some form of cardiovascular disease, including coronary artery disease (23%), hypertension (46%), dilated cardiomyopathy (5%), prior stroke or transient ischemic attack (16%), and diabetes (11%). In short, this technique has wider applicability than approaches that require considerably more skill for isolation of the PVs. It will be necessary to demonstrate the ability to consistently replicate the results of Pappone and colleagues before widespread adaptation of this technique can be advocated.

COMPLICATIONS

RF catheter ablation of AF has a relatively low risk of serious complications; no major complications, including death, stroke, or other thromboembolic events, have occurred in our extensive experience.[9,11] Small, nonhemodynamically significant pericardial effusions may occur in up to 4% of patients. Only a few patients have required pericardiocentesis for cardiac tamponade. Only one case of atrioesophageal fistula has been recently observed in our series (0.05%), in a patient who had several RF applications on the posterior LA; a similar case was reported by the Michigan group.[12] Atrioesophageal fistula is very rare, but its occurrence is dramatic and devastating. We now recommend lower RF energy applications when ablating on the left atrial posterior wall. The course of the esophagus is quite variable relative to the PVs, and some electrophysiologists lower RF energy to 50 to 60 W and temperature to 52°C to 55°C during ablation of the posterior wall, especially near the left PVs. PV occlusion has been reported to occur rarely, despite a circumferential approach.[48,49] Postablation left atrial tachycardias resulting from macroreentry or focal mechanisms have been reported in 5% to 20% of patients.[50] Although these arrhythmias are self-limited in some patients, repeated ablation procedures are required in others.

Troubleshooting the Difficult Case

Because the circumferential PV isolation technique is anatomically guided and devoid of electrical mapping, problems during the procedure itself are usually limited to catheter navigation about the PVs (Table 17–5). The generation of an accurate electroanatomic map that is true to the cardiac anatomy is essential for this procedure. Strict attention to defining the PV ostia and atrial appendage may require the use of fluoroscopy and venography in cases of uncertainty. Review of preprocedural cardiac MRI or CT images will identify unusual anatomic features beforehand. The most recent generation of electroanatomic mapping systems allows for importation of 3-D CT or MRI images for direct comparison with the electroanatomic map. Residual high electrogram amplitudes within the atrial segments bounded for isolation may indicate incomplete ablation lines. The thoroughness of the lines should be reviewed, and segments of the ablation lines may need to be repeated.

References

1. Wyse DG, Waldo AL, DiMarco JP, et al.: A comparison of rate control and rhythm control in patients with atrial fibrillation. N Engl J Med 347:1825-1833, 2002.
2. Cox JL, Canavan TE, Schuessler RB, et al.: The surgical treatment of atrial fibrillation. II: Intraoperative electrophysiologic

mapping and description of the electrophysiologic basis of atrial flutter and atrial fibrillation. J Thorac Cardiovasc Surg 101:406-426, 1991.

3. Swartz JF, Pellersels G, Silvers J, et al.: A catheter-based curative approach to atrial fibrillation in humans [abstract]. Circulation 90(Suppl I):I-335, 1994.

4. Haissaguerre M, Jais P, Shah DC, et al.: Right and left atrial radiofrequency catheter therapy of paroxysmal atrial fibrillation. J Cardiovasc Electrophysiol 7:1132-1134, 1996.

5. Pappone C, Oreto G, Lamberti F, et al.: Catheter ablation of paroxysmal atrial fibrillation using a 3D mapping system. Circulation 100:1203-1208, 1999.

6. Pappone C, Rosanio S, Oreto G, et al.: Circumferential radiofrequency ablation of pulmonary vein ostia. Circulation 102:2619-2628, 2000.

7. Pappone C, Oreto G, Rosanio S, et al.: Atrial electroanatomic remodeling after circumferential radiofrequency pulmonary vein ablation: Efficacy of an anatomic approach in a large cohort of patients with atrial fibrillation. Circulation 103:2539-2544, 2001.

8. Pappone C: Atrial fibrillation: A curable condition? Eur Heart J 23:514-517, 2002.

9. Pappone C, Rosanio S, Augello G, et al.: Mortality, morbidity, and quality of life after circumferential pulmonary vein ablation for atrial fibrillation: Outcomes from a controlled nonrandomized long-term study. J Am Coll Cardiol 42:185-197, 2003.

10. Pappone C: Pulmonary vein isolation for atrial fibrillation. In Zipes DP, Jalife J. Cardiac Electrophysiology: From Cell to Bedside, 4th ed. Philadelphia: Saunders, 2004.

11. Pappone C, Santinelli V, Manguso F, et al.: Pulmonary vein denervation enhances longterm benefit after circumferential ablation for paroxysmal atrial fibrillation. Circulation 109:327-334, 2004.

12. Pappone C, Oral H, Santinelli V, et al.: Atrio-esophageal fistula as a complication of percutaneous transcatheter ablation of atrial fibrillation. Circulation 109:2724-2726, 2004.

13. Oral H, Scharf C, Chugh A, et al.: Catheter ablation for paroxysmal atrial fibrillation: Segmental pulmonary vein ostial ablation vs. left atrial ablation. Circulation 108:2355-2360, 2003.

14. Haissaguerre M, Shah DC, Jais P, et al.: Electrophysiological breakthroughs from the left atrium to the pulmonary veins. Circulation 102:2463-2465, 2000.

15. Natale A, Pisano E, Shewchik J, et al.: First human experience with pulmonary vein isolation using a through-the-balloon circumferential ultrasound ablation system for recurrent atrial fibrillation. Circulation 102:1879-1882, 2000.

16. Oral H, Knight BP, Tada H, et al.: Pulmonary vein isolation for paroxysmal and persistent atrial fibrillation. Circulation 105:1077-1081, 2000.

17. Shah DC, Haissaguerre M, Jais P, et al.: Electrophysiologically guided ablation of the pulmonary veins for the curative treatment of atrial fibrillation. Ann Med 32:408-416, 2000.

18. Tada H, Oral H, Wasmer K, et al.: Pulmonary vein isolation: Comparison of bipolar and unipolar electrograms at successful and unsuccessful ostial ablation sites. J Cardiovasc Electrophysiol 13:13-19, 2002.

19. Tada H, Oral H, Knight BP, et al.: Randomized comparison of bipolar versus unipolar plus bipolar recordings during segmental ostial ablation of pulmonary veins. J Cardiovasc Electrophysiol 13:851-856, 2002.

20. Oral H, Ozaydin M, Tada H, et al.: Mechanistic significance of intermittent pulmonary vein tachycardia in patients with atrial fibrillation. J Cardiovasc Electrophysiol 13:645-650, 2002.

21. Oral H, Knight BP, Ozaydin M, et al.: Segmental ostial ablation to isolate the pulmonary veins during atrial fibrillation: Feasi-

bility and mechanistic insights. Circulation 106:1256-1262, 2002.

22. Marrouche NF, Dresing T, Cole C, et al.: Circular mapping and ablation of the pulmonary vein for treatment of atrial fibrillation: Impact of different catheter technologies. J Am Coll Cardiol 40:464-474, 2002.

23. Oral H, Knight BP, Ozaydin M, et al: Segmental ostial ablation to isolate the pulmonary veins during atrial fibrillation: feasibility and mechanistic insights. Circulation 106(10):1256-1262, 2002.

24. Marrouche NF, Martin DO, Wazni O, et al.: Phased-array intracardiac echocardiography monitoring during pulmonary vein isolation in patients with atrial fibrillation: Impact on outcome and complications. Circulation 107:2710-2716, 2003.

25. Oral H, Knight BP, Tada H, et al.: Pulmonary vein isolation for paroxysmal and persistent atrial fibrillation. Circulation 105: 1077-1081, 2002.

26. Jais P, Shah DC, Takahashi A, et al.: Long-term follow-up after right atrial radiofrequency catheter treatment of paroxysmal atrial fibrillation. Pacing Clin Electrophysiol 21:2533-2536, 1998.

27. Garg A, Finneran W, Mollerus M, et al.: Right atrial compartmentalization using radiofrequency catheter ablation for management of patients with refractory atrial fibrillation. J Cardiovasc Electrophysiol 10:763-771, 1999.

28. Natale A, Leonelli F, Beheiry S, et al.: Catheter ablation approach on the right side only for paroxysmal atrial fibrillation therapy: Long-term results. Pacing Clin Electrophysiol 23:224-233, 2000.

29. Scharf C, Sneider M, Case I, et al.: Anatomy of the pulmonary veins in patients with atrial fibrillation and effects of segmental ostial ablation analyzed by computed tomography. J Cardiovasc Electrophysiol 14:150-155, 2003.

30. Kato R, Lickfett L, Meininger G, et al.: Pulmonary vein anatomy in patients undergoing catheter ablation of atrial fibrillation: Lessons learned by use of magnetic resonance imaging. Circulation 107:2004-2010, 2003.

31. Jais P, Haissaguerre M, Shah DC, et al.: A focal source of atrial fibrillation treated by discrete radiofrequency ablation. Circulation 95:572-576, 1997.

32. Chen SA, Hsieh MH, Tai CT, et al.: Initiation of atrial fibrillation by ectopic beats originating from the pulmonary veins: Electrophysiological characteristics, pharmacological responses, and effects of radiofrequency ablation. Circulation 100:1879-1886, 1999.

33. Shah DC, Haissaguerre M, Jais P: Catheter ablation of pulmonary vein foci for atrial fibrillation: PV foci ablation for atrial fibrillation. Thorac Cardiovasc Surg 47(Suppl 3):352-356, 1997.

34. Shah D, Haissaguerre M, Jais P, et al.: Left atrial appendage activity masquerading as pulmonary vein potentials. Circulation 105:2821-2825, 2002.

35. Hwang C, Karagueuzian HS, Chen PS: Idiopathic paroxysmal atrial fibrillation induced by a focal discharge mechanism in the left superior pulmonary vein: Possible roles of the ligament of Marshall. J Cardiovasc Electrophysiol 10:636-648, 1999.

36. Wu TJ, Ong JJ, Chang CM, et al.: Pulmonary veins and ligament of Marshall as sources of rapid activations in a canine model of sustained atrial fibrillation. Circulation 103:1157-1163, 2001.

37. Chen PS, Chou CC: Coronary sinus as an arrhythmogenic structure. J Cardiovasc Electrophysiol 13:863-864, 2002.

38. Chen PS, Wu TJ, Hwang C, et al.: Thoracic veins and the mechanisms of non-paroxysmal atrial fibrillation. Cardiovasc Res 54:295-301, 2002.

39. Oral H, Ozaydin M, Chugh A, et al.: Role of the coronary sinus in maintenance of atrial fibrillation. J Cardiovasc Electrophysiol 14:1329-1336, 2003.

40. Lin WS, Tai CT, Hsieh MH, et al.: Catheter ablation of paroxysmal atrial fibrillation initiated by non-pulmonary vein ectopy. Circulation 107:3176-3183, 2003.

41. Arora R, Verheule S, Scott L, et al.: Arrhythmogenic substrate of the pulmonary veins assessed by high-resolution optical mapping. Circulation 107:1816-1821, 2003.

42. Mandapati R, Skanes A, Chen J, et al.: Stable microreentrant sources as a mechanism of atrial fibrillation in the isolated sheep heart. Circulation 101:194-199, 2000.

43. Jalife J, Berenfeld O, Mansour M: Mother rotors and fibrillatory conduction: A mechanism of atrial fibrillation. Cardiovasc Res 54:204-216, 2002.

44. Ernst S, Ouyang F, Lober F, et al.: Catheter-induced linear lesions in the left atrium in patients with atrial fibrillation. J Am Coll Cardiol 42:1271-1282, 2003.

45. Ouyang F, Bansch D, Ernst S, et al.: Complete isolation of the left atrium surrounding the pulmonary vein: New insights from the double-Lasso technique in paroxysmal atrial fibrillation. Circulation 110:2090-2096, 2004.

46. Lemola K, Oral H, Cheung P, et al.: Is pulmonary vein isolation necessary during left atrial ablation for atrial fibrillation. Heart Rhythm 1:S10, 2004.

47. Stabile G, Turco P, La Rocca V, et al.: Is pulmoary vein isolation necessary for curing atrial fibrillation? Circulation 108:657-660, 2003.

48. Vasamreddy CR, Jayam V, Bluemke DA, Calkins H: Pulmonary vein occlusion: An unanticipated complication of catheter ablation of atrial fibrillation using the anatomic circumferential approach. Heart Rhythm 1:78-81, 2004.

49. Saad EB, Marrouche NF, Saad CP, et al.: Pulmonary vein stenosis after catheter ablation of atrial fibrillation: Emergence of a new clinical syndrome. Ann Intern Med 138:634-638, 2003.

50. Mesas CE, Pappone C, Lang CCE, et al.: Left atrial tachcyardia after circumferential pulmonary vein ablation for atrial fibrillation. J Am Coll Cardiol 44:1071-1079, 2004.

Catheter Ablation of Atrioventricular Nodal Reentrant Tachycardia

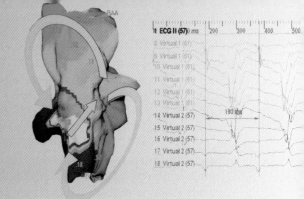

18

Ablation of Atrioventricular Nodal Reentry by the Anatomic Approach

Hugh Thomas McElderry • G. Neal Kay

Key Points

■ Diagnosis of atrioventricular (AV) nodal reentry is based on earliest retrograde activation at the near apex of the triangle of Koch, usually with the ability to dissociate atrium and ventricle from the tachycardia, and the response to ventricular pacing maneuvers.

■ The target for ablation is the slow pathway located between the coronary sinus ostium and the tricuspid valve.

■ Cryoablation may be useful. Electroanatomic mapping is optional. Catheter location and navigation systems are useful, as are long preformed sheaths.

■ Sources of difficulty include ablation near the His bundle or compact AV node, the presence of multiple slow pathways, and nonspecific ablation end points.

The most common paroxysmal supraventricular tachycardia (SVT) is atrioventricular (AV) nodal reentry, which accounts for more than 50% of all SVT cases in adults. Atrioventricular nodal reentrant tachycardia (AVNRT) is more common in females than males and is relatively uncommon in infants and young children. The electrocardiogram typically reveals P waves that are either absent or can be seen distorting the terminal portion of the QRS (Fig. 18–1), suggesting to early investigators that the atria and ventricles are activated simultaneously. Esophageal and intracardiac recordings in patients with this arrhythmia later confirmed these findings and demonstrated that a long septal right atrium-to-His bundle (AH) interval and a short His-to-atrial (HA) interval were typical of AVNRT (Fig. 18–2). Evidence supporting a reentrant mechanism in AVNRT was provided by Denes et al.,[1] who demonstrated that initiation of tachycardia was dependent on attainment of a critical delay in the AH interval, and by observations that dual conduction pathways are typical of patients with AVNRT. Additional support for the presence of dual conduction pathways through the AV node was presented by Rosen et al.,[2] who demonstrated the presence of two distinct sets of PR intervals on the surface electrocardiogram of a patient with AVNRT. Based on these observations, typical AVNRT was initially thought to involve reentrant activation within the AV node, with antegrade conduction via a slowly conducting (slow) pathway and retrograde conduction over a more rapidly conducting (fast) pathway. Since the demonstration that selective slow AV nodal pathway ablation can be achieved without compromising fast pathway conduction, the preponderance of evidence has suggested that the reentrant circuit includes perinodal atrial tissue or inputs in addition to the AV node proper. Further observations suggest that AVNRT has several variants, often involving more than just two AV nodal pathways. This chapter reviews the present state of knowledge regarding typical (slow-fast) AVNRT and the anatomic approach to its ablation. The variants of AV nodal reentry and intracardiac electrogram guidance to ablation of these arrhythmias are described in Chapter 19.

Anatomy

THE ATRIOVENTRICULAR NODE

The AV node proper is located in the right atrium, within Koch's triangle. In adults, the AV node is usually 5 to 7 mm in length and 2 to 5 mm wide and lies immediately beneath the right atrial endocardium.[3] The size and shape of the node show considerable variation, however. As depicted in Figure 18–3, the septal leaflet of the tricuspid valve is actually the anterior boundary of Koch's triangle. The superior boundary of this region is the membranous interventricular septum, representing the apex of the triangle. The posterior border of the triangle is the tendon of Todaro, and the inferior boundary is the ostium of the coronary sinus (CS). Figure 18–4 shows fluoroscopic views of Koch's triangle in the left anterior oblique (LAO) and right anterior oblique

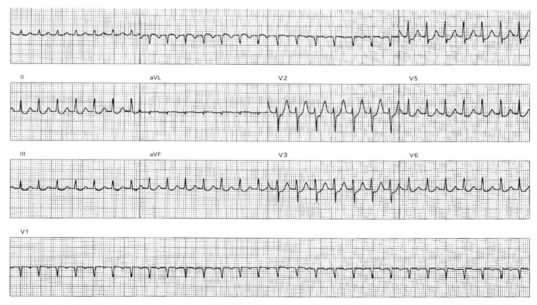

FIGURE 18–1. A 12-lead electrocardiogram of typical slow-fast atrioventricular nodal reentry tachycardia (AVNRT).

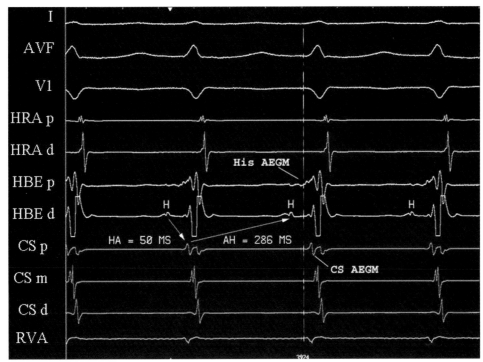

FIGURE 18–2. Typical slow-fast. Surface leads I, AVF, and V1 were recorded simultaneously with bipolar intracardiac electrograms from the right atrium proximal (HRA p) and distal (HRA d) electrode pairs; His bundle electrogram proximal (HBE p) and distal (HBE d) electrode pairs; coronary sinus (CS) proximal (p), middle (m), and distal (d) electrode pairs; and the right ventricular apex distal (RVA) electrode pairs. Note that anterograde conduction occurs with a long conduction (AH) interval of 286 msec with retrograde conduction having a short (HA) interval of 50 msec. The earliest atrial electrogram (AEGM) is recorded near the His *(vertical line)*.

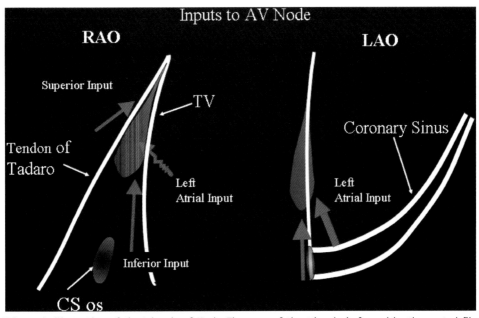

FIGURE 18–3. Schematic illustration of the triangle of Koch. The apex of the triangle is formed by the central fibrous body at the junction of the septal leaflet of the tricuspid valve and the tendon of Todaro, which extends from the eustachian valve inferiorly to the central fibrous body superiorly. The base of the triangle is bounded by the ostium of the coronary sinus. Atrial inputs to the atrioventricular (AV) node may come from three directions: (1) superiorly, from fibers parallel to the tendon of Todaro; (2) inferiorly, from fibers between the tricuspid annulus and the coronary sinus ostium (CSos); and (3) leftward, by fibers extending from the left atrium and muscular coat of the coronary sinus. LAO, left anterior oblique view; RAO, right anterior oblique view; TV, tricuspid valve.

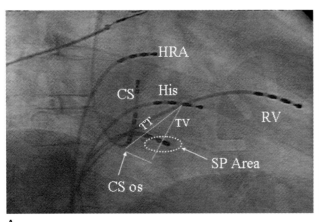
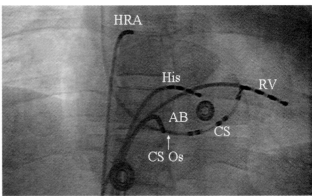

A   B

FIGURE 18–4. A, Right anterior oblique view of catheter positions for anatomically guided slow pathway ablation. The *fine lines* delineate the estimated location of the triangle of Koch. The *dotted circle* indicates common target areas for slow pathway ablation (SP area). **B,** Left anterior oblique view of the same catheter positions. AB, ablation catheter; CS, coronary sinus catheter; His, His catheter; HRA, high right atrial catheter; RV, right ventricular catheter; TV, tricuspid valve; TT, tendon of Todaro.

(RAO) projections. The CS is marked by the CS catheter, and the apex of Koch's triangle is approximated by the electrode pair from which the His bundle electrogram is recorded. The blood supply to the AV node is derived from the right coronary artery in 90% of patients. Innervation to the node primarily arises from the cardiac plexus surrounding the aortic arch.[3]

A degree of confusion has been introduced into the electrophysiologic literature regarding the terminology of the triangle of Koch. For example, the superior portion of the triangle has sometimes been termed "anterior," and the inferior portion has been termed "posterior." In reality, the terms superior or cephalad more accurately describe the apex of the triangle, whereas the terms inferior or caudal better describe the base of the triangle. The perinodal region that is associated with slow pathway conduction is located inferior (caudal) to the compact AV node in the triangle of Koch. Radiofrequency (RF) ablation of the slow pathway is usually directed to the myocardial fibers that lie between the tricuspid annulus and the anterior lip of the CS ostium. In contrast, the fast pathway fibers approach the compact AV node from a posterior and superior direction in the region of the tendon of Todaro.

ATRIAL INPUTS TO THE ATRIOVENTRICULAR JUNCTION

A current model of AV nodal reentry places great emphasis on the role of the atrial inputs to the AV node in the physiology of AVNRT. Although other theories exist that consider longitudinal dissociation within the AV node or anisotropic conduction, the AV nodal input model does much to explain the response of AV nodal physiology to ablation. This model is used throughout this chapter, with the understanding that no single model is conclusively proven.

Much of the available anatomic information concerning atrial inputs to the AV junction is derived from animal models, particularly from rabbit and canine hearts.[3-5] In the human heart, the model includes atrial input to the AV node from three main sources: superior, inferior, and left atrial. The superior and inferior inputs are believed to be critical to the development of typical slow-fast AV nodal reentry. In this model, as shown schematically in Figure 18–3, the compact AV node receives atrial input from transitional cells approaching superiorly from the region of the limbus of the fossa ovalis in the right atrium and from a deep group of transitional cells that approach the node from the left atrial side of the interatrial septum.[3-5] This superior input may insert into the common AV bundle distal to most of the compact AV node, and is believed to be the fast pathway. This input is the preferred conduction to the AV node, because ablation severely alters AV nodal conduction. The inferior input is via transitional cells that are found in the region between the tricuspid annulus and the CS ostium and approach the AV node from the region of the CS ostium.[6] This input is believed to be the source of the slow pathway. The inferior input represents transitional fibers that probably are not a discrete bundle but multiple strands. This may explain the occurrence of multiple slow pathways, often seen in the clinical setting. Extensions of this inferior input (also referred to as the posterior input) have been described that reach along the tricuspid annulus (rightward posterior extension) and along the mitral annulus (left posterior extension). These extensions may play a role in slow-slow and fast-slow variants of AV nodal reentry (Chapter 19).

The presence of additional inputs to the AV junction was suggested by Hirao and others who showed that combined fast and slow pathway ablation in dogs resulted in only a 4% incidence of complete heart block.[7-9] Differential atrial pacing has been used by several groups as evidence for both posterior and left atrial inputs to the AV.[8,9] The role of these inputs in the genesis of AV nodal reentry are not known.[7-13] Wu et al.[13] used optical mapping in dogs to document the presence of intermediate pathways connecting the atria to the AV junction. They found that antero-grade conduction over an intermediate pathway smoothed the transition from the fast pathway to the slow pathway, resulting in a continuous AV nodal function curve. This finding could explain the continuous AV nodal function curve seen in some patients with AVNRT.

Pathophysiology

AV nodal reentry requires longitudinal dissociation of AV nodal conduction, either functionally or anatomically, to create a reentrant circuit. Direct evidence in support of an anatomic separation of the slow and fast pathways has been provided by patients undergoing operative dissection of the perinodal atrial myocardium for cure of AVNRT.[14-30] In these studies, surgical dissection eliminated either the fast or the slow pathway, leaving the alternative conduction pathway intact. The data suggest that the fast conducting fibers are located superiorly, extending from the AV node toward the tendon of Todaro and foramen ovale; that is, they form the superior input to the AV node. The slowly conducting fibers were shown to be located inferiorly, extending toward the compact AV node, along the tricuspid annulus, from the direction of the CS ostium, consistent with the inferior input to the AV node. A schematic representation of antegrade and retrograde conduction through the fast and slow pathways is shown in Figure 18–5.

These distinct patterns or pathways for conduction are designated the fast and slow pathways based on distinct electrophysiologic properties. First, conduction through the fast pathway is more rapid than through the slow pathway. Second, the effective refractory period (ERP) of the antegrade fast pathway is usually longer than that of the slow pathway.[28,29] There are many exceptions to this observation, a

fact with great practical importance for the demonstration of slow pathway conduction. Third, the retrograde fast pathway of patients with AVNRT typically has nondecremental conduction properties. For example, programmed ventricular stimulation is usually associated with prolongation of the ventricu-lar-to-His conduction interval with minimal change in the HA interval. This is often in contrast to patients without AVNRT, in whom the retrograde HA inter-val is typically decremental. Finally, the fast and slow pathways often have quantitatively differing responses to autonomic and pharmacologic manipu-lations. For example, adrenergic stimulation tends to shorten the ERP of the fast pathway (both antegrade and retrograde) to a greater extent than that of the slow pathway.[7-9] The administration of isoprotere nol usually enhances antegrade and retrograde fast pathway conduction when slow pathway conduction predominates at rest. Conversely, for patients with high catecholamine states, slow pathway conduction may not be demonstrable if the ERP of the fast pathway is less than that of the slow pathway. In these individuals, the use of a β-adrenergic blocking agent such as propranolol or esmolol tends to prolong the ERP of the antegrade fast pathway to a greater extent than for the slow pathway, allowing demonstration of slow pathway conduc-tion. Although retrograde fast pathway conduction tends to result in earliest retrograde atrial activation at the apex of Koch's triangle, whereas retrograde slow pathway conduction activates the base of the triangle near the CS ostium, there are exceptions to this rule.

CIRCUIT FOR REENTRY

AV nodal reentrant beats have been demonstrated to involve antegrade conduction over the inferior input to the node or slow pathway with retrograde atrial activation via the superior superficial fibers or fast pathway.[31,32] A schematic representation of the reen-trant circuit is shown in Figure 18–6. In this concep-tualization, antegrade conduction is carried over the inferior input (possibly the right posterior extension) to approach the AV node from a caudal-to-cranial direction within the triangle of Koch. In detailed recordings, the earliest electrograms are recorded within the proximal CS or between the CS and the tri-cuspid annulus. This is consistent with the location of the rightward posterior extension.[32] The tendon of Todaro forms a line of block preventing right atrial activation from occurring until conduction reaches the apex of the triangle of Koch and exits via the fast pathway. The CS musculature is activated proximally within the triangle of Koch, leading to the proximal-to-distal CS conduction. Passage of the wavefront

A Retrograde Conduction Over the Fast AV Nodal Pathway

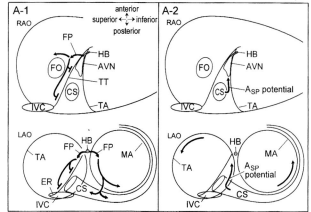

B Retrograde Conduction Over the Slow AV Nodal Pathway

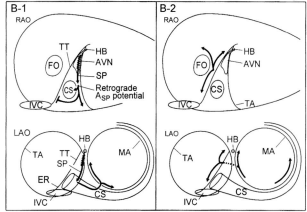

C Sinus Rhythm   D Sinus Rhythm

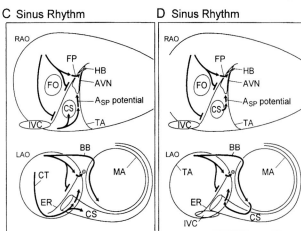

FIGURE 18–5. Proposed patterns of atrial activation during retrograde conduction over the fast atrioventricular (AV) nodal pathway (**A**), retrograde conduction over the slow AV nodal pathway (**B**), and sinus rhythm (**C** and **D**). *A-1,* During slow-fast atrioventricular nodal reentrant tachycardia (AVNRT), retrograde fast pathway (FP) conduction activates both sides of the interatrial septum *(left anterior oblique [LAO] projection).* Activation of the right side of the septum occurs superior to the tendon of Todaro (TT) and may not be able to reenter the triangle of Koch *(right anterior oblique [RAO] projection).* Activation of the left side of the septum propagates to the left atrial myocardium adjacent to the mitral annulus (MA), which activates the coronary sinus (CS) myocardial coat *(LAO projection).* Activation along the CS myocardium proceeds rightward to the CS ostium. AVN, atrioventricular node; ER, eustachian ridge; FO, fossa ovale; HB, His bundle; IVC, inferior vena cava; TA, tricuspid annulus. *A-2,* The CS ostium activates the right atrium and the transitional cell fibers within the triangle of Koch. Activation of this tissue in the posterior-anterior direction generates the A$_{SP}$ potential. *B-1,* Retrograde slow pathway (SP) activation propagates posteriorly along the posterior extension of the AVN to the tissue generating the A$_{SP}$ potential. Block along the eustachian valve/ER may confine this activation within the triangle of Koch *(RAO projection).* The CS musculature is then activated, which propagates the impulse leftward and activates the left atrial myocardium 1.5 to 3 cm from the CS ostium *(LAO projection).* *B-2,* Left atrial activation proceeds leftward and rightward to the septum and propagates across the interatrial septum to activate the right atrium (superior to the TT). **C,** During sinus rhythm, the septal right atrial impulse propagates across the anterior portion of the TT along the transitional cells, comprising the fast pathway. The low current from these cells may not be able to activate the atrial myocardium in the anterior portion of the triangle of Koch. Activation along the crista terminalis (CT) activates the musculature of the CS and the tissue between the TA and the CS ostium, generating the A$_{SP}$ potential in the posterior-to-anterior direction. This accounts for the late timing of the A$_{SP}$ potential during sinus rhythm. BB, Bachmann's bundle. **D,** In patients who exhibit a marked delay in the timing of the A$_{SP}$ potential during sinus rhythm, left atrial activation may activate the CS musculature, which then activates the tissue generating the A$_{SP}$ potential. From: Otomo K, Wang Z, Lazzara R, Jackman WM. Atrioventricular nodal reentrant tachycardia: electrophysiological characteristics of four forms and implications for the reentrant circuit. In: Zipes DP, Jalife J, eds. Cardiac Electrophysiology: From Cell to Bedside. 3rd ed. Philadelphia, Pa: WB Saunders Co; 2000; 504-521.

through the fast pathway then activates the right and left sides of the atrial septum. There are several possible routes by which the wavefront can then reenter the inferior AV nodal input; however, conduction down the left atrial septum may be common (see Fig. 18–6).

THE UPPER AND DISTAL COMMON PATHWAYS

The reentry circuit involving fast and slow pathways must have proximal and distal continuities to be com-

plete. The anatomic basis and functional properties of these continuities are unsettled, but certain electrophysiologic behaviors have led to speculation about the upper and lower common pathways that join fast and slow pathway conduction. Debate over the presence of an upper and lower common pathway, and whether the reentrant circuit is purely intranodal or contains extranodal atrial inputs, is still unsettled.[14,25-32] Evidence for the existence of an upper common pathway proximal to fast and slow fibers located within the AV node has been suggested by

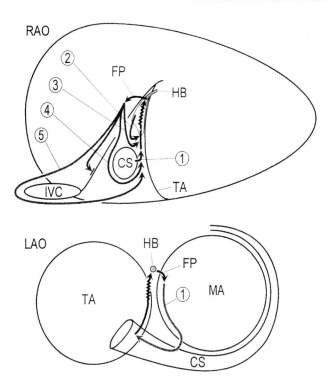

FIGURE 18–6. Possible reentrant circuits for slow-fast atrioventricular nodal reentry. Five potential circuits are shown. Retrograde conduction occurs over the fast pathway (FP) with the eustachian ridge forming a line of block into the triangle of Koch from the right atrium. In this hypothesized circuit, the retrograde atrial impulse propagates down the left atrial septum to activate the slow pathway through the proximal coronary sinus (CS) best seen in the left anterior oblique (LAO) view. HB, His bundle; IVC, inferior vena cava; MA, mitral annulus; RAO, right anterior oblique projection; TA, tricuspid annulus. *(From Lockwood D, Otomo K, Wang Z, et al.: Electrophysiologic characteristics of atrioventricular nodal reentrant tachycardia: Implications for reentry circuits. In Zipes DP, Jalif J (eds.): Cardiac Electrophysiology: From Cell to Bedside, 4th ed. Philadelphia: WB Saunders, 2004, pp 537-557, with permission.)*

the finding of AV Wenckebach block during atrial pacing at a pacing rate slower than that of AVNRT.[20] However, this finding is only seen in a minority of patients, and other significant supporting evidence for the existence of an upper common pathway is lacking.

The existence of a distal common pathway, located proximal to the His bundle in the lower region of the AV node, is more widely accepted. Miller et al.[14] recorded the HA interval during AVNRT and during ventricular pacing in 28 patients with this arrhythmia. The HA interval during pacing exceeded the HA interval during AVNRT in 19 (68%) of 28 patients by a mean of 25 msec, suggesting the presence of AV nodal tissue between the His bundle and the distal turnaround of the fast and slow pathways. In addition, VA Wenckebach block occurred at a ventricular

pacing rate slower than that of AVNRT in 2 patients. The spontaneous occurrence of 2:1 AV block proximal to the His bundle during AVNRT also strongly supports the existence of a distal common pathway (see Chapter 19).[15,16]

NECESSITY OF THE ATRIUM IN THE REENTRANT CIRCUIT

The initial experimental evidence suggesting that some atrial myocardium is required to maintain the reentrant circuit in human AVNRT came from mapping studies at the time of surgery. These studies showed that cure of AVNRT can be produced by placing ablative lesions in the perinodal atrial myocardium, as much as 10 mm or more from the compact AV node.[15-32] More recent studies using optical mapping techniques have confirmed the presence of anatomically separate regions with slow and fast conduction properties and identified the existence of intermediate regions located between the slow and fast regions. This technique has also established that the perinodal atrial tissue and transitional cells are indeed involved in the reentry circuit.[10,30] Histologic analysis has shown that these regions of the slow and fast pathways are not discrete, specialized myocardial fibers. Rather, these perinodal regions merge into the compact AV node and have differing conduction velocities and refractory periods. Therefore, it may be overly simplistic to consider separate atrial and AV nodal components to the reentry circuit, because the tissues more closely approximate an electrical and anatomic continuum.

CLINICAL VARIANTS OF ATRIOVENTRICULAR NODAL REENTRY TACHYCARDIA

At least four types of AVNRT have been described: (1) slow-fast, (2) fast-slow, (3) slow-slow, and (4) left variant slow-fast.[32] By far the most commonly encountered form is slow-fast AVNRT. These variants are described in Chapter 19. Ablation of slow pathway function is curative for all variants of AV nodal reentry. Slow pathway ablation or modification can be achieved either by the anatomic approach described in this chapter or with guidance from intracardiac electrograms (see Chapter 19).

Diagnosis and Differential Diagnosis

The diagnostic criteria for typical slow-fast AV nodal reentry are given in Table 18–1. On the surface elec-

---

TABLE 18–1

Diagnostic Criteria for Typical (Slow-Fast) Atrioventricular Nodal Reentrant Tachycardia

Dual AV nodal physiology present (typically)

Initiation of tachycardia dependent on critical AH interval

Earliest retrograde atrial activation in tachycardia at His bundle*
  Ventricular postpacing interval >115 msec longer than tachycardia cycle length

Difference between VA interval in supraventricular tachycardia and VA interval in ventricular pacing at tachycardia cycle length >85 msec

HA interval in tachycardia < HA interval with ventricular pacing

Ability to dissociate atrium and ventricle from tachycardia (usually)

Exclude atrial tachycardia and reciprocating tachycardia

*Eccentric coronary sinus activation may occur in tach, simulating a left-sided accessory pathway.
AH, right atrium-to-His-bundle activation; AV, atrioventricular; HA, His-bundle-to-atrium activation; VA, ventricle-to-atrium activation.

TABLE 18–2

Features of Dual Atrioventricular Nodal Physiology or Slow Pathway Conduction

Dual AV Nodal Physiology

>50 msec increase in A2-H2 interval with decrease of ≤10 msec in A1-A2

>50 msec increase in AH interval with 10 msec decrease in atrial pacing interval

Abrupt change in slope of AV nodal conduction curve without "jump" (especially in children)

Slow Pathway Conduction

Stable PR interval > paced P-P interval without Wenckebach block in absence of isoproterenol

Stable VA interval > RR interval with ventricular pacing (retrograde slow pathway)

AH interval >200 msec

---

trocardiogram, slow-fast AV nodal reentry most commonly manifests as a regular, narrow complex tachycardia with no clear P waves evident (see Fig. 18–1). The presence of a P wave can be inferred in many patients, however, by the presence of a pseudo r' wave in lead V_1 or pseudo Q or S waves in the inferior leads. These patterns represent the superimposed P wave within the QRS complex and are best recognized by comparing the morphologies in sinus rhythm and in tachycardia. Bundle branch aberrancy is uncommon in AV nodal reentry, and the tachycardia rate may be highly influenced by the state of autonomic tone.

By intracardiac recordings, no one finding alone is diagnostic of AVNRT (see Table 18–1). The diagnosis of slow-fast AV nodal reentry by intracardiac recordings usually rests on the demonstration of a regular SVT with earliest concentric atrial activation at the His bundle. The HA times are typically short at 25 to 90 msec (average, 50 msec), and VA times are usually less than 60 msec (see Fig. 18–2).[32] The VA times may be longer than 60 msec, however, and in 6% of patients retrograde atrial activation is eccentric, with earliest activation in the middle to distal CS.[33] Occasionally, AV block to the ventricles may be noted during tachycardia but VA block to the atrium is exceedingly rare. In most patients, antegrade dual AV nodal physiology is present and tachycardia onset depends on achieving a critical AH interval. The criteria for dual AV nodal physiology are listed in Table 18–2. Although typical of patients with AVNRT, discontinuous AV nodal physiology can be initially demonstrated with programmed atrial stimulation in only 60% to 85% of patients in whom this arrhythmia is inducible.[34,35] Failure to demonstrate dual AV nodal physiology may be a result of similar refractory periods of the fast and slow pathways, a functional refractory period of the atrium that limits A_1A_2 coupling intervals at the AV node, block in the fast pathway during the drive train, or the presence of intermediate AV nodal pathways.[36] Although the electrogram pattern is highly characteristic (see Fig. 18–2), the diagnosis requires confirmation by pacing maneuvers.

In the absence of bystander accessory pathways, the tachycardia is not reset by premature ventricular stimuli delivered during His refractoriness. Similarly, atrial extrastimuli may not advance the tachycardia even when very premature (Fig. 18–7). Typical slow-fast AV node reentry produces a V-A-V response to termination of entrainment by ventricular pacing. The ventricular postpacing interval is more than 115 msec longer than the tachycardia cycle length because the ventricle acts as a "bystander" in the tachycardia. The long postpacing interval is caused by the time needed for the signal to travel retrogradely in the His-Purkinje system, engage the AV node, and return back antegrade down the His-Purkinje system to the ventricular pacing site. The VA times during ventricular pacing are more than 85 msec longer than those in tachycardia. The

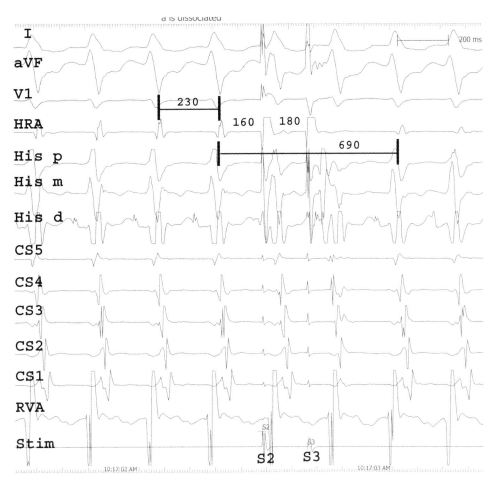

FIGURE 18–7. Failure to advance atrial activation of slow-fast atrioventricular (AV) nodal reentry with double atrial extrastimuli. The tachycardia cycle length is 230 msec. Atrial extrastimuli (S2, S3) are delivered at coupling intervals of 160 and 180 msec. The tachycardia is unperturbed, with the atrial and ventricular activation falling on time after the extrastimuli. CS, coronary sinus electrode pairs (CS5, proximal; CS1, distal); d, distal; HBE, His bundle; HRA, high right atrium; p, proximal; RVA, right ventricular apex; Stim, stimulation channel.

response to parahisian pacing is a prolongation of the VA time with loss of His capture that is equal to the prolongation in the stimulus-to-His interval. In addition, there is no change in atrial activation sequence, and the HA interval remains constant.[36] Other features suggestive of typical AV nodal reentry are the occurrence of antegrade or retrograde AV block at paced cycle lengths equal to the tachycardia cycle length immediately after termination of the tachycardia demonstrating 1:1 conduction.

DIFFERENTIAL DIAGNOSIS

The differential diagnosis of typical AV nodal reentry includes atrial tachycardia arising from the atrial septum, reciprocating tachycardias using septal bypass tracts, and accelerated junctional tachycardias.[36] The diagnosis of atrial tachycardia is supported by a V-A-A-V response to termination of ventricular entrainment and an eccentric atrial activation sequence. A variable HA interval in tachycardia is characteristic of atrial tachycardia but uncommon for AV nodal reentry. After abrupt termination of ventricular pacing with entrainment of the tachycardia, the next beat of AVNRT typically occurs at a cycle

length somewhat longer than that of the tachycardia due to the presence of decremental slow pathway conduction. However, this beat typically has the same HA interval as during spontaneous tachycardia. Reciprocating tachycardias using septal bypass tracts are diagnosed by the ability to advance atrial activation during His refractoriness and by the response to parahisian pacing (see Chapter 19 for examples). For AV reciprocating tachycardias, the ventricular post-pacing interval in tachycardia is less than 115 msec longer than the tachycardia cycle length, and the VA intervals with ventricular pacing are less than 85 msec longer than those in tachycardia.

In patients with AV nodal reentry and eccentric CS activation, AV nodal reentry may be misdiagnosed as a left-sided accessory pathway (Fig. 18–8). The diagnosis of AV nodal reentry is established by (1) the demonstration of dual AV nodal physiology, (2) the ability to also induce AVNRT with concentric atrial activation or variable patterns of retrograde atrial activation in most patients, (3) absence of retrograde VA conduction without isoproterenol, (4) inability to advance the atrium with premature ventricular stimuli during His refractoriness (may require left ventricular pacing), (5) demonstration of only

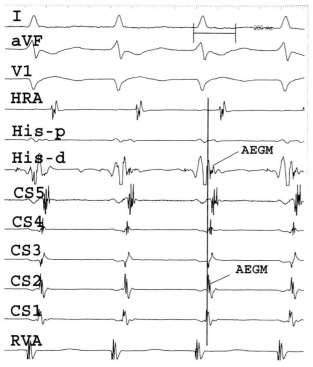

FIGURE 18–8. Eccentric atrial activation sequence during slow-fast atrioventricular nodal reentry. The onset of the earliest atrial electrogram (AEGM) is designated by the *vertical line* and occurs at the distal coronary sinus (CS1). The atrial electrogram at the His is slightly later. I, aVF, and V1 are surface electrocardiographic leads. CS, coronary sinus; d, distal; His, His bundle; HRA, high right atrium; p, proximal; RVA, right ventricular apex.

decremental retrograde VA conduction, and (6) the ability to dissociate the atrium and ventricle from the tachycardia.[33] Features differentiating AVNRT from reciprocating tachycardias are listed in Table 18–3.

A source of confusion can be the differentiation of an accelerated junctional rhythm from slow-fast AVNRT. Both tachycardias have a short and constant HA conduction interval with a retrograde atrial activation sequence at the apex of the triangle of Koch. Accelerated junctional tachycardias are often relatively slow but overlap in rate with slow-fast AVNRT, especially in elderly patients. The demonstration of classic transient entrainment clearly defines the tachycardia as AVNRT.

Mapping

Before mapping and ablation, it is essential to perform a thorough baseline study to confirm the diagnosis and to establish end points for ablation. The inability to reinitiate a previously easily-inducible tachycardia is an important end point, although in some patients the tachycardia is difficult to induce and not reproducible. In such patients, the demonstration of modified slow pathway function may be the only end point. This of course requires the

TABLE 18–3		
Differentiating Atrioventricular Nodal Reentrant Tachycardia from Septal Orthodromic Reciprocating Tachycardia		
Maneuver	**Septal ORT**	**AVNRT**
Parahisian pacing	No change in Stim-A with loss of His capture	Increased Stim-A with loss of His capture
Premature ventricular stimuli during His refractoriness	Advances atrial activation Terminates tachycardia without conduction to atrium	Unable to advance atrial activation
Ventricular PPI minus TCL	<115 msec	>115 msec
VA during ventricular pacing at TCL minus VA during tachycardia	<85 msec	>85 msec
VA with pacing at ventricular base vs at ventricular apex	VA shorter with pacing at base	VA shorter with pacing at apex
Retrograde VA conduction	Nondecremental	Decremental
Atrial or ventricular pacing at TCL	1:1 conduction present	Wenckebach conduction may occur
VA dissociation during tachycardia	Not possible	Possible
VA interval in tachycardia	>65-70 msec	Typically <65-70 msec
HA interval in tachycardia	Fixed	May be variable

HA, His-bundle-to-atrium; PPI, postpacing interval; Stim-A, interval from ventricular stimulus to atrial electrogram; TCL, tachycardia cycle length; VA, ventricular-atrial.

demonstration of dual AV nodal physiology at baseline (see Table 18–2). This may be accomplished by the construction of an AV nodal function curve. The A_1A_2 interval is plotted on the X axis and the A_2H_2 interval on the Y axis (Fig. 18–9A). A A_2H_2 "jump" of 50 msec or more in response to a 10-msec decrease in

the A_1A_2 interval is considered evidence of dual AV nodal pathway conduction.

Rapid atrial pacing is then performed, starting at a rate slightly faster than that of the sinus node and increased gradually until AV Wenckebach block is observed. The development of a PR interval that is

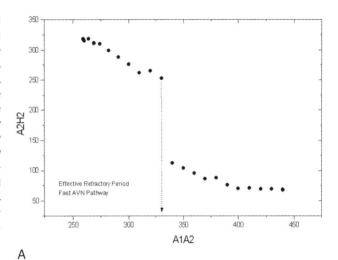

FIGURE 18–9. Dual atrioventricular nodal (AVN) physiology and slow pathway conduction. **A,** AVN function curve produced during programmed atrial stimulation from the high right atrium. The A2H2 interval in response to a premature atrial stimulus is plotted on the Y-axis against the A1A2 coupling interval recorded in the His bundle electrogram (in milliseconds). Note that at an A1A2 interval of 330 msec there is a marked increase in the A2H2 interval, indicating block in the fast AVN pathway and conduction over the slow AVN pathway. **B,** The effect of slow AVN pathway ablation on the PR:RR sign. Before slow pathway (SP) ablation *(top panel)*, rapid atrial pacing produces a stimulus-to-conducted QRS interval that exceeds the atrial pacing cycle length *(arrows)*. After ablation *(bottom panel)*, rapid atrial pacing results in A-V Wenckebach block; the stimulus-to-conducted-QRS interval never exceeds the atrial pacing cycle length.

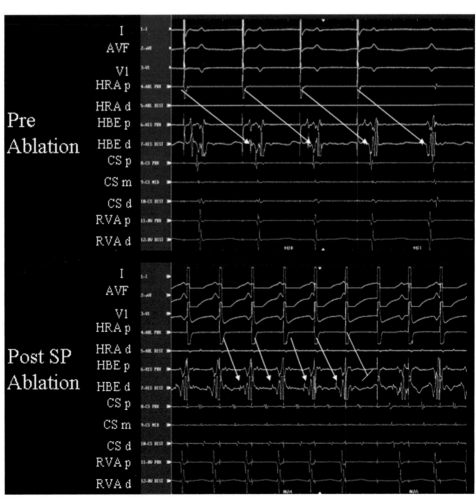

greater than the atrial pacing cycle length is a strong indicator of antegrade slow pathway conduction (see Fig. 18–9B).[37] For this sign to be meaningful, the PR interval should exceed the RR interval with rapid atrial pacing during stable 1:1 AV conduction. Repeated rapid atrial pacing near the Wenckebach cycle length may be necessary for induction of the tachycardia.

Next, careful attention is given to retrograde VA conduction. During programmed ventricular stimulation, a retrograde VA conduction curve may be constructed with attention to the site of earliest atrial activation. In addition, incremental ventricular pacing is performed to evaluate the sequence of retrograde atrial activation and the VA and HA intervals. In contrast to typical slow-fast AVNRT, slow-slow and fast-slow AVNRT are most often induced by ventricular pacing. Retrograde slow pathway conduction is commonly manifested by a VA conduction interval that exceeds the ventricular pacing cycle length (RP > RR sign). Isoproterenol is infused to allow assessment of antegrade and retrograde conduction during adrenergic stimulation and to facilitate the induction of AVNRT (if necessary).

For patients in whom a discontinuous AV nodal function curve cannot be demonstrated during programmed atrial stimulation, pharmacologic treatment may be necessary to unmask it. If the fast pathway conduction is suppressed in the baseline state, as evidenced by a long AH interval at all atrial pacing rates or by VA block during ventricular pacing, isoproterenol is infused. Isoproterenol usually facilitates fast pathway conduction in such cases, often allowing recognition of dual AV nodal pathways and induction of AVNRT. Occasionally, atropine must also be administered in such patients. If AVNRT is noninducible with these measures, programmed atrial stimulation with $S_1S_2S_3$ may be effective for demonstrating dual AV nodal pathways or AVNRT. Lessening of sedation, hyperventilation, and hand grip exercises may facilitate tachycardia induction.

Occasionally, sustained AVNRT cannot be induced in patients with a history of sustained SVT despite these maneuvers. If, however, two AV nodal echo beats are induced, there is evidence for a complete reentrant circuit, and catheter ablation of the slow AV nodal pathway can be justified. If no beats or only a single AV nodal echo beat is induced, catheter ablation of the slow pathway can be justified if the PR interval exceeds the RR interval during rapid atrial pacing. In the absence of two or more AV nodal echo beats or a PR interval greater than the RR interval, prudence would dictate against empiric slow AV nodal pathway ablation.

ANATOMIC LOCALIZATION OF THE SLOW PATHWAY

Once slow pathway conduction can be reproducibly demonstrated and the diagnosis of AVNRT is confirmed, the ablation catheter is positioned along the tricuspid annulus immediately anterior to the CS ostium (see Fig. 18–4). Although the technique is described as an anatomic approach to ablation, it does in fact make use of some intracardiac electrograms to guide ablation. The RAO view is especially useful for positioning of catheters, because it best displays Koch's triangle in profile. The optimal RAO angulation results in placement of the CS catheter perpendicular to the long axis of the heart and perpendicular to the plane of the fluoroscopic image. The target zone for ablation is the isthmus of tissue between the tricuspid valve annulus and the ostium of the CS (Table 18–4). Positioning of the catheters is best performed during sinus rhythm, because the atrial and ventricular deflections in the tricuspid annulus electrogram are more easily discerned. The ablation catheter should have a distal electrode 4 or 5 mm in length and should have a deflectable distal segment. The length of the deflecting segment of the ablation catheter that has proved most effective has ranged from 2.0 to 3.0 inches. The ablation catheter is advanced into the right ventricle, moved inferiorly so that it lies anterior to the ostium of the CS, and then withdrawn toward the tricuspid annulus until the distal pair of electrodes records a small atrial deflection and a large ventricular deflection. Although there are many exceptions, the proximal electrode pair typically records a larger atrial than ventricular deflection. The ratio of atrial to ventricular electrograms (A/V ratio) recorded from the distal electrode pair in sinus rhythm may range from approximately 0.7:1 to 1:5. The atrial electrogram at successful locations usually has multiple components and is rarely

TABLE 18–4
Targets for Slow Pathway Ablation
Tissue between CS os and tricuspid annulus at level of CS os; may also need to target tissue slightly superior to os
Mouth of CS os and proximal 1 cm of CS
A/V ratio = 0.7:1 to 0.25:1
Interval from AEGM at His bundle to AEGM at ablation electrode ≥20 msec
Sites producing junctional rhythm with 1:1 retrograde conduction during RF delivery

AEGM, atrial electrogram; A/V ratio, atrial-to-ventricular electrogram ratio; CS, coronary sinus; RF, radiofrequency energy.

sharp or of high frequency, as is the signal recorded from the CS (Fig. 18–10). In addition, the risk of AV block is higher when the onset of the atrial electrogram on the ablation catheter occurs less than 20 msec after the atrial electrogram on the His recording.[38,39]

Our convention for describing the position of the ablation catheter in the region of Koch's triangle is to divide the length of the tricuspid annulus into 12 segments, with site 1 located at the apex of the triangle near the central fibrous body, site 10 located at the most inferior extent (floor) of the CS ostium, and site 12 located more caudally, as the tricuspid annulus begins to curve toward the free wall of the right atrium (Figs. 18–11 and 18–12). The most common site for effective ablation of slow pathway conduction is along the tricuspid annulus immediately anterior to the CS ostium (sites 8 through 10). The slow pathway is successfully ablated at these sites in approximately 95% of patients with AVNRT. Elimination of slow pathway conduction may sometimes require that the catheter be repositioned along the tricuspid annulus inferior to the CS ostium (sites 11 and 12). If ablation of the slow pathway is not successful at these locations, the ablation catheter is then moved superior to the CS ostium, along the tricuspid annulus (site 7). In a very small percentage of patients, elimination of slow pathway conduction requires application of RF energy at other sites, such as in the ostium of the CS, against the interatrial septum immediately superior to the CS ostium, or more cephalad along the tricuspid annulus (sites 5 or

6). The risk of AV block is related to how superiorly RF energy is applied in Koch's triangle. In general, sites more than half way between the CS ostium and the His catheter carry a much higher incidence of AV block (see Fig. 18–11). If it is believed necessary to ablate sites closer to the AV node, cryoablation with "ice mapping" may be considered, because it is associated with a lower incidence of AV nodal block (Fig. 18–13).[40] For patients who are very risk averse, RF current should not be applied to sites more superior than site 7.

FAST PATHWAY LOCALIZATION

The technique of selective fast AV nodal pathway ablation has been abandoned in all but selected instances in favor of slow pathway ablation. There are two overriding advantages of the slow pathway ablation technique. First, the risk of complete AV block is significantly lower with slow pathway ablation. Rates of complete heart block ranging from 8% have been reported with fast pathway ablation, compared with less than 1% in our experience with

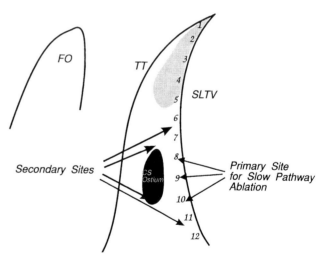

FIGURE 18–11. Schematic diagram of Koch's triangle used for slow pathway ablation. Koch's triangle is bounded anteriorly by the septal leaflet of the tricuspid valve (SLTV), posteriorly by the tendon of Todaro (TT), superiorly by the central fibrous body, and inferiorly by the coronary sinus (CS) ostium. The tricuspid annulus is divided into 12 sites, with site 1 being located at the apex of the triangle and site 10 at the level of the inferior extent of the CS ostium. Sites 11 and 12 are located inferior to the level of the CS ostium. The most common sites for ablation of the slow atrioventricular nodal pathway are along the tricuspid annulus immediately anterior to the CS ostium (sites 8 through 10). Less commonly, application of radiofrequency current may be effective in ablating slow pathway conduction at other sites immediately superior or inferior to the CS ostium, or along the tricuspid annulus at sites 7 and 8 or 11 and 12. FO, fossa ovale.

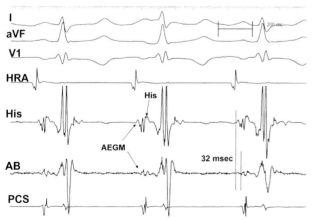

FIGURE 18–10. Atrial electrogram (AEGM) from the distal ablation electrodes (AB) at site of successful slow pathway ablation. The AEGM has multiple components and the atrial-ventricular electrogram ratio (A/V ratio) is 1:7. The onset of the ablation AEGM is 32 msec later than the onset of the His bundle (His) atrial electrogram *(vertical lines),* suggesting a low likelihood of inducing atrioventricular block at this site. I, aVF, and V1 are surface electrocardiographic leads. HRA, high right atrium; PCS, proximal coronary sinus.

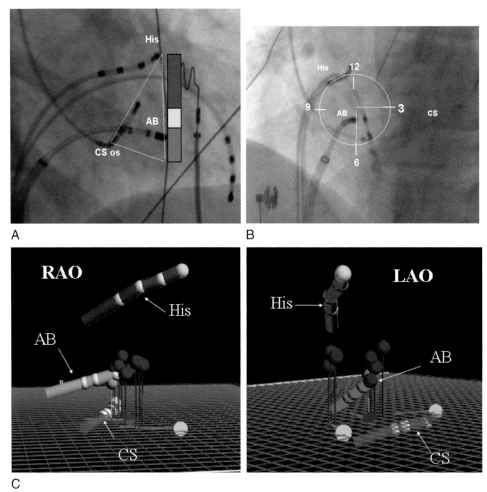

FIGURE 18–12. Limits of anatomic sites for slow pathway ablation. **A,** Right anterior oblique (RAO) view of ablation catheter (AB) at level of the coronary sinus (CS) os near the tricuspid annulus. The estimated location of the triangle of Koch is delineated as in Figure 18-4. The superior to inferior limits of the green marker correspond to sites 8 through 12 in Figure 18-11 and are the safest and most effective region for slow pathway ablation. The yellow marker corresponds to sites 6 and 7; at these sites, caution is warranted due to increased risk of atrioventricular (AV) block. The red marker corresponds to sites 1 through 5; AV nodal injury should be expected with ablation at these sites. **B,** In the left anterior oblique (LAO) view, appropriate sites of ablation may be approximated by envisioning a clock face with the His catheter at 12 o'clock and the CS os at 6 o'clock. The slow pathway usually is ablated at the 4, 5, or 6 o'clock positions. Between 3 and 4 o'clock, the risk of AV block is increased, corresponding to the yellow area in **A.** At sites superior to 3 o'clock, AV nodal injury is expected. **C,** Use of LocaLisa (Medtronic, Minneapolis, Minn.) nonfluoroscopic catheter navigation system in slow pathway ablation. Computer renderings of the diagnostic (CS, His) and ablation (AB) catheters are shown in a virtual three-dimensional space. The red spheres represent sites of radiofrequency energy delivery. In the LAO view, the more anterior group of ablation sites were ineffective. The ablation catheter rests in the site of successful delivery that ultimately eliminated all slow pathway conduction and prevented tachycardia induction. Multiple energy deliveries were needed in this area to prevent tachycardia despite frequent generation of junctional rhythm.

selective slow pathway ablation. The second major advantage of slow pathway ablation is the avoidance of a prolonged PR interval after the procedure. Fast pathway ablation can leave the patient with a very long PR interval (related to residual AV conduction over the slow pathway). If the RP interval is less than the PR interval during slow pathway conduction, patients may complain of symptoms similar to those encountered with VVI pacing (pseudopacemaker syndrome).[41]

The site for fast pathway ablation is proximal and slightly superior to the site at which the largest His potential is recorded. After recording of the maximal His potential, the ablation catheter is withdrawn until an A/V ratio greater than 1 is recorded. The target site may have no discernible His bundle recording or, more commonly, a small His potential (<100 µV in amplitude).[42] The site of earliest atrial activation in tachycardia has not proved to be a useful target. The earliest atrial activation is difficult

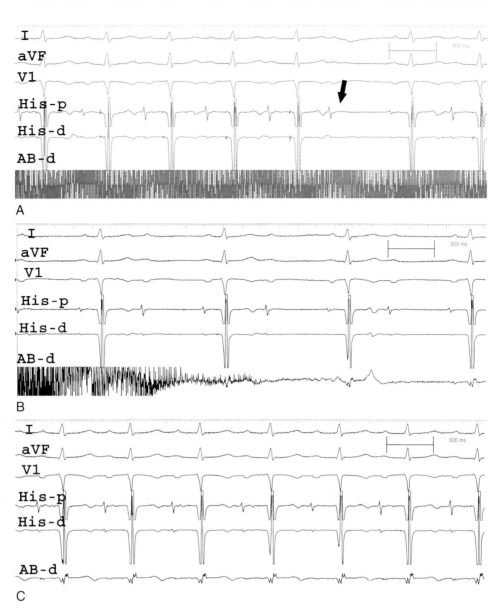

FIGURE 18–13. Reversible atrioventricular (AV) block with cryoablation for AV nodal reentry. In this patient, radiofrequency energy to elicit junctional rhythm was associated with catheter positions midway between the coronary sinus os and the His catheter (His). Retrograde ventricular-atrial (VA) block during junctional rhythm was noted. During cryoablation to this site (**A**), AV block occurred *(arrow)*. The ablation was immediately discontinued (**B**), but 2:1 AV block also occurred. Note return of electrograms on the ablation catheter (AB), consistent with melting of the ice ball. Less than 2 minutes later (**C**), there is return of 1:1 conduction. Tachycardia remained noninducible after this lesion, and the patient had no AV block in follow-up. I, aVF, and V1 are surface electrocardiographic leads. d, distal; p, proximal.

to determine due to overlap with the local ventricular electrogram, and the actual atrial activation is recorded away from the insertion of the input with the AV node.

Ablation

Several investigators have examined the role of temperature and impedance monitoring and the effect of power output titration on initial success and tachycardia recurrence. Using fixed power output in 35 patients with AVNRT, Strickberger et al.[43] showed that the steady-state electrode-tissue interface temperature during successful applications of energy was $48.5 \pm 3.3°C$, compared with $46.8 \pm 5.5°C$ in unsuccessful applications. The change in mean impedance did not differ between successful and unsuccessful applications of RF energy. In this study, there were no recurrences of AVNRT during 114 ± 21 days of follow-up. Calkins et al.[34] examined the relationship of electrode temperature and recurrent tachycardia in 201 patients undergoing AVNRT ablation. In this group of patients, no relation was found between the likelihood of tachycardia recurrence and peak electrode temperature during RF ablation. Finally, Epstein et al.[44] used a closed-loop, temperature-feedback energy source in a series of 39 patients with AVNRT and retrospectively compared their results with those of 43 patients undergoing RF ablation of AVNRT with a non–temperature-guided energy source. Procedural success was the same in both groups, as were the number of RF applications and the procedure duration. There was a significant difference in fluoroscopic duration and in the formation of coagulum, in favor of temperature control.

In our laboratory, RF current is delivered using a 4-mm-tip catheter in a unipolar configuration from the distal electrode of the ablation catheter toward a pair of dispersive electrode pads placed over the posterior thorax. RF current is delivered with an initial power of 50 W for 60 seconds. Impedance is carefully monitored, and RF energy is halted with any sudden rise in impedance or any evidence of AV block. In temperature control mode, target temperatures of 55°C to 60°C are typical, with maximal power of 50 to 60 W for 60 seconds. The use of cooled ablation systems or large-tip catheters and high-output generators is rarely (if ever) needed and is more likely to be contraindicated due to a higher risk of AV block. Catheter position is continuously monitored by fluoroscopy or real time 3-D catheter localization. The electrocardiogram is continuously monitored for the presence of an accelerated junctional rhythm which typically occurs at the effective slow pathway ablation site. In addition, retrograde VA block during RF ablation indicates a risk for AV block and must be monitored carefully (see Chapter 19). If retrograde block occurs, RF delivery is discontinued immediately, the conduction status is assessed, and the catheter position is re-evaluated. RF should also be immediately terminated if PR prolongation or antegrade AV block occurs during delivery.

An accelerated junctional rhythm is not specific to slow pathway ablation, because it is routinely observed during intentional ablation of the AV node, as well as with intentional fast pathway ablation. After each RF current application, programmed atrial stimulation or rapid atrial pacing, or both, are performed to determine the presence or absence of slow pathway conduction or inducible AVNRT. If these characteristics remain, the catheter is repositioned and RF current is applied at a slightly different position.

PREDICTORS OF ATRIOVENTRICULAR BLOCK WITH ABLATION

The rate of the junctional rhythm during ablation has not been demonstrated to be a reliable indicator of impending AV block.[38] The occurrence of VA block during junctional rhythm is more useful; however, it serves a sensitive but not a specific indicator. In a study by Hintringer et al.,[38] only 23% of episodes of VA block during junctional rhythm were associated with impaired antegrade conduction in a series of 58 patients. Despite its low specificity, the occurrence of retrograde block with junctional rhythm must be

heeded and RF terminated. Hintringer also systematically studied the intervals between His atrial electrograms and proximal CS atrial electrograms during retrograde conduction and found no association with AV block. In this study, only an interval of less than 20 msec between the ablation atrial electrogram and the His atrial electrogram was predictive of AV block with RF.[38] A/V ratio, presence of a slow pathway potential, atrial electrogram fractionation, and number of RF lesions were not predictive. An increased incidence of AV block may be present if pacing from the ablation catheter produces stimulus-to-His intervals that are shorter in the slow pathway region than in the anteroseptal and midseptal regions.

IMPORTANCE OF ACCELERATED JUNCTIONAL RHYTHM DURING SLOW PATHWAY ABLATION

Our data and that of others suggest that an accelerated junctional rhythm is to be expected with successful ablation of slow pathway conduction.[34,35,45-47] Indeed, among 127 patients in whom this phenomenon was carefully studied, the RF current application that was effective in eliminating slow pathway conduction was associated with an accelerated junctional rhythm in 120 patients (94%).[48] In another study designed to characterize the difference between junctional ectopy associated with successful versus unsuccessful RF ablation of AVNRT, junctional ectopy was seen more frequently (100% versus 65%) and for a longer duration (7.1 ± 7.1 versus 5.0 ± 7.0 seconds) during successful applications.[49] Because the absence of junctional ectopy during RF ablation corresponds to an ineffective ablation site, it is our practice to terminate the application of RF current at a given site if an accelerated junctional rhythm is not observed within 10 to 15 seconds. It should be emphasized that observation of an accelerated junctional rhythm is not specific to ablation of the slow pathway, because it is routinely induced during intentional AV nodal ablation and is thought to be a response to thermal injury of the compact AV node or perinodal inputs of the slow and fast pathway.

END POINTS FOR SLOW ATRIOVENTRICULAR NODAL PATHWAY ABLATION

It is clear that delivery of RF current at the sites along the tricuspid annulus discussed earlier can eliminate inducible AVNRT without eliminating all evidence of slow pathway conduction.[45,46,50] In most patients who no longer have inducible AVNRT after application of RF current in the slow pathway region but who demonstrate a residual discontinuous AV nodal function curve and *single* AV nodal echo beats, AVNRT

TABLE 18–5

End Points for Delivery of Radiofrequency Energy

Tachycardia rendered noninducible
  Elimination/modification of slow pathway function

Jump with single echoes only (previously inducible)

PR interval prolongation (persistent)

Transient antegrade atrioventricular block after RF (caution warranted for further ablation)

TABLE 18–6

Effect of Slow Pathway Ablation on Atrioventricular Conduction

Parameter	Preablation	Postablation	P
Sinus CL (msec)	769 ± 172	688 ± 170	.10
AH interval (msec)	69.3 ± 18.5	71.7 ± 27	NS
Antegrade ERP fast (msec)	360.9 ± 100.2	342.2 ± 90	.09
Retrograde ERP fast (msec)	296.3 ± 118	290.0 ± 79.2	NS
AV Wenckebach rate (bpm)	179.2 ± 65.5	175.4 ± 73.4	NS
VA Wenckebach rate (bpm)	188.3 ± 47.2	194.1 ± 45.4	NS

AH, atrium-to-His-bundle; AV, atrium-to-ventricle; CL, cycle length; ERP, effective refractory period; NS, not significant; VA, ventricle-to-atrium.

does not recur during a follow-up of several years. Therefore, elimination of all evidence of slow pathway conduction and single echo beats is not a necessary requirement for a successful slow pathway ablation procedure. However, in those patients who do have total elimination of slow pathway function, the recurrence rate of AV nodal reentry may be incrementally less.[45,46,50] Residual evidence of slow AV nodal pathway conduction is the strongest predictor of recurrent AVNRT after an apparently successful slow pathway ablation procedure.[45,46,50] Although it probably represents the ideal situation, any incremental reduction in tachycardia recurrence from total slow pathway elimination must be carefully weighed against the risk of complications from extensive ablation to achieve this goal. Additionally, the absence of junctional tachycardia during RF application also predicts an increased risk of recurrent tachycardia.[45,46,50] Other end points for slow pathway ablation are noninducibility of tachycardia, persistent PR prolongation after ablation, and heart block lingering after ablation (Table 18–5).

THE EFFECT OF SLOW PATHWAY ABLATION ON RESIDUAL ATRIOVENTRICULAR NODAL CONDUCTION

The effect of slow pathway ablation on residual AV nodal conduction is shown in Table 18–6. As our data and that of others demonstrate, selective ablation of the slow pathway by application of RF current along the tricuspid annulus, caudal to the expected location of the compact AV node, eliminates the typical discontinuous AV conduction curve without impairing fast pathway function.[43,51] In many cases, the ERP of the fast pathway actually shortens after slow pathway ablation.[43,51] The mechanism of shortening was investigated by Natale et al.,[51] who compared changes in the fast pathway ERP with and without autonomic blockade both before and after RF ablation of the slow pathway. Before ablation, autonomic

blockade did not alter the ERP of the fast pathway. After ablation, the fast pathway ERP was shortened in both groups of patients, but there was no difference in the degree of shortening between patients with and without autonomic blockade.

In another study designed to look at changes in fast pathway ERP after slow pathway ablation, Strickberger et al.[43] found that the fast pathway ERP was shortened only after complete loss of slow pathway conduction (loss of dual AV nodal physiology and absence of echo beats). These observations led the authors to suggest that changes in fast pathway ERP after RF ablation of the slow pathway were secondary to a withdrawal of electrotonic inhibition of the fast pathway by the slow pathway. In general, retrograde fast pathway conduction is not influenced by slow pathway ablation. However, if the ablation site is moved more superiorly (closer to the AV node), antegrade slow pathway ablation may be associated with elimination of retrograde fast pathway conduction. If the ablation site is in the usual inferior location (at the level of the CS ostium), retrograde conduction remains intact in the fast pathway and continues to be associated with a nondecremental HA interval.

SLOW PATHWAY ABLATION OF MULTIPLE ANTEROGRADE ATRIOVENTRICULAR NODAL PATHWAYS

Multiple "slow" anterograde AV nodal pathways, as demonstrated by the discontinuous AV nodal function curve, may be present in up to 5% of patients with AVNRT. Whether these pathways represent discrete, anatomically distinct circuits or are functionally present because of nonuniform anisotropy is unclear. Frequently, multiple slow pathways (whether functional or anatomic) are in close proximity within Koch's triangle. Tai et al.[52] found that 42% of a series of 26 patients with multiple slow pathways had elimination of the multiple pathways with RF ablation at one site. In that series and others, it was noted that slow pathways with longer conduction times have a more inferior location in Koch's triangle when compared with locations producing a shorter AH interval. In patients with multiple slow pathways, RF ablation of the fast pathway may be associated with persistently inducible AVNRT, with anterograde conduction over a second slowly conducting pathway. Therefore, the presence of a discontinuous AV nodal function curve suggestive of multiple slow pathways should be considered an indication for catheter ablation of the slow pathway. As discussed earlier, elimination of all evidence of dual AV nodal physiology is not necessary for permanent "cure" of AV nodal reentry. AV nodal "jumps" without echoes, or with single echo beats only, are accepted end points for ablation.

Clinical Outcomes

THE UNIVERSITY OF ALABAMA AT BIRMINGHAM EXPERIENCE

Between June 10, 1990, and January 1, 2005, a total of 2333 patients with AVNRT were referred to the clinical electrophysiology laboratory at the University of Alabama at Birmingham for catheter ablation. There were 1627 females (70%) and 707 males (30%), ranging in age from 7 to 93 years (mean, 47.8 ± 17.1 years). The clinical arrhythmia was typical AV nodal reentry (slow-fast) in 97% of patients, atypical AV nodal reentry (fast-slow or slow-slow) in 1% of patients, and both typical and atypical forms of AV nodal reentry in 1% of patients. The demonstration of dual AV nodal pathways required the administration of isoproterenol, isoproterenol plus atropine, or esmolol in 19% of patients. The intent of AV nodal modification was to selectively ablate the slow AV nodal pathway. The slow pathway was selectively ablated in 2317 (99%) of 2329 patients in whom the procedure was attempted. In our entire series of 2333 patients, the mean fluoroscopic exposure time was 12.5 minutes. The success rates from other reported trials are also excellent, at greater than 95%.[35,45,47]

Follow-up

AVNRT recurred in 1.7% of patients who had an initially successful procedure, more commonly in patients with slow-slow AVNRT. Overall, 99.7% had long-term elimination of AVNRT without antiarrhythmic medications. Several patients complained of rapid palpitations that were documented to be sinus rhythm or premature atrial and ventricular depolarizations; management in these cases consisted of reassurance.

Complications

The total complication rate was 0.5%. Six patients developed complete AV block, with three cases occurring among our first 50 patients. Pericardial tamponade occurred in three patients and was managed with percutaneous drainage without long-term sequelae. Two patients developed groin hematomas, and one developed a femoral artery pseudoaneurysm, requiring surgical repair. One patient developed a deep vein thrombosis that was treated with long-term anticoagulation.

RATIONALE FOR THE ANATOMIC APPROACH

Several investigators have reported that activation of the slow pathway is associated with the inscription of discrete electrical potentials, often referred to as "slow pathway potentials" or "slow potentials."[53-55] In these studies, the presence of a slow potential was used to locate the slow pathway, as a site to target RF energy. Specific targeting of the slow pathway should minimize the number of RF lesions needed for curative therapy. The origin of these potentials is uncertain, however, and they are not specific to the slow pathway region. In addition, prolonged mapping and verification of slow pathway potentials may add to the length of a case and increase fluoroscopic exposure to the patient. McGuire et al.[53] concluded that these potentials were produced by asynchronous activation of muscle bundles at various sites in Koch's triangle in blood-perfused porcine and canine hearts. The electrogram morphology has been variously described as either sharp and rapid or slow and broad with a low amplitude, and the timing of slow pathway potentials during the cardiac cycle has been reported either to closely follow local atrial activation near the CS ostium or to span the AH interval. Such potentials are specific neither to Koch's triangle nor to patients with AVNRT.[54] Niebauer et al.[54] investigated the prevalence of slow pathway potentials at various sites in the atrium in patients with and without AVNRT. There was no difference in the number or morphology of "slow potentials" in the posteroseptal area in patients with and without AVNRT. In addition, slow pathway potentials were found at locations outside Koch's triangle—at the anterior, posterior, and lateral aspects of the tricuspid valve annulus—in a minority of patients with and without AVNRT. These data support the notion that slow pathway potentials are not specific to individuals with AVNRT and may occur in regions of the right atrium where transitional cells are not thought to be found. Despite these observations, the probability of recording putative slow pathway potentials at the site of effective slow pathway ablation is quite high, probably in excess of 90% of cases.[35,55]

The specificity of these deflections to predict an effective ablation site is likely to be much lower, however. In our experience, the recording of electrograms compatible with slow pathway potentials at a site along the tricuspid annulus does not necessarily predict successful RF ablation of the slow pathway. In addition, slow pathway conduction can also be eliminated by the delivery of RF current at sites that do not record putative slow pathway potentials. Nevertheless, fractionated atrial electrograms are usually recorded at sites along the tricuspid annulus that have other characteristics predictive of successful slow pathway ablation. Therefore, we prefer to refer to these characteristic signals as "fractionated atrial electrograms" rather than imply a discrete specialized conduction pathway.

FAST PATHWAY ABLATION AND CONTEMPORARY ROLE

The practice of fast pathway ablation was largely abandoned before the widespread use of temperature monitoring, so most of the data describe only energy titration to effect. RF energy is delivered at the target site starting at low levels of 5 to 10 W. The ideal result from ablation is the elimination of retrograde fast pathway function only, although antegrade fast pathway function is frequently modified as well. RF energy is titrated upward until target energies or target temperatures are achieved. In the absence of selective retrograde fast pathway ablation determined by repeated programmed stimulation, RF deliveries are continued until a 50% increase in the PR interval results. Other end points for RF delivery are an increase of greater than 50% in VA conduction time and noninducible AV nodal reentry.[42]

The indications for fast pathway ablation are limited to those patients in whom antegrade fast pathway function is absent or severely impaired before ablation. In most patients with prolonged pre-ablation PR intervals, slow pathway modification

remains effective and carries a low incidence of heart block.[56] In patients with a clear absence of antegrade fast pathway function, however, slow pathway ablation may result in complete heart block. In this situation, targeting of the retrograde fast pathway function is advisable. Similarly, ablation of the slow pathway may not be desirable in patients with evidence of impaired fast pathway conduction. These patients are usually elderly and have relatively slow AVNRT (typically 100 to 150 beats per minute). In these individuals, ablation of the slow pathway results in mandatory AV conduction via the fast pathway and may result in AV Wenckebach block during rest. Although the development of AV Wenckebach block during sleep or rest has not been symptomatic in our experience, the potential for impaired residual AV conduction should be suspected in these individuals after successful slow pathway ablation. Compromised fast pathway function is likely in patients who previously had an unsuccessful attempt at fast pathway ablation with persistent AVNRT. In these individuals, slow pathway ablation may result in high-degree AV block because of impairment of fast pathway conduction related to the previous fast pathway ablation attempt. Indeed, in our experience, three episodes of AV block occurred in patients with previous ablation attempts. Therefore, for patients who have had recurrence of conduction or primary failure of an ablation attempt involving either the slow or the fast pathway, it is probably wise to confine further ablation efforts to the pathway originally targeted for ablation.

Of 2329 patients undergoing ablation for AV nodal reentry at our institution, only 4 were targeted for fast pathway ablation. The fast pathway was successfully ablated in all 4 patients. In these patients, the fast pathway was chosen for selective ablation because of inability to reliably demonstrate slow pathway conduction in 2 patients, recurrence of AV nodal reentry after a previous slow pathway ablation procedure in 1 patient, and concerns regarding the functional status of the antegrade fast pathway in 1 patient.

Troubleshooting the Difficult Case

Failure to achieve junctional rhythm with RF ablation may be the most common difficulty encountered with ablation of AV nodal reentry (Table 18–7). As previously stated, most instances of AVNRT can be successfully ablated at the typical slow pathway region on the tricuspid valve annulus at the level of the CS

TABLE 18-7

Troubleshooting the Difficult Case

Problem	Causes	Solutions
No junctional rhythm during RF	Wrong ablation site	Try CS os or proximal CS; ablate higher on septum
	Low temperature/current delivery	Use sheath to improve catheter contact and reduce impedance
	Left-sided variant	Map left paraseptal mitral annulus
VA block during junctional rhythm	Too near AV node/His	Deliver RF lower on septum, use cryoablation, pace atrium during RF to follow antegrade conduction
	Slow-slow variant	Confirm variant, pace atrium during RF to follow antegrade conduction
	Absence of retrograde fast pathway	Confirm diagnosis and retrograde conduction status
Nonspecific end points	Poorly inducible tachycardia	Monitor for junctional rhythm and modified slow pathway function
	Absence of dual AV nodal physiology	Monitor for junctional rhythm with RF, thorough baseline study, noninducibility
Multiple AV nodal jumps and echoes after ablation	Multiple slow pathways	Reassess inducibility after each ablation
PR prolongation or AV block with RF	Delivery near AV node/His	Ablate lower on septum; use cryoablation
	Injury to AV nodal artery	Lower energy, cryoablation
	Absence of antegrade fast pathway	Ablate retrograde fast pathway
Catheter instability	Excessive torque or short reach	Use long sheath with septal angulation; change catheter

AV, atrioventricular; CS, coronary sinus; RF, radiofrequency ablation; VA, ventricular-atrial.

ostium or just superior to it. If ablation at these sites is unsuccessful, the next step should be to re-evaluate the diagnosis. Once the diagnosis is confirmed, alternative sites of ablation are considered. Sites lower on the tricuspid annulus expose the patient to little risk and should be explored. We have found ablation within the proximal CS to be particularly beneficial if application of RF current in the usual position between the tricuspid annulus and the CS ostium does not result in an accelerated junctional rhythm. The application of RF in the region of the proximal CS, extending up to 2 cm from the ostium, is most likely to be helpful for patients with slow-slow AVNRT. Particular caution should be used for patients in whom all evidence of retrograde VA conduction is neither at the apex of Koch's triangle nor at the proximal CS. In such patients, in whom all retrograde conduction occurs in the middle of Koch's triangle, a left-sided approach should be considered if RF application in the usual slow pathway position along the tricuspid annulus is ineffective in eliminating slow pathway conduction. Although the evidence for left atrial extensions of the AV node and their involvement in AVNRT is convincing, ablation in the left atrium to treat AVNRT is only rarely required.

Several reports of left-sided ablation to treat AVNRT are present in the literature, although these are limited to case reports and small case series.[57-59] It has been suggested that patients with eccentric retrograde atrial activation represent a subset of patients in whom ablation at the mitral valve annulus within the left atrium is necessary to eliminate AVNRT.[60] This has likewise been our experience, and we do not advocate ablation in the left atrium to treat AVNRT except in rare circumstances. Only after failing to eliminate slow pathway conduction at these sites do we consider ablation closer to the compact AV node. At these more superior sites, cryoablation offers the distinct advantages of catheter stability, small lesion size, and, most importantly, reversibility of ablation effects.

The occurrence of VA block at sites producing junctional rhythm with RF ablation of slow-fast AV nodal reentry portends induced heart block. If retrograde block of junctional rhythm occurs, a new catheter position, further from the AV node, should be tried. Cryoablation does not produce junctional rhythm but allows for reversibility of the ablation effects at these sites. For slow-slow and fast-slow variants of AV nodal reentry, retrograde block of junctional rhythm may not carry the same implications of impending heart block, and ablation may be continued. The use of low-energy ablation and atrial pacing to monitor antegrade AV conduction during ablation may be helpful.

The end points for ablation may be nonspecific, especially if tachycardia or dual AV nodal physiology is not readily demonstrable. A careful baseline study before ablation to best define dual AV nodal physiology and slow pathway function is essential in this situation. As described, elimination of all evidence of slow pathway conduction is not a necessary requirement for a successful slow pathway ablation procedure. Residual AV nodal "jumps" with single echoes constitute an acceptable end point if the tachycardia was previously inducible. This end point is especially important for patients with multiple slow pathways, in whom total elimination of all slow pathway function could lead to extensive and unnecessary ablation. In patients who are without reproducible or inducible tachycardia but in whom the diagnosis is certain, empiric modification of slow pathway function may be the only reasonable end point. Other potential problems and solutions are listed in Table 18–7.

References

1. Denes P, Wu D, Dhingra RC, et al.: Demonstration of dual AV nodal pathways in patients with paroxysmal supraventricular tachycardia. Circulation 48:549-555, 1973.
2. Rosen KM, Mehta A, Miller RA: Demonstration of dual atrioventricular nodal pathways in man. Am J Cardiol 33:291-294, 1974.
3. Bharati S: Anatomic-morphologic relations between AV nodal structure and function in the normal and diseased heart. In Mazgalev TN, Tchou PJ (eds.): Atrial AV Nodal Physiology: A View from the Millennium. Armonk, N.Y.: Futura, 2000, pp 25-48.
4. Paes de Carvalho AF, de Almeida D: Spread of activity through the atrioventricular node. Circ Res 8:801-809, 1960.
5. Anderson RH, Janse MJ, van Capelle FJL, et al.: A combined morphological and electrophysiological study of the atrioventricular node of the rabbit heart. Circ Res 35:909-922, 1974.
6. McGuire MA: What is the slow AV nodal pathway? In Mazgalev TN, Tchou PJ (eds.): Atrial-AV Nodal Physiology: A View from the Millennium. Armonk, N.Y.: Futura, 2000, pp 183-198.
7. van Capelle FJL, Janse MJ, Varghese PJ, et al.: Spread of excitation in the atrioventricular node of isolated rabbit hearts studied by multiple micro-electrode recording. Circ Res 31:602-616, 1972.
8. Janse MJ: Influence of the direction wave front on A-V nodal in isolated hearts of rabbit. Circ Res 25:439-449, 1969.
9. Hirao K, Scherlag BJ, Poty H, et al.: Electrophysiology of the atrio-A-V nodal inputs and exits in the normal dog heart: Radiofrequency ablation using an epicardial approach. J Cardiovasc Electrophysiol 8:904-915, 1997.
10. Young C, Lauer MR, Liem LB, et al.: Demonstration of a posterior atrial input to the atrioventricular node during sustained

11. Fujimuar O, Guiraudon GM, Yee R, et al.: Operative therapy of atrioventricular node reentry and results of an anatomically guided procedure. Am J Cardiol 64:1327-1332, 1989.
12. Gonzalez MD, Contreras LJ, Cardona F, et al.: Demonstration of a left atrial input to the atrioventricular node in humans. Circulation 106:2930-2934, 2002.
13. Wu J, Olgin J, Zipes DP, et al.: Mechanisms underlying the reentrant circuit of atrioventricular nodal reentrant tachycardia in isolated canine atrioventricular nodal preparation using optical mapping. Circ Res 88:1189-1195, 2001.
14. Miller JM, Rosenthal ME, Vassallo JA, et al.: Atrioventricular nodal reentrant tachycardia: Studies on upper and lower "common pathways." Circulation 75:930-940, 1987.
15. Wellens HJJ, Wesdorp JC, Duren DR: Second degree block during reciprocal atrioventricular nodal tachycardia. Circulation 53:595-599, 1976.
16. Bauernfeind RA, Wu D, Denes P, et al.: Retrograde block during dual pathway atrioventricular nodal reentrant paroxysmal tachycardia. Am J Cardiol 42:499-505, 1978.
17. Jackman WT, Beckman KJ, McClelland JH, et al.: Participation of atrial myocardium (posterior septum) in AV nodal reentrant tachycardia: Evidence for resetting by atrial extrastimuli [abstract]. Pacing Clin Electrophysiol 14:646, 1991.
18. Keim S, Werner P, Jazayeri M, et al.: Localization of the fast and slow pathways in atrioventricular nodal reentrant tachycardia by intraoperative ice mapping. Circulation 86:919-924, 1992.
19. McGuire MA, Lau KC, Johnson DC, et al.: Patients with two types of atrioventricular junctional (AV nodal) reentrant tachycardia. Circulation 83:1232-1246, 1991.
20. Kay GN, Epstein AE, Plumb VJ: Evidence for posterior input of both fast and slow AV nodal pathways in patients with AV nodal reentrant tachycardia [abstract]. Circulation 85:1675-1688, 1992.
21. Josephson ME, Kastor JA: Paroxysmal supraventricular tachycardia: Is the atrium a necessary link? Circulation 54:430-435, 1976.
22. Sung RJ, Waxman HL, Saksena S, et al.: Sequence of retrograde atrial activation in patients with dual atrioventricular nodal pathways. Circulation 64:1059-1067, 1981.
23. Holman WL, Ikeshita M, Lease JG, et al.: Alteration of antegrade atrioventricular conduction by cryoablation of periatrioventricular nodal tissue. J Thorac Cardiovasc Surg 88:67-80, 1984.
24. Cox JL, Holman WL, Cain ME: Cryosurgical treatment of atrioventricular node reentrant tachycardia. Circulation 76:1329-1336, 1987.
25. Ross DL, Johnson DC, Dennis R, et al.: Curative surgery for atrioventricular junctional ("AV nodal") reentrant tachycardia. J Am Coll Cardiol 6:1383-1392, 1985.
26. Pritchett ELC, Anderson RW, Benditt DG, et al.: Reentry within the atrioventricular node: Surgical cure with preservation of atrioventricular conduction. Circulation 60:440-446, 1979.
27. McGuire MA, Bourke JP, Robotin MC, et al.: High resolution mapping of Koch's triangle using sixty electrodes in humans with atrioventricular junctional (AV nodal) reentrant tachycardia. Circulation 88:2315-2328, 1993.
28. Wu D, Denes P, Dhingra R, et al.: Clinical electrocardiographic and electrophysiological observations in patients with paroxysmal supraventricular tachycardia. Am J Cardiol 41:1045-1051, 1978.
29. Surawicz Z, Reddy C, Prystowsky E (eds.): Tachycardias. Boston, Mass.: Martinus Nijhoff, 1984.
30. Olgin JE, Ursell P, Kao AK, et al.: Pathological findings following slow pathway ablation for AV nodal reentrant tachycardia. J Cardiovasc Electrophysiol 7:625-631, 1996.

anterograde slow pathway conduction. J Am Coll Cardiol 31:1615-1621, 1998.

31. Gamache MC, Bharati S, Lev M, et al.: Histopathological study following catheter guided radiofrequency current ablation of the slow pathway in a patient with atrioventricular nodal reentrant tachycardia. Pacing Clin Electrophysiol 17:247-251, 1994.

32. Lockwood D, Otomo K, Wang Z, et al.: Electrophysiologic characteristics of atrioventricular nodal reentry tachycardia: Implications for the reentrant circuits. In Zipes DP, Jaliffe J (eds.): Cardiac Electrophysiology from Cell to Bedside, 4th ed. Philadelphia: Saunders, 2004, pp 537-557.

33. Hwang C, Martin D, Goodman J, et al.: Atypical atrioventricular node reciprocating tachycardia masquerading as tachycardia using a left-sided accessory pathway. J Am Coll Cardiol 30:218-225, 1997.

34. Calkins H, Prystowsky E, Berger RD, et al., and the ATAKR Multicenter Investigators Group: Recurrence of conduction following radiofrequency catheter ablation procedures: Relationship to ablation target and electrode temperature. J Cardiovasc Electrophysiol 7:704-712, 1996.

35. Jackman WM, Beckman KJ, McClelland JH, et al.: Treatment of supraventricular tachycardia due to atrioventricular nodal reentry by radiofrequency catheter ablation of slow-pathway conduction. N Engl J Med 327:313-318, 1992.

36. Josephson MD: Supraventricular tachycardias. In Josephson, ME: Clinical Cardiac Electrophysiology: Techniques and Interpretations, 3rd ed. Philadelphia: Lippincott Williams & Wilkins, 2002, pp 168-271.

37. Baker JH II, Plumb VJ, Epstein AE, et al.: PR/RR interval ratio during rapid atrial pacing: A simple method for confirming the presence of slow AV nodal pathway conduction. J Cardiovasc Electrophysiol 7:287-294, 1996.

38. Hintringer F, Hartikainen J, Davies W, et al.: Prediction of atrioventricular block during radiofrequency ablation of the slow pathway of the atrioventricular node. Circulation 92;3490-3496, 1995.

39. Tebbenjohanns J, Pfeiffer D, Schumacher B, et al.: Impact of the local atrial electrogram in AV nodal reentrant tachycardia: Ablation versus modification of the slow pathway. J Cardiovasc Electrophysiol 6:245-251, 1995.

40. Skanes AC, Dubuc M, Klein GJ, et al.: Cryothermal ablation of the slow pathway for the elimination of atrioventricular nodal reentrant tachycardia. Circulation 102:2856-2860, 2000.

41. Langberg JJ, Kim Y-N, Goyal R, et al.: Conversion of typical to "atypical" atrioventricular nodal reentrant tachycardia after radiofrequency catheter modification of the atrioventricular junction. Am J Cardiol 69;503-508,1992.

42. Lai L-P, Lin J-L, Huang SK. Ablation of atrioventricular nodal reentrant tachycardia with the anterior approach: Is it obsolete in the year 2000? In: Radiofrequency catheter ablation of cardiac arrhythmias. Huang SKS, Wilber DJ (eds). Oxford: Future Publishing, 2000, pp 415-421.

43. Strickberger SA, Daoud E, Niebauer M, et al.: Effects of partial and complete ablation of the slow pathway on fast pathway properties in patients with atrioventricular nodal reentrant tachycardia. J Cardiovasc Electrophysiol 5:645-649, 1994.

44. Epstein LM, Jung S, Lee RJ, et al.: Slow AV nodal pathway ablation utilizing a unique temperature controlled radiofrequency energy system. Pacing Clin Electrophysiol 20:664-670, 1997.

45. Kay GN, Epstein AE, Dailey SM, et al.: Selective radiofrequency ablation of the slow pathway for the treatment of atrioventricular nodal reentrant tachycardia. Circulation 85:1675-1687, 1992.

46. Lee MA, Morady F, Kadish A, et al.: Catheter modification of the atrioventricular junction with radiofrequency energy for control of atrioventricular nodal reentry tachycardia. Circulation 83:827-835, 1991.

47. Wathen M, Natale A, Wolfe K, et al.: An anatomically guided approach to atrioventricular node slow pathway ablation. Am J Cardiol 70:886-889, 1992.

48. Jentzer JH, Goyal R, Williamson BD, et al.: Analysis of junctional ectopy during radiofrequency ablation of the slow pathway in patients with atrioventricular nodal reentrant tachycardia. Circulation 90:2820-2826, 1994.

49. Wang X, McClelland JH, Beckman KJ, et al.: Accelerated junctional rhythm during slow pathway ablation. Circulation 84(Suppl):II-582, 1991.

50. Baker JH II, Plumb VJ, Epstein AE, et al.: Predictors of recurrent atrioventricular nodal reentry after selective slow pathway ablation. Am J Cardiol 73:765-769, 1994.

51. Natale A, Klein G, Yee B, et al.: Shortening of fast pathway refractoriness after slow pathway ablation. Circulation 89:1103-1108, 1994.

52. Tai CT, Chen SA, Chiang CE, et al.: Multiple anterograde atrioventricular node pathways in patients with atrioventricular node reentrant tachycardia. J Am Coll Cardiol 28:725-731, 1996.

53. McGuire MA, de Bakker JMT, Vermeulen JT, et al.: Origin and significance of double potentials near the atrioventricular node. Circulation 89:2351-2360, 1994.

54. Niebauer MJ, Daoud E, Williamson B, et al.: Atrial electrogram characteristics in patients with and without atrioventricular nodal reentrant tachycardia. Circulation 92:77-81, 1995.

55. Haissaguerre M, Gaita F, Fischer B, et al.: Elimination of atrioventricular nodal reentrant tachycardia using discrete slow potentials to guide application of radiofrequency energy. Circulation 85:2162-2175, 1992.

56. Sra JS, Jazayeri MR, Blanck Z, et al.: Slow pathway ablation in patients with atrioventricular node reentrant tachycardia and a prolonged PR interval. J Am Coll Cardiol 24:1064-1068, 1994.

57. Sorbera C, Martin C, Woolf P, et al.: Atrioventricular nodal reentry tachycardia: Slow pathway ablation using the transseptal approach. Pacing Clin Electrophysiol 23:1343-1349, 2000.

58. Jais P, Haissaguerre M, Shah D, et al.: Successful radiofrequency ablation of a slow atrioventricular nodal pathway on the left posterior atrial septum. Pacing Clin Electrophysiol 22:525-527, 1999.

59. Altemose GT, Scott LR, Miller JM: Atrioventricular nodal reentrant tachycardia requiring ablation on the mitral annulus. J Cardiovasc Electrophysiol 11:1281-1284, 2000.

60. Tondo C, Otorno K, Jackman WT, et al.: Atrioventricular nodal reentry tachycardia: Is the reentrant circuit always confined in the right atrium. J Am Coll Cardiol 27:159A, 1996.

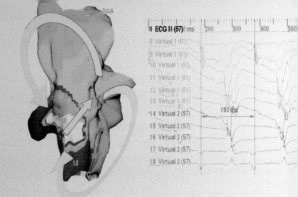

19

Ablation of Atrioventricular Nodal Reentrant Tachycardia and Variants Guided by Intracardiac Recordings

Mario D. González • *Jaime Rivera*

Key Points

- Mechanism of atrioventricular nodal reentrant tachycardia (AVNRT) is reentry involving the fast and slow atrioventricular (AV) nodal pathways.

- The typical slow-fast form of AVNRT is diagnosed by the presence of a long atrium-to-His bundle (AH) interval (>180 msec) during tachycardia, with the earliest retrograde atrial activation localized at the level of the superior part of the triangle of Koch, just behind the tendon of Todaro (fast pathway or anterior approach to the AV node).

- The fast-slow variant has a short AH interval during tachycardia (<180 msec), and early retrograde atrial activation is localized near the coronary sinus (CS) ostium or in the proximal portion of the CS.

- The slow-slow variant has a long AH interval (>180 msec), with early retrograde atrial activation as in the fast-slow form of AVNRT.

- The left-sided variant is similar to the slow-fast type, but slow pathway conduction cannot be eliminated from the right atrium or CS.

- The ablation target for all variants is the antegrade or retrograde slow pathway.

- Catheter navigation systems are useful to label sites of interest. Electroanatomic mapping systems are optional, and cryoablation may be used for selected cases.

- The acute success rate is almost 100%, with a 1% to 2% rate of recurrence. The rate of complications (AV block) is approximately 0.5%.

Atrioventricular nodal reentrant tachycardia (AVRNT) is the most common form of supraventricular tachycardia studied in the electrophysiology laboratory.[1] Although AVNRT can have a benign course, it can also result in disabling symptoms. AVNRT is more frequent in women than in men, and it is more prevalent among the middle-aged population, although it is found in all age groups. A review of the last 200 patients studied in our laboratory revealed a mean age of 49 ± 17 years (range, 17 to 85 years); 149 (74%) of these patients were females. Eleven patients (6%) presented with syncope. In three (1.5%), sustained AVNRT was induced during an electrophysiology study performed to investigate the cause of syncope. Syncope did not recur after elimination of 1:1 slow atrioventricular (AV) nodal pathway conduction.

Catheter ablation eliminates AVNRT in most patients with a low risk of complications.[2] Therefore, it is now offered as a first-line therapy to symptomatic patients and to those who cannot tolerate or do not wish to take antiarrhythmic agents.[3] In addition, patients with high-risk occupations may undergo catheter ablation as first-line therapy. The anatomic approach to ablation of AV nodal reentry is covered in Chapter 18. This chapter focuses on the ablation of AVNRT and its variants as guided by intracardiac electrograms. All forms of AV nodal reentry can be treated by the anatomic or the electrogram-guided approach. Readers who are interested in AV nodal reentry should read both chapters, because the information contained in them is complementary, to minimize redundancy.

Pathophysiology

The concept of reentry involving the AV node has evolved with the acquisition of new knowledge about the specialized conduction system of the heart. The fundamental studies of a century ago by Gaskell,[4] His Jr.,[5] and Tawara[6] formed the basis for the present understanding of the anatomy and physiology of the AV node. Mines, in 1913,[7] was the first to describe the existence of dual conduction properties in the AV node of the electric ray using properly timed stimuli. He attributed the reciprocating rhythm he induced to the presence of two regions in the specialized conduction system, each with different conduction and recovery properties. Moe et al.[8] later demonstrated the existence of two different AV nodal conducting pathways underlying AVNRT. The fast AV nodal pathway (or β pathway) was found to have a longer refractory period than the slow AV nodal pathway (or α pathway). These different properties facilitate the onset and maintenance of AVNRT. Mendez and Moe[9] found that the two AV nodal pathways located in the upper portion of the AV node in the rabbit communicated with a final (lower) common pathway. Denes et al.[10] were the first to describe the presence of dual AV nodal pathways in patients with AVNRT. Dual AV nodal pathways can be demonstrated using single atrial extrastimuli of increasing prematurity (Fig. 19–1) or during decremental atrial stimulation (Fig. 19–2).

Dual AV nodal physiology is a normal behavior of the human AV node. This physiology indicates two

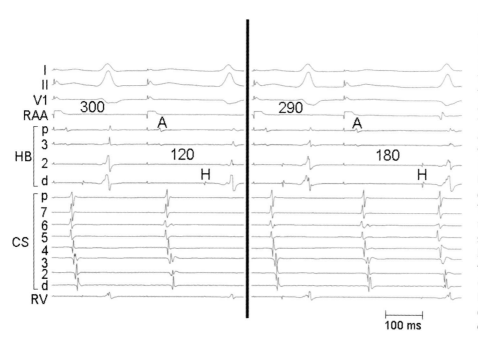

FIGURE 19–1. Demonstration of dual atrioventricular (AV) nodal pathways. Single extrastimuli of progressively shorter coupling intervals (S_2) were delivered from the right atrial appendage (RAA) at a basic drive of 600 ms (S_1). A "jump" or sudden increase of the atrium-to-His bundle (AH) interval from 120 ms (left panel) to 180 ms (right panel) occurs following shortening of the atrial extrastimulus from 300 to 290 ms. The atrial extrastimulus in the right panel conducts through the slow AV nodal pathway followed by retrograde conduction through the fast AV nodal pathway (echo beat). CS, coronary sinus; HB, His bundle; RV, right ventricle; p, proximal; d, distal; A, atrial electrogram; H, His recording.

100 ms

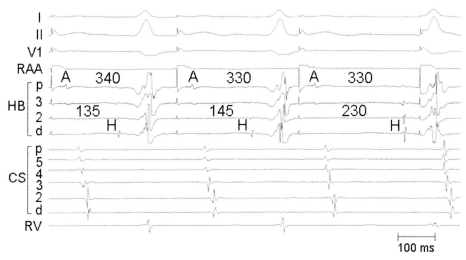

FIGURE 19–2. Demonstration of dual atrioventricular (AV) nodal pathways during decremental atrial stimulation. A decrease in the cycle length of stimulation from the right atrial appendage (RAA) from 340 to 330 msec results in prolongation of the AH interval from 135 to 145, and 230 msec. Abbreviations as per Figure 19-1.

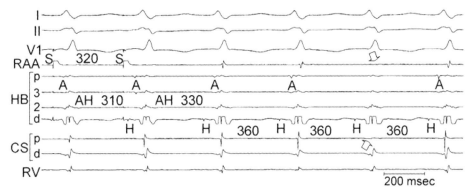

FIGURE 19–3. Induction of sustained slow-fast atrioventricular nodal reentrant tachycardia (AVNRT). Rapid atrial pacing at a cycle length of 320 ms results in sustained AVNRT following a critical prolongation of the AH interval (330 msec). The cycle length of the tachycardia was 360 msec. The third tachycardia complex fails to conduct to the atrium *(open arrows)* without perturbation of the tachycardia. CS, coronary sinus; HB, His bundle; RAA, right atrial appendage; RV, right ventricle. *(From Gonzalez MD, Contreras L, Cardona F, et al. V-A block during atrioventricular nodal reentrant tachycardia: Reentry confined to the AV node. Pacing Clin Electrophysiol 26:775-778, 2003, with permission.)* Abbreviations as per Figure 19-1.

or more populations of AV nodal cells with different refractoriness and conduction times but does not imply the presence of AVNRT. Dual AV nodal physiology can be demonstrated in patients without AVNRT who are studied for other arrhythmias.[11,12] Consistent with these observations, we found similar incidences of dual AV nodal physiology in patients with and without AVNRT. A jump of 50 msec or longer was present in 82% (164/200) of patients with AVNRT and in 79% (158/200) of patients without AVNRT; this difference was not statistically significant. The magnitude of the "jump" however, was greater in patients with AVNRT (87 ± 6 versus 59 ± 7 msec, $P < .05$).

Considerable disagreement still exists among investigators regarding the nature of the slow and fast AV nodal pathways. Two current theories suggest that these pathways represent longitudinal dissociation of conduction within the AV node or, alternatively, that they comprise the structural inputs

into the AV node. Before the advent of surgical and catheter ablation, the slow and fast AV nodal pathways were believed to be part of the AV node, representing regions with different electrophysiologic properties (i.e., longitudinal dissociation). In fact, several experimental and clinical observations support an intranodal location of these AV nodal pathways and the reentrant circuit supporting AVNRT. [13-16] In patients with AVNRT, under certain conditions, atrial activation close to the AV node can be dissociated from the reentrant circuit without interruption of the tachycardia (Fig. 19–3).[16] This observation, although uncommon, suggests that reentry confined to the AV node can indeed sustain AVNRT.

The first clinical study documenting different exits from the AV node during retrograde fast and slow AV nodal pathway activation was published by Sung et al.[17] Earliest atrial activation during retrograde AV nodal conduction can occur in the upper or lower portion of the triangle of Koch, depending on whether the fast or the slow AV nodal pathway is activated. These observations and the results of surgical and catheter ablation of the anterior or posterior approaches to the AV node[18-23] led to the conclusions that the fast and slow AV nodal pathways have an extranodal component and that the atrium is required to sustain AVNRT. However, the portion of the atrium that is involved in the reentrant circuit remains elusive.

Some discrepancies may be explained in part by our incomplete knowledge of the anatomy of the AV node and its extensions. The original description of the AV node, made by Tawara in 1906,[6] is unfortunately quite different from what is frequently presented in textbooks. One common misconception is to consider the AV node a rounded structure located at the apex of the triangle of Koch. In contrast, the original description by Tawara included posterior extension of the AV node reaching both the mitral and tricuspid annuli.[6] Becker and Anderson[24] confirmed and expanded the pioneer work of Tawara. Inoue and Becker[25] clearly demonstrated the presence of rightward and leftward posterior extensions of the AV node in human hearts. Importantly, they showed that the rightward posterior extension reaches the ostium of the coronary sinus (CS), and the leftward extension reaches the mitral annulus (Fig. 19–4).

More recently, a functional left atrial input to the AV node, proceeding from the mitral annuls, was demonstrated in humans.[26] This left atrial (mitral annulus) input to the AV node probably represents the electrophysiologic counterpart of the leftward extension of the AV node. Therefore, in addition to the anterior and posterior approaches to the AV node, the mitral annulus provides an input for activation proceeding from the left atrium (Fig. 19–5). Whether these inputs actively participate in the various forms of AVNRT by providing entrance and exit sites in a reentry that involves the atrium,[27] or whether they merely represent the exit points for activation proceeding from an "intranodal" circuit sustaining AVNRT, is unknown.[16] Consistent with the clinical observation of "intranodal" reentry,[16] different forms of AVNRT can be contained within the transitional cells of the posterior AV nodal input in a rabbit heart[28] due to functional dissociation of cellular activation.[29]

Diagnosis and Differential Diagnosis

Three different forms of AVNRT are observed: slow-fast, slow-slow, and fast-slow AVNRT. In a single

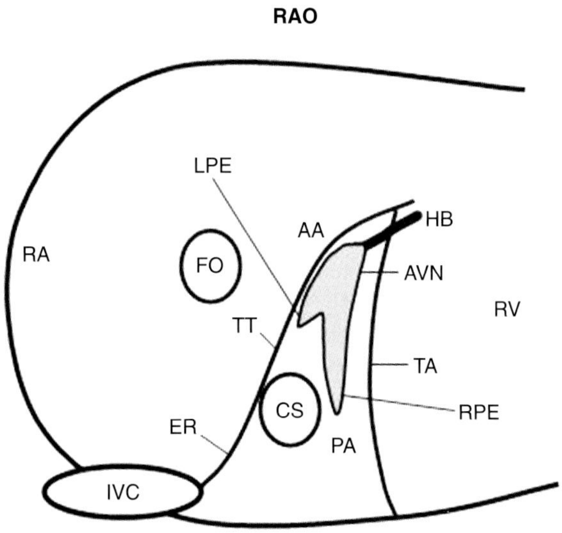

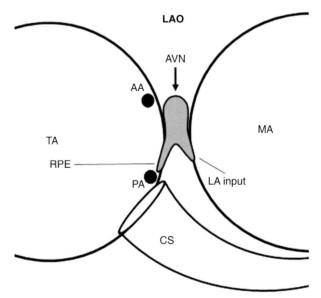

FIGURE 19–4. Schematic representation of atrioventricular (AV) node inside the triangle of Koch as viewed from the right anterior oblique projection (RAO). The boundaries of the triangle of Koch are defined by the tendon of Todaro (TT), the tricuspid annulus (TA), and the ostium of the coronary sinus (CS). The anterior approach (AA) and the posterior approach (PA) to the AV node (AVN) are shown. The rightward posterior extension (RPE) and leftward posterior extension (LPE) of the AV node is shown as if the AV septum has been removed. ER, Eustachian ridge; FO, fossa ovalis; IVC, inferior vena cava; RA, right atrium; RV, right ventricle.

FIGURE 19–5. Schematic representation of AV node (AVN) as viewed from the left anterior oblique projection (LAO). The AVN is shown above the coronary sinus (CS) along with the mitral annulus (MA), and the tricuspid annulus (TA). The anterior approach (AA) and the posterior approach (PA) are represented by solid circles. The left atrial input (LA input) to the AVN node is shown. The rightward extension reaches the coronary sinus. The leftward inferior extension reaches the mitral annulus. *(Modified from Gonzalez MD, Contreras LJ, Cardona F, et al.: Demonstration of a left atrial input to the atrioventricular node in humans. Circulation 106:2930-2934, 2002, with permission.)*

patient one, two, or all three forms may be present at different times during the electrophysiology study. There are no electrophysiologic findings that alone are absolutely diagnostic of AVNRT; the diagnosis is made on the weight of typical features and the exclusion of atrial tachycardias and septal accessory AV pathways (Table 19–1). Electrophysiologic variables in different forms of AV nodal reentry are given in Table 19–2.

SLOW-FAST AVNRT

The typical form, or slow-fast variant, occurred in 168 (84%) of our 200 patients. The electrocardiogram obtained during tachycardia can suggest the diagnosis, because the retrograde P wave superimposed on the terminal portion of the QRS gives rise to a pseudo–right bundle branch block pattern (Fig. 19–6). The tachycardia cycle length averages 359 ± 68 msec (range, 235 to 640 msec). The antegrade limb of the tachycardia is the slow AV nodal pathway, with an atrium-to-His bundle (AH) interval longer than 180 msec (range, 190 to 540 msec; mean, 314 ± 67 msec).

Earliest retrograde atrial activation in the slow-fast form is recorded posterior (in anatomic description) and leftward of the catheter recording proximal His bundle activation.[12] The presence of retrograde fast AV nodal pathway conduction either before or during adrenergic stimulation is a requirement for the induction of slow-fast AVNRT. This is in contrast to the other forms of AVNRT, in which retrograde fast AV nodal pathway conduction may be absent. Retrograde fast AV nodal pathway conduction needs to be differentiated from retrograde conduction over an anteroseptal accessory AV pathway. This can be done by parahisian pacing at the beginning of the procedure (Fig. 19–7 and 19–8).[30] A short VA time of less than 60 msec usually excludes reciprocating tachycardias. Induction of

TABLE 19–1

Diagnostic Criteria of Atrioventricular Nodal Reentrant Tachycardia and Variants

Slow-Fast

Dual AV nodal physiology in most but not all cases

Long AH interval (>180 msec) during tachycardia

Initiation tachycardia dependent on critical AH interval during antegrade slow pathway conduction

Earliest retrograde atrial activation in tachycardia behind the tendon of Todaro, posterior and to the left of the His bundle

Exclude atrial tachycardia and reciprocating tachycardia by appropriate maneuvers

Slow-Slow

Same as for slow-fast variant except for early retrograde atrial activation near the CS ostium*

Fast-Slow

Short AH interval during tachycardia (<180 msec)

Initiation dependent on critical HA interval during retrograde slow pathway conduction

Early retrograde atrial activation near the CS ostium or in the proximal portion of the CS*

AH interval during atrial pacing at TCL >40 msec longer than AH interval in tachycardia

Left-Sided

Same as for slow-fast variant except for the following:
Inability to ablate slow pathway from right atrium or CS
Short HA interval (<15 msec) may be present
Double response to atrial extrastimulus may be present

*The sequence of CS activation may simulate the presence of a posteroseptal or left-sided accessory pathway.
AH, atrium-to-His bundle; AV, atrioventricular; CS, coronary sinus; HA, His bundle-to-atrium; TCL, tachycardia cycle length.

TABLE 19–2

Electrophysiologic Variables of Different Forms of Atrioventricular Nodal Reentrant Tachycardia

Variable	Slow-Fast	Slow-Slow	Fast-Slow
TCL	359 ± 68 (235-640)	413 ± 64 (330-565)	331 ± 63 (250-440)
AH	315 ± 66 (190-540)	277 ± 75 (185-465)	90 ± 39 (35-160)
HA	42 ± 13 (20-140)	139 ± 34 (90-205)	243 ± 65 (125-405)
Site of earliest retrograde atrial activation	Posterior and to the left of the catheter recording His bundle activation	At the CS ostium or in the CS up to 1.1 ± 0.5 cm from the ostium	At the CS ostium or in the CS up to 1.5 ± 0.7 cm from the ostium

AH, atrium-to-His bundle; CS, coronary sinus; HA, His bundle-to-atrium; TCL, tachycardia cycle length.

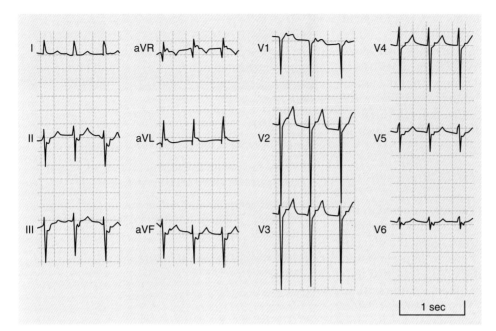

FIGURE 19–6. Electrocardiogram during slow-fast atrioventricular nodal reentrant tachycardia. This tracing was obtained in a 76-year-old man with palpitations and syncope. Retrograde P waves at the end of the QRS complex in V1 give rise to a pseudo right bundle branch block pattern. The QRS also shows left ventricular hypertrophy and a left anterior hemiblock unrelated to the tachycardia.

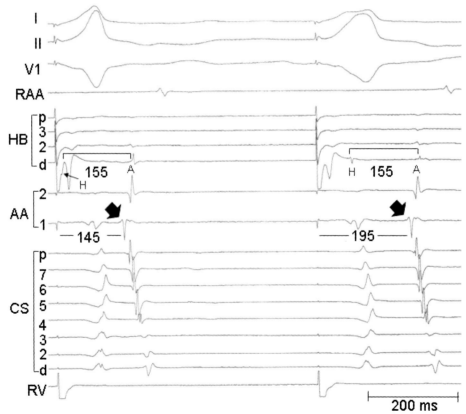

FIGURE 19–7. Parahisian pacing in a patient with retrograde conduction through the fast atrioventricular (AV) nodal pathway. The mapping catheter is located in the region of the anterior approach (AA, *arrow*) corresponding to the atrial exit site of the fast AV nodal pathway. The first stimulus captures both the His and the ventricle. The second stimulus captures only the ventricle. Note that the HA interval remains constant (155 msec) but the VA interval shortens during His capture (from 195 to 145 msec) due to earlier atrial activation with earlier His bundle activation. This observation demonstrates that retrograde conduction occurs over the AV node and not over an accessory AV pathway. In addition, earliest retrograde atrial activation was recorded from the anterior approach indicating that the fast, not the slow, AV nodal pathway was responsible for retrograde conduction. Abbreviations as per Figure 19-1.

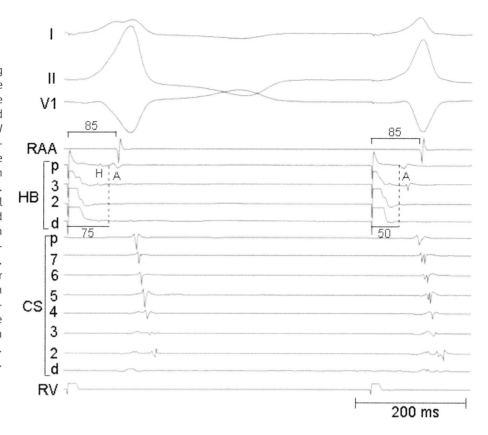

FIGURE 19–8. Parahisian pacing in a patient with retrograde conduction through both the atrioventricular (AV) node and a right anterior accessory AV pathway. The first stimulus captures only the ventricle and the second stimulus captures both the ventricle and the His bundle. Activation at the right atrial appendage (RAA) shows a fixed VA interval (85 msec) in both complexes indicating the presence of an accessory AV pathway. Atrial activation is advanced near the His bundle (HB) region (from 75 to 50 msec) and in the coronary sinus (CS) during His bundle capture indication conduction over the fast AV nodal pathway. Abbreviations as per Figure 19-1.

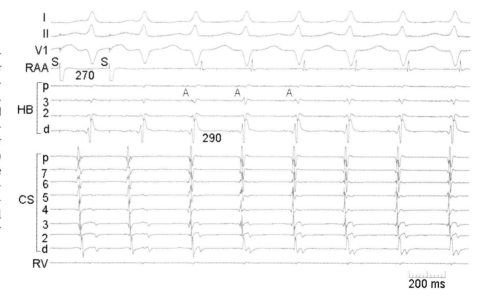

FIGURE 19–9. Induction of sustained slow-fast atrioventricular nodal reentrant tachycardia following rapid atrial stimulation. An atrial electrogram recorded from the proximal pair of electrode (HBp) of the catheter located in the His bundle (HB) region precedes activation in the proximal coronary sinus (CS) consistent with retrograde conduction over the fast AV nodal pathway. Abbreviations as per Figure 19-1.

this tachycardia is usually accomplished by delivering atrial extrastimuli or rapid atrial stimulation (Fig. 19–9). Regardless of the maneuver used, induction of slow-fast AVNRT from the atrium requires antegrade block over the fast AV nodal pathway, with antegrade conduction over the slow AV nodal pathway allowing retrograde conduction over the fast AV nodal pathway (Fig. 19–10). Less commonly, ventricular stimulation can also induce slow-fast

AVNRT. Local atrial activation near the exit site of the fast AV nodal pathway can be recorded using closely spaced electrodes (see Fig. 19–10). The site of earliest retrograde atrial activation is critical to differentiate slow-fast from slow-slow AVNRT, because the HA intervals can overlap in these two forms of tachycardia. In our population, the HA interval in the slow-fast form was 41.6 ± 13.4 msec (range, 20 to 140 msec).

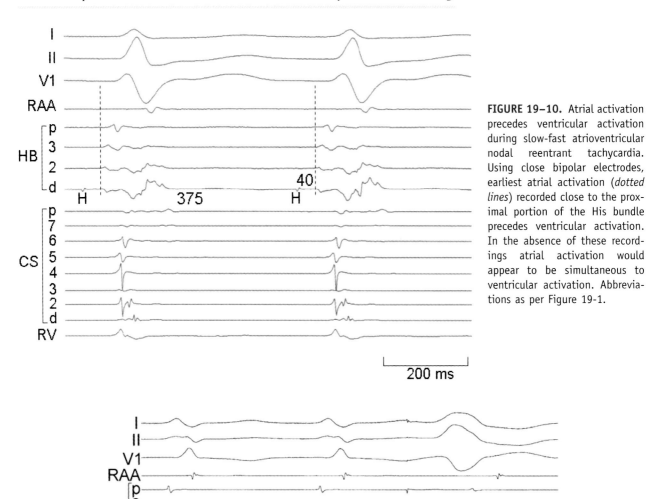

FIGURE 19–10. Atrial activation precedes ventricular activation during slow-fast atrioventricular nodal reentrant tachycardia. Using close bipolar electrodes, earliest atrial activation (*dotted lines*) recorded close to the proximal portion of the His bundle precedes ventricular activation. In the absence of these recordings atrial activation would appear to be simultaneous to ventricular activation. Abbreviations as per Figure 19-1.

FIGURE 19–11. Entrainment of slow-fast atrioventricular nodal reentrant tachycardia by a late ventricular extrastimulus (s). A single ventricular extrastimulus delivered during tachycardia (cycle length 360 msec) advances both retrograde His bundle (H) and retrograde atrial (A) activation by 10 msec. Note that the sequence of atrial activation during tachycardia and following ventricular stimulation are identical. (*From Gonzalez MD, Contreras L, Cardona F, et al.: V-A block during atrioventricular nodal reentrant tachycardia: Reentry confined to the AV node. Pacing Clin Electrophysiol 26:775-778, 2003, with permission.*) Abbreviations as per Figure 19-1.

Entrainment of the tachycardia by late ventricular extrastimuli is critical to confirm the diagnosis. A common lower pathway is not present in most patients with slow-fast AVNRT. Therefore, a ventricular extrastimulus that minimally advances retrograde His bundle activation will also advance retrograde atrial activation, with an identical atrial sequence as that observed during tachycardia (Fig. 19–11). Interestingly, many patients with slow-fast AVNRT have a concurrent arrhythmia. In 12 (7%) of 168 patients, in addition to AVNRT, we induced AV reentrant tachycardia using an accessory AV pathway. A focal atrial tachycardia was present in 15 (9%) of 168

patients and originated from the following sites: crista terminalis (10), CS ostium (1), fast AV nodal pathway region (2), and mitral annulus–aorta junction (2).[31] Another important finding is that slow-fast AVNRT can be associated with other forms of AVNRT (Fig. 19–12). For example, 2% of patients also had slow-slow AVNRT, 2% had fast-slow AVNRT, and in 1% the three forms coexisted in the same patient.

SLOW-SLOW AVNRT

Slow-slow AVNRT occurred in 22 (11%) of 200 patients with AVNRT. In this form of reentry, a slow

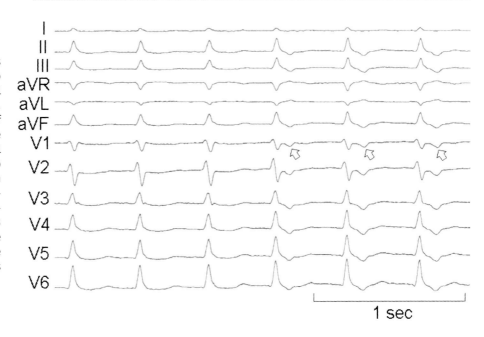

FIGURE 19–12. Spontaneous conversion of slow-fast into slow-slow atrioventricular nodal reentrant tachycardia (AVNRT). During the first 3 complexes of slow-fast AVNRT, the P waves are superimposed to the terminal portion of the QRS giving rise to a pseudo right bundle branch block pattern. Spontaneous transition from slow-fast into slow-slow AVNRT during the last 3 complexes, results in a negative P wave following the QRS in the inferior and precordial leads *(arrows)*.

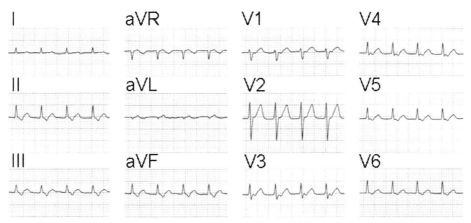

FIGURE 19–13. Electrocardiogram during slow-slow atrioventricular nodal reentrant tachycardia. Negative P waves are recorded in inferior and precordial leads after the QRS complexes followed by a long PR interval. The morphology and polarity of the P waves suggest earliest atrial activation in the proximal coronary sinus. The differential diagnosis includes an atrial tachycardia and orthodromic AV reentrant tachycardia using a postero-septal accessory AV pathway.

AV nodal pathway is used as the antegrade limb, and another slow AV nodal pathway as the retrograde limb (Fig. 19–13). The electrocardiogram during tachycardia shows characteristic negative P waves in inferior and precordial leads, typical of earliest retrograde atrial activation in the proximal CS (see Fig. 19–13).[32] This tachycardia can be induced by atrial or ventricular stimulation (Fig. 19–14) and frequently requires administration of isoproterenol. *The earliest site of retrograde atrial activation near the CS ostium (see Fig. 19–14) is what characterizes slow-slow AVNRT, and not necessarily the HA interval.* As previously mentioned, although the HA interval is usually longer than that recorded during slow-fast AVNRT, an overlap in the HA intervals between these two forms of AVNRT is frequently observed.[12] In our patients,

the range of HA during slow-slow and slow-fast AVNRT was 90 to 205 msec and 20 to 140 msec, respectively.

The earliest site of retrograde atrial activation was found in the right atrium near the anterior edge of the CS ostium or just inside the CS (mean distance from the ostium, 1.1 ± 0.5 cm). The tachycardia cycle length was 413 ± 64 msec; the AH interval was 277 ± 75 msec; the HA interval was 139 ± 33 msec (range, 90 to 205 msec); and the shortest HA interval (measured at the earliest atrial activation site during tachycardia) was 100 ± 42 msec.

Characteristic of this form of AVNRT is the presence of a lower common pathway.[33] In other words, there is a portion of the AV node that is distal to, and not part of, the reentrant circuit that sustains this

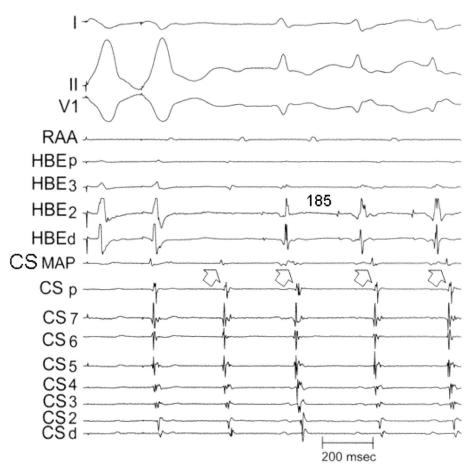

FIGURE 19–14. Induction of slow-slow atrioventricular nodal reentrant tachycardia (AVNRT) using ventricular stimulation. Rapid ventricular pacing induced sustained slow-slow AVNRT (AH interval 185 msec) following retrograde conduction over the slow AV nodal pathway. Earliest retrograde atrial activation *(arrows)* was recorded from the mapping catheter (MAP) positioned just inside the coronary sinus. Abbreviations as per Figure 19-1.

form of tachycardia. The presence of a lower common pathway is demonstrated by comparison of the HA interval during tachycardia to the earliest atrial activation site, with the HA interval observed during ventricular pacing at the same cycle length as the tachycardia. In patients with slow-slow AVNRT, the HA interval during ventricular pacing (measured from the end of the His bundle deflection) is longer than that recorded during tachycardia (Fig. 19–15A). This tachycardia needs to be differentiated from atrial tachycardia and from AV reentrant tachycardia using a concealed posteroseptal accessory AV pathway.

As in the slow-fast form, pre-excitation of the atrium during slow-slow AVNRT only follows ventricular extrastimuli that advance retrograde His bundle activation. However, because of the presence of a lower common pathway, retrograde His bundle activation needs to be advanced more than 15 msec[33] before retrograde atrial activation is also advanced. In contrast, during AV reentrant tachycardia, late ventricular extrastimuli can advance retrograde atrial activation even when retrograde His bundle activation is not altered, as long as ventricular activation near the earliest atrial activation site is advanced. An atrial tachycardia with 1:1 AV conduction can be differentiated from AVNRT by comparing the sequence of atrial activation during tachycardia with that observed during ventricular pacing at a cycle length identical to that of the tachycardia. An atrial tachycardia has a different sequence of atrial activation than that observed during ventricular pacing with 1:1 VA conduction and may demonstrate a V-A-A-V response after ventricular pacing. In patients with AVNRT and long retrograde conduction times, a V-A-A-V response may still occur (see Fig. 19–15B). This happens when the retrograde VA interval exceeds the paced RR interval and atrial activation precedes ventricular activation during tachycardia.

FAST-SLOW AVNRT

The fast-slow form of AVNRT occurred in 16 (8%) of our 200 patients with AVNRT. In this form of reentry, the fast AV nodal pathway is used as the antegrade limb and one or more slow AV nodal pathways as the retrograde limb. The electrocardiogram obtained during tachycardia shows a PR interval that is shorter than the RP interval (long RP tachycardia) (Fig. 19–16). This tachycardia closely resembles the slow-slow form and is not simply the reverse of slow-fast AVNRT. Similar to the slow-slow form, fast-slow AVNRT can be induced by atrial or ventricular

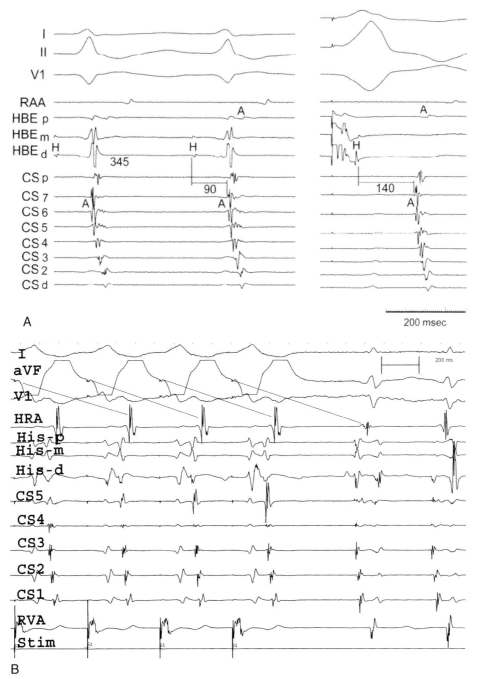

FIGURE 19–15. Demonstration of a lower common pathway in patients with atrioventricular (AV) nodal reentrant tachycardia using the retrograde slow AV nodal pathway. **A,** The HA during tachycardia measured from the beginning of the His deflection to the earliest atrial activation site in the proximal coronary sinus (CS_7) was 90 msec. During ventricular stimulation at the same cycle length of the tachycardia (345 msec) the HA interval measured from the end of the His deflection to the earliest atrial activation site was 140 msec, consistent with a common lower pathway distal to the reentrant circuit supporting the tachycardia. *(Reproduced with the permission from Curtis AB, Gonzalez MD: Supraventricular tachycardia. In Naccarelli GV, Curtis AB, Goldschlager NF (eds.): Electrophysiology Self-Assessment Program. Bethesda, MD, American College of Cardiology, 2000.)* **B,** V-A-A-V response following ventricular stimulation in another patient with AV nodal reentry. Because of very long VA intervals that exceed the paced R-R interval, the atrial activation for any paced beat is actually associated with the second ventricular complex back, not the one that immediately precedes it *(lines)*. In addition, atrial activation precedes ventricular activation during tachycardia. CS, coronary sinus with 5 proximal and 1 distal; d, distal; His, His bundle; HRA, high right atrium; m, mid; p, proximal; RVA, right ventricular apex; Stim, stimulation. *(Figure courtesy of Dr. Mark A. Wood.)*

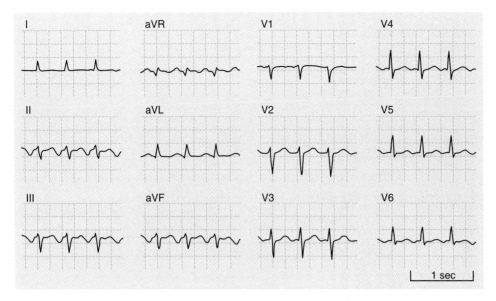

FIGURE 19–16. Electrocardiogram during fast-slow atrioventricular nodal reentrant tachycardia. Negative P waves in inferior and precordial leads are recorded before the QRS complexes with a PR shorter than the RP interval, giving rise to a long RP tachycardia pattern.

stimulation, frequently during administration of isoproterenol. In addition, the presence of a lower common pathway results in an HA interval during tachycardia that is shorter than that observed during ventricular stimulation.[33] Because of the short PR interval associated with antegrade conduction over the fast AV nodal pathway, the electrocardiogram shows a longer RP than PR interval, with negative P waves in inferior leads consistent with early atrial activation close to the CS ostium (see Fig. 19–16).[32] With forms of AV nodal reentry that have long RP intervals, the AH interval during atrial pacing at the tachycardia cycle length exceeds the AH interval in tachycardia by greater than 40 msec. For AV reciprocating tachycardias the difference in the values of these intervals is 20 to 40 msec, and for atrial tachycardias it is less than 20 msec.

Catheter Ablation of Slow-Fast AVNRT

ABLATION OF ANTEGRADE SLOW ATRIOVENTRICULAR NODAL PATHWAY CONDUCTION

Ablation of the slow AV nodal pathway is the current approach to eliminate slow-fast AVNRT. Appropriate diagnosis and ablation require positioning of multipolar catheters in the following regions: proximal His bundle, proximal CS, right ventricular septum, and right atrium. An electrophysiologic study is initially performed to determine antegrade and retrograde AV nodal conduction in the basal state and during

administration of isoproterenol. The conduction properties of the fast and slow AV nodal pathways are defined before and after ablation. Once the correct diagnosis is established, the infusion of isoproterenol is interrupted, the tachycardia is terminated, and the properties of the AV node are documented. The patient is sedated to reduce catheter movements during the ablation procedure.

Ablation of antegrade conduction over the slow AV nodal pathway can be accomplished using either a pure anatomic approach, a pure electrophysiologic approach, or, most commonly, a combination of both methods. The anatomic approach is described in Chapter 18.[20,34-36]

Two electrophysiologic approaches were described by Jackman[23] and Haissaguerre[21] and their colleagues. These approaches, although they use different activation potentials, both reduce the number of radiofrequency (RF) current applications by identifying critical components of the reentrant circuit. Jackman described a sharp late potential following a low-amplitude atrial potential near the CS ostium during sinus rhythm and suggested that this potential represents the atrial connection of the slow AV nodal pathway (Fig. 19–17). Consistent with this concept, during retrograde slow AV nodal conduction, the sequence is inverted and the sharp potential precedes the atrial electrogram. This potential is usually recorded anterior (in front of) or just inside the CS ostium (Figs. 19–18 and 19–19). The slow potential described by Haissaguerre is usually recorded at sites slightly superior to the site where the potential described by Jackman is observed. The Haissaguerre potential becomes delayed and of lower amplitude at rapid rates of stimulation, consistent with AV nodal properties.[21] The locations

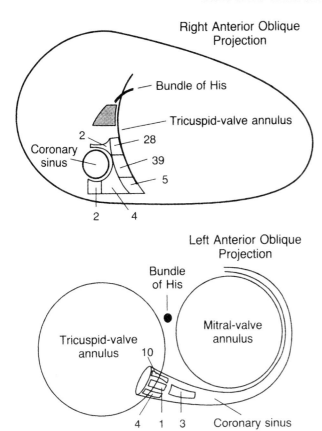

FIGURE 19-17. Sites of successful ablation of slow pathway conduction using an electrophysiologic approach. A potential consistent with activation of the atrial end of the slow pathway was used as a target for ablation. The numbers indicate the number of successful ablations in each region. The shaded region indicates the area of retrograde fast pathway conduction. *(From Jackman WM, Beckman KJ, McClelland JH, et al. Treatment of supraventricular tachycardia due to atrioventricular nodal reentry by radiofrequency catheter ablation of slow-pathway conduction. N Engl J Med 327:313-318:1992, with permission.)*

TABLE 19-3
Electrogram-Guided Targets for Slow Pathway Ablation
Late atrial activation potentials (atrial end of the slow pathway), usually located in front of or at the anatomic anterior edge of the CS
Earliest retrograde atrial activation site during slow-slow or fast-slow AVNRT

AVNRT, atrioventricular nodal reentrant tachycardia; CS, coronary sinus.

where these two potentials can be recorded frequently overlap.[37] The targets for slow pathway ablation are given in Table 19-3.

These potentials may represent activation of transitional cells[38] as they approach the AV node or activation of the rightward inferior extension of the AV node described by Inoue and Becker[25] and by Tawara.[6] In addition, these potentials are present in individuals with and without AVNRT.[38,39] These potentials facilitate catheter ablation of antegrade slow AV nodal pathway conduction, reducing the number of RF energy applications required to eliminate AVNRT.

The mapping and ablation catheter (4-mm-tip electrode) is advanced through the femoral vein and positioned between the tricuspid annulus and the CS ostium. Mapping from the distal and proximal pairs of electrodes is performed using bipolar recordings

(30 to 500 Hz). Unipolar electrograms (0.5 to 500 Hz) are simultaneously obtained from the two distal electrodes, including the 4-mm-tip electrode. To facilitate catheter stability, a long sheath with slight septal angulation is frequently used to maintain good tissue contact. The right and left anterior oblique projections are used to document the position of the tip of the ablation catheter in relation to the catheters recording proximal His bundle activation and proximal CS activation, respectively. The CS ostium can be much larger than what may be suggested by the catheter positioned in the CS. Therefore, before proceeding with ablation, we use the mapping catheter to explore the size and location of the CS ostium. Lesions delivered above the superior edge of the CS ostium are more likely to result in AV block. The previously described potentials associated with slow AV nodal pathway activation can be found between the tricuspid annulus and the anatomic anterior edge of the CS ostium. If ablation of these potentials is unsuccessful, we withdraw the catheter slowly to the CS ostium and deliver ablation at the anatomic anterior edge of the CS ostium. If that is also unsuccessful, we perform ablation inside the proximal CS with the catheter pointing toward the left ventricle (counterclockwise rotation). Application of RF energy on the mitral annulus,[39-41] using the trans-septal approach, was required in our experience in only 1 (0.5%) of 200 patients. Noninduction of AVNRT was achieved in all of our patients, and elimination of 1:1 antegrade conduction over the slow pathway occurred in 98% of patients.

It is advisable to initially use low power (20 to 30 W) to test for unwanted effects such as prolongation of the AH interval. After 15 seconds, the power can be gradually increased up to 50 W. During RF delivery, the impedance is continuously monitored, because a drop in impedance is a better indicator of tissue temperature than the tip electrode temperature is.

During catheter ablation of the slow AV nodal pathway, a junctional rhythm is frequently induced (Fig. 19-20). Although a junctional rhythm is not

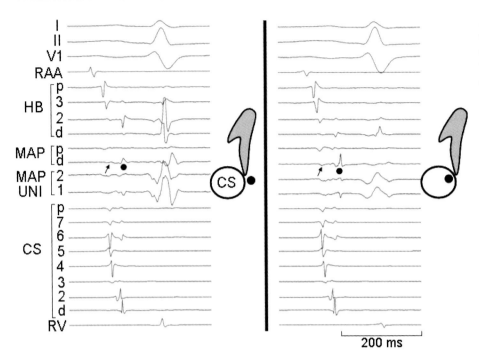

FIGURE 19–18. Electrograms recorded near the coronary sinus ostium and the rightward posterior (inferior) extension of the atrioventricular (AV) node. Bipolar and unipolar (UNI) recordings obtained from the mapping catheter (MAP) just before ablation of the slow AV nodal pathway. Late activation potentials (*dots*) believed to represent slow pathway activation and following local atrial activation (*arrows*) are recorded in front of the anterior edge of the coronary sinus ostium (CS, left panel) and just inside the coronary sinus (right panel). Abbreviations as per Figure 19-1.

200 ms

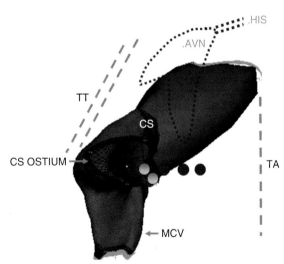

RAO VIEW

FIGURE 19–19. Recording sites of late atrial activation potentials. Anatomical reconstruction of the coronary sinus (CS) was obtained with the NavX system (Endocardial Solutions, St. Paul, Minn.) in the right anterior oblique (RAO) view. The approximate location of the atrioventricular node (AVN) with its extensions and the His bundle are shown. These potentials, believed to signal the atrial connection to the slow AV nodal pathway, were recorded in front and just inside of the anterior edge of the coronary sinus ostium. MCV, middle cardiac vein; TA, tricuspid annulus; TT, tendon of Todaro.

specific, it is more commonly elicited at successful than at unsuccessful sites. During RF current delivery, we closely monitor the AH interval during sinus rhythm and retrograde conduction during junctional beats. Energy delivery must be rapidly interrupted if a junctional beat fails to conduct retrogradely to the atrium (Fig. 19–21), because this reflects damage to the AV node. In some cases, successful ablation of slow AV nodal pathway conduction can be achieved in the absence of junctional beats during RF energy application.[42] More frequently, however, successful ablation is heralded by a junctional rhythm that gradually abates during ablation.[43]

Ablation is considered successful if the tachycardia cannot be reinduced even during administration of isoproterenol and 1:1 antegrade conduction over the slow AV nodal pathway is eliminated. Not uncommonly, AH interval jumps and single slow-fast AV nodal echo beats may still be inducible after successful ablation. These echo beats are most likely the result of conduction over a different slow AV nodal pathway than the one required to sustain AVNRT.

CRYOABLATION TO ELIMINATE AVNRT

Cryoablation has been introduced to reduce the risk of AV block during catheter ablation of AVNRT.[44] This is a new technology, and we have had less clinical experience with it than with RF catheter ablation. Therefore, at the present time we can not compare the advantages and disadvantages of these two different technologies.

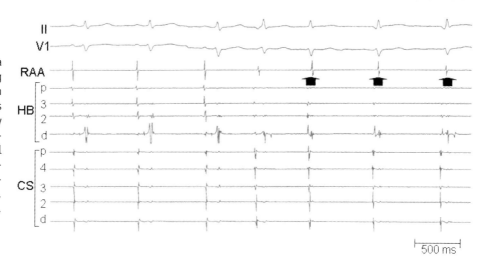

FIGURE 19–20. Induction of a junctional rhythm during radiofrequency application between the tricuspid annulus and the ostium of the coronary sinus. One to one retrograde conduction over the fast AV nodal pathway (arrows) implies preserved normal of AV nodal function during energy delivery. Abbreviations as per Figure 19-1.

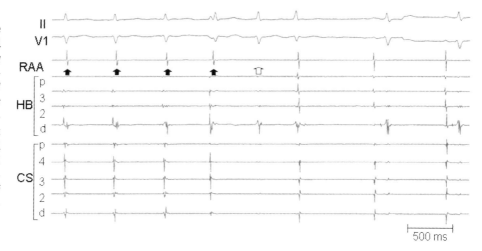

FIGURE 19–21. Retrograde block over the fast AV nodal pathway during radiofrequency application. One to one retrograde conduction over the fast AV nodal pathway during catheter ablation *(filled arrows)* is followed by sudden retrograde block manifested by absence of atrial activation *(open arrow)*. Rapid discontinuation of energy application resulted in preservation of AV nodal conduction. Abbreviations as per Figure 19-1.

During tissue cooling, the initial reduction of tip electrode temperature to –30°C is associated with a reversible lesion (cryomapping), allowing time to discontinue cryoenergy application if an adverse effect is observed. This is the main advantage of cryoablation over RF ablation, in which irreversible AV block can occur even if lesion delivery is rapidly terminated. The appearance of a junctional rhythm observed during the heating produced by RF current application is *not* observed during cryoablation. Another advantage of cryoablation is that the catheter adheres to the endocardial surface at a temperature of –70°C; therefore, fluoroscopy is not needed to check the position of the catheter once this temperature has been reached. During cryomapping (–30°C) and cryoablation, the conduction properties of the fast and slow AV nodal pathways are continuously checked using atrial stimulation. Termination of AVNRT during tissue cooling, abolition of 1:1 AV conduction over the slow AV nodal pathway, and inability to reinduce AVNRT are markers of success. Continuous monitoring of the AH interval is important, because the lesion becomes larger when

the temperature is lowered from –30°C to –70°C and can affect AV nodal conduction even though it was not altered at –30°C.

The choice between cryoablation and RF ablation needs to be determined on an individual basis. Patients with previous ablation near the fast AV nodal pathway region and those with a short distance between the proximal His bundle and the roof of the CS ostium may benefit from cryoablation, because they are at higher risk of AV block. Another subgroup of high-risk patients comprises those with a prolonged AH interval in the basal state.

ATRIOVENTRICULAR BLOCK DURING OR AFTER CATHETER ABLATION

In our experience, AV block occurred in 1 (0.5%) of 200 patients during RF current delivered between the midportion of the CS ostium and the tricuspid annulus. In this one patient, a rapid junctional rhythm was induced, associated with retrograde VA block; despite rapid termination of energy application, the patient developed permanent AV block requiring pacemaker implantation. Rare cases of delayed AV block have also been documented despite preserved AV conduction at the end of the procedure.[45,46]

Therefore, patients with transient AH prolongation and those requiring multiple applications need close and prolonged observation after the procedure. The induction of a junctional rhythm during application of RF current in the region of the slow AV nodal pathway is a desirable response that occurs at effective ablation sites. However, the induction of a fast junctional rhythm or sudden retrograde block during junctional rhythm can be associated with AV block.[47,48] Damage to the AV nodal artery, which is located between the tricuspid annulus and the CS ostium, may explain the occurrence of AV block even when applications are delivered far from the compact AV node.[49]

ABLATION OF SLOW ATRIOVENTRICULAR NODAL PATHWAY IN PATIENTS WITH ABNORMAL ATRIAL-VENTRICULAR CONDUCTION

It is important to determine the conduction properties of the fast and slow AV pathways before catheter ablation. Patients with delayed conduction or prolonged refractoriness of the fast AV nodal pathway have an increased risk of AV block after ablation of the slow AV nodal pathway. However, two reports have documented a lack of detrimental effect of catheter ablation in such patients despite preexisting abnormal AV conduction.[50,51] This clinical finding confirmed experimental observations in the canine heart showing that ablation of the anterior and posterior inputs rarely results in complete AV block.[52] This favorable effect of slow AV nodal pathway ablation despite an abnormal fast AV nodal pathway may be explained by several factors. One possibility is that in these patients the left atrial (mitral annulus) input[26] preserves AV nodal conduction despite damage to the right-sided inputs. Another possibility is that, before ablation, conduction via the posterior input (slow AV nodal pathway) prolongs the refractory period of the anterior input (fast AV nodal pathway) due to concealed retrograde conduction of the fast pathway, the so-called linking phenomenon.[53] There is evidence that antegrade conduction over the fast AV nodal pathway frequently improves after ablation of the slow AV nodal pathway.[54,55] However, in an individual patient it is impossible to predict whether AV conduction will improve or worsen after ablation of the slow AV nodal pathway. Therefore, the higher risk of AV block in these patients should be weighed against the benefit of eliminating the arrhythmia before ablation is attempted.

Catheter Ablation of Slow-Slow and Fast-Slow AVNRT

ABLATION OF RETROGRADE SLOW ATRIOVENTRICULAR NODAL PATHWAY CONDUCTION

Elimination of slow-slow and fast-slow AVNRT requires elimination of the slow AV nodal pathway that is used for retrograde conduction. This pathway is frequently different from the slow AV nodal pathway used for antegrade conduction.

During ablation of AVNRT, it is not necessary to eliminate all slow pathway conduction to prevent recurrence.[56-58] For slow-fast AVNRT, we attempt to eliminate 1:1 antegrade conduction over the slow AV nodal pathway in all patients, to eliminate reinduction of tachycardia. In contrast, in patients with slow-slow or fast-slow AVNRT, elimination of retrograde 1:1 slow AV nodal pathway conduction is the primary goal.

Ablation is directed at the site of the earliest retrograde atrial activation, which is most frequently between the tricuspid annulus and CS ostium in fast-slow AVNRT and along the anterior aspect of the proximal CS in slow-slow AVNRT (Figs. 19–22 and 19–23).[59] Frequently, antegrade and retrograde slow pathway conduction pathways are ablated at different sites.[60] Mapping and ablation can be performed during tachycardia or during ventricular pacing to eliminate 1:1 retrograde slow AV nodal pathway conduction in these patients. Initially, mapping is performed in the lower portion of the triangle of Koch, between the CS ostium and the tricuspid annulus, followed by mapping in the proximal portion of the CS. The site of earliest retrograde atrial activation is targeted for ablation. If ablation is performed in the proximal CS, low voltage (20 W) is initially used. The energy output is progressively increased while the impedance is monitored. Successful ablation results in elimination of retrograde conduction over the slow AV nodal pathway (Fig. 19–24).

Patients with slow-slow or fast-slow AVNRT frequently lack retrograde conduction over the fast AV nodal pathway. Therefore, during RF current application, junctional beats may have no retrograde conduction over the fast AV nodal pathway (Fig. 19–25), preventing assessment of AV nodal function during delivery of energy. In these patients, we deliver short applications of RF energy and evaluate AV nodal conduction between applications. Alternatively, overdrive atrial pacing may allow continuous monitoring of antegrade AV conduction during ablation.

FIGURE 19–22. Site of earliest retrograde atrial activation site during ventricular pacing in a patient with slow-slow atrioventricular nodal reentrant tachycardia. Radiographs in the right anterior oblique (RAO) and left anterior oblique (LAO) projections showing the position of the mapping catheter (MAP) inside the proximal portion of the coronary sinus, approximately 1.5 cm from the ostium. Multipolar catheters are positioned in the coronary sinus (CS), right atrial appendage (RAA), His bundle (HB), and right ventricle (RV).

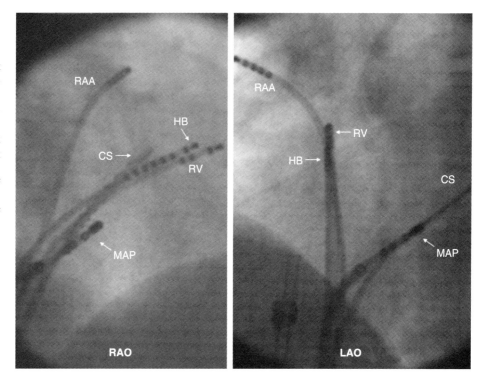

FIGURE 19–23. Recording of earliest retrograde atrial activation site during ventricular pacing in a patient with slow-slow atrioventricular nodal reentrant tachycardia. Earliest bipolar and unipolar (UNI) recording from the mapping catheter (arrows) were obtained in the proximal portion of the coronary sinus (CS MAP) as shown in Figure 19–22. Abbreviations as per Figure 19-1.

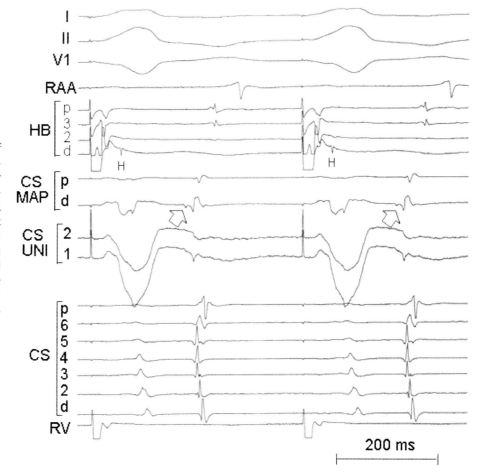

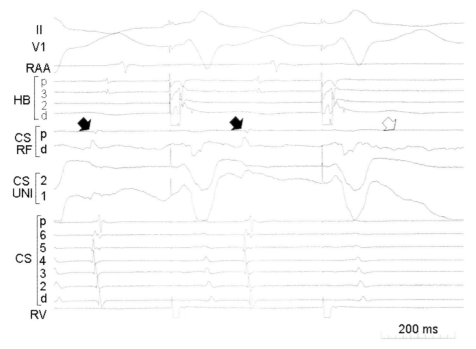

FIGURE 19–24. Retrograde block of slow atrioventricular (AV) nodal pathway conduction during radiofrequency current ablation. During delivery of radiofrequency current in the proximal coronary sinus (CS RF) the first two ventricular paced complexes are followed by retrograde conduction through the slow AV nodal pathway *(filled arrows)*. Retrograde block over the slow AV nodal pathway is observed following the third ventricular paced complex *(open arrow)*. UNI, unipolar. Abbreviations as per Figure 19-1.

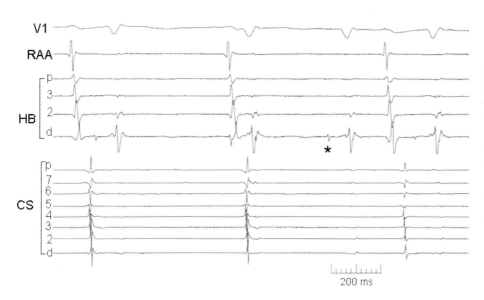

FIGURE 19–25. Junctional beat without retrograde VA conduction. Patients with slow-slow and fast-slow AVNRT frequently lack retrograde conduction over the fast AV nodal pathway. During ablation of the slow AV nodal pathway, junctional beats may show no retrograde conduction despite preserved AV nodal function. Abbreviations as per Figure 19-1.

CATHETER ABLATION OF "LEFT-SIDED" AVNRT

Rarely, extensive ablation from the right atrium and CS fails to eliminate slow pathway function. In these patients, the slow pathway can sometimes be eliminated by ablation at the posterior mitral annulus[12] (Fig. 19–26). At these sites, the tachycardia is usually reset by left atrial extrastimuli, indicating proximity to the reentrant circuit. At successful left-sided ablation sites, junctional rhythm is observed, as with ablation of "conventional" slow-fast AVNRT. In these patients, the left posterior extension of the AV node may form the slow pathway. The presence of a short HA interval (≤15 msec) and the occurrence of a antegrade double-response to atrial pacing are sometimes noted in patients with this AVNRT variant.

Troubleshooting the Difficult Case

The ablation of AV nodal reentry is usually straightforward, but problems can arise (Table 19–4). Induction of AV nodal reentry is infrequently a problem. AV nodal reentry is usually greatly influenced by

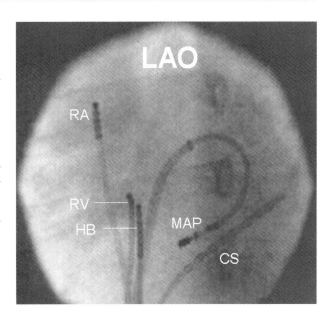

FIGURE 19–26. Catheter position at site of successful ablation in a patient with the left sided variant of slow-fast AV nodal reentry. Intracardiac tracings and diagnostic maneuvers were consistent with slow-fast AV nodal reentry but all attempts at ablation of slow pathway conduction from the right atrium and proximal coronary sinus were unsuccessful. Left anterior oblique (LAO) projection. The mapping catheter was introduced into the left atrium through a preformed sheath following trans-septal puncture. The catheter was positioned parallel to the mitral annulus with its tip at the inferior para-septal region. At this ablation site junctional rhythm occurred, slow pathway function was eliminated, and tachycardia rendered non-inducible. CS, coronary sinus catheter; HB, His bundle catheter; MAP, mapping/ablation catheter; RA, right atrial catheter; RV, right ventricular catheter.

TABLE 19–4

Troubleshooting Difficult Cases

Problem	Causes	Solution
Difficult to induce AVNRT	Retrograde fast AV nodal pathway block due to catheter manipulation Increased vagal tone due to sedation Fast and slow AV nodal pathways with similar conduction properties	Avoid catheter contact with the fast AV nodal pathway region Administration of isoproterenol and atropine Atrial burst pacing resulting in long-short cycles, atrial and ventricular programmed stimulation
Poor catheter stability	Prominent eustachian ridge	Use long sheath with septal angulation and apply clockwise rotation
Prolonged AH interval before AVNRT ablation	Absent or prolonged conduction over the fast AV nodal pathway Prolonged refractoriness of the fast AV nodal pathway resulting in conduction over the slow pathway in sinus rhythm	High risk of complete AV block, implant pacemaker Decision to ablate should be taken on an individual basis; consider cryoablation
Unable to obtain a junctional rhythm during RF delivery	Inadequate ablation catheter contact Inaccurate mapping	Use of long sheaths; assess inducibility of AVNRT after each application, because successful slow pathway ablation can occur in the absence of a junctional rhythm Continue mapping including proximal CS, consider left-sided approach
Change to a different form of AVNRT	One, two, or three different forms of AVNRT can coexist in the same patient	Ablation of antegrade and retrograde slow AV nodal pathway conduction frequently requires RF lesions delivered at different sites

AH, atrium-to-His-bundle; AV, atrioventricular; AVNRT, atrioventricular nodal reentrant tachycardia; CS, coronary sinus; RF, radiofrequency energy.

autonomic tone. Reduced sedation, hyperventilation, isoproterenol, and atropine may facilitate induction. Catheter stability is sometimes problematic but is usually remedied by the use of a long sheath with slight septal angulation. The use of a catheter with adequate "reach" adds to catheter stability. If no junctional rhythm is apparent with RF ablation between the tricuspid annulus and the CS ostium, mapping of the proximal CS may identify slow pathway potentials and provide successful ablation. As noted earlier, patients with absent or poor antegrade fast pathway function are at risk for heart block after slow pathway ablation. The status of the antegrade fast pathway should be documented before ablation. If fast pathway function is poor and the decision is to proceed with ablation, AV conduction must be closely monitored during ablation. Cryoablation is probably safer than RF ablation in these patients.

References

1. Wu D, Denes P, Amat-Y-Leon F, et al.: Clinical, electrocardiographic and electrophysiologic observations in patients with paroxysmal supraventricular tachycardia. Am J Cardiol 41:1045-1051, 1978.
2. Morady F: Catheter ablation of supraventricular arrhythmias: State of the art. Pacing Clin Electrophysiol 27:125-142, 2004.
3. Blomstrom-Lundqvist C, Scheinman MM, Aliot EM, et al.: ACC/AHA/ESC guidelines for the management of patients with supraventricular arrhythmias: Executive summary. J Am Coll Cardiol 42:1493-1531, 2003.
4. Gaskell WH: On the innervation of the heart, with especial reference to the heart of the tortoise. J Physiol 4:43-127, 1883.
5. His W Jr: Die Thätigkeit des embryonalen Herzens und deren Bedeutung für die Lehre von der Herzbewegung beim Erwachsenen. Arb Med Klin Leipzig 1:14-49, 1983.
6. Tawara S: The conduction system in the mammalian heart: An anatomico-histological study of the atrioventricular bundle and the Purkinje fibers. Verlag Von Gustav Fischer in Jena, 1906, pp 3-7.
7. Mines GR: On dynamic equilibrium of the heart. J Physiol 46:349-382, 1913.
8. Moe GK, Preston JB, Burlington H: Physiologic evidence for a dual A-V transmission system. Circ Res 4:357-375, 1956.
9. Mendez C, Moe GK: Demonstration of a dual AV nodal conduction system in the isolated rabbit heart. Circ Res 19:378-393, 1966.
10. Denes P, Wu D, Dhingra RC, et al.: Demonstration of dual A-V nodal pathways in patients with paroxysmal supraventricular tachycardia. Circulation 48:549-555, 1973.
11. Hazlitt HA, Beckman KJ, McClelland JH, et al.: Prevalence of slow AV nodal pathway potentials in patients without AV nodal reentrant tachycardia [abstract]. J Am Coll Cardiol 21:281A, 1993.
12. Lockwood D, Otomo K, Wang Z, et al.: Electrophysiologic characteristics of atrioventricular nodal reentrant tachycardia: Implications for the reentrant circuits. In Zipes DP, Jalife J (eds.): Cardiac Electrophysiology: From Cell to Bedside. Philadelphia: Saunders, 2004, pp 537-557.
13. Mignone RJ, Wallace AG: Ventricular echoes: Evidence for dissociation of conduction and reentry within the AV node. Circ Res 19:638-649, 1996.
14. Josephson ME, Kastor JA: Paroxysmal supraventricular tachycardia: Is the atrium a necessary link? Circulation 54:430-435, 1976.
15. Loh P, de Bakker JMT, Hocini M, et al.: Reentrant pathway during ventricular echoes is confined to the atrioventricular node: High-resolution mapping and dissection of the triangle of Koch in isolated, perfused canine heart. Circulation 100:1346-1353, 1999.
16. Gonzalez MD, Contreras L, Cardona F, et al.: V-A block during atrioventricular nodal reentrant tachycardia: Reentry confined to the AV node. Pacing Clin Electrophysiol 26:775-778, 2003.
17. Sung RJ, Waxman HL, Saksena S, et al.: Sequence of retrograde atrial activation in patients with dual atrioventricular nodal pathways. Circulation 64:1059-1067, 1981.
18. Haïssaguerre M, Warin JF, Lemetayer P, et al.: Closed chest ablation of retrograde conduction in patients with atrioventricular nodal reentrant tachycardia. N Engl J Med 320:426-433, 1989.
19. Epstein LM, Scheinman MM, Langberg JJ, et al.: Percutaneous catheter modification of the atrioventricular node: A potential cure for atrioventricular nodal reentrant tachycardia. Circulation 80:757-768, 1989.
20. Jazayeri MH, Hempe SL, Sra JS, et al.: Selective transcatheter ablation of the fast and slow pathways using radiofrequency energy in patients with atrioventricular nodal reentrant tachycardia. Circulation 85:1318-1328, 1992.
21. Haïssaguerre M, Gaita F, Fisher B, et al.: Elimination of atrioventricular nodal reentrant tachycardia using discrete slow potentials to guide application of radiofrequency energy. Circulation 85:2162-2175, 1992.
22. Ross DL, Johnson DC, Denniss AR, et al.: Curative surgery of atrioventricular junctional ("AV nodal") reentrant tachycardia. J Am Coll Cardiol 6:1383-1392, 1985.
23. Jackman WM, Beckman KJ, McClelland JH, et al.: Treatment of supraventricular tachycardia due to atrioventricular nodal reentry by radiofrequency catheter ablation of slow pathway conduction. N Engl J Med 327:313-318, 1992.
24. Becker AE, Anderson RH: Morphology of the human atrioventricular junctional area. In: Wellens HJJ, Lie KI, Janse MJ (eds.): The Conduction System of the Heart: Structure, Function, and Clinical Implications. Leiden, Germany: HE Stenfert Kroese BV, 1976, pp 263-286.
25. Inoue S, Becker AE: Posterior extensions of the human compact atrioventricular node: A neglected anatomic feature of potential clinical significance. Circulation 97:188-193, 1998.
26. Gonzalez MD, Contreras LJ, Cardona F, et al.: Demonstration of a left atrial input to the atrioventricular node in humans. Circulation 106:2930-2934, 2002.
27. Yamabe H, Shimasaki Y, Honda O, et al.: Demonstration of the exact anatomic tachycardia circuit in the fast-slow atrioventricular nodal tachycardia. Circulation 104:1268-1273, 2001.
28. Patterson E, Scherlag BJ: Longitudinal dissociation within the posterior AV nodal input of the rabbit. Circulation 99:143-155, 1999.
29. Gonzalez MD, Scherlag BJ, Mabo P, Lazzara R: Functional dissociation of cellular activation as a mechanism of Mobitz type II atrioventricular block. Circulation 87:1389-1398, 1993.
30. Hirao K, Otomo K, Wang X, et al.: Para-Hisian pacing: A new method for differentiating retrograde conduction over an accessory AV pathway from conduction over the AV node. Circulation 94:1027-1035, 1996.
31. Gonzalez MD, Contreras LJ, Jongbloed MRM, et al.: Left atrial tachycardia originating from the mitral annulus-aorta junction. Circulation 110:3187-3192, 2004.
32. Waldo AL, Maclean AH, Karp RB, et al.: Sequence of retrograde atrial activation of the human heart: Correlation with P wave polarity. Br Heart J 39:634-640, 1977.
33. Heidbuchel H, Jackman WM: Characterization of subforms of AV nodal reentrant tachycardia. Europace 4:316-329, 2004.
34. Taylor GW, Kay NG: Selective slow pathway ablation for treatment of AV nodal reentrant tachycardia. In Huang SK, Wilber DJ (eds.): Radiofrequency Catheter Ablation of Cardiac Arrhythmias. Armonk, N.Y.: Futura, 2000, pp 423-461.
35. Scheinmann MM, Huang S: The NASPE prospective catheter ablation registry. Pacing Clin Electrophysiol 23:1020-1028, 2000.

36. Strickberger A, Morady F: Catheter ablation of atrioventricular nodal reentrant tachycardia. In Zipes D, Jalife J (eds.): Cardiac Electrophysiology: From Cell to Bedside. Philadelphia: Saunders, 2004, pp 1028-1035.

37. McGuire MA, Bourke JP, Robotin MC, et al.: High resolution mapping of Koch's triangle using sixty electrodes in humans with atrioventricular junctional ("AV nodal") reentrant tachycardia. Circulation 88:2315-2328, 1993.

38. de Bakker JMT, Coronel L, McGuire MA, et al.: Slow potentials in the atrioventricular junctional area of patients operated for atrioventricular nodal tachycardias and in isolated porcine hearts. J Am Coll Cardiol 23:709-715, 1994.

39. Altemose GT, Scott LR, Miller JM: Atrioventricular nodal reentrant tachycardia requiring ablation on the mitral annulus. J Cardiovasc Electrophysiol 11:1281-1284, 2000.

40. Jais P, Haïssaguerre M, Shah DC, et al.: Successful radiofrequency ablation of a slow atrioventricular nodal pathway on the left posterior atrial septum. Pacing Clin Electrophysiol 22:525-527, 1999.

41. Sorbera C, Cohen M, Woolf P, et al.: Atrioventricular nodal reentry tachycardia: Slow pathway ablation using the transseptal approach. Pacing Clin Electrophysiol 23:1343-1349, 2000.

42. Hsieh MH, Chen SA, Tai CT, et al.: Absence of junctional rhythm during successful slow-pathway ablation in patients with atrioventricular nodal reentrant tachycardia. Circulation 98:2296-2300, 1998.

43. Wagshal AB, Crystal E, Katz A: Patterns of accelerated junctional rhythm during slow pathway catheter ablation for atrioventricular nodal tachycardia: Temperature dependence, prognostic value, and insights into the nature of the slow pathway. J Cardiovasc Electrophysiol 11:244-254, 2000.

44. Skanes AC, Dubuc M, Klein GJ, et al.: Cryothermal ablation of the slow pathway for the elimination atrioventricular nodal reentrant tachycardia. Circulation 102:2856-2860, 2000.

45. Gaita F, Riccardi R, Calo L: Importance and implications of the occurrence of AV block following radiofrequency ablation. Heart 79:534-535, 1998.

46. Elhag O, Miller HC: Atrioventricular block occurring several months after radiofrequency ablation for the treatment of atrioventricular nodal reentrant tachycardia: A report of two cases. Heart 79:616-618, 1998.

47. Thakur RK, Flein GJ, Yee R: Junctional tachycardia: A useful marker during radiofrequency ablation for AV node reentrant tachycardia. J Am Coll Cardiol 22:1706-1710, 1993.

48. Jentzer J, Goyal R, Williamson B, et al.: Analysis of junctional ectopy during radiofrequency ablation of the slow pathway in patients with atrioventricular node reentrant tachycardia. Circulation 90:2820-2826, 1994.

49. Lin JL, Huang SK, Lai LP, et al.: Distal end of the atrioventricular nodal artery predicts the risk of atrioventricular block during slow pathway catheter ablation of atrioventricular nodal re-entrant tachycardia. Heart 83:543-550, 2000.

50. Sra JS, Jazayeri MR, Blank Z, et al.: Slow pathway ablation in patients with atrioventricular nodal reentrant tachycardia and a prolonged PR interval. J Am Coll Cardiol 24:1064-1068, 1994.

51. Basta MN, Krahn AD, Klein GJ, et al.: Safety of slow pathway ablation in patients with atrioventricular nodal reentrant tachycardia and a long fast pathway effective refractory period. Am J Cardiol 80:155-159, 1997.

52. Hirao K, Scherlag BJ, Poty H, et al.: Electrophysiology of the atrio-AV nodal inputs and exits in the normal dog heart: Radiofrequency ablation using an epicardial approach. J Cardiovasc Electrophysiol 8:904-915, 1997.

53. Gonzalez MD, Greenspon AJ, Kidwell GA: Linking in accessory pathways: Functional loss of antegrade pre-excitation. Circulation 83:1221-1231, 1991.

54. Strickberger SA, Daoud E, Niebauer M, et al.: Effects of partial and complete ablation of the slow pathway on fast pathway properties in patients with atrioventricular nodal tachycardia. J Cardiovasc Electrophysiol 5:645-649, 1994.

55. Natale A, Klein G, Yee R, et al.: Shortening of fast pathway refractoriness after slow pathway ablation: Effects of autonomic blockage. Circulation 89:1103-1108, 1994.

56. Lindsay BD, Chung MK, Gamache MC, et al.: Therapeutic end points for the treatment of atrioventricular node reentrant tachycardia by catheter-guided radiofrequency current. J Am Coll Cardiol 22:733-740, 1993.

57. Hummel JD, Strickberger SA, Williamson BD, et al.: Effect of residual slow pathway function on the time course of recurrences of atrioventricular nodal reentrant tachycardia after radiofrequency ablation of the slow pathway. Am J Cardiol 75:628-630, 1995.

58. Manolis AS, Wang PJ, Estes NA 3rd: Radiofrequency ablation of slow pathway in patients with atrioventricular nodal reentrant tachycardia: Do arrhythmia recurrences correlate with persistent slow pathway conduction or site of successful ablation? Circulation 90:2815-2819, 1994.

59. Wang Z, Otomo K, Shah N, et al.: Slow/slow and fast/slow atrioventricular nodal reentrant tachycardia use anatomically separate retrograde slow pathways [abstract]. Circulation 100:I-65, 1999.

60. Wang Z, Otomo K, Arruda M, et al.: Ablation of slow/slow atrioventricular nodal reentrant tachycardia: Evidence for multiple slow pathways [abstract]. J Am Coll Cardiol 33:166A, 1999.

Catheter Ablation of Accessory Atrioventricular Connections

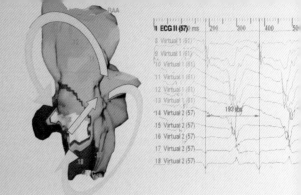

PART VI

20

Ablation of Free Wall Accessory Pathways

Mark A. Wood

Key Points

■ The atrioventricular annulus is mapped for atrial or ventricular accessory pathway (AP) insertion sites or the AP itself.

■ Ablation targets include the earliest site of atrial or ventricular activation by the AP, sites of AP potentials, and sites of electrogram polarity reversal (left free wall APs).

■ Special equipment includes preformed sheaths (especially for the trans-septal approach) and multielectrode "halo" mapping catheters (right free wall). Catheter navigation systems are useful, and electroanatomic mapping is optional.

■ Sources of difficulty are misdiagnosis of atrioventricular nodal reentry with eccentric atrial activation or atrial tachycardia as orthodromic reciprocating tachycardia, catheter stability (especially with right free wall APs), and epicardial APs.

Free wall locations are the most common positions for accessory pathways (APs) in clinical practice. Right and left free wall APs account for 10% to 20% and 50% to 60% of all APs, respectively.[1] These pathway locations each present distinct challenges to the electrophysiologist. Left free wall APs are amenable to ablation with the highest success rates and lowest incidences of recurrence. The left heart location is less accessible, however, necessitating arterial or trans-septal approaches. In contrast, right free wall APs are readily approached from simple venous access but have the lowest acute success rates and highest incidences of recurrence.

Anatomy

The anatomy of the tricuspid annulus is different from that of the mitral annulus.[2-4] The hinge of the mitral atrioventricular annulus is a well-formed and distinct cord of fibrous tissue around the annulus (Fig. 20–1A). This accretion of fibrous tissue is interposed between the atrial and ventricular myocardiums. On the ventricular side of the mitral annulus, basal cords of ventricular myocardium may descend in a curtain-like fashion from the mitral hinge to insert into the trabeculations on the ventricular wall. These cords may limit catheter mobility beneath the valve during attempts at left free wall AP ablations. In the limited human histologic descriptions of left free wall APs, the atrial connection is usually discrete and near to the annulus.[2,3] The pathways then skirt the annulus on its epicardial aspect and may cross at variable depths within the epicardial fat pad (see Fig. 20–1B). The ventricular insertion usually branches into multiple connections with the ventricle that may be displaced away from the annulus, toward the apex.[2,3] The histologically determined length of an AP is typically 5 to 10 mm, with a maximal diameter of 0.1 to 7 mm.[5] The left-sided epicardial atrioventricular groove is shallow but contains the left circumflex artery near the annulus and the coronary sinus (CS) more remote from the annulus. Although the CS is useful for quickly mapping the mitral valve area, it runs an average of 10 to 14 mm on the atrial side of the true annulus.[6] This separation from the annulus is more pronounced in the proximal 20 mm of the CS. Therefore, during catheter mapping, the CS location and electrograms are best regarded as gross estimates of the true AP location on the annulus. The anterior limit of the left free wall is anatomically well demarcated by the aortic-mitral valve continuity, which rarely, if ever, contains AP connections. The exact location of this continuity is difficult to recognize by fluoroscopy alone. The posterior limit of the left free wall is anatomically continuous with the posteroseptal area and is arbitrarily defined on fluoroscopy.

In contrast to the mitral annulus, the tricuspid valve annulus is less well formed and frequently discontinuous.[2,3] The right atrial and right ventricular myocardiums tend to overlap or fold over one another as they insert on the tricuspid annulus (see Figure 20–1A). Right free wall APs may cross discontinuities in the less distinct fibrous annulus or skirt the epicardial aspect of the annulus, as do left free wall APs.[2,3] The less developed tricuspid annulus and acute angulation of the tricuspid leaflets toward the ventricle make catheter positions along the right free wall unstable. Fluoroscopic definition of the right free wall is difficult because there are no clear landmarks for guidance.

Because of the association of Ebstein's anomaly with right-sided APs, the anatomy of this condition merits special consideration.[7] In this disorder, the tricuspid valve leaflets are tethered to the ventricular wall for variable distances from the annulus. This contributes to catheter instability during mapping of the tricuspid annulus. Although not anatomically displaced, the true tricuspid annulus may be poorly developed, with extensive discontinuities of the fibrous architecture.[3] Electrograms recorded from the annulus in Ebstein's anomaly may be of low amplitude and fragmented due to the disorganized tissue.[8] This fragmentation adds to the difficulty in mapping the tricuspid annulus in this condition. APs in Ebstein's anomaly are often multiple and may skirt the epicardial aspect of the annulus or pass subendocardially through gaps in the fibrous annulus.[2,3]

A complete description of free wall accessory atrioventricular connections must also include those resulting from connections of the ventricle to the CS musculature, the ligament of Marshall, and the atrial appendage. Mahaim-type atriofascicular connections are described Chapter 23. The venous wall of the CS is surrounded by a continuous sleeve of atrial myocardium that extends for 25 to 51 mm from the CS ostium.[9] This muscle is continuous with the right atrial myocardium proximally but is usually separated from the left atrium by adipose tissue. This separation may be bridged by strands of striated muscle, however, producing electrical continuity between the CS musculature and the left atrium (Fig. 20–2 and 20–3). These connections, which can be broad and very extensive, are reported in up to 80% of hearts in autopsy series.[9] Electrical continuity of the CS musculature with the ventricle is less common, but, if present, it may provide the substrate for reciprocating tachycardias.[10] Ventricular connections may

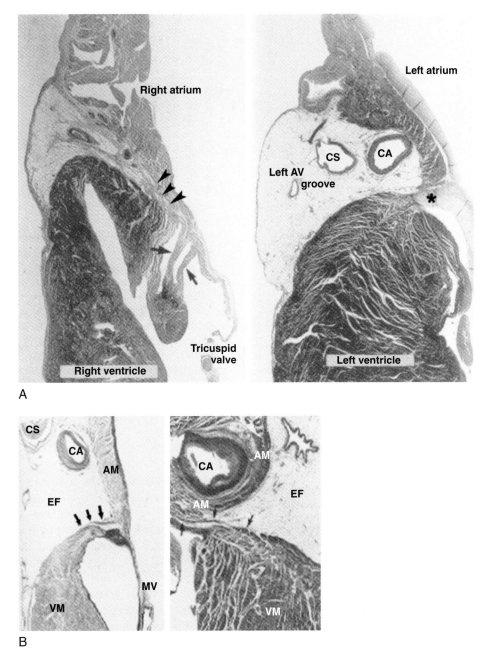

FIGURE 20–1. A, Histologic sections of the tricuspid (left panel) and mitral valve (right panel) annuli through the free walls. Along the tricuspid annulus, the atrial and ventricular myocardium fold over one another separated by a poorly defined fibrous component (*arrowheads*). The *arrows* show 2 cords supporting the base of the valve leaflet. In the right panel, the distinct fibrous component to the mitral annulus creates a well formed hinge (*asterisk*) for the mitral valve and separates the atrial and ventricular myocardium. Note the relation of the circumflex coronary artery (CA) and coronary sinus (CS) to the mitral annulus. AV, atrioventricular. *(From Ho SY, Anderson RH: Anatomy of accessory pathways. In Farre J, Moro C [eds.]: Ten Years of Radiofrequency Catheter Ablation. Armonk, N.Y.: Futura, 1998, pp 149-163, with permission.)* **B**, Histologic sections of the mitral annulus in patients with a left posterior accessory pathway (left panel) and a left lateral accessory pathway (right panel). In each case, the accessory pathways (*arrows*) cross in the epicardial fat pad (EF) on the epicardial aspect of the annulus fibrosis. Note the distant location of the coronary sinus (CS) to the accessory pathway in the left panel. In the right panel atrial myocardium (AM) encircles the circumflex coronary artery (CA). MV, mitral valve; VM, ventricular myocardium. *(From Becker A, Anderson R, Durrer D, et al.: The anatomic substrates of Wolff-Parkinson-White syndrome: A clinicopathologic correlation in seven patients. Circulation 57:870-879, 1978, with permission.)*

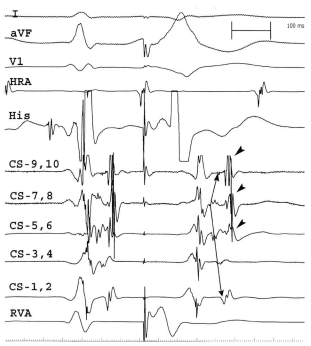

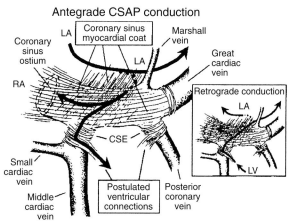

FIGURE 20–2. Coronary sinus (CS) potentials recorded during mapping of left lateral accessory pathway. The first complex represents orthodromic reciprocating tachycardia with earliest atrial activation at CS-7,8. The second complex is a premature ventricular stimulus which reverses the sequence of ventricular activation along the CS. This separates the atrial and ventricular potentials without altering the atrial activation sequence. After the ventricular electrogram on the CS tracings, there are low amplitude, low frequency "far field" atrial potentials (*arrows*). After the atrial potentials on CS 5,6 through CS 9,10, there are large high frequency amplitude CS musculature potentials (*arrowheads*) that are activated in a proximal to distal sequence. This is interpreted as activation of the proximal CS atrium by the accessory pathway with atrial conduction proximally to the point of connection to the CS musculature. The CS musculature then conducts proximally to distally along a portion of the CS catheter. CS-9,10: proximal CS; CS-1,2: distal CS; HRA: high right atrium; RVA: right ventricular apex.

FIGURE 20–3. Schematic for possible anatomic basis of connections between the coronary sinus musculature and left ventricular myocardium (LV). The coronary sinus musculature may form extensions (CSE) over the proximal portions of the middle and posterior cardiac veins. If connections between the coronary sinus musculature and the left (LA) or right (RA) atrial myocardium exist as well, the substrate for reciprocating tachycardias is formed. *(From Sun Y, Arruda M, Otomo K, et al.: Coronary sinus-ventricular accessory connections producing posteroseptal and left posterior accessory pathways: Incidence and electrophysiologic identification. Circulation 106:1362-1367, 2002, with permission.)*

result from CS musculature extensions over the middle cardiac vein, posterior cardiac vein, or AV groove branch of the distal left circumflex artery (Fig. 20–3). Ventricular connections with the CS are described in 3% to 6% of hearts at autopsy.[10] Sun et al.[10] reported that 36% of patients (most with previously failed ablation) who had left posterior or left posteroseptal AV connections actually used the CS musculature as the intermediary between the atrium and ventricle in reciprocating tachycardias.

The ligament of Marshall is a vestigial fold of pericardium that carries the vein of Marshall from its origin as a branch of the distal CS to its termination near the left superior pulmonary vein. This structure may also contain bundles of muscle fibers that are continuous with the CS musculature. These fibers may end blindly, or they may insert directly into the left atrial musculature at the inferior interatrial pathway.[11] With proximal connections between the CS musculature and the ventricle, the ligament of Marshall can support AV reciprocating tachycardia.[11]

Another unusual form of AV connection is a direct epicardial muscular continuity between the atrial appendage and the ventricle.[12-14] Several reports of connections between the right atrial appendage and ventricle are available, whereas left-sided connections appear even more rare.[14] The developmental basis for these connections is unknown. Because of epicardial ventricular insertions more than 1 cm apical to the annulus and atrial origins within the atrial appendage, endocardial mapping of the annulus for conventional APs is perplexing.[12,13] For left-sided connections, mapping of the anterior coronary venous branches may demonstrate the earliest ventricular activation.[14] At surgical division of one such right-sided connection, a broad band of myocardium under the epicardial fat pad was noted from the base of the atrial appendage to the base of the right ventricle.[12] Case reports describe successful catheter ablation of these connections from the right atrial appendage.[13]

Pathophysiology

DIAGNOSIS

As with APs at other locations, free wall APs may participate in reciprocating tachycardias or undergo bystander activation during tachycardias mechanistically unrelated to the presence of the AP. Free wall APs have been associated with specific electrophysiologic characteristics.[15] Compared with septal and left free wall locations, right free wall APs are less likely to demonstrate retrograde conduction, to participate in reciprocating tachycardias, and to be associated with inducible atrial fibrillation.[15] Pathways in the right free wall may be more likely to demonstrate decremental antegrade conduction than those in other locations. Compared with right free wall pathways, left free wall APs are more likely to demonstrate decremental retrograde conduction and have longer retrograde refractory periods.[15]

Surface electrocardiographic (ECG) localization of manifest free wall APs is imperfect and becomes less accurate if minimal preexcitation is present (QRS <120 msec).[16] ECG algorithms for AP localization are most accurate for the diagnosis of left free wall APs compared with all other locations, achieving at least 90% sensitivity and almost 100% specificity.[16-20] In using any localization algorithm, one must be aware of the portion of the QRS on which the algorithm is based. Some algorithms use only the first 20 to 60 msec of the delta wave, whereas others are based on the morphology or polarity of the entire QRS complex.[18-21] Provided that significant preexcitation is present, all left free wall APs should demonstrate a positive delta wave in V_1, with the R wave greater than the S wave (R > S) in lead V_1 or V_2 at the latest (Fig. 20–4). A negative delta wave in lead I, aVL, and/or V6 is pathognomonic of a left lateral pathway. As the pathway location moves from posterior to lateral to anterior, the delta waves in the inferior leads, especially aVF and III, change from negative to isoelectric to positive in polarity.

As opposed to left free wall APs, the ECG diagnosis of right free wall APs is the least accurate and least consistent among algorithms,[16-18,20] with a sensitivity of 80% to 90% and a specificity of 90% to 100%. Confusion may arise in the interpretation of a positive delta wave in V_1 as indicating a left-sided AP (Fig. 20–5). This is diagnostic of a left free wall AP only if R > S; a positive delta wave with R < S in V_1 is consistent with a right free wall AP or a minimally preexcited left free wall AP. A negative delta wave in V_1 is consistent with a septal AP. Therefore, most algorithms identify right free wall APs by a positive initial delta wave in V_1 but a late transition to R > S in the precordial leads at V_3 or later, coupled with leftward orientation to the initial delta wave, such as delta wave positivity in lead I or aVL.[18-20] As the pathway location moves from the right superior free wall to the right middle and right inferior free wall, the delta wave in inferior leads aVF and II changes from positive to isoelectric to negative.[18-20] A useful algorithm for AP localization that is based on the initial 20 msec of the delta wave is shown in Figure 20–6.

The location of the AP can also be inferred from the surface ECG, from the polarity of the retrograde P waves during orthodromic reciprocating tachycardia (ORT).[22,23] A negative P wave in lead I is highly suggestive of a left free wall location, with a 95%

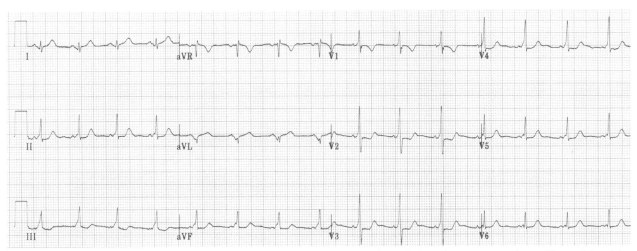

FIGURE 20–4. Twelve lead ECG in sinus rhythm from a patient with a manifest left lateral accessory pathway. The positive delta wave in V1 with R > S wave indicates a left free wall location. The negative delta waves in leads I and aVL are pathognomonic of a left free wall position. The positive delta waves in leads II, III and aVF suggest a position anterolateral on the annulus.

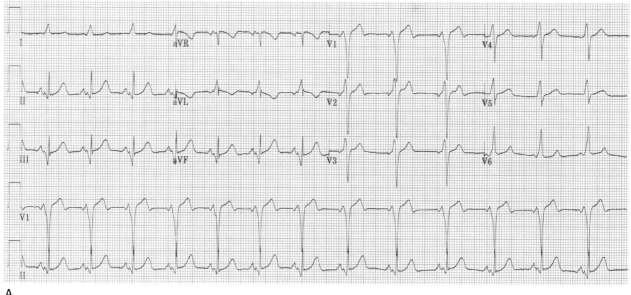

A

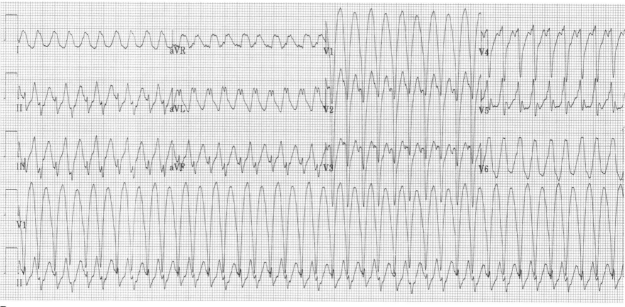

B

FIGURE 20–5. A, Twelve lead ECG in sinus rhythm from a patient with a manifest right free wall accessory pathway. The delta wave is positive in lead V1, however, the transition to R > S wave in the precordial leads does not occur until V5 indicating a right free wall location. The delta waves are negative in leads II, III and aVF indicating a position inferiorly on the right ventricular free wall. **B,** ECG from the same patient during antidromic reciprocating tachycardia using the right free wall pathway. The QRS complex is fully preexcited.

positive predictive value.[23] A negative P wave in lead V1 is highly suggestive of a right-sided AP. The presence of a positive retrograde P wave in lead I suggests a right free wall AP with a positive predictive value of 99%.[23] For either right or left free wall APs, the presence of negative P waves in all three inferior leads indicates an inferior location, whereas positive P waves in these leads indicate a superior location. Isoelectric or biphasic P waves in any of the inferior leads suggest a middle free wall location.[22]

At electrophysiologic testing, the hallmark of any ORT is the demonstration of obligatory 1:1 atrial and ventricular activation for persistence of the tachycardia (Table 20–1).[24] The diagnosis of ORT using a free wall AP also requires an eccentric atrial activation sequence earliest along the right or left atrial free wall. Coupled with such an eccentric atrial activation sequence, ORT is highly suggested by demonstration of the shortest QRS-to-atrium time greater than or equal to 60 msec, constant ventricle-to-atrium times

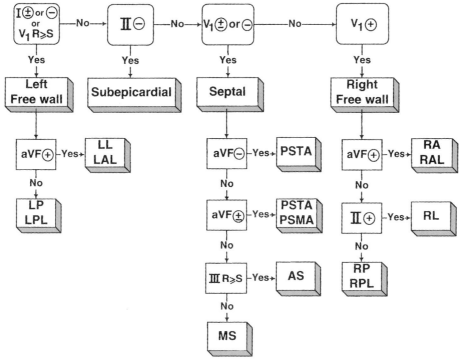

FIGURE 20–6. Algorithm for accessory pathway localization by surface ECG. This algorithm is based on the polarity of the first 20 msec of the delta wave. Left free wall pathways are readily identified by an isoelectric or negative delta wave in lead I or an R > S wave in V1. Note that with right free wall pathways, the initial component of the delta wave is positive in V1 but with R < S wave. Right free wall pathways are identified by a late transition to R > S usually in V3 or later. LAL, left anterolateral; LL, left lateral; LP, left posterior; LPL, left posterolateral; MS, midseptal; PSMA, posteroseptal mitral annulus; PSTA, posteroseptal tricuspid annulus; RA, right anterior; RAL, right anterolateral; RL, right lateral. *(From Arruda MS, McClelland J, Wang X, et al.: Development and validation of an ECG algorithm for identifying accessory pathway ablation site in Wolff-Parkinson-White syndrome. J Cardiovasc Electrophysiol 9:2-12, 1998, with permission.)*

despite changes in the tachycardia cycle length, and the ability to advance atrial activation by a premature ventricular stimulus delivered during His bundle refractoriness.[24] The last finding indicates the presence of an AP but does not prove participation in the tachycardia. A preexcitation index greater than 70 msec is consistent with a left lateral AP.[25] The preexcitation index is the difference between the tachycardia cycle length and the longest coupling interval of a right ventricular apical premature stimulus that advances the atrium.[25] *Diagnostic* of a free wall pathway is prolongation of the QRS-to-atrium time during reciprocating tachycardia (and usually of the tachycardia cycle length as well) by 35 to 40 msec or longer with ipsilateral bundle branch block.[24,26] Left anterior fascicular block also prolongs the QRS-to-atrium time in patients with left free wall APs.[26] Coupled with an eccentric atrial activation sequence, the ability to reproducibly terminate the tachycardia with a premature ventricular stimulus delivered during His bundle refractoriness also proves an ORT. Parahisian pacing techniques consistently indicate the presence of retrograde conduction over right free

wall APs.[27] The response of left free wall APs to parahisian pacing is more complex. In about 25% of cases of left free wall APs, parahisian pacing is consistent with retrograde conduction over only the AV node.

The diagnostic features of antidromic reciprocating tachycardia are given in Table 20–1. Preexcited reciprocating tachycardias may use the AV node or a second AP as the retrograde limb. There are no surface ECG features that are diagnostic of antidromic tachycardia, but the diagnosis is excluded by demonstration of other than a 1:1 atrial-to-ventricular relationship.

DIFFERENTIAL DIAGNOSIS

ORTs using free wall APs must be differentiated from atrial tachycardias arising from near the AV valve annuli or, rarely, from the CS musculature.[28] Differentiation between atrial tachycardia and ORT is best accomplished by dissociating the ventricles from the tachycardia. The demonstration of a V-A-A-V

TABLE 20–1

Diagnostic Criteria

Orthodromic Tachycardia

Obligatory 1:1 AV relationship with earliest atrial activation on AV free wall

Shortest V-to-A time ≥60 msec

Constant V-to-A conduction times despite TCL variations

Advance atrial activation during His refractoriness (proves pathway presence but not participation in tachycardia)

Pre-excitation index >70 msec (left lateral AP)

Ipsilateral bundle branch block prolongs His (or V)-to-A time (and usually TCL) by ≥35 msec*

Reproducible tachycardia termination by premature ventricular stimuli during His refractoriness without conduction to atrium†

Antidromic Tachycardia

Obligatory 1:1 AV relationship with earliest ventricular activation on free wall

QRS morphology in tachycardia consistent with maximal preexcitation

Tachycardia QRS morphology reproduced by atrial pacing near pathway insertion

Each limb of tachycardia circuit supports conduction at TCL

Advance ventricular activation by atrial extrastimuli near insertion with advancement of subsequent His and atrial activation†

Changes in V-to-His interval precede changes in TCL

Exclusion of ventricular tachycardia and bystander participation, especially AV nodal reentry (His-to-A time in tachycardia ≤70 msec consistent with AV nodal reentry)

*Proves free wall AP-mediated tachycardia.
†Proves AP-mediated tachycardia.
A, atrium; AP, accessory pathway; AV, atrioventricular; His, bundle of His; TCL, tachycardia cycle length; V, ventricle.

response after termination of ventricular pacing that *entrains* the atrium excludes an ORT and confirms an atrial tachycardia.[29] The ability to initiate the tachycardia with ventricular pacing, initiation with a critical atrium-to-ventricle (AV) or ventricle-to-atrium (VA) interval, or advancement of the same atrium activation sequence with premature ventricular stimuli during His refractoriness are all consistent with an ORT rather than AV nodal reentry.[24]

Approximately 6% of cases of AV nodal reentry are associated with an eccentric atrial activation sequence that is earliest in the posterior or distal CS,

with the shortest VA times being longer than 60 msec (Fig. 20–7).[30] This pattern is easily confused with ORT using a left-sided concealed AP, both at electrophysiologic testing and on the surface ECG, because the retrograde P wave during atrioventricular nodal reentrant tachycardia (AVNRT) is negative in leads I and aVL and positive in V_1. The eccentric atrial activation sequence is usually demonstrated with ventricular pacing as well. The keys to the diagnosis of AVNRT with eccentric atrial activation are (1) the demonstration of dual AV nodal physiology, (2) the ability to also induce "typical" AV nodal reentry with concentric atrial activation or variable patterns of retrograde atrial activation in most patients, (3) absence of retrograde VA conduction without isoproterenol, (4) inability to advance the atrium with premature ventricular stimuli during His refractoriness (may require left ventricular pacing), (5) demonstration of only decremental retrograde VA conduction, and (6) the ability to dissociate the atrium and ventricle from the tachycardia.[30] Standard slow pathway ablation in the posteroseptal right atrium eliminates the tachycardia in these cases.

The differential diagnosis of an antidromic tachycardia includes ventricular tachycardia and bystander AP participation. Ventricular tachycardia should be diagnosed by the dissociation of the atrium from the tachycardia or a variable His-to-atrium timing relationship without alteration of the tachycardia cycle length. Antidromic tachycardia is diagnosed by demonstrating an obligatory 1:1 A/V relationship during tachycardia, reproduction of tachycardia QRS morphology by atrial pacing at the presumed AP insertion site, and advancement of the ventricular *and* subsequent atrial activation by a premature atrial stimulus near the AP site (see Table 20–1).[24]

Bystander participation of the AP is best recognized by dissociation of AP conduction from the tachycardia. The demonstration of a His-to-atrium interval of 70 msec or less indicates AV nodal reentry with bystander AP rather than an antidromic reciprocating tachycardia.[24]

Mapping

The most widely used approaches to mapping of free wall APs rely on identification of the earliest ventricular activation during antegrade AP conduction and earliest retrograde atrial activation during ORT (Table 20–2). However, mapping based on electrogram morphology rather than timing can be per-

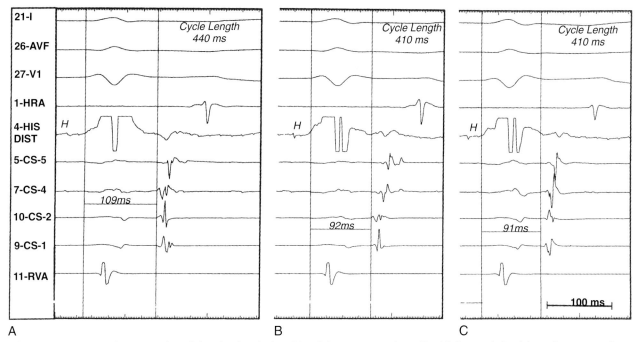

FIGURE 20–7. Eccentric retrograde atrial activation during AV nodal reentrant tachycardia. All figures derived from the same patient. **A,** Earliest atrial activation occurs in the mid coronary sinus. **B** and **C,** The atrial activation is recorded more distally in the coronary sinus in the same study. In each case there are long ventricular to atrial (VA) conduction times of >90 msec. This eccentric atrial activation and long ventricular-atrial times are readily confused with orthodromic reciprocating tachycardia using a left free wall pathway. CS-1, distal coronary sinus; CS-5, proximal coronary sinus; H, His electrogram; His Dist, distal His; HRA, high right atrium; RVA, right ventricular apex. *(From Hwang C, Martin D, Goodman J, et al.: Atypical atrioventricular node reciprocating tachycardia masquerading as tachycardia using a left-sided accessory pathway. J Am Coll Cardiol 30:218-225, 1997, with permission.)*

formed in some situations. Both unipolar and bipolar recordings are helpful. Unipolar recordings from the electrode tip provide information on local activation through electrogram timing and morphology. Bipolar recordings from the distal electrode pair reflect timing and more clearly demonstrate the electrogram components and AP potentials.

LEFT FREE WALL ACCESSORY PATHWAYS

Mapping of left free wall APs is facilitated by multi-electrode recordings from a CS catheter; however, the anatomic distance from the true mitral annulus limits the accuracy of CS mapping alone to identify target sites for ablation. Left free wall APs can be ablated without the use of CS catheters at highly experienced centers with no compromise in the success rate.[31] For most practitioners, however, the CS catheter is standard, along with right atrial, His, and right ventricular catheters. Mapping and ablation may be performed by the transaortic (retrograde) approach or the trans-septal approach. The transaortic approach is directed at sites beneath the mitral annulus and therefore targets the AP ventricular insertion. For the transaortic approach, the catheter is

always prolapsed across the aortic valve, to prevent perforation of the leaflets or entry into the coronary arteries. The catheter most readily crosses the aortic valve with the "J" of the deflected catheter tip opening to the right of the fluoroscopy screen (anteriorly) in the right anterior oblique view. After entering the left ventricular cavity, the "J" curvature is maintained on the catheter tip and the catheter is rotated in a counterclockwise direction to turn the catheter tip posteriorly toward the annulus. The catheter then can be opened slightly to engage a sub-annular position, or it can be withdrawn to cross over the annulus into the left atrium. The catheter tip is either moved incrementally in steps beneath the annulus or made to slide along the mitral annulus for mapping before being dropped down beneath the annulus for energy delivery (Fig. 20–8). It is often difficult to achieve stable catheter positions for the far lateral and anterolateral mitral annulus with the transaortic approach.

The trans-septal approach is primarily directed at mapping the atrial side of the annulus or the mitral annulus itself. As opposed to the transaortic approach, in which the ablation electrode is perpendicular to and beneath the annulus, the trans-septal

TABLE 20–2

Target Sites

Left Free Wall

Presumed AP potential

Delta-VEGM ≤0 msec (antegrade conduction)

VEGM-AEGM ≤40 msec (retrograde conduction)

AEGM-VEGM ≤40 msec (antegrade conduction)

AEGM amplitude >0.4 mV

QRS-AEGM interval ≤70 msec (retrograde conduction)

Isoelectric VEGM-AEGM interval ≤5 msec (retrograde conduction)

Site of AEGM polarity reversal

Right Free Wall

Presumed AP potential

Delta-VEGM ≤ − 10 msec

AEGM amplitude >1 mV

AEGM-VEGM ≤40 msec (antegrade conduction)

QRS-AEGM interval ≤70 msec (retrograde conduction)

Isoelectric VEGM-AEGM interval ≤5 msec (retrograde conduction)

AEGM, atrial electrogram; AP, accessory pathway; Delta, delta wave onset; QRS, QRS onset; VEGM, ventricular electrogram.

approach is directed at positions on or above the annulus, with the electrodes parallel to the annulus (Fig. 20–9).[1,34] After passing through the atrial septum, the catheter is directed laterally with a large sweeping curve, to direct the tip back toward the atrial septum. With the aid of preformed sheaths, the catheter tip is made to slide along the annulus by advancing and withdrawing the catheter (see Fig. 20–9). Although catheter mobility is greater, catheter stability may be more problematic than with the transaortic approach.

The decision regarding use of the transaortic or trans-septal approach is based on physician familiarity and certain patient characteristics. Because the two approaches are complementary, it is best for the physician to be familiar with both techniques. The trans-septal approach is favored in the presence of peripheral vascular disease, aortic valve disease or prosthesis, or small ventricular chambers. In children weighing less than 30 kg, the transaortic approach may be associated with frequent valve trauma.[33] The trans-septal approach provides better access to far lateral and anterolateral AP locations. The trans-

septal approach may be contraindicated in the presence of distorted cardiac anatomy such as congenital heart disease, pneumonectomy, kyphoscoliosis, or severe dilation of the aorta or right atrium.

The characteristics of electrograms at successful ablation sites have been studied extensively for left free wall APs.[34-39] Most of these data are derived from early experience with ablation by the transaortic approach and have not been reproduced for the trans-septal approach. Five electrogram characteristics have been described as useful in predicting successful ablation sites when mapping antegrade AP activation by the transaortic approach: (1) delta wave-to-ventricle (V) interval, (2) atrial electrogram amplitude, (3) electrogram stability, (4) local AV electrogram interval, and (5) presence of a presumed AP potential. The delta-to-V interval should be measured from the onset of the delta wave to the peak or intrinsicoid deflection of bipolar mapping electrograms.[36,37,40] For unipolar electrograms, the maximal negative dV/dt reflects local ventricular activation.[40] The absence of a QS morphology in the unipolar electrogram indicates a site with a less than 10% chance of ablation success.[40] Pacing from near the AP insertion accentuates the degree of preexcitation. For left free wall APs, a delta-to-V time less than or equal to 0 msec is usually recorded at successful ablation sites, with average intervals of only −2 to −10 msec (Fig. 20–10).[35,37,41]

The atrial electrogram amplitude at successful sites should be greater than 0.4 to 1 mV, or the A/V ratio should be greater than 0.1 by the transaortic approach. The small atrial electrogram amplitude indicates the subannular position of the catheter. The absence of any atrial electrogram suggests a position too far from the annulus. For trans-septal mapping, an A/V ratio equal to 1 is sought along the mitral annulus.[32] Greater and lesser ratios indicate atrial and ventricular displacement of the catheter, respectively. Electrogram stability is defined as less than 10% change in the atrial and ventricular electrogram amplitudes or A/V ratio over 5 to 10 cardiac cycles.[35,37,39]

The transaortic approach usually provides good catheter stability because the catheter is "wedged" beneath the mitral valve. For the trans-septal approach, stability can be assessed by consistent electrogram amplitudes, catheter motion concordant with the CS catheter, and, when on the atrial side of the annulus, consistent "PR" segment elevation on the unipolar electrogram.[13] The last finding also indicates sufficient catheter contact with the atrial myocardium. Local AV intervals of 40 msec or less should be sought, with average intervals of 25 to 50 msec reported for successful ablation sites (see Fig. 20–10).[38,39] The AV intervals for left free wall APs are

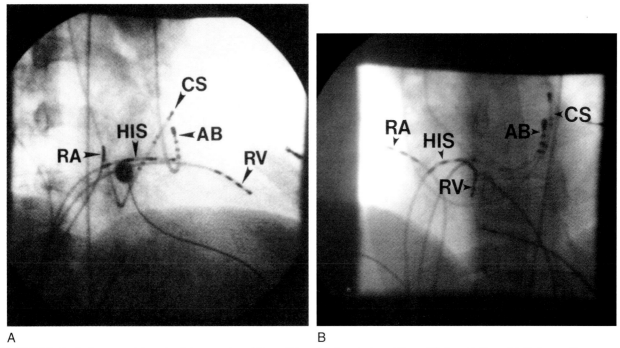

FIGURE 20–8. Catheter positions in right anterior oblique (**A**) and left anterior oblique (**B**) for ablation of left free wall accessory pathway by the retrograde transaortic approach. AB, ablation catheter; CS, coronary sinus catheter; His, His catheter; RA, right atrial catheter; RV, right ventricular catheter.

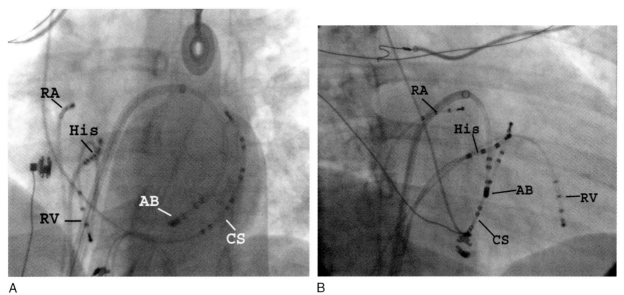

FIGURE 20–9. Catheter positions for trans-septal approach to ablation of left free wall accessory pathway. **A**, Left anterior oblique view showing the preformed trans-septal sheath (SL2 Swartz Sheath Daig Corp) crossing the foramen ovale and used to position the ablation catheter (AB) along the proximal mitral annulus. CS, coronary sinus catheter; His, His catheter; RA, right atrial catheter; RV, right ventricular apical catheter. From this position, the ablation catheter can be easily advanced to move proximally on the annulus and withdrawn to move distally. **B**, Right anterior oblique view of catheter positions. The ablation catheter has been moved slightly more distally. Note the tip of the ablation catheter is slightly on the ventricular side of the CS.

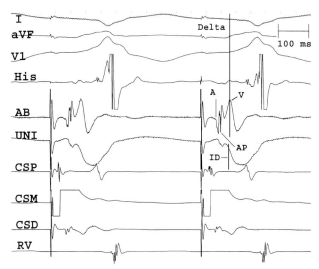

FIGURE 20–10. Mapping antegrade left free wall accessory pathway (AP) activation during pacing from the middle coronary sinus (CSM). The onset of the delta wave (Delta) is marked by the vertical line on the surface electrocardiographic leads (top 3 tracings). On the bipolar distal ablation electrodes (AB), the onset of the local atrial electrogram (A) and local ventricular electrogram (V) are marked. The local atrium-to-ventricle A-V interval is 25 msec and the peak of the local bipolar ventricular electrogram coincides with delta wave onset (Delta-V = 0). The intrinsicoid deflection (ID) of the unipolar electrogram (UNI) precedes delta wave onset by about 5 msec. The unipolar ventricular ablation electrogram is entirely negative (QS morphology) and fuses with the atrial electrogram. A discrete high frequency electrogram between the atrial and ventricular components represents a possible AP potential. CSD, distal coronary sinus; CSP, proximal coronary sinus; RV, right ventricle.

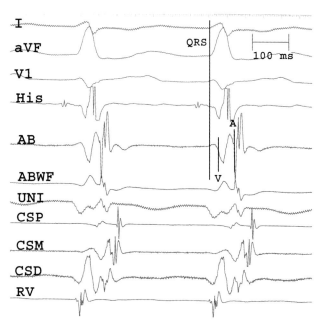

FIGURE 20–11. Electrograms from successful ablation site during mapping of retrograde accessory pathway (AP) conduction in orthodromic reciprocating tachycardia. The distal coronary sinus is earliest on this catheter. The QRS onset (QRS) to local atrial electrogram (**A**) interval on the ablation catheter is 68 msec and is shown by the vertical lines. The local ventricular (**V**) to atrial interval on the ablation electrodes is 40 msec. Note the isoelectric morphology of the atrial component of the electrogram on the wide filtered ablation electrogram (ABWF) representing the atrial insertion point of the AP (see text). Abbreviations per Figure 10.

longer than for other AP locations, and the times at successful sites overlap with those at unsuccessful sites. The local AV times alone, therefore, have limited specificity in identifying successful ablation sites for left-sided APs.

Finally, the recording of a presumed AP potential has been used to define appropriate ablation sites. The ability to record AP potentials may be influenced by the catheter approach used to map the annulus. Presumed AP potentials are defined as discrete, high-frequency potentials that occur between the atrial and ventricular electrograms and at least 10 msec before the onset of the delta wave (see Fig. 20–10).[34-36,38,42] The amplitude of AP potentials ranges from 0.5 to 1 mV.[35] The validation of a signal as a true AP potential is a tedious process and is not practical in the clinical setting. It is probably for this reason that "AP potentials" are reported at 35% to 94% of successful ablation sites and at up to 72% of unsuccessful sites.[35,36,38,42,43] The recording of larger AP potentials in the CS than along the mitral annulus suggests the presence of an epicardial AP.[44]

For mapping of retrograde AP conduction during ORT or ventricular pacing, electrogram characteristics reported to identify successful sites include (1) catheter stability, (2) presence of a presumed AP potential, (3) continuous electrical activity, and (4) the local VA interval.[34,35,39] These data are derived largely from studies of ablation from the transaortic approach. Catheter stability is defined as for mapping of antegrade conduction. The presence of a presumed AP potential is reported at only 37% to 67% of successful ablation sites during retrograde AP conduction mapping.[34,35,39] It is possible that AP potentials are obscured by the large ventricular electrogram with the transaortic approach. The QRS-onset-to-local-atrial electrogram (QRS-A) interval is usually 70 msec or less in the absence of a left ventricular conduction delay (Fig. 20–11).[34,35] The local VA interval at successful ablation sites is typically 25 to 50 msec.[34,35,39] At very short VA intervals, the atrial electrogram may be inscribed on the terminal portion of the ventricular electrogram. Continuous electrical activity (<5 msec isoelectric interval between V and A electrograms) and the "pseudo-disappearance" of the atrial electrogram into the ventricular electrogram are manifestations of extremely short VA times.[34,37] One group has reported successful ablation by pace-mapping beneath the mitral annulus with the ablation catheter and measuring the stimulus-to-atrial times recorded on the CS catheter.[45] The site producing the shortest stimulus-to-atrial interval should be at the ventricular insertion of the AP. The average stimulus-to-atrial interval at successful sites was 46 ± 15 msec.[45]

The predictive accuracy of any single electrogram characteristic for identifying a successful ablation site rarely exceeds 30%. The electrogram must satisfy three or four criteria to achieve 60% to 80% predictive values.[37,42] Multivariate predictors of successful ablation sites are given in Table 20–3.

One problem with mapping retrograde atrial activation times is the difficulty in discriminating between atrial and ventricular components of the electrograms. This problem may be addressed in several ways. One method is to compare the electrogram recorded on the ablation catheter while simultaneously pacing the atrium and the ventricle with the electrogram recorded during ventricular pacing alone (Fig. 20–12).[46]

Another approach to unmasking distinct components of antegrade and retrograde electrograms exploits the oblique course of AP conduction across the atrioventricular annulus.[47] For left free wall APs, the ventricular insertion is usually more proximal in the CS than the atrial insertion.[47,48] When the ventricular insertion of the AP is activated by a wavefront conducting in the same direction as the oblique AP propagation, the VA intervals recorded on mapping electrodes are short and may overlap (Figs. 20–13 and 20–14). By reversing the direction of wavefront activation, the local VA intervals may be prolonged if conduction over the AP "backtracks" past ventricular sites previously activated. The same separation of components of antegrade conducted electrograms is possible by reversing the direction of activation of the atrial AP insertion. For left lateral APs, pacing of the basal posteroseptal right ventricle provides "counterclockwise" activation of the ventricular insertion (from the left anterior oblique perspective), whereas pacing of the high right ventricular outflow tract near the pulmonic valve provides a "clockwise" activation of the ventricular insertion. Because the ventricular AP insertion tends to be more proximal along the CS than the atrial insertion, the VA intervals are typically prolonged by clockwise activation with right ventricular outflow tract pacing. A change in local VA times of greater than 15 msec is considered to represent a significant change in the activation wavefront. For reversing atrial activation wavefronts of left free wall APs, CS pacing proximal and distal to the site of earliest retrograde atrial activity is used. For antegrade mapping, pacing distal to the atrial insertion should provide a counterclockwise activation wave-

TABLE 20–3

Multivariate Predictors of Successful Left Free Wall Ablation Sites by the Transaortic Approach

Authors (Ref. No.)	AP Potential	EGM Stability	Delta-V Interval (msec)	A Amplitude	Local AV Interval (msec)	Local VA Interval (msec)	Best Positive Predictive Value (%)
Hindricks et al. (36)	+	—	Value not Specified	—	—	—	70
Bashir et al. (37)	+	—	10	—	—	—	20-25
Chen et al. (35)	+	<10% change in EGM amplitude	0	A >1 mV	—	—	62
Cappato et al. (38)	+	—	≤0	A/V ratio ≥0.1	≤40	—	87
Xie et al. (39)	+	—	≤0	—	≤30	≤30	67
Villacastin et al. (34)	+	—	—	—	—	Pseudodisappearance	59

A, atrial electrogram; AP, accessory pathway; AV, atrium-to-ventricle; Delta, delta wave onset; EGM, electrogram; V, ventricular electrogram; VA, ventricle-to-atrium; –, not reported.

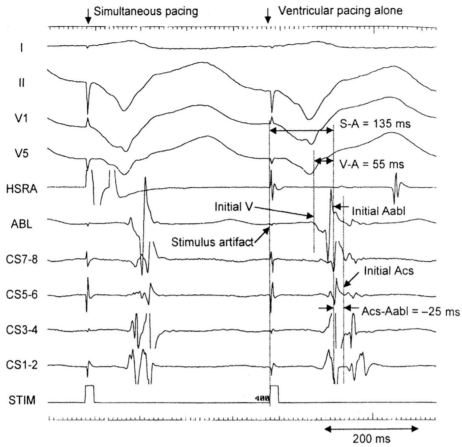

FIGURE 20–12. Use of simultaneous atrial and ventricular pacing to discriminate components of mapping electrograms in a patient with left sided accessory pathway. The penultimate beat of the drive train comprises simultaneous atrial and ventricular pacing (labeled). The atrial electrogram is advanced relative to the ventricular electrogram and precedes it. No electrical activity follows the ventricular activation in this beat. The last beat of the drive comprises only ventricular pacing. Retrograde conduction over the accessory pathway is evident by atrial activation now following the ventricular electrograms. By comparing the electrograms from the 2 cardiac cycles the atrial and ventricular components of the electrograms are more apparent. Aabl, onset local retrograde atrial electrogram on the ablation catheter; ABL, ablation; Acs, onset local atrial electrogram recorded on the coronary sinus; CS1-2, distal coronary sinus; CS7-8, proximal coronary sinus; HRSA, high septal right atrium; S-A, interval between stimulus artifact (Stim) and local atrial electrogram; V-A, interval between local ventricular and atrial electrograms. *(From Nakao K, Seto S, Iliev II, et al.: Simultaneous atrial and ventricular pacing to facilitate mapping of concealed left-sided accessory pathways. Pacing Clin Electrophysiol 25:922-928, 2002, with permission.)*

front and the longest AV intervals. The target sites are AP potentials or just to the side of the earliest site of atrial or ventricular activation predicted to be the mid-AP site by changes in the local electrogram times. Note that this technique does not target the sites of the shortest AV or VA times.

A useful technique to ablation of left free wall pathways from the trans-septal approach is to identify the point of atrial electrogram polarity reversal when mapping the annulus.[49] This vectorial technique obviates the need to measure VA intervals. Through trans-septal access, the ablation electrode bipole is oriented parallel to the axis of the annulus. Wide-bandpass electrogram filtering is set to 0.5 to 500 Hz to accentuate the directional characteristics of the electrogram polarity. The bipole is then moved proximally and distally, parallel to the annulus, during ORT, and the polarity of the atrial electrogram is noted. With the tip electrode negative and the proximal electrode positive, the atrial electrogram will be predominantly negative at catheter positions on the annulus proximal to the atrial insertion (Fig. 20–15). At positions distal to the atrial insertion, the direction of the atrial activation wavefront is reversed relative to the bipole, and the atrial electrogram is predominantly positive. The point at which the atrial electrogram becomes isoelectric marks the atrial insertion and the site for ablation. The positive predictive value of electrogram reversal for identifying the successful ablation site is 75%.[49] To be effective, this technique requires that the mapping bipole remain parallel with axis of atrial activation on the annulus.

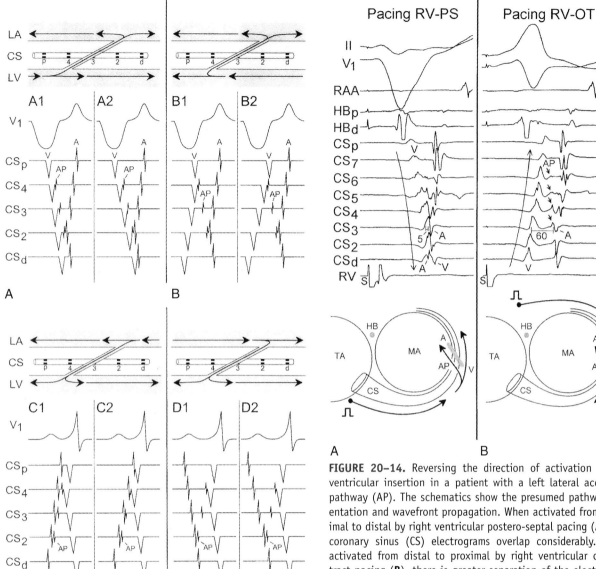

FIGURE 20–13. Activation of oblique accessory pathways. Schematic of antegrade and retrograde activation of an oblique left free wall accessory pathway (AP) from opposing directions. **A** and **B** demonstrate activation of the ventricular insertion from the proximal to distal and distal to proximal directions, respectively. **C** and **D** represent activation of the atrial insertion from the distal to proximal and proximal to distal directions, respectively. Note the separation of the components of the electrograms when the AP is activated from the direction opposite to the direction of conduction over the pathway. A, atrial potential; CS, coronary sinus; d, distal; LA, left atrium; LV, left ventricle; p, proximal; V, ventricular potential. *(From Kenichiro O, Gonzalez M, Beckman K, et al.: Reversing the direction of paced ventricular and atrial wavefronts reveals an oblique course in accessory AV pathways and improves localization for catheter ablation. Circulation 104:550-556, 2001, with permission.)*

FIGURE 20–14. Reversing the direction of activation of the ventricular insertion in a patient with a left lateral accessory pathway (AP). The schematics show the presumed pathway orientation and wavefront propagation. When activated from proximal to distal by right ventricular postero-septal pacing (**A**), the coronary sinus (CS) electrograms overlap considerably. When activated from distal to proximal by right ventricular outflow tract pacing (**B**), there is greater separation of the electrogram components and definition of an AP potential. HB, his bundle; MA, mitral annulus; RAA, right atrial appendage; S, stimulus artifact; TA, tricuspid annulus. *(From Kenichiro O, Gonzalez M, Beckman K, et al.: Reversing the direction of paced ventricular and atrial wavefronts reveals an oblique course in accessory AV pathways and improves localization for catheter ablation. Circulation 104:550-556, 2001, with permission.)*

RIGHT FREE WALL ACCESSORY PATHWAYS

Mapping and ablation of right free wall APs is often more difficult than for left-sided APs because of the absence of a venous structure paralleling the tricuspid annulus and because of catheter instability. To facilitate rapid localization of right free wall APs, it is often useful to employ circular multielectrode "halo" catheters positioned near the tricuspid annulus (Fig. 20–16). Use of this catheter or, rarely, of 2-French (2F) mapping catheters positioned in the

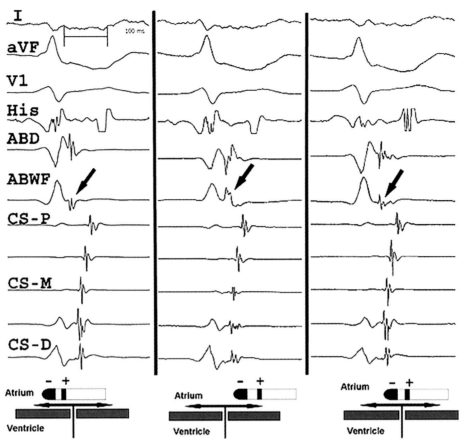

FIGURE 20–15. Atrial electrogram polarity reversal during mapping of orthodromic reciprocating tachycardia using a left free wall accessory pathway. **Left Panel,** During reciprocating tachycardia, the distal bipolar ablation electrograms are displayed with standard (ABD) filtering at 30-500 Hz and wide filtering (ABWF) at 0.5-500 Hz. In this panel the electrode is parallel to the annulus and proximal to the site of atrial accessory pathway (AP) insertion. The atrial component of the ABWF electrogram (*arrow*) is negative. **Center Panel,** The distal electrode pair has been moved distal to the site of the AP insertion, represented by the positive atrial component to the ABWF electrogram. **Right Panel,** When the electrode pair is directly over the atrial insertion of the AP, the atrial component to the ABWF electrogram is isoelectric as the wavefront spreads away from the electrode pair in 2 opposing directions. The schematics at the bottom of the tracings illustrate the relation of the electrodes to the atrial insertion site. CS, coronary sinus; D, distal; M, mid; P, proximal.

right coronary artery represents the closest equivalent to a CS mapping for the right side of the heart.[8] Catheter mapping from the subclavian or right internal jugular approach is sometimes more productive than from the femoral approach. As for trans-septal access to the left side of the heart, the use of preformed sheaths to direct the ablation catheter to specific locations on the tricuspid annulus is helpful. The sheaths allow for placement of the mapping catheter parallel to the annulus for mapping, as with the trans-septal approach to left APs (see Fig. 20–16).

Because of the relative infrequency of right free wall APs, multivariate analyses of electrogram characteristics specific to this site that predict successful ablation are not available. Presumably, the stability and AP criteria defined for left APs are applicable. For ablation along the tricuspid annulus, a 1:1 A/V ratio is usually sought.[41,50] Most series have also used

retrograde VA times of 40 msec or less as a criterion for radiofrequency (RF) delivery. The timing of local ventricular activation before delta wave onset is usually earlier than for left APs (Fig. 20–17). Haissaguerre et al.[41,50] found that the local ventricle preceded delta wave onset by 18 ± 10 msec for right APs and 2 ± 6 msec for left APs at successful sites. The average AV time was 28 ± 7 msec for right-sided APs. In children, the local AV times were 11 to 26 msec, and delta-to-ventricular electrogram intervals of –28 msec to –52 msec at sites of successful right free wall AP ablation in five patients.[51] If it is difficult to discriminate the components of the local electrograms, reversal of the activating wavefronts may be useful, as described earlier.[47] For right free wall APs, opposing ventricular wavefronts are produced by pacing the right ventricle near the annulus, anterior and posterior to the site of earliest retrograde AP conduction. Opposing atrial activation is produced by pacing

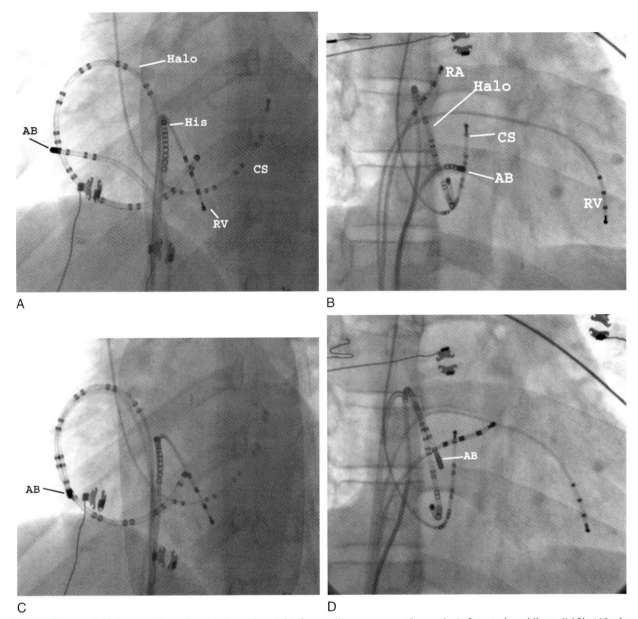

FIGURE 20–16. Catheter positions for ablation of a right free wall accessory pathway. **A**, Left anterior oblique (LAO) 40° view showing the 20 electrode "halo" catheter parallel to the tricuspid annulus and the ablation (AB) catheter near to electrodes 11 and 12 along the free wall. The His, right ventricular apical (RV) and coronary sinus (CS) catheters are shown. **B**, Right anterior oblique (RAO) 30° view of the same catheter positions as in **A**, except the His catheter is replaced by a right atrial (RA) catheter. Note that the ablation catheter tip is to the ventricular side of the halo catheter. **C**, LAO 40° view with the ablation catheter now placed parallel to the tricuspid annulus. **D**, RAO 30° view of catheter positions in **C**.

on either side of the presumed atrial insertion. Parahisian pacing reliably identifies retrograde right free wall AP conduction.[27]

For both right and left free wall pathways, it is my opinion that computerized *mapping* of electrical activation is optional. This is because there are usually relatively few points of electrical interest. Electroanatomic mapping systems have been shown to dramatically reduce fluoroscopic exposure to pediatric patients, however.[51] The catheter *navigation* capabilities of computerized systems are very

helpful, because they allow the operator to precisely return to sites of interest (Fig. 20–18).

Ablation

Before ablation energy delivery, it is essential to obtain the most stable catheter position possible. Catheter dislodgement before completion of the abla-

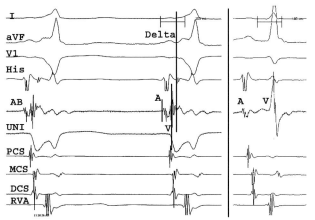

FIGURE 20–17. Electrograms from the site of successful ablation of a right free wall accessory pathway. **Left Panel:** On the distal ablation bipole (AB) there is continuous electrical activity with the local ventricular electrogram (V) preceding the delta wave (Delta) onset by 25 msec. The local atrial (A)-to-ventricular (V) electrogram interval is 38 msec. The unipolar distal ablation electrogram (UNI) has a QS morphology. **Right Panel:** After ablation, the ablation electrogram shows prolongation of the AV times but the morphology of the local atrial electrogram is unchanged. Abbreviations as per Figure 20-15.

tion lesion may transiently suppress AP function, allowing future recovery. Catheter stability is enhanced by the use of preformed sheaths and catheters with sufficient curvature or reach to access the target site. Cardiac motion can be minimized during ablation by discontinuing the use of isoproterenol and by rapid ventricular pacing at rates of 120 beats per minute or greater. With ventricular pacing to entrain reciprocating tachycardias, the ablation catheter is less subject to dislodgement on termination of the arrhythmia. Adequate sedation should be established before RF delivery, because the patient may move in response to pain. Marking of the catheter site with computerized navigation systems or by fluoroscopy may allow return to successful sites despite catheter dislodgement (see Fig. 20–18). Standard 4-mm-tip RF catheters are usually adequate for free wall APs.

The target temperatures for right and left free wall APs is typically 60°C to 65°C.[52] Favorable ablation sites should not be abandoned until temperatures >50°C to 55°C are achieved. For impedance monitoring, a 5- to 10-ohm (Ω) decrease in impedance usually signifies tissue heating. The energy needed to reach the target temperature varies with catheter location. Low blood flow positions beneath the mitral or tricuspid annulus may require little energy due to the absence of convective cooling. Loss of AP function should occur within 1 to 6 seconds after RF energy delivery.[53] Longer times to success may be associated with higher recurrence rates. Endocardial cryoablation is effective for free wall AP ablation and

offers the advantage of complete catheter stability due to adherence to the tissue during ablation.[54] I favor the 6-mm tip size for larger cryolesions. After successful ablation, thorough electrophysiologic testing should be undertaken to document the complete elimination of AP function and to exclude other mechanisms of tachycardias.

For resistant APs, irrigated catheters may prove successful by delivering greater energies.[55] For irrigated systems, target temperatures of 50°C with 50 W maximal power may safely eliminate 94% of APs after failed conventional RF delivery.[55] Use of passively cooled large-tip catheters with high-output generators may also result in larger lesions.

Epicardial left free wall APs may require ablation from within the CS (Table 20–4).[44,55-61] Epicardial APs account for 4% of all left free wall APs and 10% of failed ablations.[44] Before CS ablation, CS angiography is recommended to delineate the anatomy, exclude diverticula, and assess possible damage to the CS from the ablation. Also, coronary angiography should be performed to determine the proximity of the ablation site to the left circumflex artery. Initial experience included non–temperature-controlled ablation in a small series of patients (see Table 20–4). Mural thrombus in the CS was reported in one series.[57] More recently, temperature control has been used for ablation of APs.[55] Within the CS target temperatures of 60°C with power limits of 20 to 30 W have been used.[55] For resistant epicardial APs, irrigated RF ablation within the CS may be effective. For irrigated catheters, the target temperature is 50°C with maximal power of 20 to 30 W delivered for 60 seconds at effective sites.[55] No complications were reported in small series of patients. Cryoablation in the CS has been used effectively and may carry a lesser risk of injury to the circumflex coronary artery than RF ablation does.[61] Right and left epicardial APs may also be ablated by direct epicardial mapping achieved by percutaneous pericardial access (Fig. 20–19).[62]

Clinical Results

LEFT FREE WALL ACCESSORY PATHWAYS

The rates of success for left free wall AP ablation are the highest of any AP location and are typically greater than 90% (Table 20–5).[32,49,63-76] In the largest reported single-center series, 96% of 388 patients with left free wall APs were successfully ablated by the trans-septal approach.[63] The recurrence rates for left free wall APs are the lowest of any location, at 2% to

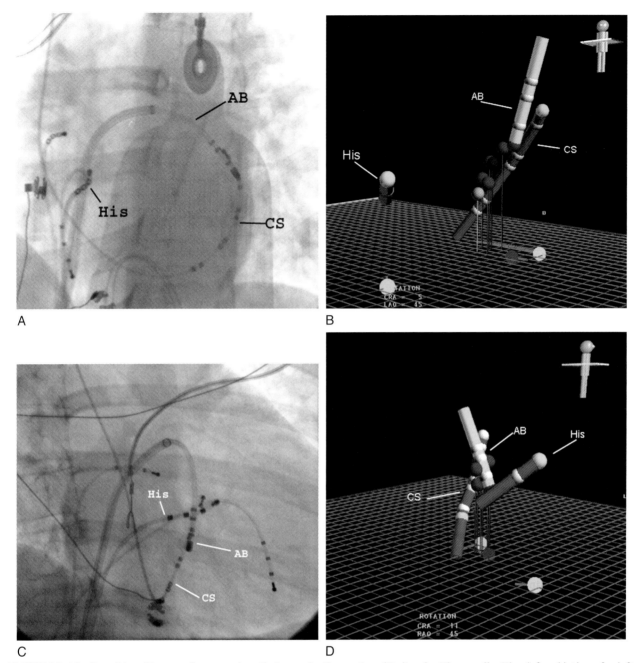

FIGURE 20–18. Use of LocaLisa non-fluoroscopic catheter navigation system (Medtronic, Minneapolis, Minn.) for ablation of a left free wall accessory pathway. **A**, Left anterior oblique (LAO) fluoroscopic view of the ablation catheter (AB) in the far lateral free wall near coronary sinus (CS) electrodes 3 and 4. **B:** Comparable LAO representation of the ablation catheter, His and distal six CS electrodes in the non-fluoroscopic navigation system. The red spheres indicate sites of radiofrequency delivery with the dark red marker being the successful site. **C:** RAO fluoroscopic view of catheter positions as in **A. D**, RAO non-fluoroscopic navigation system view comparable to **C**. In both **C** and **D** the ablation catheter is seen slightly on the ventricular side of the coronary sinus catheter.

5%.[32,49,63-65] Recurrences are more likely with concealed APs, delivery of transiently effective pulses, or need for more than five lesions for acute success.[53,66-68] The success rates for ablation by the transaortic and trans-septal approaches appear to be similar in direct comparisons (Table 20–6).[69-76] These studies usually report similar total procedure times, fluoroscopy times, and rates of crossover to the other approach. Overall, complication rates appear to be similar, but some studies have found a trend toward a higher rate of complications with the transaortic approach.[71,73] In comparative trials, there are no fea-

TABLE 20–4

Catheter Ablation of Left Free Wall Accessory Pathways from within the Coronary Sinus

Authors (Ref. No.)	Energy Type	No. of Patients	Maximal Power	Target Temperature	Duration (sec)	Success (No./Total)	Complications
Wang et al. (56)	RF	5	Not reported	Power control	—	5/5 (100%)	Not reported
Haissaguerre et al. (57)	RF	7	30 W	Power control	60	6/7 (85%)	CS mural thrombus (2 patients)
Giorgberidze et al. (58)	RF	5	Not reported	Power control	—	3/5 (60%)	None
Langberg et al. (59)	RF	2	28 ± 9 W	Power control	—	2/2 (100%)	Not reported
Cappato et al. (60)	RF	6	Not reported	Power control	—	6/6 (100%)	None
Yamane et al. (55)	Irrigated RF	7	30 W maximum	50° C	60	7/7 (100%)	Stenosis or irregularity cardiac veins (2 patients)
Gaita et al. (61)	Cryoablation	1	NA	−75° C	240	1/1 (100%)	None

CS, coronary sinus; NA, not applicable; RF, radiofrequency; —, not reported.

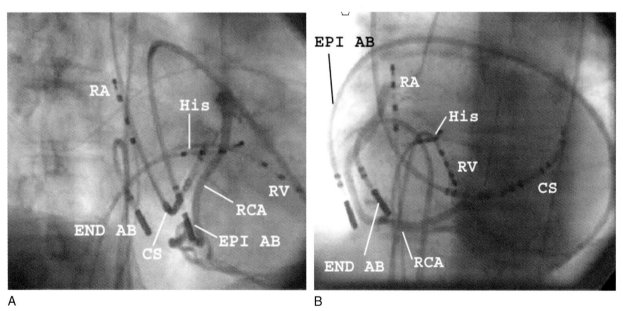

A   B

FIGURE 20–19. Percutaneous epicardial catheter approach to ablation of an epicardial right inferior free wall pathway. **A,** In this RAO view the epicardial ablation catheter (EPI AB) enters the pericardial space from subxyphoid access and encircles the heart from posterior to anterior to reach the site of successful ablation. Attempts at ablation from the endocardial catheter (END AB) failed. The right coronary artery (RCA) is visualized by angiography and is very near the epicardial ablation catheter. **B,** Same catheter positions shown in LAO view. His, His catheter; RA, right atrial catheter; RV, right ventricular catheter. *(Courtesy of Dr. K. Shivkumar.)*

TABLE 20-5

Results of Trans-septal Ablation for Left Free Wall Accessory Pathways

Author (Ref. No.)	No. of Patients	Success (%)	Compl. (%)	Recurrence (%)	X-over (%)	Flouro Time (min)	Procedure Time (hr)	Comments
De Ponti et al. (63)	388	96	1.2	1.2	2	—	—	Complication rate includes ablation of atrial tachycardias
Swartz et al. (32)	76	97	2	2	0	63 ± 47	4.9 ± 2.2	Complication rate includes other pathway locations
Fisher & Swartz (49)	26	100	0	0	0	25 ± 10.5	2.8 ± 0.9	Vectorial 3-D mapping
Yip et al. (64)	49	92	4	4	4	22.5 ± 15.2	1.7 ± 0.05	Preformed trans-septal sheaths
Manolis et al. (65)	31	100	0	3	0	76 ± 48	5.4 ± 1.9	"W sign" used for mapping

Compl., complications; Fluoro, fluoroscopy; X-over, crossover to transaortic approach; —, not reported.

TABLE 20-6

Comparison of Transaortic and Trans-septal Ablation Procedures

Author (Ref. No.)	Approach	No. of Patients	Success (%)	Recurrence (%)	Compl. (%)	X-over (%)	Procedure Time (Range)	Fluoro Time (Range) (min)	Comments
Deshpande et al. (69)	TA	42	95	—	4.7	4.7	244 ± 82 min	51 ± 22	—
	TS	58	75	—	3.4	24	268 ± 88 min	53 ± 22	
Lesh et al. (70)	TA	89	85	—	6.7	12	220 ± 13 min	44 ± 4	—
	TS	33	85	—	6.1	12	205 ± 13 min	45 ± 5	
Natale et al. (71)	TA	49	88	4	4	6	—	42 ± 29	—
	TS	31	100	0	0	0	—	34 ± 18	
Saul et al. (72)	TA	50	40	—	—	14	3.3 (2-9.5) hr*	52 (18-259)	Pediatric patients
	TS	13	100	—	—	0	4.3 (2-6) hr*	58 (14-197)	
Manolis et al. (73)	TA	50	87	11	8	10	7.1 ± 2.4 hr*	121 ± 81*	—
	TS	23	96	4	0	17	5.5 ± 2.1 hr*	81 ± 57	
Vora et al. (74)	TA	13	100	16	8	0	—	38 ± 30*	Nonrandomized pediatric patients
	TS	36	100	0	3	0	—	61 ± 45	
Ma et al. (75)	TA	50	100	0	0	4	77 ± 20 min	12 ± 7	Randomized study (abstract)
	TS	50	96	0	0	0	81 ± 19 min	13 ± 8	
Montenero et al. (76)	TA	10	100	—	—	—	—	45 ± 10	Pediatric patients
	TS	18	100	—	—	—	—	23 ± 1	
Katritsis et al. (96)	TA	23	87	4	0	13	156 ± 58 min*	37 ± 25*	Single catheter for both approaches
	TS	21	90	5	0	5	119 ± 39 min	22 ± 21	

*$P < .05$ transaortic vs trans-septal
Compl., complications; Fluoro, fluoroscopy; TA, transaortic approach; TS, trans-septal approach; X-over, crossover to other approach; —, not reported.

tures that predict the success of one approach or the other.[70] Because the techniques are complementary, it is to the operator's advantage to be familiar with both, allowing crossover should one approach fail. Because arterial access is required for the retrograde transaortic approach, vascular complications may be more common with this technique.[71,73] The success rates for ablation of concealed left APs by the transaortic approach are lower in some reports, possibly because of the smaller atrial electrograms recorded with this approach.

The success rates for right free wall AP ablation are the lowest of any AP location, averaging about 90% but ranging from 66% to 100% (Table 20–7).[32,41,51,66,77,78] In the largest series of 92 patients with right free wall APs, the success rate was 90%.[77] The lower success rate is attributed in general to greater catheter instability for right free wall locations. The recurrence rates are higher for right free wall APs than for other locations, ranging from 9% to 16.7% (see Table 20–7).[32,41,66,77,78] The right free wall location is a predictor of recurrence in some studies.[77] Notably, one center reported 100% success and no recurrences of right free wall APs in 21 children with ablation using an electroanatomic catheter mapping system.[51] The success rates are lower still for patients with Ebstein's anomaly. In the largest reported series of 100 such patients, 52 had right free wall APs.[79] The initial success rate for these pathways was 79%, with a 32% recurrence rate. In another report of 21 patients with Ebstein's anomaly, only 76% of patients had elimination of all right-sided APs.[8] In these patients, acute success was predicted by a body surface area less than or equal to $1.7\,m^2$, a mild degree of tricuspid regurgitation, and mild severity of Ebstein's anomaly.[79] Only body surface area predicted long-term success, however.

COMPLICATIONS

The complication rate for the transaortic approach to left-sided APs ranges from 0% to 8% and is typically less than 4%.[32,49,63-65,69-76] Half of all complications are vascular related due to arterial access and include hematomas, dissections, pseudoaneurysms, and atrioventricular fistulas.[80,81] Almost unique to the transaortic approach is damage to the aortic or mitral valve. Aortic valve damage occurs in up to 30% of pediatric patients undergoing a retrograde ablation technique.[33] Aortic leaflet perforation and catheter entrapment in the mitral valve apparatus have been reported.[82,83] The latter may require transesophageal echocardiography to direct the extraction, and surgical removal has been necessary. By removing the CS catheter, the mitral annulus may be relaxed, facilitating catheter removal. Dissection or thrombosis of the left main coronary artery has resulted from catheter trauma or energy delivery in the artery.[84] There is a 2% risk of thromboembolic events due to thrombus formation on the catheter, despite anticoagulation or dislodgment of aortic debri.[85] A 1.5% risk of tamponade, stroke, pericardial effusion, or cardiac perforation is reported for ablations at all locations. The risk of complications is higher for patients older than 65 years of age.[86]

The reported incidence of complications with the trans-septal approach is 0% to 6% in adults and 0% to 25% in pediatric series.[32,49,63-65,74,87,88] The trans-septal approach greatly reduces the incidence of vascular complications but introduces potential complications from atrial septal puncture. In large series of trans-septal procedures performed in the catheterization laboratory, the incidence of major complications related to access was 1.3% and included tamponade (1.2%), embolization (0.08%),

TABLE 20–7				
*Success Rates for Right Free Wall Accessory Pathways**				
Authors (Ref. No.)	No. of Patients	Acute Success (%)	Recurrence (%)	Comments
Calkins et al. (77)	92	90	14	Power-controlled ablation
Swartz et al. (32)	12	67	16.7	Power-controlled ablation
Jackman et al. (78)	14	100	9	Power-controlled ablation
Lesh et al. (66)	21[†]	80	11.8	Power-controlled ablation
Haissaguerre et al. (41)	32	93.7	11	—
Drago et al. (51)	21	95	0	Pediatric series with electroanatomic mapping

*Non-Ebstein's anomaly series.
[†]No. of accessory pathways.

and death (0.08%).[89] Thermal injury to the circumflex artery is also possible.

There is limited experience with ablation within the CS. To date, only mural thrombus or venous branch stenosis has been reported.[57] There remain the theoretical but genuine risks of perforation, catheter adhesion, or coronary artery injury, however.

Complications from right free wall AP ablation are rare and are less common than for other AP locations.[32,41,66,78,90] Cardiac perforation may rarely occur, as may pulmonary embolism. Stenosis of a marginal right coronary artery branch was reported in a child with Ebstein's anomaly.[91] Mapping of the right coronary artery can lead to arterial injury or thrombosis.

Troubleshooting the Difficult Case

The most common causes of failed AP ablations are inability to access the target site (25% of cases), catheter instability (23%), mapping errors due to oblique AP orientation (11%), epicardial AP (8%), and recurrent atrial fibrillation (3%).[92] These problems and possible solutions are listed in Table 20–8. Misdiagnosis of the arrhythmia mechanism is more common for left than for right free wall APs. For left free wall APs, the diagnosis of ORT may be mimicked by atrioventricular nodal reentry with eccentric atrial activation or by atrial tachycardias arising from the CS musculature or the ligament of Marshall.[11,28,30] These arrhythmias can be recognized by the presence of decremental retrograde conduction only and by the ability to dissociate the ventricle from the tachycardia. It should be noted that, during retrograde atrioventricular nodal conduction in patients without APs, the far lateral to anterolateral CS is frequently activated in a distal to proximal sequence.[93] This results from rapid conduction over Bachmann's bundle and may be confused with retrograde conduction over an AP. Parahisian pacing maneuvers validate the presence of retrograde right free wall AP conduction with consistency, but left free wall APs may be missed.[27]

Difficulties with mapping may occur if no favorable ablation sites are found. If both antegrade and retrograde AP conduction are present, it may be useful to map conduction in the opposite direction to that which is problematic (i.e., map retrograde conduction if antegrade mapping fails).[92] It should be remembered that most APs have an oblique course, and the atrial and ventricular insertions can be several centimeters apart. If no early antegrade or retrograde sites are found for left free wall APs in the CS, direct mapping of the mitral annulus should be performed, because the CS is usually anatomically removed from the course of the AP. It is possible to place multielectrode "halo" catheters along the mitral annulus through trans-septal access for difficult cases. Altering of the direction of AP antegrade or retrograde activation may make the electrogram components more apparent and reveal AP potentials.[47] This approach can be used for right free wall APs as well. Changing the approach of the mapping catheter to access sites of interest may be needed. For left APs, changing from transaortic to trans-septal mapping, or vice versa, may be helpful. For right-sided APs, changing from the femoral to a subclavian or internal jugular approach can be tried. If the AP demonstrates slow antegrade or retrograde conduction, the usual timing criteria used to identify successful ablation sites may not be applicable. In such cases, the earliest activation sites should be sought. Mapping of electrogram polarity reversal is particularly helpful in this situation, because this technique is independent of electrogram timing.[49] The use of 2F multielectrode catheters to map the CS branches or the right coronary artery can be tried.[94] For complex cases, the use of electroanatomic mapping systems can be valuable. The occurrence of frequent atrial fibrillation may preclude mapping, especially for retrograde-only APs. In such cases, small incremental doses of ibutilide (0.1 mg to maximum 1 to 2 mg) may prevent atrial arrhythmias without altering AP conduction.

Poor catheter mobility and stability are the most common reasons for failed AP ablations.[92] Catheter stability can be enhanced by using preformed sheaths, or different catheter curvatures and shaft stiffnesses, or by changing the approach to the ablation site (e.g., transaortic to trans-septal). Rapid pacing or the use of cryothermic energy may also stabilize the catheter during ablation.

RF ablation may also fail due to the inability to deliver sufficient current or to achieve satisfactory temperatures at the target site. If low current delivery is a problem, cooled ablation electrodes can be used.[55] If satisfactory temperatures cannot be reached, the use of large (8-mm) electrodes and high-output generators should be considered after poor catheter contact is excluded as a source of the problem.

The inability to ablate an AP from endocardial approaches suggests an epicardial location.[44] Further attempts at endocardial ablation slightly away from the annulus may occasionally be successful for pathways inserting off the annulus. Left free wall epicardial APs may be recognized by earliest activation times or large AP potentials recorded in the CS or in a venous tributary. Coronary muscular connections

TABLE 20–8

Troubleshooting the Difficult Case

Problem	Causes	Solution
Misdiagnosis	Atrioventricular nodal reentry with eccentric atrial activation	Demonstrate only decremental retrograde conduction, dissociate atrium and/or ventricle from tachycardia
	Atrial tachycardia near atrioventricular annulus or from CS musculature	Dissociate ventricle from tachycardia
No early or favorable target sites	Poor catheter mobility	Use preformed sheaths or "halo" catheter, change catheter reach or stiffness
	CS distant from mitral annulus	Map mitral annulus directly
	Unable to discriminate component electrograms	Map AP conduction in opposite direction, change approach of mapping catheter (e.g., transaortic to trans-septal), reverse direction of AP activation wavefront, map electrogram polarity reversal, simultaneous pacing
	Long AP conduction times	Map electrogram polarity reversal or shortest times with electroanatomic mapping system
	Epicardial AP location	Map CS and venous branches, map right coronary artery, epicardial mapping by pericardial access, map atrial appendages or ventricle apical to atrioventricular annulus
	Ligament of Marshall connection	Map left atrium anterior to left superior pulmonary vein
	Ebstein's anomaly	Simultaneous atrial and ventricular pacing or atrial or ventricular premature stimuli to separate fractionated electrograms, map right coronary artery, use computerized mapping system
Unsuccessful energy delivery	Poor catheter stability and/or contact	Use preformed sheaths, change catheter curvature, reach or stiffness; change catheter approach to ablation site (e.g., femoral to subclavian for right-sided AP); rapid pacing during ablation, use cryoablation
	Low temperatures with radiofrequency ablation	Improve catheter contact; use high-output generator and large-tip catheter
	Low current delivery with radiofrequency ablation	Lower system impedance (additional skin patches); use irrigated or cooled radiofrequency catheter; use cryoablation
	Epicardial AP	Ablation in CS or tributary with cryoablation or cooled radiofrequency; percutaneous epicardial ablation
	Wrong location	Continued mapping, map polarity reversal, map AP conduction in alternate direction, map for epicardial AP, consider unusual AP locations

AP, accessory pathway; AV, atrioventricular; CS, coronary sinus.

to the ventricle are typically mapped to the proximal middle cardiac vein or a posterior venous branch.[10] Ablation within the CS or venous branch may be necessary. For these applications, cryoablation provides the greatest safety, followed by irrigated-tip RF ablation and, finally, noncooled RF ablation. Epicardial mapping and ablation via percutaneous pericardial access provides another approach to epicardial AV connections.[63,95]

Intra-atrial conduction block without alteration of AP conduction after ablation delivery may occur in 6.9% of attempts at left free wall AP ablation.[96] In this situation, the resulting abrupt change or reversal of the retrograde atrial activation sequence may be misinterpreted as the appearance of a new arrhythmia (Fig. 20–20). Careful mapping along the CS distal to the ablation site will reveal persistent sites of early atrial activation.

FIGURE 20–20. Intra-atrial conduction block after radiofrequency energy delivery for left lateral accessory pathway (AP). **A**, Electrograms and surface ECG tracings in orthodromic reciprocating tachycardia with earliest atrial activation in the distal coronary sinus (CS 1,2). After ablation the tachycardia cycle length is unchanged at 310 msec, but ventricle-to-atrial (VA) times are prolonged and the atrial activation is earliest in the proximal His electrogram (HIS p). The CS is now activated from proximal (CS 9,10) to distal. ABL d, ablation distal; ABL p, ablation proximal; I, F, V1, surface ECG; RVA, right ventricle. **B**, Schematic illustration of the reentry circuits before and after ablation. Before ablation, there is left atrial activation radiating proximally and distally from the AP insertion (*arrows*). After ablation, intra-atrial block results in left atrial activation only distally from the AP insertion. The wavefront crosses over the roof of the left atrium to the atrial septum and then conducts proximal to distal in the CS. The ablation catheter recorded a VA time of 40 msec distal to the site of block and the tachycardia was terminated with ablation to this site. LA, left atrium; LIPV, left inferior pulmonary vein; RA, right atrium.

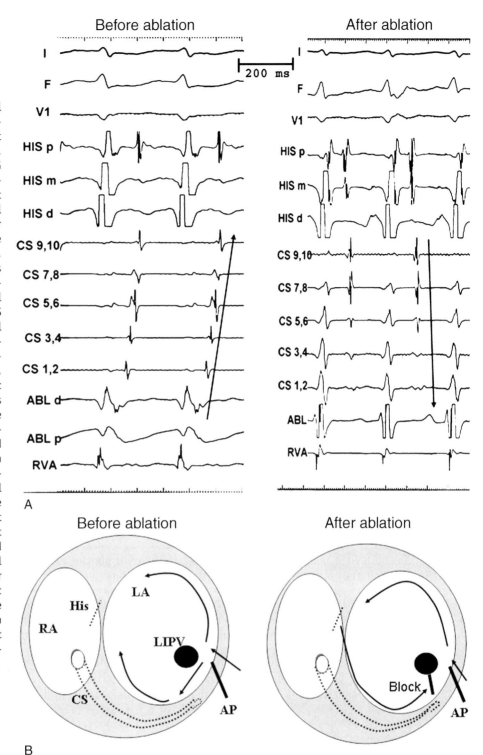

References

1. Yee R, Klein GJ, Prystowsky E: The Wolff-Parkinson-White syndrome and related variants. In Zipes D (ed.): Cardiac Electrophysiology: From Cell to Bedside, 3rd ed. Philadelphia: WB Saunders, 2000, pp 845-861.

2. Becker AE, Anderson RH: The Wolff-Parkinson-White syndrome and its anatomical substratres. Anat Rec 201:169-177, 1981.

3. Becker A, Anderson R, Durrer D, et al.: The anatomical substrates of Wolff-Parkinson-White Syndrome: A clinical correlation in seven patients. Circulation 57:870-879, 1978.

4. Anderson R, Ho S: Anatomy of the atrioventricular junctions with regard to ventricular preexcitation. Pacing Clin Electrophysiol 20:2072-2076, 1997.

5. Klein G, Hackel D, Gallagher J: Anatomic substrate of impaired conduction over an accessory atrioventricular pathway in the Wolff-Parkinson-White syndrome. Circulation 61:1249-1256, 1980.

6. Shinbane J, Lesh M, Stevenson W, et al.: Anatomic and electrophysiologic relation between the coronary sinus and mitral annulus: Implications for ablation of left-sided accessory pathways. Am Heart J 135:93-98, 1998.

7. Ho SY, Goltz D, McCarthy K, et al.: The atrioventricular junctions in Ebstein malformation. Heart 83:444-449, 2000.

8. Cappato RI, Schluter M, Weiss C, et al.: Radiofrequency current catheter ablation of accessory atrioventricular pathways in Ebstein's anomaly. Circulation 94:376-383, 1996.

9. Chauvin M, Shah D, Haissaguerre M, et al.: The anatomic basis of connections between the coronary sinus musculature and the left atrium in humans. Circulation 101:647-652, 2000.

10. Sun Y, Arruda M, Otomo K, et al.: Coronary sinus-ventricular accessory connections producing posteroseptal and left posterior accessory pathways: Incidence and electrophysiological identification. Circulation 106:1362-1367, 2002.

11. Hwang C, Peter C, Chen P: Radiofrequency ablation of accessory pathways guided by the location of the ligament of Marshall. J Cardiovasc Electrophysiol 14:616-620, 2003.

12. Milstein S, Dunnigan A, Tang C, et al.: Right atrial appendage to right ventricle accessory atrioventricular connection: A case report. Pacing Clin Electrophysiol 20:1877-1880, 1997.

13. Goya M, Takahashi A, Nakagawa H, et al.: A case of catheter ablation of necessary atrioventricular connection between the right atrial appendage and right ventricle guided by a three-dimensional electroanatomic mapping system. J Cardiovasc Electrophysiol 10:1112-1118, 1999.

14. Arruda M, McClelland J, Beckman K, et al.: Atrial appendage-ventricular connections: A new variant of preexcitation. Circulation 90:I-126, 1994.

15. De Chillou C, Rodriguez L, Schlapfer J, et al.: Clinical characteristics and electrophysiologic properties of atrioventricular accessory pathways: Importance of the accessory pathway location. J Am Coll Cardiol 20:666-671, 1992.

16. Katsouras C, Greakas G, Goudevenos J, et al.: Localization of accessory pathways by the electrocardiogram: Which is the degree of accordance of three algorithms in use? Pacing Clin Electrophysiol 27:189-193, 2004.

17. Teo W, Klein G, Guiraudon G, et al.: Predictive accuracy of electrophysiologic localization of accessory pathways. J Am Coll Cardiol 18:527-532, 1991.

18. Arruda M, McClelland J, Wang X, et al.: Development and validation of an ECG algorithm for identifying accessory pathway ablation site in Wolff-Parkinson-White Syndrome. J Cardiovasc Electrophysiol 9:2-12, 1998.

19. Chiang C, Chen S, Teo W, et al.: An accurate stepwise electrocardiographic algorithm for localization of accessory pathways in patients with Wolff-Parkinson-White Syndrome from a comprehensive analysis of delta waves and r/s ratio during sinus rhythm. Am J Cardiol 76:40-46, 1995.

20. Boersma L, Garcia-Moran E, Mont L, et al.: Accessory pathway localization by QRS polarity in children with Wolff-Parkinson-White syndrome. J Cardiovasc Electrophysiol 13:1222-1226, 2002.

21. Xie B, Heald S, Bashir Y, et al.: Localization of accessory pathways from the 12-lead electrocardiogram using a new algorithm. Am J Cardiol 74:161-165, 1994.

22. Chen S, Tai C: Ablation of atrioventricular accessory pathways: Current technique-state of the art. Pacing Clin Electrophysiol 24:1795-2809, 2001.

23. Fitzgerald DM, Hawthorne HR, Crossley GH, et al.: P wave morphology during atrial pacing along the atrioventricular ring: ECG localization of the site of origin of retrograde atrial activation. J Electrocardiol 29:1-10, 1996.

24. Josephson M: Preexcitaion syndromes. In Josephson M: Clinical Cardiac Electrophysiology: Techniques and Interpretations, 3rd ed. Philadelphia: Lippincott Williams & Wilkins, 2002, pp 322-424.

25. Miles WM, Yee R, Klein GJ, et al.: The preexcitation index: an aid in determining the mechanism of supraventricular tachycardia and localizing accessory pathways. Circulation 74:493-500, 1986.

26. Yang Y, Cheng J, Glatter K, et al.: Quantitative effects of functional bundle branch block in patients with atrioventricular reentrant tachycardia. Am J Cardiol 85:826-831, 2000.

27. Hirao K, Otomo K, Wang X, et al.: Para-Hisian pacing: A new method for differentiating retrograde conduction over an accessory AV pathway from conduction over the AV node. Circulation 94:1027-1035, 1996.

28. Pavin D, Boulmier D, Daubert J, et al.: Permanent left atrial tachycardia: Radiofrequency catheter ablation through the coronary sinus. J Cardiovasc Electrophysiol 13:395-398, 2002.

29. Knight BP, Zivin A, Souza J, et al.: A technique for the rapid diagnosis of atrial tachycardia in the electrophysiology laboratory. J Am Coll Cardiol 33:775-781, 1999.

30. Hwang C, Martin D, Goodman J, et al.: Atypical atrioventricular node reciprocating tachycardia masquerading as tachycardia using a left-sided accessory pathway. J Am Coll Cardiol 30:218-225, 1997.

31. Kuck K-H, Schluter M: Single-catheter approach to radiofrequency current ablation of left-sided accessory pathways in patients with Wolff-Parkinson-White syndrome. Circulation 84:2366-2375, 1991.

32. Swartz F, Tracy CM, Fletcher RD: Radiofrequency endocardial catheter ablation of accessory atrioventricular pathway atrial insertion sites. Circulation 87:487-499, 1993.

33. Minich LL, Snider AR, Dick M: Doppler detection of valvular regurgitation after radiofrequency ablation of accessory connections. Am J Cardiol 70:116-117, 1992.

34. Villacastin J, Almendral J, Medina O, et al.: "Pseudodisappearance" of atrial electrogram during orthodromic tachycardia: New criteria for successful ablation of concealed left-sided accessory pathways. J Am Coll Cardiol 27:853-859, 1996.

35. Chen X, Borggrefe M, Shenasa M, et al.: Characteristics of local electrogram predicting successful transcatheter radiofrequency ablation of left-sided accessory pathways. J Am Coll Cardiol 20:656-665, 1992.

36. Hindricks G, Kottkamp H, Chen X, et al.: Localization and radiofrequency catheter ablation of left-sided accessory pathways during atrial fibrillation. J Am Coll Cardiol 25:444-451, 1955.

37. Bashir Y, Heald SC, Katritsis D, et al.: Radiofrequency ablation of accessory atrioventricular pathways: Predictive value of local electrogram characteristics for the identification of successful target sites. Br Heart J 69:315-321, 1993.

38. Cappato R, Schlüter M, Mont L, Kuck K-H: Anatomic, electrical and mechanical factors affecting bipolar endocardial electrogram: Impact on catheter ablation of manifest left free-wall accessory pathways. Circulation 90:884-894, 1994.

39. Xie B, Heald SC, Camm AJ, et al.: Successful radiofrequency ablation of accessory pathways with the first energy delivery: The anatomic and electrical characteristics. Eur Heart J 17:1072-1079, 1996.

40. Barlow MA, Klein GJ, Simpson CS, et al.: Unipolar electrogram characteristics predictive of successful radiofrequency catheter ablation of accessory pathways. J Cardiovasc Electrophysiol 11:146-154, 2000.

41. Haissaguerre M, Gaita F, Marcus FI, et al.: Radiofrequency catheter ablation of accessory pathways: A contemporary review. J Cardiovasc Electrophysiol 5:532-552, 1994.

42. Calkins H, Kim Y-N, Schmaltz S, et al.: Electrogram criteria for identification of appropriate target sites for radiofrequency catheter ablation of accessory atrioventricular connections. Circulation 85:565-573, 1992.

43. Jackman WM, Friday KJ, Fitzgerald DM, et al.: Localization of left free-wall and posteroseptal accessory atrioventricular pathways by direct recordings of accessory pathway activation. Pacing Clin Electrophysiol 12:204-214, 1989.

44. Langberg JJ, Man KC, Vorperian VR, et al.: Recognition and catheter ablation of subepicardial accessory pathways. J Am Coll Cardiol 22:1100-1104, 1993.

45. Yamabe H, Shimasaki Y, Honda O, et al.: Localization of the ventricular insertion site of concealed left-sided accessory pathways using ventricular pace mapping. Pacing Clin Electrophysiol 25:940-950, 2002.

46. Nakao K, Seto S, Iliev II, et al.: Simultaneous atrial and ventricular pacing to facilitate mapping of concealed left-sided accessory pathways. Pacing Clin Electrophysiol 25:922-928, 2002.

47. Otomo K, Gonzalez M, Beckman K, et al.: Reversing the direction of paced ventricular and atrial wavefronts reveals an oblique course in accessory AV pathways and improves localization for catheter ablation. Circulation 104:550-556, 2001.

48. Tai C-T, Chen S-A, Chiang C-E, et al.: Identification of fiber orientation in left free-wall accessory pathways: Implications for radiofrequency ablation. J Intervent Cardiac Electrophysiol 1:235-241, 1997.

49. Fisher WG, Swartz JF: Three dimensional electrogram mapping improves ablation of left-sided accessory pathways. Pacing Clin Electrophysiol 15:2344-2356, 1992.

50. Haissaguerre M, Fischer B, Warin J-F, et al.: Electrogram patterns predictive of successful radiofrequency catheter ablation of accessory pathways. Pacing Clin Electrophysiol 15:2138-2145, 1992.

51. Drago F, Silvetti M, Di Pino A, et al.: Exclusion of fluoroscopy during ablation treatment of right accessory pathway in children. J Cardiovasc Electrophysiol 13:778-782, 2002.

52. Langberg JJ, Calkins H, El-Atassi R, et al.: Temperature monitoring during radiofrequency ablation of accessory pathways. Circulation 86:1469-1474, 1992.

53. Twidale N, Wang Z, Beckman KJ, et al.: Factors associated with recurrences of accessory pathway conduction after radiofrequency catheter ablation. Pacing Clin Electrophysiol 14:2042-2048, 1991.

54. Rodriguez L, Geller J, Tse H, et al.: Acute results of transvenous cryoablation of supraventricular tachycardia (atrial fibrillation, atrial flutter, Wolff-Parkinson-White syndrome, atrioventricular nodal reentry tachycardia). J Cardiovasc Electrophysiol 13:1082-1089, 2002.

55. Yamane T, Jais P, Shah D, et al.: Efficacy and safety of an irrigated-tip catheter for the ablation of accessory pathways resistant to conventional radiofrequency ablation. Circulation 102:2565-2568, 2000.

56. Wang X, McCelland J, Beckman K, et al.: Left free-wall accessory pathway ablation from the coronary sinus: Unique coronary sinus electrogram pattern. Circulation 86:I-586, 1992.

57. Haissaguerre M, Gaita F, Fischer B, et al.: Radiofrequency catheter ablation of left lateral accessory pathways via the coronary sinus. Circulation 86:1464-1468, 1992.

58. Giorgberidze I, Saksena S, Krol RB, Mathew P: Efficacy and safety of radiofrequency catheter ablation of left-sided accessory pathways through the coronary sinus. Am J Cardiol 76:359-365, 1995.

59. Langberg JJ, Man KC, Vorperian VR, et al.: Recognition and catheter ablation of subepicardial accessory pathways. J Am Coll Cardiol 22:1100-1104, 1993.

60. Cappato R, Weiss C, Brown E, et al.: Catheter ablation of manifest accessory pathways related to the coronary sinus. New Trends Arrhythmias 9:421, 1993.

61. Gaita F, Paperini L, Riccardi R, et al.: Cryothermic ablation within the coronary sinus of an epicardial posterolateral pathway. J Cardiovasc Electrophysiol 13:1160-1163, 2002.

62. Schweikert RA, Saliba WI, Tommassoni G, et al.: Percutaneous pericardial instrumentation for endo-epicardial mapping of previously failed ablations. Circulation 108:1329-1335, 2003.

63. De Ponti R, Zardini M, Storti C, et al.: Trans-septal catheterization for radiofrequency catheter ablation of cardiac arrhythmias. Eur Heart J 19:943-950, 1998.

64. Yip ASB, Chow W-H, Yung T-C, et al.: Radiofrequency catheter ablation of left-sided accessory pathways using a transeptal technique and specialized long intravascular sheaths. Jpn Heart J 38:643-650, 1997.

65. Manolis AS, Wang PJ, Estes NAM. Radiofrequency ablation of atrial insertion of left-sided accessory pathways guided by the "W sign." J Cardiovasc Electrophysiol 6:1068-1076, 1995.

66. Lesh MD, Van Hare GF, Schamp DJ, et al.: Curative percutaneous catheter ablation using radiofrequency energy for accessory pathways in all locations: Results in 100 consecutive patients. J Am Coll Cardiol 19:1303-1309, 1992.

67. Chen X, Borggrefe M, Hindricks G, et al.: Radiofrequency ablation of accessory pathways: Characteristics of transiently and permanently effective pulses. Pacing Clin Electrophysiol 15:1122-1130, 1992.

68. Langberg JJ, Calkins H, Kim Y-N, et al.: Recurrence of conduction in accessory atrioventricular connections after initially successful radiofrequency catheter ablation. J Am Coll Cardiol 19:1588-1592, 1992.

69. Deshpande SS, Bremmer S, Sra JS, et al.: Ablation of left free-wall accessory pathways using radiofrequency energy at the atrial insertion site: Transseptal versus transaortic approach. J Cardiovasc Electrophysiol 5:219-231, 1994.

70. Lesh MD, Van Hare GF, Scheinman MM, et al.: Comparison of the retrograde and transeptal methods for ablation of left free-wall accessory pathways. J Am Coll Cardiol 22:542-549, 1993.

71. Natale A, Wathen M, Yee R, et al.: Atrial and ventricular approaches for radiofrequency catheter ablation of left-sided accessory pathways. Am J Cardiol 70:114-116, 1992.

72. Saul JP, Hulse JE, De W, et al.: Catheter ablation of accessory atrioventricular pathways in young patients: Use of long vascular sheaths, the transeptal approach and a retrograde left posterior parallel approach. J Am Coll Cardiol 21:571-583, 1993.

73. Manolis AS, Wang PJ, Estes NAM: Radiofrequency ablation of left-sided accessory pathways: Transaortic versus transseptal approach. Am Heart J 128:896-902, 1994.

74. Vora AM, McMahon S, Jazayeri MR, Dhala A: Ablation of atrial insertion sites of left-sided accessory pathways in children: Efficacy and safety of transeptal versus transoartic approach. Pediatr Cardiol 18:332-338, 1997.

75. Ma C, Dong J, Yang X, et al.: A randomized comparison between retrograde and transseptal approach for radiofrequency ablation of left-sided accessory pathways. Pacing Clin Electrophysiol 18:479, 1995.

76. Montenero AS, Drago F, Crea F, et al.: Ablazione transcatetere con radiofrequenza delle tachicardie sopraventricolari in eta pediatrica: Risultati immediati e di un follow-up a medio termine. G Ital Cardiol 26:31-40, 1996.

77. Calkins H, Yong P, Miller J, et al.: Catheter ablation of accessory pathways, atrioventricular nodal reentrant tachycardia, and the atrioventricular junction: Final results of a prospective, multicenter clinical trial. Circulation 99:262-270, 1999.

78. Jackman WM, Wang X, Friday KJ, et al.: Catheter ablation of accessory atrioventricular pathways (Wolff-Parkinson-White syndrome) by radiofrequency current. N Engl J Med 324:1605-1611, 1991.

79. Reich J, Auld D, Hulse E, et al.: The pediatric radiofrequency ablation registry's experience with Ebstein's anomaly. J Cardiovasc Electrophysiol 9:1370-1377, 1998.

80. Greene TO, Huang SKS, Wagshal AB, et al.: Cardiovascular complications after radiofrequency catheter ablation of supraventricular tachyarrhythmias. Am J Cardiol 74:615-617, 1994.

81. Chen S-A, Chiang C-E, Tai C-T, et al.: Complications of diagnostic electrophysiologic studies and radiofrequency catheter ablation in patients with tachyarrhythmias: An eight-year survey of 3,966 consecutive procedures in a tertiary referral center. Am J Cardiol 77:41-46, 1996.

82. Conti JB, Geiser E, Curtis AB: Catheter entrapment in the mitral valve apparatus during radiofrequency ablation. Pacing Clin Electrophysiol 17:1681-1685, 1994.

83. Seifert MJ, Morady F, Calkins H, et al.: Aortic leaflet perforation during radiofrequency ablation. Pacing Clin Electrophysiol 14:1582-1585, 1991.

84. Kosinoki DJ, Grubb BP, Burket MW, et al.: Occlusion of the left main coronary artery during radiofrequency ablation for the Wolff-Parkinson-White syndrome. Eur J C P E 1:63-66, 1993.

85. Epstein MR, Knapp LD, Martindill M, et al.: Embolic complications associated with radiofrequency catheter ablation. Am J Cardiol 77:655-658, 1996.

86. Hindricks G: The multicentre European radiofrequency survey (MERFS): Complications of radiofrequency catheter ablation of arrhythmias. Eur Heart J 14:1644-1653, 1993.

87. Dick M, O'Conner BK, Serwer GA, et al.: Use of radiofrequency current to ablate accessory connections in children. Circulation 84:2318-2324, 1991.

88. Benito F, Sanchez C: Radiofrequency catheter ablation of accessory pathways in infants. Heart 78:160-162, 1997.

89. Roelke M, Smith AJC, Palacios IF: The technique and safety of transeptal left heart catheterization: The Massachusetts General Hospital experience with 1,279 procedures. Cathet Cardiovasc Diagn 32:332-339, 1994.

90. Calkins H, Langberg J, Sousa J, et al.: Radiofrequency catheter ablation of accessory atrioventricular connections in 250 patients. Circulation 19:1303-1309, 1992.

91. Bertram H, Bokenkamp R, Peuster M, et al.: Coronary artery stenosis after radiofrequency catheter ablation of accessory atrioventricular pathways in children with Ebstein's malformation. Circulation 103:538-543, 2001.

92. Morady F, Strickberger SA, Man KC, et al.: Reasons for prolonged or failed attempt at radiofrequency catheter ablation of accessory pathways. J Am Coll Cardiol 27:683-689, 1996.

93. Suzuki F, Tosaka T, Ashikawa H, et al.: Earlier activation of the distal than the proximal site of the coronary sinus may represent retrograde conduction through AV node: Significance of recording of far distal coronary sinus. Pacing Clin Electrophysiol 19:331-341, 1996.

94. Cappato R, Schluter M, Weiss C, et al.: Mapping of the coronary sinus and great cardiac vein using a 2-french electrode catheter and a right femoral approach. J Cardiovasc Electrophysiol 8:371-376, 1997.

95. Valderrabano M, Cesario DA, Sen J, et al.: Percutaneous epicardial mapping during ablation of difficult accessory pathways as an alternative to cardiac surgery. Heart Rhythm 3:311-316, 2004.

96. Luria DM, Nemec J, Etheridge SP, et al.: Intra-atrial conduction block along the mitral annulus during accessory pathway ablation: evidence for a left atrial "isthmus." J Cardiovasc Electrophysiol 12:744-749, 2001.

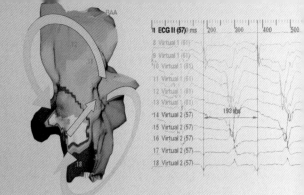

21

Ablation of Posteroseptal Accessory Pathways

Mark A. Wood

Key Points

- Mapping of posteroseptal accessory pathways (APs) may involve the inferior right and left paraseptal atrioventricular (AV) annuli, proximal coronary sinus (CS), middle cardiac vein, posterior cardiac vein, and coronary venous diverticula.

- Ablation targets are the accessory pathway potentials, the earliest atrial or ventricular activation by AP conduction for endocardial APs, and the CS muscular extension potentials and ventricular insertions for epicardial accessory AV connections.

- Angiographic catheters for injection of the CS and possibly the right coronary artery may be needed, as may preformed sheaths and apparatus for trans-septal access. Irrigated radiofrequency ablation or cryoablation systems and catheter location/navigation systems may be helpful.

- Sources of difficulty include complex anatomy possibly requiring right- and left-sided mapping, epicardial connections involving the coronary venous system and diverticula, and injury to the right coronary artery or AV nodal artery from ablation.

Posteroseptal accessory pathways (APs) are the second most common location for accessory connections and account for 25% to 30% of APs in most series.[1-4] Surgically, these connections are the most difficult to transect, owing to the complex anatomy of the posteroseptal region.[5,6] In the electrophysiology laboratory, ablation of these connections has been associated with longer procedure times, greater fluoroscopic exposure, and more radiofrequency (RF) lesions than any other location.[7,8] Ironically, these pathways are ablated with catheter-based techniques with a very high degree of success despite the potential complexity of mapping in this area.[3,4,7-11]

Anatomy

The term "posteroseptal" is inaccurate, because this region is inferior to the true atrial septum.[12-15] The term *inferoparaseptal* would be more anatomically correct; however, the posteroseptal terminology is ingrained in the literature and will be used in this chapter.

The anatomy of the posteroseptal region is more complex than for any other AP location. This area includes the pyramidal space, which represents the confluence of all four cardiac chambers and the coronary sinus (CS) in their closest proximity (Fig. 21-1).[12-15] The superior boundary of the pyramidal space is the central fibrous body. The anterior aspect is the ventricular septum and the posterior walls are formed by the convergence of the left and right atria. The tricuspid valve annulus is displaced apically 5 to

10 mm in relation to the mitral annulus. In this gap between the mitral and tricuspid annuli lies the right atrium–left ventricular sulcus. Here is the junction between the inferomedial right atrium and the posterosuperior process of the left ventricle. The right atrium in this area is separated from the left ventricle by only a thin sheet of fibrous tissue that may be readily crossed by accessory connections (Fig. 21-2).[12-15] The ostium of the CS abuts the superior margin of the right atrial–left ventricular sulcus and the paraseptal mitral annulus in the pyramidal space. This proximity may allow for the ablation of APs from the proximal CS itself in many cases. In anatomic series, the distance from the CS ostium (os) to the left margin of the posteroseptal space is 2.3 ± 0.4 cm.[12] Thus, the left boundary of the posteroseptal space is often defined as extending 2 cm from the CS os. The topography of the right posteroseptal space from the right atrial perspective includes the inferior portion of the triangle of Koch and the area around the ostium of the CS (see Fig. 21-2).[15]

APs in this region can take a variety of courses (Fig. 21-3). From the surgical literature, most of these connections are believed to be right atrial-to-left ventricular pathways skirting the atrioventricular (AV) annulus.[2,5,6,10,16] The course of such connections can be explained by the interface of the inferior medial right atrium with the posterosuperior process of the left ventricle in this region (see Fig. 21-2). AP connections may also run from the paraseptal left atrium to left ventricle and from the paraseptal right atrium to right ventricle (see Fig. 21-3).[7] In up to 20% of posteroseptal connections, the AV circuit results from CS musculature connections between the ventricle and left atrium (Fig. 21-4).[16] Of these connections, 70% are

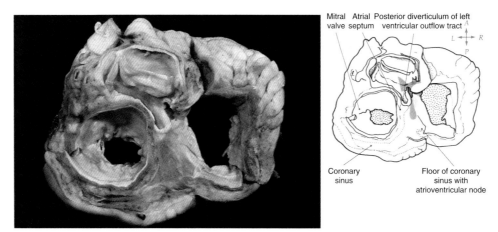

FIGURE 21-1. Anatomy of pyramidal space and posteroseptal regions in the human heart. This short axis view is cut through the level of the coronary sinus (labeled). The position of the atrioventricular node and conduction axis is illustrated in the schematic. Note the fat filled pyramidal space formed between the mitral and tricuspid annuli and above the floor of the coronary sinus. *(From Wilcox BR, Anderson RH [eds.]: Surgical Anatomy of the Heart. Edinburgh: Churchill Livingstone, 1985, p 4-5, with permission.)*

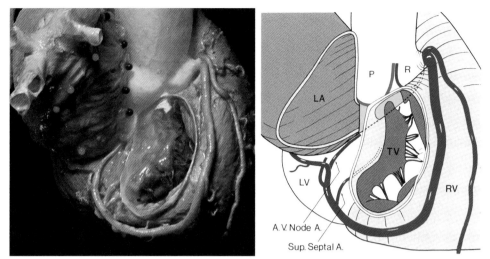

FIGURE 21–2. View of the pyramidal space and right endocardial posteroseptal region from the perspective of the right atrium. The AV nodal artery is seen in the pyramidal space and may be vulnerable to injury from ablation in the posteroseptal region. In the schematic representation of the heart, the left ventricle is white and the right ventricle is blue. Note the region of the right atrium (cut away) above the tricuspid valve that is in apposition with the superior posterior portion of the left ventricle. This area may give rise to right atrial to left ventricular accessory pathways. A, artery; LA, left atrium; LV, left ventricle; P, posterior aortic cusp; R, right aortic cusp; RV, right ventricle; Sup., superior; TV, tricuspid valve. *(From McAlpine WA: Heart and Coronary Arteries. New York: Springer-Verlag, 1975, pp 160-162, with permission.)*

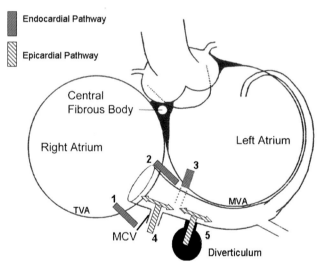

FIGURE 21–3. Schematic showing possible courses of accessory AV connections in the posteroseptal region. A short axis view of the heart is shown. MCV, middle cardiac vein; MVA, mitral valve annulus; TVA, tricuspid valve annulus. 1) right atrial to right ventricular connection crossing tricuspid annulus, 2) right atrial to left ventricular connection inserting in the posterior superior process of the left ventricle, 3) left atrial to left ventricular connection crossing the mitral annulus, 4) coronary sinus muscular extension to left ventricle over the middle (or posterior) cardiac vein, 5) coronary sinus muscular connection to diverticulum that contains muscular fibers in continuity with the left ventricle. Note that connections 4 and 5 are epicardial and connect to the atria by the coronary sinus musculature.

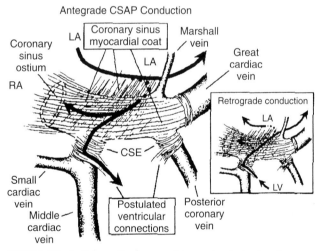

FIGURE 21–4. Schematic for possible anatomic basis of connections between the coronary sinus musculature and left ventricular myocardium (LV). The coronary sinus musculature may form extensions (CSE) over the proximal portions of the middle and posterior cardiac veins. If connections between the coronary sinus musculature and the left (LA) or right (RA) atrial myocardium exist as well, the substrate for reciprocating tachycardias is formed. *(From Sun Y, Arruda M, Otomo K, et al.: Coronary sinus-ventricular accessory connections producing posteroseptal and left posterior accessory pathways: Incidence and electrophysiologic identification. Circulation 106:1362-1367, 2002, with permission.)*

associated with normal CS anatomy. In the normal human heart, a sleeve of myocardial tissue that is continuous with the right atrial myocardium invests the proximal portion of the CS. In 2% to 3% of autopsy specimens, this myocardium forms extensions over the middle or posterior cardiac veins to the epicardial aspect of the left ventricle.[16] If the CS muscular coat also has electrical connection to the left ventricle, the circuit for an epicardial accessory AV connection is present.[17]

In 21% of patients with CS muscular extensions to the left ventricle, the connection occurs in association with a CS diverticulum.[16] These venous anomalies arise within the proximal 1.5 cm of the CS and before the middle cardiac vein in most cases; however, they can arise from the middle or posterior cardiac veins themselves (Fig. 21–5). The body of the diverticulum is typically within the epicardial layers of the posterior superior process of the left ventricle.[2] The walls of a CS diverticulum contain ventricular musculature and are often seen to contract on angiography.[16] This musculature is in continuity with the epicardial left ventricle and with the CS musculature at the mouth of the diverticulum to form the reentry circuit. CS diverticula are reported in 9% of all patients presenting for ablation; if present in patients with evidence of a posteroseptal AP, they are usually the site of the connection.[16,18,19] CS muscular extensions forming accessory AV connections may be associated with coronary venous anomalies other than diverticula.[16]

Pathophysiology

As with any AP connection, posteroseptal connections may participate in reciprocating tachycardia or be activated as a bystander. The pathways associated with permanent junctional reciprocating tachycardia (PJRT) are most commonly found in the posteroseptal location but can rarely be found in free wall locations as well.[10,11] These connections are usually concealed and exhibit slow and decremental retrograde conduction properties that result in incessant reciprocating tachycardia.[10,11]

Diagnosis and Differential Diagnosis

On the surface electrocardiogram (ECG), the distinction between right and left posteroseptal APs has been made based on the presumed site of ventricular

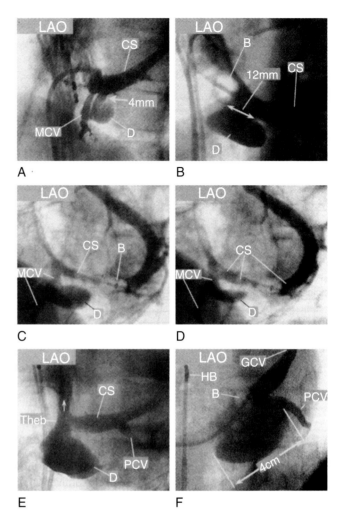

FIGURE 21-5. Coronary sinus (CS) diverticulum (D) visualized by occlusive venography. Dimensions of the anomalies are shown. In **A**, **B**, and **E** the diverticula arise from the coronary sinus. In **C** and **D** the diverticula arise from the middle cardiac vein (MVC). In **F** the diverticulum arises near the posterior cardiac vein. *(From Sun Y, Arruda M, Otomo K, et al.: Coronary sinus-ventricular accessory connections producing posteroseptal and left posterior accessory pathways: Incidence and electrophysiologic identification. Circulation 106:1362-1367, 2002, with permission.)*

insertion. This classification of the surface ECG features has limited ability to predict the site of successful ablation as right- or left-sided, however.[7,9,20,21] For those pathways considered to be right-sided, the delta wave in lead V_1 is negative to isoelectric, with abrupt transition to R > S in lead V_2 (75% of cases) or V_3 (Fig. 21–6). The delta waves are deeply negative in lead III and usually in aVF as well. Those pathways classified as left posteroseptal in location have a more variable ECG presentation, with the delta wave positive or isoelectric in V_1 and sometimes with R > S in V_1 (Fig. 21–7). Lead III is negative, but lead aVF is less

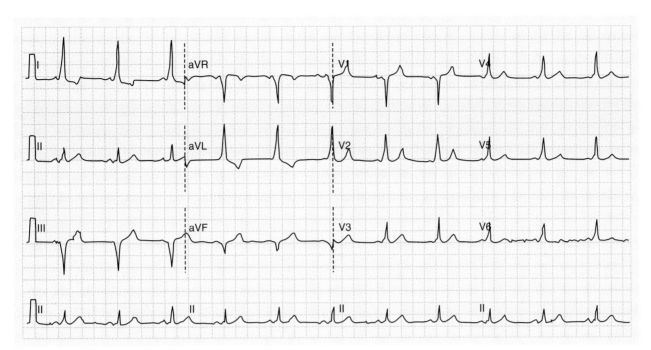

FIGURE 21–6. Surface electrocardiogram from a patient with a manifest right posteroseptal accessory pathway. Note the negative delta wave in lead V1 and abrupt transition to R > S in lead V2. In addition, the delta waves are negative in lead III and aVF but upright in II. This pathway was ablated along the posteroseptal tricuspid annulus.

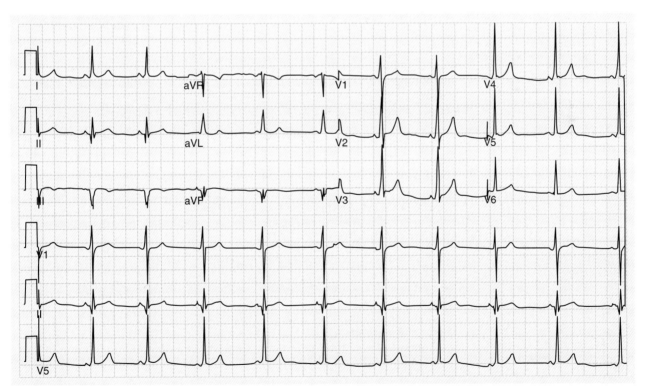

FIGURE 21–7. Surface electrocardiogram consistent with a left posteroseptal accessory pathway. The delta wave is positive in V1 and the transition to R > S is in V2. The delta waves are negative in II, II and aVF. This pathway was ablated 1 cm within the coronary sinus.

commonly negative. In either case, a negative delta wave in lead II was previously thought to be sensitive for indicating an epicardial posteroseptal connection, but larger studies demonstrated a sensitivity for this finding of about 70%.[16] During orthodromic reciprocating tachycardia (ORT), the P-wave morphology on surface ECG commonly is negative in II, III, and aVF; positive in aVR and aVL; and biphasic or isoelectric in V_1. These features do not allow discrimination of right- and left-sided APs based on P-wave morphology.[22] Of interest, with loss of preexcitation during reciprocating tachycardia or after ablation, prominent T wave inversion is often noted with posteroseptal pathways believed to reflect a cardiac memory phenomenon.[23] PJRT manifests with a distinctive ECG pattern, however. This long-RP tachycardia is present for more than 12 hours per day and has large inverted P waves in leads II, III, and aVF.[10,11]

Based on intracardiac recordings, posteroseptal pathways are diagnosed by the demonstration of antegrade and/or retrograde AP conduction with pathway insertion in the inferior right or left paraseptal region, in the proximal 2 cm of the CS including the ostium and its tributaries (Table 21–1).[8,9,19] The diagnosis of CS musculature-to-ventricular connections is based on demonstrating earlier epicardial than endocardial ventricular activation antegrade, earliest retrograde activation of CS musculature with subsequent atrial activation, and AP-like potentials representing activation of the CS muscular connections (Figs. 21–8 and 21–9; see Table 21–1).[16] Reciprocating tachycardias using posteroseptal APs must be differentiated from AV nodal reentry with an eccentric atrial activation sequence and from slow-slow AV nodal reentry with long ventricular-to-atrial (VA) times and earliest atrial activation near the CS os.[24] The differential diagnosis is best accomplished by timed ventricular stimulation during His refractoriness during tachycardia. The diagnosis of reciprocating tachycardia is made by the ability to terminate the tachycardia by premature ventricular complexes that do not conduct to the AV node or atrium and is supported by the ability to advance atrial activation during His refractoriness. The use of parahisian pacing, response of ventricular postpacing interval, comparison of His to atrium times during supraventricular tachycardia, and ventricular pacing at the

---

TABLE 21–1

Diagnostic Criteria for Posteroseptal Accessory Pathway Connections

Type of Connection	Criteria
Posteroseptal AP	Features of AP traversing pyramidal space or inserting along (1) tricuspid annulus near CS ostium, (2) proximal CS, its ostium or tributary vessels, or (3) inferior paraseptal mitral annulus VA interval prolongation 10–30 msec during ORT with ipsilateral bundle branch block
CS muscular extension— antegrade*	Rapid downstroke in unfiltered unipolar endocardial VEGM >15 msec later than onset of far-field ventricular potential at site >1 cm apical to tricuspid and mitral annuli Ventricular activation from MCV, PCV, or CS diverticulum precedes endocardial ventricular activation High-frequency potential (similar to AP potential) from CS muscular extension recorded from MCV, PCV, or CS diverticulum before ventricular activation CS muscular extension potential can be dissociated from local atrial and ventricular activity by programmed stimulation
CS muscular extension— retrograde*	Earliest high frequency potential (similar to AP potential) recorded from MCV, PCV, or CS diverticulum CS muscular extension potential followed by activation of CS muscular coat near the orifice of the vein CS muscular potentials propagate leftward, activating left atrium before right atrium (in absence of prior ablation) CS muscular extension potential can be dissociated from local atrial and ventricular activation
PJRT	Tachycardia present >12 hr/day ORT with typically concealed, slow decrementally conducting AP (>50 msec increase in VA time with tachycardia or pacing), usually in posteroseptal region Exclude fast-slow AVNRT and low septal atrial tachycardia

AP, accessory pathway; AVNRT, atrioventricular nodal reentrant tachycardia; CS, coronary sinus; MCV, middle cardiac vein; ORT, orthodromic reciprocating tachycardia; PCV, posterior cardiac vein; PJRT, permanent junctional reciprocating tachycardia; VA, ventricular-to-atrial; VEGM, ventricular electrogram.
*From reference 16.

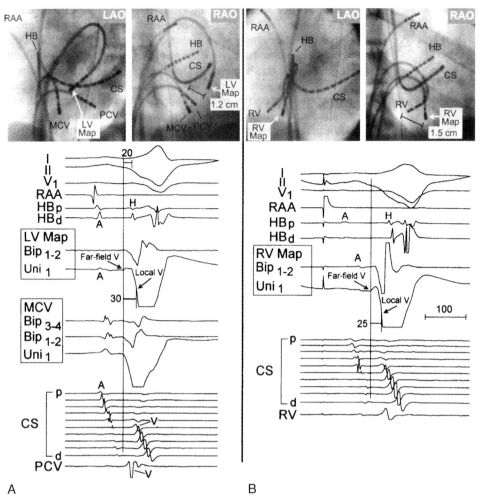

FIGURE 21–8. Intracardiac recordings from a patient with coronary sinus muscular extensions in the middle cardiac vein (MCV). **A,** The earliest ventricular activation from the left ventricular endocardium (LV Map) is far-field (vertical line) and 20 msec before the delta wave onset. The local ventricular activation (local V) is 30 msec after the far-field potential. The earliest ventricular activation is recorded from a catheter deep in the MCV. Bip, bipolar recording; Uni, unipolar recording. The catheter positions are shown. A, atrial electrogram; CS, coronary sinus; d, distal; H, His recording; HB, His bundle; I, II, V1, surface electrocardiogram; LAO, left anterior oblique; LV, left ventricle; p, proximal; PCV, posterior cardiac vein; RAA, right atrial appendage; RAO, right anterior oblique; RV, right ventricle; V, ventricular electrogram. **B,** The earliest endocardial right ventricular recording (local V) occurs 25 msec after a far-field ventricular potential with the catheter 1.5 cm from the posteroseptal tricuspid annulus. *(From Sun Y, Arruda M, Otomo K, et al.: Coronary sinus-ventricular accessory connections producing posteroseptal and left posterior accessory pathways: Incidence and electrophyisiologic identification. Circulation 106:1362-1367, 2002, with permission.)*

same cycle length are also important methods of making the differential diagnosis (Table 21–2).[25]

PJRT is diagnosed by demonstrating a slowly and decrementally conducting AP participating in incessant ORT (see Table 21–1). Approximately 80% of these pathways are located in the posteroseptal region, and they demonstrate antegrade conduction in the minority of patients.[10,11] PJRT using a posteroseptal AP must be differentiated from the fast-slow (atypical) form of AV nodal reentry and from atrial tachycardia. In PJRT, the atrial activation may be advanced or the tachycardia terminated without conduction to the atria by premature ventricular stimuli during His refractoriness. In addition, the atrial-to-His bundle (AH) interval during atrial

pacing at the tachycardia cycle length is within 20 to 40 msec of the AH interval in tachycardia in PJRT. In atypical AV nodal reentry, the difference in AH intervals is greater than 40 msec. A VAAV response to the termination of ventricular pacing with tachycardia entrainments indicates an atrial tachycardia rather than an ORT.

Mapping

The potential locations for posteroseptal APs are many, and the anatomy of this region is complex (see

TABLE 21–2

Differentiating Posteroseptal ORT from AVNRT

Maneuver	Posteroseptal ORT	AVNRT
Parahisian pacing	No change Stim-A with loss of His capture	Increased Stim-A with loss of His capture
PVC during His refractoriness	Advances atrial activation Terminates tachycardia without conduction to atrium	Unable to advance atrial activation Terminates tachycardia only with conduction to atrium
Difference between ventricular PPI and TCL	<115 msec	>115 msec
Difference between VA during ventricular pacing at TCL and VA during tachycardia	<85 msec	>85 msec
VA pacing at ventricular base vs pacing at ventricular apex	VA shorter with pacing of base	VA shorter with pacing of apex

AVNRT, atrioventricular nodal reentrant tachycardia; ORT, orthodromic reciprocating tachycardia; PPI, postpacing interval; PVC, premature ventricular complex; Stim-A, ventricular stimulus-to-atrial electrogram interval; TCL, tachycardia cycle length; VA, ventricular-to-atrial interval.

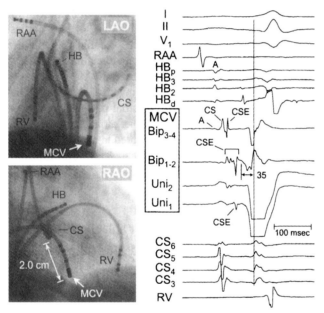

FIGURE 21–9. Recordings of antegrade coronary sinus muscular extension potentials (CSE). Abbreviations per Figure 21–8. The CSE recordings are made from the mapping catheter 2 cm deep into the middle cardiac vein. Analogous to an accessory pathway potential the CSE potentials are interposed between the atrial and ventricular electrograms and precede delta wave onset. *(From Sun Y, Arruda M, Otomo K, et al. Coronary sinus-ventricular accessory connections producing posteroseptal and left posterior accessory pathways: Incidence and electrophyisiologic identification. Circulation 106:1362-1367, 2002, with permission.)*

Fig. 21–3). For these reasons, it is best to adopt a systematic approach to mapping in this area.[2,7] Regardless of the surface ECG manifestations as right- or left-sided, most of these connections can be ablated from a right endocardial approach along the inferior paraseptal tricuspid annulus or in the proximal CS.[2,7-9] Features that suggest successful ablation from the right endocardial approach include a negative delta wave in V_1, a difference in VA time between the His recording and the earliest CS recording of less than 25 msec (validated for concealed APs), and the presence of a long-RP tachycardia (Table 21–3).[2,7,9] However, there are features that strongly predict the need for left endocardial ablation. If present, these features may justify primary left-sided mapping or an early transition to left endocardial mapping. Features associated with successful ablation from the left endocardial approach are earliest retrograde atrial activation in the mid-CS, a difference in VA time between the His electrogram and the earliest CS atrial electrogram of greater than 25 msec (validated for concealed APs), an increase in the VA time of 10 to 30 msec with left bundle branch block, R > S in V_1, and earliest retrograde atrial activation recorded greater than 15 mm from the CS ostium (see Table 21–3).[7,9] Use of this mapping strategy has been shown to reduce procedure and fluoroscopic times through the elimination of unnecessary right-sided mapping (Fig. 21–10).[7]

Some authors have suggested assessing the response of the VA interval during ORT to the development of bundle branch block as a means of predicting the need for right- or left-sided ablation.[2,7-9] If the VA interval is prolonged by less than 10 msec with ipsilateral bundle branch block, the AP is likely to be truly septal in location. Similarly, increases in the VA time of greater than 35 msec suggest a free wall location. If the VA interval increases by 10 to 30 msec with right or left bundle branch block, the pathway is considered to have, respectively, a right or left

TABLE 21-3	
Indicators of Ablation Site	
Right Side Favored	**Left Side Favored**
Difference between VA at His and earliest VA in CS <25 msec	Difference between VA at His and earliest VA in CS >25 msec
Long-RP tachycardia	Earliest retrograde atrial activation in ORT at mid-CS
Negative delta wave in V_1*	R > S wave in V_1 Earliest VA > 15 mm from CS ostium*

*From Haissaguerre M, Gaita F, Marcus FI, Clementy J: Radiofrequency catheter ablation of accessory pathways: A contemporary review. J Cardiovasc Electrophysiol 5:533–552, 1994.

CS, coronary sinus; ORT, orthodromic reciprocating tachycardia; VA, ventricular-to-atrial interval.

TABLE 21-4			
Predictors of Epicardial Atrioventricular Connection			
Finding	**Sensitivity (%)**	**Specificity (%)**	**PPV (%)**
Steep negative delta wave in lead II*	87	79	50
Steep positive delta wave in lead aVR*	61	98	88
Deep S wave in lead V_6*	70	87	57
Presence of CS diverticulum	NA	NA	NA

*From Takahashi A, Shah D, Jais P, et al.: Specific electrocardiographic features of manifest coronary vein posteroseptal accessory pathways. J Cardiovasc Electrophysiol 9:1015-1025, 1998.

CS, coronary sinus; NA, not applicable; PPV, positive predictive value.

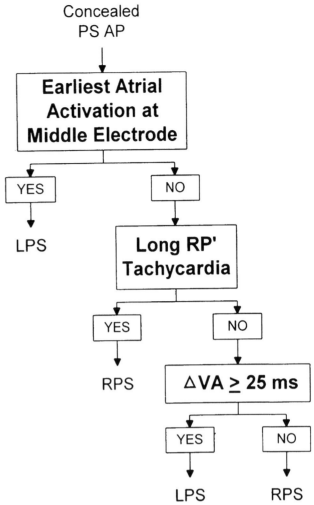

FIGURE 21–10. Algorithm for identifying the need for left endocardial ablation of concealed posteroseptal (PS) accessory pathways (AP). L, left; R, right; ΔVA, difference in ventricular to atrial conduction time between the His bundle recording and the earliest site in the coronary sinus. *(From Chiang CE, Chen S, Tai C, et al. Prediction of successful ablation on concealed posteroseptal accessory pathways by a novel algorithm using baseline electrophysiological parameters. Circulation 93:982-991, 1996, with permission.)*

ventricular insertion. The site of insertion then indicates the approach to ablation as right or left endocardial. Despite the electrophysiologic rationale for this finding, it is frequently inaccurate in predicting the site of successful ablation.[9]

If endocardial mapping fails, attention should turn to the CS.[16] Features that suggest an epicardial accessory AV connection using CS musculature include the presence of a CS diverticulum, a negative delta wave in lead II, a steep positive delta wave in aVR, and a deep S wave in V_6 (Table 21–4).[26] The combination of a steep positive delta wave in aVR and R < S in V_6 provides a 91% positive predictive value for ablation within the CS or middle cardiac vein. A negative delta wave in lead II alone has a 50% positive pre-

dictive value.[26] With these findings or failure of tricuspid annular mapping, attention should turn quickly to detailed CS angiography and thorough mapping of the proximal CS, middle and posterior cardiac veins, and any diverticulum visualized. Retrograde CS angiography can be performed with an 8-French guiding sheath introduced from the femoral, internal jugular, or subclavian vein approaches.[16]

A technique for occlusive venography has been described and is preferred by experienced centers, however.[16] A steerable, balloon-tipped, lumened catheter (Vueport, Cardima, Fremont, Calif.) is introduced into the body of the CS or great cardiac vein. After the balloon is gently inflated, 5 to 15 mL of contrast medium is slowly injected to fill the distal CS.

With continued injection, the entire venous system is filled via collaterals, and the catheter can be slowly withdrawn to enhance retrograde filling of the proximal structures (see Fig. 21–5).[16] The coronary venous system can also be visualized by injection of the left coronary artery. CS muscular connections are present in up to 21% of all patients with posteroseptal connections and in up to 47% of patients with previously failed ablation in this region.[16] CS mapping are facilitated in some cases by catheter manipulation from the right internal jugular or left subclavian vein approaches. These connections most commonly occur in the middle cardiac vein (82%), followed by the posterior cardiac vein (11%), both veins (5%), and the floor of the CS between these two veins (2%).[16] The connections are recorded from 5 to 20 mm deep into the veins.[16] The features that are diagnostic of accessory connections using coronary muscular connections with the left ventricle are given in Table 21–1.

Conventional electrogram criteria for selecting right-sided ablation sites apply: local AV and VA times of 40 msec or less and local ventricular activation greater than 15 msec before delta wave onset (Table 21–5).[1,3,4,9] For mitral annular mapping, the earliest ventricular activation before delta onset is typically later than for right-sided APs. Some authors describe a high frequency of fractionated atrial electrograms at the site of successful mapping of retrograde conduction.[9] Many authors have stressed the frequency and benefit of recording AP potentials from accessory connections in this area.[4,9,15,16] The demonstration of AP potentials may be enhanced by reversing the direction of atrial or ventricular activation at the AP insertion sites.[27] For epicardial connections, the activity of the CS muscular connections can be recorded, analogous to conventional AP connections (see Fig. 21–9).[16] The site of successful ablation is in the posteroseptal tricuspid annulus in 35% to 65%, the proximal CS in 31% to 33%, the mitral annulus in 4% to 23%, and CS diverticula in 9% to 21% of patients.[2-4,7,9] PJRT is targeted at the site of shortest VA time and by mapping for negative unipolar atrial electrograms.[10,11] The AP is located in the posteroseptal right atrium or proximal CS in 76% of cases, is in a midseptal location in 12%, and is right or left posterior or lateral in the remainder.[11]

Ablation

For ablation along the tricuspid or mitral annulus, conventional RF ablation with 4-mm-tip catheters is usually sufficient (Fig. 21–11).[3,4,7-10] Standard RF

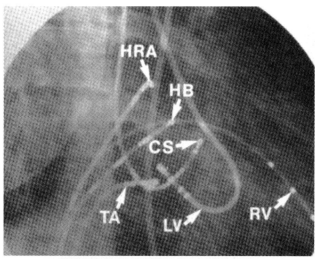

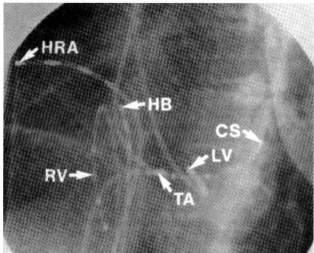

FIGURE 21–11. RAO (**top**) and LAO (**bottom**) fluoroscopic views of catheter positions for mapping the left and right posteroseptal regions. CS, coronary sinus; HB, His bundle; HRA, high right atrium; LV, left ventricle; RV, right ventricle; TA, tricuspid annulus. The LV catheter is introduced by the retrograde transaortic approach. The RV catheter is simultaneously positioned at the coronary sinus ostium. (*From Jazayeri MR, Deshpande S, Dhala A, et al. Transcatheter mapping and radiofrequency ablation of cardiac arrhythmias. Curr Probl Cardiol 6:285-396, 1994, with permission.*)

TABLE 21–5
Targets for Ablation
AP potentials
Local AV or VA ≤40 msec
Right-sided V-delta interval >15 msec
Left-sided V-delta interval >0 msec
Ventricular insertion for epicardial connections

AV, atrial-to-ventricular interval; AP, accessory pathway; VA, ventricular-to-atrial interval; V-delta, local ventricular-to-delta-wave onset.

ablation can also be delivered in the proximal 1 cm of the CS. The left endocardium can be approached by retrograde transaortic or trans-septal techniques (see Fig. 21–11). For ablation more distally in the CS or in venous tributaries or diverticulum, greater care is necessary (see Figs. 21–8 and 21–9). In these cases, conventional RF may be associated with high electrode temperatures due to venous occlusion and lack of cooling. The result may be low power delivery and limited lesion size or coagulum formation with catheter adherence to the venous wall. For these situations, the use of an irrigated catheter system may allow for greater power delivery with a lesser risk of coagulum formation. Alternatively, cryoablation may be an alternative with a low potential for vascular injury.[28]

Finally, for ablation within the CS and its proximal tributaries, the proximity of the ablation site to the right coronary artery must be considered. Based on angiography sites greater than 2 mm away from the right coronary artery may be treated with irrigated RF limited to 12 to 15 W. For sites less than 2 mm from the right coronary artery, RF energy carries a significant risk of arterial damage, and cryoablation is the modality of choice.

Not uncommonly, ablation of the atrial insertion of posteroseptal AP connections alters the retrograde activation sequence without eliminating reciprocating tachycardia. Although this situation may represent multiple APs, it is believed in many instances to result from multiple CS-to-atrial connections. In such cases, targeting the usually single ventricular insertion site may be more efficient.

Despite the complex nature of posteroseptal APs, the success rate for ablation is high, at 93% to 98%.[1,3,4,7-11,22] Complications are common to any ablation procedure for right and left endocardial approaches. Ablation within the CS, its branches, or diverticula carries the risk of venous perforation and tamponade[29] or venous occlusion.[29] Damage to the right coronary artery is also possible. Rarely, heart block has resulted from postseptal ablation, possibly from damage to the AV nodal artery. Recurrence rates are reported to be approximately 12% but range from 6% to 50%.[30-32]

Troubleshooting the Difficult Case

Sources of difficulty most frequently arise from the complex and extensive mapping required to localize APs in this region (Table 21–6). This problem can be minimized by adhering to a systematic approach to mapping. In general, mapping begins in the right endocardium unless there are signs that strongly suggest the need for a left endocardial approach (see Table 21–3). From the right endocardium, the proximal CS is mapped and venography is performed if no attractive sites are identified. If the venography is

---

TABLE 21–6

Troubleshooting the Difficult Case

Problem	Cause	Solution
No early sites	Incomplete mapping	Map proximal CS and tributaries; CS venogram for venous anomalies; map left heart
	Oblique AP course	Reverse direction of activation of AP to separate electrogram components and map AP potentials
	Epicardial AV connection	Map proximal CS tributaries, perform CS venography
	Slow and/or decremental AP conduction	Map shortest of prolonged conduction times or map AP potentials
Changing retrograde activation with ablation	Broad band atrial insertion or multiple CS musculature to atrial connections	Target ventricular insertion especially within CS venous system
Low power delivery	Low blood flow location	Use irrigated RF
	RF in CS tributary or diverticulum	Use irrigated RF; or, if near right coronary artery (<2 mm), use cryoablation
Epicardial connection near right coronary artery	Epicardial connection in proximal CS venous system	Use cryoablation

AP, accessory pathway; AV, atrioventricular; CS, coronary sinus; RF, radiofrequency.

unrevealing for diverticula or other anomalies, the left endocardium is mapped by a transaortic or transseptal technique. It may be necessary to compare the AV and VA conduction times recorded from the right and left sides to direct more detailed mapping at the site of the shorter time. Because of slow and decremental conduction of some APs in this area, conventional criteria for identifying favorable ablation sites based on short AV and VA times may not apply. In this instance, careful cataloguing of the conduction times at all sites may identify the shortest as the best site for ablation. Alternatively, AP potentials can be sought aided by reversal of the activation wavefront for the atrial and ventricular insertions. Careful CS venography should be performed early in the difficult case, because the presence of a venous anomaly usually identifies the site of the accessory connection. Changing retrograde atrial activation with ablation of CS muscular connections can cause confusion. In this instance, targeting of the ventricular insertion may be more efficient. Ablation within the CS tributary branches and diverticula may lead to excessive electrode temperatures with conventional RF catheters. The use of irrigated RF at low power settings may be required. Cryoablation is an attractive alternative to RF for ablation in the venous branches, especially when ablating near the right coronary artery. Ablation in the venous branches should be preceded by right coronary angiography to evaluate this risk.

References

1. Calkins H, Kim Y-N, Schmaltz S, et al.: Electrogram criteria for identification of appropriate target sites for radiofrequency catheter ablation of accessory atrioventricular connections. Circulation 85:565-573, 1992.
2. Jazyeri MR, Deshpande S, Dhala A, et al.: Transcatheter mapping and radiofrequency ablation of cardiac arrhythmias. Cardiology 19:285-396, 1994.
3. Calkins H, Yong P, Miller J, et al.: Catheter ablation of accessory pathways, atrioventricular nodal reentrant tachycardia, and the atrioventricular junction: Final results of a prospective, multicenter clinical trial. Circulation 99:262-270, 1999.
4. Jackman WM, Wang X, Friday KJ, et al.: Catheter ablation of accessory atrioventricular pathways (Wolff-Parkinson-White syndrome) by radiofrequency current. N Engl J Med 324:1605-1611, 1991.
5. Sealy WC, Gallagher JJ: The surgical approach to the septal area of the heart based on the experiences with forty-five patients with Kent bundles. J Thorac Cardiovasc Surg 79:542-551, 1980.
6. Sealy WC, Mikat EM: Anatomical problems with identification and interruption of posterior septal Kent bundles. Ann Thorac Surg 36:584-595, 1983.
7. Chiang C, Chen S, Tai C, et al.: Prediction of successful ablation site of concealed posteroseptal accessory pathways by a novel algorithm using baseline electrophysiological parameters. Circulation 93:982-991, 1996.
8. Dhala AA, Deshpande SS, Bremner S, et al.: Transcatheter ablation of posteroseptal accessory pathways using a venous approach and radiofrequency energy. Circulation 90:1799-1810, 1994.
9. Haissaguerre M, Gaita F, Marcus FI, Clementy J: Radiofrequency catheter ablation of accessory pathways: A contemporary review. J Cardiovasc Electrophysiol 5:533-552, 1994.
10. Haissaguerre M, Montserrat P, Warin JF, et al.: Catheter ablation of left posteroseptal accessory pathways and of long RP′ tachycardias with a right endocardial approach. Eur Heart J 12:845-859, 1991.
11. Gaita F, Haissaguerre M, Giustetto C, et al.: Catheter ablation of permanent junctional reciprocating tachycardia with radiofrequency current. J Am Coll Cardiol 25:648-654, 1995.
12. Davis LM, Byth K, Ellis P, et al.: Dimensions of the human posterior septal space and coronary sinus. Am J Cardiol 68:621-625, 1991.
13. Hood MA, Cox JL, Lindsay BD, et al.: Improved detection of accessory pathways that bridge posterior septal and left posterior regions in the Wolff-Parkinson-White syndrome. Am J Cardiol 70:205-210, 1992.
14. McAlpine WA: Heart and coronary arteries: An anatomical atlas for clinical and surgical treatment. New York: Springer-Verlag, 1975.
15. Sánchez-Quintana D, Ho SY, Cabrera JA, et al.: Topographic anatomy of the inferior pyramidal space: Relevance to radiofrequency catheter ablation. J Cardiovasc Electrophysiol 12:210-217, 2001.
16. Sun Y, Arruda M, Otomo K, et al.: Coronary sinus-ventricular accessory connections producing posteroseptal and left posterior accessory pathways. Circulation 106:1362-1367, 2002.
17. Kasai A, Anselme F, Saoudi N: Myocardial connections between left atrial myocardium and coronary sinus musculature in man. J Cardiovasc Electrophysiol 12:981-985, 2001.
18. Chiang CE, Chen SA, Yang CR, et al.: Major coronary sinus abnormalities: Identification of occurrence and significance in radiofrequency ablation of supraventricular tachycardia. Am Heart J 127:1279-1289, 1994.
19. Weiss C, Cappato R, Schluter M, et al.: Anomalies of the coronary venous system in patients with and without accessory pathways [abstract]. J Am Coll Cardiol 25:18A, 1995.
20. Chiang CE, Chen SA, Teo WS, et al.: An accurate stepwise electrocardiographic algorithm for localization of accessory pathways in patients with Wolff-Parkinson-White syndrome from a comprehensive analysis of delta waves and R/S ratio during sinus rhythm. Am J Cardiol 76:40-46, 1995.
21. Arruda M, McClelland J, Wang X, et al.: Development and validation of an ECG algorithm for identifying accessory pathway ablation site in Wolff-Parkinson-White Syndrome. J Cardiovasc Electrophysiol 9:2-12, 1998.
22. Chen S-A, Tai C-T: Ablation or atrioventricular accessory pathways: Current technique—state of the art. Pacing Clin Electrophysiol 24:1795-1809, 2001.
23. Wood MA, DiMarco JP, Haines DE: Electrocardiographic abnormalities following radiofrequency catheter ablation of accessory bypass tracts in Wolff-Parkinson-White syndrome. Am J Cardiol 70:200-204, 1992.
24. Hwang C, Martin D, Goodman J, et al.: Atypical atrioventricular node reciprocating tachycardia masquerading as tachycardia using a left-sided accessory pathway. J Am Coll Cardiol 30:218-225, 1997.
25. Miller JM, Rosenthal ME, Gottlieb CD, et al.: Usefulness of the ΔHA interval to accurately distinguish atrio-ventricular nodal reentry from orthodromic septal bypass tract tachycardias. Am J Cardiol 68:1037-1044, 1991.
26. Takahashi A, Shah D, Jais P, et al.: Specific electrocardiographic features of manifest coronary vein posteroseptal accessory pathways. J Cardiovasc Electrophysiol 9:1015-1025, 1998.

27. Otomo K, Gonzalez M, Beckman K, et al.: Reversing the direction of paced ventricular and atrial wavefronts reveals an oblique course in accessory AV pathways and improves localization for catheter ablation. Circulation 104:550-556, 2001.

28. Gaita F, Paperini L, Riccardi R, et al.: Cryothermic ablation within the coronary sinus of an epicardial posterolateral pathway. J Cardiovasc Electrophysiol 13:1160-1163, 2002.

29. Wang X, Jackman WM, McClelland J, et al.: Sites of successful radiofrequency ablation of posteroseptal accessory pathways [abstract]. Pacing Clin Electrophysiol 15:535, 1992.

30. Chen SA, Chiang CE, Tsang WP, et al.: Recurrent conduction in accessory pathway and possible new arrhythmias after radiofrequency catheter ablation. Am Heart J 125:381-387, 1993.

31. Yee R, Klein GJ, Guiraudon GM: The Wolff-Parkinson-White syndrome. In Zipes DP, Jalife J (eds.): Cardiac Electrophysiology: From Cell to Bedside. Philadelphia: WB Saunders, 1995, pp 1199-1214.

32. Calkins H, Prystowski E, Carlson M, et al.: Temperature monitoring during radiofrequency catheter ablation procedures using closed loop control. Circulation 90:1279-1286, 1994.

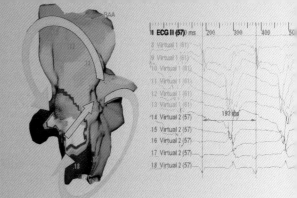

22

Catheter Ablation of Superoparaseptal ("Anteroseptal") and Midseptal Accessory Pathways

John M. Miller • Mithilesh K. Das • Anil V. Yadav • Deepak Bhakta

Key Points

- Diagnosis of superoparaseptal ("anteroseptal") and midseptal accessory pathways (APs) is made on the basis of an electrocardiographic pattern (if overt preexcitation is present) and evidence of midseptal/anteroseptal AP insertions.

- Orthodromic supraventricular tachycardia using a midseptal AP must be differentiated from atrioventricular (AV) nodal reentry and septal or parahisian atrial tachycardias.

- Mapping of superoparaseptal APs is done to locate the earliest anterograde ventricular activation near or anterior to the His bundle recording, the earliest anterograde ventricular activation-to-delta wave interval of 15 to 40 msec, and earliest retrograde atrial activation in His bundle recordings.

- Mapping of midseptal APs is done to locate the earliest anterograde ventricular activation between the coronary sinus (CS) ostium and the His recording, the earliest anterograde ventricular activation-to-delta wave interval of 15 to 25 msec, and the earliest retrograde atrial activation between the CS ostium and the His recordings. Left midseptal connections are rare.

- The ablation target is the site of earliest ventricular activation or retrograde atrial activation on the AV annulus.

- The use of preformed vascular sheaths may be helpful; catheter navigation systems are often useful to "tag" sites of interest, and cryoablation may be useful. Cooled radiofrequency ablation is rarely needed and is possibly contraindicated.

- Sources of difficulty include lack of catheter stability, proximity to normal conduction system with risk of heart block, catheter-induced mechanical block of pathway conduction, and accelerated junctional rhythm (narrow QRS) during ablation mistaken for elimination of preexcitation.

413

Atrioventricular (AV) accessory pathways (APs) are thin fibers, usually composed of typical myocardial cells, that allow electrical communication between atrium and ventricle extrinsic to the normal AV node-His bundle axis. The clinical expression of these pathways ranges from simply causing an abnormal electrocardiogram; to forming an integral component of a macroreentrant circuit incorporating atrial and ventricular myocardium, AV node and His bundle, and the AP (AV reciprocating supraventricular tachycardia [SVT]); to functioning as an alternative pathway for transmission of rapid atrial tachyarrhythmias such as flutter and fibrillation to the ventricles. Symptoms may range from none; to occasional mild palpitations; to severe palpitations accompanied by dyspnea, chest discomfort, light-headedness, and even syncope or cardiac arrest from rapidly conducted atrial fibrillation.

Since its introduction in the late 1980s, catheter ablation of APs has become a relatively routine matter in most electrophysiology laboratories. However, ablation of pathways in the so-called anterior and midseptal locations remains a challenge for even experienced operators because of the proximity of these pathways to the normal cardiac conduction system (AV node and His bundle). Inadvertent injury to these structures resulting in the need for permanent pacing, especially in a young patient, is a significant adverse outcome. Fortunately, techniques have been developed to decrease the likelihood of this complication. This chapter discusses the relevant anatomy of these pathways and the use of these techniques.

Anatomy and Nomenclature

Current nomenclature of septal pathways is undergoing modification. A reexamination of the anatomy of the AV junctions has suggested that the terminology used in the original descriptions of AP locations was anatomically inaccurate and, in some cases, frankly misleading. Most electrophysiology trainees have had the experience of asking, "Why is my attending telling me to move the catheter *anteriorly* when I see it moving toward the head?!" A reclassification of cardiac electrophysiologic anatomy has been developed to try to correct these antiquated but ingrained terms.[1] In addition, a more complete understanding of the anatomy of the atrial and ventricular septa has resulted in a "shrinking" of the atrial septum: most trainees conceive of the atrial septum as a relatively large disk comprising the intersection of two spheres compressed together. In fact,

the true muscular atrial septum is much smaller, consisting of a relatively thin rim of atrial tissue surrounding the fossa ovalis.[2-4] This has implications for how precisely one must position a needle and catheter to safely puncture the septum for left atrial access and also for evaluation and ablation of the pathways under consideration in this chapter.

In the old vernacular, "anteroseptal" pathways were regarded as being located in the apex of Koch's triangle, connecting the atrial and ventricular septa in the region of the His bundle. In the anatomically accurate nomenclature, these pathways are more properly regarded as *superoparaseptal*, because there is no atrial septum in the region anterior to the His recording location (atrial walls are separated here by the aortic root) (Fig. 22–1). These connections are thus right free wall, paraseptal pathways. Posteriorly, pathways in the region of the ostium of the coronary sinus (CS), which previously were called "posteroseptal," are in fact *posterior paraseptal*, because the CS itself is, by definition, entirely posterior to the atrial septum. Pathways located between these two boundaries of the septum have been called "midseptal" or "intermediate septal," but, because they are the only truly septal interconnections, they may simply be called *septal*. Further complicating the situation is the fact that the AV valves are not isoplanar; the tricuspid valve is slightly inferiorly displaced such that a portion of the medial right atrium is juxtaposed to subaortic left ventricular muscle, rather than right ventricle.

In the discussion that follows, we will consider that superoparaseptal ("anteroseptal") APs are located in the apex of Koch's triangle at a site from which a small His potential can usually be recorded. True septal or midseptal APs are located in the floor of Koch's triangle, between the His recording location and the anterior portion of the CS ostium.

Diagnosis and Differential Diagnosis

SUPEROPARASEPTAL ACCESSORY PATHWAYS

Superoparaseptal APs comprise 6% to 7% of all APs in most large series. About 80% of these APs exhibit anterograde conduction, and 20% are retrograde-only conducting ("concealed"); only about 5% conduct exclusively in the anterograde direction. Because these pathways connect the right atrial and right ventricular paraseptal free walls in a region that is cephalad, or superior, as well as anterior to most of the rest of the ventricular mass, an anterograde con-

FIGURE 22–1. View of atrioventricular (AV) groove from above with most of the atrial muscle removed; the right atrial rim has been rendered semi-transparent to reveal structures beneath. Note the small dimensions of the actual atrial septum (*dashed line*). True septal ("midseptal") pathways have an atrial insertion on the right or left side in this region, in which the AV node resides. Pathways in the region of the His bundle, previously called anteroseptal, in fact have free wall and not septal atrial insertions (hence "superoparaseptal" pathways).

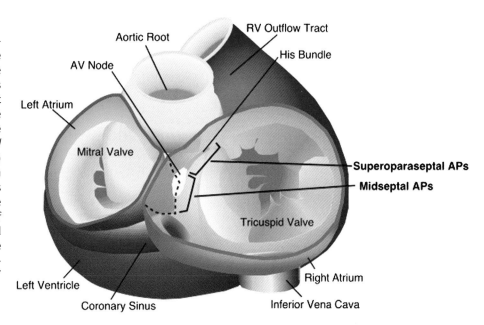

FIGURE 22–2. Electrocardiogram of superoparaseptal AP with anterograde conduction, showing a very short PR segment and positive delta waves in 1, 2, 3, aVF and lateral precordial leads.

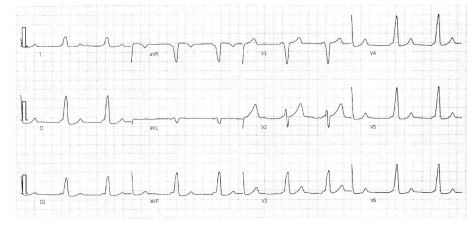

ducting pathway manifests positive delta waves in the inferior leads (II, III, and aVF) and the lateral precordial leads (V_3 through V_6); negative delta waves are present in lead V_1 and often in V_2 (Fig. 22–2). Leads I and aVL have positive delta waves (negative in aVR). During orthodromic SVT, the P wave is typically situated in the early portion of the ST segment; although retrograde, it is usually positive in the inferior leads, because much of the atrial mass is located caudad from the atrial insertion (Fig. 22–3).

MIDSEPTAL ACCESSORY PATHWAYS

Midseptal pathways account for 5% or less of all APs in most series. Approximately 85% of midseptal APs show anterograde conduction (15% are retrograde only), with only about 4% conducting anterograde only. These APs connect atrium and ventricle in a complex region that can give rise to slightly different delta wave polarities in different individuals. A typical preexcitation pattern has predominantly positive delta waves in leads I, II, aVL, and V_2 through V_6, with leads III and aVF usually having predominantly negative delta waves and aVR and V_1 having isoelectric delta waves. Variations in this pattern, especially in the inferior leads and in V_2, have been reported. During SVT, because of the more posterior location of the pathway's atrial insertion (near the compact AV node), the P wave is usually inverted in the inferior leads. Multiple APs are present in up to 25% of patients with midseptal APs.

ELECTROPHYSIOLOGIC TESTING

The electrophysiologic diagnosis of SVT incorporating a superoparaseptal or midseptal pathway is

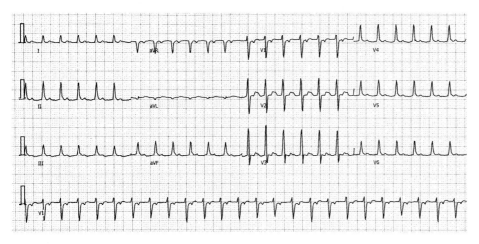

FIGURE 22–3. Electrocardiogram of supraventricular tachycardia incorporating a retrogradely-conducting superoparaseptal AP. Note the positive P waves in the inferior leads with negative P wave polarity in leads aVR and V_1.

usually relatively straightforward (Table 22–1); however, the atrial activation sequence during SVT may resemble that of normal AV nodal output (unlike the situation with left or right free wall APs, in which the atrial activation sequence during SVT is eccentric). This similarity of atrial activation can provide a diagnostic challenge in some cases. Standard diagnostic techniques, including introduction of ventricular premature extrastimuli during His refractoriness in an episode SVT, should be used to define the tachycardia mechanism. In some cases, such as when the ventricular-to-atrial interval is very short or SVT is nonsustained or noninducible, other techniques must be used to establish the presence of an AP. These include parahisian pacing, differential site ventricular pacing, comparison of His-to-atrial (HA) intervals, and entrainment of SVT.

Pacing from a location near the His bundle (parahisian pacing) can distinguish conduction over an AP from that over the AV node, as follows: at low pacing outputs, ventricular capture occurs, whereas at higher outputs, the His bundle/proximal right bundle branch are captured with the adjacent ventricular myocardium, resulting in a narrower QRS. If an AP in the regions under consideration is present, the stimulus-to-atrial interval will be identical regardless of whether the His is captured, because these APs typically conduct more rapidly than the AV node does. If there is no AP, the stimulus-to-atrial interval is longer with ventricular-only capture than when the His is captured, because with ventricular pacing the impulse must travel some distance using relatively slow myocyte-myocyte conduction before it encounters elements of the His-Purkinje network to begin activating it retrogradely. With His capture, the impulse need only traverse the AV node to activate the atrium (Fig. 22–4).[5] This technique can be used to confirm successful ablation of the AP.

Using a principle similar to that of parahisian pacing, comparison of the stimulus-to-atrial intervals observed with right ventricular apical versus basal stimulation can demonstrate the presence of an AP. The apex, though physically more distant from the atrium than the ventricular base, is nonetheless electrically closer because of the proximity of the distal right bundle branch to the pacing site. Entry into the rapidly-conducting His-Purkinje system allows a shorter stimulus-to-atrial interval during pacing from the apex than from the base. From the base, the impulse must again travel relatively slowly over some distance through ventricular myocardium before it engages the His-Purkinje system (Fig. 22–5). Fixed-rate pacing or extrastimuli during SVT can be used.[6] This technique can also be used to confirm successful AP ablation.

Comparison of the (HA) intervals observed during SVT and during ventricular pacing at the SVT cycle length can distinguish AV nodal reentry from septal pathway–dependent orthodromic SVT. The HA interval during orthodromic reciprocating tachycardia should be the same as, or slightly shorter than, the interval during ventricular pacing. The His bundle and atrium are activated in series during SVT but in parallel during pacing.[7] However, the HA during AV nodal reentry should be much shorter than that during pacing, because the His bundle and atrium are activated in parallel during SVT but in series during pacing (the opposite of the situation in AV nodal reentry).[7]

Similarly, Overdrive right ventricular apical pacing at a cycle length slightly faster than that of SVT (entrainment of SVT) can distinguish atypical AV nodal reentry from orthodromic SVT using a septal AP. If AV nodal reentry is the SVT diagnosis, the stimulus-to-atrial interval during ventricular pacing will exceed the QRS-to-atrial interval by more

TABLE 22-1

Diagnostic Criteria

Technique	Criteria
Surface ECG: sinus rhythm (in presence of preexcitation)	
Superoparaseptal APs	Delta waves predominantly positive in leads I, II, III, aVL, aVF, and V_3 through V_6; negative in aVR and V_1, and often in V_2
Midseptal APs	Delta waves predominantly positive in I, II, aVL, and V_2 through V_6; negative in III and aVF; negative or isoelectric in aVR and V_1
Surface ECG: orthodromic SVT	
	P waves (in early ST segment); may be positive in inferior leads (superoparaseptal APs)
Intracardiac recordings and electrophysiology	
	Premature ventricular extrastimulus during His refractoriness can advance atrial activation or terminate tachycardia without causing atrial activation
	ΔHA interval (SVT vs ventricular pacing) to distinguish orthodromic SVT from AV nodal reentry
	Midseptal pathways may exhibit "decremental" conduction properties (anterograde or retrograde)
	Parahisian or differential site ventricular pacing useful to prove existence of pathway, confirm its ablation (if normal retrograde AV node/His conduction intact)
Superoparaseptal APs	Earliest anterograde ventricular activation at or anterior to His recording location
	Earliest retrograde atrial activation in His bundle recording
	Small (<0.1 mV) His deflection in ablation recording
	Sensitivity to mechanical block by catheter manipulation
Midseptal APs	Earliest anterograde ventricular and retrograde atrial activation between His and coronary sinus ostium

AP, accessory pathway; AV, atrioventricular; ECG, electrocardiogram; ΔHA, difference in His-to-atrial interval; SVT, supraventricular tachycardia.

than 85 msec, and the postpacing interval will exceed the SVT cycle length by more than 115 msec. In orthodromic SVT using a septal AP, these intervals are less than the cutoff values noted. This distinction occurs because the pacing site is remote from the SVT circuit in AV nodal reentry but near or within it in orthodromic SVT.[8]

Midseptal APs occasionally present additional nuances. In some cases, these pathways have demonstrated so-called decremental conduction properties (cycle length–dependent prolongation of conduction intervals). Especially in the absence of overt preexcitation, this feature could cause confusion by suggesting conduction only through the AV node, rather than the presence of an AP.[9]

Mapping and Ablation Techniques

SUPEROPARASEPTAL ACCESSORY PATHWAYS

Ablation of APs in the region of the His bundle may be successfully and safely accomplished using the same techniques employed for APs in other locations (Table 22–2). In the presence of preexcitation, the ventricular insertion site can be targeted by searching for the earliest site of ventricular activation during sinus rhythm; atrial pacing usually is not necessary to attain maximum preexcitation, because the ventricular insertion of the AP is relatively close to the sinus node. Electrogram characteristics at successful ablation sites include (1) a ventricular activation time that precedes the surface ECG delta wave onset by 15 to 40 msec; (2) a sharp "QS" deflection on the unipolar electrogram of the ablation electrode; (3) a sharp AP potential; and (4) an almost continuous recording incorporating atrial-AP-ventricular components (Fig. 22–6). Differentiation of atrial from ventricular components of a complex recording can usually be accomplished by introducing atrial extrastimuli or burst pacing of that block in the AP. Pre–delta wave activation times are longer (i.e., earlier) in right-sided than in left-sided APs in general, and especially so with superoparaseptal APs.[10] The site with the longest (earliest) pre-delta time should be sought. (For example, even if the pre-delta time in the first site sampled is 15 msec, ablation should not be performed there until multiple other nearby sites have been sampled, none of which has a longer interval.) Fluoroscopically, this can be very close to the His bundle recording site (Fig. 22–7).

During orthodromic SVT, the site with the earliest atrial electrogram activation, often with an AP poten-

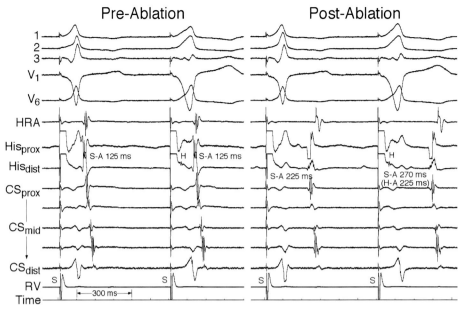

FIGURE 22–4. Parahisian pacing. In this and subsequent figures, surface leads 1, 2, 3 V$_1$ and V$_6$ are shown with intracardiac record-ings from high right atrium (HRA), His bundle proximal (prox) and distal (dist) electrode pairs, coronary sinus (CS), right ventricle (RV) near the His recording location; S denotes stimulus artifact, H the His deflection. Parahisian pacing is shown before (left panel) and after ablation (right panel). On each panel, the first complex shows His and ventricular capture, the second ventricular capture only. Before ablation, the stimulus-atrial (S-A) interval is the same regardless of whether His capture occurs because the AP is the preferred path of conduction. In the complex on the right, the apparent "H-A" interval is shorter than the S-A interval during His capture, indicating that atrial activation is occurring independent of AV nodal conduction. After successful ablation, retrograde con-duction requires His activation; the S-A interval is longer than before ablation, and increases further in the absence of His capture (complex on the right) since with pure ventricular pacing it takes longer to get to the His bundle. Once the His is activated as shown, the H-A time is the same as the S-A time during His capture.

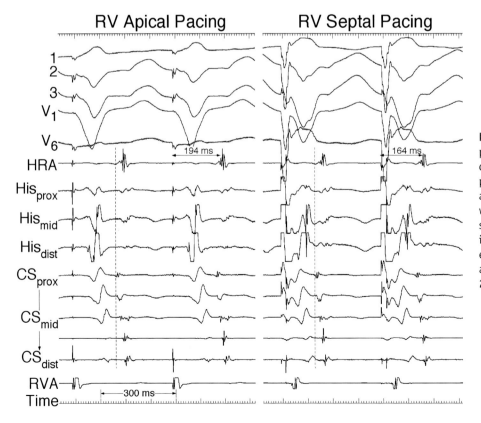

FIGURE 22–5. Differential site pacing. *Dashed lines* denote onset of atrial activation. On the left panel, RV apical pacing yields a stimulus-HRA time of 194 ms whereas RV basal pacing yields a stimulus-HRA interval of 164 ms, indicating the presence of an extranodal. RVA, right ventricular apex. Abbreviations per Figure 22–4.

TABLE 22-2

Target Sites for Ablation

Superoparaseptal	*Ventricular insertion site (in presence of preexcitation):* Ventricular activation time that precedes surface ECG delta wave onset by 15-40 msec Sharp "QS" deflection on the unipolar electrogram of the ablation electrode Presence of a sharp AP potential between atrial and ventricular electrograms, preceding delta wave onset Nearly continuous recording with atrial-AP-ventricular components Small (<0.1 mV) His deflection may be present (may be obscured by ventricular electrogram) *Atrial insertion site (in presence of retrograde conduction):* Earliest atrial electrogram Presence of a sharp AP potential between ventricular and atrial electrograms Small (<0.1 mV) His deflection may be present
Midseptal	*Ventricular insertion site (in presence of preexcitation):* Ventricular activation time that precedes the surface ECG delta wave onset by 15-40 msec Sharp "QS" deflection on the unipolar electrogram of the ablation electrode Presence of a sharp AP potential between atrial and ventricular electrograms, preceding delta wave onset Nearly continuous recording with atrial-AP-ventricular components *Atrial insertion site (in presence of retrograde conduction):* Earliest atrial electrogram Presence of a sharp AP potential between ventricular and atrial electrograms

AP, accessory pathway; ECG, electrocardiogram.

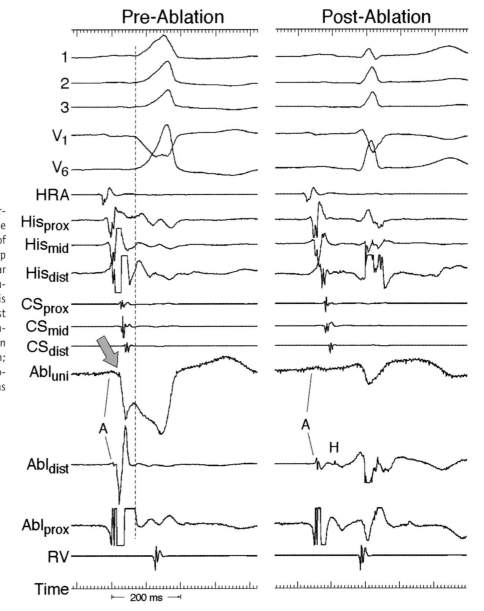

FIGURE 22-6. Site of superoparaseptal AP ablation. The *dashed line* indicates the onset of the delta wave. Note the sharp negative deflection in the unipolar electrogram (*arrow*) with a diminutive atrial electrogram that is clearly evident as such only post ablation. Note also the His potential (H) in the post-ablation recording. A, atrial electrogram; Abl, ablation catheter; uni, unipolar electrogram. Abbreviations as per Figure 22-4.

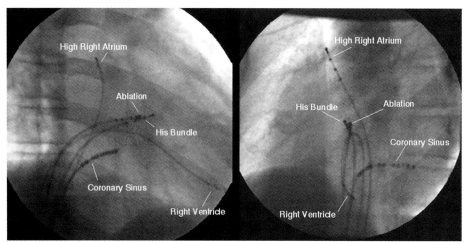

Right Anterior Oblique   **Left Anterior Oblique**

FIGURE   22–7. Fluoroscopic images of superoparaseptal AP ablation site. Catheters and views as labeled; note the near-superimposition of the ablation catheter and His recording electrodes. Ablation at this site was successful without injury to the His bundle.

tial, is the target. It is important to distinguish between the site with the *shortest ventricular-to-atrial interval* and the site with the *earliest atrial activation time;* they are often the same site, but if they are not, the site with the earliest atrial activation time is preferred. The ventricular and atrial electrograms may be almost fused during SVT or ventricular pacing; introduction of premature ventricular extrastimuli during either pacing or SVT may separate the electrogram components, allowing the operator to correctly assess the timing of atrial activation as well as relative electrogram amplitudes. Also during SVT, the amplitude of the His bundle electrogram in the ablation recording can be assessed. The AP can be safely ablated if the His deflection is less than 0.2 mV in amplitude, though there is probably less chance of injury if it is smaller still.

Ordinarily, one should ablate on the ventricular aspect of the annulus if this site is stable; atrial sites (ratio of atrial to ventricular electrogram amplitudes >0.4) may yield successful ablation but with a slightly higher risk of injury to the normal conduction system. A long vascular sheath may help stabilize the position of the catheter tip regardless of whether an atrial or a ventricular site is chosen. Some operators prefer to ablate with a catheter introduced from the internal jugular vein approach, either positioning the catheter tip on the atrial aspect or advancing it slightly across and beneath the tricuspid annulus to ablate from the ventricular aspect.

It is worth spending extra time to "fine tune" the ablation site, ensuring both the best possible timing and the morphology of the ablation electrogram as well as catheter tip stability. Delivering as few ablation applications as possible (and, consequently, doing as little damage as possible) is an important goal when ablating in the vicinity of the AV node and

His bundle. Mapping systems that can "tag" or track the location of mapping or ablation sites may be useful in guiding the operator either toward more favorable sites or away from sites that are less attractive. If the best ablation site is very close to the His bundle recording site, the His recording catheter can occasionally be advanced slightly into the ventricle, leaving the insulated portion of the catheter as a potential physical barrier overlying the His bundle itself.

Once a site has been chosen for ablation, radiofrequency (RF) energy delivery should begin at relatively low power (30 W) and low temperature (50°C to 60°C) settings but with firm catheter contact. Poor contact may result in only minimal damage but with edema formation that then distorts electrograms and may lead to an increased physical barrier to subsequent effective energy delivery. If preexcitation is present, ablation may be attempted during sinus rhythm or during atrial pacing. Unsuccessful energy applications should be stopped after no more than 15 seconds; continued energy delivery at such sites is unlikely to be beneficial but may have already caused damage to the AV node or His bundle that cannot be discerned as long as preexcitation persists. It is useful to try to ensure that normal AV node-His conduction is still intact after one or two failed ablation energy deliveries. Use of higher energies, or of large-tip catheters capable of causing more extensive damage, has practically no role in ablation of these APs; the cause of ablation failure in these APs is almost always incorrect localization or poor contact, and not inadequacy of a standard-sized RF lesion.

For concealed APs, ablation is usually performed during ventricular pacing so that loss of AP conduction can be readily monitored. However, use of this method for ablation of pathways in the vicinity of the

AV node and His bundle could result in inadvertent damage to these structures that would not be evident until after cessation of pacing (when it may be too late). Alternative methods for ablation of concealed APs in this region include ablation during sinus rhythm, during SVT, and during atrial-entrained SVT.

Ablation during sinus rhythm has the advantage of allowing monitoring for either PR prolongation or accelerated junctional rhythm, indicating damage to the normal conduction system and prompting cessation of energy delivery. However, AP ablation success cannot be assessed until ventricular pacing is performed after cessation of RF delivery.

Ablation during SVT allows monitoring of both normal conduction and ablation success (SVT terminates in retrograde limb). However, the sudden change in heart rate associated with successful ablation and cessation of SVT can lead to ablation catheter displacement and incomplete ablation.

With ablation during atrial-entrained SVT, atrial pacing is performed slightly faster than the SVT cycle length while ablation energy is delivered. When the AP conduction is ablated, SVT terminates but the heart rate does not change; therefore, the likelihood of catheter movement is decreased and complete ablation is facilitated. Because this method allows monitoring of efficacy (AP ablation) and safety (normal AV conduction) and addresses the problem of catheter movement, it is preferred.

Cryomapping and ablation have been introduced as techniques to avoid unwanted damage to the AV node and His bundle.[11,12] With cryomapping, the catheter tip is first cooled to $0°C$ at potential ablation sites; if AP conduction is lost without damage to the normal conduction elements, the catheter tip temperature can be decreased to $-80°C$ for cryoablation. Cold-induced attenuation of normal pathway conduction may be hard to appreciate because preexcitation is near-maximal in sinus rhythm or with right atrial pacing; instead, if CS pacing results in a greater degree of normal conduction (less preexcitation), application of cold to the AV node or His bundle will result in an increase in preexcitation. Such areas should be noted as sites at which ablation definitely should not be performed.

Troubleshooting the Difficult Case

Successful ablation of superoparaseptal APs poses particular challenges (Table 22–3). These APs are by definition close enough to the His bundle that a small His potential is usually recorded in the ablation signal (or sometimes first becomes evident after successful ablation). Inadvertent damage to the His

TABLE 22–3
Troubleshooting The Difficult Case

Problem	Causes	Possible Solutions
Pathway block during mapping	Catheter trauma of superficially located pathway	Careful catheter manipulation If catheter remains in same location that caused block, ablate Wait up to 1 hr for recovery
Accelerated junctional rhythm during RF application	Heating of AV node	Stop RF application immediately; reposition catheter
Right bundle branch block during RF application	Catheter positioned too distally	Reposition catheter
Unable to successfully ablate at earliest site of RA activation in SVT	Poor catheter contact	Vascular sheath; alter approach (switch to SVC or femoral vein)
	Incorrect location on right side	Continue mapping
	Left-sided atrial or ventricular pathway insertion	Map LA/LV septum; LVOT; noncoronary sinus of Valsalva
Large His potential in best ablation recording	True parahisian pathway	Use cryomapping to test sites before ablation Advance His catheter so that insulated shaft "shields" His bundle from ablation energy

AV, atrioventricular; LA, left atrium; LV, left ventricle; LVOT, left ventricular outflow tract; RA, right atrium; RF, radiofrequency; SVC, superior vena cava; SVT, supraventricular tachycardia.

bundle is the primary hazard in ablating these APs. Additional potential difficulties include AP sensitivity to catheter trauma and accelerated junctional rhythm during RF energy delivery.

These pathways are often very superficial (toward the endocardial surface), and catheter trauma results in transient block of pathway conduction in one or both directions in up to 38% of cases (Fig. 22–8).[13] If this occurs, and the catheter has moved ("grazed" the pathway as it was passing by), one can only wait and hope that pathway conduction resumes. This may take up to 30 minutes. Isoproterenol has been used by some to try to facilitate resumption of conduction; although this has been reported to be successful, the additional waiting time may have been responsible for return of AP conduction, rather than the medication, and there are no controlled studies of isoproterenol in this setting. If the catheter tip is still at the site at which trauma interrupted AP conduction, one can proceed with ablation despite lack of return of conduction after a reasonable waiting period (10 to 15 minutes). Use of mapping systems that allow tagging of sites on a three-dimensional rendering of the heart may be helpful in this regard, but only if sites with acceptable electrogram characteristics were designated as such before catheter-mediated loss of AP conduction. If catheter-induced AP block occurs and one is uncertain as to whether the catheter is still at the site that caused mechanical block, it may be appropriate to move the catheter well away from the site (i.e., its continued presence may be causing ongoing mechanical block). In this situation, tagging of the site with a mapping system can be very

helpful: if conduction returns after the catheter is moved away, the mapping reference facilitates replacement of the tip back to the same site.

Accelerated junctional rhythm during RF energy delivery (Fig. 22–9) occurs in up to 5% of patients[14] and results from heating of the His bundle. Accelerated junctional rhythm typically results in a narrow QRS complex on ECG, a finding that may erroneously suggest that the AP has been successfully ablated and that energy delivery should continue. In fact, this is exactly the wrong thing to do, because the His bundle may be undergoing destruction. The operator has only seconds to discontinue RF energy delivery before the His bundle is destroyed. If energy delivery continues, progressive acceleration of the junctional discharge rate may occur, as during intentional His bundle ablation. This can provide an important warning to the operator if the danger has not already been appreciated. Fortunately, the His bundle itself is contained within a fibrous sheath that is somewhat protective against inadvertent ablation. Of note, cryoablation does not result in accelerated junctional rhythm; however, absence of this rhythm during cryoablation should not be interpreted as lack of risk of damaging the normal conduction system.

Parahisian pathways represent a subgroup of the superoparaseptal pathways that are more closely related to the His bundle itself (His deflection >0.1 mV).[15] Despite this proximity to the His, these APs can still be ablated successfully without incurring His bundle injury, perhaps because of the insulative effect of the fibrous sheath surrounding the His

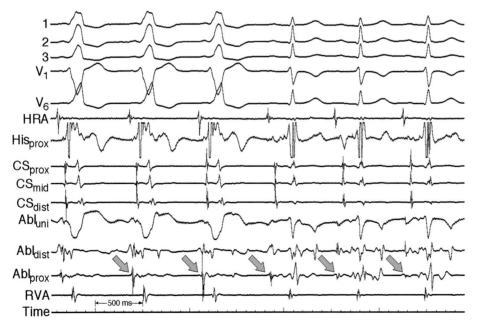

FIGURE 22–8. Mechanical block in superoparaseptal AP due to catheter manipulation. The first 3 beats show preexcitation; the last 3 do not, due to catheter trauma. *Diagonal arrows* show a changing atrial electrogram in the ablation recording, indicating unstable catheter position. Abbreviations as per Figure 22–4.

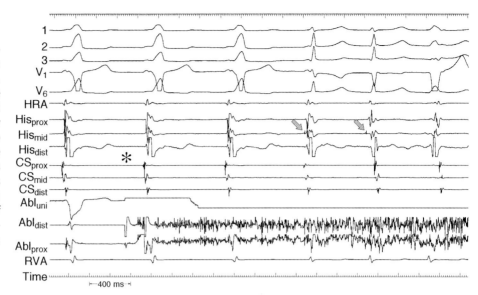

FIGURE 22–9. Accelerated junctional rhythm during ablation attempt (superoparaseptal AP). RF delivery is begun at the *asterisk*; the next 2 preexcited beats are followed by 2 narrow QRS complexes, but not due to AP ablation. Instead, these are accelerated junctional complexes caused by heating of the His bundle (*arrows*). RF application was stopped just after the end of the recording. The AP was eventually ablated with preservation of normal AV conduction.

bundle. Some authors have observed inappropriate sinus tachycardia shortly after ablation of APs in this location, presumably due to alteration of parasympathetic tone caused by the ablation.[16] This is self-limited and requires no treatment.

Rare cases have been reported in which superoparaseptal APs could be ablated only at sites other than the expected apex of Koch's triangle. These sites have included the left ventricular outflow tract[17] and the noncoronary sinus of Valsalva.[18] If several attempts at ablation in the expected right ventricular region have failed to interrupt AP conduction, one should evaluate other, less common ventricular insertion sites such as these.

Using the techniques described, superoparaseptal pathways can be successfully ablated in more than 95% of patients, with about 1% risk of heart block or other significant complications. Right bundle branch block occurs in up to 10% of cases.[14] Cryoablation has been less successful on long-term follow-up than RF ablation (up to 20% recurrence after hospital discharge)[11,12]; whether this is due to an inherent inferiority of cryoablation or simply less familiarity with the technique is not clear. Assessment of successful ablation includes standard techniques (i.e., lack of preexcitation at rest or with decremental atrial pacing, lack of any retrograde conduction, or conduction only over the AV node with cycle length–dependent prolongation of conduction time). Parahisian pacing and differential-site right ventricular pacing can also be used (see earlier discussion).

MIDSEPTAL ACCESSORY PATHWAYS

The principles of ablation of midseptal APs are similar to those for superoparaseptal APs (Fig. 22–10). Care should be taken to ablate on the ventricular side of the annulus, to avoid AV nodal damage (Fig. 22–11). Midseptal APs are successfully ablated in about 98% of cases, with an approximately 1% risk of complete AV block, although transient AV block may occur in up to 5% of patients. Junctional rhythm during RF delivery is seen in up to 50% of cases.[14]

Occasionally, ablation of midseptal APs is not successful after several RF applications on the tricuspid annulus. In most cases, this is due to poor site selection or poor electrode-endocardial contact at an appropriate site. In some cases, ablation can be successful only if it is performed from the left side of the septum. Clues to the presence of a left midseptal AP are absence of sites with pre–delta wave intervals in excess of 10 msec if preexcitation is present, absence of an AP potential at all sites on the tricuspid annulus, and relatively long local ventricular-to-atrial intervals (>60 msec) on the tricuspid annulus. Left-sided ablation may be performed using the retrograde aortic or the trans-septal approach. The surface ECG preexcitation pattern is not specific enough to suggest the necessity of a left-sided approach.[14]

APs in both superoparaseptal and midseptal regions can be safely and successfully ablated using only two electrode catheters (an ablation catheter and a right ventricular for assessing retrograde conduction).[19] Most operators prefer to use additional catheters for fluoroscopic (coronary sinus) and electrical (His bundle) reference.

Recurrence of AP conduction after apparently successful ablation occurs in up to 15% of right-sided APs, including superoparaseptal and midseptal APs.[20] Poor catheter stability is the most common

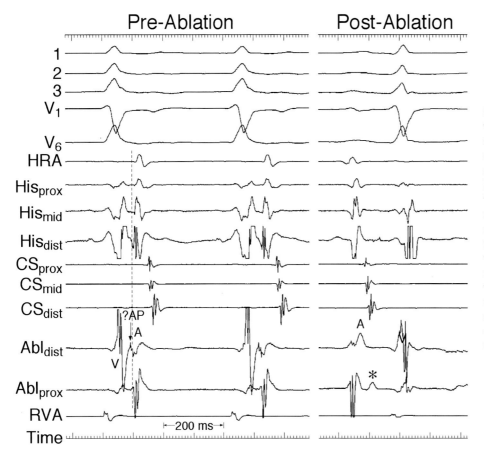

FIGURE 22–10. Site of midseptal AP ablation. The left panel shows supraventricular tachycardia incorporating a retrogradely-conducting midseptal pathway having earliest atrial activation in the distal ablation (Abl$_{dist}$) recording followed by the His region. The Abl$_{dist}$ also shows a possible AP potential between ventricular and atrial components (*small arrow*). After ablation, the ablation recordings do not show a His potential but a deflection similar to some so-called slow AV nodal pathway recordings is seen (asterisk).

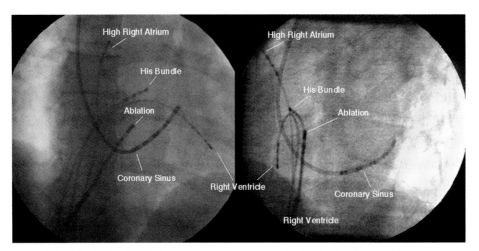

Right Anterior Oblique   Left Anterior Oblique

FIGURE 22–11. Fluoroscopic images of midseptal accessory pathway ablation site. Catheters and views as labeled. The ablation catheter is situated between the coronary sinus ostium and His recording electrodes, in the region of the compact atrioventricular (AV) node. Ablation at this site was successful without damaging the AV node.

cause (suboptimal ablation due to poor contact), although in the case of APs near the AV node and His bundle, operator timidity (unwillingness to deliver adequate energy to the area for fear of causing heart block) may be responsible for incomplete ablation. Common problems encountered in the ablation of septal pathways and their solutions are listed in Table 22–3.

Summary

Ablation of APs in the region of the normal conduction system presents special challenges to the electrophysiologist. Although differentiation of AP-related SVTs from atrial tachycardias and AV nodal reentry can sometimes be difficult, the major challenge remains avoidance of damage to the AV node and His bundle that would require permanent pacing. Fortunately, this complication can usually be avoided by careful attention to catheter positioning and monitoring of normal AV conduction.

References

1. Cosio FG, Anderson RH, Kuck KH, et al.: ESCWGA/NASPE/P experts consensus statement. Living anatomy of the atrioventricular junctions: A guide to electrophysiologic mapping. Working Group of Arrhythmias of the European Society of Cardiology. North American Society of Pacing and Electrophysiology. J Cardiovasc Electrophysiol 10:1162-1170, 1999.
2. Anderson RH, Brown NA: The anatomy of the heart revisited. Anat Rec 246:1-7, 1996.
3. Anderson RH, Brown NA, Webb S: Development and structure of the atrial septum. Heart 88:104-110, 2002.
4. Anderson RH, Webb S, Brown NA, et al.: Development of the heart: 2. Septation of the atriums and ventricles. Heart 89:949-958, 2003.
5. Hirao K, Otomo K, Wang X, et al.: Para-Hisian pacing: A new method for differentiating retrograde conduction over an accessory AV pathway from conduction over the AV node. Circulation 94:1027-1035, 1996.
6. Goldberger J, Wang Y, Scheinman M: Stimulation of the summit of the right ventricular aspect of the ventricular septum during orthodromic atrioventricular reentrant tachycardia. Am J Cardiol 70:78-85, 1992.
7. Miller JM, Rosenthal ME, Gottlieb CD, et al.: Usefulness of the delta HA interval to accurately distinguish atrioventricular nodal reentry from orthodromic septal bypass tract tachycardias. Am J Cardiol 68:1037-1044, 1991.
8. Michaud GF, Tada H, Chough S, et al.: Differentiation of atypical atrioventricular node re-entrant tachycardia from orthodromic reciprocating tachycardia using a septal accessory pathway by the response to ventricular pacing. J Am Coll Cardiol 38:1163-1167, 2001.
9. Coppess MA, Altemose GT, Jayachandran JV, et al.: Unusual features of intermediate septal bypass tracts. J Cardiovasc Electrophysiol 11:730-735, 2000.
10. Xie B, Heald SC, Camm AJ, et al.: Characteristics of bipolar electrograms during anterograde mapping: The importance of accessory atrioventricular pathway location. Am Heart J 131:720-723, 1996.
11. Gaita F, Haïssaguerre M, Giustetto C, et al.: Safety and efficacy of cryoablation of accessory pathways adjacent to the normal conduction system. J Cardiovasc Electrophysiol 14:825-829, 2003.
12. Wong T, Markides V, Peters NS, Davies DW: Clinical usefulness of cryomapping for ablation of tachycardias involving perinodal tissue. J Interv Card Electrophysiol 10:153-158, 2004.
13. Belhassen B, Viskin S, Fish R, et al.: Catheter-induced mechanical trauma to accessory pathways during radiofrequency ablation: Incidence, predictors and clinical implications. J Am Coll Cardiol 33:767-774, 1999.
14. Kuck KH, Ouyang F, Goya M, Boczor S: Ablation of anteroseptal and midseptal accessory pathways. In Zipes DP, Haïssaguerre M (eds.): Catheter Ablation of Arrhythmias, 2nd ed. Armonk, N.Y.: Futura, 2002, pp 305-320.
15. Haïssaguerre M, Marcus F, Poquet F, et al.: Electrocardiographic characteristics and catheter ablation of parahisian accessory pathways. Circulation 90:1124-1128, 1994.
16. Pappone C, Stabile G, Oreto G, et al.: Inappropriate sinus tachycardia after radiofrequency ablation of para-Hisian accessory pathways. J Cardiovasc Electrophysiol 8:1357-1365, 1997.
17. Miyauchi Y, Kobayashi Y, Morita N, et al.: Successful radiofrequency catheter ablation of an anteroseptal (superoparaseptal) atrioventricular accessory pathway from the left ventricular outflow tract. Pacing Clin Electrophysiol 27:668-670, 2004.
18. Tada H, Naito S, Nogami A, Taniguchi K: Successful catheter ablation of an anteroseptal accessory pathway from the noncoronary sinus of Valsalva. J Cardiovasc Electrophysiol 14:544-546, 2003.
19. Brugada J, Puigfel M, Mont L, et al.: Radiofrequency ablation of anteroseptal, para-Hisian, and mid-septal accessory pathways using a simplified femoral approach. Pacing Clin Electrophysiol 21:735-741, 1998.
20. Twidale N, Wang XZ, Beckman KJ, et al.: Factors associated with recurrence of accessory pathway conduction after radiofrequency catheter ablation. Pacing Clin Electrophysiol 14:2042-2048, 1991.

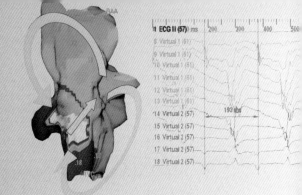

23

Ablation of Atriofascicular (Mahaim) Accessory Pathways

Henry A. Chen • Amin Al-Ahmad • Paul J. Wang

Key Points

■ Mapping of atriofascicular (Mahaim fiber) accessory pathways is directed at identifying a Mahaim potential or atrial insertion site on the tricuspid annulus or, rarely, the ventricular insertion.

■ The ablation target is usually the Mahaim fiber; alternatives are the atrial insertion on the tricuspid annulus or rarely the ventricular insertion distally in right ventricle.

■ The use of long preformed sheaths may be helpful. Specialized ablation systems are rarely necessary. Electroanatomic mapping systems are optional, but catheter location or navigation systems may be useful.

■ Sources of difficulty include ablation of the distal ventricular insertion site, localization of the atrial insertion, catheter instability during mapping, and sensitivity of the pathway to mechanical trauma.

An evolution in the understanding of a unique type of accessory pathway (AP) that demonstrates slow, decremental, and exclusively antegrade conduction, originally termed "Mahaim fiber," has occurred over several decades of histopathologic, electrophysiologic, and surgical observations.

In 1938, Mahaim and colleagues originally described pathologic findings of discrete accessory conductive pathways connecting the atrioventricular (AV) node and the ventricle.[1,2] Observation of a unique preexcitation tachycardia syndrome that demonstrated AV nodal-like slow and decremental conduction, exclusively antegrade in direction (with minimal or no preexcitation during sinus rhythm) led to the speculation of pathways that connect the AV node with the right ventricle using the fibers described by Mahaim.[3,4] The preexcited tachycardia conduction was thought to travel antegrade through the AV node and then along a Mahaim fiber to the ventricle ("nodoventricular"), to the fascicle ("nodofascicular"), or along the native conduction system to the fascicle and then over a Mahaim fiber to the ventricle ("fasciculoventricular").[4]

Later surgical and electrophysiologic observations challenged the accuracy of such an explanation.[5-8] Lack of nodal involvement was demonstrated by the persistence of preexcited tachycardia despite ablation of the AV node.[5,9] In small series of patients thought to have nodoventricular pathways, surgical ablation of the AV node failed to terminate preexcited tachycardia, whereas ablation at the right anterior epicardial tricuspid annulus successfully ended the tachycardia.[7] Others similarly observed that catheter ablation at the AV node failed to eliminate preexcitation,[5,9] but that it could be terminated by ablation at the tricuspid annulus.[10-12] Demonstrating the extranodal nature of the pathways further, Tchou et al.[6] observed in 1988 that a late-coupled right atrial extrastimulus delivered in the tachycardia cycle while the AV node was refractory could advance the timing of the subsequent QRS. Such findings have helped reshape the understanding of the anatomic and functional nature of these pathways.

Anatomy

Current concepts of the pathways have been shaped by modern surgical and electrophysiologic data. The proximal insertion of the pathway is thought to be at the atrial margin of the free wall tricuspid annulus, and the distal insertion either at the right bundle branch (RBB) or directly into ventricular myocardium—termed "atriofascicular" or "atrioventricular," respectively (Figs. 23–1, 23–2, and 23–3).[6-8,10-16] Less commonly, there are also "fasciculoventricular" APs; they originate from the His bundle or bundle branches and insert into ventricles and are not known to be associated with clinical arrhythmias.[17] Most of the atriofascicular pathways are on the right side of the heart, although there are rare cases reported of left-sided pathways.[18-20]

The atrial component of the pathway (usually located at or near the lateral, anterolateral, or posterolateral tricuspid annulus) is thought to have nodal-like properties and is largely responsible for the decremental conduction properties of the pathway.[10]

The atrial insertion connects to a long fiber, similar to the RBB, that can insert proximally into the ventricular myocardium close to the tricuspid annulus (proximal atrioventricular) or more distally into the apical ventricular myocardium (distal atrioventricular). Alternatively, it can travel along the right ventricular endocardial surface to insert into the RBB, usually in the distal third of the free wall (atriofascicular).[10] The long pathways often have a wide distal insertion, which can be up to 0.5 to 2 cm in diameter.[13] Atriofascicular pathways represent the majority of these decremental APs.

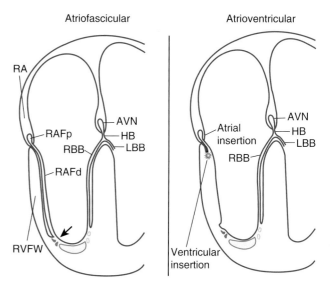

FIGURE 23–1. Schematic representation of the Mahaim atriofascicular pathway (left) and an atrioventricular connection (right). The *arrow* indicates ventricular insertion of the atriofascicular pathway in the apical right ventricular free wall close to the terminal right bundle. For the atrioventricular connection, the ventricular insertion is near to the annulus. AVN, AV node; HB, His bundle; LBB, left bundle branch; RA, Right atrium; RAFd, right atriofasciualr distal segment; RAFp, Right atriofascicular proximal insertion; RBB, right bundle branch; RVFW, right ventricular free wall. *(Modified from Jackman WM, et al. Ablation of Right Atriofascicular (Mahaim) Accessory Pathways. In Zipes DP [ed.]: Catheter Ablation of Cardiac Arrhythmias. Armonk, N.Y.: Futura, 1994, pp 187-210, with permission.)*

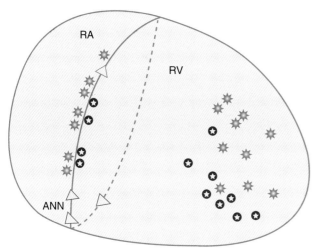

FIGURE 23–2. Pathway insertion sites (in 21 patients). In the right anterior oblique perspective, the tricuspid annulus is depicted by the *black line* and the *dotted black line* (septal aspect), the atriofascicular pathway insertions are represented by the *black stars*, the long atrioventricular pathway insertions are represented by the *white stars on black background*, and the short atrioventricular pathway insertions are represented by the *triangles*. (From Haissaguerre M, Cauchemez B, Marcus F, et al.: *Characteristics of the ventricular insertion sites of accessory pathways with anterograde decremental conduction properties. Circulation 91:1077-1085, 1995, with permission.*)

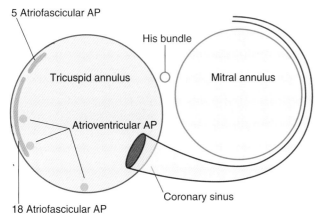

FIGURE 23–3. Schematic representation in vertical perspective of tricuspid annulus insertion sites in 26 patients. Twenty-three patients were found to have atriofascicular accessory pathways, and three were found to have atrioventricular accessory pathways. (From McClelland JH, Wang X, Beckman KJ, et al.: *Radiofrequency catheter ablation of right atriofascicular [Mahaim] accessory pathways guided by accessory pathway activation potentials. Circulation 89:2655-2666, 1994, with permission.*)

Pathophysiology

During tachycardia, conduction travels antegrade down the AP, to the RBB (typically), and retrograde back up to the His bundle, AVN, and then atrium

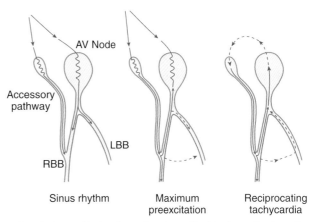

FIGURE 23–4. Mechanism of tachycardia. In sinus rhythm, the atrial signal may travel down the accessory pathway as well as the AV node. During maximum preexcitation, or antidromic reciprocating tachycardia, the signal travels antegrade down the accessory pathway. It then retrogradely activates the bundle of His and then the AVN. (From Leitch JW, Klein GJ, Yee R: *New concepts on nodoventricular accessory pathways. J Cardiovasc Electrophysiol 1:220-230, 1990, with permission.*)

(Fig. 23–4).[12] In electrophysiologic study, the RBB signal can be seen to precede the His signal during tachycardia.[12] These APs are characterized by specific electrophysiologic properties. During sinus rhythm, they demonstrate only minimal preexcitation. They conduct only in the antegrade direction and exhibit long baseline conduction time, increased conduction time with closer coupling intervals in atrial pacing, Wenckebach behavior during conduction block, and transient conduction block with adenosine.[10,21] These pathways are predominantly right-sided. A summary of eight series of patients (N = 99) demonstrated no patients with left-sided atriofascicular APs.[10-15,22,23]

Similar to the AV node, the decremental property of these APs is related to the slow rate of recovery of excitability.[24] Coexistent with the atriofascicular or atrioventricular pathways, other APs may be present, serving as the retrograde limb in the reentrant circuit. Atrioventricular nodal reentrant tachycardia (AVNRT) may be present, with the atriofascicular APs serving a "bystander" role.[12,16,25,26]

In antidromic AV reentrant tachycardia, the earliest ventricular activation is seen at the right ventricular apical catheter, with activation at or before the QRS onset (Fig. 23–5). RBB activation precedes His bundle activation. There is a short ventricular-to-atrial (VA) interval (retrograde atrial activation begins near the end of the QRS). Finally, there is progressive prolongation of antegrade conduction to eventual block with injection of adenosine.

Atrial pacing with decreasing cycle lengths prolongs the PR interval (increased decremental

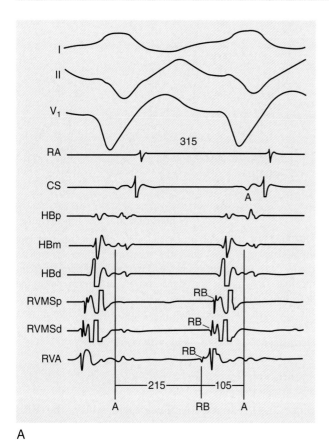

A

FIGURE 23–5. A, Intracardiac electrogram of patient in reciprocating tachycardia, demonstrating typical features: left bundle branch morphology, ventricular activation preceded by retrograde activation of right bundle branch (RB), early retrograde activation of the His bundle causing short ventriculoatrial (VA) interval, and long accessory pathway conduction time causing long AV interval. *(From McClelland JH, Wang X, Beckman KJ, et al.: Radiofrequency catheter ablation of right atriofascicular [Mahaim] accessory pathways guided by accessory pathway activation potentials. Circulation 89:2655-2666, 1994, with permission.)* **B,** Bystander Mahaim conduction during AV nodal reentry. After one beat of sinus rhythm, a premature ventricular contraction (VPD) is delivered *(arrow)* inducing AV nodal reentry. The cycle length is 310 ms. The dotted line demarcates the QRS onset. The preexcited tachycardia shows a H-A interval of approximately 50-60 ms. This is shorter than the H-A interval after the VPD which represents the H-A interval that would be expected in antidromic tachycardia. The short H-A interval in tachycardia is consistent with AV nodal reentry and bystander Mahaim preexcitation. A, atrial electrogram; CS, coronary sinus; HRA, high right atrium; RVA, right ventricular apex; V, ventricular electrogram. *(Reproduced with permission from Josephson ME. Clinical Cardiac Electrophysiology. In: Techniques and Interpretations, 3/e. Philadelphia: Lippincott Williams and Wilkins, 2002, 322-424).*

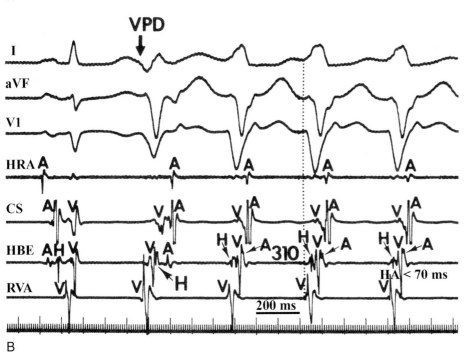

B

conduction) and widens the QRS duration (increased preexcitation) (Fig. 23–6). During rapid atrial pacing, the atrial-to-His (AH) interval is prolonged more than the AV interval. As a result, the His-to-ventricular (HV) interval shortens and the atrium-to-delta wave interval is prolonged up to the point of maximal preexcitation.[12] With atrial pacing and adenosine, the prolongation of antegrade conduction over the AP occurs between the atrial insertion and the Mahaim potential. The Mahaim potential-to-ventricle interval remains constant. Progressively faster pacing can cause prolongation of the PR and

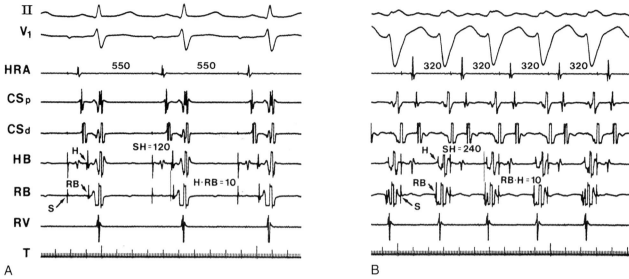

FIGURE 23–6. Atrial pacing. In **A**, atrial pacing at cycle length of 550 msec demonstrates no preexcitation in the QRS morphology, and antegrade conduction through the right bundle is suggested by the His-right bundle interval. In **B**, when the atrial pacing cycle length is shortened to 320 msec, there is maximal preexcitation with widened QRS morphology, and the sequence of His and right bundle activations is reversed. Intracardiac leads are high right atrium (HRA), proximal and distal coronary sinus (CSp and CSd, respectively), His bundle (HB), right bundle branch (RB), and right ventricular apex (RV). Surface ECG leads are II and V1. *(From Tchou P, Lehmann MH, Jazayeri M, Akhtar M: Atriofascicular connection or a nodoventricular Mahaim fiber? Electrophysiologic elucidation of the pathway and associated reentrant circuit. Circulation 77:837-848, 1988, with permission.)*

QRS intervals up to a point of maximal preexcitation, beyond which AV block occurs. Often, preexcited tachycardia can be induced when a critical pacing interval is reached or when pacing is stopped abruptly. Antidromic tachycardia is usually initiated with ventricular pacing.

Because these pathways are usually located along the tricuspid annulus, right atrial pacing commonly produces greater preexcitation than does pacing from the coronary sinus.

Similar to rapid atrial pacing, delivery of early atrial extrastimuli can cause prolongation of the PR and QRS intervals. Even shorter coupling intervals lead to a point of maximal preexcitation and then, ultimately, to AV block. If conduction then goes antegrade down the AP, supraventricular tachycardia can be initiated. This impulse travels down the AP, activates the ventricle, and then goes retrograde up the His system and AV node to the atrium.

Introduction of an atrial extrastimulus, usually from the lateral right atrium, during tachycardia can help prove both the presence of an atriofascicular or atrioventricular pathway and its participation in the reentrant circuit (Fig. 23–7). These stimuli are usually delivered late, to prevent the premature extrastimulus from conducting down the AV node.[6] The atrial extrasystole should be delivered late enough to first observe the retrograde atrial activation at the atrial septum or coronary sinus ostium before the paced atrial beat.[10] Presence of an atriofascicular pathway is suggested if this atrial extrasystole preexcites the ventricle. If it advances the atrial signal that follows the QRS (resets the tachycardia), then participation of the pathway in the reentrant circuit is also demonstrated. Mere presence of the AP without involvement in the reentrant tachycardia may occur if there are other pathways (e.g., AVNRT) and the AP acts as a bystander.

Diagnosis and Differential Diagnosis

CLINICAL PRESENTATION

Patients with Mahaim-type APs can be young in age with or without cardiac structural abnormality. There have been reported associations with Ebstein's anomaly of the tricuspid valve[27,28] as well as dual AV nodal pathways and coexistent APs.[22]

Among all APs, atriofascicular pathways are relatively uncommon, accounting for up to 2% to 3%.[11,22] The actual incidence may be greater due to potential under-reporting, because the surface electrocardiogram (ECG) during sinus rhythm may appear normal without evident preexcitation. In tachycardia,

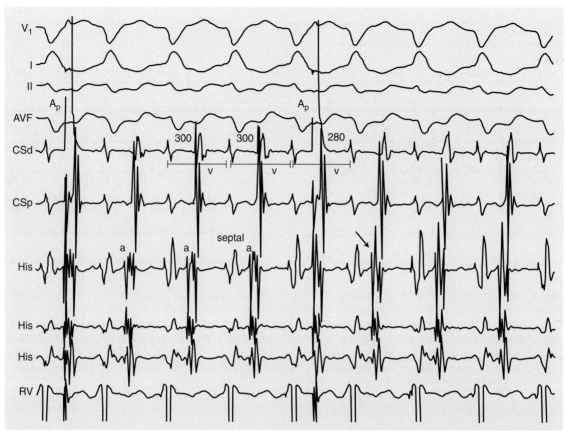

FIGURE 23-7. Introduction of atrial extrastimulus during tachycardia, timed after deflection of septal atrial electrogram. Advancement of the following QRS complex (with identical preexcited morphology) and retrograde atrial activation are displayed. The next atrial electrogram after the extrastimulus is advanced by about 30 msec (*arrow*). The ability to advance the subsequent ventricular and atrial electrograms after an early atrial extrastimulus demonstrates the participation of the Mahaim accessory pathway in the tachycardia circuit rather than atrioventricular nodal reentry. Surface ECG leads include V_1, I, II, and aVF. Intracardiac recordings are from the coronary sinus distal and proximal (CSd and CSp), His bundle (His), and right ventricular apex (RV). Septal atrial electrogram is marked with "a," and ventricular electrogram is noted with "v." *(From Grogin HR, Lee RJ, Kwasman M, et al.: Radiofrequency catheter ablation of atriofascicular and nodoventricular Mahaim tracts. Circulation 90:272-281, 1994, with permission.)*

patients with Mahaim pathways exhibit preexcitation on the surface ECG, suggestive of antidromic AV reciprocating tachycardia. The particular diagnostic findings on surface ECG, as well as in electrophysiology studies, are derived from the pathways' unique physiologic properties.

ELECTROCARDIOGRAPHIC CHARACTERISTICS

In sinus rhythm, there may be little or no evident preexcitation (Fig. 23–8A). In preexcited tachycardia, however, particular findings can be observed, such as typical or atypical left bundle branch (LBB) block morphology or a delta wave (if atrioventricular, with insertion into the ventricle near the tricuspid annulus),[13] a QRS interval of 150 msec (commonly), axis between 0 and 75 degrees, and late R wave transition at V_4 or V_5 (Fig. 23–9; see Fig. 23–8B).[29] Clues to subtle preexcitation in sinus rhythm are the absence of septal Q waves in leads I, aVL, V_5, and V_6 and the

presence of an rS complex in lead III in the setting of a narrow QRS.[30,31]

DIAGNOSIS BY INTRACARDIAC RECORDINGS

The criteria to diagnose an atriofascicular pathway by intracardiac recordings are given in Table 23–1. There should be evidence of an antegrade-only, slow, decrementally conducting AP with atrial insertion along the tricuspid annulus (usually) and ventricular insertion in the distal right bundle. For atrioventricular pathways, the insertion is usually the right ventricular free wall near the annulus. The atriofascicular pathway demonstrates decremental conduction between the atrial insertion and the AP potential as well as a fixed AP-to-ventricular interval.

During antidromic reciprocating tachycardia, an atriofascicular connection should demonstrate the following: (1) short ventricular-to-His bundle (VH) interval (in absence of RBB block); (2) earliest ven-

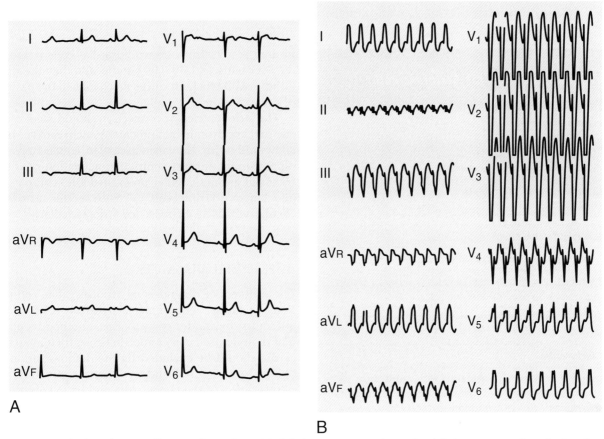

FIGURE 23–8. Surface electrocardiogram of a patient with Mahaim accessory pathway. Panel **A** demonstrates sinus rhythm. No pre-excitation is observed. Panel **B** demonstrates reciprocating tachycardia, in which left bundle branch morphology is seen. *(From Okishige K, Goseki Y, Itoh A, et al.: New electrophysiologic features and catheter ablation of atrioventricular and atriofascicular accessory pathways: evidence of decremental conduction and the anatomic structure of the Mahaim pathway. J Cardiovasc Electrophysiol 9:22-33, 1998, with permission.)*

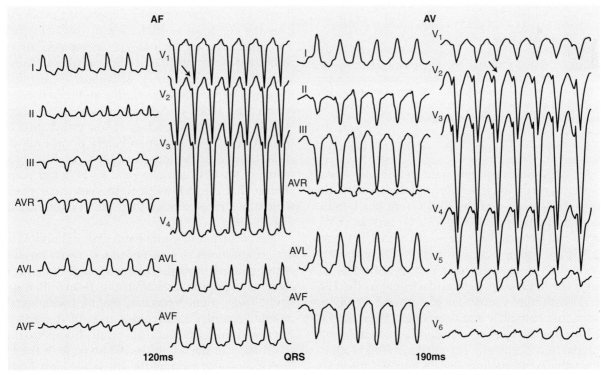

FIGURE 23–9. Surface electrocardiograms of patients with atriofascicular accessory pathway (AF, left) and atrioventricular accessory pathway (AV, right). The QRS duration is longer (190 msec) and the initial R wave in the anterior leads (*arrow*) is broader in the electrocardiogram of the atrioventricular accessory pathway. *(From Haissaguerre M, Cauchemez B, Marcus F, et al.: Characteristics of the ventricular insertion sites of accessory pathways with anterograde decremental conduction properties. Circulation 91:1077-1085, 1995, with permission.)*

TABLE 23-1

Diagnostic Criteria for Atriofascicular Accessory Pathways

Electrocardiography

LBBB morphology

QRS interval ≤150 msec (commonly)

Axis between 0 and 75 degrees

Late R > S wave transition at V_4 or V_5

Electrophysiologic study

AP conduct only in antegrade direction

AP exhibits slow, decremental conduction proximal to AP potential with fixed AP-to-V interval

Earliest ventricular activation during preexcitation at RV apex

In Tachycardia

Features of antidromic reciprocating tachycardia with ability to advance V and subsequent A activation with PAC during AV nodal refractoriness

Short VH interval (<50 msec)

Earliest ventricular activation and short postpacing interval in RV apex

RBB activation before His (in absence of RBBB)

Increased VA and VH with RBBB without change in preexcitation

VH in SVT < VH with RV pacing

HA in SVT = HA with RV pacing

A, atrium; AP, accessory pathway; HA, His bundle-to-atrial interval; LBBB, left bundle branch block; PAC, premature atrial extrastimulus; RBB(B), right bundle branch (block); RV, right ventricular; SVT, supraventricular tachycardia; V, ventricle; VA, ventricular-to-atrial interval; VH, ventricular-to-His bundle interval.

tricular activation near the right ventricular apex, with short postpacing intervals from this location; (3) retrograde activation of the RBB before His bundle activation (in absence RBB block); (4) increased VA interval and tachycardia cycle length with RBB block; (5) a VH interval in tachycardia shorter than the VH interval with right ventricular pacing; (6) a His-to-atrial (HA) interval in tachycardia equal to the HA interval with right ventricular pacing; and (7) ability to advance ventricular and subsequent atrial activation by a premature atrial stimulus delivered during AV nodal refractoriness.[31] The effects of RBB block in tachycardia are to prolong the VA and VH intervals in tachycardia and also to produce antegrade right bundle activation after His depolarization. This latter

finding results from transmyocardial conduction to the left ventricle, LBB, His bundle, and then the right bundle. RBB block produces no change in the pattern of preexcitation.

The atrioventricular connection should meet criteria for antidromic reciprocating tachycardia, but, compared with the atriofascicular connections, it demonstrates earliest ventricular activation near the tricuspid annulus, wider preexcited QRS complexes, and longer VH intervals (37 ± 9 msec for atrioventricular versus 16 ± 5 msec for atriofascicular).[13]

DIFFERENTIAL DIAGNOSIS

The differential diagnosis of atriofascicular connections includes ventricular tachycardia, LBB block aberrancy, bystander participation, and nodoventricular or nodofascicular connections. Ventricular tachycardia should be excluded by the demonstration of obligatory 1:1 atrial and ventricular activation for perpetuation of the tachycardia and by the ability to reset the ventricle and subsequent atrial activation by a premature atrial stimulus delivered during AV nodal refractoriness. Bundle branch reentry with LBB block morphology has an HV interval greater than the HV interval in sinus rhythm and His activation before RBB activation. Supraventricular tachycardia with LBB block aberrancy is proven by recording a normal or prolonged HV interval with antegrade His activation during tachycardia. Bystander participation can be demonstrated by dissociating conduction over the AP from continuation of the tachycardia. AV nodal reentry is not an uncommon finding associated with atriofascicular pathways. AVNRT with bystander pathway activation is suggested by continuation of tachycardia at the same cycle length with block in AP, HA in tachycardia shorter than HA during RV pacing, HA in tachycardia less than 70 msec, His activation before or on time with right bundle activation in absence of RBB block, fusion of the QRS complex, and a VH in tachycardia shorter than the VH with right ventricular pacing, which in turn is shorter than the HV interval (see Fig. 23-5B).[31]

The exclusion of nodoventricular and nodofascicular connections is also necessary. These rare connections arise from the AV node to insert into the right ventricular myocardium and distal RBB, respectively. These connections may manifest with narrow- or wide-complex tachycardia and AV dissociation. Narrow-complex tachycardia results from retrograde conduction in the AP to the AV node, with the His-Purkinje system forming the antegrade limb. During antidromic tachycardia, the VH interval may be short (<50 msec for nodofascicular) or intermediate (50 to

TABLE 23–2

Differential Electrophysiologic Findings for Atriofascicular Connections and LBBB Tachycardias

Connection/ Arrhythmia	Proximal Insertion	Distal Insertion	HV with Decremental Atrial Pacing	VH in Tach	Effect of RAFW PAC in Tach	AV Dissociation in Tach	HA in Tach*	QRS Fusion from Atrial Activation during Tach⁺	Sequence of His and RBB in Tach*
Atriofascicular	RA free wall	Distal RBB	Decreases then fixed	Short‡ and <VH with RV pacing	V and subsequent A advanced when septal A refractory	Not possible	= HA with RV pacing	Not possible	RBB before His
Slow atrioventricular	RA free wall	RV near TVA	Decreases then fixed	Intermed§ and >VH with RV pacing	A and subsequent V advanced when septal A refractory	Not possible	= HA with RV pacing	Not possible	RBB before His
Typical atrioventricular (antidromic tach)	RA near TVA	RV near TVA	Decreases	Intermed§ and >VH with RV pacing	V and subsequent A advanced if near insertion	Not possible	= HA with RV pacing	Not possible	Usually RBB before His
Nodoventricular	AV node	Ventricular myocardium	Decreases then fixed	>VH with RV pacing	V advanced if septal A advanced	Possible	= HA with RV pacing	Not possible	RBB before His
Nodofascicular	AV node	Distal RBB	Decreases then fixed	Short‡ and <VH with RV pacing	V advanced if septal A advanced	Possible	= HA with RV pacing	Not possible	RBB before His

TABLE 23-2

Differential Electrophysiologic Findings for Atriofascicular Connections and LBBB Tachycardias—cont'd

Connection/Arrhythmia	Proximal Insertion	Distal Insertion	HV with Decremental Atrial Pacing	VH in Tach	Effect of RAFW PAC in Tach	AV Dissociation in Tach	HA in Tach*	QRS Fusion from Atrial Activation during Tach+	Sequence of His and RBB in Tach*
Fasciculo-ventricular	His or RBB	RV myocardium	Short and fixed	Bystander only	Bystander only	Bystander only	Bystander only	Bystander only	His before RBB
Intra-myocardial VT	RV or V septum	RV or V septum	Normal or prolonged	Usually intermed§ or long	V advanced only if septal A and His advanced	Common	= HA with RV pacing	Possible	Typically RBB before His
BBR	Usually RBB antegrade	Myocardium and LBB retrograde	Usually fixed and prolonged	HV in tach ≥HV in sinus rhythm	V advanced only if septal A and His advanced	Common	= HA with RV pacing	Not possible	Typically His before RBB with H-RBB interval ≤ H-RBB interval in sinus rhythm
AVNRT with bystander atriofascicular	RA free wall	Distal RBB	Decreases then fixed	< 70 msec and/or <VH with RV pacing	Usually no effect	Possible	< HA with RV pacing	Possible	His before or on time with RBB
SVT LBBB Aberrancy	Variable depending on mechanism	Variable depending on mechanism	Fixed or prolonged	HV fixed	Variable depending on mechanism	Depends on mechanism	Depends on mechanism	Not possible	His before RBB

*Assumes no RBBB.
+Assumes absence of second accessory pathway.
†VH < 50 msec.
§VH = 50-80 msec.

A, atrium; AV, atrioventricular; AVNRT, atrioventricular nodal reentrant tachycardia; BBR, bundle branch reentry; HA, His-to-atrial interval; His, His bundle; HV, His-to-ventricular interval; LBB(B), left bundle branch (block); RA, right atrium; RAFW, right atrial free wall; RV, right ventricle; SVT, supraventricular tachycardia; tach, tachycardia; TVA, tricuspid valve annulus; V, ventricle; VH, ventricle-to-His interval; VT, ventricular tachycardia.

80 msec for nodoventricular) in the absence of RBB block.[31] These tachycardias should not be advanced by premature atrial stimulation during AV nodal refractoriness (above the level of the AP insertion) and are advanced only if the septal atrial activation is advanced. Table 23–2 lists features that differentiate fascicular and ventricular APs and LBB block tachycardias.

Mapping

Techniques for mapping and ablating these pathways have been derived from their unique properties. Because these APs conduct only in an anterograde direction without much preexcitation in sinus rhythm, mapping is usually performed during antidromic AV tachycardia, atrial pacing, or atrial extrastimuli. The techniques for mapping atriofascicular connections are as follows.

1. *Identification of site of discrete Mahaim potential at the tricuspid annulus:* This is the most commonly used technique.[10,13,15,22,32] By scanning the tricuspid annulus at the right atrial free wall with the catheter tip, one looks for the presence of AP or "Mahaim" potentials, which are very similar to His bundle potentials.[10,12,22] Distinct atrial, AP, and ventricular potentials can be found at the atrial insertion site. The Mahaim potential represents the atrial insertion site (Fig. 23–10) and provides the best site for ablation of these APs.[33,34]
2. *Atrial pace mapping at the tricuspid annulus:* Localization of the point that produces the shortest stimulus-to-preexcitation (delta wave) interval with atrial pacing can be used in an effort to identify the atrial insertion site. The major limitations of this method are the technical difficulty of positioning the catheter and distinguishing sites of similar stimulus-to-delta wave intervals.[14]
3. *Introducing an atrial extrastimulus:* Similar to atrial pace mapping, localization of the spot from which a late premature atrial extrastimulus delivered during preexcited tachycardia results in the greatest advancement of the next QRS can be used to locate the atrial insertion site. This technique involves introducing a late premature atrial extrastimulus at various spots to identify the one that provides the greatest advancement of the next QRS complex with fixed coupling interval or the site from which the longest coupled atrial extrastimulus during tachycardia causes resetting of the cycle (Fig. 23–11).[15] This method has also been found to be technically difficult and time-consuming.[11,15,35]

4. *Activation mapping of the ventricle:* The ventricular insertion site, especially those that are at the level of the tricuspid annulus, can be localized with this method.[13,36,37] For more distally inserting APs, mapping for the earliest ventricular activation is difficult. These APs tend to arborize widely into the ventricular tissue, making it difficult to completely ablate the ventricular insertion.[13] Often, only a change in the preexcitation electrogram results, rather than abolition. Nonetheless, there are a few reports of successful ablation at the ventricular insertion of the APs.[36,38]
5. *Mechanical disruption of conduction:* These APs have a particular sensitivity to mechanical trauma compared with other APs.[11,14,22] Cappato, et al.[11] demonstrated that merely applying pressure to the AP with the catheter tip easily induces conduction block (Figs. 23–12 and 23–13). This phenomenon can be used to help identify the location of the AP. The catheter tip is positioned along the tricuspid annulus, gentle pressure is exerted, and the tip is brought along the tricuspid annular groove. After induction of mechanical block (sudden loss of preexcitation or prolongation of the AV interval, suggesting the location of the tricuspid annular crossing), one waits for return of the preexcitation (which can take minutes to hours) and chooses that spot for ablation.[11,39] There are several criticisms of this technique. Namely, there is a significant amount of waiting time for the return of the preexcitation after block is induced, and, if the catheter moved after the block was formed, the spot cannot be found again until the conduction recurs. Electroanatomic mapping may help with this problem. The targets for ablation are summarized in Table 23–3.

TABLE 23–3

Target Sites

Near tricuspid annulus

Site of Mahaim fiber potential

Site of shortest atrial stimulus-to-ventricular activation

Site of greatest advancement of subsequent QRS complex after introduction of premature AES during AV node refractoriness

Sites of loss of preexcitation with catheter mechanical pressure ("bump mapping")

Ventricular insertion site

Site identified by activation mapping (atrioventricular connection)

AES, atrial extrastimulus.

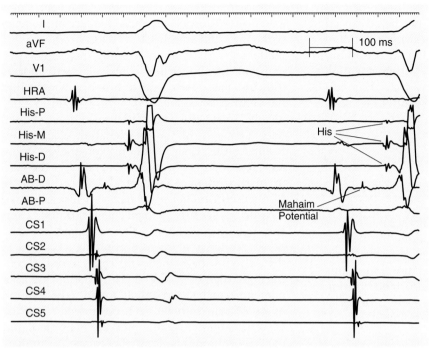

A

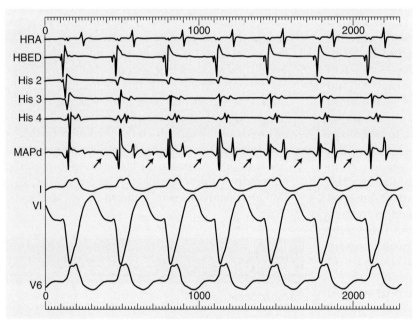

Speed: 100 mm/s

B

FIGURE 23–10. Mahaim potential. **A.** Mahaim potential (labeled) shown at high recording speed in sinus rhythm. The ablation catheter (AB) was along the inferior tricuspid valve free wall. CS, coronary sinus; CS1, proximal; CS5, distal; D, distal; HRA, high right atrium; M, mid; P, proximal. Panel **B** demonstrates tachycardia with Mahaim potentials (*arrows*). Note that both the Mahaim potentials and the His bundle activation precede the surface QRS deflection. The Mahaim potential and the His bundle potential on the HBED electrode precede ventricular activation. Note that in tachycardia but not in sinus rhythm, the ventricular activation and onset of QRS precede retrograde His bundle activation. Surface ECG leads are I, aVL, V1, and V6. Intracardiac signals are from the high right atrium (HRA), distal His bundle (HBED), mid His bundle (His 2 and 3), proximal His bundle (His 4), and right ventricular apex (MAPd). *(Panel B from Heald SC, Davies DW, Ward DE, et al.: Radiofrequency catheter ablation of Mahaim tachycardia by targeting Mahaim potentials at the tricuspid annulus. Br Heart J 73:250-257, 1995, with permission.)*

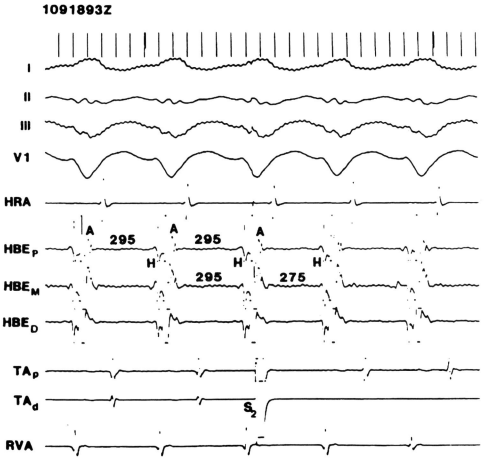

FIGURE 23–11. Locating atrial insertion site using atrial extrastimulus. After an atrial extrastimulus (S₂) is delivered in a right lateral location during tachycardia, there is AH shortening in the recording from HBEp, as the His signal is advanced 20 msec while the preceding atrial electrogram is not. This finding implies that the proximal insertion of the accessory pathway is located in a different area than the atrial insertion of the AV-node. This stimulus location also identified the site at which the latest atrial extrastimulus advanced the His deflection but not the atrial signal in the His bundle recording, implicating that catheter location as the atrial insertion of the accessory pathway. Surface ECG leads are I, II, III, and V₁. Intracardiac recordings are from the high right atrium (HRA), proximal His bundle (HBEₚ), middle His bundle (HBEₘ), distal His bundle (HBE_D), and proximal and distal tricuspid annulus (TAₚ and TA_D, respectively). RVA, right ventricular apex. *(From Klein LS, Hackett FK, Zipes DP, Miles WM: Radiofrequency catheter ablation of Mahaim fibers at the tricuspid annulus. Circulation 87:738-747, 1993, with permission.)*

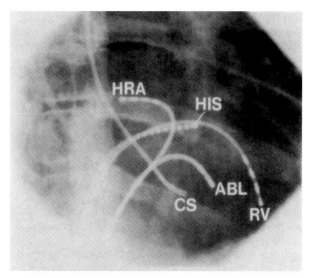

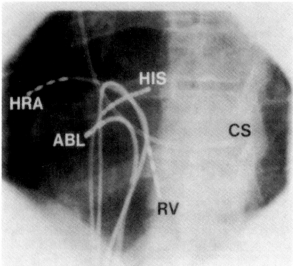

FIGURE 23–12. Catheter placement. The ablation catheter (ABL) is placed with the tip at the atrial insertion of the accessory pathway, positioned in the right posterolateral region of the tricuspid annulus. Mapping catheters include quadripolar catheters in the high right atrium (HRA) and in the right ventricular apex (RV), a decapolar catheter at the bundle of His (HIS), and a 12-polar catheter in the coronary sinus (CS). The top panel displays 30 degrees in right anterior oblique view, and the bottom panel displays 30 degrees in left anterior oblique view. *(From Cappato R, Schluer M, Weiss C, et al.: Catheter-induced mechanical conduction block of right-sided accessory fibers with Mahaim-type preexcitation to guide radiofrequency ablation. Circulation 90:282-290, 1994, with permission.)*

Ablation

Although practice variations exist, typically a femoral vein approach is used with a 7-French, 4-mm-tip electrode and a deflectable-tip catheter for mapping and ablation. Long curved sheaths may provide greater catheter stability and may help position the catheter

tip at various places along the tricuspid annulus. If the ventricle is being mapped, the catheter can cross the tricuspid annulus and be situated below the tricuspid valve. Mapping is then performed in the left anterior oblique view, with the tricuspid annulus in the center. Mapping techniques, as discussed earlier, are then performed (during tachycardia or with pacing). Most commonly, ablation is performed at the atrial insertion using mapping of discrete Mahaim pathways (Table 23–4). Loss of preexcitation during ablation is usually observed (Fig. 23–14).

Usually these APs are right-sided, traveling along the free wall tricuspid annulus to the ventricular myocardium or, more commonly, to the RBB fascicle (and there have been isolated reports of decrementally conducting left-sided APs). Although most successful ablations are in the lateral or anterolateral tricuspid annulus (80% of those reported), there have been rare cases of right atrial posterior or posteroseptal atrial insertions.[19]

Although there may be practice variations, the target temperature for ablation is usually 60°C to 70°C, which is delivered for 10 to 15 seconds while evaluating for termination of AP conduction or tachycardia. If either has been interrupted, radiofrequency ablation is usually continued for a total of 30 to 60 seconds, and the patient is monitored thereafter for recurrence. Often, radiofrequency energy produces nonsustained preexcited rhythm during ablation. This is believed to represent thermally induced automaticity from the pathway, analogous to junctional rhythm during AV nodal ablation. If the tachycardia or AP conduction does not terminate, alternative ablation sites are selected.[40]

Catheter ablation of these pathways appears to be safe and highly successful with little recurrence (see Table 23–4). Success rates for ablation of tricuspid annulus discrete potentials have been quite high.[11,39] Overall ablation success rates are approximately 90% to 95%, with approximately a 5% recurrence rate.[10-15,22,23,40,41]

Troubleshooting the Difficult Case

Mapping techniques generally offer a high probability of successful localization, and ablation is usually quite successful; however, there are specific difficulties that may arise (Table 23–5).

In some cases, it may be difficult to record a Mahaim potential. Because ventricular activation at the tricuspid annulus is not the earliest, it is not

Text continued on p. 433

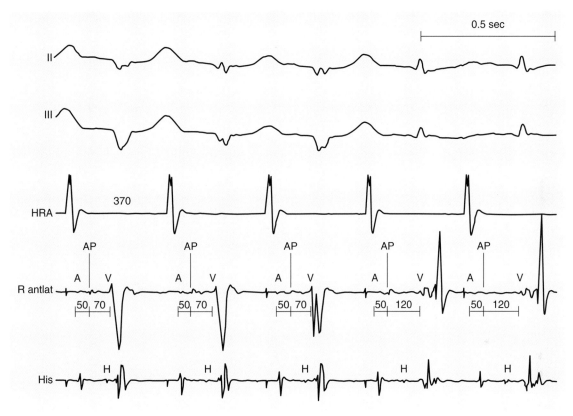

FIGURE 23–13. Mechanical disruption. During pacing at the high right atrium, preexcitation is lost (last two beats) after manipulation of the mapping catheter in the anterolateral tricuspid annulus, demonstrating mechanically-induced block in the accessory pathway. In addition, the mapping catheter continues to record accessory pathway potential (AP), localizing site of antegrade conduction block at the subannular level of the atrial input. While the A-AP interval stays constant, the AP-V interval lengthens 50 ms after the onset of mechanical disruption of the accessory pathway conduction. Surface ECG leads are II and III. Intracardiac recordings are from high right atrium (HRA), mapping catheter in right anterolateral tricuspid annulus (R antlat), and bundle of His. *(From Cappato R, Schluer M, Weiss C, et al.: Catheter-induced mechanical conduction block of right-sided accessory fibers with Mahaim-type preexcitation to guide radiofrequency ablation. Circulation 90:282-290, 1994, with permission.)*

TABLE 23–4

Electrophysiological Mapping and Ablation

Authors (Ref. No.)	Year	No. of Pts	Mapping Method	Mapping Outcome	Ablation Method	Ablation Outcome	Follow-up	Complications
Tchou et al.[6]	1988	1	A and V pacing, delivery of AES	Late AES during tachycardia preexcited V while unable to conduct through AVN, thus demonstrating RA component of AP independent of AVN	—	—	—	—
Haissaguerre et al.[37]	1990	3	V pace mapping for V insertion	—	DC energy to V insertion	100% success	12, 14, and 16 mo: no recurrence	Subclavian vein thrombosis (2 pts), pulmonary embolism (1 pt)
Klein et al.[15]	1993	4	AES during SVT Stim-delta	AFP (3 pts), AVP (1 pt)	RF to posterior and lateral TA	100% success	8 mo: no recurrent tachycardia	None
Grogin et al.[12]	1994	6	Discrete MP	AFP (4 pts), nodoventricular AP (2 pts)	AFP: RF to A side of TA (2 pts), to V side of TA (1 pt), or to distal V insertion (1 pt) Nodoventricular pathways: RF to midseptal region	100% success	Not reported	Not reported
Cappato et al.[11]	1994	11	Mechanical block at subannular TA in 8 pts (2 pts in AF)	Successful ablation in all 8 pts at subannular TA Failures: ablation at V insertion (1 pt), ablation at supra-annular TA (1 pt), mechanical block not achieved but ablated at subannular TA in SVT (1 pt)	RF to site identified by mechanical block during A pacing (6 pts) or in AF (2 pts)	Of 6 pts with ablation in A pacing, 5 had recurrence of preexcitation in 12 hr; with additional ablation next day, overall conduction was eliminated in 9 (82%) of 11 pts	9.5 ± 2.3 mo: preexcitation recurred in 1 pt	—

Study	Year	n	Mapping	Findings	Ablation	Success	Follow-up	Complications
McClelland et al.[10]	1994	23	Discrete MP	22 pts had single, discrete high-frequency AP potential at TA	RF applied to site recording AP potential (TA in 19 pts and RV free wall in 3 pts)	100% success (22 pts)	18 ± 13 mo: no tachycardia recurrence (all pts) EP study at 3.8 ± 1.7 mo (9 pts): no AP conduction	Small thrombus in superior vena cava (catheter-induced trauma)
Li et al.[23]	1994	4	Discrete MP	—	—	100% success	—	—
Heald et al.[22]	1995	21	Discrete MP	—	RF to site identified by MP at ventricular aspect of TA or if no MP, then site found by stimulus-to-delta-wave mapping	18 (90%)	9 mo: 1 recurrence (5%)	None
Haissaguerre et al.[13]	1995	21	Discrete MP	17 pts with long AP (10 with AFP, 7 with AVP) and 4 with short AVP	RF to distal or to TA sites in long AP and RF to TA in short AP patients	100% success	12 mo: no recurrence	Not reported
Brugada et al.[32]	1995	4	Discrete MP	—	RF to TA	100% success	5 mo: no recurrence	None
Okishige et al.[14]	1998	7	Proximal site: discrete MP along TA Distal site: earliest bipolar V activation relative to preexcitation signal	7 pts with AFP or AVP; 6 pts with discrete MP observed	RF to atrial or ventricular aspect of TA, localized to MP site or to site detected by S-delta mapping	100% success	19 mo: no recurrence of AP conduction	None

A, atrial; AES, atrial extrastimulus; AF, atrial fibrillation; AFP, atriofascicular pathway; AP, accessory pathway; AVP, atrioventricular pathway; DC, direct current; EP, electrophysiologic; MP, Mahaim potential; pts, patients; RA, right atrium; RF, radiofrequency energy; Stim-delta, stimulus-to-delta interval; SVT, supraventricular tachycardia; TA, tricuspid annulus; V, ventricular.

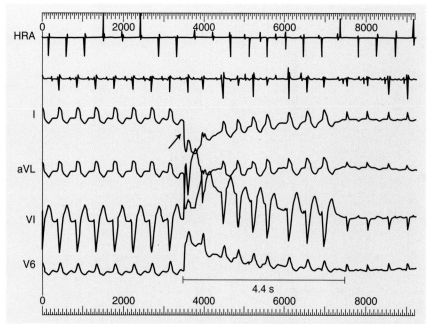

Speed: 25 mm/s

A

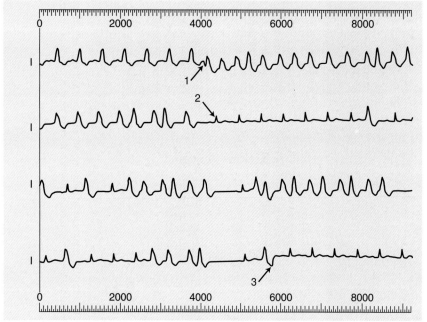

Speed: 25 mm/s

B

FIGURE 23–14. Radiofrequency energy ablation. Panel **A** displays intracardiac recordings from the high right atrium (HRA) and distal His bundle (unlabelled) as well as surface recordings from leads I, aVL, VI, and V6. After 4.4 seconds of energy delivery, there is block of Mahaim pathway conduction and resultant normalization of surface QRS complex. Panel **B** displays a continuous recording from surface ECG lead I. Typical pattern of stuttering block is demonstrated during energy application. The onset of radiofrequency energy (1) is followed by initial block in Mahaim during energy application after 9.5 seconds (2). Ectopic activity from the Mahaim pathway was observed until the end of the first 30 seconds of energy application (3). *(From Heald SC, Davies DW, Ward DE, et al.: Radiofrequency catheter ablation of Mahaim tachycardia by targeting Mahaim potentials at the tricuspid annulus. Br Heart J 73:250-257, 1995, with permission.)*

TABLE 23–5

Troubleshooting the Difficult Case

Problem	Causes	Solution
Inability to identify insertion site at TA for ablation	Absence of retrograde conduction precludes localizing spot of earliest retrograde atrial activation. Pathways with ventricular insertion distal to TA cannot be localized by evaluating for earliest ventricular activation at the TA	Map for Mahaim potentials during antidromic AVRT or atrial pacing Map for the area that provides shortest paced AV interval or greatest advance of tachycardia with PAC
Poor catheter stability	Sudden change in rhythm and heart rate Poor catheter contact	Use long sheath Use electroanatomic mapping to relocate catheter tip to previous location
Transient conduction block during mapping or ablation	High sensitivity to mechanical trauma, such as bumping catheter into AP	Use computerized catheter navigation Wait until reappearance of AP activity (may take minutes to hours)

AP, accessory pathway; AV, atrioventricular; AVRT, atrioventricular reentrant tachycardia; TA, tricuspid annulus; PAC, premature atrial contraction.

helpful to map ventricular activation at that location. Alternative methods, such as identifying the shortest stimulus-to-delta wave interval or "bump" mapping, may be necessary.

Catheter movement, particularly during a change in rhythm during ablation, may interfere with successful ablation. Catheter stability can be increased with the use of long, curved-tip sheaths. In addition, electroanatomic mapping techniques may help relocalize a catheter tip to a previous location precisely if it has moved.[42]

Finally, these pathways are very sensitive to mechanical trauma.[11,39] If a catheter bumps into it, there may be pause of AP activity, which can last from minutes to hours. The ability to relocate the AP is confounded by the time it takes to recover.

Conclusion

Current understanding of a unique type of preexcitation that exhibits nodal-like properties has evolved over the decades since Mahaim's original description of nodoventricular and nodofascicular fibers. Atriofascicular and atrioventricular pathways appear to have atrial insertion at the tricuspid annulus and insert at the RBB or proximal or apical right ventricle. The specific preexcitation characteristics can be used to localize them in mapping, which is largely done by identifying discrete Mahaim pathways. Ablation of these pathways is highly successful. Although these atriofascicular and atrioventricular pathways are relatively rare, they are unique and offer a high probability of successful ablation.

References

1. Mahaim I, Winston MR: Recherches d'lanatomic comparee et du pathologic experimental sur les connexions hautes du faisceau de His-Tawara. Cardiologia 5:189-260, 1941.
2. Mahaim I, Benatt A: Nouvelles recherches sur les connexions superieures de la branch gauche du faisceau de His-Tawara avec cloison interventriculaire. Cardiologia 1:61-76, 1938.
3. Wellens HJ: The preexcitation syndrome. In Wellens, HJ (ed.): Electrical Stimulation of the Heart in the Study and Treatment of Tachycardias. Baltimore: University Park Press, 1971, pp 97-109.
4. Anderson RH, Becker AE, Brechenmacher C, et al.: Ventricular preexcitation: A proposed nomenclature for its substrates. Eur J Cardiol 3:27-36, 1975.
5. Ellenbogen KA, et al.: Catheter atrioventricular junction ablation for recurrent supraventricular tachycardia with nodoventricular fibers. Am J Cardiol 55:1227-1229, 1985.
6. Tchou P, Lehmann MH, Jazayeri M, Akhtar M: Atriofascicular connection or a nodoventricular Mahaim fiber? Electrophysiologic elucidation of the pathway and associated reentrant circuit. Circulation 77:837-848, 1988.
7. Gillette PC, Garson A Jr, Cooey DA, et al.: Prolonged and decremental antegrade conduction properties in right anterior atrioventricular connections: Wide QRS antidromic tachycardia of left bundle block pattern without Wolff-Parkinson-White configuration in sinus rhythm. Am Heart J 103:66-74, 1982.
8. Klein GJ, Guiraudon GM, Kerr CR, et al.: "Nodoventricular" accessory pathway: Evidence for a distinct accessory atrioventricular pathway with atrioventricular node-like properties. J Am Coll Cardiol 11:1035-1040, 1988.
9. Bhandari A, Morady F, Shen EN, et al.: Catheter-induced His bundle ablation in a patient with reentrant tachycardia associated with a nodoventricular tract. J Am Coll Cardiol 4:611-616, 1984.
10. McClelland JH, Wang X, Beckman KJ, et al.: Radiofrequency catheter ablation of right atriofascicular (Mahaim) accessory pathways guided by accessory pathway activation potentials. Circulation 89:2655-2666, 1994.
11. Cappato R, Schluer M, Weiss C, et al.: Catheter-induced mechanical conduction block of right-sided accessory fibers with Mahaim-type preexcitation to guide radiofrequency ablation. Circulation 90:282-290, 1994.

12. Grogin HR, Lee RJ, Kwasman M, et al.: Radiofrequency catheter ablation of atriofascicular and nodoventricular Mahaim tracts. Circulation 90:272-281, 1994.

13. Haissaguerre M, Cauchemez B, Marcus F, et al.: Characteristics of the ventricular insertion sites of accessory pathways with anterograde decremental conduction properties. Circulation 91:1077-1085, 1995.

14. Okishige K, Goseki Y, Itoh A, et al.: New electrophysiologic features and catheter ablation of atrioventricular and atriofascicular accessory pathways: Evidence of decremental conduction and the anatomic structure of the Mahaim pathway. J Cardiovasc Electrophysiol 9:22-33, 1998.

15. Klein LS, Hackett FK, Zipes DP, Miles WM: Radiofrequency catheter ablation of Mahaim fibers at the tricuspid annulus. Circulation 87:738-747, 1993.

16. Haissaguerre M, Capos J, Marcus FI, et al.: Involvement of a nodofascicular connection in supraventricular tachycardia with VA dissociation. J Cardiovasc Electrophysiol 5:854-862, 1994.

17. Prystowsky EM, Miles WM, Heger JJ, Zipes DP: Preexcitation syndromes: Mechanisms and management. Med Clin North Am 68:831-893, 1984.

18. Hluchy J, Schlegelmilch P, Schickel S, et al.: Radiofrequency ablation of a concealed nodoventricular Mahaim fiber guided by a discrete potential. J Cardiovasc Electrophysiol 10:603-610, 1999.

19. Johnson CT, Brooks C, Jaramillo J, et al.: A left free-wall, decrementally conducting, atrioventricular (Mahaim) fiber: Diagnosis at electrophysiological study and radiofrequency catheter ablation guided by direct recording of a Mahaim potential. Pacing Clin Electrophysiol 20:2486-2488, 1997.

20. Tada H, Nogami A, Naito S, et al.: Left posteroseptal Mahaim fiber associated with marked longitudinal dissociation. Pacing Clin Electrophysiol 22:1696-1699, 1999.

21. Ellenbogen KA, Rogers R, Old W: Pharmacological characterization of conduction over a Mahaim fiber: Evidence for adenosine sensitive conduction. Pacing Clin Electrophysiol 12:1396-1404, 1989.

22. Heald SC, Davies DW, Ward DE, et al.: Radiofrequency catheter ablation of Mahaim tachycardia by targeting Mahaim potentials at the tricuspid annulus. Br Heart J 73:250-257, 1995.

23. Li HG, Klein GJ, Thakur RK, Yee R: Radiofrequency ablation of decremental accessory pathways mimicking "nodoventricular" conduction. Am J Cardiol 74:829-833, 1994.

24. Lee PC, Kanter R, Gomez-Marin O, et al.: Quantitative assessment of the recovery property of atriofascicular/atrioventricular-type Mahaim fiber. J Cardiovasc Electrophysiol 13:535-541, 2002.

25. Beurrier D, Brembilla-Perrot B, Bragard MF: Radiofrequency catheter ablation of a nodoventricular Mahaim tract. Herz 21:314-319, 1996.

26. Kottkamp H, Hindricks G, Shenasa H, et al.: Variants of preexcitation–specialized atriofascicular pathways, nodofascicular pathways, and fasciculoventricular pathways: Electrophysiologic findings and target sites for radiofrequency catheter ablation. J Cardiovasc Electrophysiol 7:916-930, 1996.

27. Gallagher JJ, Smith WM, Kasell JH, et al.: Role of Mahaim fibers in cardiac arrhythmias in man. Circulation 64:176-189, 1981.

28. Ellenbogen KA, Ramirez NM, Packer DL, et al.: Accessory nodoventricular (Mahaim) fibers: A clinical review. Pacing Clin Electrophysiol 9:868-884, 1986.

29. Bardy GH, Fedor JM, German LD, et al.: Surface electrocardiographic clues suggesting presence of a nodofascicular Mahaim fiber. J Am Coll Cardiol 3:1161-1168, 1984.

30. Sternick EB, Timmermans C, Sosa E, et al.: The electrocardiogram during sinus rhythm and tachycardia in patients with Mahaim fibers: The importance of an "rS" pattern in lead III. J Am Coll Cardiol 44:1626-1635, 2004.

31. Josephson ME: Preexcitation syndromes. In Josephson ME: Clinical Cardiac Electrophysiology: Techniques and Interpretations, 3rd ed. Philadelphia: Lippincott Williams & Wilkins, 2002, pp 322-424.

32. Mounsey JP, Griffith MJ, McComb JM: Radiofrequency ablation of a Mahaim fiber following localization of Mahaim pathway potentials. J Cardiovasc Electrophysiol 5:432-437, 1994.

33. Brugada J, Martinez-Sanchez J, Kuzmicic B: Radiofrequency catheter ablation of atriofascicular accessory pathways guided by discrete electrical potentials recorded at the tricuspid annulus. Pacing Clin Electrophysiol 18:1388-1394, 1995.

34. Miles WM: Bundle branch and Mahaim fiber ablation: Technique and results. In Second International Symposium on Interventional Electrophysiology in the Management of Cardiac Arrhythmias. July 1994.

35. Okishige K, Strickberger A, Walsh E: Catheter ablation of the atrial origin of a decrementally conducting atriofascicular accessory pathway by radiofrequency current. J Cardiovasc Electrophysiol 2:465-475, 1991.

36. Miller JM, Harper GR, Rothman SA, Hsia HH: Radiofrequency catheter ablation of an atriofascicular pathway during atrial fibrillation: A case report. J Cardiovasc Electrophysiol 5:846-853, 1994.

37. Haissaguerre M, Warin JF, Le Metayer P, et al.: Catheter ablation of Mahaim fibers with preservation of atrioventricular nodal conduction. Circulation 82:418-427, 1990.

38. Haissaguerre M, et al.: Nature of the distal insertion site of Mahaim fibers as defined by catheter ablation [abstract]. Eur Soc Cardiol 1993.

39. Belhassen B, Viskin S, Fish R, et al.: Catheter-induced mechanical trauma to accessory pathways during radiofrequency ablation: Incidence, predictors and clinical implications. J Am Coll Cardiol 33:767-774, 1999.

40. Tomassoni G, et al.: Ablation of right free wall and atriofascicular accessory pathways. In Singer I (ed.): Interventional Electrophysiology. Philadelphia: Lippincott Williams & Wilkins, 2001, pp 193-236.

41. Miller JM, Olgin JE: Catheter ablation of free-wall accessory pathways and "Mahaim" fibers. In Zipes DP, Haissaguerre M (eds.): Catheter Ablation of Arrhythmias. Armonk, N.Y.: Futura, 2002, pp 277-303.

42. Worley S: Use of a real-time three-dimensional magnetic navigation system for radiofrequency ablation of accessory pathways. Pacing Clin Electrophysiol 21:1636-1645, 1998.

43. Leitch JW, Klein GJ, Yee R: New concepts on nodoventricular accessory pathways. J Cardiovasc Electrophysiol 1:220-230, 1990.

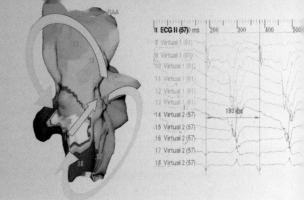

24

Special Problems in Ablation of Accessory Pathways

Basilios Petrellis • Allan C. Skanes • George J. Klein
Andrew D. Krahn • Raymond Yee

Key Points

- The approach to the difficult accessory pathway ablation is, first, to exclude "cognitive" ablation failure by confirming the tachycardia diagnosis and re-evaluating the electrograms.

- Second, use systematic approach to identify contributing technical factors, such as pathway-related factors (including location and atypical configuration) and associated cardiac structural abnormalities.

- Finally, devise an appropriate strategy. This may include optimizing pathway localization, adjusting the ablation approach to improve stability and tissue contact, and changing the ablation modality (conventional versus saline-cooled radiofrequency ablation or cryothermy).

The atrioventricular (AV) groove is normally composed of fibrous tissue devoid of electrical conductive properties; this commits ventricular activation to proceed over the specialized AV conduction tissue, the His-Purkinje system. Accessory pathways (APs) are considered a remnant of incomplete separation of the atrial and ventricular myocardium by the annulus fibrosus during cardiogenesis. The resulting myocardial bridges are capable of electrical conduction that may facilitate early ventricular activation and provide the arrhythmogenic substrate for AV reentrant tachycardia.

Because of its low risk and high efficacy, catheter ablation is first-line therapy for symptomatic patients with APs.[1-5] Ablation of APs was historically achieved first by surgical dissection and subsequently by direct current energy applied through transvenous catheters. The first successful catheter ablation of an AP using radiofrequency (RF) energy was performed in 1984.[6]

Although successful pathway elimination is achieved in more than 95% of cases, primary success is occasionally elusive, resulting in lengthy procedures or multiple attempts. Furthermore, AP conduction may return after initial success. This chapter aims to outline problems that may be encountered during ablation of APs and to propose practical solutions.

General Considerations

The incidence of successful elimination and recurrence after RF catheter ablation of APs has been well documented.[2-4,7-11] Initial ablation success is highest for left-sided pathways (97%) and is lower for right-sided (88%) and septal connections (89%). Recurrence is also less frequent at left free wall locations (5%) than at the right free wall (17%) and septum (11%).

Failed RF catheter ablation of APs is most frequently related to technical difficulties or misdiagnosis (Table 24–1). Other factors include the coexistence of structural cardiac abnormalities, atypical pathway configuration, and high-risk AP locations, such as those adjacent to the AV node or within the coronary sinus (CS).

INABILITY TO HEAT

Technical considerations such as catheter instability or difficult access may give rise to poor endocardial contact, leading to insufficient energy delivery and local heat production at the ablation target. This problem is more frequently encountered with right-

TABLE 24–1
Causes of Failed Catheter Ablation of Accessory Pathways
Inability to heat
Catheter instability, poor tissue contact, difficult access to target site
Pathway location beyond range of RF lesion size (e.g., epicardial location)
Misdiagnosis
Misinterpretation of electrophysiologic data
Previous ablation, low-amplitude or distorted electrogram recordings
Incomplete electrophysiology study, inaccurate pathway localization, incomplete mapping
Multiple tachycardia mechanisms (e.g., AP with AVNRT or ectopic tachycardia, pathway-to-pathway tachycardia)
Associated structural cardiac abnormalities
Ebstein's anomaly
Persistent left-sided superior vena cava
Atypical pathway configuration
Multiple APs
Oblique APs
Epicardial APs
Atypical AP connections
High-risk AP location
Adjacent to the AV node: midseptal or anteroseptal pathway (risk of inadvertent AV block)
Epicardial APs: accessible within the coronary sinus or associated with diverticulum (risk of arterial stenosis—circumflex artery or distal right coronary branches)

AP, accessory pathway; AV, atrioventricular; AVNRT, atrioventricular nodal reentrant tachycardia; RF, radiofrequency energy.

sided APs due to a less clearly defined anatomic groove delineating the tricuspid annulus. Poor energy delivery, indicated by a low power output of the RF generator during temperature-controlled RF ablation, may achieve the desired tip-tissue interface temperature but does not provide adequate depth of energy penetration for elimination of AP conduction. Tissue contact and catheter access to the target site are often improved by the use of long, preformed intravascular sheaths or deflectable ablation catheters of varying reach, curve, and tip size, which are designed in a variety of configurations to allow access to all locations on either the tricuspid or the mitral annulus.

Energy delivery is further enhanced by the use of saline-irrigated (cooled-tip) or passively cooled large-tip catheters, which infuse normal saline during RF delivery. Because interfacial heating is reduced, coagulum formation and char at the catheter tip are prevented, allowing the point of maximal heating to be shifted into the tissue rather than focused at the tissue surface. Deeper conductive heating produces deeper tissue lesions.

Catheter stability may be compromised if ablation is performed during orthodromic AV reentrant tachycardia. Ablation during tachycardia is sometimes necessary if retrograde fusion during ventricular pacing obscures the pathway location in patients with concealed APs. Abrupt heart rate slowing on RF-induced termination of tachycardia frequently results in catheter dislodgement, preventing full-duration RF current delivery at the successful site. Entrainment of the tachycardia by ventricular pacing during ablation overcomes this potential problem.[12] While maintaining retrograde activation over the AP, entrainment prevents an abrupt change in ventricular rate, allowing a stable catheter position during pathway ablation for continued RF energy delivery despite tachycardia termination.

MISDIAGNOSIS

Misinterpretation of electrophysiologic data, by failure or inability to recognize atrial or ventricular activation sequence or AP potentials prohibits accurate pathway localization. Appropriate interpretation of data may be precluded by factors attributable to the AP, such as overlapping electrograms, which are often seen with multiple and right free wall pathways (Fig. 24–1), or distorted low-amplitude electrograms at the site of RF lesions in patients with a previously unsuccessful ablation attempt.

Incomplete mapping may prevent accurate localization, a point of particular relevance to posteroseptal APs. If thorough mapping at the posteroseptal region on the right fails to identify a successful ablation site, careful mapping of the CS and the left posteroseptal region is essential. In the event that an epicardial pathway is suspected, CS angiography may identify a coexistent CS diverticulum or aneurysm.

A complete initial electrophysiology study is necessary to exclude an unrecognized or unexpected tachycardia mechanism, because APs, atrioventricular nodal reentrant tachycardia (AVNRT), and ectopic tachycardias infrequently coexist. Furthermore, successful AP ablation may lead to the emergence of a latent AP, causing symptom recurrence and need for

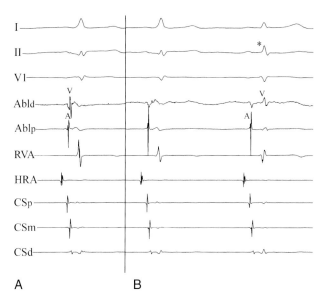

FIGURE 24–1. Misinterpretation of electrophysiologic data may lead to ablation failure. *A,* Mapping of a right posterior free wall accessory pathway during sinus rhythm. The ablation catheter (Abl) is located at the atrial aspect of the tricuspid annulus (6 o'clock position, LAO 30° projection). At first inspection, only an atrial electrogram appears to be recorded. Closer inspection reveals balanced atrial (A) and ventricular (V) electrograms confirming an annular catheter position. The earlier atrial electrogram is recorded proximally (Ablp) and the ventricular electrogram distally (Abld). Electrogram fusion is frequently observed with right-sided accessory pathways and misinterpretation can result in failure to identify the successful ablation site. *B,* Radiofrequency current application at this site eliminated pathway conduction demonstrated by loss of pre-excitation (*asterisk*) and separation of the previously fused A and V electrograms. Abl, ablation catheter (d, distal; p, proximal); CS, coronary sinus (p, proximal; m, mid; d, distal); HRA, high right atrium; RVA, right ventricular apex.

a repeat procedure. A repeat diagnostic study after presumed successful pathway ablation is strongly recommended to exclude this possibility.

A number of published series have identified factors associated with difficult or failed ablation and recurrence of AP conduction. In a retrospective analysis, Morady et al.[13] identified six factors contributing to a failed or prolonged ablation session. In the failure group, the proportion of APs located at the right free wall was significantly greater than in the overall group (29% versus 16%), with right anterolateral and right posterolateral locations specifically over-represented.

Of the six factors identified, problems related to catheter manipulation and inaccurate pathway localization accounted for the majority of cases (48% and 26%, respectively). Other contributing factors included the presence of an epicardial pathway (5%), recurrent atrial fibrillation interfering with mapping

(3%), unusual AP anatomy (1.5%), and procedure-related vascular complications (3%) preventing an ablation attempt.

PROBLEMS RELATED TO CATHETER MANIPULATION

Inability to guide the ablation catheter to the endocardial target, catheter instability and/or inadequate tissue contact contributed to failed or prolonged ablation in 48% of Morady's patients.[13] Successful pathway elimination was achieved in some cases by a change in the ablation approach. Specifically, for left-sided pathways, a retrograde aortic approach was switched to a trans-septal approach; for pathways located on the right, an inferior vena cava approach was switched to a superior vena cava approach. In other cases, the use of a long guiding sheath, multiple operators, or ablation catheters of varying distal configurations during tip deflection proved to be successful.

INACCURATE PATHWAY LOCALIZATION

Inaccurate pathway localization may lead to RF energy application at inappropriate sites, a problem that was encountered in two circumstances.[13] The first occurred when the surface electrocardiogram (ECG) suggested right posteroseptal preexcitation but subsequent successful ablation was achieved at the left posteroseptal region. In the second type, failure was observed during ablation of unrecognized oblique APs caused by disparate atrial and ventricular insertions at the AV junction. As a result, ventricular insertion sites did not correspond to the site of earliest retrograde atrial activation during ventricular pacing or orthodromic tachycardia. Similarly, atrial insertion sites were not identified by the earliest anterograde ventricular activation during preexcitation. Success was ultimately achieved by identifying the atrial or ventricular insertion sites on their corresponding side of the annulus or by ablating a midportion of the pathway itself, as identified by AP potentials.

OTHER FACTORS

Epicardial APs were identified in a small number of patients in whom successful elimination was achieved by application of RF energy within the CS after failure at the corresponding endocardial site.[13] In these patients, prominent AP potentials recorded within the CS were absent or of small amplitude at the endocardial surface. An unusual AP course was identified in one patient, in whom the ventricular insertion was at the anterior wall of the right ventricle, 2 cm from the tricuspid annulus. Delivery of RF current at this site eliminated pathway conduction and confirmed its atypical ventricular insertion.

Similar findings were reported by Xie et al.[14] Primary ablation failure was observed in 10% of patients and was associated with catheter instability, epicardial pathway course, and a right-sided location, particularly in midseptal and anteroseptal positions. Recurrence was seen in 6% during a mean follow-up period of 20 months and was predicted by a right free wall location, time to conduction block after onset of RF current greater than 12 seconds, poor ablation electrogram stability, and inability to deliver the desired temperature despite maximum power output, a reflection of poor electrode-tissue contact.

Twidale et al.[15] reported recurrence in 8% of patients during a mean follow-up period of 8.5 months. Again recurrence was more frequent with anteroseptal, right free wall, and posteroseptal connections (12% to 14%), and concealed pathways recurred more frequently (16%) than manifest pathways (5.5%). In addition to the time to conduction block from onset of RF, a strong predictor for pathway recurrence was failure to record an AP potential at the ablation site, a difference attributable to less accurate pathway localization.

Specific Challenges

ABLATION OF EPICARDIAL ACCESSORY PATHWAYS

Coronary Sinus and Epicardial Accessory Pathways

The CS originates at its ostium within the right atrium and extends distally to the valve of Vieussens, where it receives the great cardiac vein. Other major tributaries include the left obtuse marginal vein, the posterior left ventricular vein (PCV), the middle cardiac vein (MCV), and the right coronary vein, also known as the small cardiac vein (Fig. 24–2).[16]

The CS provides a conduit for catheter access, permitting mapping of left-sided APs adjacent to the mitral annulus and of posteroseptal (paraseptal) APs traversing the inferior pyramidal space. Moreover, it provides a means of access to epicardial areas of the myocardium for potential ablation of epicardial pathways.

A myocardial coat around the CS is present in all individuals.[17,18] It is composed of bands of muscle arising from the right and left atrial walls[19] and extends in most cases to, and occasionally beyond, the great cardiac vein. Electrical continuity therefore exists between both atria and this muscular sleeve.[20]

The tributaries of the CS are usually devoid of a myocardial coat. Nonetheless, sleeve-like muscular extensions covering the terminal portions of the MCV and PCV are present in 3% and 2% of hearts, respec-

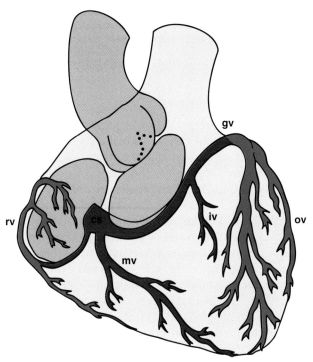

FIGURE 24-2. Schematic representation of the coronary venous system. gv, great cardiac vein; iv, inferior left cardiac vein; mv, middle cardiac vein; ov, obtuse left cardiac vein; rv, right cardiac vein.

tively,[17] potentially serving as connections between the ventricle and the CS and completing a CS-AP connection (Fig. 24-3).

The association of CS diverticula with posteroseptal and left posterolateral APs is well documented.[21-24] Myocardial fibers found within diverticula frequently connect the ventricle with the CS musculature. Other anatomic anomalies, such as fusiform or bulbous enlargement of the CS tributaries, have also been reported to be associated with such connections.

Sun et al.[25] identified a CS AP in 36% of 480 patients with posteroseptal or left posterior APs. During antegrade AP conduction, the presence of a CS AP was established by the recording of ventricular activation at the MCV, PCV or neck of a CS diverticulum earlier than endocardial ventricular activation. At the same site, a high-frequency potential was recorded before the earliest recorded far-field ventricular potential. This high-frequency potential, analogous to an AP potential, was generated by the muscular extension of the CS myocardial coat, which formed a connection to the epicardial surface of the ventricle.

Retrograde angiography in patients with CS AP demonstrated a CS diverticulum in only 21% of cases, most frequently extending from the CS and the MCV. Fusiform or bulbous venous enlargement was identified in 9% of patients, but CS anatomy was normal in the remaining 70%, suggesting that most CS APs occur without a diverticulum or other venous anomaly.

FIGURE 24-3. Schematic for possible anatomic basis of connections between the coronary sinus musculature and left ventricular myocardium (LV). The coronary sinus musculature may form extensions (CSE) over the proximal portions of the middle and posterior cardiac veins. If connections between the coronary sinus musculature and the left (LA) or right (RA) atrial myocardium exist as well, the substrate for reciprocating tachycardias is formed. *(From Sun Y, Arruda M, Otomo K, et al.: Coronary sinus-ventricular accessory connections producing posteroseptal and left posterior accessory pathways: Incidence and electrophysiological identification. Circulation 106:1362-1367, 2002, with permission.)*

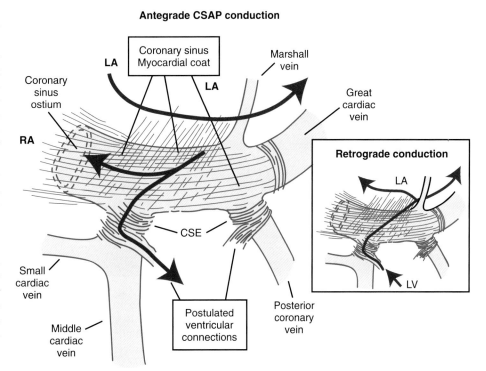

Because of their epicardial location, successful ablation of these APs is accomplished only by RF current delivered within the CS or by direct percutaneous catheter access to the pericardial space. Specific ECG features have been described to identify manifest pathways requiring such an approach.[26] A negative delta wave in lead II predicts a successful ablation site within the CS or MCV with a sensitivity of 87%, but with a relatively low specificity (79%) and positive predictive value (50%). However, a steep positive delta wave in lead aVR and a deep S wave in lead V_6 (R ≤ S) yields high specificity and positive predictive values, 99% and 91% respectively, for a successful ablation site within the CS. These ECG findings, along with a difficult or previously failed ablation attempt, suggest that contrast definition of the coronary venous anatomy and subsequent detailed mapping may prove helpful in identification of a successful epicardial ablation target.

RF ablation within the coronary venous system has been shown to be successful and safe for the elimination of epicardial APs (Fig. 24–4).[27-35] Reports of CS injury after RF catheter ablation are infrequent, possibly because of the lack of clinical sequelae and symptoms of CS stenosis. Nevertheless, RF current delivery within the vein has been associated with endoluminal thrombosis, stenosis, perforation leading to pericardial tamponade, and damage to adjacent structures. The proximity of the right coronary artery and its AV nodal branch with the proximal MCV, and crossover points of the left anterior descending and left circumflex arteries with the great cardiac vein, represent potential sites of susceptibility for coronary artery spasm or myocardial infarction during RF ablation.[36-38] Selective coronary angiography to delineate the relation of a prospective ablation site to the coronary arteries is prudent before RF current application within the CS. Luminal patency may also be reassessed after ablation. Irrigated RF ablation may be safer in this situation than noncooled RF, due to the lower incidence of impedance rises and coagulum formation. Cryoablation may be the modality of choice for these cases.

Cryothermal ablation within the CS has been successfully employed to eliminate epicardial posterolateral APs.[39] Cryolesions are associated with less endothelial disruption and thrombus formation than RF lesions. Furthermore, the safety of cryothermal ablation adjacent to the coronary arteries has been demonstrated by extensive surgical experience[40] and by recent catheter-based studies using animal models.[41,42] A percutaneous epicardial approach using RF energy has also been successfully employed for elimination of posteroseptal APs associated with CS diverticula after multiple failed transvenous ablation attempts.[43,44]

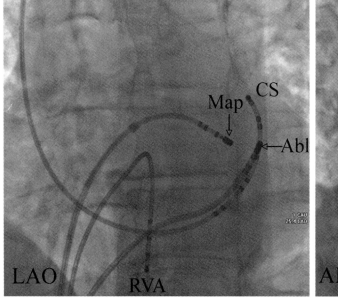
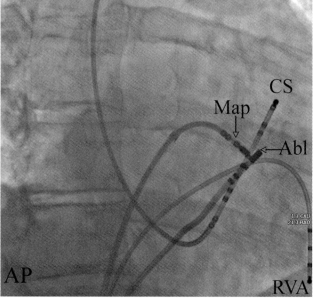

A   B

FIGURE 24–4. Radiofrequency ablation within the coronary sinus, fluoroscopic images in LAO (**A**) and AP (**B**) projections. Endocardial RF current delivered adjacent the mitral annulus (Map) where local myocardial activation was optimal failed to eliminate accessory pathway conduction. An ablation catheter (Abl) positioned within the coronary sinus identified a discrete accessory pathway potential. Low power (15 W) RF current delivery at this site resulted in permanent pathway elimination within seconds of application. Abl, coronary sinus ablation catheter; CS, coronary sinus; Map, endocardial ablation catheter; RVA, right ventricular apex.

Atrial Appendage-to-Ventricular Accessory Pathways

The majority of reported epicardial APs occur adjacent to a CS diverticulum, the MCV, or the great cardiac vein.[45] The atrial appendage-to-ventricular pathway is a recognized variant of AP connections that is characterized by an epicardial course connecting the atrial appendage and the ventricular base, most frequently on the right side. RF energy at endocardial sites may be ineffective, resulting in failure of ablation or recurrence of pathway conduction.

The first histologic documentation of this pathway type was at autopsy after the sudden death of a pediatric patient with known Wolff-Parkinson-White syndrome.[46] A band-like muscular structure extending from the underside of the right atrial appendage to the right ventricle was identified during dissection of the right AV groove (Fig. 24–5). Internally, this structure corresponded to a pouch with a muscular wall that coursed through the epicardial fat and ultimately continued into the ventricular myocardium approximately 5 mm from the annular insertion of the tricuspid valve.

Features suggestive of this pathway variant include (1) a preexcitation pattern indicative of a right anterior or right anterolateral pathway; (2) retrograde atrial activation recorded earlier in the right atrial appendage than at the tricuspid annulus; (3) a relatively long ventricular-to-atrial (VA) conduction time during tachycardia, consistent with a long epicardial AP course and earliest ventricular activation

recorded more than 1 cm apical to the tricuspid annulus; (4) failed or transient loss of pathway conduction with RF delivery at the tricuspid annulus; and (5) the need for high-energy delivery within the appendage to achieve permanent pathway elimination.

Arruda et al.[47] reported 3 bidirectional APs, each with an atrial insertion at the atrial appendage, representing fewer than 0.5% of cases in their series of 646 patients undergoing catheter ablation for the Wolff-Parkinson-White syndrome. After unsuccessful RF catheter ablation, pathway conduction was eliminated in two patients by surgical separation of the atrial appendage from the ventricle at a site distant to the annulus, on the left side in one patient and on the right in the other. RF current eliminated conduction in the third patient when delivered to the tip of the right atrial appendage. Similarly, Milstein et al.[48] observed a bridge of tissue crossing from the base of the right atrial appendage into the fat pad overlying the base of the right ventricle at least 10 mm distal to the tricuspid annulus at surgery. Transection of this tissue resulted in loss of preexcitation.

Successful RF catheter ablation was also reported by Soejima[49]; however, application of RF current within the appendage was limited by frequent impedance rises when a 4-mm-tip electrode ablation catheter was used. High-energy delivery and elimination of impedance rise was achieved by substitution of an 8-mm large-tip ablation catheter. Similar advantages are afforded by saline-irrigated catheters.

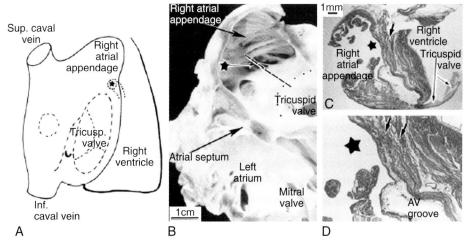

FIGURE 24–5. **A,** Diagram showing the location of an accessory connection joining the floor of the right atrial appendage (*star*) to the supraventricular crest. **B,** The heart is sectioned in a plane to show the 4 cardiac chambers from a posterior perspective. The broken line marks the level of the histologic sections shown in panels **C** and **D**. Note the distance between the pouch (*star and arrow*) and the hinge of the tricuspid valve (*dotted line*). **C,** This section through the atrioventricular junction shows the pouch (*star*) overlying the superior wall of the right ventricle and the band of accessory tissue (*arrow*). **D,** This magnification of the pouch reveals the muscular band (*arrows*) from the wall of the pouch to the ventricular myocardium. *(From Heaven DJ, Till JA, Ho SY: Sudden death in a child with an unusual accessory connection. Europace 2:224-227, 2000, with permission.)*

Nonfluoroscopic three-dimensional mapping has also facilitated catheter ablation.[50] In our laboratory, this approach was used in a patient with three prior unsuccessful ablation attempts. The baseline 12-lead ECG was suggestive of a right-sided AP (Fig. 24–6). At electrophysiology study, earliest atrial activation occurred within the right atrial appendage during orthodromic reentrant tachycardia and ventricular pacing (Fig. 24–7). Initial ablation attempts were made using a 4-mm-tip electrode ablation catheter, but successful pathway elimination within the right atrial appendage was achieved with a saline-irrigated catheter. Adding complexity to a technically challenging case was the presence of a broad pathway insertion or muscle "band" that acted like multiple discrete APs. This feature had undeniably contributed to the failure of previous attempts. Electroanatomic mapping proved invaluable by allowing remapping of earliest retrograde atrial activation after ablation of successive pathway "strands."

Epicardial elimination of an atrial appendage-to-ventricular pathway was reported in a patient who had undergone multiple unsuccessful endocardial attempts.[51] Transcutaneous instrumentation via a subxiphoid puncture permitted insertion of a 7-French (7F) deflectable catheter into the epicardial space. Epicardial mapping using a three-dimensional electroanatomic mapping system assisted localization of the earliest atrial activation and an AP potential at the anterior aspect of the heart. Delivery of low-power RF current at 20 W permanently eliminated pathway conduction without recurrence.

ABLATION OF ACCESSORY PATHWAYS ASSOCIATED WITH STRUCTURAL CARDIAC ABNORMALITIES

APs are commonly associated with a variety of structural heart disorders, including Ebstein's anomaly, a persistent left superior vena cava, hypertrophic cardiomyopathy, and L-transposition of the great vessels. Ebstein's anomaly, although rare, is the most common congenital heart disease associated with the Wolff-Parkinson-White syndrome.[52]

Ebstein's Anomaly

Ebstein's anomaly is characterized by apical displacement of the tricuspid valve into the right ventricle, with atrialization of the area of right ventricle between the true tricuspid annulus and the anomalous attachments of the septal and posterior leaflets. The atrialized right ventricle is thinned and dilated, and the remainder of the ventricular chamber is diminished in size. Associated cardiac anomalies include a patent foramen ovale, atrial and ventricular septal defects, and right ventricular outflow tract obstruction.

Approximately 20% to 30% of patients with Ebstein's anomaly experience AV reciprocating tachycardia,[53,54] and the presence of preexcitation with atrial tachyarrhythmias is associated with sudden cardiac death. Right bundle branch block pattern is typically present due to posteroseptal conduction delay, and its absence should raise suspicion of the presence of an AP.

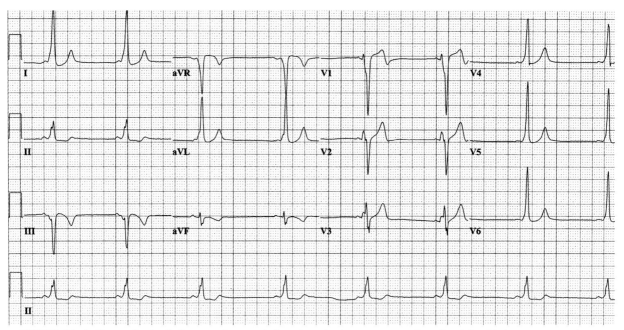

FIGURE 24–6. The twelve-lead electrocardiogram during sinus rhythm was suggestive of a right-sided accessory pathway.

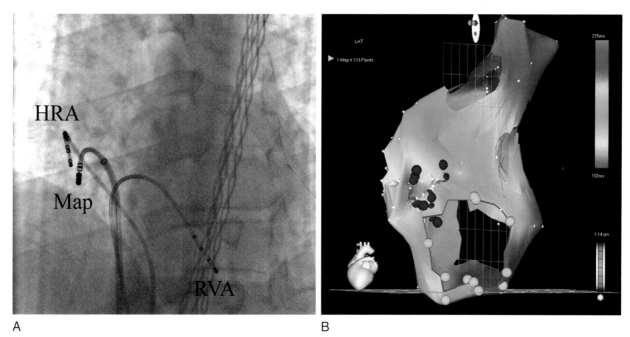

FIGURE 24-7. A, The mapping catheter identifies the site of successful pathway elimination within the right atrial appendage (LAO projection). Elimination of conduction was achieved using a saline irrigated ablation catheter allowing higher energy delivery producing a larger, deeper lesion. **B,** Electroanatomic right atrial activation map constructed during right ventricular pacing (LAO projection). Earliest retrograde atrial activation was localized to the right atrial appendage (red area). Brown markers indicate ablation sites. Light blue markers outline the tricuspid annulus. HRA, high right atrium; Map, ablation catheter; RVA, right ventricular apex.

Accessory AV connections associated with Ebstein's anomaly are usually right-sided and located along the dysplastic portion of the tricuspid annulus,[54] where abnormal endocardial electrograms are frequently recorded.[53] These connections, along with difficulty localizing the true AV groove fluoroscopically, the presence of multiple AV connections in up to 50% of patients,[52,54,55] and the presence of significant tricuspid regurgitation, hinder precise pathway localization and impair catheter stability and tissue contact. These factors ultimately account for the lower reported rates of success compared with catheter ablation of pathways not associated with this malformation. RF catheter ablation is not limited by previous surgical intervention, because successful pathway elimination has been achieved in patients presenting with cardiac arrhythmias after tricuspid valve replacement.[56,57]

Cappato et al.[55] reported their experience of RF catheter ablation in 21 patients with symptomatic AV reciprocating tachycardia and Ebstein's anomaly. Of the 34 APs identified, all were right-sided, with the majority located in the posteroseptal (9), posterior (10), and posterolateral (10) positions. Normal endocardial electrograms were recorded at all sites along the tricuspid annulus with successful abolition of all APs in 10 patients. In the remaining 11 patients, continuous fragmented electrical activity with multiple

spikes was recorded along the surface of the atrialized ventricle in the posteroseptal and posterolateral regions permitting conventional endocardial AP localization in only 1 patient. In all other patients, epicardial mapping via the right coronary artery was attempted. Selective right coronary angiography was performed to assess vessel size and an anatomic course confined to the AV groove. An over-the-wire system was used to advance a 2F multipolar catheter to map AP potentials and earliest anterograde ventricular or retrograde atrial activation during slow withdrawal of the catheter. The intracardiac mapping catheter was then positioned at the endocardial site that best matched the anatomic location and electrogram configuration recorded by the epicardial electrode pair, and RF energy was delivered. With this approach, APs were eliminated in 5 patients but did not assist pathway localization or could not be performed due to an adverse vessel course in the remaining patients.

Overall, Cappato et al.[55] reported successful AP ablation in 76% of patients, compared to their experience of 95% success for right-sided pathways in the absence of Ebstein's anomaly. Factors identified that contributed to lower success included (1) abnormal and ill-defined tricuspid annulus anatomy with resultant catheter instability and poor tissue contact and (2) recording of fractionated activation potentials at the atrialized ventricle, impairing the ability to identify AP potentials and the site of earliest antegrade ventricular and retrograde atrial activation.

In another reported series of five patients,[58] the importance of localization of the "electrical" AV ring, where balanced atrial and ventricular electrograms were recorded, was emphasized. The inferiorly displaced anatomic annulus was initially mapped and found to be devoid of balanced electrograms with short AV intervals or AP potentials. Repositioning of the ablation catheter at the true annulus, guided anatomically by insertion of a guide wire into the right coronary artery, identified electrograms where successful RF pathway elimination was achieved in each patient. All of the AV connections were located in the right posterior and posterolateral region.

Reich et al.[59] reported their pediatric experience of RF ablation in Ebstein's anomaly, which included 59 patients with AP-mediated arrhythmias. Multiple APs occurred in 33% of the patients, and the pathways were right-sided in 96%. Acute success was achieved for 79% of right free wall pathways and 89% of right septal pathways. The reported rate of complications was low and included one patient who required permanent pacemaker implantation due to the development of complete heart block. Coronary artery occlusion after AP ablation has been reported in two pediatric patients with Ebstein's anomaly.[60]

Electroanatomic mapping techniques may facilitate pathway localization after failed conventional mapping.[61] Construction of a right atrial activation map permits demarcation of the "electrical" AV junction, where balanced atrial and ventricular electrograms are recorded at the endocardium. This approach is analogous to use of the right coronary artery as an anatomic landmark but eliminates the need for coronary arterial instrumentation and its associated risks.

Persistent Left Superior Vena Cava

Failure of involution of the left cardinal vein during embryologic development results in a persistent left superior vena cava (LSVC). It is the most common systemic venous anomaly, occurring with an incidence of 0.5% in the general population[62] and in 4% of patients with congenital heart disease.[63] Associated cardiac anomalies include atrial septal defect, tetralogy of Fallot, AV canal defect, and partial anomalous pulmonary venous connection.[64]

In its pure form, the LSVC enters the left atrium between the appendage and the left pulmonary veins, providing direct transvenous access to the left side of the heart. Rarely, it is accompanied by complete absence of the right superior vena cava, permitting right heart access only by the femoral approach. Alternatively, an anastomosis with the CS results in an LSVC-to-CS fistula that acts as a conduit for systemic venous return to the right atrium. The CS in this instance is significantly dilated due to increased blood flow. Infrequently, atresia of the CS ostium results in absence of a connection to the right atrium; consequently, coronary venous blood is directed systemically, to the left subclavian vein.

CS anomalies frequently coexist with AV APs,[65,66] occurring more frequently in patients with AP-mediated tachycardia (4.7%) than in patients with AVNRT (0.6%). Such abnormalities include vertical CS angulation, hypoplasia, narrowing, and persistent LSVC-to-CS fistula. Furthermore, CS abnormalities are anatomically related to the location of the APs and frequently preclude CS catheterization.

Although echocardiographic examination may demonstrate CS dilatation, the presence of an LSVC-to-CS fistula is usually first discovered during CS instrumentation at electrophysiology study. When advanced, a left subclavian venous catheter travels in an anomalous inferior course in the left chest to the posterior aspect of the heart. Alternatively, passage of the catheter from the CS to the left subclavian vein is observed when the catheter is introduced via a femoral or right jugular vein approach (Fig. 24–8). The inability to advance the catheter into the CS should raise suspicion of associated atresia of the CS ostium.

Although asymptomatic, the presence of an LSVC-to-CS fistula may complicate catheter ablation of left-sided pathways. The cavernous nature of the vessel may prohibit precise pathway localization due to excessive motion and poor electrode contact of the CS mapping catheter. Alternatively, the CS may be located at a site distant to the mitral annulus. Successful pathway ablation requires a modified approach.[67-71] Ultimately, if the CS cannot be used to guide ablation, a single-catheter technique with careful mapping of the mitral annulus is obligatory.

ABLATION OF PATHWAYS WITH ATYPICAL CONFIGURATION

Multiple Accessory Pathways

The reported incidence of multiple APs is 3% to 15%.[52,72-80] APs have been defined as multiple when they are separated at the AV junction by 1 to 3 cm based on an approximation of distance during catheter mapping; however, it is difficult to differentiate multiple pathways from those with broad atrial or ventricular insertions or an oblique course. Multiple pathways are typically located unilaterally and are most frequently two in number. Clinical variables associated with their presence include Ebstein's

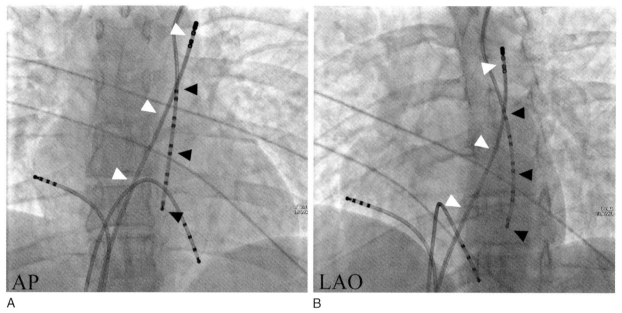

FIGURE 24–8. Fluoroscopic images of a persistent left superior vena cava and associated coronary sinus fistula in the AP (**A**) and LAO (**B**) projections. An anomalous inferior course in the left chest to the posterior aspect of the heart is identified as a decapolar mapping catheter is advanced from the left subclavian vein (*black arrows*). A deflectable catheter advanced via the ostium into the coronary sinus from the inferior vena cava (*white arrows*) confirms the presence of a fistulous connection. The cavernous nature of the coronary sinus is suggested by the distance separating the catheters, indicated by *arrows*. Unsuccessful passage of a guide wire from the right subclavian vein to the right atrium confirmed associated absence of a right superior vena cava.

anomaly[52,73,77-80] and a history of preexcited reciprocating tachycardia.[52,78,80] Several reports also suggest a higher incidence in patients with right free wall and posteroseptal AV connections,[52,74,77-79] possibly related to the presence of multiple discontinuities in the tricuspid annulus fibrosus.[81,82]

Notable electrophysiologic properties distinguish patients with multiple APs from those with a single pathway. Multiple pathways provide the substrate for complex reentrant circuits, potentially resulting in multiple atrial wavefronts and the development of atrial fibrillation during reciprocating tachycardia. In addition, shorter AP effective refractory periods and measured R-R intervals during atrial fibrillation (<250 msec) are a reflection of superior AP conduction in these patients. The combination of enhanced pathway conduction with more frequent occurrence of atrial fibrillation potentially increases the risk of deterioration into ventricular fibrillation and sudden cardiac death.[78-80,83,84]

Multiple APs are identified during the electrophysiologic study by (1) the occurrence of different patterns of preexcitation during atrial pacing or atrial fibrillation with different delta-wave morphologic and ventricular activation patterns; (2) different sites of atrial activation during right ventricular pacing or orthodromic reciprocating tachycardia; (3) preexcited tachycardia using a second pathway as the retro-

grade limb of the circuit; (4) mismatch between the atrial and ventricular ends of the AP as assessed by comparing antidromic and orthodromic reciprocating tachycardia (mismatch distance >1 cm); and (5) change from orthodromic to antidromic reciprocating tachycardia, or vice versa.[72,78] Some pathways cannot be identified during the baseline study and become evident only during RF ablation after successful interruption of the dominant pathway.

Several published series have demonstrated safe and efficacious elimination of multiple pathways with success rates of 86% to 98%.[74-76,78] Many reports have shown rates of success equivalent to those in patients possessing a single pathway, but others have not.[75,77,79] Predictably, however, procedure duration, radiation exposure time, and number of ablation pulses have been significantly greater.[74,75,76,79] A higher rate of recurrent pathway conduction is also reported, ranging from 8% to 12%.[74,75,77-79]

From a practical standpoint, failure to recognize the existence of multiple pathways may result in primary ablation failure or recurrent tachycardia. A multipolar CS mapping catheter imparts detailed information on VA timing in addition to atrial and ventricular activation at multiple sites along the mitral annulus. This is invaluable during ablation of left-sided pathways, which are most frequently located at the posterior and lateral regions of the AV junction, within reach of the CS catheter. Therefore, subtle activation changes during ablation are easily recognizable (Fig. 24–9). Mapping of the tricuspid annulus with a multielectrode catheter is less convenient but can be achieved with a multipolar "halo" catheter positioned near the tricuspid annulus. Brief current applications in the presence of multiple pathways may be erroneously considered ineffective if subtle activation changes, such as prolongation of local VA timing or changes in surface delta-wave morphology, are unrecognized.

In order to reduce primary ablation failure, the following key points must be emphasized: (1) apparent failure of current application at a site of optimal electrogram timing and morphology should raise suspicion of the presence of multiple APs; (2) commitment to a full-duration current application at such a site should be undertaken with careful scrutiny of local VA timing or delta-wave morphologic changes; and (3) meticulous remapping of the AV junction should be undertaken to identify any new site of early activation or presence of an AP potential, indicative of a distinct pathway. The procedure described earlier should be repeated until elimination of all pathways is achieved. Again, the importance of careful observation during RF application in such cases cannot be overemphasized.

Despite a meticulous approach, recurrent tachycardia may occur. Recurrent tachycardia, although most commonly caused by recurrence of AP conduction, should raise the possibility of other tachycardia mechanisms. Recurrence of clinical symptoms due to AP conduction occurred in 4.2% of cases in a series of 1280 patients who underwent ablation of an AP.[85] Manifestation of a previously unrecognized pathway caused symptom recurrence in 0.7% of patients and was subsequently ablated at an anatomic site distinct from the initial target. These "dormant" pathways were usually concealed and not identified at the time of initial study, suggesting intermittent conduction. Recurrence of tachycardia may also occur because of transient interruption of conduction, either by mechanical pressure of the mapping catheter or by delivery of RF current. These findings strongly support the recommendation for a complete diagnostic electrophysiology study with isoproterenol to confirm elimination of pathway conduction after apparently successful ablation.

Oblique Accessory Pathways

Atrioventricular APs are usually regarded as following a course perpendicular to the AV groove, producing the shortest local ventriculoatrial interval at

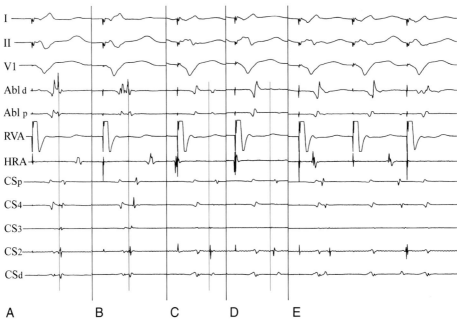

FIGUER 24–9. Radiofrequency ablation of multiple concealed accessory pathways. The ablation catheter is positioned adjacent the mitral annulus at the site of earliest recorded retrograde atrial activation (*vertical line*) during right ventricular pacing. Panels *A* to *D* demonstrate the intracardiac recordings preceding each current application. With successive pathway elimination, subtle changes in local VA interval and retrograde atrial activation sequence is observed. A total of four accessory pathways were identified with separate atrial insertions along the posterolateral and lateral mitral annulus. The development of ventriculoatrial block heralded success (Panel E). Abl, ablation catheter (d, distal; p, proximal); CS, coronary sinus (p, proximal; d, distal); HRA, high right atrium; RVA, right ventricular apex.

the site of the pathway during orthodromic AV reentrant tachycardia or ventricular pacing. Appropriately, this site is considered a favorable target for AP ablation.[86,87] However, studies suggest that APs frequently follow an oblique course.[88-91]

Jackman et al.[88,89] identified AP potentials associated with left free wall and posteroseptal APs using a multipolar mapping catheter inserted into the CS. By mapping AP potentials along the length of the CS, an oblique course was established in 87% of left-sided pathways; the atrial insertion was identified 4 to 30 mm (median, 14 mm) proximal (posterior) to its corresponding ventricular insertion.

Oblique APs are also identified by a change of the local VA or AV interval as a result of reversing the direction of paced ventricular and atrial wavefronts.[90] Such a change in local activation was observed in 87% of patients with a single left- or right-sided AP presenting for catheter ablation. Local atrial and ventricular activation was recorded using a multipolar (20-electrode) catheter placed in the CS or positioned around the tricuspid annulus in patients with a right free wall AP. Based on the site of earliest recorded retrograde atrial activation, two ventricular pacing sites were selected on either side, to produce a clockwise and counterclockwise wavefront to the AP. Similarly, two atrial pacing sites were selected to reverse the atrial wavefront along the annulus surrounding the site of earliest recorded anterograde ventricular activation.

A ventricular wavefront propagating from the direction of the ventricular end produced a short local-VA interval, because activation along the AP proceeded to the earliest atrial activation site simultaneously with the ventricular wavefront (Fig. 24–10A, CS 2). Consequently, the ventricular potential often masked the AP potential and overlapped the atrial electrogram, masking earliest atrial activation. Conversely, a wavefront propagating in the opposite direction resulted in a longer local-VA interval, because the ventricular wavefront had to pass the site of earliest atrial activation before reaching the ventricular end of the AP (see Fig. 24–10B, CS 2). This countercurrent wavefront was found to expose the AP potential and the atrial activation sequence, allowing identification of an appropriate ablation target. Similarly, atrial pacing in the direction of the atrial end resulted in a short local-AV interval (see Fig. 24–10C, CS 4), and a countercurrent wavefront lengthened the local-AV interval, exposing the AP potential and ventricular activation sequence (see Fig. 24–10D, CS 4).

In a study of concealed left-sided APs, Yamabe et al.[91] compared the ventricular insertion site with the corresponding atrial insertion, which was identified at the site of earliest recorded retrograde atrial

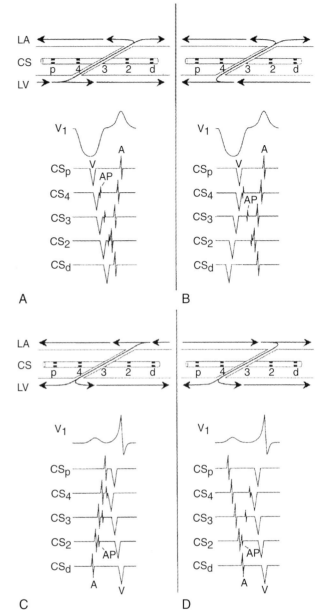

FIGUER 24–10. Activation of oblique accessory pathways. Schematic of antegrade and retrograde activation of an oblique left free wall accessory pathway (AP) from opposing directions. **A** and **B** demonstrate activation of the ventricular insertion from the proximal to distal and distal to proximal directions, respectively. **C** and **D** represent activation of the atrial insertion from the distal to proximal and proximal to distal directions, respectively. Note the separation of the components of the electrograms when the AP is activated from the direction opposite to the direction of conduction over the pathway. A, atrial potential; CS, coronary sinus; d, distal; LA, left atrium; LV, left ventricle; p, proximal; V, ventricular potential. *(From Otomo K, Gonzalez MD, Beckman KJ, et al.: Reversing the direction of paced ventricular and atrial wavefronts reveals an oblique course in the accessory AV pathways and improves localization for catheter ablation. Circulation 104:550-556, 2001, with permission.)*

activation within the CS. The ventricular insertion was identified at the site of shortest measured stimulus-to-atrial (Stim-A) interval during pacing delivered at mapping sites under the mitral valve leaflet. In 49% of patients, a number of observations indicated an oblique pathway course. First, the site of the shortest Stim-A interval did not to coincide fluoroscopically with the site at which the earliest retrograde atrial activation was recorded. In these patients, the Stim-A interval at the shortest Stim-A site was significantly shorter than that at the corresponding ventricular side of earliest retrograde atrial activation. Second, during tachycardia, the interval between the onset of the surface QRS and the retrograde atrial electrogram (QRS-A interval) was longer at the shortest Stim-A site than at the site of earliest retrograde atrial activation. In all patients, elimination of pathway conduction was achieved by a single application of RF energy to the ventricular side of the mitral annulus at the site of the shortest identified Stim-A interval.

Successful elimination of pathway conduction can be achieved by application of RF current at or anywhere between the atrial and ventricular insertion sites, although targeting of an isolated AP potential is associated with the highest rate of ablation success (Fig. 24–11).[2,86,92] Oblique AV APs provide a challenge to ablation because of the inherent difficulties in identifying AP potentials due to obscured or overlapping electrograms and disparate myocardial insertions at the AV junction. An assumption of a perpendicular pathway course may lead to an inappropriate or suboptimal ablation site, underscoring the importance of selecting an ablation site guided by the appropriate data. Specifically, the atrial insertion site is best identified by the earliest recorded atrial activation during retrograde mapping, and the ventricular insertion site is best identified by the earliest recorded ventricular activation during anterograde mapping on the corresponding side of the annulus. Ablation here or at sites where discrete AP potentials are recorded will most likely yield success.

Atypical Accessory Pathways

Failure of RF catheter ablation may be caused by the complexity of the AP course. Pathways with an atypical course and those with connections to the His-Purkinje system are considered AP variants (Fig. 24–12 and Table 24–2). The differential diagnosis of these connections is discussed in Chapter 23.

One anatomically distinct pathway variant is an epicardial connection extending between the atrial appendage and the ventricular base.[46-48] In such cases, the AP traverses the epicardial fat from an atrial insertion at the floor of the left or right atrial

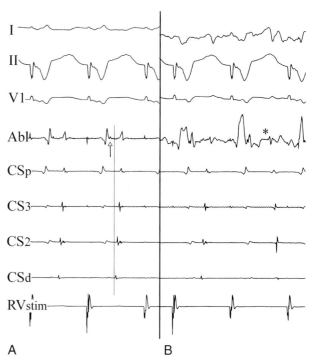

FIGURE 24–11. Intracardiac recordings during mapping and ablation of an oblique left-sided atrioventricular accessory pathway. Panel *A* shows an ablation catheter (Abl) positioned at the atrial aspect of the mitral annulus recording of retrograde activity during ventricular pacing. A discrete accessory pathway potential is recorded between the ventricular and atrial electrograms (*arrow*). Note that earliest retrograde atrial activation is recorded at the distal coronary sinus (*vertical line*), significantly earlier than recorded at the site of the ablation catheter. Atrial activation recorded at the ablation catheter coincides with activation at the proximal coronary sinus. Panel *B* shows within seconds of RF current application at this site, permanent elimination of accessory pathway conduction occurred indicated by a change in atrial activation sequence (*asterisk*). Following ablation, the discrete accessory pathway potential adjacent the ventricular electrogram was no longer recorded. Abl, ablation catheter; CS, coronary sinus (p, proximal; d, distal); RVstim, right ventricular apex.

appendage to the base of the ventricle, usually at a site distant to the tricuspid or mitral annulus. Endocardial RF current application at the AV junction is either unrewarding or results in only transient elimination of pathway conduction. Mapping within the atrial appendage allows recording of retrograde atrial activation earlier than at the tricuspid annulus and may also identify the presence of an AP potential. Conventional mapping at annular locations will fail to identify an atrial or ventricular insertion site, leading to ablation failure.

Similarly, posteroseptal and left posterior APs may require ablation via the CS because of their epicardial location. Failure of RF energy at the endocardium

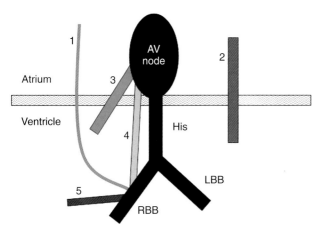

FIGURE 24–12. Schematic of variant endocardial accessory AV connections. 1) Atriofascicular pathway, 2) Atrioventricular pathway, 3) Nodoventricular pathway, 4) Nodofascicular pathway, 5) Fasciculoventricular pathway.

TABLE 24–2
Accessory Pathway Variants
Accessory pathways with His-Purkinje connections
Atriofascicular
Atrium-His
Nodoventricular, nodofascicular
Fasciculoventricular
Accessory pathways with atypical course
Epicardial accessory pathways Coronary sinus Atrial appendage to ventricle
Other

should prompt a search within the CS for identification of high-frequency potentials, analogous to AP potentials, and atrial and ventricular activation occurring earlier than at the corresponding endocardial site. Successful elimination may be achieved by cautious application of RF current or by cryothermal ablation.

Rarely, an AP with a truly atypical course is encountered. This is best exemplified by an anteroseptal AP with a ventricular insertion at the outflow tract region, reported by our institution in 1992.[93] More than 10 years later, an anatomically identical pathway was encountered. An atypical AP, more specifically an atypical ventricular insertion site, was suggested by the surface ECG during preexcited atrial fibrillation. The preexcitation pattern did not conform to typical pathways at the AV ring but was suggestive of right ventricular outflow tract preexcitation, exhibiting left bundle branch block morphology with an inferior axis (Fig. 24–13).

In both instances, the AP course was confirmed by the standard electrophysiology study using pacing maneuvers and careful mapping to accurately identify the atrial and ventricular insertion sites. The ventricular insertion site of our most recent case was identified by earliest ventricular activation recorded at the anterior septal right ventricular outflow tract during CS pacing, where local activation preceded the surface delta wave by 10 msec (Fig. 24–14). The atrial insertion was precisely localized to a site adjacent the AV node in the right anterior septum off the tricuspid annulus (1 o'clock position, left anterior oblique 30-degree projection), where the shortest stimulus-to-delta wave interval was identified (Fig. 24–15). Cryothermic mapping (reversible loss of pre-

excitation without AV block) confirmed the atrial insertion site when cooled to –30°C, and RF current application at this site resulted in permanent pathway elimination.

Although uncommon, these examples illustrate the importance of a complete electrophysiology study and accurate interpretation of all available data. If endocardial mapping or ablation at the AV ring is unrewarding, consideration should be given for the presence of an atypical AP. In these instances, endocardial mapping at sites off the AV ring or within the CS may prove invaluable.

New Technologies

SALINE-COOLED RADIOFREQUENCY ABLATION

RF energy is typically delivered in a unipolar fashion to the myocardial surface via the electrode tip of an ablation catheter. The passage of alternating current through the tissues to a large dispersive patch applied to the patient's skin produces resistive heat at the tip-tissue interface. Conductive heating from the catheter tip through the tissue results in a thermal gradient within the adjacent myocardium. Tissue heating to more than 50°C results in irreversible myocardial tissue damage[94,95] and the production of permanent RF ablation lesions.

The temperature recorded at the tip-tissue interface is the most accurate predictor of RF lesion volume. As interface temperature is increased, deeper ablation lesions are produced. However,

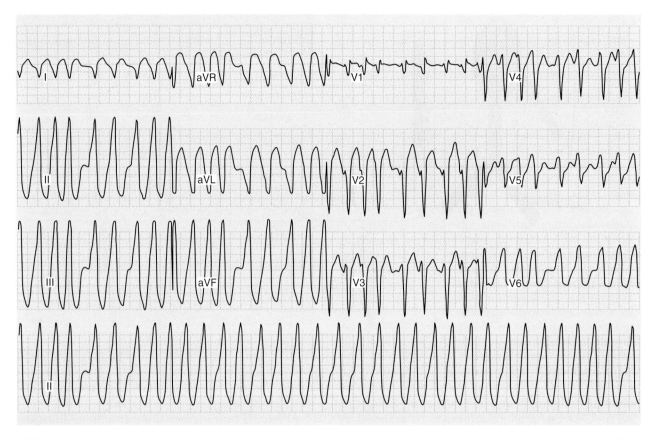

FIGURE 24–13. Twelve-lead ECG recorded during preexcited atrial fibrillation. An unusual preexcitation pattern with precordial R wave transition suggesting a right-sided accessory pathway but QS complexes in leads I and aVL consistent with a left lateral pathway. The left bundle branch block QRS morphology with inferior axis is suggestive of right ventricular outflow tract pre-excitation.

at an interface temperature of 100°C, plasma boiling and coagulum formation at the catheter tip results in a sudden impedance rise, loss of thermal conductivity, and loss of effective tissue heating.[96] Tip temperature monitoring aims to prevent excessive interfacial heating and loss of efficacy of energy delivery.

Power delivery is another important determinant of RF lesion size and is limited during conventional RF ablation by a tip-tissue interface temperature of 100°C. Greater RF energy delivery can be achieved by the use of saline-irrigated (cooled-tip) catheters. Cooling the electrode tip with infused normal saline reduces interfacial heating and shifts the point of maximal heating into the tissue rather than focusing it at the tissue surface.[97,98] As a result, deeper conductive heating occurs and produces deeper tissue lesions, an attribute essential for targets beyond the range of conventional RF lesions, such as epicardial APs. Large (8- to 10-mm) ablation electrodes provide a similar effect through passive convective cooling of the electrode by local blood flow.

CRYOTHERMAL ABLATION

Cryoablation was first used as an alternative to surgical dissection of arrhythmic substrates during arrhythmia surgery in the 1970s. Evolution of cryoablation technologies has yielded catheter-based delivery systems providing a novel ablation modality and an alternative to RF energy for transvenous catheter ablation. Since its introduction, percutaneous cryoablation has been shown to be safe and effective for the treatment of supraventricular arrhythmias and atrial fibrillation.[99-102] In addition, properties unique to cryothermy offer potential advantages over RF energy in selected clinical applications.[103,104]

The clinical effects of cryothermy are achieved by cooling tissue to subzero temperatures. A cryoablation console controls the delivery of pressurized nitrous oxide gas from a storage cylinder to the tip of the ablation catheter; the gas then expands and causes cooling. The amount of heat and the speed at which it is removed allows for a permanent or transient effect in the target cells.

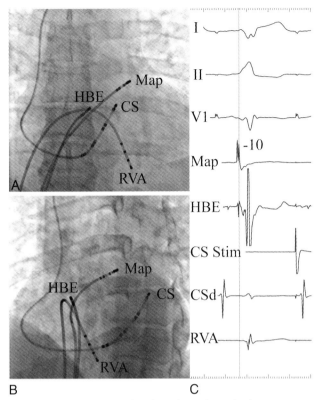

FIGURE 24–14. Ventricular insertion site of the accessory pathway in the anteroposterior (**A**) and left anterior oblique (**B**) projections identified by earliest ventricular activation during coronary sinus pacing. Intracardiac electrograms (**C**) indicate ventricular activation at the ablation catheter preceding the surface delta wave by 10 ms. CS, coronary sinus (stim, pacing site; d, distal); HBE, His bundle electrogram; Map, ablation catheter; RVA, right ventricular apex.

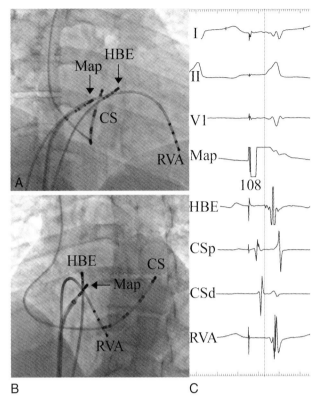

FIGURE 24–15. Atrial insertion site of the accessory pathway in the right anterior oblique (**A**) and left anterior oblique (**B**) projections identified during stimulus-to-delta pace mapping. Note the anatomical proximity of the accessory pathway to the site of the recorded His bundle electrogram. Intracardiac electrograms (**C**) indicate the shortest stimulus-to-delta interval identified (108 ms) at the site of successful elimination of accessory pathway conduction during ice mapping and radiofrequency ablation. CS, coronary sinus (p, proximal; d, distal); HBE, His bundle electrogram; Map, ablation catheter; RVA, right ventricular apex.

When tissue is cooled to −20°C, the formation of extracellular ice results in a hyperosmotic extracellular environment, forcing an outward shift of intracellular fluid. This leads to cell shrinkage, causing damage to the cell membrane and intracellular constituents. On rewarming, reversal of these effects results in cell swelling and disruption of the cell membrane. If the tissue is cooled to −40°C or lower, intracellular ice formation leads to irreversible destruction of intracellular organelles and cellular membranes, with ensuing cell death.

If cooling is limited to milder temperatures, the tissue effects at the cellular level are fully reversible. At temperatures between 0 and −10°C, loss of membrane transport capability and ion pump function occurs, prohibiting tissue depolarization and conduction. Reversible loss of electrophysiologic function during cooling permits testing of the functionality of a prospective ablation target before the creation of a permanent destructive lesion. This unique property of cryothermy is commonly known as "ice mapping."

Cryothermy also affords exceptional electrode tip-tissue interface stability during mapping and ablation due to "cryoadherence." As the temperature is reduced below 0°C, progressive ice formation at the catheter tip causes its adherence to the adjacent tissue, ensuring secure contact of the tip to the target site during respiration and cardiac motion. Furthermore, cryolesions are associated with less endothelial disruption and thrombus formation than RF lesions are,[105,106] and the safety of cryothermal ablation adjacent to coronary arteries has been demonstrated by extensive surgical experience and recent catheter-based studies using animal models.[41,42]

IMPACT OF LOCATION ON ABLATION OF ACCESSORY PATHWAYS

The location of an AP may dictate the need for special consideration of the ablation approach to reduce potential complications. By definition, septal APs have an atrial insertion located within the triangle of Koch. Anteroseptal and midseptal pathways course near the septum in close anatomic relationship to the His bundle and AV node. As a result, surgical division or RF catheter ablation is associated with an increased risk of AV block, reported to occur in up to 36% of patients.[107-109] Not infrequently, ablation of such pathways is postponed in the absence of drug-refractory symptoms or a short antegrade effective refractory period and rapidly conducted atrial fibrillation.

This difficulty notwithstanding, several studies have demonstrated effective RF interruption of these pathways with preservation of AV nodal conduction.[110-114] Conventional RF energy with step-up power titration has been successful with a low incidence of AV block.[113] Placement of a His bundle recording catheter as a reference point allows estimation of the distance between the ablation target and the AV node. Once a suitable target without a His bundle recording is identified, RF energy may be delivered, commencing at a power setting of 10 W. If pathway interruption has not occurred after 10 to 15 seconds, the power is increased by 5 W every 10 to 15 seconds, with continuous attention given to the earliest recognition of AV nodal impairment (development of atrium-to-His [AH] interval prolongation or AV block), accelerated nodal rhythm, or catheter displacement. Ablation commencing with a low power setting has been recommended by several authors to achieve the desired result while producing the smallest possible lesion.[111-113] The success of this approach and the frequently observed temporary conduction block after catheter-induced mechanical trauma suggest a superficial subendocardial location of these pathways.

An alternative and possibly safer approach for elimination of septal pathways is cryoablation. The well-established properties of cryothermy, including reversibility, small discrete lesion size, and cryoadherence, make this ablation modality particularly suitable if lesions are required adjacent the AV node. Stability secures accurate lesion placement, and reversibility allows functional testing of the target before ablation, a combination that makes inadvertent permanent AV block an unlikely complication (Fig. 24–16). This technology intuitively offers significant advantages over RF energy in this setting.

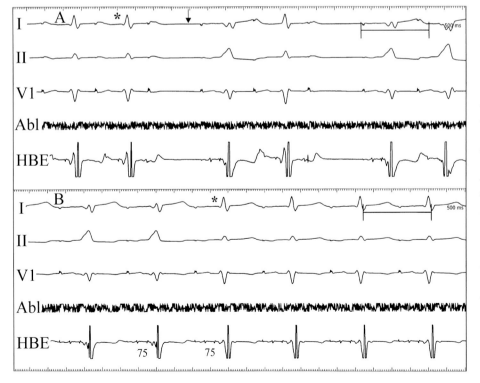

FIGURE 24–16. Cryoablation of an anteroseptal accessory pathway. Panel *A* shows during ice mapping (−30° C) at the atrial insertion site, intermittent loss of preexcitation (*asterisk*) and transient AV block (*arrow*) is observed with return of conduction at rewarming. In panel *B* further ice mapping identified a site where loss of preexcitation occurred without AV block (*asterisk*) prior to permanent pathway elimination. Note that the AH interval (75 msec) remains unchanged with loss of preexcitation. Abl, ablation catheter; HBE, His bundle electrogram.

Epicardial APs also warrant special consideration. Posteroseptal and left posterolateral pathways may be accessible only via the CS or by intra-pericardial access. Application of RF current within the CS has been reported to be safe and successful; however, vascular complications including venous thrombosis, stenosis, perforation, tamponade, and arterial injury infrequently occur. Thorough mapping and the use of high standards in accepting suitable electrograms for ablation, including identification of AP potentials, can minimize complications by reducing the number of required RF current pulses. Risk may also be reduced by the use of lower delivered energy and temperature-guided ablation with conventional RF. Irrigated cooled-tip catheters may facilitate ablation by allowing delivery of higher energy within the confined space of the CS, preventing the impedance rises that may be observed with conventional catheters. Furthermore, selective coronary arterial angiography may reduce arterial injury by defining the anatomic relation of the ablation target to the coronary vessels.

The complications associated with RF energy delivery within the CS are all but eliminated when cryoablation is used. Cryothermy has been safely and successfully employed within the CS for elimination of posterolateral epicardial APs.[39] Preservation of the endothelial surface, less thrombus formation, and safe application adjacent to the coronary arteries are potential benefits offered by this modality compared with RF energy.

Failure to eliminate AP conduction with conventional RF often prompts substitution with a saline-irrigated catheter.[115] Ablation failure may relate to AP anatomy, such as a broad pathway insertion or an epicardial location. Conversely, suboptimal energy delivery may be contributory, as can occur with catheter instability or poor tissue contact. In these circumstances, successful ablation is often accomplished by enhanced delivery of RF energy to the tissue, which in turn produces larger and deeper endomyocardial lesions. However, the benefits of saline-irrigated RF ablation are not without risk. Higher energy delivery may permit subendocardial tissue temperature to rise above 100°C. Plasma boiling and tissue desiccation at these temperatures, frequently accompanied by an audible pop, may result in crater formation and wall rupture, particularly in thin-walled cavities such as the atria or outflow tracts. Accordingly, saline-irrigated RF ablation should be used judiciously, with power limited to 30W[116,117] and at temperatures not exceeding 45°C,[118-120] to reduce the risk of "steam pop" and perforation.

Approach to the Patient Requiring Repeat Ablation

Primary failure or recurrent tachycardia after initial ablation success may necessitate a repeat ablation procedure. Patients may be referred from other laboratories or may undergo a subsequent attempt at the same institution. In any case, a systematic approach to identifying contributing factors and formulation of an appropriate ablation strategy are essential to improve the likelihood of success (Table 24–3).

Although the most frequent causes of primary ablation failure are technical, the contribution of "cognitive" failure must not be underestimated. Inaccurate pathway localization and tachycardia misdiagnosis are the next most common causes of failed ablation.[13] Consequently, a thorough review of all available information, including the clinical history, the 12-lead ECG during sinus rhythm and tachycardia, and findings of the initial electrophysiology study, is essential. Accompanying correspondence from the referring physician may document relevant technical information, including difficult target site access, catheter instability, or perinodal ablation.

Confirmation of the tachycardia diagnosis is the single most critical step in the management of repeat ablation. This is achieved only by completion of a full repeat diagnostic electrophysiology study. New findings, incongruent with preceding data, may provide grounds for a previously failed attempt. If the tachycardia mechanism is verified, localization of the AP and repeat ablation should be undertaken. *Importantly, maximal preexcitation during sinus rhythm and lack of tachycardia inducibility should raise suspicion of previous inadvertent AV nodal injury, particularly in the setting of anteroseptal or midseptal APs.* Consequently, demonstration of intact AV nodal function during the baseline study is crucial, because the anterograde conducting AP may represent the only electrical connection between the atrium and ventricle, and its elimination will result in complete AV block and pacemaker dependence.

Instability and difficult target site access may be overcome by the use of purpose-specific long intravascular sheaths, ablation catheters of different reach or distal configuration, an alternative ablation approach (e.g., retrograde aortic versus trans-septal), or attempt by a second operator. Larger and deeper ablation lesions produced by saline-irrigated catheters may allow elimination of epicardial APs or permit delivery of RF energy within a confined space, such as the CS. In addition, cryothermy may afford a

TABLE 24–3

Approach to Failed Ablation at the Site of an "Ideal" Electrogram

Re-evaluate electrogram interpretation

Presence of far-field activity on the electrogram before the rapid deflection suggests need for more accurate pathway localization
   Use a unipolar electrogram to help determine ideal timing compared with the rapid deflection of the bipolar electrogram

Possible misinterpretation of closely approximated A and V electrograms
   Assess and compare local A and V activation during sinus rhythm and A or V pacing
   Brush back and forth from A to V to clarify timing of A and V activation (especially at the right free wall, where A and V may be superimposed*)
   Pacing maneuvers to dissociate the putative AP potential from A and V electrograms (useful in the presence of fractionated electrograms)

Instability

Remap using a long sheath or different catheter curve to improve stability

Consider an alternative approach: SVC vs IVC, retrograde aortic vs trans-septal

Entrainment during AVRT to prevent dislodgement with RF termination of tachycardia

Cryoablation

Consider an alternative target

Posteroseptal pathways
   May be left sided or epicardial—possibly accessible via the coronary sinus

Atypical accessory pathways and non-annular AV pathways
   Map at sites away from the AV annulus (e.g., appendage, outflow tract)

High-risk target

Ablation target adjacent to the AV node or within the coronary sinus
   Consider cryothermal ablation

Unrecognized change

Possible multiple accessory pathways
   Commit to full-duration energy application if subtle changes in electrogram timing or QRS morphology are observed, then remap and repeat

Transient elimination of AP conduction

   Time to elimination is a good indicator of ablation catheter proximity to the pathway
Instability—as above

Multiple accessory pathways
   Carefully re-evaluate preexcitation pattern or retrograde atrial activation sequence

"Deep" or epicardial location
   Consider using a saline-irrigated catheter

*See Figure 24-1.

A, atrium; AP, accessory pathway; AV, atrioventricular; AVRT, atrioventricular reentrant tachycardia; IVC, inferior vena cava; RF, radiofrequency energy; SVC, superior vena cava; V, ventricle.

degree of safety for ablation targets in high-risk locations, such as those adjacent the AV node or within the CS and its branches.

Fortunately, failure to eliminate AP conduction and recurrence of tachycardia after apparently successful ablation are infrequent outcomes of therapeutic intervention for AV reentrant tachycardia. In these cases, perseverance and patience usually prevail.

References

1. Hindricks G: The Multicentre European Radiofrequency Survey (MERFS). Complications of radiofrequency catheter

ablation of arrhythmias: The Multicentre European Radiofrequency Survey (MERFS) of the Working Group on Arrhythmias of the European Society of Cardiology. Eur Heart J 14:1644-1653, 1993.

2. Jackman WM, Wang X, Friday KJ, et al.: Catheter ablation of atrioventricular accessory pathways (Wolff-Parkinson-White syndrome) by radiofrequency current. N Engl J Med 324:1605-1611, 1991.

3. Kuck KH, Schluter M, Geiger M, et al.: Radiofrequency current catheter ablation of accessory atrioventricular pathways. Lancet 337:1557-1561, 1991.

4. Lesh MD, Van Hare GF, Schamp DJ, et al.: Curative percutaneous catheter ablation of using radiofrequency energy for accessory pathways in all locations: Results in 100 consecutive patients. J Am Coll Cardiol 19:1303-1309, 1992.

5. Calkins H, Yong P, Miller JM, et al.: Catheter ablation of accessory pathways, atrioventricular nodal reentrant tachycardia, and the atrioventricular junction: Final results of a prospective, multicentre clinical trial. Circulation 99:262-270, 1999.

6. Borgreffe M, Budde T, Podczeck A, et al.: High frequency alternating current ablation of an accessory pathway in humans. J Am Coll Cardiol 10:576-582, 1987.

7. Schluter M, Geiger M, Siebels J, et al.: Catheter ablation using radiofrequency current to cure symptomatic patients with tachyarrhythmias related to an accessory atrioventricular accessory pathway. Circulation 84:1644-1661, 1991.

8. Calkins H, Langberg J, Sousa J, et al.: Radiofrequency catheter ablation of accessory atrioventricular connections in 250 patients: Abbreviated therapeutic approach to Wolff-Parkinson-White syndrome. Circulation 85:1337-1346, 1992.

9. Warin JF, Haissaguerre M, D'ivernois, et al.: Catheter ablation of accessory pathways: Technique and results in 248 patients. Pacing Clin Electrophysiol 13:1609-1614, 1990.

10. Kay GN, Epstein AE, Dailey SM, et al.: Role of radiofrequency ablation in the management of supraventricular arrhythmias: Experience in 760 consecutive patients. J Clin Electrophysiol 4:372-389, 1993.

11. Leather RA, Leitch JW, Klein GJ, et al.: Radiofrequency catheter ablation of accessory pathways: A learning experience. Am J Cardiol 68:1651-1655, 1991.

12. Li HG, Klein GJ, Zardini M, et al.: Radiofrequency catheter ablation of accessory pathways during entrainment of AV reentrant tachycardia. Pacing Clin Electrophysiol 17:590-594, 1994.

13. Morady F, Strickberger SA, Man KC, et al.: Reasons for prolonged or failed attempts at radiofrequency catheter ablation of accessory pathways. J Am Coll Cardiol 27:683-689, 1996.

14. Xie B, Heald SC, Camm AJ, et al.: Radiofrequency catheter ablation of accessory atrioventricular: Primary failure and recurrence of conduction. Heart 77:363-368, 1997.

15. Twidale N, Wang XZ, Beckman KJ, et al.: Factors associated with recurrence of accessory pathway conduction after radiofrequency catheter ablation. Pacing Clin Electrophysiol 14:2042-2048, 1991.

16. Ho S, Sánchez-Quintana D, Becker AE: A review of the coronary venous system: A road less travelled. Heart Rhythm 1:107-112, 2004.

17. Lüdinghausen VM, Ohmachi N, Boot C: Myocardial coverage of the coronary sinus and related veins. Clin Anat 5:1-15, 1992.

18. Chauvin M, Shah DC, Haissaguerre M, et al.: The anatomic basis of connections between the coronary sinus musculature and the left atrium in humans. Circulation 101:647-652, 2000.

19. Ho SY, Sánchez-Quintana D, Cabrera JA, Anderson RH: Anatomy of the left atrium: Implications for radiofrequency ablation of atrial fibrillation. J Cardiovasc Electrophysiol 10:1525-1533, 1999.

20. Antz M, Otomo K, Arruda M, et al.: Electrical conduction between the right atrium and the left atrium via the musculature of the coronary sinus. Circulation 98:1790-1795, 1998.

21. Gerlis LM, Davies MJ, Boyle R, et al.: Pre-excitation due to accessory sinoventricular connections associated with coronary aneurysms: A report of two cases. Br Heart J 53:314-322, 1985.

22. Segni ED, Siegal A, Katzenstein M, et al.: Congenital diverticulum of the heart arising from the coronary sinus. Br Heart J 56:380-384, 1986.

23. Guiraudon GM, Guiraudon CM, Klein GJ, et al.: The coronary sinus diverticulum: A pathologic entity associated with Wolff-Parkinson-White syndrome. Am J Cardiol 62:733-735, 1988.

24. Ho SY, Russell G, Roland E: Coronary venous aneurysms and accessory atrio-ventricular connections. Br Heart J 60:348-351, 1988.

25. Sun Y, Arruda M, Otomo K, et al.: Coronary sinus-ventricular accessory connections producing posteroseptal and left posterior accessory pathways: Incidence and electrophysiological identification. Circulation 106:1362-1367, 2002.

26. Takahashi A, Shah DC, Jais P, et al.: Specific electrocardiographic features of manifest coronary vein posteroseptal accessory pathways. J Cardiovasc Electrophysiol 9:1015-1025, 1998.

27. Haissaguerre M, Gaita F, Fischer B, et al.: Radiofrequency catheter ablation of left lateral accessory pathways via the coronary sinus. Circulation 86:1464-1468, 1992.

28. Beukema WP, Van Dessel PF, Van Hemel NM, Kingma JH: Radiofrequency catheter ablation of accessory pathways associated with a coronary sinus diverticulum. Eur Heart J 15:1415-1418, 1994.

29. Villacastin J, Merino JL, Almendral J, et al.: Radiofrequency ablation of a posteroseptal accessory pathway associated with coronary sinus diverticulum. Rev Esp Cardiol 48:638-641, 1995.

30. Kleinman D, Winters SL: Successful catheter ablation of an inferoseptal accessory pathway within the coronary sinus in a patient with a previously unsuccessful attempt at surgical interruption: Coronary sinus ablation for Wolff-Parkinson-White syndrome. J Electrocardiol 29:55-60, 1996.

31. Takatsuki S, Mitamura H, Ieda M, Ogawa S: Accessory pathway associated with an anomalous coronary vein in a patient with Wolff-Parkinson-White syndrome. J Cardiovasc Electrophysiol 12:1080-1082, 2001.

32. Kusano KF, Morita H, Fujimoto Y, et al.: Catheter ablation of an epicardial accessory pathway via the middle cardiac vein guided by monophasic action potential recordings. Europace 3:164-167, 2001.

33. Davidson NC, Cooper MJ, Ross DL: Radiofrequency catheter ablation of a posteroseptal accessory pathway with two diverticula of the coronary sinus. Circulation 104:240-241, 2001.

34. Lewalter T, Yang A, Schwab JO, Lüderitz B: Accessory pathway catheter ablation inside the neck of a coronary sinus diverticulum. J Cardiovasc Electrophysiol 14:1386, 2003.

35. Hussin A, Sanders P, Kistler PM, et al.: Accessory pathway in left inferoposterior diverticulum masquerading as left posterior pathway due to conduction over coronary sinus to left atrium connection. J Cardiovasc Electrophysiol 14:403-406, 2003.

36. Hartzler GO, Giorgi LV, Diehl AM, Hamaker WR: Right coronary spasm complicating electrode catheter ablation of a right lateral accessory pathway. J Am Coll Cardiol 6:250-253, 1985.

37. Chatelain P, Zimmermann M, Weber R, et al.: Acute coronary occlusion secondary to radiofrequency catheter ablation of a left lateral accessory pathway. Eur Heart J 16:859-861, 1995.

38. de Paola AA, Leite LR, Arfelli E: Mechanical reperfusion of acute right coronary artery occlusion after radiofrequency catheter ablation and long term follow-up angiography. J Invasive Cardiol 15:173-175, 2003.

39. Gaita F, Paperini L, Riccardi R, Ferraro A: Cryothermic ablation within the coronary sinus of an epicardial posterolateral accessory pathway. J Cardiovasc Electrophysiol 13:1160-1163, 2002.

40. Klein GJ, Harrison L, Ideker RF, et al.: Reaction of the myocardium to cryosurgery: Electrophysiology and arrhythmogenic potential. Circulation 59:364-372, 1979.

41. Skanes AC, Jones DL, Teefy P, et al.: Safety and feasibility of cryothermal ablation within the mid- and distal coronary sinus. J Cardiovasc Electrophysiol 15:1319-1323, 2004.

42. Yagi T, Nakagawa H, Khammar GS, et al.: Safety and efficacy of cryo-ablation in the canine coronary sinus [abstract]. Circulation 104:II-620, 2001.

43. Saad EB, Marrouche NF, Cole CR, Natale A: Simultaneous epicardial and endocardial mapping of a left-sided posteroseptal accessory pathway associated with a large coronary sinus diverticulum: Successful ablation by transection of the diverticulum's neck. Pacing Clin Electrophysiol 25:1524-1526, 2002.

44. Sapp J, Soejima K, Couper G, Stevenson W: Electrophysiology and anatomic characterization of an epicardial accessory pathway. J Cardiovasc Electrophysiol 12:1411-1414, 2001.

45. Anderson RH, Ho SY: Anatomy of the atrioventricular junctions with regard to ventricular preexcitation. Pacing Clin Electrophysiol 20:2072-2076, 1997.

46. Heaven DJ, Till JA, Ho SY: Sudden death in a child with an unusual accessory connection. Europace 2:224-227, 2000.

47. Arruda M, McClelland J, Beckman K, et al.: Atrial appendage-ventricular connections: A new variant of preexcitation [abstract]. Circulation 90:I-126, 1994.

48. Milstein S, Dunnigan A, Tang C, Pineda E: Right atrial appendage to right ventricle accessory atrioventricular pathway: A case report. Pacing Clin Electrophysiol 20:1877-1880, 1997.

49. Soejima K, Mitamura H, Miyazaki T, et al.: Catheter ablation of accessory atrioventricular connection between right atrial appendage to right ventricle: A case report. J Cardiovasc Electrophysiol 9:523-528, 1998.

50. Goya M, Takahashi A, Nakagawa H, Iesaka Y: A case of catheter ablation of accessory atrioventricular connection between the right atrial appendage and right ventricle guided by a three-dimensional electroanatomic mapping system. J Cardiovasc Electrophysiol 10:1112-1118, 1999.

51. Lam C, Schweikert R, Kanagaratham L, Natale A: Radiofrequency ablation of a right atrial appendage-ventricular accessory pathway by transcutaneous epicardial instrumentation. J Cardiovasc Electrophysiol 11:1170-1173, 2000.

52. Colavita PG, Packer DL, Pressley JC, et al. Frequency, diagnosis and clinical characteristics of patients with multiple accessory atrioventricular pathways. Am J Cardiol 59:601-606, 1987.

53. Kastor JA, Goldreyer BN, Josephson ME, et al.: Electrophysiologic characterization of Ebstein's anomaly of the tricuspid valve. Circulation 52:987-995, 1975.

54. Smith WM, Gallagher JJ, Kerr CR, et al.: The electrophysiologic basis and management of symptomatic and recurrent tachycardia in patients with Ebstein's anomaly of the tricuspid valve. Am J Cardiol 49:1223-1234, 1982.

55. Cappato R, Schluter M, Weiss C, et al.: Radiofrequency current catheter ablation of accessory atrioventricular pathways in Ebstein's anomaly. Circulation 94:376-383, 1996.

56. Kocheril AG, Rosenfeld LE: Radiofrequency ablation of an accessory pathway in a patient with corrected Ebstein's anomaly. Pacing Clin Electrophysiol 17:986-990, 1994.

57. Ai T, Horie M, Washizuka T, et al.: Successful radiofrequency current catheter ablation of accessory atrioventricular pathway after tricuspid replacement in Ebstein's anomaly. Jpn Circ J 62:791-793, 1998.

58. Okishige K, Azegami K, Goseki Y, et al.: Radiofrequency ablation of tachyarrhythmias in patients with Ebstein's anomaly. Int J Cardiol 60:171-180, 1997.

59. Reich J, Auld D, Hulse JE, et al.: The pediatric radiofrequency ablation registry's experience with Ebstein's anomaly. J Cardiovasc Electrophysiol 9:1370-1377, 1998.

60. Bertram H, Bökenkamp R, Peuster M, et al.: Coronary artery stenosis after radiofrequency catheter ablation of accessory atrioventricular pathways in children with Ebstein's malformation. Circulation 103:538-543, 2001.

61. Ai T, Ikeguchi S, Watanuki M, et al.: Successful radiofrequency current catheter ablation of accessory atrioventricular pathway in Ebstein's anomaly using electroanatomic mapping. Pacing Clin Electrophysiol 25:374-375, 2002.

62. Steinberg I, Dubilier W, Lucas D: Persistence of left superior vena cava. Dis Chest 24:479-488, 1953.

63. Fraser RS, Dvorkin J, Rossall RE, Eidem R: Left superior vena cava: A review of associated congenital heart lesions, catheterisation data, and roentgenologic findings. Am J Med 31:771-776, 1961.

64. Bjerregaard P, Laursen HB: Persistent left superior vena cava. Acta Paediatr Scand 69:105-108, 1980.

65. Chiang CE, Chen SA, Yang CR, et al.: Major coronary sinus abnormalities: Identification of occurrence and significance in radiofrequency ablation of supraventricular tachycardia. Am Heart J 127:1279-1289, 1994.

66. Weiss C, Cappato R, Willems S, et al.: Prospective evaluation of coronary sinus anatomy in patients undergoing electrophysiology study. Clin Cardiol 22:537-543, 1999.

67. Ma CS, Hu D, Fang Q, et al.: Catheter ablation of a left-sided accessory pathway with a left superior vena cava. Am Heart J 130:613-615, 1995.

68. Takatsuki S, Mitamura H, Ieda M, Ogawa S: Accessory pathway associated with an anomalous coronary vein in a patient with Wolff-Parkinson-White syndrome. J Cardiovasc Electrophysiol 12:1080-1082, 2001.

69. Kursaklioglu H, Kose S, Barcin C, et al.: Radiofrequency catheter ablation of a left lateral accessory pathway in a patient with persistent left superior vena cava. Heart Dis 4:162-165, 2002.

70. Chiou CW, Chen SA, Chiang CE, et al.: Radiofrequency catheter ablation of paroxysmal supraventricular tachycardia in patients with congenital heart disease. Int J Cardiol 50:143-151, 1995.

71. O'Callaghan WG, Colavita PG, Kay GN, et al.: Persistent left superior vena cava: Localization of site of ectopic atrial pacemaker and associated atrioventricular accessory pathway. Am Heart J 111:1200-1202, 1985.

72. Gallagher JJ, Sealy WC, Kasell J, Wallace AG: Multiple accessory pathways in patients with the pre-excitation syndrome. Circulation 54:571-591, 1976.

73. Iwa T, Magara T, Watanabe Y, et al.: Interruption of multiple accessory pathways in patients with the Wolff-Parkinson-White syndrome. Ann Thoracic Surg 30:313-325, 1980.

74. Chen SA, Chiang CE, Chiou CW, et al.: Reappraisal of radiofrequency ablation of multiple accessory pathways. Am Heart J 125:760-771, 1993.

75. Yeh SJ, Wang CC, Wen MS, et al.: Radiofrequency ablation in multiple accessory pathways and the physiologic implications. Am J Cardiol 15:1174-1180, 1993.

76. Wang LX, Ding YS, Hu DY: Endocardial mapping and radiofrequency catheter ablation of multiple atrioventricular accessory pathways. Chin Med J 107:83-87, 1994.

77. Iturralde Torres P, Lara S, Picos Bovio E, et al.: Radiofrequency ablation in multiple accessory pathways. Arch Inst Cardiol Mex 66:390-399, 1996.

78. Huang JL, Chen SA, Tai CT, et al.: Long-term results of radiofrequency catheter ablation in patients with multiple accessory pathways. Am J Cardiol 78:1375-1379, 1996.

79. Iturralde P, Guevara-Valdivia M, Rodríguez-Chàvez L, et al.: Radiofrequency ablation of multiple accessory pathways. Europace 4:273-280, 2002.

80. Weng KP, Wolff GS, Young ML: Multiple accessory pathways in paediatric patients with Wolff-Parkinson-White syndrome. Am J Cardiol 91:1178-1183, 2003.

81. Verduyn Lunel AA: Significance of annulus fibrosis of heart in relation to AV conduction and ventricular activation in cases of Wolff-Parkinson-White syndrome. Br Heart J 34:1263-1271, 1972.

82. Becker AE, Anderson RH, Durrer D, Wellens HJ: The anatomic substrates of Wolff-Parkinson-White syndrome. Circulation 57:870-879, 1978.

83. Klein GJ, Bashore TM, Sellers TD, et al.: Ventricular fibrillation in the Wolff-Parkinson-White syndrome. N Engl J Med 301:1080-1085, 1979.

84. Teo WS, Klein GJ, Guiraudon GM, et al.: Multiple accessory pathways in the Wolff-Parkinson-White syndrome as a risk factor for ventricular fibrillation. Am J Cardiol 67:889-891, 1991.

85. Schluter M, Cappato R, Ouyang F, et al.: Clinical recurrences after successful accessory pathway ablation: The role of "dormant" accessory pathways. J Cardiovasc Electrophysiol 8:1366-1372, 1997.

86. Silka MJ, Kron J, Halperin BD, et al.: Analysis of local electrogram characteristics correlated with successful radiofrequency catheter ablation of accessory atrioventricular accessory pathways. Pacing Clin Electrophysiol 15:1000-1007, 1992.

87. Swartz JF, Tracy CM, Fletcher RD: Radiofrequency endocardial catheter ablation of accessory atrioventricular pathway atrial insertion sites. Circulation 87:487-499, 1993.

88. Jackman WM, Friday KJ, Yeung-Lai-Wah JA, et al.: New catheter technique for recording left free-wall accessory atrioventricular pathway activation: Identification of pathway fiber orientation. Circulation 78:598-611, 1988.

89. Jackman WM, Friday KJ, Fitzgerald DM, et al.: Localization of left free-wall and posteroseptal accessory atrioventricular pathways by direct recording of accessory pathway activation. Pacing Clin Electrophysiol 12:204-214, 1989.

90. Otomo K, Gonzalez MD, Beckman KJ, et al.: Reversing the direction of paced ventricular and atrial wavefronts reveals an oblique course in the accessory AV pathways and improves localization for catheter ablation. Circulation 104:550-556, 2001.

91. Yamabe H, Shimasaki Y, Honda O, et al.: Localization of the ventricular insertion site of concealed left-sided accessory pathways using ventricular pace mapping. Pacing Clin Electrophysiol 25:940-950, 2002.

92. Calkins H, Kim YN, Schmaltz S, et al.: Electrogram criteria for identification of appropriate target sites for radiofrequency catheter ablation of accessory atrioventricular accessory connections. Circulation 85:565-573, 1992.

93. Teo WS, Guiraudon G, Klein GJ, et al.: A unique preexcitation pattern related to an atypical anteroseptal accessory pathway. Pacing Clin Electrophysiol 15:1696-1701, 1992.

94. Nath S, Haines DE: Biophysics and pathology of catheter energy delivery systems. Prog Cardiovasc Dis 37:185-204, 1995.

95. Haines DE: The biophysics of radiofrequency catheter ablation in the heart: the importance of temperature monitoring. Pacing Clin Electrophysiol 16:586-591, 1993.

96. Haines DE, Verow AF: Observations on electrode tissue interface temperature and effect on electrical impedance during radiofrequency ablation of ventricular myocardium. Circulation 82:1034-1038, 1990.

97. Nakagawa H, Yamanashi WS, Pitha JV, et al.: Comparison of in vivo tissue temperature profile and lesion geometry for radiofrequency ablation with a saline-irrigated electrode versus temperature control in a canine thigh muscle preparation. Circulation 91:2264-2273, 1995.

98. Demazumder D, Mirotznik MS, Schwartzman D: Biophysics of radiofrequency ablation using an irrigated electrode. J Intervent Cardiol Electrophysiol 5:377-389, 2001.

99. Skanes AC, Dubuc M, Klein GJ, et al.: Cryothermal ablation of the slow pathway for the elimination of atrioventricular nodal reentrant tachycardia. Circulation 102:2856-2860, 2000.

100. Dubuc M, Khairy P, Rodriguez-Santiago A, et al.: Catheter cryoablation of the atrioventricular node in patients with atrial fibrillation: A novel technology for ablation of cardiac arrhythmias. J Cardiovasc Electrophysiol 12:439-444, 2001.

101. Rodriguez LM, Geller C, Tse HF, et al.: Acute results of transvenous cryoablation of supraventricular tachycardia (atrial fibrillation, atrial flutter, Wolff-Parkinson-White syndrome, atrioventricular nodal tachycardia). J Cardiovasc Electrophysiol 13:1082-1089, 2002.

102. Lanzotti ME, De Ponti R, Tritto M, et al.: Successful treatment of anteroseptal accessory pathways by transvenous cryomapping and cryoablation. Ital Heart J 3:128-132, 2002.

103. Skanes AC, Klein GJ, Krahn AD, Yee R: Advances in energy delivery. Coron Artery Dis 14:15-23, 2003.

104. Skanes AC, Yee R, Krahn AD, Klein GJ: Cryoablation of atrial arrhythmias. Cardiac Electrophysiol Rev 6:383-388, 2002.

105. Ayala-Paredes F, Sturmer ML, Macle L, et al.: Catheter-based cryothermal versus radiofrequency ablation: Morphometric lesion characteristics [abstract]. Pacing Clin Electrophysiol 25:663, 2002.

106. Khairy P, Chauvet P, Lehmann J, et al: Lower incidence of thrombus formation with cryoenergy versus radiofrequency catheter ablation. Circulation 107(15):2045-2050, 2003.

107. Gallagher JJ, Selle JG, Sealy WC, et al.: Intermediate septal accessory pathways (IS-AP): A subset of preexcitation at risk for complete heart block/failure during WPW surgery [abstract]. Circulation 74(Suppl II):II-387, 1986.

108. Epstein AE, Kirklin JK, Holman WL, et al.: Intermediate septal accessory pathways: Electrocardiographic characteristics, electrophysiologic observations and their surgical implications. J Am Coll Cardiol 17:1570-1578, 1991.

109. Yeh SJ, Wang CC, Wen MS, et al.: Characteristics and radiofrequency ablation therapy of intermediate septal accessory pathways. Am J Cardiol 73:50-56, 1994.

110. Kuck KH, Schluter M, Gursoy S: Preservation of atrioventricular nodal conduction during radiofrequency catheter ablation of midseptal accessory pathway. Circulation 86:1743-1752, 1992.

111. Schluter M, Kuck KH: Catheter ablation from right atrium of anteroseptal accessory pathways using radiofrequency current. J Am Coll Cardiol 19:663-670, 1992.

112. Haissaguerre M, Marcus F, Poquet F, et al.: Electrocardiographic characteristics and catheter ablation of para-Hisian accessory pathways. Circulation 90:1124-1128, 1994.

113. Tai CT, Chen SA, Chiang CE, et al.: Electrocardiographic and electrophysiologic characteristics of anteroseptal, midseptal and para-Hisian accessory pathways: Implication for radiofrequency catheter ablation. Chest 109:730-740, 1996.

114. Gatzoulis K, Apostolopoulos T, Costeas X, et al.: Paraseptal accessory connections in the proximity of the atrioventricular node and the His bundle: Additional observations in relation to the ablation technique in a high risk area. Europace 6:1-9, 2004.

115. García-García J, Almendral J, Arenal A, et al.: Irrigated tip catheter ablation in right posteroseptal accessory pathways resistant to conventional ablation. Pacing Clin Electrophysiol 25:799-803, 2002.

116. Skrumeda LL, Mehra R: Comparison of standard and irrigated radiofrequency ablation in the canine ventricle. J Cardiovasc Electrophysiol 9:1196-1205, 1998.

117. Mittleman RS, Huang SKS, De Guzman WT, et al.: Use of saline infusion electrode catheter for improved energy delivery and increased lesion size in radiofrequency catheter ablation. Pacing Clin Electrophysiol 18:1022-1027, 1995.

118. Wharton JM, Wilber DJ, Calkins H, et al.: Utility of tip thermometry during radiofrequency ablation in humans using an internally perfused saline cooled catheter [abstract]. Circulation 96:I-318, 1997.

119. Barold HS, Jain MK, Dixon-Tulloch E, et al.: What is the optimal temperature limit for the temperature-controlled cooled radiofrequency ablation? [abstract]. Circulation 98:I-644, 1998.

120. Barold HS, Jain MK, Dixon-Tulloch E, et al.: A comparison of temperature-controlled cooled tip versus standard temperature-controlled radiofrequency ablation in left ventricular myocardium [abstract]. Circulation 98:I-644, 1998.

Catheter Ablation of Ventricular Tachycardia

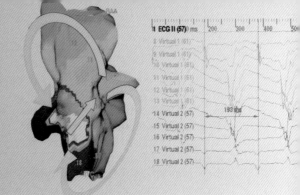

1 ECG II (57) ms   200   300   400   50m
8 Virtual 1 (61)
9 Virtual 1 (61)
10 Virtual 1 (61)
11 Virtual 1 (61)
12 Virtual 1 (61)
13 Virtual 1 (61)
14 Virtual 2 (57)   193 ms
15 Virtual 2 (57)
16 Virtual 2 (57)
17 Virtual 2 (57)
18 Virtual 2 (57)

PART VII

25

Ablation of Ventricular Outflow Tract Tachycardias

Sanjay Dixit • David Lin • Francis E. Marchlinski

Key Points

▪ Mapping of ventricular outflow tract tachycardias includes the right or left ventricular outflow tract, aortic cusps, pulmonary artery, and possibly epicardial mapping.

▪ The ablation targets are the site of earliest activation and/or the site of identical pace mapping.

▪ Electroanatomic mapping systems are often useful. Noncontact mapping may be helpful for nonsustained tachycardias. Irrigated radiofrequency ablation catheters or large-tip catheters may be needed. Coronary angiographic catheters may be needed to visualize coronary arteries.

▪ Sources of difficulty include tachycardias that are noninducible or nonsustained, electrocardiographic localization based on ECG morphology, and ablation near the coronary arteries or His bundle.

Ventricular tachycardias (VTs) are usually observed in the setting of structural heart disease.[1,2] However, in 10% of the patients presenting with VT, the routine diagnostic modalities demonstrate no myocardial damage.[1] These arrhythmias have been called idiopathic ventricular tachycardias (IVTs), and they consist of various subtypes that have been defined by their clinical presentation (e.g., repetitive monomorphic tachycardias, exercise-induced sustained ventricular arrhythmias) and/or their underlying mechanism (e.g., adenosine-sensitive triggered arrhythmias, β-blocker–dependent automatic arrhythmias, intrafascicular or interfascicular reentrant arrhythmias).[3-5] Importantly, the mechanistically different subgroups of IVT favor certain anatomic locations within the heart and hence manifest specific electrocardiographic (ECG) patterns which help to identify their site of origin.

Outflow tract tachycardias comprise a subgroup of IVTs that are predominantly localized in and around the right and left ventricular outflow tracts (RVOT and LVOT, respectively). Lerman et al.[6,7] elegantly demonstrated that the mechanism underlying this group of arrhythmias appears to be triggered activity due to delayed afterdepolarizations that are determined by intracellular calcium release (load). The release of calcium is negatively affected by adenosine, which thus inhibits the afterdepolarizations and their clinical manifestations and these arrhythmias are typically "adenosine sensitive."

In a group of 122 patients who underwent ablation of IVT at our center between January 1999 and December 2003, using the site of successful ablation and/or the earliest activation marked on the magnetic electroanatomic map (MEAM) as the gold standard, the site of origin was localized to the RVOT region in 88 patients (72%). Of the remaining 34 patients, 14 manifested fascicular VT, 9 had a site of origin localized to the aortic cups and/or the left ventricular (LV) epicardium, and in 11 the site of origin of clinical arrhythmia was localized to the endocardium of the basal LV.[8] Therefore, the majority of outflow tract tachycardias in our series were found to originate in the RVOT, which is in concurrence with other reports.[1,5]

This chapter describes briefly the common features of outflow tract tachycardias as a group and then focuses more specifically on the various sites of origin for illustrating the effect of anatomic location on ECG morphology. It then outlines strategies that we have used for ablation based on the site of origin in the outflow tract region.

Clinical Presentation

In general, outflow tract tachycardias manifest at a relatively early age. Lerman et al.[9] found equal distribution of the tachycardia between the two sexes. In our experience, VT originating in the RVOT shows a predilection for females (69.6%), whereas LVOT is predominantly seen in males (8 of 11 patients).[8,10]

The typical presentation of these arrhythmias consists of "salvos" of paroxysmal ventricular ectopic beats and nonsustained VT; however, sustained tachycardia is not uncommon. Most patients (48% to 80%) experience palpitations. Presyncope and lightheadedness may also be observed (28% to 50%). True syncope is infrequently seen (overall incidence, <10%), and these rhythm disorders are rarely life-threatening (there is only one case of documented fatality by cardiac arrest).[11-13] However, in a recent case series by Haissaguerre et al.,[14] ventricular ectopic beats with morphology and intracardiac localization suggesting a site of origin in the RVOT region were shown to consistently initiate ventricular fibrillation in a selected group of patients with Brugada and long QT syndrome. Outflow tract tachycardias are typically provoked by exercise, and treadmill testing can reproduce the clinical VT in most patients.[11,15,16] The arrhythmia may occur during the acceleration of heart rate with exercise or during the recovery phase of exercise, suggesting that there is a combination of critical heart rate and endogenous catecholamine release that potentiates the rhythm disturbance.[17] Other triggers for inducing or enhancing the arrhythmia include stress, anxiety, and stimulants such as caffeine. In females, outflow tachycardias are more often observed during premenstrual and perimenopausal periods and with gestation, suggesting the role of hormonal influences. Our own experience suggests that, in female patients, a hormonal trigger for outflow tract tachycardia initiation is more common than exercise.[18]

LACK OF STRUCTURAL HEART DISEASE

Absence of structural heart disease is the rule with these arrhythmias. Structural heart disease has been traditionally assessed in most studies with the use of ECGs, chest radiographs, echocardiography, radionuclide imaging/stress testing, and cardiac catheterization. A more recent study using cine magnetic resonance imaging (MRI) in patients with RVOT tachycardia showed evidence for right ventricular (RV) outflow abnormalities (focal wall thinning, diminished systolic wall thickening, and abnormal systolic wall motion localized to the anterior and lateral RVOT).[19] However, these findings were not corroborated in another study using similar imaging techniques.[20] Researchers have also attempted to analyze the cardiac sympathetic innervation of ventricles in these patients, using ^{123}I-meta-iodobenzylguanidine (^{123}I-MIBG) scintigraphy and have inconsistently found regional deficiencies in sympathetic innervation.[21-24] Therefore, it can be concluded that, although subtle abnormalities cannot be ruled out, overt structural heart disease is lacking in the setting of outflow tract tachycardia.

Anatomy

Outflow tract tachycardia, as the name implies, tends to originate primarily from the outflow tract of either ventricle, and in these regions they are further localized to even narrower zones. For example, in our series, the majority of RVOT tachycardias (≥80%) originated in the superior, septal, and anterior aspect (under the pulmonic valve),[10] whereas LVOT tachycardias were localized predominantly to the medial aspect of the basal LV (septal-parahisian region, aortomitral continuity, and superior mitral annulus), the epicardial region of the LV above the aortic valve, and

the left and right aortic cusps.[8] If the outflow tract regions of both ventricles together are analyzed, as is illustrated in Figure 25–1, it is obvious that most of the outflow tachycardias originated from a fairly narrow anatomic zone. The relative proximity of the LVOT and RVOT areas was further reinforced by our observations in autopsied human hearts. A probe advanced from the superoanterior and septal aspect of RVOT (under the pulmonic valve) toward the LV initially was seen to overlie the basal LV epicardium and superior aspect of the left interventricular septum (Fig. 25–2). If advanced further, the probe extended toward the aortomitral continuity and superior mitral annulus, all the sites to which the majority of outflow tract tachycardias have been localized.[25]

This predisposition of outflow tract tachycardias (90%) to a specific region in the heart raises an interesting question with regard to the tissue characteristics, which may favor triggered activity and arrhythmogenesis in the area. We have noticed that most outflow tract VTs originate in perivalvular tissue, which may be anatomically predisposed to fiber disruption. Whether it is a normal anatomic finding seen in all people or is an exclusive developmental anomaly manifested in a selected group, not unlike bypass tracts, remains to be determined. It is, of course, possible that a subclinical process

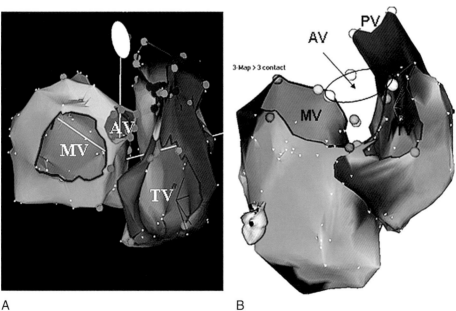

A   B

FIGURE 25–1. Depicts the anatomic relationship between the outflow tract regions of the right and left ventricles on magnetic electro-anatomic mapping generated endocardial shells. In panel **A,** the aortic valve (AV) sits perpendicular and in panel **B,** it is oriented parallel to the plane of the pulmonic valve (PV). In our opinion, this change in AV orientation is age related with the former seen more commonly in older patients as the aortic arch begins to unfold. These variations may influence the characteristics of pace maps and/or arrhythmias originating from aortic cusps, especially the right coronary cusp. See text for details. MV, mitral valve; TV, tricuspid valve.

Common sites of origin of outflow tract tachycardias

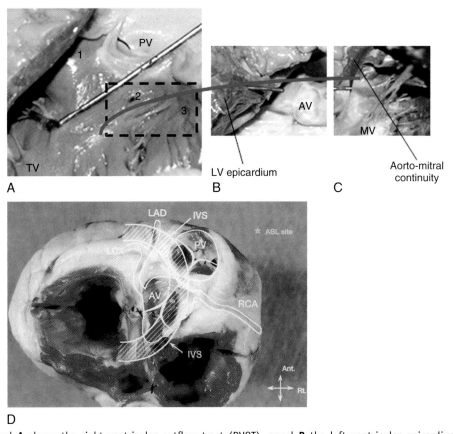

FIGURE 25-2. Panel **A** shows the right ventricular outflow tract (RVOT), panel **B** the left ventricular epicardium adjacent to the anterior RVOT above the aortic valve (AV), and panel **C,** aorto-mitral continuity and medial and superior aspect of the mitral valve (MV). Sites in the RVOT endocardium under the pulmonic valve (PV) from posterior to anterior are labeled 1, 2, and 3. The *rectangle* represents common areas of RVOT tachycardia sites; the *interrupted line* illustrates the natural course of a probe advanced into the anterior RVOT (site 3) which overlies the LV epicardium and the supero-medial aspect of the MV. These areas are also common sites of origin of outflow tract tachycardias underscoring the proximity of the RVOT and basal LV. **D,** View of the outflow tract in a pig heart. AV, aortic valve; IVS, interventricular septum; LAD, left anterior descending artery; LCX, left circumflex artery; PV, pulmonic valve; RCA, right coronary artery. The myocardium of the septal subendocardial region (*hatched semicircular area*) is located beneath the coronary cusps. *(Panel D is from Hachiya H, Aonuma K, Yamauchi Y, et al.: How to diagnose, locate, and ablate coronary cusp ventricular tachycardia. J Cardiovasc Electrophysiol 2002;13:551-556, with permission.)*

(myocarditis/pericarditis) may enhance fiber disruption or cause local dysautonomic changes predisposing the tissue to triggered activity and arrhythmogenesis. Of note, a small percentage of outflow tract tachycardias can be seen in other anatomic locations, including the lateral and inferolateral aspect of mitral annulus, the RV inflow region, the midventricular septum, and the inferoapical area of the LV. In a recent report of seven patients with RVOT tachycardia, the earliest intracardiac activation was demonstrated above the plane of the pulmonic valve. However, in most of these cases, successful ablation was still performed in the superior RVOT under the valve plane.[1,26-29]

Diagnosis

ELECTROCARDIOGRAPHIC PATTERNS AND ANATOMIC LOCATION

From the foregoing discussion, it would seem that, given the relatively narrow anatomic zone from which outflow tract tachycardias arise, they should manifest broadly similar ECG characteristics. Nevertheless, outflow tract tachycardias in fact manifest a variety of ECG morphologies, including left or right bundle branch block patterns, diverse axes (left, inferior, right, leftward), and various patterns of precordial transition (early, late, or none). However, ECG morphologies are predictable based on anatomic location, and recognition of specific ECG features may serve as a useful tool to accurately localize the site of origin of the clinical arrhythmia. Using pace mapping under electroanatomic mapping guidance (see later discussion), we have characterized specific ECG features from different aspects of RVOT, basal LV, and aortic cusps that have allowed us to develop algorithms that are useful in accurately localizing clinical VT originating from this region. The following sections discuss in more detail these site-specific ECG features.

Clinical Arrhythmias from Right Ventricular Outflow Tract

The RVOT region is defined superiorly by the pulmonic valve and inferiorly by the superior margin of the RV inflow tract (tricuspid valve). The interventricular septum and the RV free wall constitute its medial and lateral aspects, respectively. We have used the following protocol for constructing electroanatomic maps of this region. The plane of the pulmonic valve is defined to outline the superior limit of the RVOT. The mapping catheter is advanced superiorly in the RVOT until no discrete bipolar electrograms are seen in the distal electrode pair. The catheter is then retracted until electrograms in the distal electrode pair reappear and pacing results in capture of the RVOT endocardium. This marks the level of the pulmonic valve, and at this level three distinct points are acquired and tagged to construct the valve plane. Next, under electroanatomic mapping and fluoroscopic guidance, a detailed electroanatomic map of the entire RVOT and RV is constructed by acquiring multiple ($\geq$75) points during sinus rhythm.

In an earlier study, based on specific ECG morphologies identified during pace mapping, we divided the septal RVOT into nine anatomic sites to facilitate the description of the catheter position (Fig. 25–3A). However, because of the predilection for clinical arrhythmias from superior RVOT, we attempted to further characterize the ECG features of pace maps from this region in 14 patients. To accomplish this, the superiormost sites in a posterior to anterior distribution were assigned numbers 1, 2, and 3 and their counterpart locations along the free wall of superior RVOT were also assigned numbers 1, 2, and 3 (see Fig. 25–3B). The mapping catheter was positioned serially at each of these sites, which were tagged and labeled on the electroanatomic map and paced at diastolic threshold (cycle length, 400 to 500 msec) for 10 to 20 uninterrupted captured beats. A 12-lead ECG during pacing from each site was acquired. The ECG

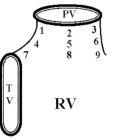 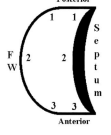

Right Anterior Oblique View   Coronal View: from above PV

A   B

FIGURE 25–3. Schematic representation of the right ventricular outflow tract (RVOT). Panel **A** shows the locations of the 9 standard mapping sites along the septal RVOT in right anterior oblique projection. Sites 1 through 3 represent the first row of sites beneath the pulmonic valve. Panel **B** depicts RVOT viewed coronally from above the PV. Sites 1 (most posterior) through 3 (most anterior) along the septum and FW are shown. See text for details.

was specifically analyzed for (1) QRS amplitude and duration in all limb leads; (2) presence of "notching" of R waves in the inferior leads II, III, and/or aVF; (3) QRS transition pattern in the precordial leads (change from a QS/rS pattern to an RS/Rs pattern) with a change at or beyond lead V_4 defined as a late transition; and (4) QRS morphology in limb lead I. We used limb lead II as representative of all the inferior leads, to quantify the differences in R wave amplitude and QRS duration of pace maps from septal and free wall sites.[30]

Figure 25–4 shows the pace maps from all six locations in the superior RVOT. The pace maps from septal sites manifest monophasic R waves in the inferior leads, which are taller and narrower when compared with those seen in the counterpart free wall locations (Fig. 25–5A). Likewise, the duration of the R wave in lead II at septal sites is narrower than that of the R wave at free wall sites (see Fig. 25–5B). The contour of the R wave in the inferior leads is also helpful in differentiating septal and free wall locations in the superior RVOT. Typically, R waves from free wall sites demonstrate characteristic "notching," which is uncommon in R waves from septal locations. Notching of the R wave was seen in 40 (95.2%) of 42 free wall sites and in only 12 (28.6%) of the 42 septal locations ($P \leq .05$). Another feature that can distinguish pace maps from septal and free wall sites in superior RVOT is the QRS transition pattern in the precordial leads (late versus early; see Fig. 25–4). A late precordial transition was observed in 40 free wall sites (95.2%) and in only 9 septal locations (21.4 %; $P \leq .05$). Importantly, only 4 (9.5%) of 42 septal sites demonstrated both a late precordial transition and notching in the inferior leads, in contrast to 39 (92.9%)

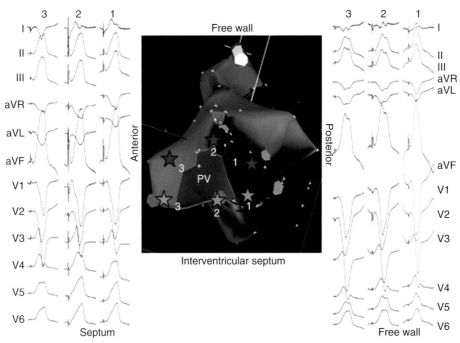

FIGURE 25–4. Twelve lead ECG pace maps from sites 1, 2 and 3 along the septum and free wall (FW) of RVOT showing characteristic features. Sites are labeled on the magnetic electroanatomic map (MEAM) in the center of the figure and over each pace map. The MEAM of the RVOT is shown in a coronal projection and was acquired during sinus rhythm. The 3-D shape of the RVOT is evident from MEAM and the cartoon at the bottom of the figure. All pace maps show left bundle branch block morphology and inferior frontal plane axis. Differences in R-waves in inferior leads (II, III and aVF) between the FW and septal pace maps are seen (broader, shorter and notched for the FW sites). Also, the precordial transition pattern for the FW site shows later transition (R to S ratio [1 by precordial leads V_4] when compared with the septal locations. Changes in lead 1 when moving from more anterior and leftward, site 3, (negative QRS) to the more posterior and rightward, site 1, (positive QRS) are also shown.

of 42 free wall sites ($P \leq .05$). We also evaluated the QRS morphology in limb lead I, during pace mapping at posterior (site 1) and anterior (site 3) locations along the septum and free wall in the RVOT (see Fig. 25–4). In general, for both the free wall and septal posterior locations (site 1), the QRS in lead I manifested a positive polarity (r waves). In comparison, anterior sites (site 3) along the septum and the free wall demonstrated a negative polarity (qs pattern). Sites midway between the anterior and posterior locations (site 2) along the septum and the free wall demonstrated either a biphasic or a multiphasic QRS morphology (qr/rs pattern), or an isoelectric segment preceding the q or r wave.[29]

We also analyzed ECG morphologies of RVOT tachycardias in 28 patients and found that all arrhythmias originating from septal locations lacked notching of R waves in inferior leads. In comparison, all tachycardias originating from the free wall sites in the superior RVOT demonstrated notching. Late precordial transition was seen in 6 (85.7%) of the 7 free wall tachycardias and only 2 (9.5%) of 21 tachycardias originating from septal locations. All spontaneous arrhythmias originating from site 3 had a qs pattern in lead I with a net negative QRS polarity. In comparison, all tachycardias originating from

site 1 demonstrated an R wave with a net positive QRS polarity. All of the remaining spontaneous arrhythmias (13 patients) originated from septal site 2 and demonstrated a biphasic or multiphasic QRS morphology (10 patients) or an isoelectric segment preceding a small rs or qr (3 patients) in lead I. Table 25–1 summarizes the criteria that we use to localize clinical VT originating from the superior RVOT region, and Figure 25–6 shows ECG morphologies of clinical arrhythmias from various superior RVOT sites.

RVOT arising from above the pulmonic valve has been described in a series of 24 patients.[29] In these patients, VT is believed to arise from strands of myocardial tissue extending over the pulmonary artery in a fashion analogous to arrhythmogenic myocardium extending over the pulmonary veins. The tachycardias had left bundle branch block morphology with intermediate, right, or vertical frontal plane axes. Precordial transition occurred in V_2 or later. Compared with RVOT arising below the pulmonic valve, VT arising from above the valve had greater R-wave amplitude in the inferior leads. The values overlapped greatly between the two groups, however, and no ECG feature reliably separated the two patterns. The successful ablation site was 0.5 to

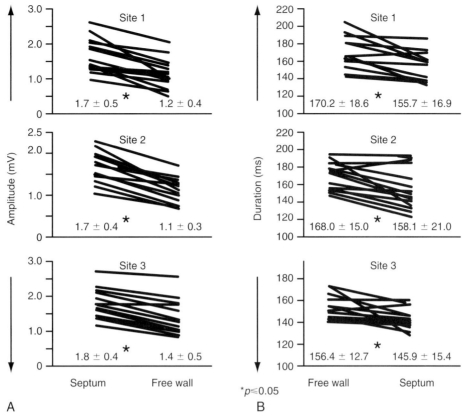

FIGURE 25-5. Comparison of QRS amplitude and width in lead II during pace mapping from septal and free wall (FW) sites. Panel **A** compares amplitude of the R-wave in limb lead II between sites 1, 2 and 3 along the septum and the FW. Each line represents R-wave amplitude (mV) at the same sites between the septum and the FW for each patient. The mean R wave amplitude for the different sites are also shown in the figure. At each site, the mean R wave amplitude in the septum was significantly greater than that in the FW. Panel **B** compares duration of the R-wave in limb lead II between sites 1, 2 and 3 along the septum and the FW. Each line represents R wave duration (msec) at the same site in the septum and the FW for each patient. The mean R-wave duration for the different sites are also shown in the figure. At each site, the mean R wave width of the FW pace-maps was significantly greater than that of the septal pace-maps.

TABLE 25-1

Electrocardiographic Characteristics of Pace Maps from Various Superior RVOT Sites

Item	SEPTAL RVOT SITES			FREE WALL RVOT SITES		
	Posterior (Site 1)	Middle (Site 2)	Anterior (Site 3)	Posterior (Site 1)	Middle (Site 2)	Anterior (Site 3)
Morphology in lead I	R, Rs	rs, qrs	qs, rS	R, Rs	rs, qrs	qs, rS
Notch in inferior leads	−	−	−	+	+	+
Precordial transition	≤V$_3$	≤V$_3$	≤V$_3$	≥V$_4$	≥V$_4$	≥V$_4$

≤, transition earlier than or equal to; ≥, transition later than or equal to; RVOT, right ventricular outflow tract.

2.1 cm above the pulmonic valve. At the successful ablation site, a sharp presystolic electrical potential was noted in VT in most patients. In sinus rhythm, the successful ablation site often recorded a small far-field atrial potential. Ablation was delivered with a standard 4-mm-tip radiofrequency catheter with a target temperature of 55°C for 60 to 90 seconds. All

24 patients were successfully ablated without complication or recurrence in follow-up.

Clinical Arrhythmias from Basal Left Ventricle

The basal LV constitutes ventricular myocardium bordering the mitral valve and encompasses a wide

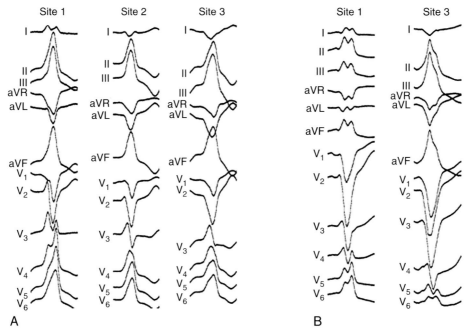

FIGURE 25–6. Shows the unique ECG morphologies that help in distinguishing site of origin of the clinical arrhythmia in the superior RVOT. Panel **A** shows the ECG morphologies of spontaneous arrhythmias from septal sites 1, 2 and 3 and panel **B** depicts ECG morphologies of spontaneous arrhythmias from free wall (FW) sites 1 and 3. All the FW sites show notching in inferior leads and late precordial transition (≥V₄). In comparison, all the septal sites lack both notching of inferior leads and late precordial transition. For both the septal and FW locations of the clinical arrhythmias, lead I helps in distinguishing anterior and leftward location (site 3; negative polarity) from posterior and leftward location (site 1; positive polarity). Site 2, which lies in between, manifests multiphasic polarity in lead I (Panel A; see text for details).

area, including septum and anterior, lateral, and inferior walls.[9,10] The aortic valve typically sits at the superiormost and medial aspect of this region, distorting its otherwise circular shape. To create the electroanatomic map of this region, we recommend the following protocol.

At the outset, planes of mitral and aortic valves are defined. For outlining the mitral valve, the mapping catheter is positioned in the basal LV such that the distal electrode pair records a large ventricular electrogram preceded by a smaller or equal size atrial electrogram. In this orientation, three different points (medial, lateral, and superior or inferior) are acquired to create the mitral valve plane. Next, the catheter is retracted into the aorta and then advanced down to the aortic valve, where the individual cusps (left, right, and noncoronary), as determined by distinct catheter locations on orthogonal fluoroscopy, are tagged. The catheter is then readvanced into the LV, and multiple points (≥100) are acquired to create an endocardial shell. To develop ECG criteria for localizing basal LV VT, we performed pace mapping in a series of patients from four or more locations in this region, including the septal-parahisian region and the aortomitral continuity as well as superior, superolateral, and lateral mitral annular locations, using

the pacing protocol described earlier for the RVOT. In general, pace maps from medial sites (septal-parahisian region and aortomitral continuity) show a mean QRS duration of 134 ± 28 msec, initial negative forces in lead V₁ (QS or Qr complexes for septal-parahisian region and qR complexes for aortomitral continuity sites), and predominantly positive forces (R or Rs morphology) in lead I. Additionally, pace maps from the septal-parahisian region manifest an early precordial transition pattern (reversal of the ratio of Q to R waves occurring earlier than or in V₃). In comparison, pace maps from lateral basal LV sites (superolateral and lateral mitral annulus) demonstrate a mean QRS duration of 182 ± 18 msec, have a right bundle branch block morphology (R and/or Rs) in lead V₁, and are associated with a late precordial transition pattern (reversal of ratio of R to Q waves in V₅ or later) or lack of precordial transition path. Also for these sites, lead I demonstrates an rS or qs morphology.[8]

Details of the pace maps from individual locations along the basal LV are shown in Figure 25–7. In general, most medial basal LV sites demonstrate the narrowest complexes, with the most positive complexes in lead I, whereas superolateral mitral annulus locations demonstrate the widest complexes, with the

FIGURE 25–7. Representation of pace maps from various basal left ventricle (LV) locations. In a lateral to medial distribution paced sites include lateral, superolateral, superior mitral annulus (Lat, Sup Lat, and Sup MA respectively), aorto-mitral continuity (AMC) and Septal-Parahisian region (S-P). Magnetic electroanatomic map (MEAM) of LV in postero-anterior projection is shown in the center. QRS morphology in leads I , II , V1 (*arrow heads*) and precordial transition pattern (*rectangles*) help in distinguishing site of origin of the pace maps.

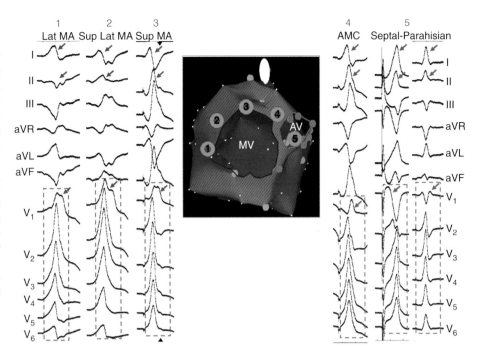

TABLE 25–2

Electrocardiographic Characteristics of Pace Maps from Various Basal Left Ventricular Sites

Item	Septal-parahisian	AMC	Superior MA	Superolateral MA	Lateral MA
Lead I	R or Rs	Rs or rs	rs or rS	rS or QS	rS or rs
Lead V_1	QS or Qr	qR	R or Rs	R or Rs	R or Rs
Precordial transition*	Early	None	None	None	None or late
Ratio of QRS in leads II and III	>1	≤1	≤1	≤1	>1

*Reversal of Q to R and vice versa ≤V_3 (early) and ≥V_5 (late).
≤, transition earlier than or equal to; ≥, transition later than or equal to; AMC, aortomitral continuity; MA, mitral annulus.

least positive forces in lead I. Also, except for septal-parahisian sites, which consistently demonstrate left bundle branch block morphology and early precordial transition patterns, pace maps from all other sites in this region manifest right bundle branch block morphology. Additionally, "qR" morphology in lead V_1 is *pathognomonic* for pace maps from aortomitral continuity locations (see Fig. 25–7).

Of the 122 patients who underwent ablation of IVT (both RV and LV) at our center over a 5-year period, the site of origin of clinical tachycardias in 12 patients was localized to basal LV endocardium based on MEAM-guided ablation, as follows: septal-parahisian region (2 patients), aortomitral continuity (4 patients), superior mitral annulus (3 patients), and superolateral mitral annulus (3 patients) (Fig. 25–8). Using the previously described ECG criteria (Table 25–2), a blinded observer was able to accurately predict the site of origin of clinical tachycardia in 10

(83%) of the 12 cases, attesting to the clinical utility of our algorithm for localizing basal LV VT.

Clinical Arrhythmias from the Aortic Cusps and Surrounding Epicardium

The aortic valve, with the left and right cusps occupying positions adjacent to the left and right coronary, respectively, forms the centerpiece of the heart. It is increasingly recognized that the aortic cusps and the sinus of Valsalva can also provide a site of origin of IVT.[31-34] Recognition of this fact may have important clinical implications, because radiofrequency ablation inside the aortic cusps is feasible and is associated with high success rates for curing IVT originating from the region.

To determine unique ECG characteristics, we performed pace mapping of the right coronary cusp, left

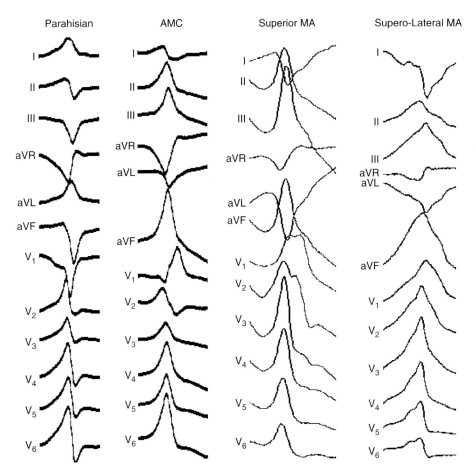

FIGURE 25–8. Typical ECG morphologies of clinical arrhythmias shown originating from basal left ventricle (LV) region that were localized based on site of successful ablation on magnetic electroanatomic mapping to the parahisian region, aorto-mitral continuity (AMC), superior mitral annular (MA) location and supero-lateral MA location. QRS morphology in leads I and V_1, together with the ratio of QRS complexes in leads II / III and precordial transition pattern, can reliably distinguish medial from lateral locations in this region (see text for details).

coronary cusp, and noncoronary cusp in a total of 20 patients with structurally normal hearts using the same protocol as described earlier for the RVOT. The catheter position in relation to the individual aortic cusps was confirmed using one or more of the following imaging modalities: phased-array intracardiac ultrasound, biplane fluoroscopy, and electroanatomic mapping (Figs. 25–9, 25–10, and 25–11).

Anatomic Considerations

To conceptualize the correct approach to catheter ablation in this region, it is important to understand the anatomic relations between the aortic cusps and their surrounding structures.[35,36] The pulmonic valve and adjoining RVOT region typically are located anteriorly and sit slightly superior to and rightward of the aortic valve. The posterior septal aspect of the superior RVOT typically lies adjacent to the right coronary cusp, whereas the anterior septal aspect tends to be situated at the junction of the right and left cusp or anterior to the medial aspect of the latter.[36] Furthermore, given the frequent convex, crescent shape of the area just below the pulmonic valve, a leftward direction can also be observed for

the most posterior and anterior aspect of the RVOT septum.[30]

Mapping Technique

As in the previous studies, a standard 12-lead ECG configuration was used to acquire pace maps. Using a retrograde approach via the femoral artery, we positioned a 7-French deflectable mapping catheter in the aortic root and manipulated it toward individual valve cusps. The catheter location at each valve cusp was confirmed by various imaging modalities, as described earlier. Pacing at each site was performed as described previously, and the ECGs of pace maps were analyzed with respect to morphology, amplitude, and duration in all leads and the precordial transition pattern.

Morphology

Lead V_1 was found to be the most useful in distinguishing the various sites. Left coronary cusp pacing consistently produced a multiphasic component resembling an "M"- or "W"-shaped QRS complex.[34] Right coronary cusp pacing demonstrated a QS or QR type pattern with a predominantly negative vector in

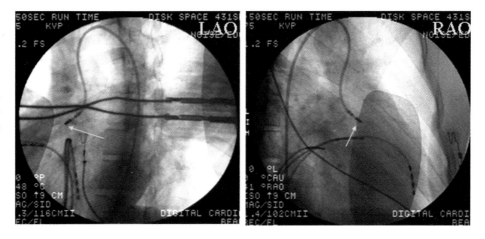

FIGURE 25–9. Typical left and right anterior oblique fluoroscopic projections (LAO and RAO respectively) showing the mapping catheter (*yellow arrow*) by the right coronary cusp.

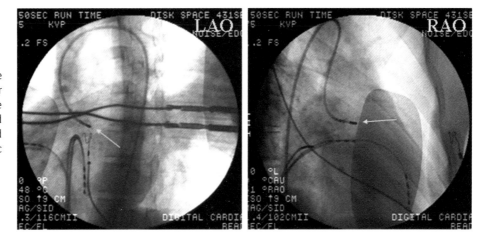

FIGURE 25–10. This figure shows the mapping catheter (*yellow arrow*) positioned at the left coronary cusp in left and right anterior oblique (LAO and RAO respectively) fluoroscopic projection.

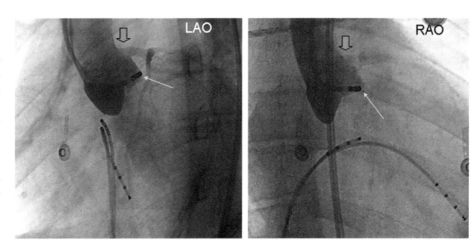

FIGURE 25–11. A representative aortogram depicting the tip of the mapping catheter (*yellow thin arrow*) by the left coronary cusp and its proximity to the takeoff of the left main coronary artery (*thick light blue arrow*). The ablation catheter tip is 4mm and the electrodes are spaced 5mm apart. LAO, left anterior oblique; RAO, right anterior oblique.

V_1 (Fig. 25–12). Pacing the noncoronary cusp resulted universally in capture of the atrium. This probably occurred because of the close proximity of the noncoronary cusp to both left and right atria. The question often raised is how one can differentiate VT arising from the aortic cusps from VT arising from the RVOT region. Because of the proximity of the RVOT septum to the aortic cusps, especially the right coronary cusp, ECG features among these sites often overlap, and differences are subtle. The RVOT is anterior, superior, and leftward of the aortic valve. Ouyang et al.[34] reported that the r wave duration in V_1 and V_2 tended to be broader when VT originated from the aortic valve cusps than when it arose from the RVOT septum. Furthermore, an R wave duration of longer than 50% of the total QRS duration or an R/S amplitude ratio greater than 30% in V_1 or V_2 also favored an aortic cusp location.

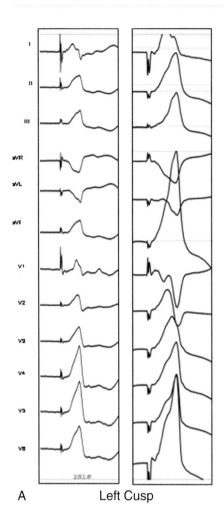

A   Left Cusp

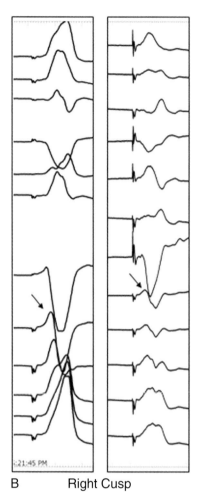

B   Right Cusp

FIGURE 25–12. Panel **A** shows two different examples of pacing from the left coronary cusp. The first example shows "M-shaped" pattern in V1 whereas it is more "W-shaped" in the second example (*arrows*). In both cases, the overall axis is inferiorly directed, with a multiphasic QRS in V1 and a transition by lead V2 or earlier. Panel **B** shows two examples of a typical pattern with pacing from the right coronary cusp. As with the left coronary cusp, the axis is inferiorly directed. However, with the right coronary cusp, the transition in the precordial leads is later, (≥V3) with a left bundle branch block type pattern.

Amplitude and Duration

In our series, evaluation of the amplitude of the R wave in inferior leads and the width of the QRS interval was inconsistent, and an absolute value of these measures could not be used to differentiate cusp pace maps. However, the QRS duration in general was wider with right coronary cusp pacing than with left coronary cusp pacing. In our experience, the mean QRS duration for pace maps from the left coronary cusp was 142 msec (range, 108 to 180 msec), whereas for right coronary cusp pace maps it was 164 msec (range, 141 to 241 msec). Because the left coronary cusp lies on the same cranial plane as the right coronary cusp, the inferior lead morphology (inferior axis) does not differ significantly between the cusps and therefore is not useful as a differentiating factor.

Precordial Transition

Analysis of the R-wave transition demonstrated that, for pace maps from left coronary cusp, precordial transition occurred in V_2 or earlier in 16 of 20 patients, whereas for right coronary cusp pace maps the pre-cordial transition was most commonly after V_2 (18/20 patients). The electrocardiographic features of coronary cusp VTs are listed in Table 25–3.

OTHER ELECTROCARDIOGRAPHIC LOCALIZATION CRITERIA

An algorithm for the localization of outflow tract VTs by surface ECG has been published.[37] However, there may be difficulties in the universal applicability of such algorithms due to overlap in certain ECG features between VT sites, varying patient characteristics, cardiac rotation, and so on.[37] In addition, a ratio of time to R-wave peak and total QRS duration greater than 0.54 in the precordial leads has been used as a useful indicator of an epicardial origin to outflow tract VTs.

DIAGNOSIS BY INTRACARDIAC RECORDINGS

The criteria for diagnosis of outflow tract VTs are given in Table 25–4. The criteria include the general features of VT and evidence of a triggered or auto-

TABLE 25–3

Electrocardiographic Features of Aortic Cusp Ventricular Tachycardias

ECG Feature	Right Coronary Cusp	Left Coronary Cusp
V_1	QS or QR predominantly negative	Multiphasic "M" or "W" configuration
Precordial transition	$\geq V_3$	$\leq V_2$

$\leq$, transition earlier than or equal to; $\geq$, transition later than or equal to.

TABLE 25–4

Diagnostic Criteria

General features of ventricular tachycardia

Evidence of triggered or automatic mechanism (typically)
  Adenosine sensitive
  Noninducible by PES or initiated with burst pacing
  Absence of entrainment

Earliest activation in RVOT, LVOT, AMC, or pulmonary artery

AMC, aortomitral continuity; LVOT, left ventricular outflow tract; PES, programmed electrical stimulation; RVOT, right ventricular outflow tract.

matic mechanism. The tachycardias are mapped to the characteristic locations described earlier.

THE DECISION TO ABLATE OUTFLOW TRACT TACHYCARDIAS

The various treatment options for outflow tract tachycardia are determined mostly by the burden of the disease.[5] Because the arrhythmia is not life-threatening, electrophysiologists have the luxury of fine-tuning the treatment strategy for individual patients. If symptoms are infrequent and relatively mild, treatment is not mandated. Ablation of outflow tract tachycardias has been traditionally reserved for patients with prolonged incapacitating symptoms for whom pharmacologic treatment with β-blockers, calcium channel blockers, and class I and/or class III antiarrhythmics has failed.[11,15,21,31,38-41] Because the population with this arrhythmia is younger and generally healthy otherwise and quality of life is a significant issue for them, the majority of patients in this group at our center, when offered the choice between antiarrhythmic agents and ablation, have opted for the latter.

TABLE 25–5

Target Sites

Site of earliest ventricular activation typically >30 msec before QRS onset

Site of $\geq 11/12$ pace map

Mapping

The favored technique for successful ablation consists of localization of the site of origin using earliest intracardiac activation or pace mapping or both (Table 25–5). Careful analysis of the 12-lead ECG during tachycardia is very useful and in our experience can guide catheter localization to within 0.5 to 1 cm of the site of successful ablation.[8,10,26,27,30] Although biplane fluoroscopy permits reasonable catheter localization, use of electroanatomic mapping further enhances precise localization by permitting three-dimensional reconstruction of intracardiac anatomy. In addition, if the endocardial shell is constructed during the tachycardia, then the site of earliest activation can also be visualized.[8,10,42] Other investigators have reported high success rates during RVOT tachycardia ablation using the EnSite 3000 noncontact mapping system (Endocardial Solutions, St. Paul, Minn.). A potential advantage of this system is its ability to map and localize nonsustained rhythms, including isolated ventricular ectopic beats.[43]

Typically for ablation, the mapping catheter is advanced to the area of interest as suggested by the 12-lead ECG, and pace mapping is performed at the diastolic threshold and at a rate similar to the tachycardia cycle length. The goal is to achieve an identical match (all 12 leads) between the clinical arrhythmia and the pace map, including subtle features such as notches in the QRS complexes in various leads. In the absence of a good match, the catheter should be repositioned with subtle movements in the area of interest. Diligent mapping is important, because inability to achieve an identical match is usually associated with unsuccessful outcome. Figure 25–13 depicts the native tachycardia and an identical pace map, which was performed from the left coronary cusp. This was also the site of successful ablation.

Activation mapping can also be used to map the site of origin.[26,27,42,44] Typically, the site of successful ablation precedes onset of QRS by approximately 30 msec on a bipolar electrogram; if unipolar recording is performed at this location, it should have a "QS" morphology.[44] However, given the size of the catheter

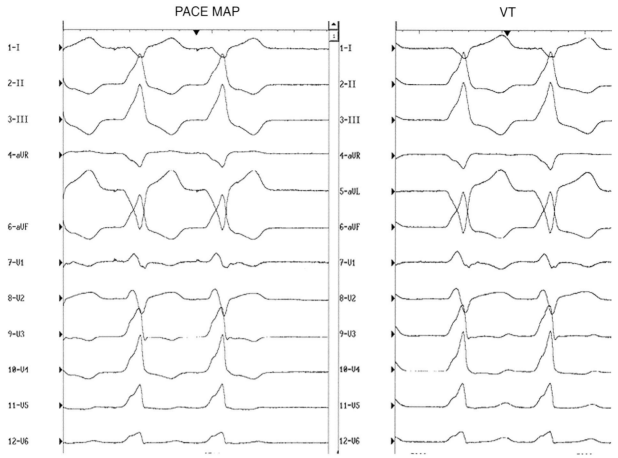

FIGURE 25–13. Clinical arrhythmia shown originating from basal left ventricle (*in right panel*) and pace map (*in left panel*), which was obtained from the left coronary cusp. The pace map at this site is a perfect match and a single radiofrequency ablation from this location terminated the tachycardia.

tip (4 to 8 mm), the site of earliest recording is not always the true site of origin and may not consistently result in successful ablation. Therefore, it is imperative to confirm an identical pace map at the site of earliest activation before ablating.[40,45]

In the event that the arrhythmia does not occur spontaneously or in response to programmed stimulation, isoproterenol is administered in incremental doses until there is an augmentation in the heart rate from baseline by at least. This sometimes requires doses of ≥10 μg/min, which in our experience are well tolerated. Because of the unpredictable nature of triggered activity, tachycardia induction may not always happen at peak heart rates; instead, it may manifest as the heart rate is slowing down after isoproterenol infusion is discontinued.[5] Aminophylline or epinephrine infusion may also enhance triggered activity and arrhythmia induction, and phenylephrine has been suggested to stimulate aortic cusp VTs (see later discussion). The triggered activity usually emanates from a narrow area (2 to 4 mm). Because of rapid conduction from the site of origin, however, a much larger area may be interpreted as

having early activation unless meticulous attention is paid to electrogram analysis. A large endocardial area of early ventricular activation may also represent the breakthrough point for an epicardial focus.

Ablation

Because the focus of the tachycardia is typically small in area, the site usually can be targeted using a 4-mm-tip ablation catheter in either temperature- or power-controlled mode. Our preference is temperature-control mode, with the typical settings for targeting RVOT and basal LV endocardium being 40 to 50 W, a temperature not to exceed 55°C, and a duration of up to 60 seconds.[8,10] For ablation in the aortic cusp region, we prefer to start at a lower power setting (10 to 15 W) and augment in steps of 5 to 10 W to achieve catheter tip temperatures of 45°C to 50°C, targeting an impedance drop of 5 ohms (Ω) or greater.[44] It may be necessary to perform a coronary angiogram to delineate the proximity of a site of origin in the aortic cusp region to the coronary vessels. In general, delivery of radiofrequency energy within 1 cm of the coronary artery ostia is to be avoided. In certain locations, such as the anteroseptal aspect of superior RVOT or the ventricular aspect of superolateral and lateral mitral annulus sites, the catheter tip may be snugly surrounded by myocardium, causing poor blood flow and resulting in rapid achievement of target temperatures with low power output and minimal impedance drop. In such a scenario, switching to a larger tip or an irrigated catheter tip may be necessary to deliver effective energy.[44] Although it is safe to ablate from most locations in RVOT and basal LV with various catheter types, care must be exercised if the tachycardia originates close to the superior septum in the vicinity of the His bundle. In two of our initial four patients with LVOT tachycardia, a prominent His deflection was seen at the site of ideal pace maps; in both of these patients, ablation therapy was deferred because of

the high risk of causing atrioventricular block.[10] Another area of the LVOT that requires special consideration in terms of ablation technique is the LV epicardium. It is impossible to achieve an ideal pace map for these tachycardias endocardially.[25] Options include the introduction of a low-profile, deflectable, multipolar catheter (with or without a sheath) into the branches of the coronary sinus (Fig. 25–14) and pacing from above the aortic valve in the region of the left coronary sinus (or both).[46] We have also used the pericardial approach for successful basal LV tachycardia ablation, following the technique described by Sosa et al.[47,48] Because of the proximity of the epicardial coronary vessels, there are some additional risks involved with this strategy, and our practice has been to perform coronary angiography routinely before ablating. Others have suggested using intravascular ultrasound.[5] Catheter visualization in some of these locations is enhanced by the use of phased-array intracardiac ultrasound, which in expert hands can accurately show the catheter-tissue interface and lesion creation in real time.[44,50,51]

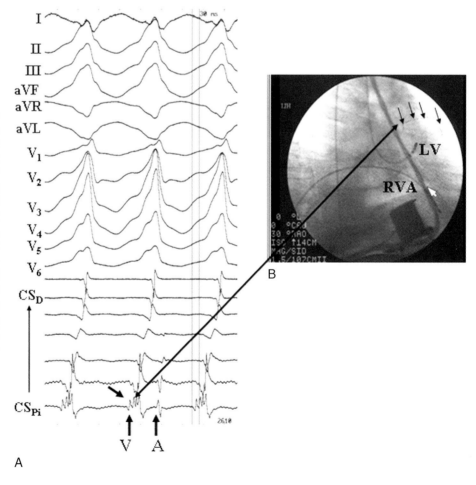

FIGURE 25–14. Panel **A** shows 12 lead ECG and recordings from the anterior branch of coronary sinus (CS) using a 2-French multielectrode mapping catheter (*arrows* on the fluoroscopic image) during tachycardia and recordings from the proximal poles of CS catheter are earliest. This was also the site for best pace map. Panel **B** shows fluoroscopic image that was obtained in the right anterior oblique (RAO) projection. Also seen in the image are catheters at the right ventricular apex (RVA) and the left ventricle (LV) endocardium under the aortic valve.

Clinical Outcomes and Complications

Radiofrequency ablation, if done with attention to energy settings and the coronary anatomy, is a safe treatment option with an overall success rate of 90% to 95%. In our opinion, ablation therapy may be considered first-line therapy in patients as an alternative to pursuing pharmacologic management. Some of the more common complications during RVOT/LVOT tachycardia ablations include development of complete and/or right bundle branch block and aortic regurgitation.[51,52] A single case of death has been reported and on autopsy was shown to have occurred from a linear tear and hemopericardium in the RVOT.[43] There is also a report of a left main coronary artery occlusion during ablation of LVOT tachycardia originating beneath the aortic valve.[52]

Troubleshooting the Difficult Case

Common problems and potential solutions to the ablation of outflow tract VTs are listed in Table 25–6. Because of the triggered or automatic mechanism underlying most of these arrhythmias, noninducibility of the arrhythmia is a frequent obstacle. High-dose isoproterenol, hand grip exercises, and intravenous aminophylline can all be tried to facilitate tachycardia onset. Phenylephrine infusion has been described to facilitate onset of aortic cusp VTs.[53] Patience is often the key to success. Even limited amounts of ectopy may allow for pace mapping or noncontact mapping. Noninducibility and infrequent ectopy are also problematic for defining end points for ablation. For RVOT especially, local conduction from the focus may be very rapid, presenting a large area with early activation. Meticulous electrogram analysis and use of unipolar electrograms are essential to defining the earliest site. Sites near coronary arteries may risk injury to these vessels. Coronary angiography is recommended in such cases, to define the proximity of the ablation catheter to the coronary artery. Sites near the His bundle or major fascicles may also risk injury to the conduction system. Cyroablation may offer less risk of collateral injury to these structures.

Despite appropriate target sites, ablation lesions may fail to terminate the tachycardia or prevent initiation. In the RVOT, a large area of early activation may be present, and the best site for ablation may not be easily distinguished from nearby sites. Careful electrogram analysis and pace mapping may be remedial. An epicardial focus or a focus removed from the site of mapping may also produce favorable

---

TABLE 25–6

Troubleshooting the Difficult Case

Problem	Causes	Solution
Tachycardia noninducible and rare spontaneous ectopy	Triggered or automatic mechanism	High-dose isoproterenol, and/or use aminophylline or phenylephrine (coronary cusp VTs) Pace map ectopy Use noncontact mapping
Large area of earliest activation	Rapid local conduction near site of origin (usually RVOT)	Use pace mapping Careful electrogram analysis, and use unipolar electrograms Electroanatomic mapping
	Origin epicardial or remote from mapping sites	Map epicardium or contralateral outflow tract sites
Best sites near coronary artery or His bundle	Origin in LVOT or septum	Coronary angiography before and after ablation Possibly use cryoablation
Ablation at favorable sites fails	Large area early activation (usually RVOT)	See above
	Epicardial focus	Map epicardium (percutaneous or by coronary veins)
	Incomplete mapping	Reanalyze maps, expand area of mapping
	Insufficient lesion size	Use irrigated or large-tip ablation catheter

LVOT, left ventricular outflow tract; RVOT, right ventricular outflow tract; VT, ventricular tachycardia.

electrograms endocardially but be resistant to endocardial ablation. Thorough endocardial mapping and possibly mapping of the contralateral outflow tract may reveal even more favorable ablation targets. Epicardial mapping by the percutaneous approach or via the coronary veins may be necessary. Cooled ablation systems may be required to enhance energy delivery and lesion size in areas of low blood flow.

Conclusion

In summary, outflow tract tachycardias are thought to be caused by adenosine-sensitive triggered activity. They are augmented by exercise and other adrenergic influences. The 12-lead ECG during the arrhythmias manifests site-specific characteristics that facilitate their localization. These arrhythmias, in general, are not life-threatening and therefore can initially be managed conservatively. However, radiofrequency ablation is a more definitive treatment option, and it can be curative in more than 90% of cases with a low risk (≤1%) of serious complications. Although it is typically reserved for patients who have failed or are intolerant to therapy with antiarrhythmic agents, ablation is an attractive initial treatment strategy in selected patients.

References

1. Lerman BB, Kenneth SM, Markovitz SM: Mechanisms of idiopathic left ventricular tachycardia. J Cardiovasc Electrophysiol 8:571-583, 1997.
2. Daliento L, Turrini P, Nava A, et al.: Arrhythmogenic right ventricular cardiomyopathy in young versus adult patients: Similarities and differences. J Am Coll Cardiol 25:655-664, 1995.
3. Froment R, Gallavardin L, Cahen P: Paroxysmal ventricular tachycardia: A clinical classification. Br Heart J 15:172, 1953.
4. Brooks R, Burgess JH: Idiopathic ventricular tachycardia: A review. Medicine (Baltimore) 67:271-294, 1988.
5. Lerman BB, Stein SM, Markowitz SM, et al.: Ventricular tachycardia in patients with structurally normal hearts. In Zipes DP, Jalife J (eds.): Cardiac Electrophysiology: From Cell to Bedside. Philadelphia: Saunders, 1999, pp 640-656.
6. Lerman BB: Response of nonreentrant catecholamine-mediated ventricular tachycardia to endogenous adenosine and acetylcholine: Evidence for myocardial receptor-mediated effects. Circulation 87:382-390, 1993.
7. Lerman BB, Belardinelli L, West GA, et al.: Adenosine-sensitive ventricular tachycardia: Evidence suggesting cyclic AMP-mediated triggered activity. Circulation 74:270-280, 1986.
8. Dixit S, Lin D, Zado E, Marchlinski F: Identification of distinct electrocardiographic patterns from basal left ventricle: Distinguishing medial and lateral sites of origin. Heart Rhythm 1:S104, 2004.
9. Lerman BB, Stein KM, Markowitz SM: Idiopathic right ventricular outflow tract tachycardia: A clinical approach. Pacing Clin Electrophysiol 19:2120-2137, 1996.
10. Callans DJ, Menz V, Schwartzman D, et al.: Repetitive monomorphic tachycardia from the left ventricular outflow tract: Electrocardiographic patterns consistent with a left ventricular site of origin. J Am Coll Cardiol 29:1023-1027, 1997.
11. Buxton AE, Waxman HL, Marchlinski FE, et al.: Right ventricular tachycardia: Clinical and electrophysiologic characteristics. Circulation 68:917-927, 1983.
12. Proclemer A, Ciani R, Feruglio GA: Right ventricular tachycardia with left bundle branch block and inferior axis morphology: Clinical and arrhythmological characteristics in 15 patients. Pacing Clin Electrophysiol 12:977-988, 1989.
13. Lemery R, Brugada P, Della Bella P, et al.: Non ischemic ventricular tachycardia: Clinical course and long-term follow-up in patients without clinically overt heart disease. Circulation 79:990-999, 1989.
14. Haissaguerre M, Extramania F, Hocini M, et al.: Mapping and ablation of ventricular fibrillation associated with long QT and Brugada syndrome. Circulation 108:925-928, 2003.
15. Mont L, Seixas T, Brugada P, et al.: Clinical and electrophysiologic characteristics of exercise-related idiopathic ventricular tachycardia. Am J Cardiol 68:897-900, 1991.
16. Lerman BB, Stein K, Engelstein ED, et al.: Mechanism of repetitive monomorphic ventricular tachycardia. Circulation 92:421-429, 1995.
17. Hayashi H, Fujiki A, Tani M, et al.: Role of sympathovagal balance in the initiation of idiopathic ventricular tachycardia originating from right ventricular outflow tract. Pacing Clin Electrophysiol 20:2371-2377, 1997.
18. Marchlinski FE, Deely MP, Zado ES: Gender specific triggers for right ventricular outflow tract tachycardias: Am Heart J 139:1009-1013, 2000.
19. Mehta D, Davies MJ, Ward DE, Camm AJ: Ventricular tachycardias of right ventricular origin: Markers of subclinical right ventricular disease. Am Heart J 127:360-366, 1994.
20. Carlson MD, White RD, Trohman RG, et al.: Right ventricular outflow tract ventricular tachycardia: Detection of previously unrecognized anatomic abnormalities using cine magnetic resonance imaging. J Am Coll Cardiol 24:720-727, 1994.
21. Markowitz SM, Litvak BL, Ramirez de Arellano EA, et al.: Adenosine sensitive ventricular tachycardia: Right ventricular abnormalities delineated by magnetic resonance imaging. Circulation 96:1192-1200, 1997.
22. Gill JS, Hunter GJ, Gane J, et al.: Asymmetry of cardiac [123I] meta-iodobenzylguanidine scans in patients with ventricular tachycardia and "clinically normal" heart. Br Heart J 59:6-13, 1993.
23. Mitrani RD, Klein LS, Miles WM, et al.: Regional cardiac sympathetic denervation in patients with ventricular tachycardia in the absence of coronary artery disease. J Am Coll Cardiol 22:1344-1353, 1993.
24. Wichter T, Hindricks G, Lerch H, et al.: Regional myocardial sympathetic dysinnervation in arrhythmogenic right ventricular cardiomyopathy: An analysis using 123I-meta-iodobenzyl-guanidine scintigraphy. Circulation 89:667-683, 1994.
25. Dixit S, Marchlinski FE: Clinical characteristics and catheter ablation of left ventricular outflow tract tachycardia. Curr Cardiol Rep 3:305-313, 2001.
26. Jadonath RL, Schwartzman DS, Preminger MW, et al.: Utility of 12-lead electrocardiogram in localizing the origin of right ventricular outflow tract tachycardia. Am Heart J 130:1107-1113, 1995.
27. Movsowitz C, Schwartzman DS, Callans DJ, et al.: Idiopathic right ventricular outflow tract tachycardia: Narrowing the anatomic location for successful ablation. Am Heart J 131: 930-936, 1996.
28. Delacey WA, Nath S, Haines DE, et al.: Adenosine and verapamil sensitive tachycardia originating from the left ventricle:

Radiofrequency catheter ablation. Pacing Clin Electrophysiol 15:2240-2244, 1992.

29. Sekiguchi Y, Aonuma K, Takahashi A, et al.: Electrocardiographic and electrophysiologic characteristics of ventricular tachycardia originating within the pulmonary artery. J Am Coll Cardiol 45:887-895, 2005.

30. Dixit S, Gerstenfeld EP, Callans DJ, Marchlinski FE: Electrocardiographic patterns of superior right ventricular outflow tract tachycardias: Distinguishing septal and free wall sites of origin. J Cardiovasc Electrophysiol 13:1-7, 2003.

31. Griffith MJ, Garratt CJ, Rowland E, et al.: Effects of intravenous adenosine on verapamil-sensitive "idiopathic" ventricular tachycardia. Am J Cardiol 73:759-764, 1994.

32. Storey J, Iwasa A, Feld G: Left ventricular outflow tract tachycardia originating from the right coronary cusp: Identification of location of origin by endocardial noncontact activation mapping from the right ventricular outflow tract. J Cardiovasc Electrophysiol 13:1050-1053, 2002.

33. Kanagaratnam L, Tomassoni G, Schweikert R, et al.: Ventricular tachycardias arising from the aortic sinus of Valsalva: An under-recognized variant of left outflow tract ventricular tachycardia. J Am Coll Cardiol 37:1408-1414, 2001.

34. Ouyang F, Fotuhi P, Ho SY, et al.: Repetitive monomorphic ventricular tachycardia originating from the aortic sinus cusp. J Am Coll Cardiol 39:500-508, 2002.

35. Yacoub M, Kilner P, Birks E, Misfeld M: The aortic outflow and root: A tale of dynamism and crosstalk. Ann Thorac Surg 68:S37-S43, 1999.

36. Lerman BB, Wesley RC, DiMarco JP, et al.: Antiadrenergic effects of adenosine on His-Purkinje automaticity: Evidence for accentuated antagonism. J Clin Invest 82:2127-2135, 1988.

37. Ito H, Tada H, Naito S, et al.: Development and validation of an ECG algorithm for identifying the optimal ablation site for idiopathic ventricular outflow tract tachycardia. J Cardiovasc Electrophysiol 14:1280-1286, 2003.

38. Goy JJ, Tauxe F, Fromer M, et al.: Ten-years follow-up of 20 patients with idiopathic ventricular tachycardia. Pacing Clin Electrophysiol 13:1142-1147, 1990.

39. Gill JS, Ward D, Camm AJ: Comparison of verapamil and diltiazem in the suppression of idiopathic ventricular tachycardia. Pacing Clin Electrophysiol 15:2122-2125, 1992.

40. Gill JS, Mehta D, Ward DE, et al.: Efficacy of flecainide, sotalol and verapamil in the treatment of right ventricular tachycardia in patients without overt cardiac abnormality. Br Heart J 68:392-397, 1992.

41. Wilber DJ, Baerman J, Olshanky B, et al.: Adenosine-sensitive ventricular tachycardia: Clinical characteristics and response to catheter ablation. Circulation 87:126-134, 1993.

42. Gepstein L, Hayam G, Ben-Haim SA: A novel method for non-fluoroscopic catheter-based electroanatomic mapping of the heart: In vitro and in vivo accuracy results. Circulation 95:1611-1622, 1997.

43. Friedman PA, Asirvatham SJ, Grice S, et al.: Noncontact mapping to guide ablation of right ventricular outflow tract tachycardia. J Am Coll Cardiol 39:1808-1812, 2002.

44. Marchlinski FE, Lin D, Dixit S, et al.: Ventricular tachycardia from the aortic cusps: Localization and ablation. In Raviele A (ed.): Cardiac Arrhythmias 2003. Proceedings of the 8th International Workshop for Cardiac Arrhythmias, Venice 2003. Milan: Springer-Verlag Italia, 2004, pp 357-370.

45. Coggins DL, Lee RJ, Sweeney J, et al.: Radiofrequency catheter ablation as a cure for idiopathic tachycardia of both left and right ventricular origin. J Am Coll Cardiol 23:1333-1341, 1994.

46. Stellbrink C, Diem B, Schaurte P, et al.: Transcoronary venous radiofrequency catheter ablation of ventricular tachycardia. J Cardiovasc Electrophysiol 8:916-921, 1997.

47. Sosa E, Scanavacca M, d'Avila A, et al.: Nonsurgical transthoracic epicardial catheter ablation to treat recurrent ventricular tachycardia occurring late after myocardial infarction [see comment]. J Am Coll Cardiol 35:1442-1449, 2000.

48. Dixit S, Narula N, Callans DJ, Marchlinski FE: Electroanatomic mapping of human heart: Epicardial fat can mimic scar. J Cardiovasc Electrophysiol 14:1128, 2003.

49. Ren J, Marchlinski FE, Callans DC, et al.: Intracardiac Doppler echocardiographic quantification of pulmonary flow velocity: An effective technique for monitoring pulmonary vein narrowing during focal atrial fibrillation ablation. J Cardiovasc Electrophysiol 13:1076-1081, 2002.

50. Dixit S, Ren J-F, Callans DJ, et al.: Favorable effect of pulmonic vein isolation by partial circumferential ablation on ostial flow velocity. Heart Rhythm 1:262-267, 2004.

51. Zhu D, Maloney JD, Simmons TE, et al.: Radiofrequency catheter ablation for management of symptomatic ventricular ectopic activity. J Am Coll Cardiol 26:843-849, 1995.

52. Friedman PL, Stevenson WG, Bihl JA, et al.: Left main coronary artery occlusion during radiofrequency catheter ablation of idiopathic outflow tract tachycardia. Pacing Clin Electrophysiol 20:1184, 1997.

53. Cole RC, Marrouche NF, Natale A: Evaluation and management of ventricular outflow tract tachycardia. Card Electrophysiol Rev 6:442-447, 2002.

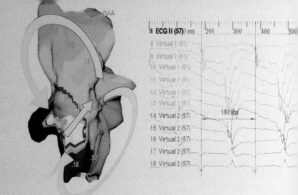

26

Ablation of Idiopathic Left Ventricular Tachycardia

Akihiko Nogami

Key Points

- The mechanism of idiopathic left ventricular tachycardia (VT) is reentry.

- Diagnosis is based on demonstration of right bundle branch block and superior axis configuration (common type); right bundle branch block and inferior axis configuration (uncommon type); or a relatively narrow QRS and inferior axis configuration (rare type), together with dependence on left ventricular fascicular activation and verapamil sensitivity (termination or slowing of the tachycardia).

- Ablation targets are the diastolic potential in the descending limb of the fascicular circuit or the presystolic fused Purkinje potential at the VT exit.

- A multipolar electrode mapping catheter may be useful. Specialized mapping systems or irrigated ablation are rarely necessary.

- The success rate of ablation is greater than 95% for the superior axis configuration (common type) and greater than 75% for the inferior axis configuration (uncommon type). The success rate for VTs with relatively narrow QRS and inferior axis configuration (rare type) is unclear.

Sustained monomorphic ventricular tachycardia (VT) is most often related to myocardial structure heart disease, including healed myocardial infarction and cardiomyopathies. However, no apparent structural abnormality is identified in approximately 10% of all sustained monomorphic VTs in the United States[1] and 20% of those in Japan.[2] These VTs are referred to as "idiopathic." Idiopathic VTs usually occur in specific locations and have specific QRS morphologies, whereas VTs associated with structural heart disease have a QRS morphology that tends to indicate the location of the scar. Idiopathic VT comprises multiple discrete subtypes that are best differentiated by their mechanism, QRS morphology, and site of origin. The most common idiopathic VT originates from a focus in the outflow tract of the right ventricle, and its mechanism is most likely triggered activity. In idiopathic left VT, three types of VT exist: verapamil-sensitive left VT (reentry), VT with a focal origin in the distal left posterior fascicle (abnormal automaticity), and left ventricular outflow tract VT (triggered activity, reentry, or automaticity). This chapter focuses on the assessment and nonpharmacologic treatment of verapamil-sensitive idiopathic left VT.

Pathophysiology

CLASSIFICATION

Verapamil-sensitive fascicular VT is the most common form of idiopathic left VT. It first was rec-

ognized as an electrocardiographic entity in 1979 by Zipes et al.,[3] who identified the characteristic diagnostic triad: (1) induction with atrial pacing, (2) right bundle branch block (RBBB) and left-axis configuration, and (3) manifestation in patients without structural heart disease. In 1981, Belhassen et al.[4] were the first to demonstrate the verapamil sensitivity of the tachycardia, a fourth identifying feature. Ohe et al.[5] reported another type of this tachycardia, with RBBB and a right-axis deviation, in 1988. More recently, Shimoike et al.[6] described the upper septal form of this tachycardia. According to the QRS morphology, verapamil-sensitive left fascicular VT can be classified into three subgroups: (1) left posterior fascicular VT, whose QRS morphology exhibits an RBBB configuration and a superior axis (Fig. 26–1); (2) left anterior fascicular VT, whose QRS morphology exhibits an RBBB configuration and right-axis deviation (Fig. 26–2); and (3) upper septal fascicular VT, whose QRS morphology exhibits a narrow QRS configuration and normal or right-axis deviation (Fig. 26–3). Left posterior fascicular VT is common, left anterior fascicular VT is uncommon, and left upper septal fascicular VT is very rare.

SUBSTRATE AND ANATOMY

The anatomic basis of this tachycardia has provoked considerable interest. Some data suggest that the tachycardia may originate from a false tendon or fibromuscular band in the left ventricle.[7-9] Suwa et al.[8] described a false tendon in the left ventricle of a patient with idiopathic VT in whom the VT was eliminated by surgical resection of the tendon. Using transthoracic and transesophageal echocardiography,

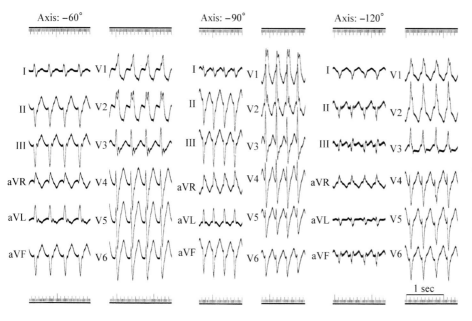

FIGURE 26–1. Twelve-lead ECGs of verapamil-sensitive left posterior fascicular VTs. Three different VTs are shown. *(From Nogami A: Idiopathic left ventricular tachycardia: Assessment and treatment. Card Electrophysiol Rev 6:448-457, 2002.)*

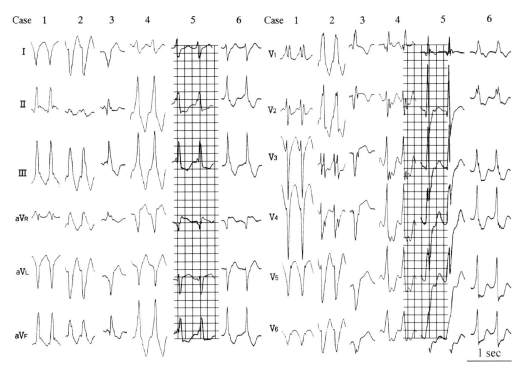

FIGURE 26–2. Twelve-lead ECGs of verapamil-sensitive left anterior fascicular VTs in 6 patients. *(From Nogami A, Naito S, Tada H, et al.: Verapamil-sensitive left anterior fascicular ventricular tachycardia: Results of radiofrequency ablation in six patients. J Cardiovasc Electrophysiol 9:1269-1278, 1998.)*

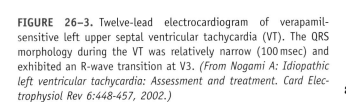

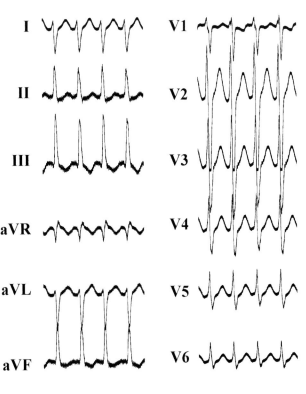

FIGURE 26–3. Twelve-lead electrocardiogram of verapamil-sensitive left upper septal ventricular tachycardia (VT). The QRS morphology during the VT was relatively narrow (100 msec) and exhibited an R-wave transition at V3. *(From Nogami A: Idiopathic left ventricular tachycardia: Assessment and treatment. Card Electrophysiol Rev 6:448-457, 2002.)*

Thakur et al.[9] found false tendons extending from the posteroinferior left ventricle to the basal septum in 15 of 15 patients with idiopathic left VT but in only 5% of control patients. Maruyama et al.[10] reported a case with the recording of sequential diastolic potentials bridging the entire diastolic period and a false tendon extending from the midseptum to the inferoapical septum. Lin et al.[11] found that 17 of 18 patients with idiopathic VT had this fibromuscular band but also found it in 35 of 40 control patients. They concluded that the band was a common echocardiographic finding and was not a specific arrhythmogenic substrate for this tachycardia, although they could not exclude the possibility that the band was a potential substrate of the VT. Small fibromuscular bands, trabeculae carneae, and small papillary muscles cannot be detected by echocardiography. The Purkinje networks in these small anatomic structures are important when considering the reentry circuit of verapamil-sensitive left posterior fascicular VT. This circuit is not completely defined but may comprise only fascicular tissue or fascicular tissue and ventricular myocardium.

MECHANISM

The mechanism of verapamil-sensitive left VT is reentry, because it can be induced, entrained, and terminated by programmed ventricle or atrial stimulation. To confirm its reentry circuit and the mechanism, my colleagues and I performed left ventricular septal mapping using an octapolar electrode catheter in 20 patients with left posterior fascicular

VT[12] (Fig. 26–4). In 15 of 20 patients, two distinct potentials, P1 and P2, were recorded during the VT at the midseptum (Fig. 26–5). Although the mid-diastolic potential (P1) was recorded earlier from the proximal rather than the distal electrodes, the fused presystolic Purkinje potential (P2) was recorded earlier from the distal electrodes. During sinus rhythm, recording at the same site demonstrated P2, which was recorded after the His-bundle potential and before the onset of the QRS complex; however, the sequence of the P2 was the reverse of that seen during the VT. At the initiation of the VT by ventricular extrastimulation, retrograde conduction of the P2 was observed (Fig. 26–6). VT could be entrained from the atrium (Fig. 26–7) and from the ventricle. Entrainment pacing from the atrium or ventricle captured P1 orthodromically and reset the VT (Figs. 26–8 and 26–9). The interval from the stimulus to P1 was prolonged as the pacing rate increased. The effect of verapamil on P1 and P2 is shown in Figure 26–10. The intravenous administration of 1.5 mg of verapamil significantly prolonged the cycle length of the VT, from 305 to 350 msec. Both the P1-P2 and P2-P1 intervals were proportionally prolonged after verapamil administration. However, the interval from P2 to the onset of the QRS complex remained unchanged. This study demonstrated that P1 is a critical potential in the circuit of the verapamil-sensitive left posterior fascicular VT and suggested the presence of a macroreentry circuit involving the normal Purkinje system and abnormal Purkinje tissue with decremental properties and verapamil sensitivity. Although P1 has proved to be a critical potential in

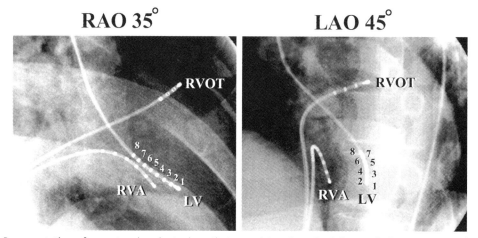

FIGURE 26–4. Representation of an octapolar electrode catheter positioned at the left ventricular septum as viewed fluoroscopically in the right oblique (RAO) and left oblique (LAO) projections. The distance between electrodes 1 and 8 of the octapolar electrode catheter was approximately 25 mm. LV, left ventricle; RVA, right ventricular apex; RVOT, right ventricular outflow tract. *(From Nogami A, Naito S, Tada H, et al.: Demonstration of diastolic and presystolic Purkinje potential as critical potentials on a macroreentry circuit of verapamil-sensitive idiopathic left ventricular tachycardia. J Am Coll Cardiol 36:811-823, 2000.)*

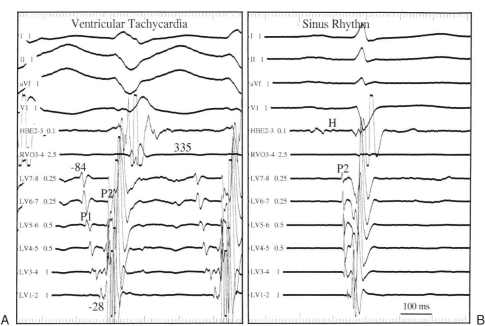

FIGURE 26–5. Intracardiac recordings from an octapolar electrode catheter. **A,** During left posterior fascicular VT, a diastolic potential (P1) and a presystolic Purkinje potential (P2) were recorded. While P1 was recorded earlier from the proximal rather than the distal electrodes, P2 was recorded earlier from the distal rather than the proximal electrodes. **B,** During sinus rhythm, recording at the same site demonstrated the P2, is now recorded before the onset of the QRS complex and is earliest on the proximal electrodes. HBE, His bundle; RVO, right ventricular outflow; LV, left ventricle; 7-8, proximal bipole; 1-2, distal bipole; H, His. *(From Nogami A, Naito S, Tada H, et al.: Demonstration of diastolic and presystolic Purkinje potential as critical potentials on a macroreentry circuit of verapamil-sensitive idiopathic left ventricular tachycardia. J Am Coll Cardiol 36:811-823, 2000.)*

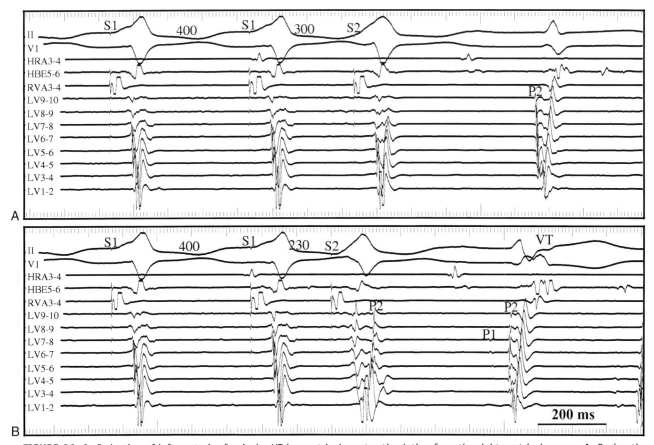

FIGURE 26–6. Induction of left posterior fascicular VT by ventricular extrastimulation from the right ventricular apex. **A,** During the basic drive (S1) and at a coupling interval of 300 msec (S2), sharp electrical potentials (P2) were recorded just before the ventricular electrograms. These potentials were recorded earlier from the proximal than the distal electrodes. **B,** When the coupling interval was decreased to 280 msec, the activations of P2 were delayed and the sequence of P2 was reversed, resulting in initiating ventricular tachycardia. This sequence may be interpreted as development of antegrade unidirectional block in the fascicle generating P2 which is now activated by a distal connection with the fascicle generating P1. Abbreviations per Figure 26–5.

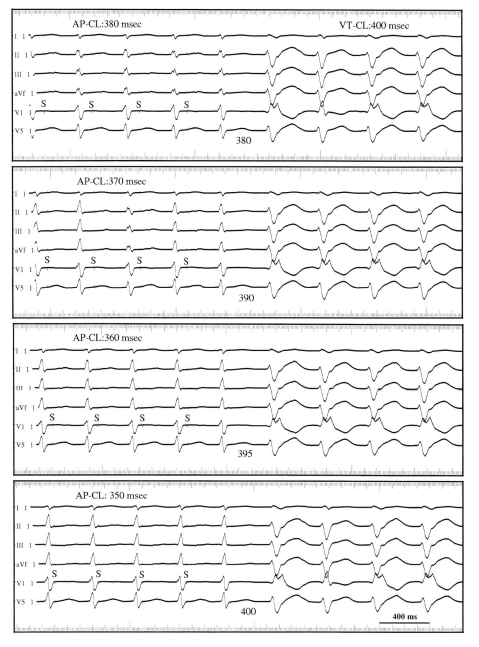

FIGURE 26–7. Surface ECGs showing entrainment pacing from the high right atrium during left posterior fascicular VT. The QRS morphology exhibited constant fusion and progressive fusion. The subsequent VT had been reset because the interval between the last entrained QRS and VT was less than the VT cycle length. The interval between the last captured QRS and VT was prolonged with shortening of the pacing cycle length presumably due to decremental conduction within the reentry circuit. AP, atrial pacing; CL, cycle length; S, pacing stimulus.

the VT circuit, whether the left posterior fascicle or Purkinje fiber (P2) is involved in the retrograde limb of the reentrant circuit remains unclear.[10,13] Ouyang et al.[14] suggested that idiopathic left VT reentry might be a small macroreentry circuit consisting of one anterograde Purkinje fiber with a Purkinje potential, one retrograde Purkinje fiber with retrograde Purkinje potential, and the ventricular myocardium as the bridge.

CIRCUIT DIAGRAM

The hypothesized VT circuit is depicted in Figure 26–11. In this circuit, P1 represents the activation potential in the distal portion of the specialized Purkinje tissue; it has decremental properties and verapamil sensitivity. P2 represents the activation of the left posterior fascicle or Purkinje fiber near the left posterior fascicle. P2 comprises the retrograde limb of the reentrant circuit in VT. P1 represents the antegrade limb of the circuit in VT and may represent longitudinal dissociation of the posterior fascicle, contiguous tissue coupled to the fascicle (false tendon), or ventricular myocardium interposed in the circuit. There is a distal link (network) between P1 and P2, and ventricular myocardium may act as a proximal bridge.

During sinus rhythm, the activation goes from P2 to P1 at the point of the fusion; therefore, P1 is buried in the local ventricular activation (see Fig. 26–11A). During VT, P1 and P2 activate in the reverse direc-

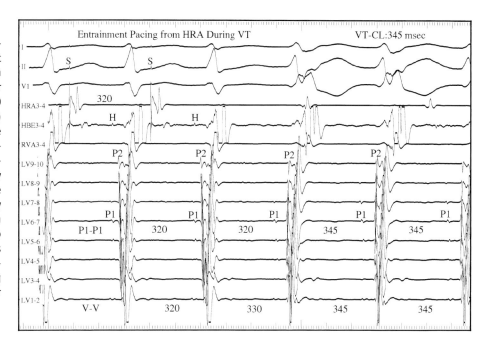

FIGURE 26–8. Intracardiac recordings during entrainment pacing from the high right atrium during left posterior fascicular VT. Right atrial pacing (CL: 320 msec) during VT (CL: 345 msec) resulted in a narrowing of the QRS width without VT interruption. While the diastolic potential (P1) was orthodromically captured, the presystolic Purkinje potential (P2) was antidromically captured. The activation sequence of P2 was identical to that observed during sinus rhythm. CL, cycle length; H, His-bundle electrogram; S, pacing stimulus. Abbreviations per Figure 26–5.

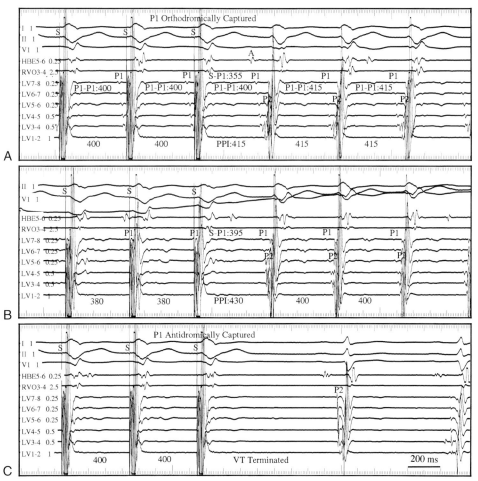

FIGURE 26–9. Concealed entrainment by pacing from the VT exit site. During left posterior fascicular VT, the earliest ventricular electrogram with the fused Purkinje potential (P2) was recorded from the distal two electrodes. **A,** Pacing from the distal two electrodes at a cycle length and a starting coupling interval of 400 ms captured P1 orthodromically and produced QRS configurations similar to that of the VT. The postpacing interval (PPI) (S-P2) was equal to the VT cycle length. **B,** Pacing from the VT exit site at a cycle length of 380 ms also captured P1. A diastolic potential was simultaneously observed with a pacing artifact from LV7-8. The pacing stimulus P1 interval was prolonged. **C,** Pacing from the VT exit at a cycle length of 400 ms but with a starting coupling interval of 300 ms terminated the VT. A diastolic potential was not observed during pacing because it might have been captured antidromically and masked in the ventricular electrogram. P1 = diastolic potential; P2 = presystolic Purkinje potential; S = pacing stimulus. *(From Nogami A, Naito S, Tada H, et al.: Demonstration of diastolic and presystolic Purkinje potential as critical potentials on a macroreentry circuit of verapamil-sensitive idiopathic left ventricular tachycardia. J Am Coll Cardiol 36:811-823, 2000.)*

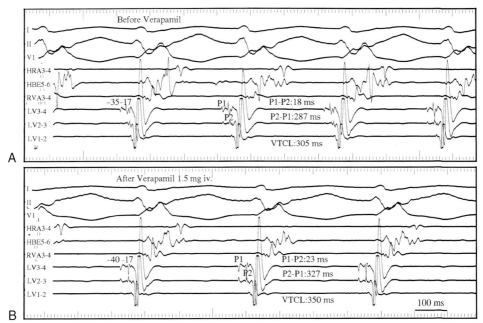

FIGURE 26-10. Effect of verapamil on the circuit of the left posterior fascicular VT. Intravenous administration of 1.5 mg of verapamil significantly prolonged the cycle length of the VT from 305 ms (**A**) to 350 ms (**B**). Both the P1-P2 and P2-P1 intervals were prolonged by similar proportions after verapamil, however, the greatest absolute prolongation is from P2 to P1. However, the interval from P2 to the onset of the QRS complex remained unchanged. HRA, high right atrium; VTCL, cycle length of ventricular tachycardia. Abbreviations per Figure 26-5. *(From Nogumi A, Naito S, Tada H, et al.: Demonstration of diastolic and presystolic Purkinje potential as critical potentials on a macroreentry circuit of verapamil-sensitive idiopathic left ventricular tachycardia. J Am Coll Cardiol 36:811-823, 2000.)*

tion (see Fig. 26–11B). This explains why the activation sequences of P2 are reversed during sinus rhythm and VT. During concealed entrainment from the VT exit (e.g., at a cycle length of 400 msec as in Fig. 26–9A), P2 and P1 are activated orthodromically and the antidromic wavefront blocks, presumably in the connection between P1 and P2 (see Fig. 26–11C). The orthodromic wavefront of the preceding (n – 1)th beat also blocks in the connection between P1 and P2 because it encounters the refractoriness created by the antidromic wavefront from the (n)th pacing impulse. The orthodromic wavefront from the last pacing impulse continues the tachycardia with resetting. During entrainment pacing with a shorter cycle length (e.g., at 380 msec as in Fig. 26–9B), the distal portion of P1 activates antidromically, and the antidromic wavefront blocks at the middle portion of P1 in the area of slow conduction (Fig. 26–11D). The orthodromic wavefront from the last pacing impulse continues and resets the tachycardia. However, the interval from the last pacing stimulus to the orthodromically activated P1 is prolonged because of rate-dependent conduction delay in the area of slow conduction. During entrainment pacing with an even shorter cycle length or a shorter starting coupling interval (e.g., at a starting coupling interval of 300 msec as in Fig. 26–9C), P1 activates antidromically, and the antidromic wavefront blocks at the proximal portion of P1 in the area of slow conduction

(Fig. 26–11E). However, the orthodromic wavefront from the previous paced beat also blocks. It blocks independent of either the collision with, or refractoriness secondary to, the previous antidromic wavefront. Because both the antidromic and the orthodromic wavefronts of the same beat are blocked, the VT is interrupted. Radiofrequency (RF) catheter ablation results in elimination of the conduction between P1 and P2.

Diagnostic Criteria

SURFACE ELECTROCARDIOGRAM

Based on the QRS morphology, verapamil-sensitive fascicular VT can be classified into three subgroups. The 12-lead electrocardiogram (ECG) of the left posterior fascicular VT exhibits an RBBB and a superior axis (left-axis deviation or northwest axis) (see Fig. 26–1). This is the common type of verapamil-sensitive fascicular VT and may account for up to 90% of cases. The uncommon type of this VT is a left anterior fascicular VT whose QRS morphology exhibits an RBBB configuration and right-axis deviation (see Fig. 26–2).[5,15] The last type of VT is an upper septal fascicular VT, whose QRS morphology exhibits

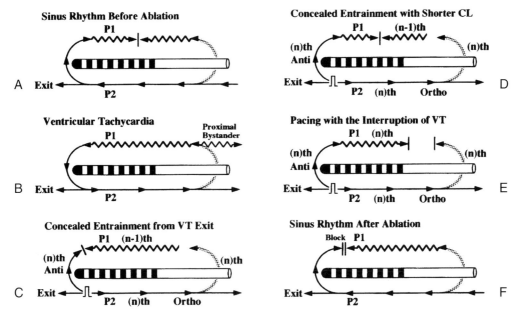

FIGURE 26–11. Schematic representation of the mechanism of left posterior fascicular VT. See the text for a discussion. Anti, antidromic wavefront; CL, cycle length; ortho, orthodromic wavefront; P1, diastolic potential; P2, presystolic Purkinje potential; VT, ventricular tachycardia. The *dotted lines* indicate the ventricular myocardium as the bridge between P1 and P2. The undulating line represents a zone of slow conduction. *(From Nogami A, Naito S, Tada H, et al.: Demonstration of diastolic and presystolic Purkinje potential as critical potentials on a macroreentry circuit of verapamil-sensitive idiopathic left ventricular tachycardia. J Am Coll Cardiol 36:811-823, 2000.)*

a relatively narrow QRS configuration and normal or right-axis deviation (see Fig. 26–3).[6] This type of VT is very rare.

INTRACARDIAC ELECTROGRAMS

With left posterior fascicular VT, the earliest ventricular activation is recorded from the apical septum, and diastolic potentials are recorded from the midseptum (see Fig. 26–5). His activation follows QRS onset by 5-30 msec.[16] During sinus rhythm, recording from the same site demonstrates the Purkinje potentials after the His-bundle potential and before the onset of the QRS complex.

With left anterior fascicular VT, the earliest ventricular activation is recorded from the anterolateral left ventricle (Fig. 26–12), and diastolic potentials are recorded from the midseptum (Fig. 26–13). There have been several reports that describe a left VT with an RBBB configuration, right-axis deviation, and a different mechanism. Yeh et al.[17] reported four cases with an RBBB configuration and right-axis deviation. This VT was adenosine sensitive and was successfully ablated from the anterobasal left ventricle. The chest leads exhibited an atypical RBBB configuration with wide "R" morphology. Crijns et al.[18] reported a rare case of interfascicular reentrant VT with an RBBB configuration and right-axis deviation. In their patient, the VT circuit used the anterior fascicle as the anterograde limb and the posterior fascicle as the retrograde limb. Interfascicular VT usually has a

His-bundle potential recorded in the diastolic phase during the VT, as well as posterior fascicular potentials. However, it may be difficult to distinguish between interfascicular VT and intrafascicular VT (verapamil-sensitive left anterior fascicular VT).[15] The diagnostic criteria for left VTs are given in Table 26–1.

TABLE 26–1

Diagnostic Criteria for Left Ventricular Tachycardia

Characteristic surface ECG appearance: RBBB and superior axis configuration (common type); RBBB and inferior axis configuration (uncommon type); narrow QRS and inferior axis configuration (rare type)

Tachycardia dependence on left ventricular fascicular reentry
  Purkinje potentials and diastolic potentials preceding ventricular activation
  Changes in tachycardia rate preceded by similar changes in Purkinje and diastolic potentials
  His activation follows QRS onset (short positive HV in rare type)
  Induction and entrainment with ventricular and/or atrial pacing

Verapamil-sensitive termination or slowing of tachycardia due to conduction slowing or block in fascicular system

ECG, electrocardiogram; RBBB, right bundle branch block.

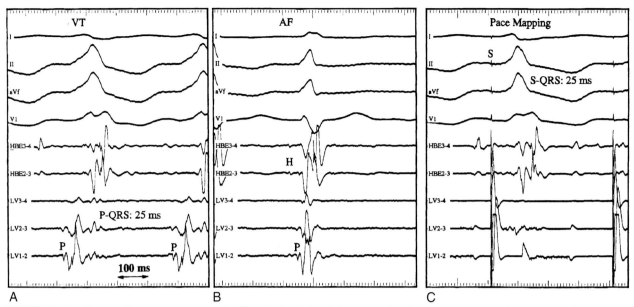

FIGURE 26–12. Intracardiac electrograms at the VT exit site during left anterior fascicular VT. **A,** During the VT, the Purkinje potential preceded the QRS (P-QRS) by 25 msec. **B,** During the basal rhythm (atrial fibrillation [AF]), a Purkinje potential was recorded after the His-bundle potential (H) and before the QRS complex. **C,** Pace mapping at that site produced a similar QRS complex with an interval between the pacing stimulus and QRS (S-QRS) of 25 msec, equal to the P-QRS interval during the VT. The RF current delivered at that site terminated the VT, however, the VT was still induced. *(From Nogami A, Naito S, Tada H, et al.: Verapamil-sensitive left anterior fascicular ventricular tachycardia: Results of radiofrequency ablation in six patients. J Cardiovasc Electrophysiol 9:1269-1278, 1998.)*

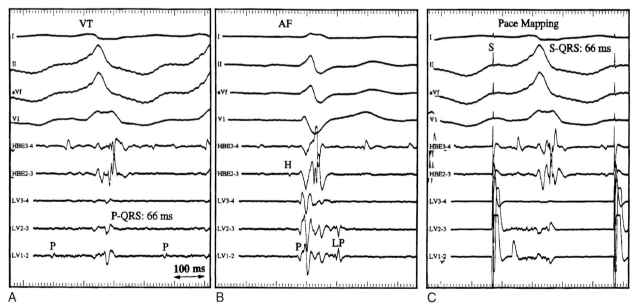

FIGURE 26–13. Intracardiac electrograms at the zone of slow conduction during left anterior fascicular VT. **A,** During the VT, the Purkinje potential (P) preceded the QRS (P-QRS) by 66 ms. **B,** During atrial fibrillation, a Purkinje potential was recorded after the His-bundle potential (H) and before the QRS complex, and a late potential (LP) was also recorded after the QRS complex. **C,** Pace mapping at that site produced a similar QRS complex with an interval between the pacing stimulus and QRS (S-QRS) of 66 ms, equal to the P-QRS interval during the VT. The RF current delivered at that site terminated the VT and suppressed the reinduction of the VT. *(From Nogami A, Naito S, Tada H, et al.: Verapamil-sensitive left anterior fascicular ventricular tachycardia: Results of radiofrequency ablation in six patients. J Cardiovasc Electrophysiol 9:1269-1278, 1998.)*

The differential diagnosis includes supraventricular tachycardias with bifascicular block aberrancy. With left upper septal fascicular VT, the retrograde activation of the His bundle is recorded before the onset of the QRS complex (Fig. 26–14). If there is retrograde ventriculoatrial conduction during the tachycardia, it mimics atrioventricular nodal reentry tachycardia or atrioventricular reciprocating tachycardia. The response of these tachycardias to verapamil and the ability to initiate and entrain them by atrial pacing may also lead to diagnostic confusion. To avoid a misdiagnosis, recognition of the retrograde sequence of the His-bundle activation and measurement of a shorter His-to-ventricular (HV) interval during the tachycardia than in sinus rhythm is important. An earlier potential than the His-bundle potential is recorded from the left ventricular upper septum, where the left bundle potential is recorded during sinus rhythm. VT can be slowed or terminated by the intravenous administration of verapamil; however, it is unresponsive to β-blockers or Valsalva maneuvers. Class Ia and class Ic drugs are also effective. Rare cases of adenosine responsiveness occur but only if the tachycardia shows catecholamine dependency.

In bundle branch reentry the His activation precedes activation of the left bundle to produce a right bundle branch block QRS morphology. In idiopathic left VT, the HV interval is shortor negative and follows left fascicular activation.

Mapping and Ablation

RF catheter ablation may be considered a potential first-line therapy for patients with idiopathic VT, because these VTs can be eliminated by ablation in a high percentage of patients.

LEFT POSTERIOR FASCICULAR VENTRICULAR TACHYCARDIA

Conventional left ventricular septal mapping using a multipolar electrode catheter is useful in patients with left posterior fascicular VT.[12] Two distinct potentials, P1 and P2, can be recorded during the VT from the midseptum (see Fig. 26–5). Because the diastolic potential (P1) has been proven to be a critical potential in the VT circuit, this potential can be targeted to cure the tachycardia. Nakagawa et al.[16] first reported the importance of Purkinje potentials in the ablation of this VT, and Tsuchiya et al.[19] reported the significance of a late diastolic potential and emphasized the role of late diastolic and presystolic potentials in the VT circuit. However, the successful ablation sites

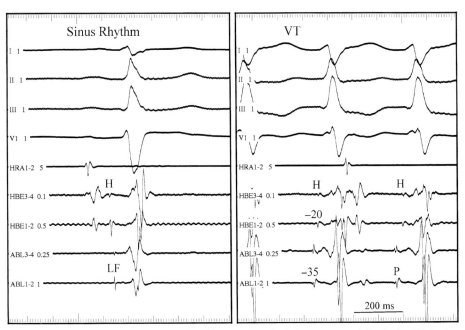

Figure 26–14. Intracardiac electrograms at the successful ablation site of a left upper septal fascicular VT. During the VT, there was a retrograde activation of the His-bundle (H). The activation sequence of the His-bundle potentials was reverse to that during sinus rhythm. The H-V interval is short during the VT. The VT was successfully ablated at the left ventricular upper septum. At that site, a left bundle branch (LF) potential was recorded during sinus rhythm and the potential preceded the QRS by 35 msec during the VT. The RF application eliminated the VT without making left bundle branch block or atrio-ventricular block. *(From Nogami A: Idiopathic left ventricular tachycardia: Assessment and treatment. Card Electrophysiol Rev 6:448-457, 2002.)*

identified by these two research groups were different. Whereas Nakagawa's ablation sites were at the apical-inferior septum of the left ventricle, Tsuchiya's ablation sites were at the basal septal regions close to the main trunk of the left bundle branch. These findings suggest that any P1 during VT can be targeted for catheter ablation. We usually target the apical third of the septum, to avoid the creation of left bundle branch block (LBBB) or atrioventricular block (Fig. 26–15).

In our study, P1 was recorded during the VT in 15 of 20 patients. RF ablation was successfully performed at this site in all 15 patients. During energy application, the P1-P2 interval was gradually prolonged, and the VT was terminated by block between P1 and P2 (Fig. 26–16). After termination of the tachycardia, the P1 was noted to occur after the QRS complex during sinus rhythm, whereas the P2 was still observed before the QRS complex. Figure 26–17 shows the potentials during sinus rhythm before and after the successful ablation. After successful ablation, the P1 occurred after the QRS complex, with an identical activation sequence to that observed during the VT. Figure 26–11F explains why P1 appears after ablation in the mid-diastolic period and with the same activation sequence as during the VT. When the distal segment of P1 is ablated, the P1 activation proceeds orthodromically around the circuit and subsequently blocks from a proximal to distal direction during sinus rhythm. The P1 that appears after ablation exhibits decremental properties during atrial pacing and/or ventricular pacing (Fig. 26–18), and the intravenous administration of verapamil significantly prolongs the His-to-P1 interval during sinus rhythm (Fig. 26–19). Pace mapping at the successful ablation site is usually not good, because the selective pacing of P1 is difficult and there is an antidromic activation of the proximal P1 potential. Pace mapping after successful ablation is sometimes better than before ablation, because the antidromic activation of P1 is blocked.[20]

In the remaining 5 of our 20 patients, the diastolic potential (P1) could not be detected, and a single fused P2 was recorded only at the VT exit site. Successful ablation was performed at this site in all 5 patients. We can speculate that the circuit in these patients may have involved less of the Purkinje system or that the area of slow conduction may not have been close to the endocardial surface. The targets for catheter ablation are given in Table 26–2.

LEFT ANTERIOR FASCICULAR VENTRICULAR TACHYCARDIA

Figure 26-2 shows the 12-lead ECGs of verapamil-sensitive left anterior fascicular VTs that we experienced.[15] The mean cycle length of the VT was 390 ±

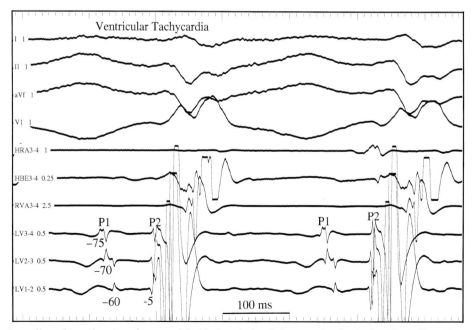

FIGURE 26–15. Recordings from the site of successful ablation during left posterior fascicular VT. A diastolic potential (P1) and presystolic Purkinje potential (P2) were recorded in the mid-septal area. The proximal 2 electrodes of the ablation catheter (LV) recorded the diastolic potential (P1) 15 ms earlier than the distal pair of electrodes. HBE, His bundle electrogram; RVA, right ventricular apex. HRA, high right atrium. Abbreviations per Figure 26–5. *(From Nogami A, Naito S, Tada H, et al.: Demonstration of diastolic and presystolic Purkinje potential as critical potentials on a macroreentry circuit of verapamil-sensitive idiopathic left ventricular tachycardia. J Am Coll Cardiol 36:811-823, 2000.)*

FIGURE 26–16. An application of radiofrequency current delivered during left posterior fascicular VT. During the energy application, the P1-P2 interval gradually prolonged and the VT was terminated by block between P1 and P2. After the ablation, the P1 occurred after the QRS complex during sinus rhythm. ABL, ablation catheter; H, His recording; RF, radiofrequency current. *(From Nogami A, Naito S, Tada H, et al.: Demonstration of diastolic and presystolic Purkinje potential as critical potentials on a macroreentry circuit of verapamil-sensitive idiopathic left ventricular tachycardia. J Am Coll Cardiol 36:811-823, 2000.)*

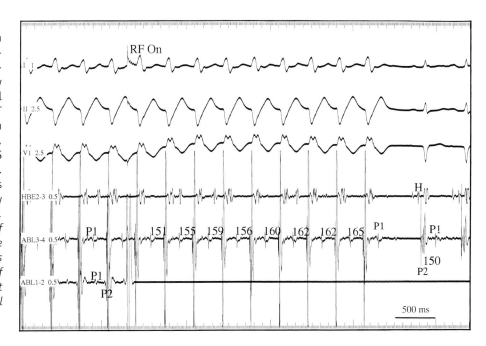

FIGURE 26–17. Intracardiac recordings during sinus rhythm before and after the successful ablation of left posterior fascicular VT. **A,** Before the ablation, no diastolic potential was observed during sinus rhythm. **B,** After the ablation, the P1 occurred after the QRS complex. The activation sequence of P1 was identical to that observed during the VT shown in Figure 26–15. *(From Nogami A, Naito S, Tada H, et al.: Demonstration of diastolic and presystolic Purkinje potential as critical potentials on a macroreentry circuit of verapamil-sensitive idiopathic left ventricular tachycardia. J Am Coll Cardiol 36:811-823, 2000.)*

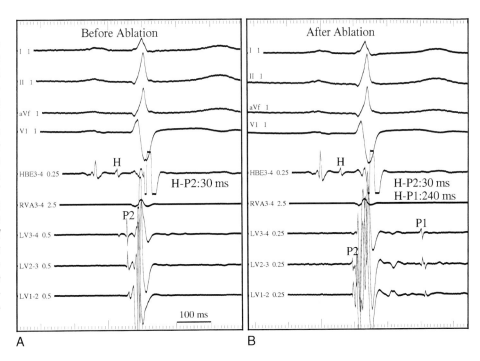

62 msec, and the mean electrical axis during the VT was 120 ± 16 degrees. Patient no. 3 also had a typical left posterior fascicular VT. Left ventricular endocardial mapping during left anterior fascicular VT identified the earliest ventricular activation in the anterolateral wall of the left ventricle. RF current delivered to this site suppressed the VT in three patients (patients 1, 2, and 3; the distal type). The fused Purkinje potential was recorded at that site and preceded the QRS complex by 20 to 35 msec, with pace mapping exhibiting an optimal match between the paced rhythm and clinical VT. In the remaining three patients, RF catheter ablation at the site of the earliest ventricular activation was unsuccessful. In these patients, a Purkinje potential was recorded in the diastolic phase during the VT at the midanterior left ventricular septum. The Purkinje potential preceded the QRS during VT by 56 to 66 msec, and catheter ablation at these sites was successful (patients 4, 5, and 6; the proximal type).

Figure 26–12 shows the intracardiac recording from the VT exit (anterolateral wall) in patient no. 4. The Purkinje potential preceded the QRS (P-QRS interval) by 25 msec during the VT, and pace

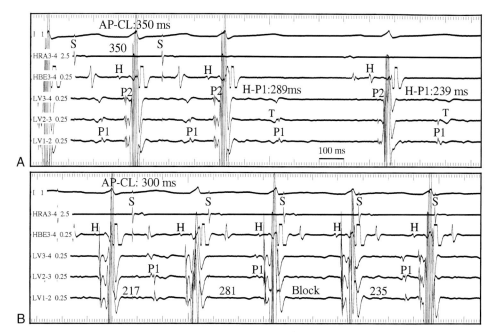

FIGURE 26–18. Decremental properties of P1, which occurred after the QRS complex. Intracardiac recordings during right atrial pacing after successful ablation of left posterior fascicular VT. **A,** The H-P1 interval increased during right atrial pacing at a cycle length of 350 msec. **B,** At a cycle length of 300 msec, the P1 demonstrated a Wenckebach-type block pattern. T, T wave repolarization artifact. Abbreviations per Figure 26–5. *(From Tada H, Nogami A, Naito S, et al.: Retrograde Purkinje potential activation during sinus rhythm following catheter ablation of idiopathic left ventricular tachycardia. J Cardiovasc Electrophysiol 9:1218-1224, 1998.)*

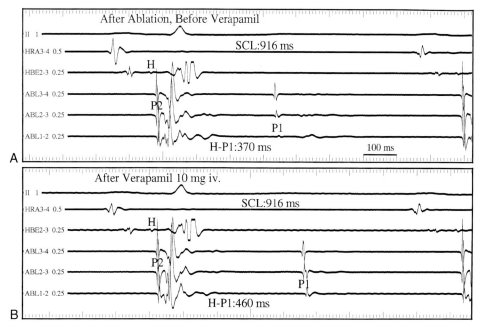

FIGURE 26–19. Verapamil-sensitivity of P1, which occurred after the QRS complex. **A,** The His to P1 interval (H-P1) during sinus rhythm was 370 msec. **B,** The H-P1 interval significantly prolonged after the intravenous administration of 10 mg of verapamil. SCL, sinus cycle length. *(From Tada H, Nogami A, Naito S, et al.: Retrograde Purkinje potential activation during sinus rhythm following catheter ablation of idiopathic left ventricular tachycardia. J Cardiovasc Electrophysiol 9:1218-1224, 1998.)*

mapping at that site produced a similar QRS complex with an interval between the pacing stimulus and QRS (S-QRS) of 25 msec, equal to the P-QRS interval during VT. RF current delivered at this site terminated the VT; however, the VT was still induced. Figure 26–13 shows the intracardiac recordings from patient 4 at the zone of slow conduction during the VT. The ablation catheter was positioned in the midseptal area, where the diastolic Purkinje potential was recorded. The Purkinje potential was recorded during the VT. Pace mapping at that site produced a

similar QRS complex, with an S-QRS interval of 66 msec, equal to the P-QRS interval during the VT. RF current delivered at this site terminated the VT and suppressed the reinduction of the VT. There was a significant difference in the 12-lead ECGs between the distal type (patients 1 through 3) and the proximal type (patients 4 through 6) of this tachycardia. Whereas the distal type of left anterior fascicular VT exhibited a "QS" or "rS" morphology in leads I, V_5, and V_6, the proximal type exhibited an "RS" or "Rs" morphology in those leads.

TABLE 26–2

Targets for Ablation

Diastolic potential (P1) in the antegrade limb of the VT circuit (midseptum). The earliest diastolic potential (P1) is not needed. The distal third of P1 potentials is usually targeted, to avoid the creation of LBBB or atrioventricular block (P1 − QRS = 28 to 130 msec)

Presystolic fused Purkinje potential (P2) at the VT exit (apical septum), if diastolic potential (P1) could not be recorded

Pace mapping (a perfect QRS match during pace mapping is not needed)

Anatomic linear ablation to transect the involved middle to distal left fascicular tract

LBBB, left bundle branch block; VT, ventricular tachycardia.

LEFT UPPER SEPTAL FASCICULAR VENTRICULAR TACHYCARDIA

Figure 26-14 shows the intracardiac electrograms at the successful ablation site of the upper septal fascicular VT. This VT was successfully ablated at the left ventricular upper septum. At this site, a left bundle branch potential was recorded during sinus rhythm, and the potential preceded the QRS by 35 msec during the VT. An RF application eliminated the VT without creating an LBBB or atrioventricular block. The 12-lead ECG configuration in a case reported by Shimoike et al.[6] was different from ours. Their case showed LBBB configurations and a normal axis during the VT. However, the QRS width was narrow, and the successful ablation site was similar to ours.

RADIOFREQUENCY ENERGY DELIVERY AND THE END POINT OF ABLATION

With catheter ablation of verapamil-sensitive idiopathic left VT, no special mapping or ablation system is typically needed. We usually use a 7-French quadripolar steerable electrode catheter with a 4-mm tip and 2-mm interelectrode spacing between the distal two electrodes. RF energy is delivered using maximum power of 40 W and a maximum electrode-tissue interface temperature of 60°C to 65°C. We deliver RF energy during the tachycardia of left posterior and anterior fascicular VTs. If the VT is terminated or slowed within 15 seconds, additional current is applied for another 60 to 120 seconds. If the test RF current is ineffective, ablation is directed to a more proximal site with the earlier diastolic potential. If the mid-diastolic potential cannot be detected, RF current is applied at the VT exit site showing a single fused presystolic Purkinje potential. With upper septal fascicular VT, we deliver RF energy for 30 to 60 seconds during sinus rhythm to avoid atrioventricular block. We perform catheter ablation in this region using a low power output (i.e., 10 W), which can gradually be increased while carefully monitoring for development of a junctional rhythm or atrioventricular block.

After the ablation, programmed stimulation should be repeated. Other than the noninducibility of VT, there are several electrophysiologic findings that can serve as end points of RF applications for left posterior fascicular VT. After ablation of the distal attachment between P1 and P2, P1 appears after the QRS complex (see Figs. 26–11F and 26–17). However, this phenomenon is not sufficient for an end point, because this only indicates conduction block in the direction from P2 to P1. This unidirectional block can be seen during the baseline state[14] or after an insufficient RF application.[20] Figure 26–20 shows an example of residual conduction from P1 to P2. After the first RF application, the VT became noninducible and P1 appeared after the QRS complex during sinus rhythm. However, 1 hour after the first RF application, a premature ventricular complex was observed and its QRS morphology was similar to that observed during the VT. The activation sequence of P2 before the premature ventricular complex was different from that during sinus rhythm but identical to that during the VT. This means that there was residual unidirectional conduction from P1 to P2. During isoproterenol infusion, an incessant form of nonsustained VT was initiated, and it was successfully ablated by additional RF applications at this site.[20] To confirm the creation of bidirectional block between P1 and P2, we do atrial pacing with various cycle lengths after the ablation (Fig. 26–21). If there is residual conduction from P1 to P2, a premature ventricular complex (i.e., ventricular echo beat) with a similar QRS morphology as that observed during the VT can be repeatedly observed.

SUCCESS AND RECURRENCE RATES

Our experience at the time of this writing includes 60 patients with left posterior fascicular VT, 8 patients with left anterior fascicular VT, and 2 patients with left upper septal fascicular VT. The success and recurrence rates are 96.7% and 5%, respectively, for left posterior fascicular VT; 87.5% and 12.5% for left anterior fascicular VT; and 100% and 0% for left upper septal fascicular VT.

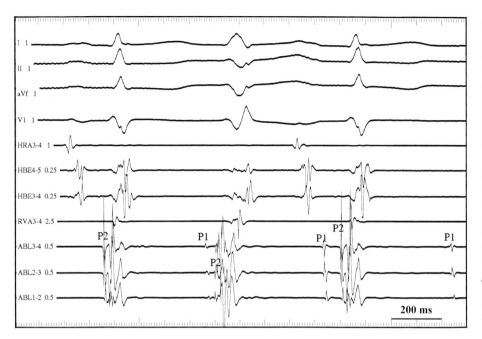

FIGURE 26–20. Intracardiac recordings from the site of catheter ablation obtained during sinus rhythm one hour after the first radiofrequency application. The premature ventricular complex was observed and its QRS morphology was similar to that during the VT. The activation sequence of P2 before the premature ventricular complex was different from that during sinus rhythm, but identical to that during the VT. *(From Tada H, Nogami A, Naito S, et al.: Retrograde Purkinje potential activation during sinus rhythm following catheter ablation of idiopathic left ventricular tachycardia. J Cardiovasc Electrophysiol 9:1218-1224, 1998.)*

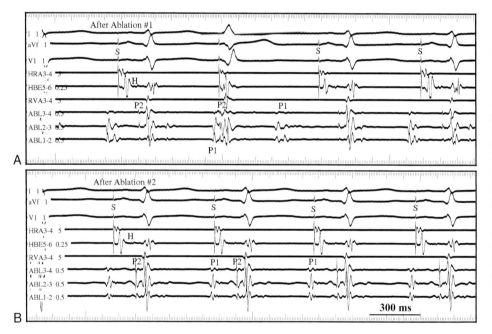

FIGURE 26–21. Confirmation of bi-directional block between P1 and P2 after the ablation. **A,** During atrial pacing (S), the premature ventricular complex with a similar QRS morphology as that during the VT was repeatedly observed. The activation sequence of P2 before the premature ventricular complex was different from that during sinus rhythm. **B,** After the additional RF application, this ventricular echo beat was abolished.

Complications

Aside from the complications that may result from any left ventricular electrophysiologic procedure (e.g., thrombophlebitis, damage to the femoral artery, ventricular perforation), the only complication that has been associated with catheter ablation of idiopathic left VT has been LBBB and atrioventricular block. Tsuchiya et al.[19] reported that 2 patients (12.5%) had transient LBBB after ablation in their series of 16 patients. They targeted the left basal

septum, and the LBBB disappeared within 10 minutes without VT recurrence. In our experience, 1 (1.4%) of 70 patients had a transient atrioventricular block. This patient had a left posterior fascicular VT, and the diastolic potential (P1) at the midseptum was targeted for the ablation. Before the ablation, the patient had catheter-induced RBBB. Approximately 15 seconds into the RF delivery, the VT terminated, and second-degree atrioventricular block was observed. The atrioventricular block disappeared immediately after discontinuation of the RF energy delivery.

Troubleshooting the Difficult Case

Common problems encountered with left VT ablation and their solutions are given in Table 26–3. Inability to reliably induce VT is a formidable obstacle to successful ablation. Isoproterenol enhances or facilitates induction of sustained VT in 60% to 70% of those patients without inducible sustained VT at baseline. Catheter mapping sometimes mechanically suppresses the conduction in the VT circuit ("bump" phenomenon). In such cases, a ventricular echo beat during sinus rhythm or atrial pacing is useful (see Figs. 26–20 and 26–21). If premature ventricular complexes with a similar QRS morphology to that observed during the VT are repeatedly seen, activation mapping can be performed. If no ventricular echo beats are inducible, the empiric anatomic approach can be an effective strategy for ablation of left posterior fascicular VT. First, the VT exit site is sought by pace mapping during sinus rhythm, and RF energy is delivered to that site. Second, a linear lesion is placed at the midseptum, perpendicular to the long axis of the left ventricle, approximately 10 to 15 mm proximal to the VT exit. During anatomic linear ablation, P1 suddenly appears after the QRS complex if the ablation site is on the descending limb of the VT circuit (Fig. 26–22).

If a good electrogram is not found at the septum, one possible reason is poor catheter contact with the

---

TABLE 26–3

Troubleshooting the Difficult Case

Problem	Causes	Solution
Unable to induce VT	Adrenergic dependency	Use isoproterenol
	"Bump" phenomenon during mapping	Find ventricular echo beat with a similar QRS morphology as that observed during the VT
		Use pace mapping and the anatomic approach
Unable to find a good electrogram	Poor catheter contact	Improve the contact with a different catheter or approach, use multipolar mapping catheter
Poor catheter stability	Excessive heart motion during the VT	Ablate during sinus rhythm, change catheter reach and stiffness, use cryoablation
	Frequent ventricular premature beats during the RF application	Use verapamil IV (after which the noninducibility of VT becomes invalid as an end point), use cryoablation or overdrive pacing

RF, radiofrequency energy; VT, ventricular tachycardia.

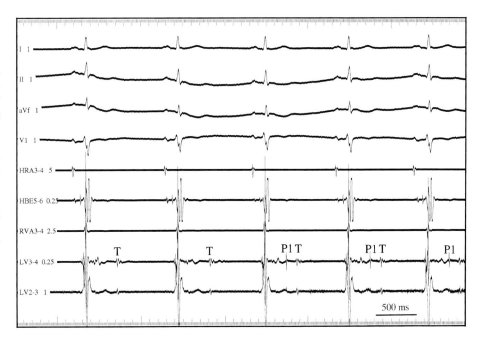

FIGURE 26–22. Anatomical linear approach during sinus rhythm in left posterior fascicular VT. A linear lesion is placed at the mid-septum perpendicular to the long axis of the left ventricle, approximately 10 to 15 mm proximal to the site of the best QRS match by pace mapping. During anatomical linear ablation, P1 suddenly appears after the QRS complex, if the ablation site is on the descending limb of the VT circuit. P1, diastolic potential; T, T wave repolarization artifact.

septum. Figure 26–23 shows examples of poor and good catheter contact with the midseptum. The left anterior oblique fluoroscopic view is used to guide the catheter toward the septum, and the right anterior oblique view to guide the catheter posteriorly and toward the apical third of the septum.

If ablation catheter stability is poor during the VT due to excessive heart motion, RF energy can be delivered during sinus rhythm. However, even during sinus rhythm, frequent ventricular premature beats (with a similar QRS morphology to that observed during the VT) and VT are sometimes induced during the RF energy application. In such cases, intravenous administration of verapamil is effective for suppressing the ventricular premature beats and VT during the RF energy application. However, after such an infusion, the noninducibility of the VT becomes invalid as an end point for the ablation. Cryoablation of left VT has not been reported but may be effective given the superficial

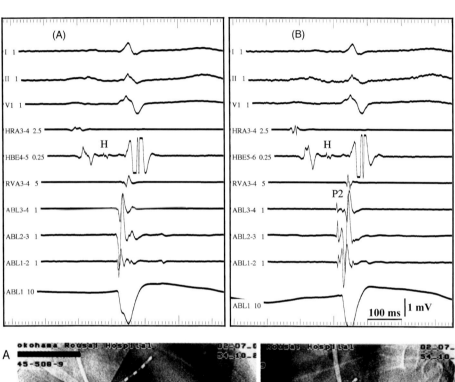

FIGURE 26–23. Representation of poor catheter contact (**A**) and good catheter contact (**B**) to the mid-septum. The left anterior oblique (LAO) fluoroscopic view is used to guide the catheter toward the septum. When the catheter has good contact with the septum, significant Purkinje potentials (P2) can be recorded after the His-bindle potential (H) and before the onset of the QRS complex. The right anterior oblique (RAO) view is used to guide the catheter posteriorly and toward the apical third of the septum.

RAO   LAO

nature of the reentrant circuit. Cryoablation may offer the advantages of no induction of premature ventricular complexes and extreme catheter stability during ablation.

References

1. Lerman BB, Stein KM, Markowitz SM: Mechanism of idiopathic ventricular tachycardia. J Cardiovasc Electrophysiol 8:571-583, 1997.

2. Okumura K, Tsuchiya T: Idiopathic left ventricular tachycardia: Clinical features, mechanism and management. Card Electrophysiol Rev 6:61-67, 2002.

3. Zipes DP, Foster PR, Troup PJ, Pedersen DH: Atrial induction of ventricular tachycardia: Reentry versus triggered automaticity. Am J Cardiol 44:1-8, 1979.

4. Belhassen B, Rotmensch HH, Laniado S: Response of recurrent sustained ventricular tachycardia to verapamil. Br Heart J 46:679-682, 1981.

5. Ohe T, Shimomura K, Aihara N, et al.: Idiopathic sustained left ventricular tachycardia: Clinical and electrophysiological characteristics. Circulation 77:560-568, 1988.

6. Shimoike E, Ueda N, Maruyama T, Kaji Y: Radiofrequency catheter ablation of upper septal idiopathic left ventricular tachycardia exhibiting left bundle branch block morphology. J Cardiovasc Electrophysiol 11:203-207, 2000.

7. Gallagher JJ, Selle JG, Svenson RH, et al.: Surgical treatment of arrhythmias. Am J Cardiol 61:27A-44A, 1988.

8. Suwa M, Yoneda Y, Nagao H, et al.: Surgical correction of idiopathic paroxysmal ventricular tachycardia possibly related to left ventricular false tendon. Am J Cardiol 64:1217-1220, 1989.

9. Thakur RK, Klein GJ, Sivaram CA, et al.: Anatomic substrate for idiopathic left ventricular tachycardia. Circulation 93:497-501, 1996.

10. Maruyama M, Terada T, Miyamoto S, Ino T: Demonstration of the reentrant circuit of verapamil-sensitive idiopathic left ventricular tachycardia: Direct evidence for macroreentry as the underlying mechanism. J Cardiovasc Electrophysiol 12:968-972, 2001.

11. Lin FC, Wen MS, Wang CC, et al.: Left ventricular fibromuscular band is not a specific substrate for idiopathic left ventricular tachycardia. Circulation 93:525-527, 1996.

12. Nogami A, Naito S, Tada H, et al.: Demonstration of diastolic and presystolic Purkinje potential as critical potentials on a macroreentry circuit of verapamil-sensitive idiopathic left ventricular tachycardia. J Am Coll Cardiol 36:811-823, 2000.

13. Kuo JY, Tai CT, Chiang CE, et al.: Is the fascicle of left bundle branch involved in the reentrant circuit of verapamil-sensitive idiopathic left ventricular tachycardia? Pacing Clin Electrophysiol 26:1986-1992, 2003.

14. Ouyang F, Cappato R, Ernst S, et al.: Electroanatomic substrate of idiopathic left ventricular tachycardia: Unidirectional block and macroreentry within the Purkinje network. Circulation 105:462-469, 2002.

15. Nogami A, Naito S, Tada H, et al.: Verapamil-sensitive left anterior fascicular ventricular tachycardia: Results of radiofrequency ablation in six patients. J Cardiovasc Electrophysiol 9:1269-1278, 1998.

16. Nakagawa H, Beckman KJ, McClelland JH, et al.: Radiofrequency catheter ablation of idiopathic left ventricular tachycardia guided by a Purkinje potential. Circulation 88:2607-2617, 1993.

17. Yeh SJ, Wen MS, Wang CC, et al.: Adenosine-sensitive ventricular tachycardia from the anterobasal left ventricle. J Am Coll Cardiol 30:339-345, 1997.

18. Crijns HJ, Smeets JL, Rodriguez LM, Meijer A: Cure of interfascicular reentrant ventricular tachycardia by ablation to anterior fascicle of the left bundle branch. J Cardiovasc Electrophysiol 6:486-492, 1995.

19. Tsuchiya T, Okumura K, Honda T, et al.: Significance of late diastolic potential preceding Purkinje potential in verapamil-sensitive idiopathic left ventricular tachycardia. Circulation 99:2408-2413, 1999.

20. Tada H, Nogami A, Naito S, et al.: Retrograde Purkinje potential activation during sinus rhythm following catheter ablation of idiopathic left ventricular tachycardia. J Cardiovasc Electrophysiol 9:1218-1224, 1998.

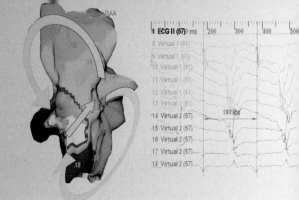

27

Ablation of Ventricular Tachycardia in Coronary Artery Disease

David J. Callans

Key Points

- The mechanism of ventricular tachycardia (VT) in coronary artery disease is reentry within the infarct scar zone.

- Diagnosis is made by tachycardia persistence independent of both supraventricular and His-Purkinje activation (except for bundle branch reentry).

- Ablation targets include presystolic electrical activity within the infarct zone that demonstrates concealed entrainment and a reproducible relationship to the VT circuit. For substrate ablation, linear lesions are created through presumed VT exit sites determined by pace mapping.

- Three-dimensional mapping systems are essential for linear ablation and often helpful for entrainment mapping. Irrigated ablation catheters may be helpful.

- The acute success rate for individual VT morphologies is greater than 90%; however, new morphologies may develop in follow-up.

Ablation for ventricular tachycardia (VT) in patients after myocardial infarction (MI) is important, not for its relative frequency, but for the profound influence this procedure has on quality of life.[1,2] Most patients who undergo VT ablation have implantable cardioverter defibrillators (ICDs) and have had frequent episodes leading to ICD shocks. Those patients who present with uniform tolerated VT typically receive ICDs after successful ablation. The reason is that, even after the most complete form of substrate modification, subendocardial resection, there is a significant residual risk of sudden cardiac death (2.1% per year).[3] This is consistent with the observation from the Electrophysiologic Study Versus Electromagnetic Monitoring (ESVEM) study that presentation with uniform tolerated VT does not predict presentation with recurrent tolerated VT, as opposed to cardiac arrest.[4] Antiarrhythmic therapy, although commonly used to compliment ICD therapy in patients with recurrent VT, is incompletely successful in preventing VT episodes and may cause important cardiac and noncardiac side effects. Although ablation is properly viewed as adjuvant therapy, most patients with frequent VT episodes have a single morphology (or a few dominant morphologies), and successful ablation significantly reduces the frequency of VT recurrence in follow-up.

Anatomy

The typical anatomic substrate for uniform VT is extensive healed infarction with resultant left ventricular (LV) dysfunction. The extent of myocardial necrosis, infarct involvement of the interventricular septum, and degree of LV dysfunction are the most important determinants of arrhythmia risk after MI. Patients with tolerated sustained VT have more extensive infarction, more frequent aneurysm formation, and more pronounced LV dysfunction than do patients with nonsustained supraventricular tachycardia or sudden cardiac death.[5] Contemporary emphasis on revascularization whenever appropriate and medical therapy to prevent LV remodeling has decreased the incidence of VT after MI to approximately 1%.[6] Nonetheless, this decreased incidence may be balanced by an increased prevalence as improved therapies prolong life in patients after MI.

Pathophysiology

The electrophysiologic substrate for VT gradually develops during the first 2 weeks after MI, and, once established, it appears to remain indefinitely. During the infarct healing process, necrotic myocardium is replaced with fibrous tissue. This results in a reduction in the number of gap junctions connecting surviving myocytes. In addition, there are likely to be molecular changes induced by the infarct that change the composition and function of remaining gap junctions.[7] Because of abnormalities in cellular coupling, conduction is slow and discontinuous, despite the fact that normal sodium-dependent action potentials are recorded from living myocytes within the infarct zone. These conduction abnormalities provide the electrophysiologic substrate for VT.[8,9] Endocardial recordings from sites of VT origin during sinus rhythm consistently demonstrate low-amplitude, prolonged, multicomponent potentials[5] (Fig. 27–1). The individual components of fractionated electrograms are generated by individual "islets" of

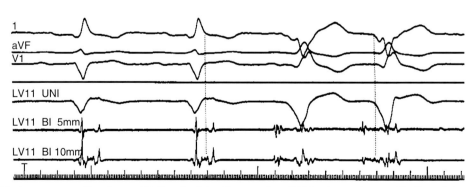

FIGURE 27–1. Electrogram recording from a VT site of origin. Three surface ECG leads are shown with three intracardiac recordings from a catheter positioned within the infarct zone. During sinus rhythm, a fractionated, multicomponent signal is recorded; the final component of this electrogram is recorded after the end of the surface QRS. During VT (final two beats of the tracing), isolated diastolic potentials are observed, preceding the QRS by 90 msec. *(From Josephson ME: Clinical Cardiac Electrophysiology: Techniques and Interpretations, 3rd ed. Philadelphia: Lippincott Williams & Wilkins; 2002, with permission.)*

myocyte groups, which are isolated from neighboring cells by ingrowth of fibrous tissue. The duration of the local electrogram represents the abnormally slow, fractionated conduction within the electrode field of view.

Although the relationship between inducible VT and spontaneous VT is poorly understood, inducible VT signifies the presence of an anatomic VT substrate and confirms increased susceptibility for arrhythmic events.[10] In addition to the presence of the anatomic substrate, spontaneous VT may occur only if a specific trigger is provided, such as premature ventricular complexes, ischemia, or heart failure.[11-14]

The mechanism for most cases of monomorphic sustained VT in coronary artery disease is reentry in the setting of the conduction abnormalities provided by the anatomic substrate of the infarct (Fig. 27–2). The evidence leading to this conclusion is listed in Table 27–1. Reentrant circuits appear to have a fairly consistent relation to the anatomic substrate (Fig. 27–3). A discrete, protected zone of slow conduction is contained within the dense infarct and proves important for many mapping techniques (see later discussion). The exit site of the circuit is consistently located at the border zone of the dense infarct. This corresponds to the onset of the QRS complex in VT. In some cases, the protected zone is bounded by scar and an anatomic structure such

as the mitral valve annulus. This observation is the foundation of many substrate ablation strategies, also discussed later. Nonreentrant mechanisms can also cause VT in patients with healed MI. Repetitive monomorphic nonsustained VT may occur in this setting and may even arise from the infarct zone (Fig. 27–4).

The relationship between the VT and the underlying infarct substrate is not as clearly defined for polymorphic ventricular arrhythmias. The observations that 80% of patients with sudden cardiac death have

TABLE 27–1

Observations Supporting Reentry as the Mechanism of Ventricular Tachycardia in Healed Infarction

Induction and termination of VT with programmed ventricular stimulation

Site-specificity of induction

Inverse relation between the extrastimulus coupling interval and onset of the first tachycardia beat

Continuous electrical activity demonstrated to be related to VT initiation and maintenance

Response to programmed stimulation during VT: resetting with fusion, entrainment

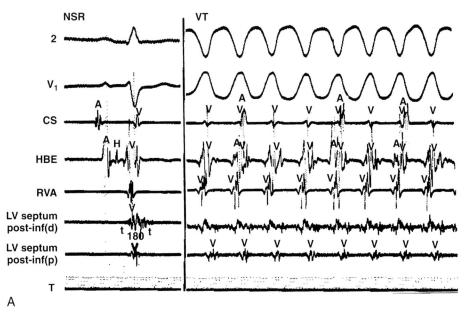

FIGURE 27–2. Observations supporting a reentrant mechanism for VT in the setting of healed infarction. **A,** Continuous electrical activity: Electrogram recordings from the infarct (LV septum post-inf (d) and (p)) during sinus rhythm and VT. Continuous activity is demonstrated in the LV recording during VT. This is consistent with a reentrant mechanism, with activation of some portion of the circuit throughout the entire cycle length, all within the field of view of a single recording site. *(From Josephson ME, Horowitz LN, Farshidi A: Continuous local electrical activity: A mechanism of recurrent ventricular tachycardia. Circulation 57:659-665, 1978, by permission of the American Heart Association.)* *Continued*

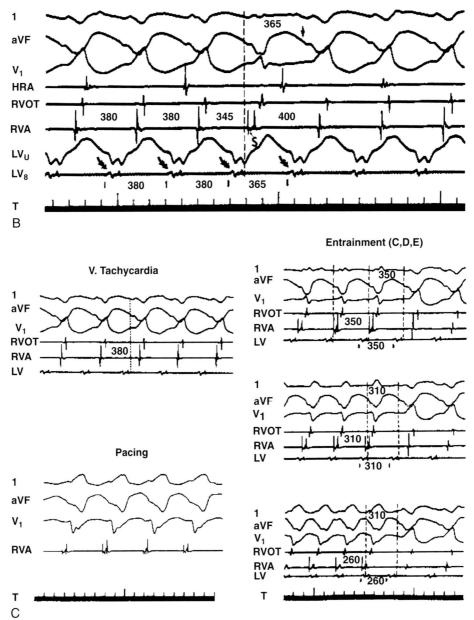

FIGURE 27–2, cont'd. B, Resetting with fusion: Surface ECG and intracardiac recordings during VT. A single extrastimulus is delivered from the RV apex after the inscription of the LV electrogram at the site of origin and the onset of the surface QRS. Nonetheless, surface fusion is observed, and the tachycardia is reset—i.e. the return cycle beat occurs earlier in time (345 + 400 msec <380 + 380 msec) than it would have had the extrastimulus not been delivered. This is inconsistent with a focal mechanism and suggests reentry within a circuit with a distinct entrance and exit site. *(From Almendral JM, Rosenthal ME, Stamato NJ, et al.: Analysis of the resetting phenomenon in sustained uniform ventriular tachycardia: Incidence and relation to termination. J Am Coll Cardiol 8:294-300, 1986, with permission).* **C,** Entrainment with progressive fusion: Surface ECG and intracardiac recordings during VT, RV apical pacing and entrainment at 3 different cycle lengths. Entrainment at faster cycle lengths changes the nature of the surface ECG fusion to more greatly resemble the paced QRS morphology. *(From Almendral JM, Gottlieb CD, Rosenthal ME, et al.: Entrainment of ventricular tachycardia: Explanation for surface electrocardiographic phenomena by analysis of electrograms recorded within the tachycardia circuit. Circulation 77:569, 1988, by permission of the American Heart Association.)*

underlying coronary heart disease and the consistent increment in risk of sudden death after MI represent strong indications of this relationship. Nonetheless, ablation therapy has not previously been possible for polymorphic VT, because the location of the responsible circuit or circuits relative to the infarct anatomy could not be established. However, recent reports by Szumowski et al.[15] have demonstrated that ablation can target the mechanism of initiation of polymorphic VT in well-selected patients.

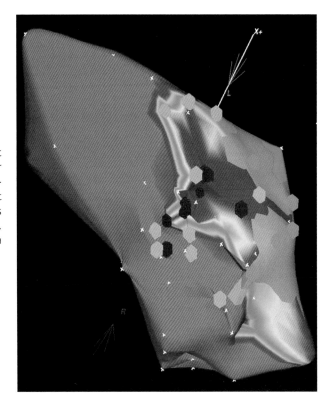

FIGURE 27–3. Relationship of the VT circuit and the infarct anatomy. View of a electroanatomic voltage map in an inferior infarct (*red color* signifies electrogram voltage <0.5 mV, identifying the dense infarct). On top of the voltage map, entrainment mapping was performed at multiple sites to demonstrate sites within (*dark blue dots*) and outside (*light blue dots*) of the circuit. The onset of the QRS corresponded to the exit of the circuit from the infarct scar.

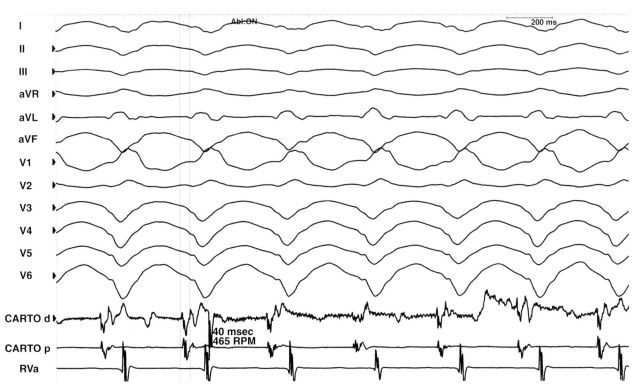

FIGURE 27–4. Repetitive monomorphic VT in the setting of healed infarction. This right bundle, right axis VT was mapped to the center of an inferior infarction, but the infarct was not particularly dense. The recordings on the ablation channel represent the earliest site within the endocardium. Despite the fact that this site was only slightly presystolic, a perfect pacemap was demonstrated at this site and application of RF resulted in prompt termination of the VT. Non-reentrant forms of VT can occur, even within the infarct, and characteristics of successful ablation sites can be markedly different than for reentrant VTs.

Reproducible arrhythmia triggers responsible for the initiation of polymorphic VT have been found in small patient groups with frequent arrhythmia episodes. Furthermore, typical electrocardiographic signatures and anatomic locations for these triggers exist, facilitating pattern recognition and mapping. The global importance of this strategy to more generalized groups of patients after MI remains to be determined.

Diagnosis

In patients who present with sustained VT, the diagnosis is often made by analysis of the electrocardiogram (ECG). Because VT is a wide-complex tachycardia, driven by the ventricles, atrioventricular dissociation may be evident. Several algorithms deal with the subject of differential diagnosis of wide-complex tachycardias.[16-18] All are based on the concept that VT originates in diseased myocardium, potentially away from the conduction system, whereas supraventricular arrhythmias with aberrancy arise from the healthy His-Purkinje system. Because of this fact, supraventricular tachycardia with aberrancy has to resemble either right or left bundle branch block and has rapid initial forces, but VT can arise from anywhere in the ventricle and therefore can have any possible QRS morphology and slow initial forces. Nonetheless, the predictive value of these observations and the algorithms can be negatively affected by the presence of antiarrhythmic drugs, electrolyte imbalances, or preexisting conduction system disease. More difficult members of the differential diagnosis include atrial flutter with 1:1 conduction (Fig. 27–5) and preexcited tachycardias. Review of stored electrograms provides essential diagnostic information regarding the etiology of tachycardias that result in ICD therapy delivery (Fig. 27–6). The morphology of the ICD electrogram is rather specific[19]; although supraventricular tachycardia with right bundle branch block (i.e., ipsilateral from the ICD lead, changing the vector with which it is activated) can change the electrogram morphology,[20] and in most instances this is diagnostic of VT. Furthermore, each different VT morphology produces a different electrogram morphology; therefore, careful review of stored electrograms before consideration of VT ablation can help to determine how many different VT morphologies are clinically relevant. Correlation of ICD electrograms recorded during induced VT morphologies with those from spontaneous episodes can also help to determine clinical relevance.

TABLE 27–2
Diagnostic Criteria for Ischemic Scar-Related Ventricular Tachycardia
Tachycardia independent of atrial and AV nodal activation
Activation of His-Purkinje system follows ventricular myocardial activation (exception: bundle branch reentry) Dissociation His-Purkinje system from tachycardia HV shorter in tachycardia than in sinus rhythm if 1:1 relationship
Meets criteria for reentrant tachycardia
Exclusion of preexcited tachycardias

AV, atrioventricular; HV, His bundle-to-ventricle interval.

The electrophysiologic criteria for diagnosing VT related to ischemic heart disease are given in Table 27–2. In general, the diagnosis is confirmed by the demonstration that the tachycardia is not dependent on atrial, atrioventricular nodal, or His-Purkinje activation. The occurrence of bundle branch reentry is an exception. Tachycardias related to prior MI usually meet the classic criteria for a reentrant mechanism.

Decision-Making Process for Ablation

The number of patients considered for ablation is relatively small compared with the denominator of patients with ventricular arrhythmias. Morady et al.[21] estimated that 10% of patients with VT are appropriate candidates for VT ablation; this number may be significantly smaller with modern post-MI therapy. This chapter considers the risk-benefit analysis of VT in ICD recipients with frequent symptomatic VT. Ablation alone (without ICD therapy) is considered by some investigators to be primary therapy for VT in patients who present with tolerated VT; however, chiefly because coronary heart disease is progressive and unpredictable, most agree that ablation therapy is palliative and adjunctive to ICD therapy.[22]

The typical patient considered for VT ablation has frequent VT episodes resulting in ICD shocks due to rapid VT or ineffective antitachycardia pacing (ATP) or has severe symptoms (palpitations, presyncope) despite effective ATP. Every attempt should be made to optimize pharmacologic and ATP therapy in such patients.[23-28]

The next important consideration in deciding about the relative merits of VT ablation is deciding

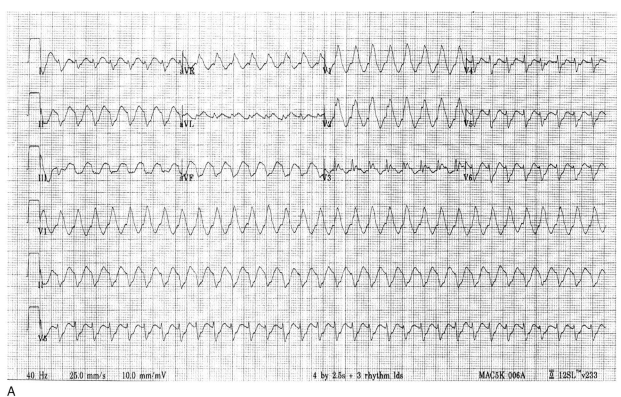

A

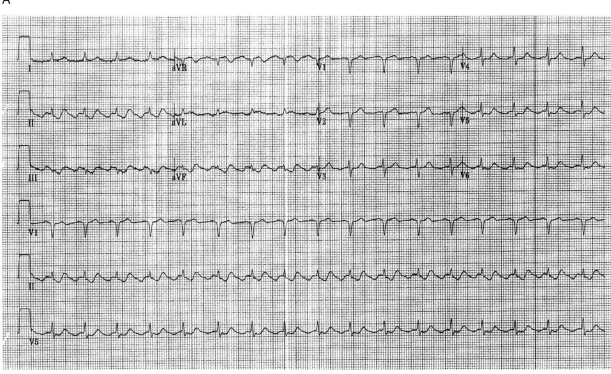

B

FIGURE 27–5. Atrial flutter with 1:1 conduction. **A,** The first ECG was recorded when an elderly woman without structural heart disease presented to the emergency room with chest pain. She had a history of atrial fibrillation, and was treated with propafenone. A wide complex tachycardia with a QRS morphology and axis consistent with VT is shown. **B,** The second ECG, however, shows atrial flutter with a narrow QRS; the atrial flutter cycle length is identical to the cycle length of the wide complex tachycardia. She was treated with catheter ablation of atrial flutter and continuation of propafenone.

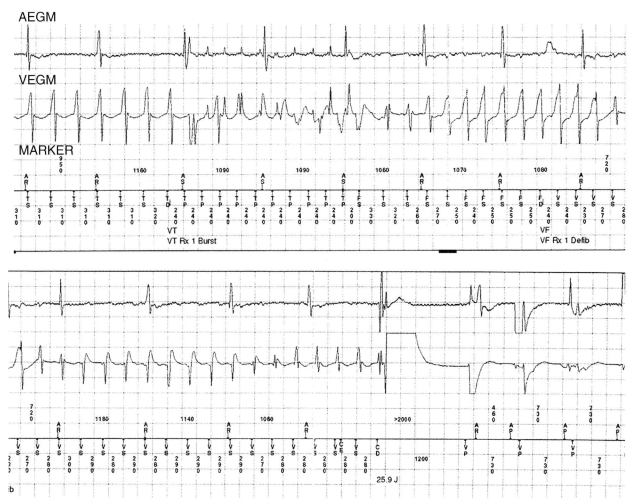

FIGURE 27–6. Electrograms recorded during ICD therapy. From top to bottom, recordings from the atrial (AEGM) and ventricular (VEGM) leads and device annotation (MARKER). The tracing begins with uniform VT (cycle length 310 msec) diagnosed by AV dissociation and an electrogram morphology different from that recorded in sinus rhythm. Antitachycardia pacing (VT Rx 1 Burst) is unsuccessful and accelerates the VT rate, resulting in detection in the VF zone, and a shock is delivered (CD).

the number of clinically relevant VT morphologies. In patients with large infarctions, multiple VT morphologies are typically induced with programmed stimulation. Although programmed stimulation identifies "what is possible," many of these morphologies may not be clinically relevant (i.e., they may not ever occur spontaneously). Often, the decision regarding which morphologies to ablate is made on the basis of the tachycardia cycle length (TCL) and the reproducibility of induction (slower, reproducibly induced VTs are thought more likely to be recurrent). Nonetheless, the gold standard for preprocedural planning is careful review of the ICD electrograms recorded during spontaneous VT episodes. As discussed earlier, the electrograms inscribed during VT episodes are fairly specific: different electrogram morphologies signify different VT morphologies (Fig. 27–7). Despite this fact, VT morphologies may be "paired" and represent different exit sites from the same circuit.[29] Still, ablation is more favorable if it is

limited to a small number of spontaneous VT morphologies, and it is less attractive as this number increases.

Finally, the patient's medical condition must be taken into account. Patients with end-stage heart failure may be intolerant of protracted procedures. Peripheral vascular disease may limit vascular access and increase the risks of complications. The patient must also be willing to accept the risk of major complications such as stroke.

Mapping

Independent of the strategy employed, the concept guiding VT ablation is similar to that for other arrhythmia substrates. Detailed mapping should precede ablation to minimize radiofrequency energy

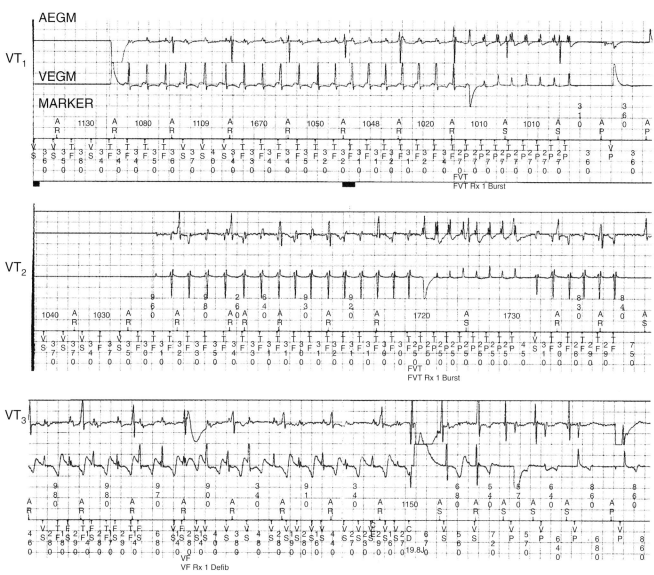

FIGURE 27–7. Multiple VT morphologies documented by stored electrograms during ICD therapy episodes collected during a single follow up visit. The recordings are arranged (top to bottom) with atrial (AEGM) and ventricular (VEGM) recordings (tip to ring) and annotation (MARKER). The ventricular electrogram recorded on each tracing is different in morphology, signifying distinct VT morphologies. In the bottom tracing, T wave oversensing is seen during VT, leading to double counting and false detection in the VF zone, leading to ICD shock.

(RF) delivery and the incidence of lesion-associated side effects (particularly stroke and heart failure). Several strategies are helpful in mapping VT in the setting of healed MI, depending on the arrhythmia presentation: (1) entrainment mapping for hemodynamically tolerated VT, (2) substrate mapping for unstable VT, and (3) mapping of triggers for polymorphic VT. Each of these strategies will be considered in turn.

ENTRAINMENT MAPPING

Entrainment refers to pacing during a reentrant arrhythmia to transiently accelerate the arrhythmia to the pacing cycle length, restoring the unchanged

tachycardia at the conclusion of pacing. Entrainment involves continuous resetting of the circuit; the paced wavefront enters the circuit during the time period of the excitable gap and exits after one revolution via the normal circuit exit. Because of this, the QRS during entrainment is a fusion of cardiac activation from the pacing site and from the tachycardia circuit. Seminal work by Waldo's research group[30-33] as well as others[34-36] developed the concept of entrainment (originally in atrial flutter), applied it to the circumstances of post-MI VT, and used it to demonstrate important properties of reentrant circuits. The concept at the heart of entrainment mapping for ablation of VT is targeting of a single site that will destroy the VT circuit. This site must be located not only within the circuit, but also in a protected and relatively narrow isthmus or channel. Although many of the mapping strategies to determine these characteristics were developed by previous investigators, a computer model and ablation verification study by Stevenson et al.[37,38] helped to crystallize understanding of these relationships (Fig. 27–8). Detailed mapping is performed during stable VT based on activation and response to pacing at multiple sites during VT (Table 27–3). The location of the protected isthmus is within the infarct zone and is typically predicted by bipolar electrogram voltages of 0.5 mV or less.[39,40] This anatomic construct provides for both the slow conduction necessary for the circuit and its narrow geometry (i.e., bounded by inexcitable areas) so that point RF lesions can abolish the circuit.

Before entry into the electrophysiology laboratory, knowledge of the patient's coronary anatomy and infarction pattern should be ascertained by review of coronary angiography, positron-emission tomography (PET), or magnetic resonance imaging (MRI) findings. This knowledge may help in selecting areas of interest for mapping and may influence the interpretation of ECGs. In addition, programmed ventricular stimulation is usually performed to initiate the clinical tachycardia and to determine the number of VT morphologies that are inducible. The process of entrainment mapping then proceeds in several steps (Fig. 27–8b). First, the general location of the VT circuit can be determined by analysis of the 12-lead ECG morphology during spontaneous and induced VTs (Table 27–4).[41,42] Under the best of circumstances,

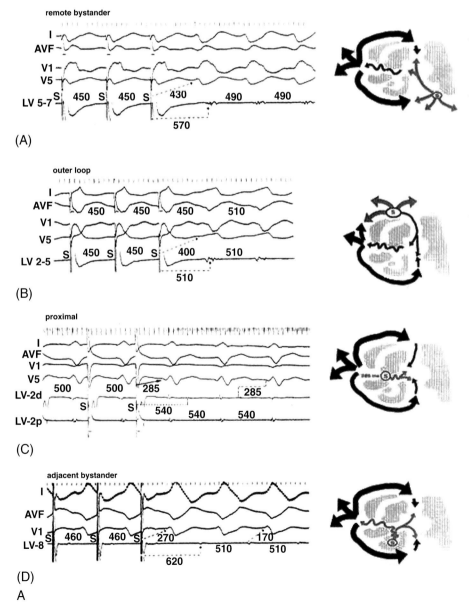

(A)

(B)

(C)

(D)

A

FIGURE 27–8. Panel A, Computer model of VT within inexcitable infarct scar (*grey stippled areas*, right panels), demonstrating the response to entrainment with pacing at different sites within the circuit. The circuit is depicted as a "figure of eight" activation utilizing a central common pathway with slow conduction. Pacings from remote bystander areas *(A)* will show some degree of fusion, and the return cycle is longer than the VT cycle length (by twice the conduction time from the site to the VT circuit). Pacing from outer loop sites *(B)* will show manifest entrainment, as the pacing site has access to recruit areas away from the circuit, as it is not bounded by the infarct. The return cycle length equals the tachycardia cycle length. Pacing from sites within the central pathway *(C)* demonstrate concealed entrainment with a stimulus to ECG equal to the electrogram to QRS during VT; the return cycle measured at this electrogram is equal to the VT cycle length. Pacing from adjacent bystander sites *(D)* result in concealed entrainment, but the return cycle is longer than the VT cycle length (by twice the conduction time from the site to the VT circuit). *(From Stevenson WG: Catheter ablation of ventricular tachycardia. In Zipes DP, Jalife J (eds.): Cardiac Electrophysiology: From Cell to Bedside, 3rd ed. Philadelphia: Saunders, 2004, p 1091, with permission.)*

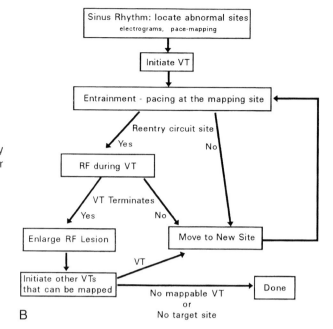

FIGURE 27–8, Panel B, Strategy for ablation of VT guided by entrainment mapping. **Panel C,** algorithm to determine catheter position relative to reentry VT circuit (see text for details).

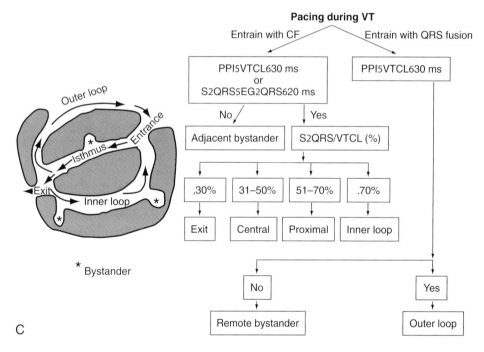

this exercise resolves the area of VT origin to approximately 4 cm². This technique has been recently reviewed.[42] Briefly, VT morphologies are examined for bundle branch pattern and axis, in the context of infarct location. Left bundle morphologies typically originate from the intraventricular septum (or, rarely in patients with coronary disease, from the right ventricle); right bundle morphologies originate from the parietal LV. Superior axis VT arises from the inferior LV (the inferior wall or inferior portion of the septum) and inferior axis VT from the superior LV (anterior wall or superior septum).

The precordial R wave transition helps to determine the site of origin in an apex-to-base dimension. VTs with positive R waves across the precordium arise from the mitral annulus, a posterior structure; VTs with negative QRS complexes across the precordium arise from the apex, which is an anterior site. VTs with a rightward axis usually arise from the lateral wall, or from the apex. However, ECG localization is very difficult in patients with anterior infarction and right bundle VT morphologies, because there are no consistent discriminating features between apical lateral versus septal sites of

TABLE 27-3

Targets for Ablation

Entrainment mapping strategy: ideal target sites are within the infarct (bipolar voltage <0.5 mV) and have components inscribed early in diastole (<70% of the VT cycle length before onset of the QRS)

Entrainment pacing from these target sites results in the following:

   Concealed entrainment on pace mapping

   Return cycle length = VT cycle length ± 30 msec

   Stimulus-to-QRS onset during pacing = electrogram − QRS during VT ± 20 msec

Substrate mapping strategy: "anchor points" for linear lesions are determined by pace mapping to match VT morphologies in the infarct border zone. Linear ablation is applied through these anchor points from the dense scar (<0.5 mV) to normal tissue (>1.5 mV) or anatomic barrier

Mapping triggers for polymorphic VT: Pace mapping at sites to match the surface ECG morphology of trigger beats. Sites typically display early Purkinje activation, both in sinus rhythm and during trigger PVCs.

ECG, electrocardiogram; PVCs, premature ventricular complexes; VT, ventricular tachycardia.

TABLE 27-4

Localization of the Ventricular Tachycardia Circuit by ECG

ECG Feature	Localization
Bundle branch morphology	
Right	Parietal LV
Left	LV Septum or right ventricle
Frontal plane axis	
Superior	LV inferior wall or inferior septum
Inferior	LV anterior wall or anterior septum
Right	LV lateral wall or apex
Precordial transition (R > S)	
Early ≤ V_3	Basal
Late ≥ V_4	Apical LV
Concordant upright	Mitral valve annulus
Concordant negative	apex
QRS upstroke	
Slurred	Epicardial

LV, left ventricle.

origin. Recent work by Patel et al.[43] demonstrated that relative timing of right ventricular apical activation may distinguish these sites. In the future, this question may be able to be resolved before the procedure by review of far-field (i.e., similar to the surface QRS) and near-field electrogram recordings from implanted defibrillators.

Programmed stimulation is performed to induce all "clinically relevant" VT morphologies and assess for hemodynamic tolerance. Different investigators have defined clinical relevance in different ways; variables to be considered include matching induced to spontaneous morphologies (on the surface ECG or ICD electrograms) and cycle length. There is some precedent to using a cutoff of 270 msec, which has been used in determining efficacy after surgical ablation and for some trials of catheter ablation as well.[44] In addition, slow VT tends to recur more frequently than rapid VT. Programmed stimulation typically yields more VT morphologies than have occurred spontaneously. Studies that have focused on induction of all possible morphologies of uniform VT yield an average of three to four morphologies per patient.[44,45] However, different morphologies are often related in "pairs" and can be ablated with the same lesion set.[29] An example of this is the left bundle/left superior and right bundle/right superior

axis VT pair commonly observed in inferior infarction, which both use the "mitral isthmus." In this case, the right bundle branch morphology tachycardia exits toward the lateral wall and the left bundle branch block morphology exits toward the septum.

Second, detailed activation mapping (and voltage mapping if applicable) is performed. If the patient is in hemodynamically stable VT, mapping is directed toward sites within the infarct zone that have high-frequency, isolated components that occur in mid-diastole and drive, rather than follow, the VT QRS. This relationship can be determined by observing a constant electrogram-to-QRS relationship with spontaneous alterations in cycle length or during the return cycle after pacing from a distant source (Fig. 27-9).[35] If the patient is in sinus rhythm due to poorly tolerated VT, mapping can proceed by pace mapping to generally reproduce the VT QRS morphology, starting at sites suggested by the ECG analysis that show fractionated potentials occurring after the end of the QRS. During pacing in sinus rhythm, sites of abnormal stimulus-to-QRS intervals (>40 msec, and ideally >70 msec) are noted.

Third, the relation of the individual site to the circuit is assessed with pacing at that site during VT (Fig. 27-10; see Fig. 27-8). If the patient is in sinus rhythm, VT must be induced at this point. Important

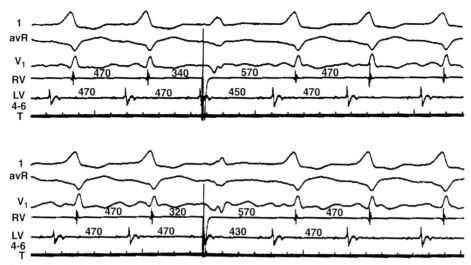

FIGURE 27–9. Relationship of diastolic potentials to the circuit. Surface ECG and intracardiac recordings from the RV and the LV within the infarct during sustained VT. The LV recording has a small component that precedes the surface QRS by 156 msec. Extrastimuli delivered from the RV apex reset the tachycardia and orthodromically capture the electrogram component. The electrogram to QRS interval is the same during the return cycle beats as during spontaneous VT. This consistent relationship to the circuit confirms that this electrogram site is early, rather than a remote bystander. *(From Josephson ME: Clinical Cardiac Electrophysiology: Techniques and Interpretations, Recurrent Ventricular Tachycardia, 2nd ed. Philadelphia: Lippincott Williams & Wilkins, 1993, with permission.)*

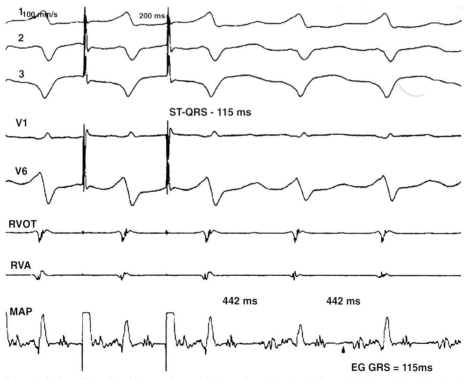

FIGURE 27–10. Characteristics of the "perfect map" for ablation of ventricular tachycardia. The optimal single ablation site for VT has the following characteristics: 1) entrainment from the site will produce an exact match of the spontaneous VT QRS in all 12 leads, 2) the return cycle (the duration from the pacing stimulus to the first non-paced beat, measured at the pacing site) will equal the VT cycle length, and 3) the stimulus (ST) to QRS will equal the electrogram (EG) to QRS. *(From El-Shalakany A, Hadjis T, Papageorgiou P, et al.: Entrainment/mapping criteria for the prediction of termination of ventricular tachycardia by single radiofrequency lesion in patients with coronary artery disease. Circulation 99:2283, 1999, by permission of the American Heart Association.)*

technical considerations include pacing just faster (usually by 20 msec) than the TCL at a current just sufficient to reliably capture the VT; some investigators insist that unipolar pacing should be used, to prevent the confounding influence of anodal capture at high output.[45] If the site is within the VT circuit and within a relatively protected zone of slow conduction, the following characteristics should be observed (see Fig. 27–10). First, the surface 12-lead ECG during entrainment pacing from this site should match that recorded during spontaneous VT. This is sometimes referred to as "entrainment with concealed fusion" or "concealed entrainment."[36] As discussed earlier, entrainment pacing from outside the protected isthmus produces a fusion QRS. If the pacing site is within a protected zone within the circuit, both the pacing site and the activation of the circuit from the pacing site are equivalently activating the heart via the VT exit site, so that no electrocardiographic fusion is observed. After pacing is stopped, the electrogram at the pacing site should again be activated one TCL after the last pacing stimulus. This follows from the idea that, if this site is within the circuit, after the last pacing stimulus the stimulated wavefront will traverse the VT circuit to again reach this site. A return cycle or postpacing interval (PPI) longer than the TCL indicates pacing from a bystander site. The formal way of expressing this concept is that the PPI should equal the TCL ± 30 msec. The PPI may be difficult to measure due to artifact on the ablation channel from pacing. This problem may be overcome by measuring the PPI from the proximal ablation electrodes after pacing from the distal electrode. This technique is well correlated with the true PPI but usually introduces some error. The PPI can also be estimated by comparing the interval of the two cycles after pacing to twice the TCL or by using a sophisticated "N + 1" method reported by Soejima et al.[46] Finally, the orthodromically captured electrogram components should keep identical relationships during pacing and spontaneous VT. In other words, the stimulus-to-QRS (S-QRS) interval during pacing should equal the electrogram-to-QRS interval during VT ± 20 msec. When expressed as a percentage of the TCL, the S-QRS interval also localizes the pacing site within the reentrant circuit (see Fig. 27–8C). Sites with S-QRS less than 30% of the TCL are considered to be near the circuit exit site, whereas those of more than 70% of the TCL are within an inner loop.

Stevenson et al.[37] provided the first "field testing" of these concepts in a unique study using VT termination during RF to assess the importance of the characteristics described earlier. RF lesions were more likely to terminate VT at sites that demonstrated concealed entrainment, a PPI approximating the TCL,

and an S-QRS greater than 60 msec but less than 70% of the TCL. Concealed entrainment alone was not sufficient to guide ablation, because 25% of sites where concealed entrainment was demonstrated were found to be bystander sites by analysis of the PPI and the S-QRS compared with the electrogram-QRS relationship. Sites with isolated diastolic potentials or continuous electrical activity were also demonstrated to be successful ablation targets; this observation was expanded in subsequent work by other investigators.[47,48] Ablation at sites that demonstrated combinations of these favorable characteristics (entrainment with concealed fusion, PPI, S-QRS interval, and isolated diastolic potentials or concealed entrainment) resulted in VT termination in 35% of applications, compared with 4% when these characteristics were absent. VT termination did not consistently correlate with elimination of that morphology in this study; this potential dichotomy is discussed later.

Subsequent work addressed the question of why these "ideal" characteristics were not absolutely predictive of successful VT ablation sites. Theoretically, three possibilities exist: either the lesion is not effective (considered in detail in a later section), the protected isthmus is broader than the volume of a single lesion, or mapping was insufficiently detailed. In a study by Bogun et al.,[40] the predictive value of combination of these favorable characteristics for VT termination increased to 70% to 90%; the most favorable of these characteristics was an isolated mid-diastolic potential that could not be dissociated from the tachycardia with pacing techniques. El-Shalakany et al.[49] demonstrated uniform success of ablation at a single site if all of the following were fulfilled: (1) an exact QRS match in all 12 leads during entrainment, (2) PPI less than 10 msec different from the TCL, and (3) S-QRS within 10 msec of the electrogram-to-QRS interval and less than 70% of the TCL. These studies strengthen the conceptual model and emphasize that successful VT ablation can be performed with ablation at a very limited number of sites using this strategy.

In order to apply entrainment mapping techniques, VT must be reproducibly inducible, hemodynamically well tolerated to allow prolonged mapping during VT, and stable (i.e., not accelerating or changing to different VT morphologies) during entrainment. This applies to a minority of patients with VT, estimated at approximately 10%[21]; however, this population is reasonably well represented in the population of patients with large infarcts and frequent VT recurrences. Strategies to improve hemodynamic tolerance during VT to facilitate mapping include the use of antiarrhythmic drugs to slow the VT rate (intravenous procainamide during the procedure or oral amiodarone before it), triggered atrial pacing during VT to provide atrioventricular synchrony, and blood pressure support with dopamine or intraaortic balloon counterpulsation.

SUBSTRATE MAPPING

The prerequisite conditions for entrainment mapping are often not met in contemporary patients referred for catheter ablation. In a consecutive series of patients referred for ablation for clinically tolerated VT, up to 25% could not be treated successfully with entrainment mapping techniques.[50] The primary reason for procedural failure was the inability to induce sustained, tolerated VT to allow detailed entrainment mapping.

The development of a new strategy for ablation of unstable VT was based on experience from surgical ablation of VT. Surgical ablation established the obligate relationship of the VT circuit and the infarct anatomy. Subendocardial resection prevented recurrent VT in more than 90% of patients who survived surgery.[51] Importantly, extension of the surgical lesion outside the visible infarct, to anatomic barriers such as the mitral annulus, further improved results.[52]

In attempting to recapitulate the surgical experience with catheter mapping, there were two immediate problems. First, although the surgeon could directly visualize the infarct anatomy, imaging techniques to represent the infarct were necessary during catheter mapping. Cassidy et al.[53] validated the concept of using bipolar electrogram characteristics (voltage, duration) to determine the underlying substrate at individual LV sites. We hypothesized that electroanatomic mapping could display the spatial orientation of the voltage information from many endocardial sites, allowing accurate representation of the infarct anatomy (Fig. 27–11). This concept has been validated by statistical analysis of normal bipolar electrograms (similar to the logic of the Cassidy analysis), by comparison to nuclear perfusion imaging, and in a porcine model of anterior infarction.[54,55] In the animal model, infarct size and topography by voltage mapping correlated well with functional (assessed by intracardiac echocardiography) and pathologic measurements. In clinical cases, confluent sites with bipolar electrogram amplitude of 0.5 mV or less represent dense scar; areas with electrograms between 0.5 and 1.5 mV represent the infarct border zone; and electrograms greater than 1.5 mV are recorded in normal areas. The characteristics of the critical isthmus, as defined by electroanatomic mapping, have been explored in detail.[56] In patients with prior MI and VT, the average isthmus length was 31 ± 7 mm, and the width was 16 ± 8 mm. During VT, the isthmus encompasses only diastolic potentials, and conduction time through the isthmus accounts for 57% to 81% of the TCL. Excluding perimitral circuits, the isthmus is usually oriented perpendicular to the mitral annulus in the septal, anteroapical, and inferolateral locations. In this study, double potentials indicating lines of block accounted for at least one boundary of the isthmus in 94% of VTs. The majority of VTs showed a double-loop reentry pattern (see Fig. 27–8).

Second, subendocardial resection removed 5 to 8 cm² of infarct substrate; the amount of substrate modification possible with current catheter ablation technology is orders of magnitude less. We hypothesized that linear lesions, delivered from the area of dense scar through the border zone and connecting out to anatomic barriers or normal myocardium, represent the closest approximation that could be accomplished in the electrophysiology laboratory. Linear lesions are constructed of individual point RF lesions and are directed to the area of the VT circuit by iden-

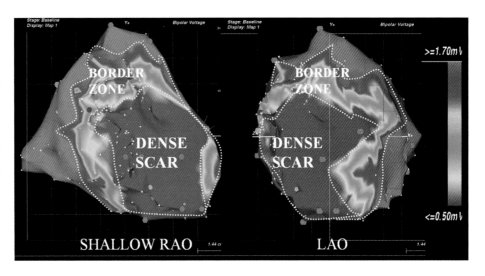

FIGURE 27–11. Electroanatomic voltage mapping. The LV endocardium is mapped in sinus rhythm to define the anatomy of the infarct scar. The color scheme is arranged so that confluent areas of *red color* correspond to the dense infarct (bipolar voltage ≤0.5 mV), *purple color* corresponds to normal tissue (bipolar voltage >1.7 mV), and the border zone in the "*rainbow*" of colors in between. Votage scale shown on right.

tifying the presumed exit site of the circuit through pace mapping to match the 12-lead ECG morphology of the targeted VT. Single-point ablation guided by analysis of individual electrograms during sinus rhythm or pace mapping has proved insufficient to guide VT ablation; ablation of regions of the border zone using multiple contiguous lesions can successfully interrupt individual VT circuits. Again, unlike surgical ablation, which can remove the substrate for all possible VT circuits, the linear ablation technique is focused on individual VT morphologies. The steps used in a linear ablation procedure are detailed in Figure 27–12.

Other investigators have modified the anatomic approach, extending linear lesions across identified isthmuses of VT circuits or between "islands" of unexcitable segments (i.e., demonstrating failure to capture at high outputs) within the infarct[57,58] or ablating all fractionated electrograms within the infarct zone. Further information regarding the ori-

entation of the VT circuit relative to the anatomy of the infarct may help to optimize anatomic ablation techniques. Arenal et al.[59] recently demonstrated the potential utility of examining the infarct anatomy for relatively high-voltage channels that may serve as preferential routes of VT circuit conduction. These channels can be identified by careful voltage mapping in sinus rhythm and could presumably be used for empiric linear ablation (although this was not performed in this study). These observations confirm preliminary results presented from our laboratory (see Fig. 27–3).[60] Channels of preferential conduction appear evident during VT mapping using unipolar, noncontact mapping systems (Fig. 27–13). Furthermore, discrete VT exit sites may correlate with sites of exit during pacing from within the infarct.[61] These observations provide further insight into the relation of the VT circuit to the infarct anatomy and may argue for linear ablation tangential, as opposed to radial, to the infarct.

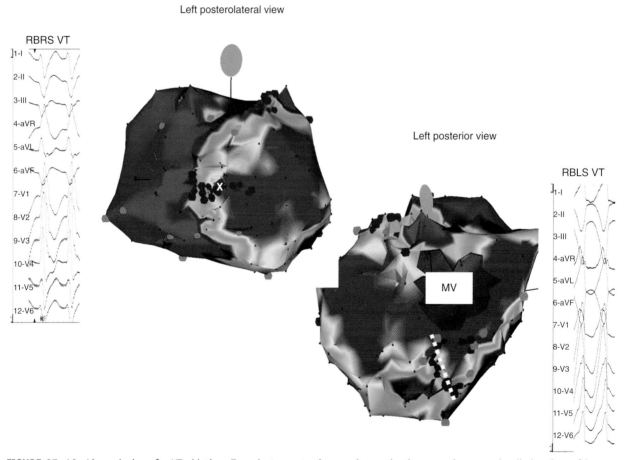

FIGURE 27–12. Linear lesions for VT ablation. Two electroanatomic mapping projections are shown to detail the sites of best pace map match for two clinical VTs with right bundle right superior axis (RBRS) and RB left superior axis (LS) morphologies. The exit site of each VT morphology is approximated by pace mapping in the infarct border zone. Using the site of closest pace map match as an "anchor," a linear lesion (red dots) is fashioned as a radial line from the dense infarct out to normal tissue or an anatomic obstacle such as the mitral annulus. MV, mitral value.

FIGURE 27–13. Noncontact mapping to demonstrate "channels" in the VT circuit. A cast of the LV is shown with a color scheme denoting isopotential mapping. Resting tissue is shown in *purple*; as sites are activated and generate negative unipolar voltage, colors from *blue to white* (depending on voltage) are displayed. Two segments of an isopotential map recorded during VT in a patient with a small basal inferior infarction (*outlined by the thick black line*). Conduction seems to enter (left panel) and exit (right panel) the infarct zone in specific zones. The exit from the infarct always occurs at the onset of the surface QRS; often there is considerable delay, perhaps due to impedance mismatch between the small mass of myocardium in the infarct and the healthy tissue outside.

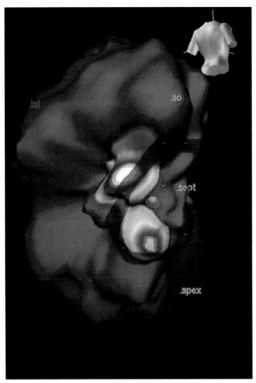 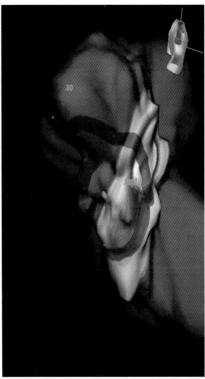

VT circuit entrance   VT circuit exit

MAPPING OF TRIGGERS FOR POLYMORPHIC VENTRICULAR TACHYCARDIA

Electrophysiologic mapping techniques cannot be applied to localization of non-uniform arrhythmias such as polymorphic VTs. Although substrate mapping could potentially be applied, this technique is typically anchored by location of a specific uniform VT morphology. Haissaguerre et al.[62] demonstrated that premature ventricular beats from relatively predictable anatomic locations may serve as the initiating events in patients with idiopathic ventricular fibrillation.

This group recently extended their original observations in patients with healed MI.[15] Five patients with MI and depressed ejection fraction were observed to have multiple episodes of polymorphic VT initiated by repetitive uniform premature beats (Fig. 27–14). Interestingly, three of the patients were treated very early after MI, at a time when automaticity in the surviving Purkinje network surrounding infarcted tissue is thought to play an important role in arrhythmogenesis. Activation and pace mapping of these inciting beats demonstrated that they consistently arose from Purkinje fibers at the infarct border. Often, Purkinje spikes had varying intervals to the earliest ventricular activation, and the morphology of successive triggering beats changed in turn. Splitting of the Purkinje signal and Purkinje-to-ventricular block also were observed. Ablation targeting these sites resulted in freedom from recurrent arrhythmias in all patients over a follow-up period of 16 ± 5 months, documented by ICD monitoring in all patients.

Ablation

Traditionally, VT mapping and ablation has been performed with 4-mm-tip catheters, using standard, temperature-controlled RF ablation. The precision of mapping, particularly as it applies to the electrode "field of view" during pacing, is better with smaller electrodes. The obvious tradeoff is the reduction in lesion size with smaller electrodes. Although only limited data are available on this issue, it is clear that this effect is even more important in infarcted tissue (Fig. 27–15).[63] As discussed later, this often limits procedural efficacy, and the use of large (8-mm) electrodes or irrigated ablation may be necessary in some cases. Typical power and temperature settings with standard 4-mm-tip catheters are similar to those used for other left-sided ablation procedures (50 W, 52° C, 60 seconds). In our laboratory, a temperature cutoff of 52° C is used, because we have observed an

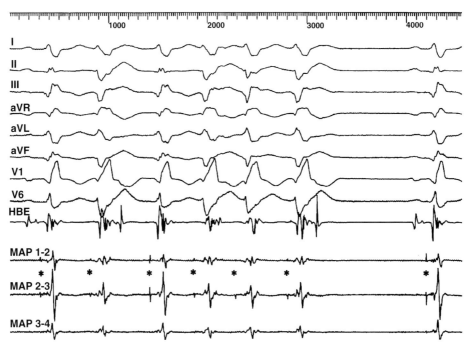

FIGURE 27-14. Mapping and ablation of Purkinje triggers of polymorphic VT. This recording was made in a patient with frequent episodes of polymorphic VT, all preceded by RBBB PVCs. In the EP lab, a run of RBBB PVCs was observed. Note the Purkinje potential (asterisk) recorded on the mapping catheter (MAP), present on PVC beats and during sinus. Both the Purkinje-ventricular interval and the morphology of the PVCs change from beat to beat. Ablation of the Purkinje system trigger resulted in freedom from recurrent polymorphic VT. *(From Szumowski L, Prashanthan S, Franciszek W, et al.: Mapping and ablation of polymorphic ventricular tachycardia after myocardial infarction. J Am Coll Cardiol 44:1700-1706, 2004, with permission.)*

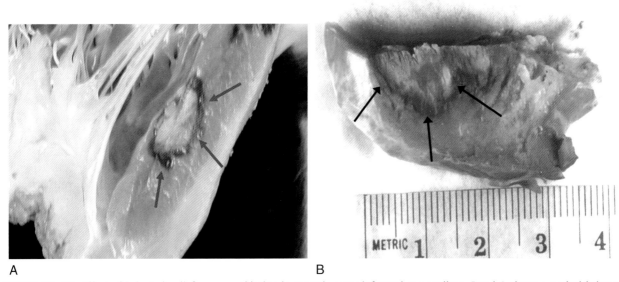

A   B

FIGURE 27-15. Effect of irrigated radiofrequency ablation in normal versus infarcted myocardium. Panel **A** shows a typical irrigated ablation lesion delivered to normal porcine ventricular myocardium. Lesions are typically 1 cm in diameter, and approximately 7 mm in depth. Irrigated ablation in infarcted tissue (Panel **B**) results in smaller lesions. Here a series of lesions were delivered to create a linear lesion. Individual lesions were 5-7 mm in diameter and 4-6 mm deep. *(B, from Callans DJ, Ren JF, Narula N, et al.: Effects of linear, irrigated-tip radiofrequency ablation in porcine healed anterior infarction. J Cardiovasc Electrophysiol 12:1037, 2001, with permission.)*

increased incidence of coagulum (without consistent evidence of impedance rise) when higher temperatures are reached. Impedance is also carefully monitored, because an excessive drop in impedance may also predict impending rise. Multiautomated RF generators (e.g., Stockert generator, Biosense Webster, Baldwin Park, Calif.) with automatic switch-off for preselected temperature and impedance parameters are helpful in this regard. Irrigated RF ablation systems may be used as the primary ablation modality or as an alternative to standard RF ablation. In a multicenter trial of an irrigated ablation catheter, it was possible to ablate all mappable VTs in 106 (75%) of 146 patients.[64] During follow-up, however, 46% of all patients experienced sustained VT recurrences. Compared with standard RF, irrigated systems may show greater efficacy in VT termination, suggesting larger lesion sizes.[63-69]

RF energy is usually applied during VT (if the tachycardia is tolerated) to determine whether ablation at a particular site leads to VT termination, verifying the site's importance in VT circuit maintenance. Although this information is critical, ablation during VT does present additional difficulties, including catheter stability at higher heart rates and on sudden VT termination. Termination during ablation is a good sign, but it is not equivalent to permanent destruction of the VT circuit. The adequacy of lesion formation can also be assessed by monitoring for impedance drop during RF delivery, electrogram amplitude reduction, and inability to pace the ablation site at 10 mA output after ablation. Programmed electrical stimulation must be repeated after apparent acute success, both to determine whether the targeted VT has been eliminated and to assess for the presence of additional VT morphologies. Some investigators argue for late followup programmed stimulation to assess efficacy,[44] because programmed stimulation during the index procedure may be less reliable as to the effects of lesion recovery and anesthesia. The end points for ablation in substrate mapping may be noninducibility of the relevant VTs or elimination of all suspected channels and/or abnormal electrograms within the infarct zone.

The success of VT ablation as a management strategy is less than completely clear. Most reports on ablation concentrate on technical details of mapping and ablation and are limited by short-term observation of highly selected patients. Nonetheless, the acute success of entrainment mapping and morphology-specific ablation is reasonable, ranging from 67% to 96% of VTs in recent published trials.[21,37,44,45,49,64,70-73] These trials represent, for the most part, "on-treatment" analysis, with "enrollment" only after tolerated VT is reproducibly induced in the laboratory.

Limited data suggest that intention-to-treat analysis yields less favorable results.[50] Clinical follow-up in these trials is typically over a 2- to 3-year horizon. Most patients (approximately 90%) have freedom from targeted VT morphologies that were successfully ablated; however, the risk of development of new clinical VTs is fairly high. Some investigators advocate ablation of all mappable VTs (i.e., rather than just the "clinical" VTs) to decrease the incidence of "new" VT morphologies in follow-up.[44,45,64] Even in these series, however, the risk of recurrence is 30% to 46%, despite multiple procedures and continued antiarrhythmic drug therapy in selected patients. The lingering effects of antiarrhythmic drugs, particularly amiodarone, during the ablation procedure is another confounding influence on intermediate-term results. In our experience, after apparently successful VT ablation, the freedom from any VT recurrence in follow-up (mean, 28 months) was higher in patients who were maintained on the same antiarrhythmic drug regimen compared with patients in whom drugs were discontinued after ablation (64% versus 32%, respectively).[74]

Another important observation in series of VT ablation is the high all-cause mortality in patients who require VT ablation after MI. Data from ablation series range from 12% to 30% mortality at 36 to 40 months, to 51% at 5 years.[45,72,73] The majority of these deaths are caused by progressive structural heart disease and refractory heart failure, although sudden, presumably arrhythmic death is also observed, arguing for adjunctive ICD therapy.

The initial experience with substrate-based VT ablation was in 16 patients with drug-refractory, unmappable VT (9 patients had healed infarction). Before ablation, patients had experienced 6 to 55 episodes of VT per month, resulting in frequent ICD shocks. Ablation was performed with a 4-mm-tip catheter and standard RF energy (up to 50 W, 52° C, 60 seconds duration). Delivery of a median of 55 RF lesions to construct four linear lesions (each through the exit site of a specific VT morphology) resulted in successful control of arrhythmia in all but one patient over a mean of 8 months of follow-up.[54] Importantly, ventricular function did not change after the procedure, despite extensive ablation in patients with advanced structural heart disease. More extensive follow-up in a larger population, including 36 patients with healed infarction, demonstrated freedom from arrhythmia recurrence in 64% and infrequent VT recurrence in 25%.[75] Even in the 11% who had frequent VT episodes (defined as more than one episode in a 3-month period), there was a considerable reduction in episodes (from a preablation mean of 30 per month) and ICD shocks after the procedure. These results were obtained largely with standard RF technology and 4-mm-tip catheters. The results of this technique with larger catheters, and particularly with irrigated-tip RF ablation, may be considerably better.

Complications

The procedural risks of VT ablation are higher than for most other electrophysiologic procedures. Potential problems include stroke, MI, cardiac perforation, aortic valve damage, catheter entrapment in the mitral apparatus, heart failure, peripheral vascular complications, and death. This is due to the inherent risk of extensive ablation in the left circulation, but, more importantly, to the presence of significant structural heart disease and comorbidities in a sick patient population. Before catheter mapping and ablation, an assessment to exclude active coronary ischemia or LV thrombus is essential. Recognized procedural risks for post-MI VT ablation include stroke (from mechanical dislodgment of atheromatous material or thrombus formation secondary to the ablation process), coronary artery embolism or injury, mechanical trauma to the aortic valve, cardiogenic shock, tamponade, heart block, and vascular complications. Cardiogenic shock may be a consequence of the

requisite prolonged duration of VT episodes required for mapping or of "stunning" of healthy myocardium due to ablation of adjacent infarcted myocardium.[63] In the 1998 North American Society of Pacing and Electrophysiology (NASPE; now called the Heart Rhythm Society) Prospective Catheter Ablation Registry,[76] significant procedural complications were observed in 3.8% of patients, but this statistic was not specific to patients with post-MI VT. A recent multicenter trial reported a more realistic incidence of 8% major complications (including death in 2.7%) and 6% minor complications.[64] Obviously, the incidence of complications varies greatly with operator experience as well as patient comorbidities, particularly peripheral or cerebral vascular disease and active ischemia.

Troubleshooting the Difficult Case

There are several factors that can make a procedure more difficult than initially expected. First, even in patients with VT that has been well tolerated clinically, there are instances in which only poorly tolerated VT is induced or the VT is noninducible. As

TABLE 27–5

Troubleshooting the Difficult Case

Problem	Causes	Solution
Unmappable VT		
Poor hemodynamic stability during VT	Ventricular dysfunction	Slow VT rate with drugs; support blood pressure with atrial pacing, pressors, balloon pump; use noncontact mapping, substrate mapping, optimize filling pressures
Noninducible	Autonomically or ischemically mediated	Programmed stimulation on dopamine or isoproterenol, substrate mapping during sinus rhythm, linear ablation
Ineffective RF delivery		
	Small lesion size	Irrigated RF ablation or large-tip catheter and high-output generator
	Poor catheter contact	Change catheter reach, stiffness, change approach (e.g., trans-septal from retrograde aortic)
	Low current delivery	Irrigated RF ablation
	Wide isthmus	Linear lesion or irrigated catheter
	Wrong site	Continue mapping
	Misdiagnosis	Consider bundle branch or fascicular reentry
Diffuse area of early activation	Intramural or epicardial site of origin	Transcutaneous pericardial approach for epicardial mapping, map RV septum

RF, radiofrequency; RV, right ventricular; VT, ventricular tachycardia.

discussed earlier, substrate mapping during sinus rhythm can be performed if the VT is unmappable, but most strategies require at least documentation of the 12-lead ECG morphology to provide some aspect of the VT circuit to target. Other strategies, such as empiric ablation based on the infarct anatomy, the presence of relatively high-voltage conducting channels, or ablation of fractionated potentials within the infarct, may be utilized. Although these strategies may be effective, they cannot be verified if it is impossible to induce VT in the first place.

Second, repeated ablation lesions can fail to produce the desired effect of VT termination or elimination. There are two possibilities in this circumstance. The most likely is inadequate power delivery. This can be recognized in temperature-control mode by achieving target temperature at very low power settings (often just a few watts). In this situation, there is also minimal change in the electrogram recorded by the distal ablation electrode after ablation. In my opinion, the temptation to increase the temperature limit should be avoided, because of the increased risk of thromboemboli. Instead, more power can be safely delivered if irrigated ablation is used. Irrigated RF lesions are routinely larger than standard RF lesions, particularly in infarcted tissue, because more current can be delivered if the limitation of high temperature at the catheter-tissue interface is removed.[63-69] The only problem with this situation, which is frequently encountered in our practice, is the lack of irrigated catheters that can be used with magnetic electroanatomic mapping. A second reason for apparently ineffective ablation is inaccuracies in mapping. Reliance solely on activation mapping data provided by sophisticated three-dimensional mapping systems may leave one particularly susceptible to this error. These systems can easily identify the earliest activation in the chamber mapped. Apparent "early" activation due to bystander sites needs to be discerned with entrainment mapping techniques. In addition, VT that comes from a source outside the chamber being evaluated (right ventricular, intramural, epicardial) often cannot be ablated at the site of earliest activation in that chamber. Careful attention to unipolar electrogram morphologies, or the diffuse nature of early activation, may be helpful in this regard (Fig. 27–16).

Techniques for transcutaneous epicardial ablation, developed by Sosa et al.[77] initially for treatment of VT in the setting of chagasic cardiomyopathy, may be helpful in selected patients with healed infarction.[78,79] Initially this seemed contrary to the conventional wisdom, formed largely with the surgical ablation experience, that VT circuits were primarily endocardial. Nonetheless, even if the majority of the circuit is endocardial, it is conceivable that individual vulnerable circuit sites may be epicardial or intramyocardial. Experience with this technique may be helpful in selected patients.

Some of the uncertainties of VT mapping and ablation may be resolved with improved imaging capabilities. Intracardiac echocardiography and MRI may be helpful in providing more anatomically relevant imaging during VT ablation, allowing real-time visualization of catheter contact and the relationship with the infarct scar, as well as validation of lesion creation. The impact of these adjunctive modalities is presently being assessed.

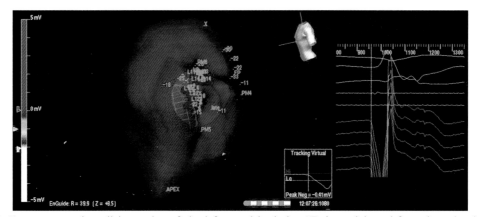

FIGURE 27–16. Noncontact endocardial mapping of the left ventricle during VT that originated from the epicardium. In the left panel, a cast of the LV is shown with a color scheme denoting isopotential mapping. Resting tissue is shown in *purple*; as sites are activated and generate negative unipolar voltage, colors from *blue to white* (depending on voltage) are displayed. At the onset of the surface QRS, there is a diffuse area (*light blue*) of the LV activated at the same time. In the right panel, selected unipolar recordings are compared to the surface QRS. The peak negative dV/dT in all recordings occurs after the onset of the surface QRS. Both of these observations suggest that the recorded sites are not the true origin of the VT. This VT was later mapped and successfully ablated using a transcutaneous approach to the pericardial space.

Summary

Ablation of VT in the setting of healed MI can have a profound influence on clinical care in patients with frequent recurrence or incessant VT. Such patients typically receive multiple ICD shocks, and often multiple attempts at antiarrhythmic therapy have failed. VT ablation is more technically difficult and is subject to a higher risk of complications than many other ablation procedures. Operators should have considerable experience with VT mapping techniques (both entrainment and substrate mapping) before embarking on these procedures, especially in patients with severe structural heart disease. The results of VT ablation in terms of elimination of targeted VT morphologies are fairly favorable; however, the disease process after index infarction is progressive, and new VT circuits can develop over time. VT ablation is palliative at present because of this consideration; optimally, ICD therapy is concurrently employed to prevent against the residual risk of sudden cardiac death. It is hoped that ongoing research will address this limitation, specifically whether new technology and understanding can allow development of true substrate modification to prevent both present and future VT circuits.

References

1. Strickberger SA, Man KC, Daoud EG, et al.: A prospective evaluation of catheter ablation of ventricular tachycardia as adjuvant therapy in patients with coronary artery disease and an implantable cardioverter-defibrillator. Circulation 96:1525, 1997.
2. Calkins H, Bigger JT Jr, Ackerman SJ, et al.: Cost-effectiveness of catheter ablation in patients with ventricular tachycardia. Circulation 101:280, 2000.
3. Sarter BH, Finkle JK, Gerszten RE, Buxton AE: What is the risk of sudden cardiac death in patients presenting with hemodynamically stable sustained ventricular tachycardia after myocardial infarction? J Am Coll Cardiol 28:122, 1996.
4. Caruso AC, Marcus FI, Hahn EA, et al.: Predictors of arrhythmic death and cardiac arrest in the ESVEM trial. Electrophysiologic Study Versus Electromagnetic Monitoring. Circulation 96:1888, 1997.
5. Josephson ME: Clinical Cardiac Electrophysiology: Techniques and Interpretations, 3rd ed. Philadelphia: Lippincott Williams & Wilkins, 2002.
6. de Bakker JM, Janse MJ: Pathophysiological correlates of ventricular tachycardia in hearts with a healed infarct. In Zipes DP, Jalife J (eds.): Cardiac Electrophysiology: From Cell to Bedside, 3rd ed. Philadelphia: Saunders, 2000, pp 415-421.
7. Peters NS, Coromillas J, Severs NJ, Wit AL: Disturbed connexin43 gap junction distribution correlates with the location of reentrant circuits in the epicardial border zone of healing canine infarcts that cause ventricular tachycardia. Circulation 95:988, 1997.
8. de Bakker J, van Capelle F, Janse M, et al.: Reentry as a cause of ventricular tachycardia in patients with chronic ischemic heart disease: Electrophysiologic and anatomic correlation. Circulation 77:589, 1988.
9. de Bakker J, van Capelle F, Janse M, et al.: Slow conduction in the infarcted human heart: "Zigzag" course of activation. Circulation 88:915, 1993.
10. Buxton AE, Lee KL, DiCarlo L, et al.: Electrophysiologic testing to identify patients with coronary artery disease who are at risk for sudden death. Multicenter Unsustained Tachycardia Trial Investigators. N Engl J Med 342:1937, 2000.
11. Echt DS, Liebson PR, Mitchell LB, et al.: Mortality and morbidity in patients receiving encainide, flecainide, or placebo. The Cardiac Arrhythmia Suppression Trial. N Engl J Med 324:781, 1991.
12. Gomes JA, Mehta D, Ip J, et al.: Predictors of long-term survival in patients with malignant ventricular arrhythmias. Am J Cardiol 79:1054, 1997.
13. Exner DV, Pinski SL, Wyse DG, et al.: Electrical storm presages nonsudden death: The Antiarrhythmics Versus Implantable Defibrillators (AVID) Trial. Circulation 103:2066, 2001.
14. Wyse DG, Friedman PL, Brodsky MA, et al.: Life-threatening ventricular arrhythmias due to transient or correctable causes: High risk for death in follow-up. J Am Coll Cardiol 38:1718, 2001.
15. Szumowski L, Prashanthan S, Franciszek W, et al.: Mapping and ablation of polymorphic ventricular tachycardia after myocardial infarction. J Am Coll Cardiol 44:1700-1706, 2004.
16. Wellens HJ, Bar FW, Lie KI: The value of the electrocardiogram in the differential diagnosis of a tachycardia with a widened QRS complex. Am J Med 64:27, 1978.
17. Kindwall KE, Brown J, Josephson ME: Electrocardiographic criteria for ventricular tachycardia in wide complex left bundle branch block morphology tachycardias. Am J Cardiol 61:1279, 1988.
18. Antunes E, Brugada J, Steurer G, et al.: The differential diagnosis of a regular tachycardia with a wide QRS complex on the 12-lead ECG: Ventricular tachycardia, supraventricular tachycardia with aberrant intraventricular conduction, and supraventricular tachycardia with anterograde conduction over an accessory pathway. Pacing Clin Electrophysiol 17:1515, 1994.
19. Callans DJ, Hook BG, Marchlinski FE: Use of bipolar recordings from patch-patch and rate sensing leads to distinguish ventricular tachycardia from supraventricular rhythms in patients with implantable cardioverter defibrillators. Pacing Clin Electrophysiol 14:1917, 1991.
20. Sarter BH, Hook BG, Callans DJ, Marchlinski FE: Effect of bundle branch block on local electrogram morphologic features: Implications for arrhythmia diagnosis by stored electrogram analysis. Am Heart J 131:947, 1996.
21. Morady F, Harvey M, Kalbfleisch S, et al.: Radiofrequency catheter ablation of ventricular tachycardia in patients with coronary artery disease. Circulation 87:363, 1993.
22. Callans DJ, Josephson ME: Ventricular tachycardia in patients with coronary artery disease. In Zipes DP, Jalife J (eds.): Cardiac Electrophysiology: From Cell to Bedside, 3rd ed. Philadelphia: Saunders, 2004, pp 569-574.
23. Wathen MS, Sweeney MO, DeGroot PJ, et al.: Shock reduction using antitachycardia pacing for spontaneous rapid ventricular tachycardia in patients with coronary artery disease. Circulation 104:796, 2001.
24. Pacifico A, Hohnloser SH, Williams JH, et al.: Prevention of implantable-defibrillator shocks by treatment with sotalol: D,L-Sotalol Implantable Cardioverter-Defibrillator Study Group. N Engl J Med 340:1855, 1999.
25. Dorian P, Borggrefe M, Al-Khalidi H, et al.: Placebo-controlled randomized clinical trial of azimilide for prevention of

ventricular tachyarrhythmias in patients with an implantable cardioverter defibrillator. Circulation 110:3646-3654, 2004.

26. Julian DG, Prescott RJ, Jackson FS, Szekely P: Controlled trial of sotalol for one year after myocardial infarction. Lancet 1:1142, 1982.

27. Camm AJ, Pratt CM, Schwartz PJ, et al.: AzimiLide post Infarct surVival Evaluation (ALIVE) Investigators. Mortality in patients after a recent myocardial infarction: A randomized, placebo-controlled trial of azimilide using heart rate variability for risk stratification. Circulation 109:990, 2004.

28. The Atrial Fibrillation Follow-up Investigation of Rhythm Management (AFFIRM) Investigators: A comparison of rate control and rhythm control in patients with atrial fibrillation. N Engl J Med 347:1825, 2002.

29. Fitzgerald DM, Friday KJ, Yueng-Lai-Wah JA, et al.: Myocardial regions of slow conduction participating in the reentrant circuit of multiple ventricular tachycardias: Report on ten patients. J Cardiovasc Electrophysiol 2:193, 1991.

30. Callans DJ, Hook BG, Josephson ME: Comparison of resetting and entrainment of uniform sustained ventricular tachycardia: Further insights into the characteristics of the excitable gap. Circulation 87:1229, 1993.

31. Henthorn RW, Okumura K, Olshansky B, et al.: A fourth criteria for transient entrainment: The electrogram equivalent of progressive fusion. Circulation 77:1003, 1988.

32. Okumura K, Henthorn RW, Epstein AE, et al.: Further observation on transient entrainment: Importance of pacing site and properties of the components of the reentry circuit. Circulation 72:1293, 1985.

33. Okumura K, Olshansky B, Henthorn RW, et al.: Demonstration of the presence of slow conduction during sustained ventricular tachycardia in man: Use of transient entrainment of the tachycardia. Circulation 75:369, 1987.

34. Almendral JM, Gottlieb CD, Rosenthal ME, et al.: Entrainment of ventricular tachycardia: Explanation for surface electrocardiographic phenomena by analysis of electrograms recorded within the tachycardia circuit. Circulation 77:569, 1988.

35. Fontaine G, Frank R, Tonet J, et al.: Identification of a zone of slow conduction appropriate for ventricular tachycardia ablation: Theoretical considerations. Pacing Clin Electrophysiol 12:262, 1989.

36. Morady F, Kadish AH, Rosenheck S, et al.: Concealed entrainment as a guide for catheter ablation of ventricular tachycardia in patients with prior myocardial infarction. J Am Coll Cardiol 1917:678, 1991.

37. Stevenson W, Khan H, Sager P, et al.: Identification of reentry circuit sites during catheter mapping and radiofrequency ablation of ventricular tachycardia late after myocardial infarction. Circulation 88:1647, 1993.

38. Stevenson WG, Friedman PL, Sager PT, et al.: Exploring postinfarction reentrant ventricular tachycardia with entrainment mapping. J Am Coll Cardiol 1929:1180, 1997.

39. Stevenson WG, Weiss JN, Weiner I, et al.: Fractionated endocardial electrograms are associated with slow conduction in humans: Evidence from pace mapping. J Am Coll Cardiol 13:369, 1989.

40. Bogun F, Bahu M, Knight BP, et al.: Comparison of effective and ineffective target sites that demonstrate concealed entrainment in patients with coronary artery disease undergoing radiofrequency ablation of ventricular tachycardia. Circulation 95:183, 1997.

41. Miller JM, Marchlinski FE, Buxton AE, Josephson ME: Relationship between the 12-lead electrocardiogram during ventricular tachycardia and endocardial site of origin. Circulation 77:759, 1988.

42. Josephson ME, Callans DJ: Using the twelve-lead electrocardiogram to localize the site of origin of ventricular tachycardia. Heart Rhythm 2:443-444, 2005.

43. Patel VV, Rho RW, Gerstenfeld EP, et al.: Right bundle-branch block ventricular tachycardias: Septal versus lateral ventricular origin based on activation time to the right ventricular apex. Circulation 110:2582, 2004.

44. Rothman SA, Hsia HH, Cossu SF, et al.: Radiofrequency catheter ablation of postinfarction ventricular tachycardia: Long-term success and the significance of inducible nonclinical arrhythmias. Circulation 96:3499, 1997.

45. Stevenson WG, Friedman PL, Kocovic D, et al.: Radiofrequency catheter ablation of ventricular tachycardia after myocardial infarction. Circulation 98:308, 1998.

46. Soejima K, Stevenson WG, Maisel WH, et al.: The N + 1 difference: A new measure for entrainment mapping. J Am Coll Cardiol 37:1386, 2001.

47. Bogun F, Bahu M, Knight BP, et al.: Response to pacing at sites of isolated diastolic potentials during ventricular tachycardia in patients with previous myocardial infarction. J Am Coll Cardiol 30:505, 1997.

48. Bogun F, Hohnloser SH, Bender B, et al.: Mechanism of ventricular tachycardia termination by pacing at left ventricular sites in patients with coronary artery disease. J Interv Card Electrophysiol 6:35, 2002.

49. El-Shalakany A, Hadjis T, Papageorgiou P, et al.: Entrainment/mapping criteria for the prediction of termination of ventricular tachycardia by single radiofrequency lesion in patients with coronary artery disease. Circulation 99:2283, 1999.

50. Callans DJ, Zado E, Sarter BH, et al.: Efficacy of radiofrequency catheter ablation for ventricular tachycardia in healed myocardial infarction. Am J Cardiol 82:429, 1998.

51. Miller J, Kienzle M, Harken A, Josephson M: Subendocardial resection for ventricular tachycardia: Predictors of surgical success. Circulation 70:624, 1984.

52. Hargrove WC 3rd, Miller JM, Vassallo JA, Josephson ME: Improved results in the intraoperative management of ventricular tachycardia related to inferior wall infarction: Importance of the annular isthmus. J Thorac Cardiovasc Surg 92:726, 1986.

53. Cassidy DM, Vassallo JA, Miller JM, et al.: Endocardial catheter mapping during sinus rhythm: Relation of underlying heart disease and ventricular arrhythmia. Circulation 73:645, 1986.

54. Marchlinski FE, Callans DJ, Gottlieb CD, Zado E: Linear ablation lesions for control of unmappable ventricular tachycardia in patients with ischemic and nonischemic cardiomyopathy. Circulation 101:1288, 2000.

55. Callans DJ, Ren J-F, Michele J, et al.: Electroanatomic left ventricular mapping in the porcine model of healed anterior myocardial infarction: Correlation with intracardiac echocardiography and pathological analysis. Circulation 100:1744, 1999.

56. de Chillou C, Lacroix D, Klug D, et al.: Isthmus characteristics of reentrant ventricular tachycardia after myocardial infarction. Circulation 105:726, 2002.

57. Soejima K, Suzuki M, Maisel WH, et al.: Catheter ablation in patients with multiple and unstable ventricular tachycardias after myocardial infarction: Short ablation lines guided by reentry circuit isthmuses and sinus rhythm mapping. Circulation 104:664, 2001.

58. Soejima K, Stevenson WG, Maisel WH, et al.: Electrically unexcitable scar mapping based on pacing threshold for identification of the reentry circuit isthmus: Feasibility for guiding ventricular tachycardia ablation. Circulation 106:1678, 2002.

59. Arenal A, del Castillo S, Gonzalez-Torrecilla E, et al.: Tachycardia-related channel in the scar tissue in patients with

sustained monomorphic ventricular tachycardias: Influence of the voltage scar definition. Circulation 110:2568, 2004.

60. Hsia HH, Callans DJ, Kocovic D, et al.: Characterization of endocardial substrate for reentrant uniform ventricular tachycardia in man [abstract]. Pacing Clin Electrophysiol 25:611, 2000.

61. Jacobson J, Michele J, Lazar S, et al.: Characterization of arrhythmogenic substrate and ventricular tachycardia circuits with non-contact unipolar mapping in a porcine model of myocardial infarction [abstract]. J Am Coll Cardiol 45:106A, 2005.

62. Haissaguerre M, Shoda M, Jais P, et al.: Mapping and ablation of idiopathic ventricular fibrillation. Circulation 106:962, 2002.

63. Callans DJ, Ren JF, Narula N, et al.: Effects of linear, irrigated-tip radiofrequency ablation in porcine healed anterior infarction. J Cardiovasc Electrophysiol 12:1037, 2001.

64. Calkins H, Epstein A, Packer D, et al.: Catheter ablation of ventricular tachycardia in patients with structural heart disease using cooled radiofrequency energy: Results of a prospective multicenter study. Cooled RF Multi Center Investigators Group. J Am Coll Cardiol 35:1905, 2000.

65. Nakagawa H, Yamanashi WS, Pitha JV, et al.: Comparison of in vivo tissue temperature profile and lesion geometry for radiofrequency ablation with a saline-irrigated electrode versus temperature control in a canine thigh muscle preparation. Circulation 91:2264, 1995.

66. Delacretaz E, Stevenson WG, Winters GL, et al.: Ablation of ventricular tachycardia with a saline-cooled radiofrequency catheter: Anatomic and histologic characteristics of the lesions in humans. J Cardiovasc Electrophysiol 10:860, 1999.

67. Soejima K, Delacretaz E, Suzuki M, et al.: Saline-cooled versus standard radiofrequency catheter ablation for infarct-related ventricular tachycardias. Circulation 103:1858, 2001.

68. Ren JF, Callans DJ, Michele JJ, et al.: Intracardiac echocardiographic evaluation of ventricular mural swelling from radiofrequency ablation in chronic myocardial infarction: Irrigated-tip versus standard catheter. J Interv Card Electrophysiol 5:27, 2001.

69. Watanabe I, Masaki R, Min N, et al.: Cooled-tip ablation results in increased radiofrequency power delivery and lesion size in the canine heart: Importance of catheter-tip temperature monitoring for prevention of popping and impedance rise. J Interv Card Electrophysiol 6:9, 2002.

70. Kim YH, Sosa-Suarez G, Trouton TG, et al.: Treatment of ventricular tachycardia by transcatheter radiofrequency ablation in patients with ischemic heart disease. Circulation 89:1094, 1994.

71. Bogun F, Bahu M, Knight BP, et al.: Comparison of effective and ineffective target sites that demonstrate concealed entrainment in patients with coronary artery disease undergoing radiofrequency ablation of ventricular tachycardia. Circulation 95:183, 1997.

72. O'Callaghan PA, Poloniecki J, Sosa-Suarez G, et al.: Long-term clinical outcome of patients with prior myocardial infarction after palliative radiofrequency catheter ablation for frequent ventricular tachycardia. Am J Cardiol 87:975, 2001.

73. Della Bella P, De Ponti R, Uriarte JA, et al.: Catheter ablation and antiarrhythmic drugs for haemodynamically tolerated post-infarction ventricular tachycardia: Long-term outcome in relation to acute electrophysiological findings. Eur Heart J 23:414, 2002.

74. Marchlinski FE, Zado E, Callans DJ, et al.: Hybrid therapy for ventricular arrhythmia management. In Miller JM (ed.): Cardiology Clinics: Ventricular Arrhythmias. Philadelphia: Saunders, 1999, pp 391-406.

75. Alonso C, Lin D, Poku J, et al.: The role of transcatheter ablation in the prevention of sudden death. In Santini M (ed.): Sudden Death: Nonpharmacological Treatment. Rome: Adrianna Editrice, 2002.

76. Scheinman MM, Huang S: The 1998 NASPE prospective catheter ablation registry. Pacing Clin Electrophysiol 23:1020, 2000.

77. Sosa E, Scanavacca M, d'Avila A, Pilleggi F: A new technique to perform epicardial mapping in the electrophysiology laboratory. J Cardiovasc Electrophysiol 7:531, 1996.

78. Sosa E, Scanavacca M, d'Avila A, et al.: Nonsurgical transthoracic epicardial catheter ablation to treat recurrent ventricular tachycardia occurring late after myocardial infarction. J Am Coll Cardiol 35:1442, 2000.

79. Schweikert RA, Saliba WI, Tomassoni G, et al.: Percutaneous pericardial instrumentation for endo-epicardial mapping of previously failed ablations. Circulation 108:1329, 2003.

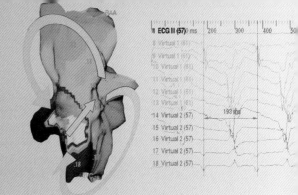

28

Ablation of Ventricular Tachycardias Associated with Nonischemic Cardiomyopathies

Mark A. Wood

Key Points

- The mechanisms of bundle branch reentry is reentry. The mechanisms ventricular tachycardia (VT) associated with right ventricular dysplasia, dilated cardiomyopathy, and Chagas' disease are reentry and possibly triggered activity.

- Ablation targets include the specialized conduction system for bundle branch reentry and sites defined by activation, entrainment, substrate, and/or pace mapping for other VTs.

- No special equipment is needed for ablation of bundle branch reentry. In other cases, computerized mapping systems are valuable, and large-tip or irrigated-tip ablation systems may be needed.

- Sources of difficulty include the following: for bundle branch reentry, ablation of broad left bundle; for right ventricular dysplasia, multiple inducible morphologies and high recurrence rates; for dilated cardiomyopathy, multiple morphologies with epicardial or intramyocardial circuits and high recurrence rates; and for Chagas' disease, epicardial foci (common).

- Success rates are 100% for bundle branch reentry and variable (often 50% to 60%) for other etiologies.

Ventricular tachycardias (VTs) may occur in any condition that results in ventricular failure or dysfunction. Ablation of VT has been most thoroughly investigated for patients with coronary artery disease, and the techniques developed from this experience are applicable to nonischemic cardiomyopathies as well. The clinical experience with ablation of VT related to nonischemic cardiomyopathies is limited, however. Like ablation of VT with coronary artery disease, VT ablation in nonischemic cardiomyopathies is almost entirely palliative and adjunctive, because most cases are also managed with implantable defibrillators and drug therapy as well. Although case reports may exist for the ablation of VT associated with a variety of nonischemic cardiomyopathies, this chapter focuses on ablation for conditions in which some systematic study has been undertaken. These conditions include bundle branch reentry (BBR), right ventricular dysplasia (RVD), dilated cardiomyopathy (DCM), and Chagas' disease.

Bundle Branch Reentry

BBR VT accounts for about 6% of sustained monomorphic VTs induced at electrophysiologic testing.[1-3] The incidence of the arrhythmia is much greater in certain patient populations.[4,5] In patients with nonischemic DCM, this mechanism may be responsible for up to 41% of inducible sustained monomorphic VTs.[1] This mechanism may be under-recognized clinically and at electrophysiologic testing. With the current trend toward early defibrillator implantation without electrophysiologic testing in patients with VTs, under-recognition is likely to continue. The diagnosis is important to make, because BBR VT is highly amenable to catheter ablation.[2]

ANATOMY

The atrioventricular (AV) node crosses the central fibrous body to become the penetrating portion of the AV bundle (Fig. 28–1). This penetrating portion of the bundle of His emerges from the central fibrous body to rest on the crest of the muscular ventricular septum.[6-8] This portion of the bundle enters the lower region of the pars membranacea, then courses for a variable distance to become the branching portion of the bundle.[6] The branching bundle lies at the lower part of the membranous ventricular septum, above the ventricular summit and below the noncoronary or posterior aortic cusp. This portion of the bundle

varies considerably in its dimensions, usually from 6.5 to 20 mm in length and 1 to 3 mm in width.[7] As it courses apically, it first gives rise to the fascicles of the left bundle branch (LBB). In general, the LBB fibers are subendocardial and very superficial. The main LBB is about 1 cm in width at its origin and extends 1 to 3 cm in length before giving rise to the posterior and anterior fascicles.[7] The main LBB first gives rise to the larger posterior fascicle and then to the smaller anterior fascicle. Fibers from these two fascicles merge at the midseptal level to form the septal branch of the left bundle.[6,7] The anterior fascicle courses along the anterior septal wall of the left ventricle to the base of the anterior papillary muscle. The posterior fascicle runs inferiorly from the His bundle to course along the posterior septum to the posterior papillary muscle. The left bundle is made up of one or more large bands of fibers, and the fascicles are networks of fine strands rather than single discrete structures. In some cases, the entire left-sided conduction system is an extensive network of fibers without discrete fascicles. In contrast, the right bundle branch (RBB) is a discrete entity formed by the continuation of the His bundle beyond the septal crest (see Fig. 28–1). As the right bundle emerges from the membranous septum, it proceeds along the lower portion of the septal band to reach the moderator band. It then reaches the anterolateral papillary muscle, where it ramifies into branches. At least the midportion of the right bundle, and sometimes its entire extent, is found intramyocardially. Mapping of the distal right bundle is often made difficult by its passage within the substance of the septomarginal trabeculation. The right bundle is usually about 50 mm long and 1 mm wide.[7]

PATHOPHYSIOLOGY

As the name indicates, BBR VT involves sustained macroreentry utilizing the bundle branches as obligatory limbs of the circuit connected proximally by the bundle of His and distally by the ventricular myocardium (Fig. 28–2).[1-3,9] At electrophysiologic testing, right ventricular premature stimuli introduced after a drive train of relatively long but constant cycle length results in retrograde conduction to the His bundle by way of the RBB.[1] At shorter coupling intervals, retrograde block occurs in the right bundle due to its longer refractory period, and retrograde conduction occurs solely over the LBB. As the coupling interval shortens even further, progressive delay in trans-septal myocardial conduction and the retrograde left bundle results in prolongation of the V_2H_2 interval. With a sufficiently long V_2H_2 interval, the right bundle may recover excitability, allowing antegrade conduction past the site of initial retro-

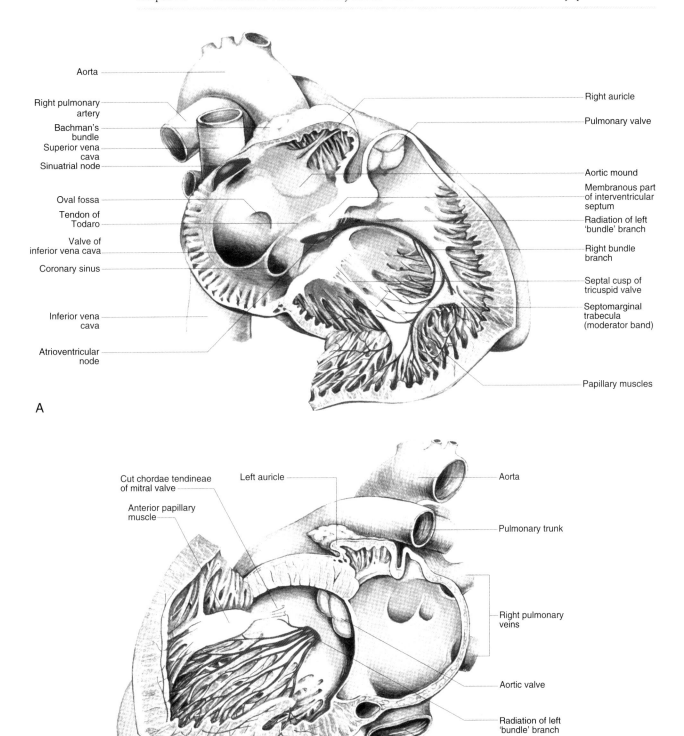

FIGURE 28–1. Anatomy of the specialized conduction system. **A,** The cord-like right bundle branch is a continuation of the bundle of His extending to the papillary muscle on the interventricular septum. **B,** The left bundle branch is short and broad before branching extensively to form the anterior and posterior fascicles. *(From Shah P: Heart and great vessels. In Standring S (ed.): Gray's Anatomy, 39th ed. Edinburgh: Elsevier, 2005, pp 995-1029, with permission.)*

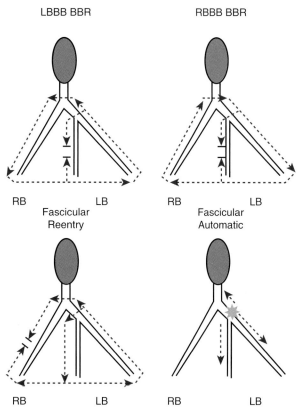

FIGURE 28–2. Schematics of reentrant circuits for bundle branch reentry (BBR), interfascicular reentry and automatic fascicular tachycardia. LB, left bundle branch; LBBB, left bundle branch block; RB, right bundle branch; RBBB, right bundle branch block. *(Modified from Tchou P, Mehdirad AA: Bundle branch reentry ventricular tachycardia. Pacing Clin Electrophysiol 18:1427-1437, 1995, with permission.)*

grade block and resulting in a reentrant beat of ventricular activation. These single BBR beats (V_3 phenomenon) are noted in 50% of patients with normal His-Purkinje conduction systems undergoing electrophysiologic testing.[9,10] With abrupt changes in cycle length, up to three consecutive BBR beats may be inducible in normal patients.[10] The rapid conduction and long refractory periods of the His-Purkinje system prevent sustained BBR in normal hearts, usually by retrograde block in the LBB.[11] In the setting of conduction delay in the His-Purkinje system, sustained BBR may occur. As described previously, the induced tachycardia would have an LBB morphology due to antegrade conduction and ventricular activation over the RBB. The left bundle branch block (LBBB) morphology is the most commonly induced and spontaneously occurring form of BBR VT.[1,12] This most likely results from the shorter LBBB refractoriness, preferential retrograde LBB conduction in most patients[1,12] and the common use of right ventricular pacing at electrophysiologic testing. BBR VT with right bundle branch block (RBBB) morphology is less

common and results from reversal of the direction of activation in the reentrant circuit (see Fig. 28–2). During right ventricular pacing, this may result from earlier retrograde block in the LBB or from recovery of retrograde RBB conduction after bilateral BBB due to the gap phenomenon.[1] Excellent detailed descriptions of the pathophysiology of BBR have been published by Blanck et al.[1,13]

In addition, interfascicular reentry involving the anterior and posterior fascicles of the LBB system has been described (see Fig. 28–2).[14-16] In this tachycardia, one of the fascicles serves as the antegrade limb and the other as the retrograde circuit. The distal link between the fascicles occurs through the ventricular myocardium. Interfascicular VT may be the clinical arrhythmia, or it may be inducible after ablation for BBR VT.[16] Finally, VT arising from automaticity in the right and left fascicular systems may occur.[16] Idiopathic left VT utilizing portions of the left fascicular systems is described in Chapter 26.

DIAGNOSIS AND DIFFERENTIAL DIAGNOSIS

Virtually all patients with BBR VT have underlying structural heart disease and evidence of His-Purkinje system disease. Dilated cardiomyopathy is present in 45% of these patients.[1] Coronary artery disease is also a frequent diagnosis. Other diagnoses associated with BBR are aortic valve replacement and muscular dystrophies.[4,5] BBR has also been described in association with mitral valve disease, Ebstein's anomaly, and hypertrophic cardiomyopathy.[17-20] BBR may occur without structural heart disease in association with fixed or functional His-Purkinje conduction delays.[13,21]

Surface Electrocardiogram

Virtually all patients with BBR VT demonstrate intraventricular conduction delays in sinus rhythm. These abnormalities may be RBBB or LBBB, but nonspecific delays are common as well. The presence of RBBB or LBBB on the electrocardiogram (ECG) may indicate conduction delay rather than complete block in a bundle branch that would preclude BBR VT. Complete antegrade bundle branch block may be present with intact retrograde conduction over the bundle to allow for BBR VT. Because ventricular activation occurs via antegrade conduction through the RBB or LBB, the ECG appearance is that of a typical RBBB or LBBB tachycardia and may be identical to the QRS morphology in sinus rhythm (Fig. 28–3). In BBR VT, an LBBB configuration is far more common and may be associated with a normal or leftward axis. Rightaxis deviation is rare and is seen only with preexisting right-axis deviation in sinus rhythm. RBBB VT

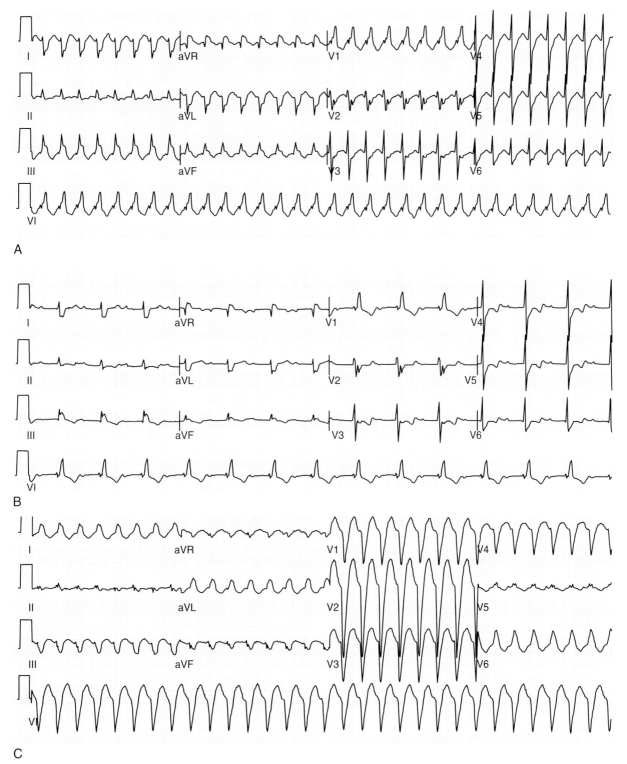

FIGURE 28–3. ECGs from the same patient during bundle branch reentry (BBR) with right bundle branch block morphology (**A**), sinus rhythm (**B**), and bundle branch reentry with left bundle branch morphology (**C**). The patient presented with sustained right bundle branch block BBR after aortic valve replacement. Note that the right bundle branch block QRS morphology in tachycardia is identical to that in sinus rhythm. The left bundle branch block BBR was induced at electrophysiologic testing.

is usually associated with a left-axis deviation, but normal and right-axis deviation may occur as well. The cycle length of BBR VT is typically short (<300msec), and the tachycardia is usually poorly tolerated hemodynamically. Interfascicular reentry has an RBBB pattern due to ventricular activation antegrade through one of the left fascicles. The direction of antegrade conduction in the left anterior or posterior fascicle determines the electrical axis.[1,16] VT from fascicular automaticity may have an LBBB or RBBB pattern, depending on the fascicle of origin.[16] In all three types of VT, the VT QRS often closely resembles the QRS in sinus rhythm, providing a clue to the diagnosis.[16]

Electrophysiologic Testing

At baseline, virtually all patients have prolongation of the His-to-ventricle (HV) interval, averaging 75 to 80msec (range, 60 to 110msec).[12,16] BBR VT has been reported in patients with a normal HV interval and ECG at baseline who demonstrated functional HV prolongation at higher rates.[21] The tachycardia is typically induced with ventricular extrastimulus testing, especially with the use of short-long-short protocols, but it may be induced with atrial pacing in some patients.[1,12] The abrupt cycle length prolongation by the long interval may result in more distal retrograde block in the His-Purkinje system, allowing more time to recover excitability in the antegrade direction. LBBB morphology VT is most commonly induced in the laboratory. Rarely, left ventricular pacing is required to induce this pattern.[1,12] RBBB morphology may be inducible in about 10% of patients but more commonly requires left ventricular pacing to initiate.[1,12] The induced BBR VT morphology may not match the clinical VT morphology (i.e., the contralateral bundle branch morphology is induced), especially if the clinical VT has an RBBB pattern (see Fig. 28–3).[1,12] Isoproterenol or class IA drug infusion (to prolong His-Purkinje conduction delays) may be needed for induction.[1] The diagnostic criteria for BBR VT are given in Table 28–1.

The QRS morphology in VT must be consistent with ventricular activation through the RBB or LBB. Each ventricular depolarization should be preceded by depolarization of the His, RBB, and LBB. For LBBB VT, RBB activation immediately precedes ventricular activation. Ventricular activation is followed by LBB activation and then activation of the His bundle (Fig. 28–4). For RBBB pattern VT, LBB immediately precedes ventricular activation, which in turn is followed by activation of the RBB and then the His. The exact timing of His and antegrade conducting bundle branch activation depends on the relative conduction velocities of each of these structures.

The HV interval during VT is characteristically similar to or slightly longer (by 10 to 20msec) than the interval in sinus rhythm. This may result from rate-related changes in conduction velocity or from anisotropic conduction during retrograde activation of the His.[22] Occasionally, the HV is shorter because the retrograde activation to the His bundle is more rapid than antegrade conduction down the bundle branch. For RBBB pattern BBR VT, the changes in HV interval from sinus rhythm may be more marked.[1] Because of the obligatory involvement of the His-Purkinje system, changes in tachycardia cycle length should be preceded by changes in the bundle-to-bundle (H-H) interval. Cycle length variation may be most common immediately after induction of the tachycardia. In addition, tachycardia induction depends on a critical degree of conduction delay in the conduction system and is terminated by block within the His-Purkinje system. The tachycardia may be advanced by premature activation of the His, RBB, or LBB. The tachycardia should be entrained from the right ventricular apex, which produces a short postpacing interval of less than 30msec.[23] BBR VT may show concealed entrainment from the atrium if AV nodal conduction is enhanced with atropine.[24]

Interfascicular reentry similarly demonstrates variations in the R-R interval preceded by changes in the H-H interval. In contrast to BBR, the HV interval in interfascicular reentry is shorter than that in sinus rhythm (Fig. 28–5).[14] Also in left interfascicular reentry, an RBBB QRS morphology should be recorded. In BBR, the His bundle activation should precede the left fascicular activation. In interfascicular reentry however, activation of the His bundle follows that of the left fascicular potentials (see Fig. 28–5).[14] Reentry can occur in opposite directions within the circuit in the same patient.[14]

Fascicular automaticity arising in the fascicular system appears to be a rare phenomenon.[16] The tachycardia may arise from either the RBB or the LBB. Clues to this diagnosis are failure to induce the tachycardia with programmed extrastimuli with, instead, dependence on catecholamines. Importantly, the HV interval as measured to the start of the QRS during tachycardia is variable. Purkinje potentials are recorded near the focus and demonstrate a short and consistent relationship to the QRS (Fig. 28–6).

Differential Diagnosis

The differential diagnosis of BBR VT includes interfascicular VT, automatic fascicular VT, idiopathic left ventricular VT, intramyocardial VT, supraventricular tachycardia with aberrancy, and atriofascicular reciprocating tachycardia. Interfascicular reentry is diagnosed by an RBBB VT pattern with an HV interval

TABLE 28–1

Diagnostic Criteria for Bundle Branch Reentry and Fascicular Tachycardias

Bundle branch reentry

QRS morphology in tachycardia demonstrates an LBBB or RBBB pattern consistent with ventricular activation through the appropriate bundle branch.

Each ventricular depolarization is preceded by His, left bundle, or right bundle activation with the appropriate sequence of activation for the tachycardia QRS morphology with stable bundle electrogram-to-ventricle intervals

Spontaneous variations in the V-V interval are preceded by similar changes in the H-H or bundle-to-bundle interval.

Tachycardia induction depends on achieving a critical conduction delay in the His-Purkinje system. The HV interval in tachycardias is typically longer than in sinus rhythm.

The tachycardia can be terminated by block in the His-Purkinje system and rendered noninducible by ablation of the RBB or LBB.

A short PPI (<30 msec) is obtained from the RVA.

Left interfascicular reentry

QRS morphology in tachycardia demonstrates an RBBB consistent with ventricular activation antegrade over the left anterior or posterior fascicle.

Each ventricular depolarization is preceded by a left fascicular potential, and activation of the His and right bundle follows left fascicular activation in tachycardia.

The HV interval is shorter than that recorded in sinus rhythm.

Tachycardia induction depends on critical delay within the left fascicular system.

The tachycardia can be terminated by block in the left fascicular system and rendered noninducible by ablation of the left anterior or posterior fascicle.

Automatic fascicular tachycardia

QRS morphology in tachycardia demonstrates a LBBB or RBBB pattern consistent with ventricular activation through the appropriate bundle branch.

Tachycardia is induced by catecholamine administration but not by programmed stimulation; classic entrainment criteria are not met.

Each ventricular depolarization in tachycardia is preceded by a Purkinje potential, and activation of the His and bundle branch occurs after Purkinje activation.

The HV interval during tachycardia as measured to the start of the QRS may be variable.

H-H, His bundle-to-His bundle; HV, His-to-ventricle; LBB(B), left bundle branch (block); RBB(B), right bundle branch (block); V-V, ventricle-to-ventricle; PPI, post pacing interval; RVA, right ventricular apex.

FIGURE 28–4. Intracardiac recordings demonstrating the sequence of activation of His-Purkinje system during bundle branch reentry. The tachycardia has a left bundle branch block morphology. The right ventricle is activated by conduction antegrade in the right bundle (RB). The RB potential precedes the ventricular activation. The right ventricular apex activation follows then retrograde activation of the left bundle (LB). The His bundle (H) is then activated to complete the circuit. Note that changes in the H-H interval are followed by similar changes in the V-V interval. The atria are in fibrillation. 1, 2, V1, surface ECG; HB, His bundle; HRA, high right atrium; RV, right ventricle. *(From Blanck Z, Sra J, Dhala A, et al.: Bundle branch reentry: Mechanisms, diagnosis and treatment. In Zipes DP, Jalife J (eds.): Cardiac Electrophysiology: From Cell to Bedside, 2nd ed. Philadelphia: Saunders, 1995, pp 878-885, with permission.)*

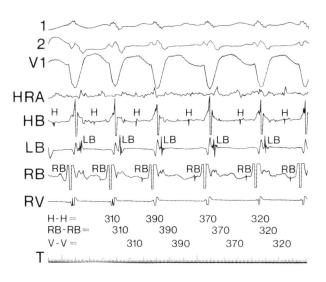

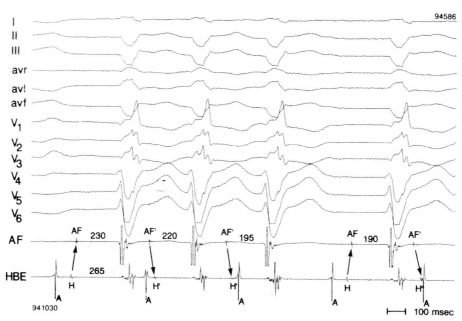

FIGURE 28–5. ECG and electrograms demonstrating interfascicular reentry. From top to bottom: all 12 surface ECG leads. The first beat is sinus rhythm with block in the anterior fascicle distal to the recording site given the left axis deviation. Two beats of interfascicular reentry follow after antergrade conduction in the posterior fascicle and retrograde activation of the anterior fascicle. After activation of the His, antegrade conduction over the left posterior fascicle activates the ventricle. Note the reversal of the sequence of activation of the His and anterior fascicle (AF) potentials during reentry. After the 2nd reentry beat retrograde conduction block occurs in the anterior fascicle. The QRS complex is identical in sinus and fascicular reentry. ', indicates retrograde activation; A, atrial electrogram; AF, anterior fascicular recording; H, His electrogram; HBE, His bundle electrogram. (From Ref. 14)

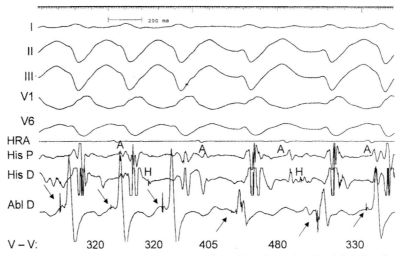

FIGURE 28–6. Electrograms of focal automatic fascicular tachycardia arising from the distal left bundle branch Purkinje system. The successful ablation site shows a sharp, discrete potential (*arrows*) preceding ventricular activation. Note the irregularity of the V-V intervals that are preceded by changes in the interval between these early potentials. I, II, III, V1, V6, surface ECG; A, atrium; ABL, ablation electrogram; D, distal; H, His bundle electrogram; HRA, high right atrium; P, proximal; V, ventricle. *(From Lopera G, Stevenson WG, Soejima K, et al.: Identification and ablation of three types of ventricular tachycardia involving the His-Purkinje system in patients with heart disease. J Cardiovasc Electrophysiol 15:52-58, 2004, with permission.)*

shorter than the HV interval in sinus rhythm and left fascicular activation before His activation.[14,16] Fascicular automaticity is catecholamine dependent, is not induced with programmed stimulation, and shows a variable HV interval in tachycardia.[16] Idiopathic left

ventricular VT has a negative or short HV interval in tachycardia and a normal baseline QRS and HV interval.[25] As with interfascicular VT, the His activation follows activation of the left fascicles, which is inconsistent with RBBB pattern BBR VT. VT arising from myocardial foci rarely produces entirely typical RBBB or LBBB patterns on surface ECG, as is expected with BBR. In addition, the His activation is usually late in the QRS complex and may be dissociated from the tachycardia.

Supraventricular tachycardias with bundle branch block aberrancy can be distinguished from BBR by the antegrade activation of both bundle branches. Reciprocating tachycardias show an obligatory 1:1 atrium-to-ventricle (A/V) relationship that is not present in BBR. AV nodal reentry may be terminated with adenosine. The ventricular postpacing interval after entrainment of the tachycardia from the right ventricular apex may differentiate BBR VT from myocardial VT and from AV nodal reentry.[23] The postpacing interval with BBR is short (<30 msec) because the RBB inserts into the ventricular apex. For myocardial VT (unless originating in the apex) and AV nodal reentry with aberrancy, the postpacing intervals greatly exceed 30 msec. An unusual form of BBR that uses the AV node as its proximal "turn-around" point has been described, as have other poorly characterized adenosine-sensitive variants of BBR (Fig. 28–7).[26,27] For atrial tachycardias, dependency on atrial activation and AV nodal conduction is diagnostic. Features differentiating BBR from other wide-complex tachycardias are listed in Table 28–2.

MAPPING

Bundle Branches

BBR VT may be prevented by ablation of either the right or left main bundle branch.[1,2,28] Even though most patients demonstrate more conduction system disease in the left bundle, the right bundle is typically the target for ablation. This is because of the technical ease of ablation of the right bundle in contrast to the difficulties involved in ablation of the left bundle. Left bundle ablation requires arterial access, increased risk of complications, and more extensive ablation to transect this broad structure. In patients with complete antegrade block in the left bundle, RBB ablation necessitates permanent pacing. Complete antegrade LBBB is likely if left bundle potentials are recorded intermittently or after the ventricular electrogram in sinus rhythm or if catheter-induced trauma to the right bundle results in transient complete heart block.[28] In these cases, LBB ablation may be preferred if there is no other indication for pacemaker or ICD implantation. Induction of complete LBBB by ablation of both the anterior and posterior fascicles is curative for patients with both BBR and interfascicular VT.

The RBB is usually easily identified along the basilar right ventricular septum.[28] After a large His

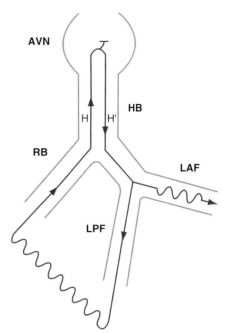

FIGURE 28–7. Proposed circuit for an unusual form of adenosine sensitive bundle branch reentry tachycardia utilizing the AV node as the proximal "turnaround" point. During the tachycardia 2 separate and adjacent His potentials are recorded without any other intervening electrograms. This represents retrograde then antegrade conduction in the His. AVN, AV node; H, retrograde His recording; H', antegrade His recording; HB, His bundle; LAF, left anterior fascicle; LPF, left posterior fascicle; RB, right bundle. *(From Markowitz SM, Stein KM, Englestein ED, et al.: A-V nodal-His-Purkinje reentry: A novel form of tachycardia. J Cardiovasc Electrophysiol 6:400-409, 1995, with permission.)*

potential is recorded, the catheter is advanced apically in the right anterior oblique view to record the RBB (Fig. 28–8). The RBB must be differentiated from the His potential in this region. The RBB is identified by the absence or minimal amplitude of an atrial electrogram and by a His-RRB interval of greater than 15 msec in sinus rhythm.[2,28] If RBB conduction delay is present, the RBB potential may be obscured by the local ventricular activation in sinus rhythm. In this case, the right bundle potential may not be identifiable in sinus rhythm and may be evident only during retrograde conduction during sustained BBR or BBR echo beats (Fig. 28–9).[29] If the RBB is not well recorded at the basilar septum, mapping of the more distal course of the RBB may be effective (Fig. 28–10).

As described earlier, the LBB arises as a broad band of fibers directed inferiorly from the bundle of His. The left main bundle is typically about 1 to 3 cm in length and 1 cm wide but shows great individual variation. Methods for recording the LBB potential have been reported.[2,28] After crossing the aortic valve,

TABLE 28–2

Differential Diagnostic Features of Bundle Branch Reentry and Related Tachycardias

Tachycardia Type	Baseline QRS	QRS in Tachycardia	HV in Tachycardia	His-Fascicular Activation	V-A Dissociation	Response to Adenosine	Response to Verapamil	V-V Changes Preceded By	Reset By	Onset Dependent On
BBR	Prolonged	Typical RBBB or LBBB	Prolonged or same as HV in sinus	LBBB VT: RB-V-LB-H; RBBB VT: LB-V-RB-H	Common	No	No	Similar change in H-H interval	Advancing His or BB	Critical delay in His-Purkinje system
Interfascicular	Prolonged	Typical RBBB	Shorter than in sinus	LBB before His	Possible	Unknown	Unknown	Similar changes in fascicular activation	Advancing left fascicular system	Critical delay in left fascicular system
Fascicular automatic	Prolonged	RBBB or LBBB	Variable	RBBB VT: LBB before His; LBBB VT: RBB before His	Possible	Unknown	Unknown	Changes in distal fascicular potentials	Advancing distal fascicular activation but not entrained	Catecholamine stimulation
Idiopathic LV VT	Normal	Typical RBBB	Negative (occurring after V)	Left fascicles or Purkinje fibers before His	Possible	Yes	Yes	Changes in presystolic P-P potential interval	Advancing left fascicular activation or P potential	Critical delay in left fascicular and/or involved myocardium

Intramyocardial VT	Normal or prolonged	Atypical BBB patterns	Negative or very short	Fascicles before His if measurable	Common	No	No			
Aberrant SVT	Normal or prolonged	Typical RBBB or LBBB	Same as in sinus or slightly prolonged	His before fascicles	AT: A > V possible; AVNRT: unlikely; AVRT: not possible	Common	Common	Changes in H-H	AT: advancing A; AVNRT: possibly advancing septal A; AVRT: advancing A or V activation	AT: critical A-A interval; AVNRT: critical AH interval; AVRT: Critical AV interval
Atriofascicular AP	Normal or minimal preexcitation	LBBB	Shorter than in sinus or negative value	RBB before His	Not possible	Yes	Yes	Changes AM or MM potential interval	Advancing atrial insertion site	Antegrade AV nodal block and critical delay in AV interval over AP

Column categories (top of table): Unrelated to His-Purkinje system; Advancing ventricular myocardium; Critical V-V coupling intervals

A, atrium; AH, atrium-to-His interval; AP, accessory pathway; AM, atrium to Mahaim potential; AVNRT, atrioventricular nodal reentrant tachycardia; AVRT, atrioventricular reciprocating tachycardia; BB(B,) bundle branch block; BBR, bundle branch reentry; H, His bundle; HV, His-to-ventricle interval; LB, left bundle; LBB(B), left bundle branch (block); LV, left ventricular; MM, Mahaim to Mahaim potential; P-P, Purkinge to Purkinge fiber; RB, right bundle; RBB(B), right bundle branch (block); SVT, supraventricular tachycardia; V, ventricle; VT, ventricular tachycardia.

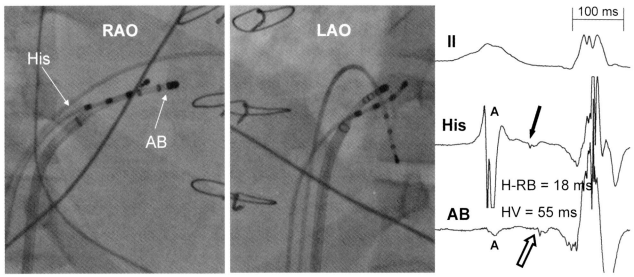

FIGURE 28–8. Right bundle branch recording. RAO and LAO views of the His and ablation (AB) catheters are shown. The far right panel shows electrograms recorded from these catheter positions. The RB recording occurs >15 msec later than the His and a very small atrial electrogram is recorded. H, His; RB, right bundle.

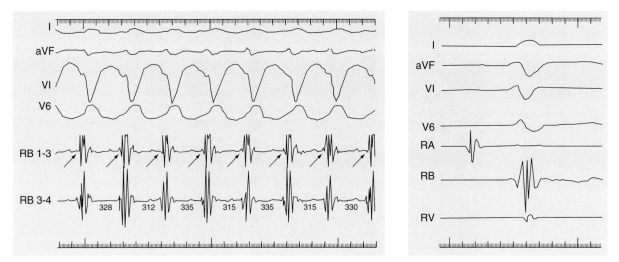

FIGURE 28–9. Inability to record antegrade right bundle potential in sinus rhythm. In sinus the right panel shows the absence of a His or right bundle (RB) potential. In bundle branch reentry however, the retrograde conduction is evident by the recording of the RB potential. *(From Wang C-W, Sterba R, Tchou P: Bundle branch reentry ventricular tachycardia with 2 distinct left bundle branch block morphologies. J Cardiovasc Electrophysiol 8:688-693, 1997, with permission.)*

the ablation catheter is directed toward the inferior apical septum, then withdrawn toward the His bundle until the LBB potential is recorded beneath the noncoronary or posterior aortic cusp (Fig. 28–11). This position is typically 1 to 1.5 cm inferior to the optimal His bundle recording site.[2,28] The LBB potential is identified by a potential-to-ventricular electrogram interval less than or equal to 20 msec, and an A/V electrogram ratio of 1:10 or less.[2,28] As mentioned, the LBB is typically a broad band that is not transected by a single RF lesion.

Left Fascicles

The left anterior fascicular network is located by extending the catheter further along the ventricular septum, toward the apex, from the area recording an LBB potential (see Fig. 28–1 and Fig. 28–11).[2,28] The left posterior fascicular network extends from the His bundle toward the inferior diaphragmatic wall (see Figs. 28–1 and 28–11). These structures are not discrete entities, and mapping is complex. Ablation of either the antegrade or the retrograde limb of the

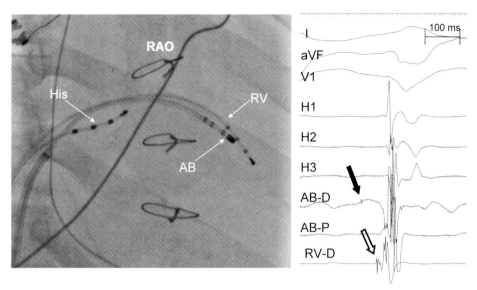

FIGURE 28–10. Recording of distal right bundle branch (RBB) potential in a patient with bundle branch reentry VT after aortic valve replacement. Neither a His nor a proximal RBB recording could be made due to septal scarring or intramyocardial course of the conduction system. The tachycardia has a left bundle branch block morphology. The distal poles of the right ventricular apical catheter (RV-D) recorded a discreet early potential at QRS onset (*open arrow*). Mapping this area with the ablation catheter (AB) revealed a small potential 25 msec before the apical potential (*solid arrow*). Ablation at this site terminated VT and prevented reinduction. I, aVF, V1, surface ECG; D, distal; H1-H3, distal to proximal His; P, proximal.

circuit should terminate the tachycardia. It may be possible to ablate "bystander" fibers within each respective fascicular system without termination of the tachycardia.[16] Although not described, determination of the postpacing intervals after entrainment at various sites may help to identify fascicular potentials that are critical to the reentry circuit. Ablation of the left main bundle would not be expected to terminate the tachycardia, because the circuit is distal to this point. Similarly, ablation of one left-sided fascicle would not be expected to prevent BBR in a patient with both interfascicular and BBR VTs. In this situation, either both left-sided fascicles or the RBB and one of the left fascicles must be ablated.

Automatic Fascicular Tachycardia

This tachycardia may arise from either the right or left distal fascicular system, and mapping is directed at identifying the earliest Purkinje potential preceding the QRS onset (see Fig. 28–6).[16] The interval between the Purkinje potential and QRS onset is short.

The target sites for ablation of BBR and related arrhythmias are listed in Table 28–3.

ABLATION

Because of the superficial nature of the His-Purkinje system in most patients, standard 4- or 5-mm-tip

TABLE 28–3
Targets for Ablation of Bundle Branch Reentry and Related Tachycardias
Bundle branch reentry
RBB usual primary target
LBB
Bundle branch reentry and interfascicular VT
RBB and left anterior or posterior fascicle
Both left anterior and posterior fascicles
Interfascicular reentry tachycardia
Left anterior or posterior fascicle
Automatic fascicular tachycardia
Site of earliest Purkinje potential associated with tachycardia

LBB, left bundle branch; RBB, right bundle branch; VT, ventricular tachycardia.

radiofrequency (RF) ablation catheters are sufficient.[12,16,28] The need for cooled ablation systems has not been described. Energy settings of 20 to 60 W with target temperatures of 60°C are reported.[12,16] For ablation of the cord-like RBB, a single RF lesion is usually effective. If the RBB cannot be identified, anatomically guided lesions or a linear ablation line placed perpendicularly to the axis of the RBB distal to the His recording may be effective.[29]

The LBB is infrequently ablated with a single RF lesion, owing to its width of about 1 cm.[7] Ablation of the LBB may require creation of a linear lesion distal to the His bundle that extends from the anterior superior septum, radiographically near the RBB in the right anterior oblique view, to the inferior basal septum. Care must be taken to avoid ablation of the His bundle itself, because the LBB can have a very short course. This linear lesion across the left septum may be used to transect both the left anterior and posterior fascicles in patients with BBR and interfascicular reentry.[28] A less extensive line can be directed at

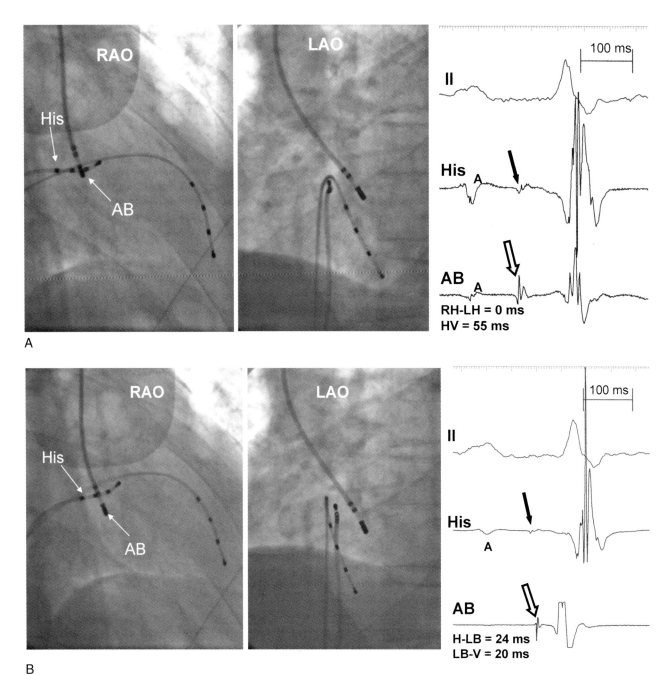

FIGURE 28–11. Recording potentials from the left sided conduction system. **A,** His recording from the left ventricle. The far right panel shows the electrograms from the right sided His catheter and the ablation catheter in the left ventricle. Note the proximity of the distal ablation electrodes to the His catheter and the equal timing of the left (LH) and right sided (RH) His potentials and the small atrial electrogram on the ablation recording. **B,** Left bundle branch recording. By advancing the ablation catheter slightly, toward the apex, the left bundle potential (*open arrow*) is identified by a timing interval 24 msec after the right sided His recording (*solid arrow*). Note the absence of an atrial electrogram on the ablation recording.

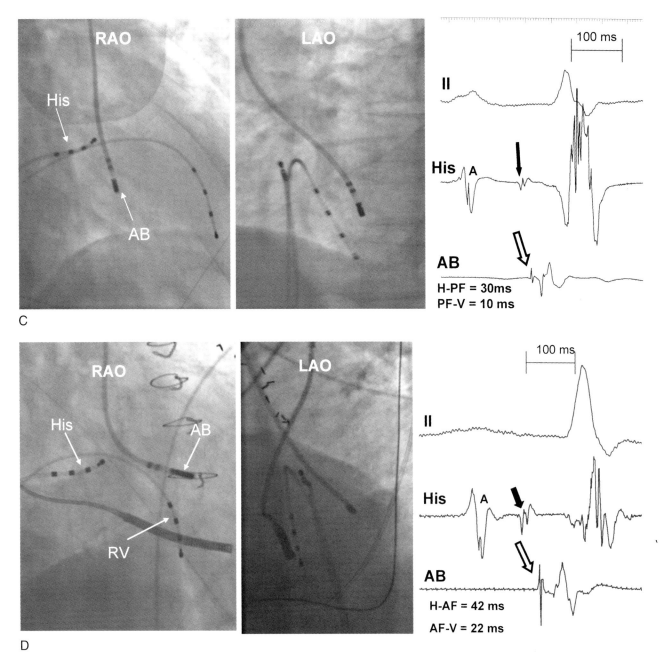

FIGURE 28–11, cont'd. C, Left posterior fascicle recording. Advancing the ablation catheter toward the inferior septum records a potential from the left posterior fascicular (PF) system that precedes the local ventricular electrogram by only 10 msec. **D,** This anterior fascicular potential is recorded directly apical from the His catheter in the mid septum. AF—anterior fascicular potential. This patient has an ICD lead in the right ventricle.

the anterior or posterior fascicular regions if ablation of single fibers is ineffective. For ablation in tachycardia, termination and noninducibility should result. In sinus rhythm, complete RBB or LBB develops with successful ablation, although the QRS changes may be subtle in patients with preexisting conduction abnormalities.[28] Electrical axis changes may be the only manifestation of fascicular ablation. Elimination of retrograde V2H2 conduction may be used as a marker of successful ablation.[1]

For automatic fascicular tachycardias, successful ablation produces automaticity followed by quiescence.[16] Because automaticity is a feature of heating from any Purkinje tissue, the patient must be rechallenged for inducibility to ensure ablation at the proper site.

After ablation, all patients should be assessed for indications for permanent pacemaker or ICD implantation, based on the status of the residual conduction system and severity of underlying structural heart disease. In addition, VT of myocardial origin may be inducible in 36% to 60% of patients after successful ablation of BBR.[12,16]

CLINICAL OUTCOMES

Acute and Long-Term Results

In the two largest series reported, the acute success rates for BBR (total 44 patients), interfascicular reentry (4 patients), and automatic fascicular tachycardia (2 patients) were all 100%.[12,16] Recurrence of these arrhythmias appears to be uncommon but has not been thoroughly documented with follow-up testing.[12,16] The long-term prognosis for these patients is more guarded, however, reflecting their underlying heart disease. Of 20 patients treated for BBR or fascicular automatic VT, Lopera et al.[16] reported need for pacing or ICD implantation in 19. Of the 14 patients who required an ICD, 7 (50%) had VT recurrences within 16 months. Five of these patients had VT of myocardial origin inducible at the time of ablation, and the recurrent VTs appeared to be different from the BBR VTs. In this series, cardiac transplantation or death from progressive heart failure occurred in 4 patients.

COMPLICATIONS

The most common complication of ablation for BBR is high-grade AV block, which is reported to occur in 10% to 30% of patients after successful ablation.[16,28]

In a recent series of 20 patients with BBR VT, 15 patients had permanent pacemakers or ICDs at the time of ablation, and 2 of the remaining 5 patients had indications for ICD implantation after ablation due to myocardial VTs.[16] Only 2 patients underwent pacemaker implantation alone for impaired AV conduction. Otherwise, complications have not been reported in the largest series of patients, but of course they may include the usual problems resulting from vascular access and left ventricular mapping.[12,16]

TROUBLESHOOTING THE DIFFICULT CASE

Problems with ablation of BBR VT are relatively uncommon and are listed in Table 28–4. Noninducibility is rarely a problem and can be addressed by infusing catecholamines or procainamide, by using short-long-short pacing protocols, and by left ventricular pacing. Inability to record electrograms from the targeted bundle branch can be overcome by mapping in VT or echo beats or by anatomically guided ablation attempts. Linear lesions are usually needed to ablate the left bundle and the left fascicles. The risk of high-grade AV block after ablation should be assessed by a thorough conduction study before ablation. Intramyocardial VTs induced during testing may require additional ablation or other forms of management. After ablation, the need for a pacemaker or ICD should be considered for all patients.

TABLE 28–4		
Troubleshooting the Difficult Case of Bundle Branch Reentry Ablation		
Problem	**Cause**	**Solution**
Unable to record RBB	RBB intramyocardial or local scarring Complete antegrade RBBB	Map/ablate LBB Anatomically guided ablation RBB Map/ablate in VT or during echo beats
Unable to ablate LBB	Broad band or multiple fibers	Linear ablation across LBB or both anterior and posterior fascicles
VT noninducible	Intermittent complete bidirectional BBB Insufficient conduction slowing	Facilitate conduction with isoproterenol Slow conduction with class IA agent (e.g., procainamide)
VT inducible after successful bundle branch ablation	Interfascicular reentry Automatic fascicular tachycardia Intramyocardial tachycardia Initial diagnosis incorrect	Ablate left anterior or posterior fascicle Ablate automatic focus Map/ablate VT or treat with ICD if appropriate Review differential diagnosis
Risk of AV block with ablation	Diffuse conduction system disease	Ablate bundle with worst conduction status Evaluate indication for pacemaker/ICD after ablation

AV, atrioventricular; BBB, bundle branch block; ICD, implantable cardiac defibrillator; LBB, left bundle branch; RBB(B), right bundle branch (block); VT, ventricular tachycardia.

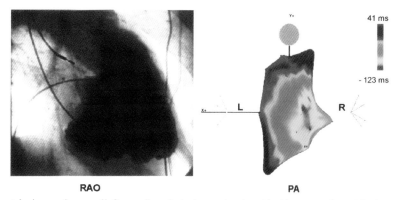

FIGURE 28–12. Right ventricular angiogram (*left panel*) and electroanatomic activation map of ventricular tachycardia from a patient with right ventricular dysplasia. The RAO angiogram shows saccular outpouchings along the tricuspid valve and diaphragmatic ventricular wall. The activation map of the right ventricle is viewed from the posterior aspect (PA) and demonstrates radial spread of activation from its source shown in *red*. (From Reithmann C, Hahnefeld A, Remp T, et al.: Electroanatomic mapping of endocardial right ventricular activation as guide for catheter ablation in patients with arrhythmogenic right ventricular dysplasia. Pacing Clin Electrophysiol 26:1308-1316, 2003, with permission.)

Right Ventricular Dysplasia

RVD is a sporadically occurring or hereditary condition involving primarily the right ventricle.[30,31] In this condition, portions of the right ventricle are replaced by fibrous and/or fatty tissue. Focal inflammation and necrosis can be seen at histologic study. The interventricular septum and left ventricle may also show involvement. The involvement of the right ventricle is usually concentrated in the anterior infundibulum, apex, and basilar inferior walls.[32] The dysplastic areas of right ventricular involvement can best be imaged by magnetic resonance imaging or right ventriculography (Fig. 28–12).[30,33]

ANATOMY AND PATHOPHYSIOLOGY

VTs are common in RVD due to the extensive myocardial fibrosis that provides the substrate for reentry.[30,31] Most patients demonstrate LBB morphology VT, and the majority have multiple VT morphologies, either spontaneous or inducible.[32-37] RBBB VT may indicate left ventricular involvement or a left septal breakthrough site. At electrophysiology study, patients with RVD have very high rates of inducible VT, and the induction is highly reproducible as well. Both clinical and nonclinical VTs are usually initiated by programmed stimulation. Up to 12 VT morphologies have been reported in a single patient.[36] In the electrophysiology laboratory, VTs in patients with RVD share many features with VTs in patients with coronary artery disease. These features include response to entrainment reflecting a reentrant basis in the majority of patients.[32] Endocardial mapping typically demonstrates broad electrograms with late high-frequency terminal deflections, consistent with slow conduction recorded in areas of dysplastic involvement.[38]

DIAGNOSIS AND DIFFERENTIAL DIAGNOSIS

The diagnostic criteria for RVD are listed in Table 28–5.[30] VTs associated with RVD must be differentiated from other etiologies of LBBB tachycardias (see Chapter 23). VT related to RVD may be confused with right ventricular outflow tract tachycardia due to the LBBB morphology in the setting of normal left ventricular function. Features distinguishing between these two conditions are listed in Table 28–6.[33] The diagnosis of RVD is usually made by clinical findings outside the electrophysiology laboratory, but right ventriculography in the laboratory may be an important maneuver.[33]

MAPPING AND ABLATION

Mapping of VT related to RVD is largely analogous to mapping of VT in coronary artery disease (Table 28–7).[32,33] Because of the reliable and reproducible inducibility of VT, entrainment and activation mapping are commonly employed.[32] Computerized mapping systems may be useful.[35] Propagation occurs in a radial pattern away from the site of earliest ventricular activation in electroanatomic maps (see Fig. 28–12).[35] Pace mapping has also been used in patients with RVD. Activation mapping demonstrates earliest ventricular electrograms averaging 38 to 112 msec before QRS onset.[33,37] With entrainment mapping, the classic entrance, exit, inner loop, outer

TABLE 28–5

Diagnostic Criteria for Right Ventricular Dysplasia*

Cardiac dysfunction and structural alterations	Depolarization abnormalities
Major	**Major**
Severe RV dilation or reduction RV ejection fraction with minimal or no LV impairment	Epsilon waves or localized prolongation (>110 msec) of the QRS in right precordial leads (V1-V3)
Localized RV aneurysms	
Severe segmental RV dilation	**Minor**
Minor	Late potentials on signal-averaged ECG
Mild global RV dilation or reduction in RV ejection fraction with normal LV function	**Arrhythmias**
	Minor
Mild segmental RV dilation	Left bundle branch type ventricular tachycardia, sustained or nonsustained
Regional RV hypokinesis	Frequent ventricular extrasystoles (>1000/24 hr)
Tissue characterization of wall	**Family history**
Major	**Major**
Fibrofatty replacement of myocardium on endomyocardial biopsy	Familial disease confirmed at necropsy or surgery
Repolarization abnormalities	**Minor**
Minor	Family history of premature sudden death (<35 years old) due to suspected RVD
Inverted T waves in right precordial leads (V₂-V₃) with age >12 yr and in absence of right bundle branch block	Family history of clinical diagnosis

*Diagnosis requires the presence of two major, one major plus two minor, or four minor criteria.
ECG, electrocardiogram; LV, left ventricle; RV, right ventricle.
From Marcus F, Towbin JA, Zareba W, et al.: Arrhythmogenic right ventricular dysplasia/cardiomyopathy (ARVD/C): A multidisciplinary study—Design and protocol. Circulation 107:2975-2978, 2003, with permission.

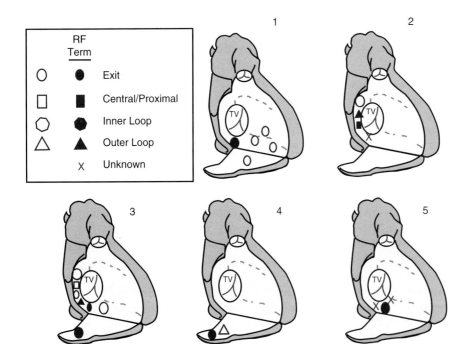

FIGURE 28–13. Sites with ventricular tachycardia circuits defined by entrainment mapping in 5 patients with right ventricular dysplasia. The exit, central/proximal, inner and outer loop locations are designated by the symbols (legend). The *solid symbols* indicate sites at which radiofrequency ablation terminated (RF Term) tachycardia. Note the clustering of sites along the tricuspid valve (TV), apex, and outflow tract. *(From Ellison KE, Friedman PL, Ganz LI, et al.: Entrainment mapping and radiofrequency catheter ablation of ventricular tachycardia in right ventricular dysplasia. J Am Coll Cardiol 32:724-728, 1998, with permission.)*

TABLE 28–6

Differentiating Right Ventricular Dysplasia from Right Ventricular Outflow Tract Tachycardia*

Feature	RVD (N = 17)	RVOT Tachycardia (N = 33)
Epsilon wave or QRS > 110 msec	30%	0%
Right precordial T-wave inversion	36%	0%
Family history of arrhythmias	53%	0%
VT mechanism in electrophysiology laboratory	Reentry	Automatic or triggered
Number of VT morphologies	Average, 1.8; range, 1-6	Single
Any major criteria for RVD	41%	0%
Any minor criteria for RVD	41%	3%
Major abnormalities on cardiac MRI	88%	6%
Minor abnormalities on MRI	12%	48%

*The values indicate the percent of patients in each group demonstrating the study feature.

MRI, magnetic resonance imaging; VT, ventricular tachycardia.

From O'Donnell D, Cox D, Bourke J, et al.: Clinical and electrophysiologic differences between patients with arrhythmogenic right ventricular dysplasia and right ventricular outflow tract tachycardia. Eur Heart J 24:801-810, 2003, with permission.

TABLE 28–7

Ablation Targets for Ventricular Tachycardia Associated with Nonischemic Cardiomyopathies (Excluding Bundle Branch Reentry)

Sites of earliest presystolic ventricular activation

Sites of concealed entrainment in tachycardia
  S-QRS − EGM-QRS < 20 msec
  PPI < 30 msec
  Concealed entrainment

Pace map sites with ≥10/12 lead match
Sites of continuous diastolic electrical activity
Electrical isthmuses defined by electroanatomic mapping for unstable VT

EGM-QRS, electrogram-to-QRS interval; PPI, postpacing interval; S-QRS, stimulus-to-QRS interval; VT, ventricular tachycardia.

CLINICAL OUTCOMES

The clinical experience with catheter ablation of VT related to RVD is limited (Table 28–8). Notable from this experience are the multiple VT morphologies inducible in most patients and the variable acute and chronic success rates.[33,36] The largest and most recently reported series of cases treated with RF ablation alone may be the most relevant. In this series of 17 RVD patients reported by O'Donnell et al.,[33] more than one morphology of VT was induced in 71% (range, 1 to 6 morphologies). Concealed entrainment was demonstrated for 15 VTs in 12 patients. Acute success, defined as absence of any inducible VT after ablation, occurred in only 41% of patients; an additional 29% of patients had elimination of the clinical VT but inducibility remained for other morphologies. After at least 12 months of follow-up, VT recurred in 47% of patients. A significant percentage of patients had ICDs at the time of ablation or have undergone placement after the procedure in contemporary reports.[32,33] Many patients remain on antiarrhythmic drugs.[32,33]

No study using RF ablation alone has reported complications from VT ablation in RVD patients. In a large series of 50 patients monitored for 16 years, Fontaine et al.[36] reported deaths and pericardial tamponade after direct current ablation in patients whose VTs were refractory to RF ablation alone.

In summary, catheter ablation may best be considered as palliative or adjunctive therapy in patients with RVD. Most patients remain on drug therapy or have an ICD implanted after ablation due to incomplete elimination of VTs, recurrent VT, or concerns for the progressive nature of the disease process.[39]

loop, and bystander sites are indentifiable.[32] Both activation and entrainment mapping usually identify the target ablation sites to be in the apex, basilar inferior wall, tricuspid valve annulus, or outflow tract (Fig. 28–13).[32] By entrainment mapping, the targets are the diastolic pathway or exit sites. Activation mapping targets the site of earliest ventricular electrical activity. Ablation is performed with standard 4-mm-tip ablation catheters with temperature control to 60°C.[33] Point and linear ablation may be needed to transect the reentrant circuit.[33] One center reported recent experience with direct current ablation to the right ventricle for cases refractory to RF ablation.[36]

TABLE 28–8

Results of Catheter Ablation for Right Ventricular Dysplasia

Authors (Ref. No.)	No. of Patients	Number of VTs	Mapping Techniques	Acute Success Rate	Complications	Recurrence Rate	Comments
Reithmann et al.[35]	5	1 clinical each, 1-2 inducible	Electroanatomic and entrainment	80% of clinical VTs	None	40% after 7 ± 3 mo	Nonclinical VTs not targeted
Ellison et al.[32]	5	3.8 average	Entrainment	42% of all morphologies	None	0% after 11-24 mo	All inducible VTs targeted
O'Donnell et al.[33]	17	1.8 average, range 1-6	Activation and entrainment	41% rendered noninducible	None	47% after 56 mo average (range, 13-92 mo)	Results compared to RVOT patients
Harada et al.[34]	7	8 VTs in 7 patients	Entrainment	100%	Not reported	0% after 19 ± 7 mo	1 patient underwent chemical ablation
Asso et al.[37]	6	7 VTs in 6 patients	Activation	66% of patients	Not reported	0% after 22 ± 6 mo	Abstract only
Haverkamp et al.[40]	14	Not reported	Activation and pace mapping	71%	None	60% after 22 ± 13 mo	Abstract only
Miljoen et al.[41]	11	12 VTs in 11 patients	Electroanatomic	75%	Not reported	50% after 9-50 mo	Abstract only
Fontaine et al.[36]	50	1-12 per patient	Not given	46% noninducible after a single procedure	2 deaths, 2 tamponade, 1 hemopericardium after DC ablation	54% after 5.4 yr average	DC ablation for patients failing RF

DC, direct current; RF, radiofrequency energy; RVOT, right ventricular outflow tract; VT, ventricular tachycardia.

Dilated Cardiomyopathy

ANATOMY AND PATHOPHYSIOLOGY

Sustained monomorphic VT is an uncommon clinical finding in patients with DCM and is infrequently induced at electrophysiologic studies.[38] Primarily for these reasons, the clinical experience with catheter ablation of VT in patients with DCM is very limited. The electrophysiologic substrate for VT in DCM appears to be heterogeneous.[42] Scarring is common and occurs as endocardial plaques and patchy areas of interstitial fibrosis.[42] In addition, variable degrees of myofiber disarray, hypertrophy, and atrophy are common. The potential mechanisms for VT in this substrate include reentry and triggered VT.[42] At electrophysiologic study, patients with DCM demonstrate less frequent abnormal endocardial electrograms than do patients with ischemic cardiomyopathy (Fig. 28–14).[42] In addition, the abnormal electrograms in patients with DCM are less likely to show fragmentation and tend to be concentrated in the basal left ventricular endocardial region. DCM patients also show a higher frequency of abnormal epicardial electrograms than do patients with coronary artery disease.[42]

MAPPING AND ABLATION

Given this wide distribution of abnormal myocardial substrate, VTs in patients with DCM may arise from the left ventricular endocardium, epicardium, midmyocardium, septum, or right ventricle.[43-46] The clinical experience with mapping of VTs in this patient group is very limited but has used activation mapping, pace mapping, and/or entrainment mapping as the inducibility, duration, and tolerance

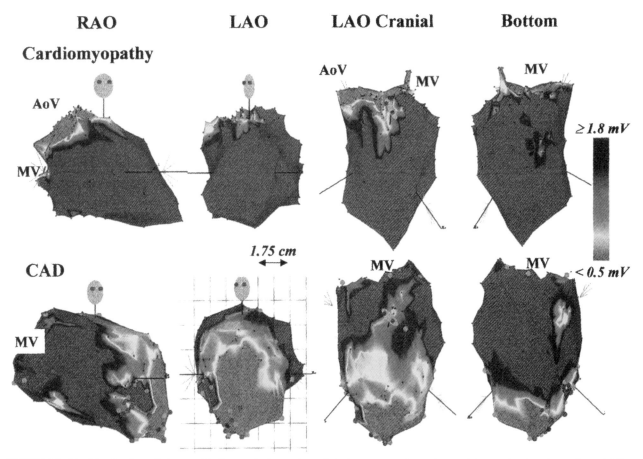

FIGURE 28–14. Distribution of abnormal left ventricular endocardial electrograms in patients with sustained tachycardia and idiopathic dilated cardiomyopathy (Cardiomyopathy, **top**) and ischemic cardiomyopathy (CAD, **bottom**). Multiple views are shown. Normal voltages (>1.8 mV) are shown in *purple* and scar (<0.5 mV) is shown in *red*. In the dilated cardiomyopathy patient, the small area of scar and abnormal electrogram voltages is confined to the base of the left ventricle near the mitral valves (MV) and aortic valves (AoV). In contrast, the patient with ischemic cardiomyopathy demonstrates an extensive apical scar over the anterior, septal, and posterior segments. *(From Hsia HH, Marchlinski FE: Characterization of the electroanatomic substrate for monomorphic ventricular tachycardia in patients with nonischemic cardiomyopathy. Pacing Clin Electrophysiol 25:1114-1127, 2002, with permission.)*

of the VTs has allowed (see Table 28–7). The reports on ablation of these arrhythmias contain small numbers of selected DCM patients.[43-45] Kottkamp et al.[43] attempted ablation for nine VTs in eight DCM patients with incessant or frequent monomorphic VTs that were reproducibly induced at testing. With the use of activation, pace, and entrainment mapping, the acute success rate was 66% with a recurrence rate of 66%. Of seven patients reported by Wilber et al.,[44] entrainment, pace, and activation mapping resulted in ablation of VT in three patients who had reproducible sustained arrhythmias but in none of the four patients with apparent nonreentrant mechanisms. The largest series was reported by Soejima et al.[45] Of 28 DCM patients with a history of recurrent sustained monomorphic VT, most had endocardial or epicardial scar by electroanatomic mapping (20 and 7 patients, respectively). Virtually all patients had ICDs implanted before or after the ablation procedure. The endocardial scars were most frequently near a valve annulus. For stable sustained VT, entrainment and activation mapping were employed. For hemodynamically unstable VT, pace mapping and substrate mapping were used to define potential exit sites. Electroanatomic mapping, entrainment mapping, and pace mapping identified 19 VT circuit isthmuses in 22 patients with intramyocardial reentry. Five patients had automatic VTs, and 2 had BBR. An epicardial isthmus was found in 7 patients and an endocardial isthmus location in 12 patients with myocardial reentry (Fig. 28–15). Ablation was performed using an irrigated-tip or 8-mm-tip catheter if initial attempts with a 4-mm-tip electrode failed. Seventy-three VTs were induced in the 22 patients. An average of 18 ± 9 lesions were delivered to endocardial ablation sites and 11 ± 8 to endocardial sites. No serious complications occurred. All VTs were ablated in 12 (54%) of 22 patients, and VT induction was modified in 4 patients (18%). Only 54% of patients were free of VT recurrence after follow-up of 348 ± 345 days. The limited acute success rate was believed to be the result of a high incidence of intramyocardial reentry circuits.

These studies suggest that scar-related reentry is the mechanism underlying sustained monomorphic VT in many patients with DCM. Automatic VT and BBR are not uncommon, however. Multiple VT morphologies are usually induced at electrophysiologic testing.[44] Electroanatomic mapping is useful to define the regions of scar and to direct pace and entrainment mapping.[45] Large-tip or irrigated-tip catheters are sometimes necessary for successful ablation.[45] Epicardial mapping and ablation also appears to be an important technique for many DCM patients.[45] Hemodynamically unstable VTs may be addressed by pace mapping or noncontact mapping and can

respond to substrate modification.[46] The limited acute success rate possibly reflects an epicardial or intramyocardial circuit in many patients. This fact and the high recurrence rate make VT ablation in DCM a palliative therapy or adjunctive to ICDs.

Chagas' Disease

Chagas' disease is a major cause of cardiac disease in Latin America and is being recognized in North America as well due to increasing emigration from endemic areas.[47] The causative organism is *Trypanosoma cruzi*, which is spread by an insect vector. Chronic heart disease develops in 10% to 40% of patients after acute infection and is manifested as DCM, heart failure, bradycardia, tachyarrhythmias, and sudden death. The diagnosis is made based on serologic testing and clinical findings.[47] Classically, patients with chronic chagasic heart disease may have RBBB, ST-segment elevation, and premature ventricular contractions on surface ECG. Left ventricular dilation, systolic dysfunction, and sometimes ventricular segmental aneurysms may be present. Sustained monomorphic VTs occurring in these patients are usually highly reproducible at electrophysiologic testing, suggesting a reentrant mechanism.[48-51] Multiple VT morphologies may be induced in individual patients.[48] Induction of sustained VT has been associated with the presence of conduction disturbances on ECG and left ventricular aneurysms (Fig. 28–16).[49,50] The arrhythmogenic potential of ventricular aneurysms is demonstrated by abolition of VT after surgical aneurysmectomy.[49]

There are limited data on catheter ablation of VTs associated with Chagas' disease.[48,50] The largest series has been reported by Tavora et al.,[50] who studied 31 patients with a history of sustained VT and chronic Chagas' disease. Activation and entrainment mapping were used to identify sites for ablation. Sites with electrograms preceding QRS onset by 30 msec or longer were sought. The VT in all patients was believed to be reentrant in nature. An endocardial site of the reentrant circuit was identified in 70% of cases. Epicardial mapping was not performed. The utility of epicardial mapping in patients with Chagas' disease was demonstrated by Sosa et al.[48] In 10 patients, an epicardial circuit was identified in 14 of 18 inducible VTs (Fig. 28–17). Epicardial ablation was performed in 6 patients. The earliest epicardial sites were 107 ± 60 msec before QRS onset. In 7 patients, epicardial mid-diastolic potentials or continuous activity was seen. Ablation was acutely successful in all patients receiving epicardial ablation, with no

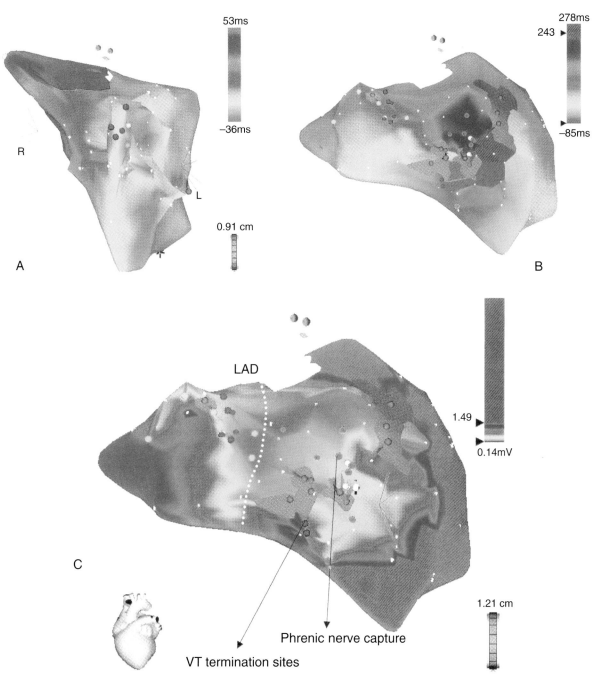

FIGURE 28–15. Endocardial (**A**) and epicardial (**B**) left ventricular activation maps from a patient with dilated cardiomyopathy and sustained ventricular tachycardia (VT). The earliest sites (*red*) in the endocardial map (**A**) are discreet suggesting a focal origin. Ablation at this site failed to terminate tachycardia. The epicardial map (**B**) was obtained for the same VT and demonstrated a large reentry circuit with a "head meets tail" sequence. The *green tags* represent areas of phrenic nerve stimulation with pacing. Panel **C** shows an epicardial voltage map from the same patient with normal voltages >1.5 mV shown in *purple* and scar (<0.14 mV) in *red*. The voltage map identified an isthmus between dense scar (*gray*). The VT was terminated by a line of radiofrequency lesions from the dense scar across the exit site and into the area of normal myocardial voltage. *(From Soejima K, Stevenson WG, Sapp L, et al.: Endocardial and epicardial radiofrequency ablation of ventricular tachycardia associated with dilated cardiomyopathy. J Am Coll Cardiol 43:1834-1842, 2004, with permission.)*

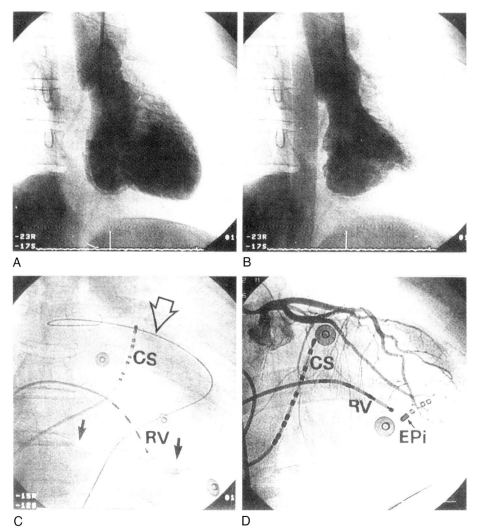

FIGURE 28–16. Right ventricular venography and catheter positions during mapping of ventricular tachycardia in a patient with Chagas' disease. RAO right ventriculogram in systole (**A**) and diastole (**B**) showing characteristic inferolateral ventricular aneurysm. **C,** Guide wire introduced percutaneously into the pericardial space for epicardial mapping. The *arrows* show radiographic contrast injected percutaneously to visualize the pericardial space. **D,** With the epicardial mapping catheter (EPi) at a potential ablation site, coronary angiography is performed to evaluate the risk of coronary artery injury from the radiofrequency energy. CS, coronary sinus catheter; RV, right ventricular endocardial catheter. *(From Sosa E, Scanavacca M, D'Avila A, et al.: Endocardial and epicardial ablation guided by nonsurgical transthoracic epicardial mapping to treat recurrent ventricular tachycardia. J Cardiovasc Electrophysiol 9:229-239, 1998, with permission.)*

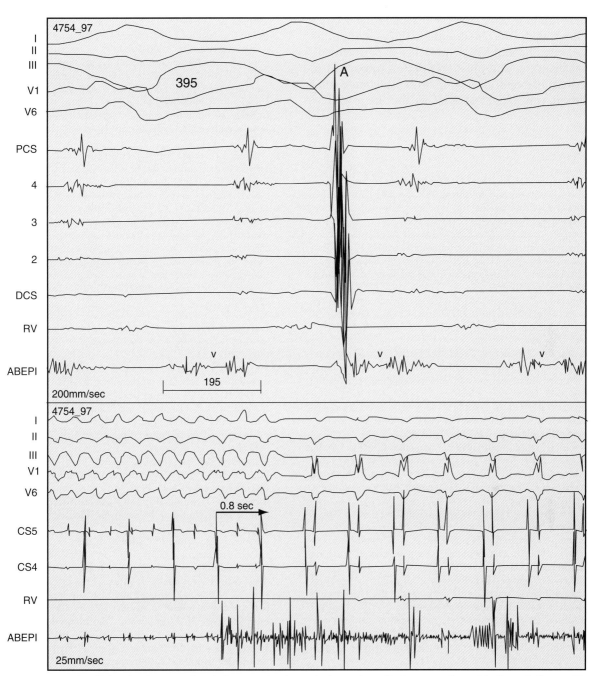

FIGURE 28–17. Epicardial activation mapping during sustained ventricular tachycardia from a patient with Chagas' disease. The top 5 tracings on each panel are surface ECG leads. **Top panel,** The epicardial ablation electrogram precedes the QRS onset by 195 msec and there is continuous electrical activity throughout diastole. The tachycardia cycle length is 395 msec. **Bottom panel,** Radiofrequency energy delivered to this site terminated the tachycardia in 0.8 seconds. 4-2, proximal to distal coronary sinus bipoles; A, atrial electrogram; ABEPI, epicardial ablation catheter; DCS, distal coronary sinus; PCS, proximal coronary sinus; RV, right ventricle; V, ventricular electrogram. *(From Sosa E, Scanavacca M, D'Avila A, et al.: Endocardial and epicardial ablation guided by nonsurgical transthoracic epicardial mapping to treat recurrent ventricular tachycardia. J Cardiovasc Electrophysiol 9:229-239, 1998, with permission.)*

recurrences reported after 5 to 9 months of follow-up. In the 4 patients undergoing endocardial ablation, the VT remained inducible. Treatment of Chagas' disease VT by chemical ablation has also been reported.[52]

These limited data suggest that ablation for VT associated with Chagas' disease may have a limited success rate of about 50%. The ability to perform epicardial mapping and ablation appears important to procedural success. The long-term outcomes after ablation in this patient population are unknown.

References

1. Blanck Z, Sra J, Dhala A, et al.: Bundle branch reentry: Mechanisms, diagnosis and treatment. In Zipes DP, Jalife J (eds.): Cardiac Electrophysiology: From Cell to Bedside, 2nd ed. Philadelphia: Saunders, 1995, pp 878-885.
2. Tchou P, Mehdirad AA: Bundle branch reentry ventricular tachycardia. Pacing Clin Electrophysiol 18:1427-1437, 1995.
3. Caceres J, Jazayeri M, McKinnie J, et al.: Sustained bundle branch reentry as a mechanism of clinical tachycardia. Circulation 79:256-270, 1989.
4. Narasimhan C, Jazayeri MR, Sra J, et al.: Ventricular tachycardia in valvular heart disease: Facilitation of sustained bundle branch reentry by valve surgery. Circulation 96:4307-4313, 1997.
5. Merino JL, Carmona JR, Fernandez Lozano I, et al.: Mechanisms of sustained ventricular tachycardia in myotonic dystrophy: Implications for catheter ablation. Circulation 98:541-546, 1998.
6. Anderson RH, Ho SY: The morphology of the specialized atrioventricular junctional area: The evolution of understanding. Pacing Clin Electrophysiol 25:957-966, 2002.
7. Bharati S, Lev M: Anatomy of the normal conduction system, disease-related changes, and their relationship to arrhythmogenesis. In Podrid PJ, Kowey PR (eds.): Cardiac Arrhythmia. Mechanisms, Diagnosis and Management. Baltimore: Williams & Wilkins, 1995, pp 1-15.
8. Shah P: Heart and great vessels. In Standring S (ed.): Gray's Anatomy, 39th ed. Edinburgh: Elsevier, 2005, pp 995-1029.
9. Akhtar M, Damato AN, Batsford WP, et al.: Demonstration of reentry within the His-Purkinje system in man. Circulation 50:1150-1162, 1974.
10. Denker S, Shenasa M, Gilbert C, et al.: Effects of abrupt changes in cycle length on refractoriness of the His-Purkinje system in man. Circulation 67:60-68, 1983.
11. Josephson M: Electrophysiologic investigation: General concepts. In Josephson M: Clinical Cardiac Electrophysiology: Techniques and Interpretations, 3rd ed. Philadelphia: Lippincott Williams & Wilkins, 2002, pp 19-67.
12. Blanck Z, Dhala A, Deshpande S, et al.: Bundle branch reentrant ventricular tachycardia: Cumulative experience in 48 patients. J Cardiovasc Electrophysiol 4:253-262, 1993.
13. Blanck Z, Jazayeri M, Dhala A, et al.: Bundle branch reentry: A mechanism of tachycardia in the absence of valvular dysfunction. J Am Coll Cardiol 22:1718-1722, 1993.
14. Crijns HJGM, Smeets JLRM, Rodriguez LM, et al.: Cure of interfascicular reentrant ventricular tachycardia by ablation of the anterior fascicle of the left bundle branch. J Cardiovasc Electrophysiol 6:486-492, 1995.
15. Berger RD, Orias D, Kasper EK, et al.: Catheter ablation of coexistent bundle branch and interfascicular ventricular tachycardias. J Cardiovasc Electrophysiol 7:341-347, 1996.
16. Lopera G, Stevenson WG, Soejima K, et al.: Identification and ablation of three types of ventricular tachycardia involving the His-Purkinje system in patients with heart disease. J Cardiovasc Electrophysiol 15:52-58, 2004.
17. Tchou P, Jazayeri M, Denker S, et al.: Transcatheter electrical ablation of the right bundle branch: A method of treating macro-reentrant ventricular tachycardia due to bundle branch reentry. Circulation 78:246-257, 1988.
18. Youboul P, Kirkorian G, Atallah G, et al.: Bundle branch reentrant tachycardia treated by electrical ablation of the right bundle branch. J Am Coll Cardiol 7:1404-1409, 1986.
19. Cohen T, Chien W, Lurie K, et al.: Radiofrequency catheter ablation for treatment of bundle branch reentry: Results and long term follow up. J Am Coll Cardiol 18:1767, 1991.
20. Andress JD, Vander Salm TJ, Huang SKS, et al.: Bidirectional bundle branch reentry tachycardia associated with Ebstein's anomaly: Cured by extensive cryoablation of the right bundle branch. Pacing Clin Electrophysiol 14:1639-1647, 1991.
21. Li Y-G, Gronefeld G, Isreal C, et al.: Bundle branch reentrant tachycardia in patients with apparent normal His-Purkinje conduction: The role of functional conduction impairment. J Cardiovasc Electrophysiol 13:1233-1239, 2002.
22. Fisher JD: Bundle branch reentry tachycardia: Why is the HV interval often longer than in sinus rhythm. The critical role of anisotropic conduction. J Intervent Card Electrophysiol 5:173-176, 2001.
23. Merino JL, Peinado R, Fernandez-Lozano I, et al.: Bundle-branch reentry and the postpacing interval after entrainment by right ventricular apex stimulation. Circulation 103:1102-1108, 2001.
24. Merino JL, Peinado R, Fernandez-Lozano I, et al.: Transient entrainment of bundle-branch reentry by atrial and ventricular stimulation. Circulation 100:1784-1790, 1999.
25. Nakagawa H, Beckman KJ, McClelland JH, et al.: Radiofrequency catheter ablation of idiopathic left ventricular tachycardia guided by a Purkinje potential. Circulation 88:2607-2617, 1993.
26. Markowitz SM, Stein KM, Englestein ED, et al.: A-V nodal-His-Purkinje reentry: A novel form of tachycardia. J Cardiovasc Electrophysiol 6:400-409, 1995.
27. Rubenstein DS, Burke MC, Kall JG, et al.: Adenosine-sensitive bundle branch reentry. J Cardiovasc Electrophysiol 8:80-88, 1997.
28. Mehdirad AA, Tchou P: Catheter ablation of bundle branch reentrant ventricular tachycardia. In Huang SKS, Wilber DJ (eds.): Radiofrequency Catheter Ablation of Cardiac Arrhythmias, 2nd ed. Armonk, N.Y.: Futura, 2000, pp 653-667.
29. Wang C-W, Sterba R, Tchou P: Bundle branch reentry ventricular tachycardia with 2 distinct left bundle branch block morphologies. J Cardiovasc Electrophysiol 8:688-693, 1997.
30. Marcus F, Towbin JA, Zareba W, et al.: Arrhythmogenic right ventricular dysplasia/cardiomyopathy (ARVD/C): A multidisciplinary study—Design and protocol. Circulation 107:2975-2978, 2003.
31. Basso C, Thiene G, Corrado D, et al.: Arrhythmogenic right ventricular cardiomyopathy: Dysplasia, dystrophy or myocarditis? Circulation 94:983-991, 1996.
32. Ellison KE, Friedman PL, Ganz LI, et al.: Entrainment mapping and radiofrequency catheter ablation of ventricular tachycardia in right ventricular dysplasia. J Am Coll Cardiol 32:724-728, 1998.
33. O'Donnell D, Cox D, Bourke J, et al.: Clinical and electrophysiologic differences between patients with arrhythmogenic right ventricular dysplasia and right ventricular outflow tract tachycardia. Eur Heart J 24:801-810, 2003.

34. Harada T, Aonuma K, Yamauchi Y, et al.: Catheter ablation of ventricular tachycardia in patients with right ventricular dysplasia: Identification of target sites by entrainment mapping techniques. Pacing Clin Electrophysiol 21:2547-2550, 1998.

35. Reithmann C, Hahnefeld A, Remp T, et al.: Electroanatomic mapping of endocardial right ventricular activation as guide for catheter ablation in patients with arrhythmogenic right ventricular dysplasia. Pacing Clin Electrophysiol 26:1308-1316, 2003.

36. Fontaine G, Tonet J, Gallais Y, et al.: Ventricular tachycardia catheter ablation in arrhythmogenic right ventricular dysplasia: A 16 year experience. Curr Cardiol Rep 2:498-506, 2000.

37. Asso A, Farre J, Zayas R, et al.: Radiofrequency catheter ablation of ventricular tachycardia in patients with arrhythmogenic right ventricular dysplasia [abstract]. J Am Coll Cardiol 25:315A, 1995.

38. Coyne RF, Marchlinski FE: Ablation of ventricular tachycardia associated with nonischemic structural heart disease. In Huang SKS, Wilber DJ (eds.): Radiofrequency Catheter Ablation of Cardiac Arrhythmias, 2nd ed. Armonk, N.Y.: Futura, 2000, pp 705-735.

39. Feld GK: Expanding indications for radiofrequency catheter ablation: Ventricular tachycardia in association with right ventricular dysplasia? J Am Coll Cardiol 32:729-731, 1998.

40. Haverkamp W, Borgreffe M, Chen X, et al.: Radiofrequency ablation in patients with sustained ventricular tachycardia and arrhythmogenic right ventricular disease [abstract]. Circulation 88:I353, 1993.

41. Miljoen H, State S, de Chillou C, et al.: Electroanatomic mapping characteristics of ventricular tachycardia in patients with arrhythmogenic right ventricular dysplasia [abstract]. J Am Coll Cardiol 45:106A, 2005.

42. Hsia HH, Marchlinski FE: Characterization of the electroanatomic substrate for monomorphic ventricular tachycardia in patients with nonischemic cardiomyopathy. Pacing Clin Electrophysiol 25:1114-1127, 2002.

43. Kottkamp H, Hindricks G, Chen X, et al.: Radiofrequency catheter ablation of sustained ventricular tachycardia in idiopathic dilated cardiomyopathy. Circulation 92:1159-1168, 1995.

44. Wilber DJ, Glascock DN, Kall JG, et al.: Radiofrequency catheter ablation of sustained ventricular tachycardia associated with idiopathic dilated cardiomyopathy [abstract]. Circulation 92(Suppl):I165, 1995.

45. Soejima K, Stevenson WG, Sapp L, et al.: Endocardial and epicardial radiofrequency ablation of ventricular tachycardia associated with dilated cardiomyopathy. J Am Coll Cardiol 43:1834-1842, 2004.

46. Marchlinski FE, Callans DJ, Gottlieb CD, et al.: Linear lesions for control of unmappable ventricular tachycardia in patients with ischemic and nonischemic cardiomyopathy. Circulation 101:1288-1296, 2000.

47. Acquatella H: Chagas' heart disease. In Crawford MH, DiMarco JP (eds.): Cardiology. London: Mosby, 2001, pp 5.13.2-5.13.4.

48. Sosa E, Scanavacca M, D'Avila A, et al.: Endocardial and epicardial ablation guided by nonsurgical transthoracic epicardial mapping to treat recurrent ventricular tachycardia. J Cardiovasc Electrophysiol 9:229-239, 1998.

49. Milei J, Pesce R, Valero E, et al.: Electrophysiologic-structural correlations in chagasic aneurysm causing malignant arrhythmias. Int J Cardiol 32:65-73, 1991.

50. Tavora MZ, Mehta N, Silva RM, et al.: Characteristics and identification of sites of chagasic ventricular tachycardia by endocardial mapping. Arq Bras Cardiol 72:451-474, 1999.

51. De Paola AA, Horowitz LN, Miyamoto MH, et al.: Angiographic and electrophysiologic substrates of ventricular tachycardia in chronic chagasic myocarditis. Am J Cardiol 65:360-363, 1990.

52. De Paola AA, Gomes JA, Miyamoto MH, et al.: Transcoronary chemical ablation of ventricular tachycardia in chronic chagasic myocarditis. J Am Coll Cardiol 20:480-482, 1992.

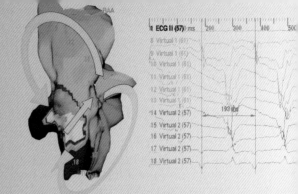

29

Ablation of Unstable Ventricular Tachycardias and Idiopathic Ventricular Fibrillation

Vivek Reddy

Key Points

■ For scar-related ventricular tachycardia (VT), substrate mapping is used to delineate the infarcted myocardial tissue. For focal ventricular fibrillation (VF), the right and left ventricles are mapped to identify the focal origin of the premature ventricular complexes (PVCs) triggering VF.

■ In scar-related VT, pace mapping may be used to identify the VT exit sites. Ablation targets also include sites identified by brief resetting/entrainment mapping, mapping of late and fractionated potentials within the infarcted tissue, latency mapping (long stimulus-to-QRS duration), and channels between regions of dense ("electrically unexcitable") scar.

■ In focal VF, if the heart is structurally normal, ablation targets include PVC triggers preceded by Purkinje potentials (in about 80% of patients) or located in a ventricular outflow tract (20% of patients). If treating after myocardial infarction, the ablation targets are PVC triggers preceded by Purkinje potentials.

■ An electroanatomic mapping system is necessary to construct a three-dimensional rendering of the ventricular geometry and infarct location. An irrigated radiofrequency ablation catheter is ideal to permit optimal mapping and ablation. Intracardiac echocardiography may facilitate trans-septal access to perform transmitral left ventricular mapping. An intra-aortic balloon pump may be used to optimize the hemodynamic state.

■ Sources of difficulty include an epicardial or deep septal location of the VT circuit and, during VF ablation, PVC triggers that are difficult to induce.

Over the past decade, significant advances have been made in the ability to perform catheter ablation of ventricular tachyarrhythmias. This is due in part to an increased understanding of the pathophysiology of these arrhythmias, and in part to improvements in technology that facilitate the catheter ablation procedure. From a procedural perspective, ventricular tachycardias (VTs) can be broadly divided into two groups: stable and unstable. In this context, a VT is considered "stable" if the ventricular chamber can be mapped during the arrhythmia of interest to permit identification of critical portions of the circuit. As described in Chapter 27, a number of investigators have established that a combination of activation and resetting/entrainment criteria can be employed to permit catheter mapping and ablation of these stable VTs with high success rates. However, in any given patient, a VT can be "unstable" because of hemodynamic intolerance during the arrhythmia of interest. In addition, the tachycardia can be "unstable" because of either nonsustained runs of the target arrhythmia or the presence of multiple morphologies of VT. Although these unstable VTs were typically not amenable to catheter ablation in the past, this chapter discusses the advances in technology and methodology that now allow for successful catheter ablation of most scar-related VTs regardless of their stability, hemodynamic or otherwise. In addition, this chapter discusses the recent demonstration that in some patients ventricular fibrillation (VF) can also be targeted for catheter ablation.

Anatomy and Pathophysiology

MECHANISM OF POST–MYOCARDIAL INFARCTION VENTRICULAR TACHYCARDIA

In most patients with a prior myocardial infarction (MI), the pathogenesis of VT is reentry in the area of the scarred myocardium.[1,2] After an MI, the tissue can be broadly divided into three zones: the dense scar, the surrounding live myocardial tissue, and the intervening "border zone." The "border zone" is not necessarily physically located only at the periphery of the scar; rather, it is located at any of the interfaces between normal tissue and scar. In this border zone, electrically active live myocardial fibrils are interspersed among the bed of infarcted, fibrotic tissue. These fibrils are characterized by abnormal electrophysiologic properties, including slower conduction velocity, and decreased cell-to-cell electrical coupling (e.g., due to altered connexin activity). As with reen-

trant circuits located in other regions of the heart, the initiation of VT depends on the development of unidirectional block and conduction that is slow enough to allow the recovery of excitability of the initially blocked region, initiating a self-perpetuating reentrant circuit. The initiators of scar-related VT are not well understood. Presumably, a well-timed premature beat or series of premature beats arises as a result of triggered activity from discrete regions of the heart, and this allows for the unidirectional block and slow conduction required to initiate reentrant VT.

To maintain the reentrant circuit once it is initiated, the wavelength of the tachycardia circuit must be short enough, or the path of the myocardial circuit long enough, so that the wavefront is constantly encountering excitable tissue. This can occur with either an anatomically determined circuit of the appropriate length or a partial anatomic barrier combined with a functional barrier. For example, a functional barrier may be caused by ischemia, electrophysiologic changes resulting from treatment with antiarrhythmic drugs, or electrolyte/pH changes (Fig. 29–1). The anatomic compartmentalization combined with altered cell-to-cell electrical coupling of the diseased tissue sets the stage for local microreentrant or macroreentrant circuits that result in VT and have the potential to culminate in VF.

Hemodynamically stable monomorphic VT circuits can be studied by careful transcatheter endocardial mapping of the electrical activity during the tachycardia. As detailed further in Chapter 27, the "anatomy" of the path of surviving myocardial tissue within the scar that comprises the VT circuit can be characterized in detail using resetting/entrainment criteria. The "exit" point of the VT circuit from the scar (often located at the border of the scarred myocardium) can be identified, and radiofrequency (RF) catheter ablation can be performed at this region to eliminate the arrhythmia. At experienced centers, this can be accomplished with high success rates (80% to 90%) and few recurrences (0% to 30%) or complications.[3-7]

However, only about 10% of patients have a sustained VT that is sufficiently hemodynamically tolerated to allow for adequate activation mapping.[8] Further, even in those patients with a stable VT that is mappable, it is almost invariably true that other unstable (i.e., "unmappable") VTs can also be induced. This is not surprising when one considers that the arrhythmogenic substrate is not a simple single circuit but rather an extensive sheet of surviving myocardial fibers in a bed of scar tissue with multiple potential entry and exit points that allow for various reentrant paths (i.e., different VTs) to be operative at any given time (Fig. 29–2).[9] From a

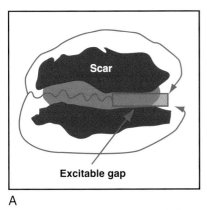
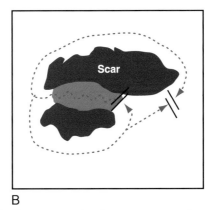
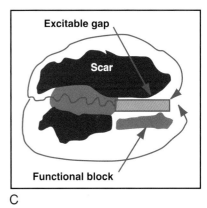

A   B   C

FIGURE 29–1. The importance of the excitable gap to maintain a reentrant tachycardia circuit. In (**A**), the wavefront traverses within the scarred tissue along a surviving tract of myocardial tissue. Conduction through this pathway is slow because of a number of potential factors including the arrangement of the myocardial fibers (side-to-side instead of end-to-end), alterations in gap junctions between myocardial fibrils, a meandering path of the tract, and slow conduction velocity at certain regions (e.g., areas of extreme wavefront curvature). The wavelength of the circuit is short enough that the leading edge of the wavefront constantly encounters excitable myocardial tissue. This "excitable gap" allows the circuit to perpetuate and manifest as VT. In (**B**), the wavelength of the tachycardia circuit is longer than the tissue tract that it must follow. The leading edge of the wavefront encountered refractory tissue so the circuit extinguished, and VT was not maintained. **C,** However, functional block can supervene in certain situations such as ischemia, increased heart rates, administration of drugs that alter conduction velocity or ventricular repolarization, electrolyte changes, acid-base imbalances, etc. In this situation, the addition of functional block to the preexisting anatomical block creates an excitable gap, allowing for sustained VT.

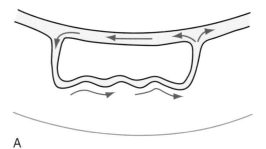

A

FIGURE 29–2. The substrate for VT in post–MI patients. Instead of a single bundle of myocardium forming the tachycardia circuit (**A**), surgical mapping studies of post-MI VT have revealed an extensive sheet of surviving myocardial fibers linked in the subendocardium through multiple "entrance" and "exit" points (**B** and **C**). This accounts for multiple potential reentrant paths (that is, different VT morphologies) at different times all originating from the same mass of infarcted tissue. *(From Downar E, Harris L, Michleborough LL, et al.: Endocardial mapping of ventricular tachycardia in the intact human heart: Evidence for reentrant mechanisms. J Am Coll Cardiol 11:783-791, 1988, with permission.)*

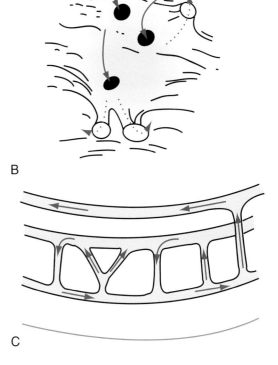

B

C

procedural perspective, it may be most appropriate to regard this substrate as a mass of arrhythmogenic tissue with multiple tracts of surviving tissue traversing through scar—many, or perhaps even most, of which might be appropriate to target for ablation to completely eliminate VT.

THE SURGICAL EXPERIENCE WITH POST–MYOCARDIAL INFARCTION VENTRICULAR TACHYCARDIA

The approach to ablation of unstable VTs developed directly from the extensive experience since the late 1970s with surgical modification of the arrhythmogenic substrate in post-MI patients. Because the reentrant circuit is most often located in the subendocardium at the junction of normal and scarred tissue, the initial surgical experience with simple aneurysmectomy was disappointing.[10,11]

However, two effective general strategies were developed over time: (1) subendocardial resection, involving surgical removal of the subendocardial layer containing the arrhythmogenic substrate in this border zone,[12-14] and (2) encircling endocardial ventriculotomy, consisting of the placement of a circumferential surgical lesion through the border zone and, presumably, interrupting potential VT circuits.[15,16] Because of its distinct advantage in destroying myocardial cells without disrupting the fibrous stroma, cryoablation has also been used, both as a stand-alone intervention during surgery and as an adjunct to subendocardial resection. Encircling cryoablation is an efficacious procedure that incorporates cryoablation into the concept of an encircling endocardial ventriculotomy.[17,18] When it is performed at experienced centers, the rate of long-term freedom from malignant VT/VF after surgery is greater than 90% (Fig. 29–3).

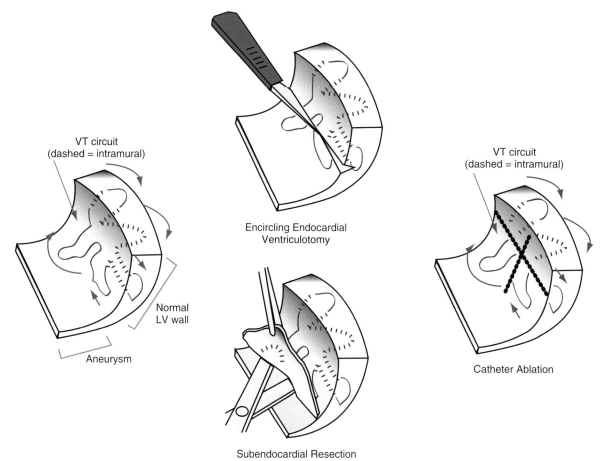

FIGURE 29–3. Surgical substrate modification to eliminate VT. The border between the normal and infarcted/aneurysmal wall contains a stylized VT circuit-predominantly endocardial, and partially intramural. The surgical procedures, subendocardial resection and ventriculotomy, are thought to either remove or transect critical endocardial portions of the VT circuit, respectively. During catheter ablation, the border zone is mapped using the electroanatomical mapping system, the putative exit site of the VT is identified by pace mapping, and catheter-based linear lesions are placed in an attempt to interrupt the circuit. Since mapping is performed during sinus rhythm instead of during VT, this allows for greater patient safety and comfort. *(From Miller J, Rothman SA, Addonizio VP: Surgical techniques for ventricular tachycardia ablation. In Singer I (ed.): Interventional Electrophysiology. Baltimore: Williams & Wilkins, 1997, pp 641-684, with permission.)*

In the early surgical experience, intraoperative mapping was initially performed to help guide the surgical resection. After open surgical bypass, multi-electrode plaques were used to precisely identify the origin of the VT. This area of endocardium was either surgically removed or surgically transected using a scalpel blade. However, VT surgery then evolved such that, in many cases, equivalent results were obtained by visualizing the scar and either simply resecting it or placing surgical cryoablation or laser ablation lesions along its border.[16-18] These "empiric" lesions are thought to eliminate critical portions of the circuit and thus render the VT noninducible (Fig. 29–4).

The effect of arrhythmia surgery on the myocardial substrate was examined in a study of 18 patients undergoing successful subendocardial resection procedures.[19] These patients had all previously sustained anterior wall MI and manifested multiple morphologies of drug-refractory monomorphic VT. During the operative procedure, a 20-electrode rectangular plaque array was used to obtain electrical data from the apical septum during VT as well as during normal sinus rhythm immediately before and immediately after resection of subendocardial tissue (Fig. 29–5). Electrograms (EGMs) could be compared from 298 (83%) of the 360 electrodes. Before resection, split EGMs were present in 130 recordings (44%) and late potentials in 81 (27%). However, the post-resection recordings revealed a complete absence of the split EGMs, as well as elimination of all of the previously recorded late potentials. The mean EGM duration

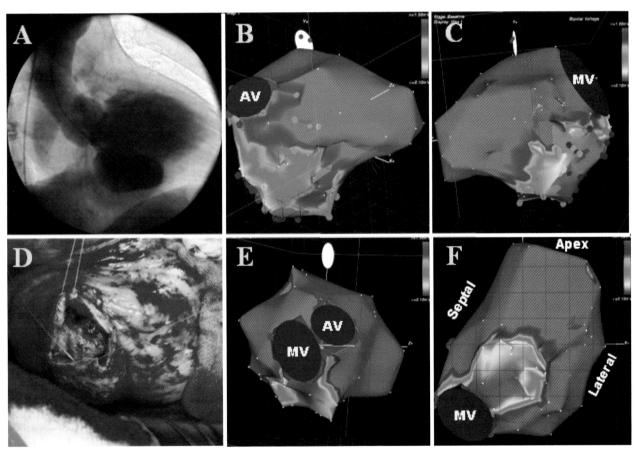

FIGURE 29–4. Electroanatomical mapping of the effect of arrhythmia surgery. **A,** Left ventriculography reveals a large infero-basal aneurysm in the setting of three-vessel coronary artery disease and clinical VT. During a pre-surgical electrophysiology study, programmed ventricular stimulation revealed easily-inducible VT. LV electroanatomical mapping was performed during sinus rhythm (using the CARTO system). The bipolar voltage amplitude maps shown in RAO-caudal (**B**) and left lateral-caudal (**C**) projections reveal a large infero-basal aneurysmal scar (gray) with EGMs containing abnormal fractionated and late potentials (not shown). During surgery (**D**), the LV was opened through the aneurysm, the aneurysm was resected, cryoablation was applied to the margins of the scar, and the ventricle was closed with the support of a patch. Months after the surgery, a repeat electrophysiology study revealed (1) a smaller homogeneous scar without evidence of fractionated and late potentials (right posterior oblique and inferior projections in **E** and **F**, respectively), (2) a more favorable ventricular geometry without an aneurysmal component, and (3) no inducible VT with programmed ventricular stimulation. The color range is set such that *purple* represents normal tissue (>1.5 mV), *red* the most severely diseased tissue (<0.1 mV), and *gray* represents pure scar with no identifiable electrical activity. AV, aortic valve; MV, mitral valve.

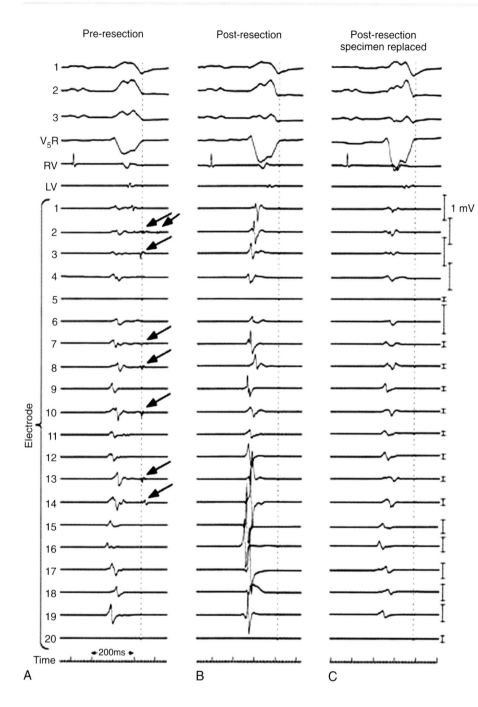

FIGURE 29–5. The electrophysiological effect of subendocardial resection surgery. Recordings were made using a 20-bipole plaque array (**A**) before and (**B**) after resection as well as after replacement of (and recording through) the resected tissue specimen (**C**). The *dotted line* in (**A**) denotes the end of the QRS complex. The split and late EGM components (*arrows*) before resection are absent in the post-resection recordings. In addition, most channels show an increase in amplitude of the remaining early EGM component, which maintains the same general morphology as before resection. After replacement of the specimen, these early EGMs appear similar to those obtained before resection, but note the absence of split and late electrograms (channels 5 and 20 did not record properly). *(From Miller JM, Tyson GS, Hargrove WC, et al.: Effect of subendocardial resection on sinus rhythm endocardial electrogram abnormalities. Circulation 91:2385-2391, 1995, with permission.)*

decreased from 112 ± 38 to 65 ± 27 msec, primarily because of the loss of these split and late potentials. Histologic studies revealed that the subendocardial tissue removed in this procedure contained bundles of surviving muscle fibrils separated by dense connective tissue. These data suggest that the direct effect of the subendocardial resection procedure is to eliminate the tissue containing these abnormal EGM components.

The significant morbidity and mortality (3% to 14%) associated with arrhythmia surgery, as well as the safety and efficacy of implantable cardioverter defibrillators (ICDs) to terminate life-threatening

VT/VF, has severely curtailed its use in general practice. However, the surgical experience provided several important lessons that are relevant for modern catheter ablation of VT: (1) critical portions of the VT circuit reside on the endocardial surface of the scar (allowing access via a percutaneous endoluminal approach); (2) the majority of VTs exit from the border of the scarred myocardium; (3) during normal sinus rhythm, the "anatomy" of the scar can be delineated by certain distinguishing endocardial EGM criteria—low voltage amplitude, prolonged EGM duration, and the presence of late potentials[20]; and (4) empiric disruption of the arrhythmogenic substrate containing these abnormal fractionated, discrete, split, or late potentials in this "border zone" area can eliminate VT.

Mapping and Ablation

There are two broad groups of strategies that one can employ to eliminate unstable VTs. The first, substrate-based catheter ablation, attempts to replicate the success of the substrate modification strategy seen with arrhythmia surgery (Table 29–1). The second relies on improvements in mapping technology that now allow one to perform rapid activation mapping during the VT or VTs of interest to identify critical portions of the circuit to target for ablation.

SUBSTRATE-BASED ABLATION OF VENTRICULAR TACHYCARDIA

This therapeutic strategy can be divided into three steps: (1) characterization of target VT morphologies, (2) delineation of the scarred myocardial substrate, and (3) identification and targeting of the arrhythmogenic myocardium—that is, those portions of the myocardial scar that are most likely to contribute to tachycardia formation. The first step is to define the many morphologies of VT that can potentially manifest from the infarct. The stimulation protocol typically includes programmed ventricular stimulation at two right ventricular (RV) sites and, if this does not induce VT, at one left ventricular (LV) site for two cycle lengths (typically 600 and 400 msec). In addition, burst pacing can also be performed until either 2 : 1 capture or a pacing cycle length of 250 msec is reached. When a VT is induced, it is pace-terminated and the stimulation protocol is continued to induce other VTs. Stimulation is continued until either the same VTs are repeatedly induced or electrical cardioversion needs to be performed to terminate VT (to minimize patient discomfort). From a safety perspective, it is important to remember that with depressed LV function, there is an increased risk of worsening congestive heart failure during the stimulation protocol. To mitigate against this, adequate time should be given between each stimulation train. Also, the empiric administration of a diuretic agent at the time of the stimulation protocol should be considered. In some patients with severely depressed ejection fraction or preexisting significant congestive heart failure, periprocedural intra-aortic balloon counterpulsation should be considered. This minimizes the adverse hemodynamic effects of the stimulation protocol as well as the remainder of the procedure; however, a second arterial puncture is required, and

TABLE 29–1

Substrate-Based Ablation of Ventricular Tachycardia

Characterize target VT morphologies

Obtain any 12-lead ECGs of spontaneous VTs

Obtain any ICD strips of spontaneous VTs

Programmed ventricular stimulation from two RV and one LV site (2 cycle lengths) and rapid ventricular pacing

Programmed stimulation from within the myocardial scar

Delineate scarred myocardial substrate

Electroanatomic mapping using a mapping catheter with the distal electrode not greater than 4 mm

F-curve (or equivalent) mapping catheter is optimal for most patients; but if ventricular chamber is markedly enlarged, consider using larger curve (e.g., J-curve)

In addition to the retrograde aortic approach, consider trans-septal mapping of the LV to facilitate mapping of ventricular chamber

Acquire LV endocardial points to a fill-threshold of ≤20 mm in normal tissue, and ≤10 mm within the abnormal tissue (bipolar voltage amplitude <1.5 mV)

If septum is involved, consider electroanatomic mapping of the RV aspect of the interventricular septum

If epicardial circuit is suspected (e.g., inferior wall MI, DCM-VT, Chagas-VT, any failed endocardial ablation attempt), pericardial electroanatomic mapping of the ventricles to the level of the atrioventricular groove

Identify "arrhythmogenic" myocardium to target for ablation

Pace mapping at the borders of the scar to regionalize the VT exit sites

Consider brief inductions of VT with mapping catheter at the optimal pace mapped sites to quickly perform entrainment maneuvers

Identify areas of late and fractionated potentials within the scarred myocardium

Pacing from within the infarcted tissue to identify sites with long stimulus-to-QRS duration (latency mapping)

Pace mapping to identify channels between areas of dense ("electrically unexcitable") scar

DCM, dilated cardiomyopathy; ECG, electrocardiogram; ICD, implantable cardioverter defibrillator; LV, left ventricle; MI, myocardial infarction; RV, right ventricle; VT, ventricular tachycardia.

the risk of vascular and embolic complications may be increased in patients with severe arterial atherosclerotic disease.

The next step involves delineation of the myocardial scar. Catheter access for LV mapping can be achieved using either a retrograde aortic approach or a trans-septal approach across the mitral valve. Typically, the mapping/ablation catheter is easily prolapsed across the aortic valve into the LV after first being deflected into a "U" shape. But occasionally it can be difficult to cross the aortic valve during retrograde aortic mapping. In this situation, it can be useful to delineate the cusps of the aortic valve by electroanatomic mapping. Then, the mapping/ablation catheter can be manipulated so that its tip is oriented to point to the center of these three cusps and then advanced directly into the ventricle.

The trans-septal puncture is reviewed in detail in Chapter 33, but several important aspects of trans-septal LV mapping bear mention. First, because abnormal ventricular anatomy is frequently encountered in patients undergoing VT ablation, atrial dilation and cardiac rotation are not uncommon and should be anticipated. Second, because these patients often have ICDs, one must be careful to not dislodge the pacing/defibrillation leads. Third, there are no trans-septal sheaths particularly suited for ventricular mapping; a simple Mullins-type curve often serves well to allow easy manipulation across the mitral valve into the LV. Fourth, as during any prolonged trans-septal access, it is prudent to maintain continuous flushing of the sheath with heparinized saline; a pump should be employed, because the ele-

vated ventricular pressures might otherwise preclude flow at times when the sheath is advanced over the catheter into the ventricular chamber proper. To save on mapping time, we typically use both the retrograde aortic and the trans-septal approach. We find that when a particular region cannot be readily mapped using one approach, temporarily switching to the alternative approach often allows facile mapping of this region. Of course, in the presence of aortic stenosis, severe arterial tortuosity, extensive aortic atheroma, or a mechanical aortic arch, the trans-septal approach alone is preferred. Conversely, a mechanical mitral valve mandates transeptal mapping.

Based on surgical mapping studies in patients with post-MI VT, there are several EGM characteristics during sinus rhythm that help to differentiate normal from abnormal myocardial tissue. Abnormal tissue is marked by EGMs of low voltage amplitude, prolonged EGM duration, and fractionated EGMs with late and split potentials (Fig. 29–6).[19,20] In the past, the difficulties in appreciating three-dimensional (3-D) anatomy using fluoroscopy alone precluded a systematic approach to targeting these abnormal EGMs.[21] However, this changed dramatically with the advent of a number of advanced 3-D cardiac mapping systems (see Chapter 8 for details): basket catheters,[22] electrode-mounted balloon catheters (EnSite, Endocardial Solutions, St. Paul,

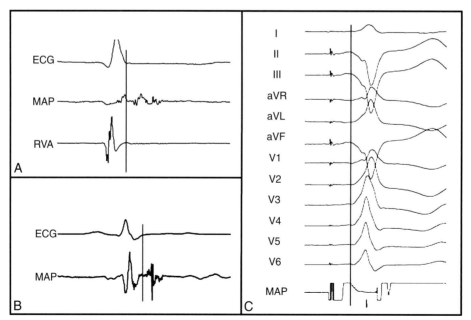

FIGURE 29–6. Abnormal electrograms. A, A normal electrogram (EGM) is recorded from a catheter placed at the right ventricular apex (RVA); it is characterized by high amplitude, short electrogram duration, and no electrical activity noted after the end of the QRS complex (vertical line). Examples of fractionated and late potentials are shown on the MAP catheter EGMs in (A) and (B). In (C), when pacing from a location at which a late potential was recorded, there is a delay between the timing of the stimulus to the beginning of the QRS complex (vertical line). This latency represents the time required for the wavefront to traverse from the surviving myocardial tissue within the infarct to the normal myocardium.

MN),[23] and electroanatomic mapping systems based on electrical impedance (LocaLisa, Medtronic, Minneapolis, MN and Navex, Endo cardial solutions, St. Paul, MN),[24] low-level magnetic fields (CARTO, Biosense Webster, Baldwin Park, CA),[25] or sonomicrometry (RPM, Boston Scientific, San Jose, CA).[26] These mapping systems serve several critical purposes during substrate mapping: (1) identification of the catheter tip during catheter mapping to minimize fluoroscopy exposure, (2) creation of electroanatomic maps to electronically depict the ventricular normal and infarcted anatomy, and (3) cataloguing of both important sites to target for ablation and the ablation sites themselves.

Most of the experimental and clinical experience with the use of electroanatomic mapping to identify the abnormal infarcted myocardium has been with magnetic electroanatomic mapping (MEAM) using the CARTO system and, to a lesser extent, with sonomicrometry-based electroanatomic mapping (SEAM) using the RPM system. Briefly, the MEAM system uses a low-intensity magnetic field to localize the mapping catheter in space with six degrees of freedom (position in the x, y, and z planes plus rotation, pitch, and yaw).[25] The accuracy of the system has been estimated at 0.8 mm and 5 degrees. Using this system to guide catheter movement, an endocardial cast of the ventricle can be constructed, and the various EGM characteristics (e.g., bipolar/unipolar EGM voltage amplitude, EGM duration) can be annotated to each displayed point. The feasibility of substrate mapping using MEAM was established in a series of experimental studies employing porcine models of healed MI (Fig. 29–7).[27,28] Detailed ventricular electroanatomic mapping during normal sinus rhythm was used to reconstruct the chamber anatomy and display the EGM characteristics. Based on values obtained in normal ventricles, delineation of the infarcted tissue by analysis of the bipolar voltage EGM amplitude was performed using a cutoff of 1.5 mV. With this bipolar voltage amplitude criterion, RF ablation lesions were placed to "tag" the borders of the scar. On gross pathologic examination, the lesions were indeed situated at the borders of the scar. These data demonstrated that the myocardial scar borders can be identified and targeted for ablation using electroanatomic mapping techniques. SEAM can also be used to perform substrate mapping (Fig. 29–8).

Additional clinical work in patients revealed that a bipolar voltage EGM amplitude cutoff of 1.5 mV also serves well to separate normal from infarcted tissue (Fig. 29–9).[29,30] Of note, some patients are not in sinus rhythm but are chronically ventricular-paced (either RV or biventricular). The effect of this change in wavefront direction on bipolar EGM amplitude and subsequent identification of myocardial infarct architecture during electroanatomic mapping was assessed at 819 LV sites during atrial or ventricular pacing in 11 post-MI patients.[31] Only 8% of sites had a bipolar EGM amplitude that was "reclassified" from abnormal (≤1.5 mV) to normal (>1.5 mV) or vice versa. Therefore, substrate maps generated using bipolar EGM amplitude provide robust representations of the infarct morphology despite variations in the direction of wavefront propagation that result from different rhythms.

Although values lower than 0.5 mV are typically arbitrarily defined as dense scar, this does not imply that this tissue contains no surviving myocardial fibrils. Indeed, this tissue often contains surviving fibrils that can be identified as split or late potentials in sinus rhythm or as mid-diastolic potentials during VT. Similarly, mapping based on bipolar EGM duration (using the MEAM system's double annotation function) has also proved capable of delineating the scarred myocardium (>50 msec in porcine or >100 msec in human ventricles).[28] Of note, because one must manually annotate the points to generate an EGM duration map, the practical utility of this approach may be limited. However, certain points that appear to be of artifactually low voltage amplitude, for example because of poor catheter-tissue contact, are often shown to be of normal EGM duration.[28] Therefore, the precise role of EGM duration mapping is still in evolution (see Fig. 29–9).

It is also important to note that any single mapped site with voltage amplitude greater than 1.5 mV (or EGM duration <50 msec in porcine or <100 msec in human ventricles) is not necessarily normal. However, although such a site may be incorrectly identified as normal (or abnormal) based on EGM criteria, use of a large number of locations to construct a map has the effect of minimizing these "outliers" and identifying the scar and border zones in a clinically useful manner. In fact, use of these arbitrary voltage amplitude cutoffs may not be the most appropriate strategy for substrate mapping. For example, in a patient with ventricular hypertrophy, it is unrealistic to expect all tissue with a bipolar EGM amplitude greater than 1.5 mV to represent normal tissue. In this setting, a reference value of 1.6 to 2.0 mV may be more appropriate as the cutoff for normal tissue.[32] Similarly, in the ventricle of a patient with dilated cardiomyopathy demonstrating a "low-voltage" electrocardiogram and superimposed scar, certain sites with a bipolar EGM amplitude of less than 1.5 mV are not likely to represent infarcted tissue. Future studies may reveal alternative means to individualize EGM criteria in a patient-specific manner. In the interim, it is prudent to employ these arbitrary EGM criteria only as a guide to the location and mor-

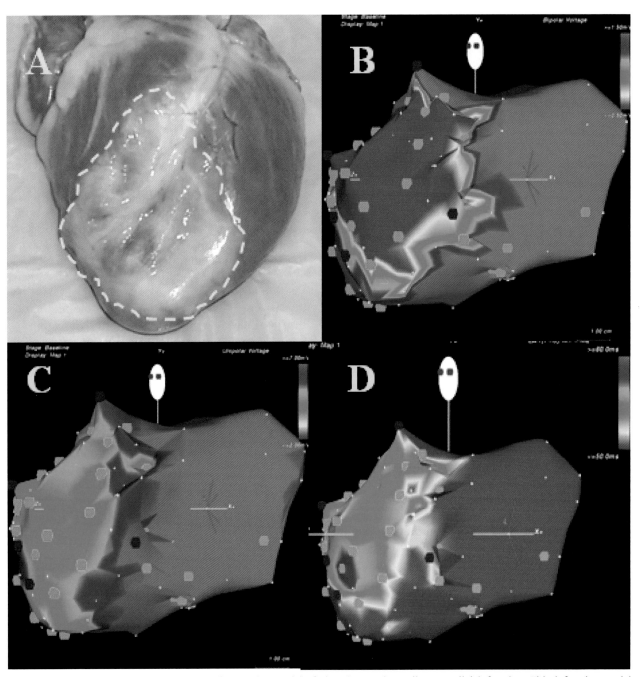

FIGURE 29–7. Electroanatomical mapping of a porcine model of chronic anterior wall myocardial infarction. This infarction model is created by injection of agarose microspheres into the mid-LAD. Eight weeks later, the electroanatomical mapping procedure is performed using the CARTO system. The transmural anterior wall infarct is visible upon gross pathological examination (**A**); the scar is outlined by the *dotted line*. In vivo electroanatomical mapping identified this anterior wall infarct by bipolar voltage amplitude criteria (**B**), unipolar voltage amplitude criteria (**C**), or bipolar electrogram (EGM) duration criteria (**D**). The projections are LAO in **B-D**; note the characteristic leftward rotation of the porcine heart. The color ranges in the bipolar voltage, unipolar voltage, and EGM duration maps are 0.5-1.5 mV, 2-7 mV, and 50-80 msec; *purple* and *red* represent normal and severely diseased tissue in the bipolar and unipolar voltage maps, respectively, while the opposite is true for the ECG duration map. The EGM duration maps were generated using the "double annotation" caliper function.

phology of the myocardial scar, and not as the final arbiter of normal versus abnormal tissue.

In an effort to translate these experimental data into clinical benefit, Marchlinski et al.[29] examined the use of electroanatomic mapping in a seminal study involving patients with drug-refractory unstable VT. They demonstrated that after identification of the infarcted myocardium using bipolar voltage amplitude criteria, catheter-based RF ablation lesions directed in a linear fashion were able to control VT

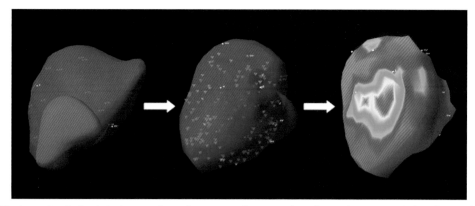

FIGURE 29–8. Electroanatomical substrate mapping using a sonomicrometry-based mapping system. Using the porcine infarct model, mapping of the LV endocardium and the ventricular epicardium (using a subxyphoid puncture pericardial approach, see later in this chapter) was performed using the RPM system. Initially, rough outlines of the chamber geometries are constructed by sweeping the catheter within the chamber. Shown is an antero-posterior projection of the LV endocardium within the ventricular epicardial shell (left). Then, contact electrograms are acquired at points sufficiently distributed across the chamber surfaces (middle). Electrogram characteristics can be displayed upon this rendering (right). An epicardial bipolar voltage amplitude map is shown with the color range from 0.5mV-1.5mV (normal tissue is purple and dense scar is red).

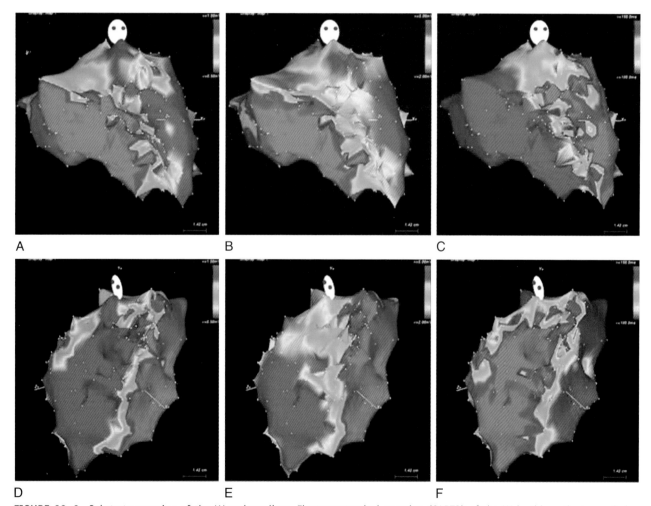

FIGURE 29–9. Substrate mapping of the LV endocardium. Electroanatomical mapping (CARTO) of the LV in this patient revealed a large anterior wall MI based on bipolar voltage amplitude (**A, D**), unipolar voltage amplitude (**B, E**) and EGM duration (**C, F**) mapping (RAO projection in **A, B, C** and LAO-cranial projection in **D, E, F**). The scale ranges from 0.5 to 1.5mV, 2 to 5mV, and 100 to 150msec in the bipolar voltage, unipolar voltage and EGM duration maps, respectively.

in nine post-MI patients. Using this high-density electroanatomic mapping system, we and others have since demonstrated that (1) a substrate-mapping strategy can be used to localize the arrhythmogenic substrate in most patients with a history of MI and sustained ventricular tachyarrhythmias, and (2) RF catheter ablation can be effectively and safely used to modify the arrhythmogenic substrate to render VT noninducible even in the presence of multiple hemodynamically unstable VT morphologies (Table 29–2).[30,33-36] Common to all of these studies is the concept of substrate mapping—that is, delineation of the infarcted myocardium based on local EGM criteria. However, there are a number of approaches to identifying and targeting the "arrhythmogenic substrate"—the third step of substrate-based VT ablation. These can be broadly divided into two categories: (1) targeting the sites of VT exit from the scarred myocardium, and (2) targeting the myocardial channels of activation within the scarred myocardium.

TARGETING THE VENTRICULAR TACHYCARDIA EXIT SITES

By definition, a reentrant rhythm is always depolarizing some quantity of myocardial tissue. Because the small mass of myocardial tissue in the protected myocardial channels within the scar contributes negligibly to the surface QRS, the QRS complex of a VT initiates when the wavefront of activation emanates from the border of the scar. Accordingly, once the myocardial scar is defined, a brief examination of the surface QRS morphology of the target VT (or VTs) can usually regionalize the VT exit site to a scar border.[37,38] The vast majority of VTs in the setting of structural heart disease originate from the LV. Accordingly, a left bundle branch block–like morphology in lead V_1 indicates that the VT is exiting from the LV septum and only rarely, from the RV proper.[39] The remaining VTs exiting from other regions of the LV typically have a right bundle branch block morphology in lead V_1. However, it should be noted that a right bundle branch morphology VT can still have a septal exit site, a situation in which the frontal plane axis is typically leftward (positive in leads I and aVL). Septal versus lateral exit for an apical LV VT with right bundle branch block–type QRS morphology can also be determined by examining the activation time to a fixed reference endocardial recording at the RV apex.[40] For any right bundle branch block–type QRS morphology created by pace mapping or VT in the setting of an apical infarct, the QRS-RV apex activation time is less than 100 msec for an apical septal origin and greater than 125 msec for an apical lateral origin. Similar values are seen in the setting of nonapical infarcts, albeit with some degree of overlap.

TABLE 29–2

Catheter Ablation of Unstable Ventricular Tachycardia

Authors (Ref. No.)	Myocardial Pathology	No. of Patients	VT Ablation Approach	Follow-up (mo)	Clinical Success (%)
Marchlinski et al.[29]	CAD, ARVC	21	Substrate-based	8 ± 7	75
Soejima et al.[33]	CAD	40	Substrate-based	10 ± 8	63
Sra et al.[34]	CAD	19	Substrate-based	7 ± 2	66
Reddy et al.[30]	CAD	11	Substrate-based	13 ± 2	82
Arenal et al.[35]	CAD	24	Substrate-based	9 ± 4	79
Kottkamp et al.[36]	CAD	28	Substrate-based	15 ± 8	64
Schilling et al.[23]	CAD, DCM	24	"Single-beat" mapping	18	64
Strickberger et al.[50]	CAD, DCM	15	"Single-beat" mapping	1	71
Della Bella et al.[51]	CAD, DCM, ARVC	17	"Single-beat" mapping	20 ± 5	59
Hsia et al.[55]	DCM	19	Substrate-based	22 ± 12	68
Soejima et al.[56]	DCM	28	Substrate-based	11 ± 9	54
Marchlinski et al.[58]	ARVC	21	Substrate-based	27 ± 22	89

ARVC, arrhythmogenic right ventricular cardiomyopathy/dysplasia; CAD, coronary artery disease; DCM, dilated cardiomyopathy; VT, ventricular tachycardia.

The ECG frontal plane axis can help differentiate a superior from an inferior exit; the former is characterized by an inferiorly directed QRS axis with positive complexes in leads II, III, and aVF, and the latter is characterized by a superiorly directed QRS axis (negative II, III, and aVF). An apical exit is characterized by predominantly negative QRS complexes in the precordial leads, whereas basal exit sites tend to be predominantly positive in these leads. Although these "rules" are helpful, a number of factors can influence the QRS complex in any given patient, including the size and location of the myocardial scar, the orientation of the heart in the thorax (horizontal versus vertical), and intrinsic conduction system disease that can modify the wavefront of activation.

Based on the ECG morphology of the VT, pace mapping is performed at the suspected borders of the scar during normal sinus rhythm to precisely localize the exit point. Unlike during VT, pacing during sinus rhythm results in omnidirectional spread of activation, which might be expected to result in a different paced-QRS morphology than the VT-QRS morphology, even with pacing from the proper exit site. However, the optimal paced-QRS morphology is often only slightly different from the target VT-QRS morphology. This is probably because, with pacing at a scar border, activation proceeding into the scar is slower and contributes little to overall ventricular activation, compared with the "orthodromic" wavefront that rapidly emanates in the opposite direction into normal tissue. Not surprisingly, less optimal matches to the pace-mapped exit sites are found with pacing along the borders of smaller scars, as opposed to larger scars.

Pace mapping is also affected by the rate, stimulus strength, and electrode polarity during pacing. At faster pacing rates, the "antidromic" wavefront of activation into the scar may contribute less to the QRS morphology than during slow pacing. In addition, ventricular repolarization may fuse into and modify the QRS morphology during faster pacing rates. Because it is difficult to predict the effects of these variables, pacing is ideally performed at a rate similar to the target VT rate. Increasing the stimulus strength can also affect the QRS morphology, presumably by capturing more distant (i.e., far-field) tissue. We typically start pacing at low output and increase the output until several QRS complexes are captured in succession. If multiple QRS morphologies are seen at varying outputs, this is indicative of a protected region (or channel) of tissue: at the lower output, only this region is captured by pacing, but at higher output, the far-field tissue is also captured. In the ideal situation, unipolar pacing would be performed, so that only the distal electrode could stimulate the myocardium and inadvertent pacing by the proximal electrode could be avoided. However, unipolar pacing can result in a larger stimulus artifact that can preclude accurate QRS morphology interpretation. And, from a practical perspective, it is unusual for bipolar and unipolar pacing morphologies to be markedly different, probably because the ablation catheter is typically not parallel to the tissue surface, resulting in lack of contact of the proximal electrode with the tissue.

As with the difficulty in trying to predict the VT exit site from the QRS morphology, it is also difficult to predict the paced-QRS morphology from different LV sites. However, in any given patient, the ECG morphology "rules" described earlier work well to predict the paced-QRS morphology of a given site in relation to another site (Fig. 29–10). That is, if a particular pacing site reveals a superior axis in the frontal QRS plane, it is fairly likely that pacing sites progressively superior to this location will reveal an intermediate and then an inferior axis in the frontal QRS plane.

Once a VT exit site is identified, linear lesions are placed using one of a number of strategies: (1) extending from the "dense scar" (defined as amplitude <0.5 mV) to anatomic boundaries or normal myocardium, (2) extending along the borders of the scar and traversing these optimal pacing sites, or (3) a pair of crossing linear lesions, one extending from the exit site into the scar and the other along the border of the scar. Lesions are typically applied at one spot until one of the following criteria is realized: (1) a decrease of the contact impedance by at least 5 ohms (Ω), (2) a reduction in the EGM voltage amplitude by at least 75%, or (3) doubling of the pace-capture threshold after ablation. Linear lesions are generated by point-to-point spot applications with interpoint distances not exceeding 10 mm, and ideally no greater than 5 mm. Because of the depth of ventricular tissue, we do not attempt to achieve, or check for, conduction block traversing these linear lesions. The strategy is not to "contain" or "isolate" the VT circuit, because this is both unlikely given current ablation technology and possibly undesirable because of potential adverse effects. Instead, these lesions are delivered to transect critical portions that are important for tachycardia maintenance.

The placement of catheter-based ablation lesions completely around the scar (mimicking the surgical procedure of partially encircling endocardial ventriculotomy) may be predicted to be of equal if not superior efficacy, potentially obviating the pace-mapping step (Fig. 29–11). This procedure could certainly be performed in some patients, but there are two aspects to this strategy that must be considered. First, generating continuous linear lesions along the

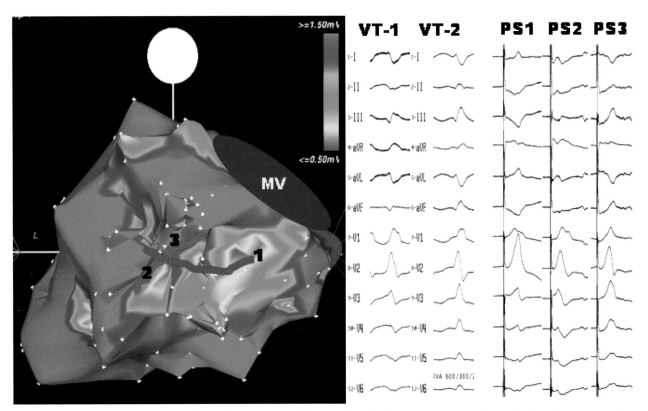

FIGURE 29–10. Substrate mapping and radiofrequency (RF) ablation. Sinus rhythm electroanatomical mapping in this post-MI patient revealed a localized postero-basal infarct as shown in this bipolar voltage map (PA projection). Two VTs were induced during programmed stimulation; note the differences in leads III and V3 V6. Pacing during sinus rhythm from site #1 (PS) was too septal to the exit sites of these two VTs—leads I and aVL are positive in the pace map but negative during the VTs. Accordingly, pacing performed from the lateral aspect of the infarct from sites #2 and #3 revealed morphologies consistent with VT-1 and VT-2. The short stimulus-QRS duration indicates that these sites represent VT exit points. (The pacing artifact caused an initial distortion of the QRS complex during pace mapping.) Pacing between sites #2 and #3 generated a QRS morphology that alternated between VT-1 and VT-2, but with a longer stimulus-QRS time; this latency likely represents a common pathway for the two VT circuits. A series of RF ablation lesions were placed in a linear fashion along the scar border incorporating these two pacing sites (represented by the *short red line*). However, programmed stimulation induced a slower VT of similar morphology to VT-1 (not shown). After placing a second linear lesion extending into the scar (represented by the intersecting *darker red line*), no VT was inducible.

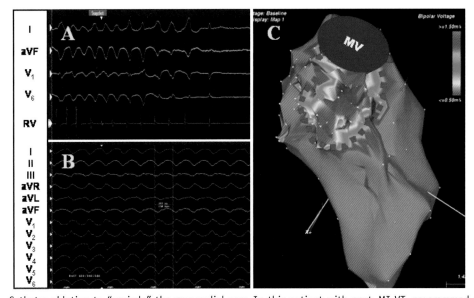

FIGURE 29–11. Catheter ablation to "encircle" the myocardial scar. In this patient with post–MI VT, programmed ventricular stimulation induced only non-sustained polymorphic VT (**A**). Repeat stimulation after infusion of intravenous Ajmaline (a Class I antiarrhythmic agent) revealed an easily inducible monomorphic VT (**B**). The bipolar voltage map (**C**) identified an infero-posterior MI (right posterior oblique caudal projection; color range from 0.5-1.5 mV). Because pace mapping identified a suboptimal "best" exit site, and because of the relatively small size of the scar, RF ablation lesions were placed along the full border of the scar (*dashed line*). VT was no longer inducible at the end of the procedure.

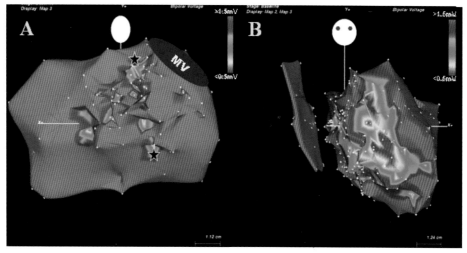

FIGURE 29–12. Post-MI scar morphologies. A range of post-MI scar morphologies are seen including small patchy scars (**A**), and large anterior wall scars with interventricular septal wall involvement (**B**). In the former situation, two VTs were induced and pace mapping revealed the exits to be located at the superior and inferior aspects of the scar (*black stars*); RF ablation lesions were placed spanning between these two sites to render VT non-inducible. In the later situation, mapping the right ventricular aspect of the septum should be considered; in this patient, the RV septum displayed normal bipolar voltage amplitude. Shown are left posterior oblique and anterior projections in **A** and **B**, respectively (bipolar voltage map; color range 0.5-1.5 mV).

entire length of the tissue can be technically difficult with larger scars. Second, the placement of multiple ablation lesions at the scar border near normal tissue has the potential to adversely affect LV function (see further discussion later in this chapter). Accordingly, a more limited cross-hair lesion set may be desirable for patients with more severe LV dysfunction.

Instead of large homogeneous infarcts, one may instead encounter patchy myocardial scars that preclude rapid identification of the VT exit zones (Fig. 29–12). These cases are particularly challenging but can still be approached using the same strategy. These patchy scars are relatively uncommon (<10% in our experience), even in the presence of severe ventricular dysfunction.

TARGETING THE MYOCARDIAL CHANNELS

Even in the setting of hemodynamically unstable VT, a number of strategies may be employed to target putative myocardial channels within the scarred tissue, including (1) resetting/entrainment mapping (in those patients with stable as well as unstable VTs), (2) ablation of split/late potentials within the scarred myocardium, (3) latency mapping, and (4) pace mapping to identify densely scarred tissue with intervening channels of activation. The most direct and reliable means to identify a channel of activation is to employ entrainment/resetting criteria (described further in Chapter 27) during VT. For hemodynamically unstable VT, this can be accomplished by first performing pace mapping at the scar border to

identify the putative exit site, followed by a brief inductions of the unstable VT to quickly perform the entrainment maneuvers and then pace-termination. This can be facilitated by the use of an intra-aortic balloon pump, both to support arterial perfusion during tachycardia and to prevent worsening heart failure after termination of the rhythm. But to perform resetting or entrainment of unstable VT, it is necessary to be able to reproducibly initiate the very same morphology of tachycardia.

Additional sites of potentially arrhythmogenic myocardium related to these resetting/entrainment sites may be identified and incorporated into the ablation strategy. For example, in addition to a VT exit site, one may identify a site deeper within the scar that demonstrates a similar QRS morphology with pace mapping during sinus rhythm, albeit with a longer stimulus-to-QRS time (latency). These regions of latency can be graphically represented to create a "latency map" (Fig. 29–13). They most likely represent surviving myocardial fibrils within the body of scar that may be critical for the target VT or other VTs arising from the arrhythmogenic mass of tissue.

Although it is true that the benefits of substrate-based VT ablation are most realized during ablation of hemodynamically unstable VT, this strategy can also be useful in ablation of stable VT.[30,41] As described earlier, the VT circuit exit site can be rapidly identified by pacing along the scar's periphery, followed by resetting/entrainment maneuvers to precisely define a critical point of the circuit (Fig. 29–14). In our experience, this frequently identifies a

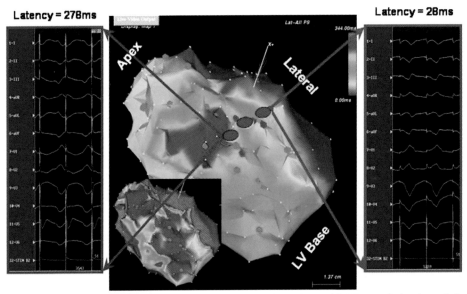

Latency = 278ms   Latency = 28ms

FIGURE 29–13. Latency mapping. Sinus rhythm substrate mapping in this patient with VT revealed a large inferior wall MI upon bipolar voltage mapping (**inset**; color range 0.5-1.5 mV). Pace mapping at various sites within/outside of the scar revealed varying degrees of delay between the pacing stimulus and the onset of the QRS complex. A latency map was generated by plotting these values onto the LV anatomical construct (**main image**; range 0-344 msec). Two examples of these pacing sites with varying degrees of latency and identical morphology to the target VT are shown. RF catheter ablation extending between these sites eliminated the VT (*red dots*).

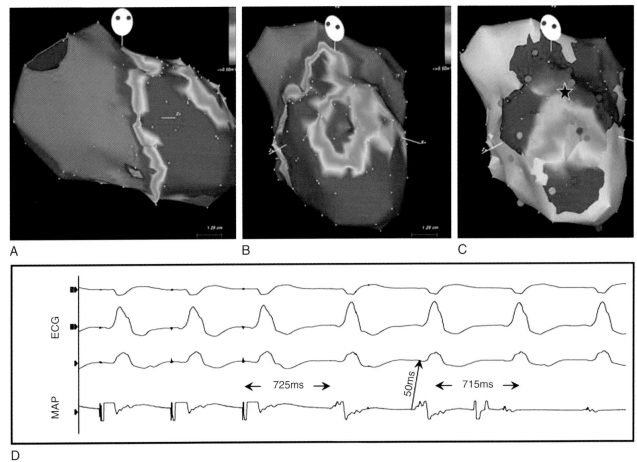

A   B   C

D

FIGURE 29–14. Role of substrate mapping in hemodynamically-stable VT. This patient with a large anterior wall MI presented with repetitive monomorphic slow VT resulting in congestive heart failure. Sinus rhythm bipolar voltage mapping revealed the large anterior infarct (RAO and LAO-cranial projections in **A** and **B**, respectively; color range 0.5-1.5 mV). Pace mapping identified a good putative exit site. Then, the VT was induced and brief activation mapping (shown in **C**) was performed. Entrainment performed at the optimal pacesite (*star* in **C**), revealed a post-pacing interval only 10 msec longer than the tachycardia cycle length, and the stimulus-QRS and EGM-QRS durations were short (**D**). RF ablation at this site eliminated the arrhythmia; in addition, further lesions were placed extending into the scar to empirically transect other potential reentrant circuits.

point at which the VT can be eliminated by a single ablation pulse. Furthermore, the duration of time that the patient is actually in VT can be minimized, optimizing both patient comfort and safety. Even hemodynamically stable VT invariably causes pulmonary congestion if it is allowed to persist for any significant period. Most importantly, because VT arises from an arrhythmogenic mass of tissue, the ablation lesions can be extended to regions deeper within the scarred myocardium to eliminate other potential VT circuits, which are often hemodynamically unstable and which may become operative at a later time.

Another strategy involves targeting of split/late potentials based on the observation that late and long-duration EGMs, despite a low sensitivity, are highly specific for identifying VT circuits.[20] This criterion requires recording high-frequency EGMs with multiple components separated by an isoelectric line, similar to the EGMs recorded at the central common pathways, inner loops, or adjacent bystander locations (Fig. 29–15). Targeting these EGMs invariably results in ablation of bystander sites that may not be operative in any VTs (e.g., a "deadend" pathway), but this approach has the advantage of placing ablation lesions at regions far from the normal tissue. Ablation at these sites would not result in any adverse effect on ventricular function. However, fractionated and late EGMs are often not identified during sinus rhythm. One potential reason is that overlapping of EGMs or a particular orientation of a line of block with respect to the activation wavefront may preclude the identification of multiple components during sinus rhythm. The sensitivity of identifying these components can be increased by changing the propagation wavefront during catheter mapping by RV pacing or LV pacing (for example, from within a ventricular branch of the coronary sinus).[35,42] From a practical perspective, this can be accomplished by pacing whenever the EGM at the site being mapped is suggestive for, but does not conclusively identify, a late potential site. As a corollary, it has also been suggested that, by performing high-density mapping of the scar, one can map channels of activation percolating into the scar in great detail.[43] Then, these channels of activation can be targeted for ablation at the borders of the scar, so that delayed or late potentials at the center of the scar are eliminated without being directly ablated. The approach is limited by the fact that (1) it does increase procedural time and technical difficulty, (2) the complexity of the arrays of myofibrillar bundles surviving within the infarcted tissue may preclude one's ability to precisely map these multiple and potentially overlapping activation pathways, and (3) this approach is unlikely to be efficacious in patients with smaller infarcts and faster VTs resulting from smaller circuits.

The alternative or "inverse" strategy to identify these protected isthmus sites is to stimulate directly within the infarcted tissue at target sites of questionable significance (i.e., at sites at which it is difficult

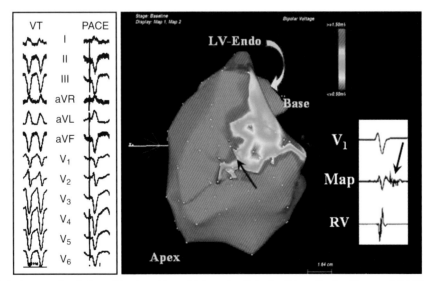

FIGURE 29–15. Substrate mapping followed by targeting of late potentials. In this patient with a post-MI VT, endocardial substrate mapping revealed a small myocardial scar without fractionated/late components and a suboptimal "best" pacing site (not shown). However, epicardial substrate mapping using the subxiphoid puncture approach (see below) revealed an infero-basal scar (color range 0.5-1.5 mV). The optimal pace map site at the apex of this epicardial scar matched the VT QRS morphology well (ECGs shown **at left**; pacing site indicated by *black arrow* in center). Also, this site demonstrated a late potential with fractionated components during sinus rhythm (**inset** at right). Catheter ablation at this site eliminated the VT.

to determine whether a late potential is present). Because of the limited myocardial tissue depolarized, activation of the isthmus contributes negligibly to the surface electrocardiogram until the wavefront of activation exits to the normal myocardium, thereby producing the observed QRS complex. Pace mapping from a site more proximally located within the isthmus should produce a QRS complex similar to the VT QRS morphology, albeit with a longer stimulus-to-QRS interval. Accordingly, the duration of the stimulus-to-QRS interval can serve as a surrogate for late potentials and can be targeted for catheter ablation to eliminate VT circuits.[44] Another approach is pace mapping to identify regions of dense scar based on the inability of pacing stimuli to capture any myocardium at a particular site (using pulses of 2-msec duration, 10-mA amplitude, and unipolar stimuli).[45] These areas of electrically unexcitable scar can delineate isthmuses for VT circuits that can be transected with ablation lesions connecting the dense scar regions to each other and to fixed anatomic barriers (such as the mitral valve).

WHICH ABLATION TARGETS OR STRATEGY SHOULD BE USED?

The relative efficacy of these various criteria to guide identification and targeting of the "arrhythmogenic" portion of the scar is unknown and will be fully appreciated only with future comparative studies. However, certain general principles can be stated. Trying to minimize the number of ablation lesions placed at the border zone would be advantageous to minimize adverse effects on LV function. Indeed, a strategy targeting late potentials is particularly attractive in patients with depressed ventricular function or congestive heart failure. Conversely, in patients with preserved ventricular function and small or patchy scars, it is not necessarily possible to identify channels of activity, and ablation lesions based in large part on pace mapping would be appropriate.

Ideally, the ablation procedure is considered complete when all VTs inducible at the beginning of the procedure have been eliminated and no additional VTs are inducible. Because the substrate modification procedure could theoretically inadvertently create new arrhythmogenic channels of activity, one is obligated to rule out this possibility. Inducibility at the end of the procedure should include one RV and one LV site. In addition, if nonsustained monomorphic VT in induced, one should consider infusion of a sympathetic agent such as isoproterenol to determine whether the VT then becomes sustained (Fig. 29–16). However, complete noninducibility is not necessarily achievable in

every patient, and particularly not in those with severe ventricular dysfunction, in whom a "sine wave–like VT" (that is, a morphologically indeterminate VT with no isoelectric segment) is often inducible with aggressive ventricular stimulation (Fig. 29–17).[30] In this situation, after all of the late potentials have been eliminated, the procedure is terminated. Common problems with ablation of unstable VT are listed in Table 29–3.

RADIOFREQUENCY ABLATION CATHETER TECHNOLOGY

An important variable to address is the type of RF ablation catheter used. In Marchlinski's seminal study,[29] one of the patients experienced a cerebrovascular accident associated with an impedance rise during RF energy delivery. The ablation catheter used in that study was a 4-mm-tip, non–temperature-controlled catheter, which has limited ability to monitor for signs of excessive heating of the electrode tip that can lead to coagulum formation. Unlike that early-generation catheter, ablation catheters are now able not only to monitor the temperature at the electrode tip but even to cool the ablation electrode in either a passive or an active fashion. Passive cooling is achieved by use of an 8-mm-tip, temperature-controlled catheter; if the distal end of the catheter is in contact with the tissue, the proximal end is cooled by the ambient blood flow to allow greater delivery of ablative energy into the tissue without excessive temperature rises.[46] However, this catheter is limited both because of its only modest cooling efficiency and because the electrode size limits the ability to perform detailed ventricular mapping. An alternative family of RF ablation catheters is the temperature-controlled saline-irrigated catheters: the 3.5-mm-tip, externally irrigated catheter (THERMO-COOL, Biosense Webster) and the 4-mm-tip, internally cooled catheter (Chili, Boston Scientific).[47] Active cooling of the ablation electrode by saline irrigation of the catheter tip has been shown to allow greater RF energy delivery into the target tissue.[48,49] Saline is constantly infused via a central lumen through the external irrigated-tip catheter at 15 to 30 mL/min during RF energy delivery or at 2 mL/min during catheter manipulation to maintain lumen patency. RF lesions are placed in 60-second intervals under power control of 35 to 70 W, with careful impedance monitoring to achieve an impedance fall of 5 to 10 Ω. Because the ablation electrode is being actively cooled, the monitored temperature is relevant only to verify that saline is actually being delivered to the catheter tip. With the externally irrigated catheter, it is our experience that the tip temperature rarely, if ever, needs to exceed 40° C, and it often does not even

FIGURE 29–16. Post-ablation inducibility of non-sustained VT. Monomorphic VT was inducible in this patient with a prior inferior wall MI (**A**). Sinus rhythm substrate mapping revealed an infero-postero-basal scar (bipolar voltage map in **B**; color range 0.4-1.5 mV), and a pace map site identical to the VT (black dot). RF ablation lesions were placed in a linear fashion incorporating this pacing site (red line in **B**). Repeat programmed stimulation induced only non-sustained VT, but of similar morphology to the sustained VT induced at baseline (**C**). However, repeat stimulation after infusion of intravenous isoproterenol caused this VT to sustain. Accordingly, additional RF lesions were placed to extend the ablation line to the mitral valve annulus; then, VT was no longer inducible at baseline or after intravenous isoproterenol infusion.

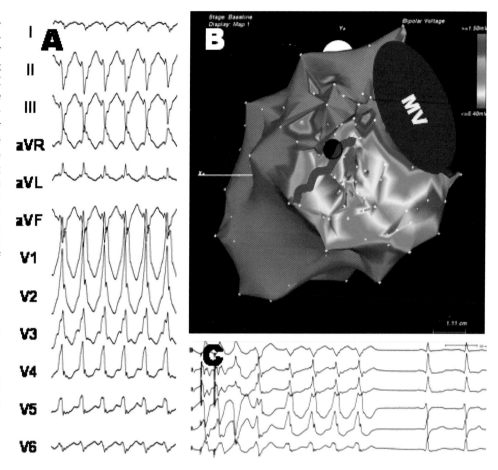

reach 37°C. It is also our empiric observation that an excessively rapid impedance fall often portends an impedance pop.

Substrate-based VT ablation is a viable strategy only if placement of the requisite multiple lesions does not adversely affect ventricular pump function. This is particularly true when use of more powerful ablation technologies, such as the saline-irrigated ablation catheter, is contemplated. Accordingly, it is imperative that ablation lesions should be largely, if not exclusively, confined to the infarcted myocardium. In clinical studies of substrate-based catheter ablation, no change in ventricular function has been noted (see later discussion of ablation complications).

CLINICAL RESULTS OF SUBSTRATE-BASED VENTRICULAR TACHYCARDIA ABLATION

Regarding the efficacy of this method, all of the published studies using a substrate-based approach have been nonrandomized studies with historical controls (see Table 29–2). Although the data are encouraging, the actual efficacy of substrate-based VT ablation is

not known and requires further study with prospective randomized clinical trials.

RAPID "SINGLE-BEAT" ACTIVATION MAPPING

Instead of the substrate-based approach, there is one mapping technology that can perform noncontact mapping of far-field EGM activity such that global chamber activation can be visualized during a single cardiac cycle (EnSite), Endocardial Solutions, St. Paul, MN.[23] As described further in Chapter 8, this system consists of a computerized electrophysiology recording system coupled to a 64-electrode, noncontact balloon catheter to create a 3-D model of the LV endocardial activation. A color-coded dynamic isopotential map derived from the virtual EGMs represents the electrical potential of each virtual EGM throughout the cardiac cycle (Fig. 29–18). Because the system theoretically requires only a single beat of VT to create an isopotential map, even hemodynamically unstable VTs are mappable. A number of investigators have assessed the use of this technology to identify and ablate hemodynamically tolerated and untolerated VTs in patients with scar-related arrhyth-

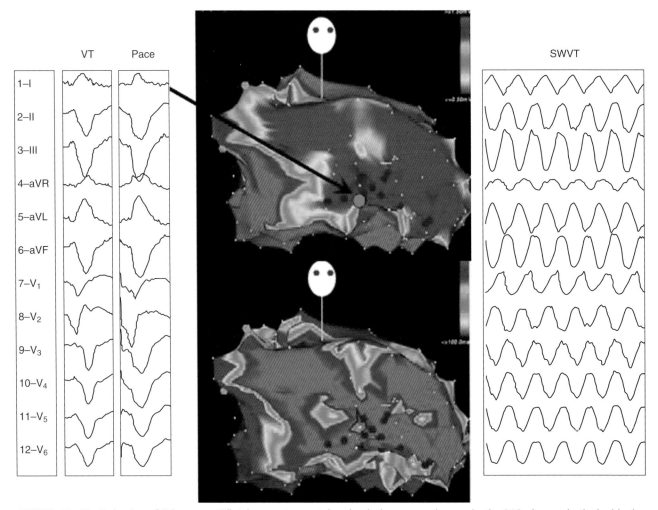

FIGURE 29–17. Induction of "sine-wave VT". A large anteroseptal and apical aneurysm is seen in the RAO view on both the bipolar voltage (*top*; color range 0.5-1.5 mV) and EGM duration (*bottom*; 100-150 msec) maps obtained during sinus rhythm. Programmed stimulation induced a hemodynamically-tolerated VT (shown at left) as well as several untolerated VTs. Pace mapping (at the site noted by the *arrow*) produced a QRS morphology similar to the tolerated VT. Concealed entrainment was noted at this point, with a post-pacing interval 25 msec greater than the VT CL. VT could not be induced when mechanical pressure was applied just inferior to this site (*green dot*). Ablation at this site eliminated the VT; additional lesions were placed in a linear fashion to incorporate pace map latency sites and fractionated potentials. Further programmed stimulation from the RV and LV induced only a sine wave-like VT (cycle length = 311ms; ECG at *right*) that rapidly degenerated into VF; note the indeterminate nature of this arrhythmia's ECG morphology. Despite the relatively slow rate, this arrhythmia could not be targeted for ablation. The clinical significance of post-ablation inducible "sine wave"-like VT (as well as inducible VF) is unclear and can only be assessed by prospective clinical trials.

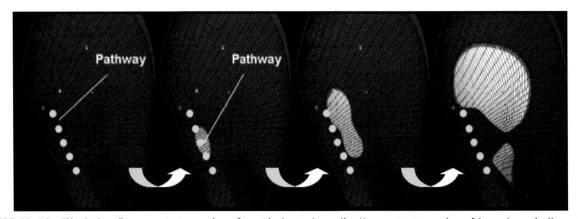

FIGURE 29–18. "Single beat" non-contact mapping of ventricular tachycardia. Non-contact mapping of hemodynamically-unstable VT is possible by analysis of a few beats, or as little as a single beat of tachycardia (EnSite; Endocardial Solutions, Inc.). The wavefront of activation is represented by white.

TABLE 29–3	
Troubleshooting Difficult Cases—Special Considerations	
Problem	**Solution**
Pre-procedural echo reveals left ventricular thrombus	Postpone procedure if possible. After anticoagulation for 4–6 wks to allow organization of the thrombus, perform procedure Consider using an epicardial approach alone
During ventricular mapping frequent PVCs complicate substrate mapping	Consider IV infusion of antiarrhythmic drugs to suppress ectopy (e.g., lidocaine)
During programmed stimulation, only polymorphic VT inducible	Consider repeat stimulation after infusion of a class I antiarrhythmic drug such as procainamide (but not if LV ejection fraction is significantly depressed)
LV mapping reveals a large septal scar	Consider RV septal mapping to assess for arrhythmogenic tissue on the right side of the septum
Unable to find suitable endocardial pacemap site or abnormal EGMs (e.g., late potentials)	Perform epicardial mapping using a subxiphoid approach If previous cardiac surgery, can use either a subxiphoid puncture approach or direct surgical subxiphoid exposure
Difficult to cross aortic valve with ablation catheter	Using electroanatomic mapping system, mark the three aortic valve cusps, then maneuver catheter tip to center of the plane to cross aortic valve Use a trans-septal approach to LV mapping
Severely depressed ventricular function (especially in association with preexisting congestive heart failure)	Aggressive patient monitoring 　Foley catheter to monitor urine output 　LA pressure monitoring—direct trans-septal sheath or Swan-Ganz catheter (wedge) Judicious use of IV diuretic agents Judicious use of IV pressor agents Consider intra-aortic balloon pump support for duration of procedure Minimize number of ablation lesions placed near normal ventricular myocardium

EGM, electrogram; IV, intravenous; LA, left atrial; LV, left ventricular; PVC, premature ventricular complex; RV, right ventricular; VT, ventricular tachycardia.

mias including post-MI VT, arrhythmogenic right ventricular cardiomyopathy/dysplasia (ARVC), and dilated cardiomyopathy (DCM).[23,50,51] After deploying the balloon catheter into the LV to record several beats of the target VT, diastolic pathways of activation are identified and targeted for ablation. However, this noncontact mapping system has several limitations: (1) the presence of the mapping balloon catheter within the ventricle can complicate one's ability to maneuver the ablation catheter to the region of interest, (2) the location accuracy of this system is inferior to that of the electroanatomic mapping system, (3) voltage amplitude maps cannot be accurately constructed from recordings of the far-field potentials,[52] and, therefore, (4) only VTs that are induced can be targeted for catheter ablation—that is, one may potentially be limited to identifying only those arrhythmogenic zones/VTs that are operative/induced during that particular procedure. The relative merits of VT ablation based on "single beat" activation mapping versus substrate mapping have not been studied in any systematic prospective manner.

OTHER SCAR-RELATED VENTRICULAR TACHYCARDIAS

Because of its frequency, most of the literature regarding scar-related reentrant VT has been devoted to the study of post-MI VT. However, reentrant VT also occurs from myocardial scar in the setting of other forms of cardiac pathology, such as DCM. As described further in Chapter 28, histologic studies of myocardial tissue from patients with DCM have revealed multiple patchy areas of interstitial and replacement fibrosis and myofibrillar disarray with variable degrees of myocyte hypertrophy and atrophy.[53] A necropsy study in patients with idiopathic DCM revealed that, despite a relative paucity of visible scar (14%), there was a high incidence of mural endocardial plaque (69% to 85%) and myocardial fibrosis (57%).[54] As with post-MI VT, the mechanism of VT related to DCM is commonly reentrant and is related to the scarred substrate. Accordingly, scar-related VT in the setting of DCM may be expected on the endocardial surface, on the epicardial surface, or in a deep intramural region of the heart. Clinical studies of VT mapping and ablation in the setting of DCM have revealed that a substrate-based approach is also useful to eliminate these arrhythmias.[32,55,56] Interestingly, the myocardial scar has been localized predominantly to two regions: the basal regions of the LV endocardial surface and the ventricular epicardium. After the myocardial scar is identified, this abnormal area can be targeted for ablation based on mapping strategies similar to those used for post-MI VT, including pace mapping and targeting of late potentials.[32,55,56]

Another pathologic state associated with scar-related VT that lends itself to a substrate mapping approach is ARVC. The precise pathophysiology of ARVC is not fully understood, but its hallmark is the presence of fibrosis and fatty infiltrate of the RV myocardium.[57] VT that occurs in the setting of ARVC usually originates from within the scarred myocardium of the RV and has a reentrant mechanism. Substrate mapping of the RV in these individuals typically reveals abnormal myocardial tissue that involves the perivalvular tricuspid valve, the pulmonic valve, or both valves.[58] The abnormal myocardium almost always involves the RV free wall, frequently the septum, and rarely the apex. A substrate-based approach is also successful in eliminating VT in these patients.[29,58]

Chronic Chagas-related cardiomyopathy is another important myocardial disease process with a high incidence of scar-related reentrant VT.[32,59] Histologic studies have again revealed myofibrillar disarray and diffuse fibrosis resulting in scar formation with two characteristic distributions: the inferolateral LV wall and the apical-septal/apical-inferior walls. The pathophysiologic mechanism of scar formation in this disease state is not fully understood, but it is thought to be a cell-mediated autoimmune reaction with autonomic denervation. As with other scar-related VTs, the mechanism of chagasic VT is reentry.[32,60] But unlike other VTs, the VT circuits in the setting of Chagas' disease have an extremely high incidence of epicardial origin.[32,61]

ARE ALL SCAR-RELATED VENTRICULAR TACHYCARDIAS LOCATED AT THE SUBENDOCARDIUM?

Because in the past only the endocardial surface of the scarred myocardium traditionally underwent catheter mapping, it was typical for little to be known regarding the electrophysiologic characteristics of the epicardial extent of the scar in any particular patient. By necessity, the infarcted substrate was typically viewed by the electrophysiologist as a two-dimensional surface with little consideration given to

its character throughout the thickness of the wall. Fortunately, in most patients with post-MI VT, the arrhythmogenic substrate is located on the endocardial surface of the heart. However, surgical mapping studies have revealed that not all VT circuits can be eliminated by endocardial ablative strategies alone. In one study, 15% of the patients undergoing arrhythmia surgery for VT required epicardial laser ablation to eliminate the target VT.[62] For reasons that are still not fully understood, most (90%) of these patients requiring epicardial ablative lesions had inferior wall MIs with no identifiable aneurysm. Therefore, only a minority of post-MI patients would require an epicardial ablation approach to eliminate their VT.

In those post-MI patients with VT for whom an endocardial approach is unsuccessful, one can perform pericardial mapping of the epicardial surface of the heart using a percutaneous subxiphoid puncture approach (see Chapter 30).[61,63] This approach has been employed to eliminate hemodynamically stable VT in a variety of clinical settings.[32,56,61,63,64] In a porcine model of healed MI, the feasibility of substrate mapping of the ventricular epicardial surface was demonstrated (Fig. 29–19).[65] Accordingly, just as with endocardial substrate mapping/ablation, epicardial substrate mapping/ablation can also be employed to eliminate VT.

It is prudent to consider an epicardial approach in patients for whom an endocardial attempt at VT ablation has failed. However, the decision as to whether to consider a primary epicardial-endocardial approach has not been studied in any prospective fashion. Epicardial mapping should certainly be considered in the setting of cardiac pathologies that appear to have a high incidence of epicardial scar (e.g., Chagas-related VT, DCM-related VT) (Fig. 29–20). The morphology of a target VT might provide additional clues as to its exit from the infarcted tissue. In a systematic study[66] of the ECG pattern of VTs eliminated from the endocardial versus epicardial surface of the heart, an epicardial origin was predicted by the following characteristics of the VT: (1) a longer pseudo-delta wave, as measured from the earliest ventricular activation to the earliest fast deflection in any precordial lead; (2) a longer intrinsicoid deflection time in lead V_2; (3) a longer "shortest RS complex," defined as the interval from the earliest ventricular activation to the nadir of the first S wave in any precordial lead; and (4) a wider QRS complex. This study concluded that an epicardial VT origin can be identified by a pseudo-delta wave of 34 msec or longer (sensitivity, 83%; specificity, 95%), an intrinsicoid deflection time of 85 msec or longer (sensitivity, 87%; specificity, 90%), and a "shortest RS complex" of 121 msec or longer (sensitivity, 76%; specificity, 85%). In relation to substrate-based VT

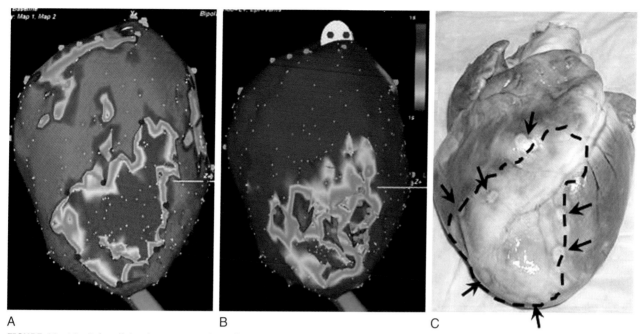

FIGURE 29–19. Epicardial substrate mapping of porcine infarcts. A porcine chronic MI model underwent epicardial electroanatomical mapping using a percutaneous subxiphoid puncture approach. Using either bipolar voltage (**A**; range 0.5-1.5 mV) or EGM duration (**B**; 50-80 msec) criteria, the epicardial extent of the myocardial scar could be mapped. Of note, sites over normal tissue with corresponding falsely-low bipolar voltage values were frequently correctly defined as normal based upon EGM duration criteria. Based solely upon the bipolar voltage electroanatomic map, RF ablation lesions were placed to "tag" the scar border (*red dots* in **A**). Gross pathological examination revealed that the ablation lesions (*black arrows* in **C**) were indeed situated at the scar periphery. The *purple-green* tube represents the pericardial access sheath.

ablation, an important caveat that must be considered is the fact that the ECG morphology addresses only the exit point of VT from the scar; little can be derived regarding the location of the critical protected portion of the circuit. For example, despite an epicardial exit, endocardial ablation may eliminate a critical portion of the circuit (and vice versa—a "narrow" QRS VT may be eliminated by epicardial ablation). Therefore, for any VT after inferior wall MI in a patient without a history of cardiac surgery, it is our practice to consider a primary combined epicardial-endocardial approach (Fig. 29–21). In patients with prior cardiac surgery, epicardial mapping can nonetheless be performed using a percutaneous[67] or surgical[68] subxiphoid approach, but this is typically reserved for patients for whom an endocardial approach has failed.

THE FUTURE OF SUBSTRATE-BASED VENTRICULAR TACHYCARDIA ABLATION

In addition to further clinical studies to refine our understanding of the optimal approach to substrate-based VT ablation, there are two technological advances in substrate mapping and ablation of scar-related VT expected over the next several years. First, the location and morphology of the infarcted

tissue can be elucidated by preprocedural computed tomography (CT) or magnetic resonance imaging (MRI). MRI is a noninvasive, nonionizing imaging modality that can provide detailed anatomic information about soft tissue with high spatial resolution. Of particular relevance to substrate mapping, delayed-enhancement contrast MRI can distinguish normal from chronically infarcted cardiac tissue with millimeter spatial resolution (Fig. 29–22).[69] By defining the scar morphology in post-MI patients, a preprocedural cardiac MRI could serve as a useful "road map" to guide substrate-based catheter ablation. Of course, MRI currently is not possible for patients with preexisting ICDs or pacemakers. However, CT imaging can also provide ventricular anatomic information with high spatial resolution, albeit with a more limited ability to discriminate scar from normal tissue. Unlike MRI, CT-based scar visualization is dependent on thinning of the ventricular wall combined with wall motion abnormality of the region of interest. With current technology, CT imaging can directly image scar tissue only in the relatively rare instance in which remotely infarcted myocardial tissue becomes partially calcified.

In the optimal scenario, 3-D cardiac MRI/CT images would be integrated with electroanatomic mapping information to guide catheter navigation to

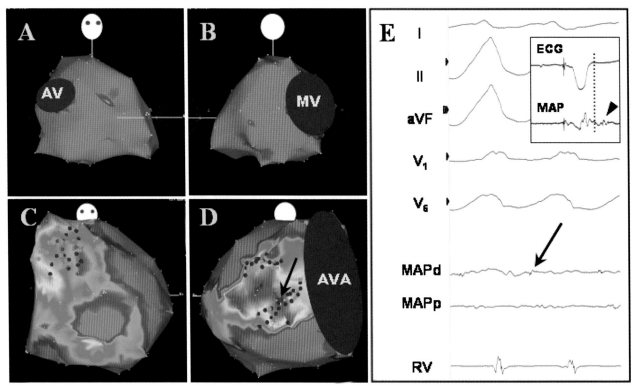

FIGURE 29-20. Substrate mapping and ablation of hemodynamically-unstable VT in a patient with dilated cardiomyopathy. This patient with dilated cardiomyopathy presented with defibrillator shocks due to fast VTs. Programmed ventricular stimulation revealed 5 hemodynamically-unstable VTs. LV endocardial substrate mapping during A-V sequential pacing (RAO and PA projections, **A** and **B**, respectively) revealed no significant patches of diseased myocardium based upon bipolar voltage criteria or EGM characteristics (fractionated/late potentials). After pericardial access using a subxiphoid puncture approach, the ventricular epicardial surface was mapped during A-V pacing (AP and PA projections, **C** and **D**, respectively). Two large patches of abnormal myocardium were identified by substrate mapping based upon both low bipolar voltage amplitude and abnormal EGM components (*blue dots* = late potentials): one right-anterior overlying the RV, and the other left-lateral overlying the LV near the atrioventricular groove. The low-voltage area overlying the RV acute margin likely represents an area of normal myocardium with overlying epicardial fat; notice the lack of late potentials at this region. At one of the late potential sites (*black arrow* in **D**; and *black arrowhead* in **E-inset**), an optimal pace map was obtained for one of the VTs. With the catheter placed at this position, VT was briefly induced (**E**); an intra-aortic balloon pump was placed for hemodynamic support. A diastolic component was noted at this site (*black arrow* in **E**), and entrainment maneuvers identified this as the exit site of the circuit. RF ablation at this site eliminated the VT. Additional RF ablation lesions were applied along areas of late potentials along the inferior and superior borders of the LV epicardial scar (**D**), and the RV epicardial scar (**C**); no further VT was inducible at the end of the procedure. AVA, atrioventricular annulus; color range 0.1-1.5 mV.

the infarct borders in real time. To accomplish this, the preacquired 3-D MRI/CT data set must be properly aligned or registered with the electroanatomic mapping system. The feasibility of this image-guided therapy paradigm was established in a series of in vitro simulation and in vivo porcine experiments.[70] In this study, preprocedural MRI scans of a chronically infarcted LV were correctly registered with MEAM to guide catheter manipulation in the ventricular chamber, as well as to guide the placement of ablation lesions at the borders of the scar (Fig. 29-23). This work established the proof-of-principle and provides an experimental basis for the use of image-guided therapy in ventricular substrate mapping. This paradigm is now being studied in the clinical setting to determine whether it can guide substrate mapping and ablation of VT in a reliable and clinically relevant manner (unpublished data, V. Reddy).

The second major advance is remote navigation technologies to facilitate and enhance ventricular mapping. One of the limitations of substrate mapping and ablation is the fact that the accuracy and detail of the ventricular map are dependent on operator skill and experience with catheter manipulation. To this end, magnetic and robotic navigation systems are being developed to allow for remote cardiac mapping.[71] When the magnetic navigation system is used in concert with a compatible elec-

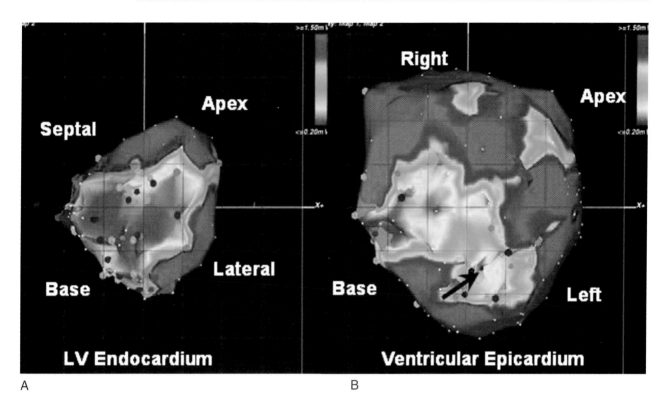

A   B

FIGURE 29–21. Combined endocardial–epicardial substrate mapping of post-MI VT. In this patient with a prior inferior wall MI, endocardial (**A**) and epicardial (**B**) substrate mapping in sinus rhythm revealed a large area of infarcted tissue (color range 0.2-1.5 mV). Extensive endocardial mapping failed to identify an isthmus site for the clinical VT. But, epicardial mapping identified a site (*arrow* in **B**) with a late potential during sinus rhythm and a diastolic component during tachycardia. Catheter ablation at this point eliminated this VT; additional RF ablation lesions at endocardial and epicardial sites of fractionated and late potentials eliminated all inducible VT.

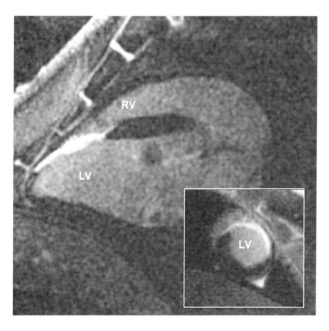

FIGURE 29–22. Contrast-enhanced MR imaging of infarcted tissue. Contrast enhancement observed relatively quickly (within tens of seconds) after injection of the MRI contrast agent, gadolinium, is related to vascular perfusion. But, delayed enhancement (defined as appearing >5 minutes after bolus injection) is selectively observed in infarcted tissue because of the relatively larger extracellular space, and therefore larger volume of distribution of gadolinium within this tissue. Long and short axis views (**main view** and **inset**, respectively) of the infarcted LV are shown after gadolinium delayed enhancement MR imaging: the infarcted interventricular septum and anterior wall are enhanced.

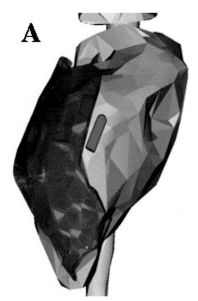
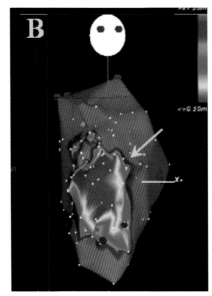
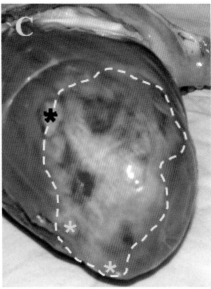

FIGURE 29–23. Image-Guided Therapy: MRI-guided catheter navigation in vivo to the myocardial infarct borders. **A,** A chronic porcine infarct model underwent MRI ~4 months after the anterior wall infarction procedure. The aorta, LV endocardium and myocardial scars were manually segmented and compiled into 3D data sets (re-compiled surface reconstructions are shown as *gray* and *brown shells*, respectively; the *green icon* represents the catheter tip). During magnetic electroanatomic mapping (MEAM), the chamber geometries were constructed without displaying the corresponding electrophysiological information. Radiofrequency ablation lesions were subsequently targeted to the borders of the scar based solely upon the registered MRI. **B,** The electroanatomical bipolar voltage map depicts the anterior wall MI (color range 0.5-1.5 mV). The ablation lesions are shown as *red dots*; the *yellow arrow* denotes the ablation lesion corresponding to the catheter position shown as a *green icon* in (**A**). **C,** The heart is inverted to visualize the endocardial surface of the heart. The corresponding lesion (*asterisk*) was noted upon gross pathological examination to be situated at the scar border; two other ablation lesions placed near the LV apex (*yellow asterisk*) were also appropriately localized to the scar borders.

troanatomic mapping system, it is possible to obtain a high-density ventricular substrate map in porcine models of healed MI (Fig. 29–24). By removing the necessity for technical skill with catheter manipulation, this methodology has the potential for both improving the efficacy of VT ablation and expanding the clinical use of the substrate mapping approach by physicians who may have less experience with ventricular substrate mapping.

Minimizing Complications

Because of the nature of the cardiac function in patients in whom substrate-based VT ablation is performed, an important potential complication of the procedure is worsening or new congestive heart failure. This can occur as a result of programmed stimulation or catheter ablation. To mitigate against worsening heart failure, programmed stimulation should be performed with an adequate pause between stimulus trains, and in patients with severe

LV dysfunction an intra-aortic balloon pump should be considered. When we use an intra-aortic balloon pump, we typically place it at the beginning of the procedure and remove it at the end, before the patient leaves the electrophysiology laboratory. Also, it is important to note that during substrate-based VT ablation, the patient is typically in sinus rhythm and not in VT throughout most of the procedure. Accordingly, this procedure is typically well tolerated even by patients with severe ventricular dysfunction.

There is also the potential for worsening ventricular function due to catheter ablation. An experimental porcine study was performed in which linear RF ablation lesions were placed along the borders of a healed MI.[72] In this study, intracardiac echocardiographic imaging revealed that linear lesions caused significant systolic dysfunction (38.5% decrease in fractional shortening) in the normal myocardium adjacent to the infarct border (1 cm from the ablation site). The mechanism of this phenomenon is unknown but is probably related to myocardial stunning resulting from microvascular dysfunction. Consistent with this hypothesis, systolic function recovered to baseline in this porcine model within 30

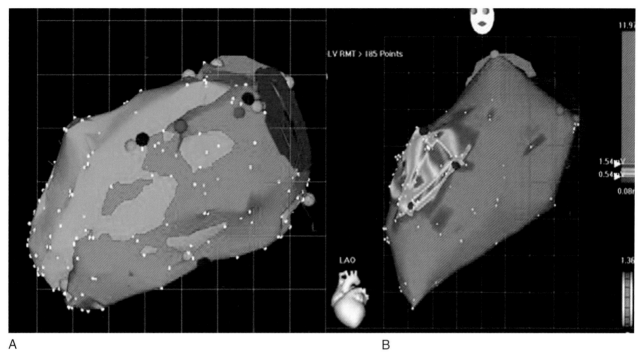

A   B

FIGURE 29–24. Remote substrate mapping using a magnetic navigation system. In the porcine chronic MI model, LV endocardial substrate mapping was performed sequentially: (1) first in the conventional fashion by manual manipulation of the mapping catheter, and (2) then remotely using a magnetic navigation system (Stereotaxis, St. Louis, MO.). The latter was performed using a prototype mapping catheter containing both a sensor to permit electroanatomical mapping and magnets to allow magnetic manipulation (Biosense Webster, Baldwin Park, Calif.). In (**A**), the manually-derived map is *blue-green* and the remotely-generated map is *purple*. A good correlation is noted between the two maps (both in terms of volume and position). In **B**, the remotely-generated bipolar voltage map (color range 0.5-1.5 mV) in this chronic porcine infarct model visualized the anterior wall MI. The RF ablation lesions placed along the borders of the scar as determined by the electroanatomical map (*red dots*) were situated at the scar borders during gross pathological examination.

minutes. Furthermore, in a separate clinical study, the impact of catheter ablation on LV function was examined in a series of 62 post-MI patients who underwent VT ablation.[73] Catheter ablation was performed using cooled RF ablation (internal or external irrigation RF ablation catheters) in 26/62 (42%) of the patients, and using a 4- or 8-mm-tip RF ablation catheter in the remainder. A mean of 25.6 ± 2.2 RF lesions (range, 3 to 89) were delivered. Digitized echocardiography performed 1 week or less before and less than 72 hours after the procedure revealed no significant changes in LV function, neither in the entire group, in the subset of patients who received more than 25 lesions, nor in the subset who received more than 40 lesions. However, the LV ejection fraction increased by more than 5% in 12/62 (19.4%) of patients and decreased (≥5%) in 14/62 (22.5%); there was no relation to the number of RF lesions or to use of a cooled RF ablation catheter. Therefore, when the ablation lesions are confined to the area of abnormal EGMs, most patients do not experience any appreciable change in LV function. Accordingly, we rarely place ablation lesions in tissue with bipolar EGM amplitudes greater than 1.0 mV.

As with all left-sided ablation procedures, it is important to minimize the risk of embolic complications by using adequate anticoagulation during and after the procedure. Our patients typically receive aspirin (325 mg) just before the procedure, and intravenous heparin is infused to achieve an activated clotting time longer than 250 seconds during the procedure. When using the trans-septal approach, an intravenous heparin bolus (5000 to 8000 units) is infused at least 5 minutes before the trans-septal puncture procedure; both the trans-septal needle and the traumatized, denuded tissue at the puncture site are extremely thrombogenic. In addition, continuous flushing of the trans-septal sheath helps prevent air or thrombotic emboli from being expelled. Because of the number of ablation lesions typically delivered during substrate-based VT ablation, cooled RF ablation technology should be strongly considered. If available, active cooling using a saline-infused RF ablation catheter is preferable; otherwise, passive cooling with an 8-mm-tip catheter is used.

Pericardial effusion resulting in cardiac tamponade is another potential complication of substrate ablation. This can occur during the trans-septal puncture procedure—a risk that is minimized by the use of intracardiac ultrasound imaging at least during "difficult" punctures. Perforation of the LV by the ablation catheter is rare because of the thickness of this chamber; in addition, when the wall is thin due to a chronic MI, the fibrous tissue is difficult to perforate. However, the thinner-walled RV may be perforated either by the ablation catheter during mapping or by the RV quadripolar pacing catheter. This is particularly prone to happen if the patient is receiving intravenous inotropic agents such as isoproterenol. Perforation of the RV related to catheter ablation has also been reported in a patient with ARVC.[47]

Damage to the aortic or mitral valves can also occur, particularly if the ablation catheters are forcibly manipulated across these structures. Damage to the coronary arteries can occur as a result of embolization from an RF ablation lesion-related thrombus. The coronary artery can also be damaged by inadvertent introduction of the ablation catheter into a coronary vessel, which could traumatize an atherosclerotic coronary plaque. This is of particular concern in patients with coronary bypass grafts, because of the difficulty in knowing the locations of the origins of these vessels. One means to avoid entering these vessels is to deflect the catheter into a "U" shape when advancing it into the ascending aorta or crossing the aortic valve, so that the catheter tip cannot enter a coronary vessel. Of course, inadvertent delivery of RF energy within the coronary artery would be disastrous.

Complications of epicardial mapping and ablation (covered in detail in Chapter 30) can be divided into those related to pericardial access and those related to ablation. Certainly, the location of the coronary arteries relative to the ablation catheter must be assessed before pericardial energy delivery. Although it is rare to find a surviving coronary vessel traversing an epicardial scar in post-MI patients, this situation is of particular concern in patients with nonischemic cardiomyopathy. In relation to substrate-based VT ablation specifically, if multiple lesions are delivered, there is an increased risk of pericardial inflammation or pericarditis. To mitigate against this complication, one can lavage the pericardial space at the end of the procedure with fresh sterile saline to minimize the presence of blood (which is proinflammatory) and then administer a one-time dose of pericardial steroids (methylprednisolone or triamcinolone, 1 to 2 mg/kg) and intravenous antibiotics (unpublished data, V. Reddy and A. d'Avila). Patients are also typically given oral nonsteroidal anti-inflammatory agents as needed. With this regimen, we have not observed any instances of significant pericarditis.

Ventricular Fibrillation

Cardiac mapping studies indicate that VF is perpetuated by reentrant or spiral waves, but little has been known regarding the initiators of these arrhythmias. Haissaguerre et al.[74] recently demonstrated that, just as atrial fibrillation can occur as the result of a focal mechanism with fibrillatory conduction, certain patients have a focal mechanism of VF that can be treated by catheter ablation.[74] After being resuscitated from recurrent (10 ± 12) episodes of primary VF, 27 patients without known structural heart disease underwent an electrophysiology procedure.[75] This group of patients was studied because of the presence of isolated PVCs of identical morphology and coupling interval (297 ± 41 msec) to the first initiating beat of VF (Fig. 29–25). Endocardial mapping revealed that these triggers initiated from the RV or LV Purkinje system in 23/27 (85%) of patients, and from the myocardium of the RV outflow tract in 4/27 (15%) of patients. The interval from the Purkinje potential to ventricular activation varied from 10 to 150 msec during the premature beat. A Purkinje potential was also seen at these same sites during sinus rhythm but preceded the QRS by only 11 ± 5 msec. RF catheter ablation at these sites eliminated the triggering PVCs and subsequent VF in most of these patients. The mean number of RF ablation lesions required to eliminate these triggers was nine.

Focal PVC triggers of VF have also been described in two other groups of patients: those with channelopathies and otherwise structurally normal hearts, and those with ischemic heart disease. Regarding the former, PVC triggers amenable to catheter ablation have been found in patients with either long QT syndrome or Brugada syndrome.[76] As for patients with other idiopathic VFs, two types of PVC triggers have been found in both of these clinical disease states: those with preceding Purkinje potentials, and those originating from the RV outflow tract.

In contrast to the scar-related reentrant VT that is seen after an MI, it has also recently been demonstrated that certain post-MI patients with drug-refractory primary VF (i.e., VF not preceded by monomorphic VT) also have PVC triggers of the arrhythmia.[77-79] These patients can be divided into those with a recent MI (<1 week) and those with remote MI (>1 month). The PVC triggers were exclusively associated with Purkinje-like potentials, and they also were successfully targeted for catheter ablation.

Common to all of these patients with VF amenable to catheter ablation is the clinical demonstration of

FIGURE 29–25. Catheter ablation of focal ventricular fibrillation (VF). **A,** In this patient with a structurally normal heart and recurrent VF, an example of monomorphic PVCs initiating VF is shown. **B,** In another patient with a structurally-normal heart and VF, catheter mapping revealed a focal site with Purkinje potentials preceding the initiating PVCs of the non-sustained polymorphic VT episode (*arrow heads*). Note that at this site, Purkinje potentials are also noted during sinus rhythm—albeit with a significantly shorter interval to the local ventricular EGM. MAP, mapping catheter; d, distal; p, proximal. (*Images courtesy of M. Haissaguerre.*)

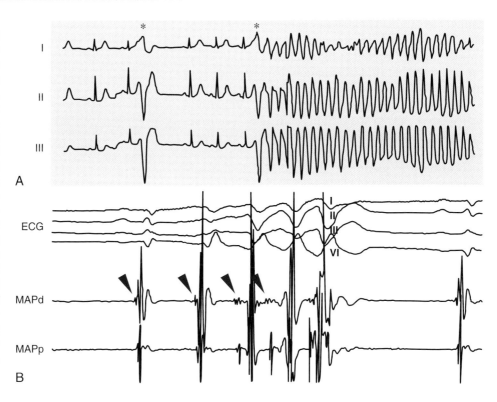

TABLE 29–4					
Catheter Ablation of Focal Ventricular Fibrillation					
Authors (Ref. No.)	Cardiac Pathology	No. of Patients	Distribution of Foci	Follow-Up (mo)	Clinical Success (%)
Haissaguerre et al.[75]	Normal	27	Purkinje = 23 RVOT = 4	24 ± 28	89
Haissaguerre et al.[76]	LQTS, Brugada	7	Purkinje = 4 RVOT = 3	17 ± 17	100
Bansch et al.[77]	CAD / MI	4	Purkinje = 4	15 ± 13	100
Marrouche et al.[78]	CAD / MI	8	Purkinje = 8	10 ± 6	88
Szumowski et al.[79]	CAD / MI	5	Purkinje = 5	16 ± 5	100

CAD, coronary artery disease; LQTS, long QT syndrome; MI, myocardial infarction; RVOT, right ventricular outflow tract.

frequent PVCs initiating the arrhythmia (Table 29–4). Despite the impressive clinical success rate of this therapeutic paradigm, an important practical limitation is the unknown frequency with which these patients can be identified. These patients might represent a highly selected cohort, thereby rendering VF ablation a rarity. Another limitation is the fact that frequent PVCs are necessary to map and target the Purkinje potentials. If frequent PVCs are absent, one is limited to pace-mapping techniques for identification of the target site (assuming that a 12-lead ECG of the pathologic PVCs is available), a technique inferior to activation mapping of the pathologic PVCs.

Further clinical experience is required to fully understand the efficacy, safety, and clinical applicability of catheter ablation of "focal" VF.

Conclusions

Until recently, hemodynamically unstable ventricular arrhythmias were not amenable to catheter ablative approaches. However, both scar-related VTs and in certain cases primary VF can now be treated with catheter ablation. The demonstration that VF can be eliminated by catheter ablation in selected patients is an exciting new option in the treatment of this sometimes intractable clinical situation. Understanding of the role of catheter ablation in primary VF will be refined with increased clinical experience. Regarding scar-related VT, a paradigm shift has occurred. Instead of only trying to identify the pathway of activation during the tachycardia of interest, the scarred myocardium is identified, and ablation lesions are strategically placed to eliminate potentially arrhythmogenic tissue. Because this substrate-based ablation strategy is performed in sinus rhythm, virtually any VT can be targeted for catheter ablation regardless of its hemodynamic effect. Indeed, a substrate-based approach to VT ablation can be employed regardless of the cardiac pathology underlying the formation of the myocardial scar. Nonrandomized studies have confirmed the effectiveness of this approach in patients with recurrent VT and ICD shocks. However, substrate-based catheter ablation of VT is a strategy in evolution, and the future will likely witness both studies to better define its clinical role and technological advances in both cardiac imaging and navigation to better guide the procedure.

Acknowledgments

The author greatly appreciates and thanks Petr Neuzil, MD PhD (Homolka Hospital, Prague, Czech Republic) for his enthusiasm and talent—thereby enabling successful outcomes in many of the cases presented herein.

References

1. Josephson ME, Horowitz LN, Farshidi A, Kastor JA: Recurrent sustained ventricular tachycardia: 1. Mechanisms. Circulation 57:431-440, 1978.
2. Downar E, Harris L, Michleborough LL, et al.: Endocardial mapping of ventricular tachycardia in the intact human heart: Evidence for reentrant mechanisms. J Am Coll Cardiol 11:783-791, 1988.
3. El-Shalakany A, Hadjis T, Papageorgiou P, et al.: Entrainment mapping criteria for the prediction of termination of ventricular tachycardia by single radiofrequency lesion in patients with coronary artery disease. Circulation 99:2283-2289, 1999.
4. Stevenson WG, Friedman PL, Kocovic D, et al.: Radiofrequency catheter ablation of ventricular tachycardia after myocardial infarction. Circulation 98:308-314, 1998.
5. Strickberger SA, Man KC, Daoud EG, et al.: A prospective evaluation of catheter ablation of ventricular tachycardia as adjuvant therapy in patients with coronary artery disease and an implantable cardioverter/defibrillator. Circulation 96:1525-1531, 1997.
6. Kim YH, Sosa-Suarez G, Trouton TG, et al.: Treatment of ventricular tachycardia by transcatheter radiofrequency ablation in patients with ischemic heart disease. Circulation 89:1094-1102, 1994.
7. Rothman SA, Hsia HH, Cossu SF, et al.: Radiofrequency catheter ablation of postinfarction ventricular tachycardia: Long-term success and the significance of inducible non-clinical tachycardias. Circulation 96:3499-3508, 1997.
8. Morady F, Harvey M, Kalbfleisch SJ, et al.: Radiofrequency ablation of ventricular tachycardia in patients with coronary artery disease. Circulation 87:363-372, 1993.
9. Downar E, Kimber S, Harris L, et al.: Endocardial mapping of ventricular tachycardia in the intact human heart: II. Evidence for multiuse reentry in a functional sheet of surviving myocardium. J Am Coll Cardiol 20:869-878, 1992.
10. Harken AH, Horowitz LN, Josephson ME: Comparison of standard aneurysmectomy and aneurysmectomy with directed endocardial resection for the treatment of recurrent sustained ventricular tachycardia. J Thorac Cardiovasc Surg 80:527-534, 1980.
11. Mason JW, Stinson EB, Winkle RA, et al.: Relative efficacy of blind left ventricular aneurysm resection for the treatment of recurrent sustained ventricular tachycardia. Am J Cardiol 49:241-248, 1982.
12. Miller JM, Kienzle MG, Harken AH, Josephson ME: Subendocardial resection for ventricular tachycardia: Predictors for surgical success. Circulation 70:624-631, 1984.
13. Garan H, Nguyen K, McGovern B, et al.: Perioperative and long-term results after electrophysiologically directed ventricular surgery for recurrent ventricular tachycardia. J Am Coll Cardiol 8:201-209, 1986.
14. Haines DE, Lerman BB, Kron IL, DiMarco JP: Surgical ablation of ventricular tachycardia with sequential map-guided subendocardial resection: Electrophysiologic assessment and long-term follow-up. Circulation 77:131-141, 1988.
15. Ostermeyer J, Breithardt G, Borggrefe M, et al.: Surgical treatment of ventricular tachycardias: Complete versus partial encircling endocardial ventriculotomy. J Thorac Cardiovasc Surg 87:517-525, 1984.
16. Miller J, Rothman SA, Addonizio VP: Surgical techniques for ventricular tachycardia ablation. In Singer I (ed.): Interventional Electrophysiology. Baltimore: Williams & Wilkins, 1997, pp 641-684.
17. Guiraudon GM, Thakur RK, Klein GJ, et al.: Encircling endocardial cryoablation for ventricular tachycardia after myocardial infarction: Experience with 33 patients. Am Heart J 128:982-989, 1994.
18. Frapier JM, Hubaut JJ, Pasquie JL, Chaptal PA: Large encircling cryoablation without mapping for ventricular tachycardia after anterior myocardial infarction: Long-term outcome. J Thorac Cardiovasc Surg 116:578-583, 1998.
19. Miller JM, Tyson GS, Hargrove WC, et al.: Effect of subendocardial resection on sinus rhythm endocardial electrogram abnormalities. Circulation 91:2385-2391, 1995.
20. Cassidy DM, Vassallo JA, Marchlinski FE, et al.: Endocardial mapping in humans in sinus rhythm with normal left ventricles: Activation patterns and characteristics of electrograms. Circulation 70:37-42, 1984.
21. Furniss S, Anil-Kumar R, Bourke JP, et al.: Radiofrequency ablation of haemodynamically unstable ventricular tachycardia after myocardial infarction. Heart 84:648-652, 2000.
22. Eldar M, Fitzpatrick AP, Ohad D, et al.: Percutaneous multielectrode endocardial mapping during ventricular tachycardia in the swine model. Circulation 94:1125-1130, 1996.
23. Schilling RJ, Peters NS, Davies DW: Feasibility of a noncontact catheter for endocardial mapping of human ventricular tachycardia. Circulation 99:2543-2552, 1999.

24. Wittkampf FHM, Wever EFD, Derksen R, et al.: LocaLisa: New technique for real-time 3-dimensional localization of regular intracardiac electrodes. Circulation 99:1312-1317, 1999.

25. Gepstein L, Hayam G, Ben-Haim SA: A novel method for non-fluoroscopic catheter-based electroanatomical mapping of the heart in vitro and in vivo accuracy results. Circulation 95:1611-1622, 1997.

26. De Groot NMS, Bootsma M, van der Velde ET, et al.: Three-dimensional catheter positioning during radiofrequency ablation in patients: First application of a real-time position management system. J Cardiovasc Electrophysiol 11:1183-1192, 2000.

27. Callans DJ, Ran J-F, Michele J, et al.: Electroanatomic left ventricular mapping in the porcine model of healed anterior myocardial infarction: Correlation with intracardiac echocardiography and pathological analysis. Circulation 100:1744-1750, 1999.

28. Wrobleski D, Houghtaling C, Josephson ME, et al.: Use of electrogram characteristics during sinus rhythm to delineate the endocardial scar in a porcine model of healed myocardial infarction. J Cardiovasc Electrophysiol 14:524-529, 2003.

29. Marchlinski FE, Callans DJ, Gottlieb CD, Zado E: Linear ablation lesions for control of unmappable ventricular tachycardia in patients with ischemic and nonischemic cardiomyopathy. Circulation 101:1288-1296, 2000.

30. Reddy VY, Neuzil P, Taborsky M, Ruskin JN: Short-term results of substrate-mapping and radiofrequency ablation of ischemic ventricular tachycardia using a saline-irrigated catheter. J Am Coll Cardiol 41:2228-2236, 2003.

31. Brunckhorst CB, Delacretaz E, Soejima K, et al.: Impact of changing activation sequence on bipolar electrogram amplitude for voltage mapping of left ventricular infarcts causing ventricular tachycardia. J Interv Card Electrophysiol 12:137-141, 2005.

32. Hsia HH, Marchlinski FE: Characterization of the electroanatomic substrate for monomorphic ventricular tachycardia in patients with nonischemic cardiomyopathy. Pacing Clin Electrophysiol 25:1114-1127, 2002.

33. Soejima K, Suzuki M, Maisel WH, et al.: Catheter ablation in patients with multiple and unstable ventricular tachycardias after myocardial infarction: Short ablation lines guided by reentry circuit isthmuses and sinus rhythm mapping. Circulation 104:664-669, 2001.

34. Sra J, Bhatia A, Dhala A, et al.: Electroanatomically guided catheter ablation of ventricular tachycardias causing multiple defibrillator shocks. Pacing Clin Electrophysiol 24:1645-1652, 2001.

35. Arenal A, Glez-Torrecilla E, Ortiz M, et al.: Ablation of electrograms with an isolated, delayed component as treatment of unmappable monomorphic ventricular tachycardias in patients with structural heart disease. J Am Coll Cardiol 41:81-92, 2003.

36. Kottkamp H, Wetzel U, Schirdewahn P, et al.: Catheter ablation of ventricular tachycardia in remote myocardial infarction: Substrate description guiding placement of individual linear lesions targeting noninducibility. J Cardiovasc Electrophysiol 14:675-681, 2003.

37. Miller JM, Marchlinski FE, Buxton AE, Josephson ME: Relationship between the 12-lead electrogram during ventricular tachycardia and endocardial site of origin in patients with coronary artery disease. Circulation 77:759-766, 1988.

38. Kuchar DL, Ruskin JN, Garan H: Electrocardiographic localization of the site of origin of ventricular tachycardia in patients with prior myocardial infarction. J Am Coll Cardiol 13:893-900, 1989.

39. Merino JL, Almendral J, Villacastin JP, et al.: Radiofrequency catheter ablation of ventricular tachycardia from the right ventricle late after myocardial infarction. Am J Cardiol 77:1261-1263, 1996.

40. Patel VV, Rho RW, Gerstenfeld EP, et al.: Right bundle branch block ventricular tachycardias: Septal versus lateral ventricular origin based on activation time to the right ventricular apex. Circulation 110:2582-2587, 2004.

41. De Chillou C, Lacroix D, Klug D, et al.: Isthmus characteristics of reentrant ventricular tachycardia after myocardial infarction. Circulation 12:105:726-731, 2002.

42. Brunckhorst CB, Stevenson WG, Jackman WM, et al.: Ventricular mapping during atrial and ventricular pacing: Relationship of multipotential electrograms to ventricular tachycardia reentry circuits after myocardial infarction. Eur Heart J 23:1131-1138, 2002.

43. Hiroshi N, Singh D, Beckman KJ, et al.: Ablation of unmappable post-MI ventricular tachycardia using substrate mapping during sinus rhythm: Predictors for a recurrence. Heart Rhythm 1:S36, 2004.

44. Brunckhorst CB, Delacretaz E, Soejima K, et al.: Identification of the ventricular tachycardia isthmus after infarction by pace mapping. Circulation 110:652-659, 2004.

45. Soejima K, Stevenson WG, Maisel WH, et al.: Electrically unexcitable scar mapping based on pacing threshold for identification of the reentry circuit isthmus: Feasibility for guiding ventricular tachycardia ablation. Circulation 106:1678-1683, 2002.

46. Langberg JJ, Gallagher M, Strickberger A, et al: Temperature-guided radiofrequency catheter ablation with very large electrodes. Circulation 88:245-249, 1993.

47. Calkins H, Epstein A, Packer D, et al: Catheter ablation of ventricular tachycardia in patients with structural heart disease using cooled radiofrequency energy. J Am Coll Cardiol 35:1905-1914, 2000.

48. Nakagawa H, Yamanashi WS, Pitha JV, et al.: Comparison of in vivo tissue temperature profile and lesion geometry for radiofrequency ablation with a saline-irrigated electrode versus temperature control in a canine thigh muscle preparation. Circulation 91: 2264-2273, 1995.

49. Nakagawa H, Wittkampf FHM, Yamanashi WS, et al.: Inverse relationship between electrode size and lesion size during radiofrequency ablation with active electrode cooling. Circulation 98:458-465, 1998.

50. Strickberger SA, Knight BP, Michaud GF, et al.: Mapping and ablation of ventricular tachycardia guided by virtual electrograms using a noncontact, computerized mapping system. J Am Coll Cardiol 35:414-421, 2000.

51. Della Bella P, Pappalardo A, Riva S, et al.: Non-contact mapping to guide catheter ablation of untolerated ventricular tachycardia. Eur Heart J 23:742-752, 2002.

52. Thiagalingam A, Wallace EM, Campbell CR, et al.: Value of noncontact mapping for identifying left ventricular scar in an ovine model. Circulation 110:3175-3180, 2004.

53. Nakayama Y, Shimizu G, Hirota Y, et al.: Extent of myocardial fibrosis and cellular hypertrophy in dilated cardiomyopathy. Am J Cardiol 10:186-192, 1988.

54. Roberts WC, Siegel RJ, McManus BM: Idiopathic dilated cardiomyopathy: Analysis of 152 necropsy patients. Am J Cardiol 60:1340-1355, 1987.

55. Hsia HH, Callans DJ, Marchlinski FE: Characterization of endocardial electrophysiological substrate in patients with nonischemic cardiomyopathy and monomorphic ventricular tachycardia. Circulation 108:704-710, 2003.

56. Soejima K, Stevenson WG, Sapp JL, et al.: Endocardial and epicardial radiofrequency ablation of ventricular tachycardia associated with dilated cardiomyopathy. J Am Coll Cardiol 43:1834-1842, 2004.

57. McKenna WJ, Thiene G, Nava A, et al.: Diagnosis of arrhyth-

mogenic right ventricular dysplasia/cardiomyopathy. Task force of the working group for myocardial and pericardial disease of the European Society of Cardiology and of the Scientific Council on Cardiomyopathies of the International Society and Federation of Cardiology. Br Heart J 71:215-218, 1994.

58. Marchlinski FE, Zado E, Dixit S, et al.: Electroanatomic substrate and outcome of catheter ablative therapy for ventricular tachycardia in setting of right ventricular cardiomyopathy. Circulation 100:2293-2298, 2004.

59. Maguire JH, Hoff R, Sherlock I, et al.: Cardiac morbidity and mortality due to Chagas' disease: Prospective electrocardiographic study of a Brazilian community. Circulation 75:1140-1145, 1987.

60. Scanavacca M, Sosa E: Electrophysiologic study in chronic Chagas' heart disease. Revista Paulista de Medicina 113:841-850, 1995.

61. Sosa E, Scanavacca M, d'Avila A, et al.: Endocardial and epicardial ablation guided by nonsurgical transthoracic epicardial mapping to treat recurrent ventricular tachycardia. J Cardiovasc Electrophysiol 9:229-239, 1998.

62. Svenson RH, Littmann L, Gallagher JJ, et al.: Termination of ventricular tachycardia with epicardial laser photocoagulation: A clinical comparison with patients undergoing successful endocardial photocoagulation alone. J Am Coll Cardiol 15:163-170, 1990.

63. D'Avila A, Scanavacca M, Sosa E, et al.: Pericardial anatomy for the interventional electrophysiologist. J Cardiovasc Electrophysiol 14:422-430, 2003.

64. Schweikert RA, Saliba WI, Tomassoni G, et al.: Percutaneous pericardial instrumentation for endo-epicardial mapping of previously failed ablations. Circulation 108:1329-1335, 2003.

65. Reddy VY, Wrobleski D, Houghtaling C, et al.: Combined epicardial and endocardial electroanatomic-mapping in a porcine model of healed myocardial infarction. Circulation 107:3236-3242, 2003.

66. Berruezo A, Mont L, Nava S, et al.: Electrocardiographic recognition of the epicardial origin of ventricular tachycardias. Circulation 109:1842-1847, 2004.

67. Sosa E, Scanavacca M, D'Avila A, et al.: Nonsurgical transthoracic epicardial approach in patients with ventricular tachycardia and previous cardiac surgery. J Interv Card Electrophysiol 10:281-288, 2004.

68. Soejima K, Couper G, Cooper JM, et al.: Subxiphoid surgical approach for epicardial catheter-based mapping and ablation in patients with prior cardiac surgery or difficult pericardial access. Circulation 110:1197-1201, 2004.

69. Kim RJ, Wu E, Rafael A, et al.: The use of contrast-enhanced magnetic resonance imaging to identify reversible myocardial dysfunction. N Engl J Med 343:1445-1453, 2000.

70. Reddy VY, Malchano ZJ, Holmvang G, et al.: Integration of cardiac MR imaging with 3-dimensional electroanatomical mapping to guide left ventricular catheter manipulation: Feasibility in a porcine model of healed myocardial infarction. J Am Coll Cardiol 44:2202-2213, 2004.

71. Faddis MN, Blume W, Finney J, et al.: Novel, magnetically guided catheter for endocardial mapping and radiofrequency catheter ablation. Circulation 106:2980-2985, 2002.

72. Callans DJ, Ren J-F, Narula N, et al.: Effects of linear, irrigated-tip radiofrequency ablation in porcine healed anterior infarction. J Cardiovasc Electrophysiol 12:1037-1042, 2001.

73. Khan HH, Maisel WH, Ho C, et al.: Effect of radiofrequency catheter ablation of ventricular tachycardia on left ventricular function in patients with prior myocardial infarction. J Interv Card Electrophysiol 2:243-247, 2002.

74. Haissaguerre M, Shah DC, Jais P, et al.: Role of Purkinje conducting system in triggering of idiopathic ventricular fibrillation. Lancet 359:677-678, 2002.

75. Haissaguerre M, Shoda M, Jais P, et al.: Mapping and ablation of idiopathic ventricular fibrillation. Circulation 106:962-967, 2002.

76. Haissaguerre M, Extramiana F, Hocini M, et al.: Mapping and ablation of ventricular fibrillation associated with long-QT and Brugada syndromes. Circulation 108:925-928, 2003.

77. Bansch D, Oyang F, Antz M, et al.: Successful catheter ablation of electrical storm after myocardial infarction. Circulation 108:3011-3016, 2003.

78. Marrouche N, Verma A, Wazni O, et al.: Mode of initiation and ablation of ventricular fibrillation storms in patients with ischemic cardiomyopathy. J Am Coll Cardiol 43:1715-1720, 2004.

79. Szumowski L, Sander P, Walczak F, et al.: Mapping and ablation of polymorphic ventricular tachycardia after myocardial infarction. J Am Coll Cardiol 44:1700-1706, 2004.

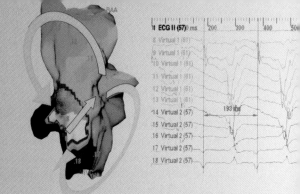

30

Epicardial Approach to Catheter Ablation of Ventricular Tachycardia

Eduardo Sosa • Mauricio Scanavacca

Key Points

- Epicardial ventricular tachycardias (VT) occur in patients with coronary artery disease and dilated cardiomyopathies.

- Epicardial VTs are suggested by pseudo-delta waves and delayed activation times on the surface electrocardiogram (ECG) and by failure of endocardial mapping/ablation.

- Percutaneous pericardial access is feasible in the electrophysiology laboratory.

- Coronary angiography is routinely performed with epicardial ablation.

- Irrigated ablation may be required.

Catheter ablation of ventricular tachycardias (VT) is still a great challenge. For several different types of supraventricular tachycardias and some idiopathic VTs, ablation is the first-line procedure due to its high success rate and low complication rate.[1,2] However, catheter ablation of atrial fibrillation[3-5] and VT, especially when associated with structural heart disease, is a complex and laborious procedure.[2] Most VTs occur because of scar-related reentry. The scar-related VT is characterized by the presence of several bundles of surviving myocardial tissue surrounded by dense scar tissue. These surviving bundles of tissue may interconnect in such a way that slow conduction is allowed and a different pathway exists to the extent that VT can occur.[2] The ability to localize and destroy the bundles of surviving tissue inside the scar constitutes the foundation for catheter-based ablation of scar-related VT. The success rate for more rare VTs, such as focal[6] or bundle-branch reentry VT,[7] depends on the ability to identify the site of origin of VT or the His branch involved in the reentry circuit.

These different targets have usually been reached from the endocardium, but the success rate from this approach has been variable.[2] The presence of epicardial circuits has been considered one of the reasons for the failure of endocardial ablation, and these circuits have been described in several types of cardiac disease in which surgical and nonsurgical techniques were used.[8-19]

The existence of epicardial VT is not a new idea. Littman et al.,[8] using epicardial laser photocoagulation during surgical ablation of 25 VTs in 10 patients, observed that VT after myocardial infarction (MI) may result from epicardial macroreentry. Slow conduction within the reentry circuit can be localized by epicardial mapping, and epicardial ablation interrupts epicardial post-MI VT. In patients with nonischemic VT, Cassidy et al.[9] and Pearlman et al.[10] suggested that abnormal, fractionated or late endocardial electrograms, or both of these together, are less frequently seen in patients with dilated cardiomyopathy (DCM) than in patients with post-MI VT, and the incidence of abnormal epicardial electrograms roughly equals the incidence of abnormal electrograms. Svenson et al.[11] described the existence of epicardial circuits in post-MI VT, suggesting that they are particularly important in inferior wall infarcts.

Several techniques to map the epicardial surface of the heart in the electrophysiology laboratory have been described. The trans-septal[12] and coronary cusp approaches[13] can be useful to map specific forms of idiopathic VT that originate in the left ventricular outflow tract. Coronary veins can be used to perform epicardial mapping, but the manipulation of the catheter is limited by the anatomic distribution of these vessels.[14] To the best of our knowledge, the subxiphoid percutaneous approach to the epicardial space is the only technique currently available that allows extensive and unrestricted mapping of the epicardial surface of both ventricles.[15,16]

At least two principal reasons explain why the epicardial VT is a matter of interest. First, as already stated, epicardial VT can be the reason for failure of endocardial VT ablation, even when modern mapping systems[17] and more powerful sources of energy, such as irrigated catheters, are used. Second, now we are able not only to reach the pericardial space but also to map and ablate epicardial VT in the electrophysiology laboratory.[16-25]

The Subxiphoid Percutaneous Approach

The subxiphoid percutaneous approach has been previously described in detail.[16] Reaching the pericardial space is easy and is performed after the multipolar catheters are positioned in the coronary sinus and right ventricular apex through the femoral venous approach, before anticoagulation is started. The pericardial space is reached by using a commercially available needle, originally developed to perform a spinal tap (Fig. 30–1). The tip of this needle is designed to reach a virtual space without damaging the spinal cord (epidural needle, 17 gauge × 3⅞ inches [9.84 cm] and × 5 inches [12.5 cm] Thin Wall (TW) with centimeter markings; Arrow International, Reading, Pa.). Because of its shape, this type of needle is considered safer for the transthoracic epicardial approach. Other types of needles can be used; however, the operator must be aware of the higher risk of perforation of the heart.

The puncture must be performed at the angle between the left border of the subxiphoid process and

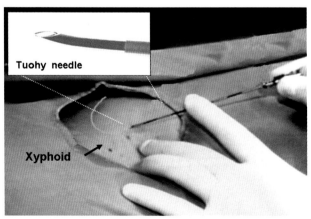

FIGURE 30–1. Technique utilized to perform subxiphoid approach. A regular Tuohy needle (*upper left corner*) is utilized to reach pericardial space.

the lowest left rib. The spatial orientation of the needle is important to determine what portion of the ventricles will be reached. The needle usually has to point toward the left shoulder, and it must be introduced more horizontally if the target is the anterior portion of the ventricles or more vertically if the diaphragmatic portion of the heart is the area of interest. After crossing the subcutaneous tissue, the needle movement should be monitored by fluoroscopy in the left anterior oblique view, at 35 to 40 degrees (Fig. 30–2). The needle must be carefully moved toward the heart silhouette until the operator can detect heart movement.

The injection of a small amount (approximately 1 mL) of contrast medium demonstrates whether the needle tip is pushing or passing through the tissue. If the diaphragm has not been reached, the contrast agent will be seen in the subdiaphragmatic area. If the needle reaches the pericardial sac, the contrast spreads around the heart and is restricted to its silhouette. The appearance of a "sluggish" layering of contrast medium indicates that the needle is correctly positioned in the pericardial space. A soft, floppy-tipped guide wire is then passed through the hollow, and an 8-French introducer is advanced. Then a regular ablation catheter is introduced into the pericardial space.

Once the catheter is inside the pericardial space, epicardial ventricular electrograms can be nicely recorded during sinus rhythm and during VT (Fig. 30–3 and 30–4). The entire surface of the heart can be mapped and eventually ablated.

From the initial report in 1996[15] until the end of 2003, this approach was performed in 215 consecutive patients with VT.[15a] VT was associated with Chagas' disease in 138 patients. Fifty were VTs occurring after inferior MI, and 15 were associated with idiopathic DCM. Twelve idiopathic VTs were included in this series. The number of inducible VTs ranged from 1.8 to 2.2 per patient. Nonmappable VTs were observed in 40% to 44% of patients. In an average of 5% of patients, only one endocardial VT was induced, and in an average of 3.5%, only one epicardial VT was induced. In a group of mappable VTs, epicardial VT was present in 25% of idiopathic DCM VTs, 32% of post-MI VTs, and 36% of chagasic VTs. Successful radiofrequency (RF) ablation (i.e., interruption and no reinduction) was obtained from the epicardium in 50% of post-MI VTs, 60% of Chagas-related VTs, and in 55% of idiopathic DCM VTs.

Epicardial VTs were defined as those VTs in which critical sites of the reentrant circuit (or the "origin" site) were located exclusively in the subepicardial tissue as suggested by entrainment maneuvers and/or those that were terminated within 10 seconds by standard RF pulses (Fig. 30–3). We are aware that, theoretically at least, critical epicardial sites could be entrained or interrupted within 10 seconds from both endocardial and epicardial surfaces, making it difficult to demonstrate the presence of a truly epicardial circuit in a given case. It is not known how often this occurs. Epicardial VT may occur in patients with idiopathic VT[17,18,25] and in those with ischemic[23,26] or nonischemic VT.[17,18,22]

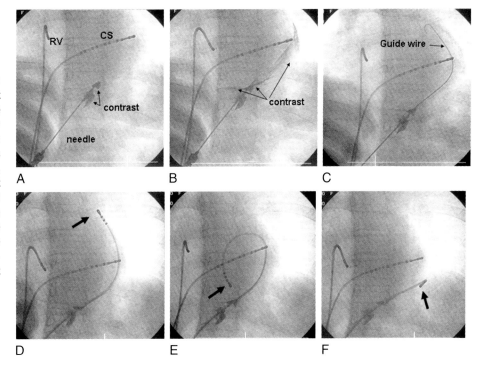

FIGURE 30–2. LAO projection shown: **A,** Injection of contrast medium to check if the needle tip is pushing or passing through the tissue. **B,** The moment in which the contrast medium is layering the heart silhouette. **C,** Guide wire around the heart silhouette correctly positioned inside the pericardial space. **D,** to **F,** Image of catheter into the pericardial space. *Arrows* indicate the epicardial catheter. CS, coronary sinus catheter; RV, right ventricular catheter.

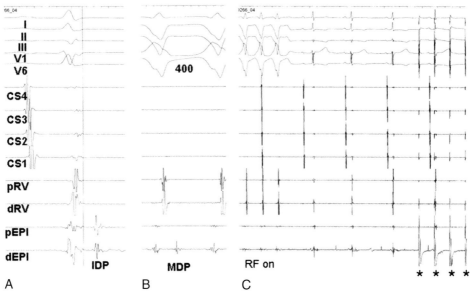

FIGURE 30–3. ECG leads I, II, III, V1 and V6 are displayed with proximal to distal coronary sinus electrograms (CS4, CS3, CS2, CS1); proximal to distal right ventricle electrograms (pRV, dRV), and proximal and distal epicardial electrograms (pEPI, dEPI). **A,** Mapping during sinus rhythms: note the presence of isolated diastolic potential (IDP). **B,** Mapping during ventricular tachycardia: note the transformation of IDP in mid-diastolic potential (MDP). **C,** RF interruption of VT. Asterisks indicate artifact of epicardial stimulation in order to avoid phrenic nerve injury.

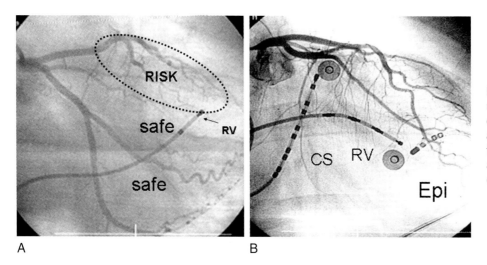

FIGURE 30–4. Avoiding coronary artery damage. **A,** Previous coronary angiography indicating areas of risk and safer areas for RF application. **B,** Coronary angiogaphy just before RF application. (See text.)

Problems Related to the Subxiphoid Epicardial Approach

Several questions are a matter of concern regarding the use of the subxiphoid epicardial approach. The first one is related to the possibility of puncture accidents. *Predictable* and *avoidable* accidents were related to a "dry" right ventricular puncture in 4.5% of 215 consecutive patients who underwent epicardial ablation.[15a] Drainable hemopericardium of 200 ± 98 mL of blood was observed in 7% of patients. These

predictable accidents were mostly related to the learning curve. One patient in this series had bleeding in the abdominal cavity from an injured diaphragmatic vessel, and blood transfusion and laparotomy were required to achieve control. This represents an *unpredictable* and *difficult to avoid* complication.

AVOIDING CORONARY ARTERY DAMAGE

One of the main concerns during epicardial mapping and ablation is to avoid coronary artery damage. In this regard, d'Avila et al.[27] reported experimental data from nine mongrel dogs in which linear and single RF lesions were applied on or near the coronary artery. The authors concluded that, in an acute model, RF application delivery above the artery may result in intimal hyperplasia and thrombosis. However, the susceptibility to damage was inversely proportional to vessel size. No endothelial lesions were present in vessels with an internal perimeter larger than 2 mm.

The chronic effects of RF lesions on epicardial coronary arteries were also analyzed by Miranda[28] in seven young pigs observed for a least 70 days after RF ablation. The results suggest that RF pulses delivered near the epicardial vessels do not provoke either MI or vascular thrombosis. The endothelium was preserved in most of the animals, but intense intimal thickening was seen in only a few animals. The reason that the presence of fat and veins interposed between the epicardial coronary arteries and the

catheter tip is related to much less intimal thickening is still unknown.

Our current approach regarding the risk of damage to coronary vessels is to obtain an angiogram before ablation in all patients. Based on analysis of the anatomy of the coronary arteries, safer versus riskier areas can be selected for epicardial ablation (Fig. 30–4 and 30–5). Depending on the location of the ablation site, another angiogram can be obtained during the procedure, just before ablation is begun (Fig. 30–6), but we do not routinely do this. As a general rule, we assume that a safe application can be delivered if the distance between the catheter tip and a visible coronary vessel is greater than 1 cm. However, if a putative critical site of the tachycardia circuit can be identified only close to a coronary artery despite extensive mapping, then, as in all

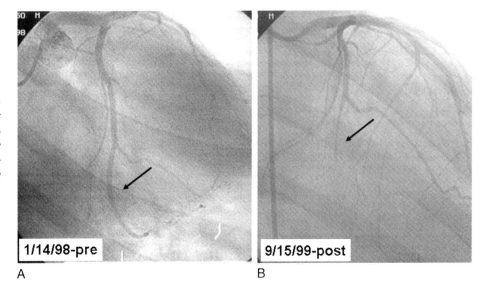

FIGURE 30–5. Coronary angiography before (**A**) and one year after epicardial ablation to control Chagas cardiomyopathy with incessant VT (**B**). The *arrows* indicate the coronary branch occluded.

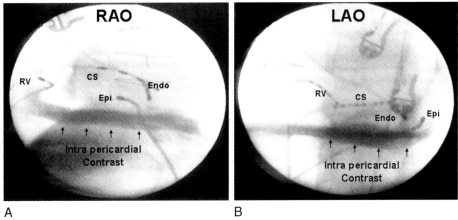

FIGURE 30–6. Right anterior oblique (RAO; **A**) and left anterior oblique (LAO; **B**) views of the heart showing the catheter position during simultaneous endocardial and epicardial mapping for VT ablation. RV, CS, Endo, and Epi: right ventricular, coronary sinus, left ventricular, and epicardial catheters respectively. Note the contrast media accumulated at the inferior wall due to dense postoperative adhesions located at the high lateral and anterior wall of both ventricles.

clinical scenarios, a risk-benefit analysis should be undertaken.

In only 1 of 215 consecutive patients, RF application caused coronary artery occlusion of a marginal branch (Fig. 30–5), resulting in non-Q wave MI with a myocardial-bound creatine kinase (CKMB) peak of 35 units/L.

EFFECTS OF EPICARDIAL FAT ON EPICARDIAL MAPPING AND ABLATION

The presence of epicardial fat interposed between the catheter tip and an epicardial target also deserves special attention. Depending on its location and amount, the fat tissue may either facilitate the efficacy of epicardial catheter ablation (by minimizing vascular damage during RF application) or diminish it (by providing an insulating cushion). d'Avila et al.[29] compared the bipolar epicardial electrograms and ventricular epicardial stimulation thresholds obtained with a 4-mm-tip ablation catheter from 44 areas without and 45 areas with epicardial fat in 10 patients during open chest surgery. They observed that epicardial fat thickness of up to 5 mm interposed between the ablation catheter and the epicardium does not alter the amplitude of the bipolar epicardial electrogram, its duration, or the epicardial ventricular stimulation threshold. In areas with a layer of epicardial fat thickness greater than 5 mm, ventricular capture was not possible even with 10-mA pulses.

The effect of epicardial fat on RF lesion formation was analyzed in animal models with the use of both standard and cool-tipped RF catheters.[30] This study suggested that fat attenuates epicardial lesion formation. The absence of blood flow in the epicardial space makes the catheter tip heat up at low power deliveries. The use of a cooled-tip ablation catheter allows for more energy to be delivered and a larger lesion to be created despite the presence of fat interposed between the catheter tip and the epicardium.

The same results[31] could be extrapolated to epicardial cryoablation. Epicardial cryoablation can create a very deep lesion, but the presence of a fat layer thicker than 5 mm strongly attenuates epicardial cryolesions. These data are important and may help to explain failures during epicardial RF ablation.

PERICARDITIS

Another potential complication seen after epicardial catheter ablation is post-procedure pericarditis. In the experimental laboratory, animals mapped and ablated intrapericardially may develop an intense pericarditis after the procedure,[32] which can be eliminated by the pericardial infusion of 2 mg/kg of triamcinolone at the end of the procedure. Such an intense pericarditis has not been seen in patients in our series. Precordial distress and pain were observed in approximately 30% of our patients. However, pericardial effusion was minimal, and the symptoms were easily controlled with regular anti-inflammatory drugs in these patients. All 29 patients in our series who had more than one epicardial procedure, ranging from 1 week to 10 months after the

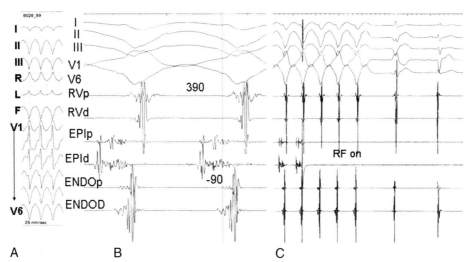

FIGURE 30–7. Shown are the electrocardiographic (ECG) patterns of inducible VT (**A**), electrogram characteristic at the ablation site (**B**), and interruption of VT (**C**) from a patient with postoperative epicardial VT. *Dotted line* indicates the onset of the QRS complex (**B**). Note the very prolonged and fractionated presystolic electrogram recorded at the epicardial ablation site. ECG leads I, II, III, V1, and V6 are displayed with proximal to distal right ventricle electrograms (RVp, RVd), proximal and distal epicardial electrograms (EPIp, EPId), and proximal (ENDOp) and distal (ENDOD) endocardial left ventricle electrograms.

first procedure, were free of pericardial effusion and pericardial adhesions.

PERICARDIAL ADHESIONS

Postoperative pericardial adhesions may represent a limitation to the percutaneous transthoracic epicardial approach. In our series, 5 patients had monomorphic VT 7 to 10 years after open chest surgery.[33] Ejection fraction was approximately 40%. Despite the presence of postoperative adhesions, all patients underwent endocardial and epicardial approaches simultaneously. In these patients, the pericardial puncture was directed to the inferior wall of the heart, where pericardial adhesions are thought to be less important than in the anterior wall. The pericardial space was entered in all patients. Fourteen VTs were induced, 8 of which were unmappable. Three of the 6 mappable VTs were successfully ablated from the endocardium, and 2 were successfully ablated from the epicardium (Fig. 30–7 and 30–8).

PHRENIC NERVE INJURY

Injury to the phrenic nerve is a rare complication of endocardial atrial RF ablation. The phrenic nerves course through the upper chest, medial to the mediastinal pleura and the apex of the right or left lung. The right phrenic nerve lies laterally to the right brachiocephalic vein and the superior vena cava. The left phrenic nerve courses along the lateral aspect of the transverse arch of the aorta. The two nerves subsequently pass anteriorly to their respective pulmonary hila and then inferiorly in a broad vertical plane along the margin of the heart between the fibrous pericardium and the mediastinal pleura. The application of RF pulses in the lateral aspect of the heart

silhouette can theoretically induce phrenic nerve injury.[34-36]

In our first 215 patients, we never observed this complication. However, we are aware that the incidence of this complication could be underestimated, because unilateral diaphragmatic paralysis usually does not cause significant shortness of breath unless other underlying pulmonary disease is present.

For prevention of phrenic nerve injury, high-output pacing (15 mA, 5 msec pulse duration) at the eventual ablation site (theoretically near the phrenic course) before RF delivery and even during RF application might be a helpful tool (Fig. 30–9; see Fig. 30–3). This is not difficult, because we usually do not apply many pulses to ablate epicardial VT.

When Should the Epicardial Approach Be Used?

There remains the question of which epicardial approach should be used, and the answer depends on the preference of the electrophysiologist. It is not clear whether one should approach only after endocardial failure or only when the electrocardiogram (ECG) of clinical VT suggests an epicardial origin of VT. As a matter of fact, the simultaneous approach may have several advantages, such as reduced cost, a better chance to map and ablate all inducible VTs, and an opportunity to acquire more expertise with the technique.

To deal with this question, we analyzed the ECG pattern obtained during endocardial and epicardial ventricular stimulation in 40 stimulated sites (Fig.

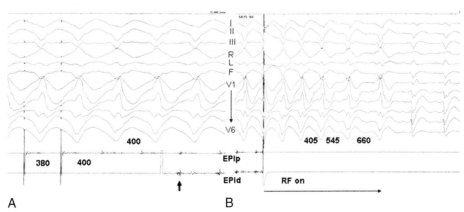

FIGURE 30–8. Panel **A,** Activation mapping during VT. Note a mid-diastolic potential (*arrows*) recorded from the distal epicardial ablation electrodes (EPId). The 12 surface ECG leads are shown. Pacing at this site reproduce the VT QRS morphology. The post pacing interval is identical to VT cycle length suggesting that this epicardial site is part of the VT circuit. Panel **B,** One radiofrequency pulse applied at this site interrupted and rendered VT non-inducible.

30–10). The differences in endocardial and epicardial QRS complex duration and shortest RS complex were not statistically significant. However, the intrinsicoid deflection time and the presence of a pseudo-delta wave were statistically different.

Comparing the same parameter for the QRS complexes of endocardial and epicardial VTs (Fig. 30–11), we observed that the intrinsicoid deflection time was longer in the epicardial VTs. Also, the specificity and

sensitivity of a deflection time longer than 97 msec for an epicardial VT were 80% and 50%, respectively. Something similar occurs with QRS duration (Fig. 30–12). QRS duration is longer in epicardial VT than in endocardial VT. A QRS complex longer than 198 msec had a specificity of 86% and a sensitivity of 69% for epicardial circuits. The shortest RS time also was longer in epicardial VT, with a sensitivity of 82% and a specificity of 57% when longer than 122 msec (see Fig. 30–11).

The presence of a pseudo-delta wave was also suggestive of an epicardial VT. This parameter had sensitivity and specificity of 80% for epicardial circuits (see Fig. 30–12). Although these ECG characteristics are subtle, an epicardial origin should be suspected if the QRS duration is longer than 200 msec and a delta wave–like pattern is present. Berruezo et al.[37] recently reported similar findings. At electrophysiologic testing, an epicardial VT may be suggested by a broad area of "early" endocardial ventricular activation (representing endocardial breakthrough), the absence of early endocardial ventricular activation or satisfactory pace maps, or the failure of ablation at the most favorable endocardial sites (Table 30–1).

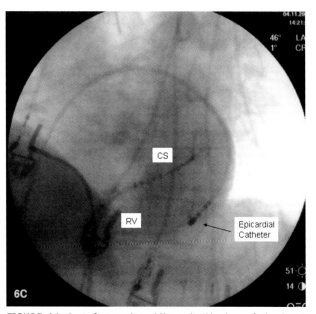

FIGURE 30–9. Left anterior oblique (LAO) view of the heart from the patient described in Figure 30–3, showing the epicardial catheter positions during VT ablation at a site with phrenic nerve stimulation. CS, coronary sinus catheter; RV, right ventricle catheter.

Conclusion

Subepicardial VT may occur in ischemic, nonischemic, and idiopathic VT. Truly subepicardial VT can preferentially be ablated from the epicardial surface. A percutaneous subxiphoid approach to the

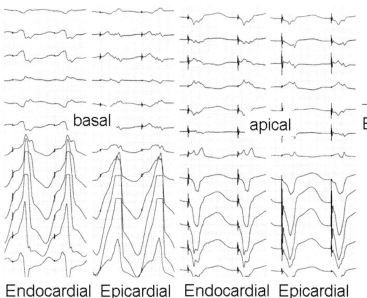

Endocardial Epicardial   Endocardial Epicardial

PDW
——————————
Endocardial:
36±34 ms

Epicardial
67±38 ms

p: <0.05

FIGURE 30–10. Examples of endocardial versus epicardial stimulated QRS complex obtained in 40 sites at the basal and apical zone of left ventricular. PDW, pseudo delta wave. (See text.) From top to bottom ECG leads I, II, III, aVR, aVL, aVF, and V1-V6.

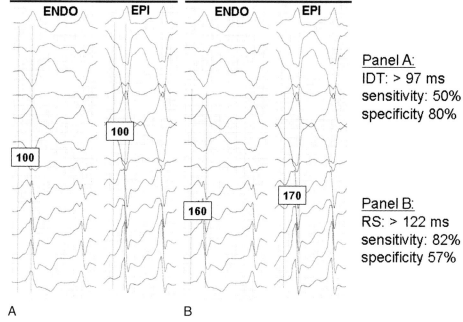

FIGURE 30–11. Twelve lead ECG obtained during spontaneous endocardial and epicardial VTs. *Dotted lines* indicate the parameter measured. The number between the *dotted lines* show the interval measured in ms in a specific case. **A,** Comparison of the intrinsicoid deflection time (IDT) in endocardial (ENDO) and epicardial (EPI) VT. **B,** Comparison of RS duration (RS). From top to bottom ECG leads I, II, III, aVR, aVL, aVF, and V1-V6.

Panel A:
IDT: > 97 ms
sensitivity: 50%
specificity 80%

Panel B:
RS: > 122 ms
sensitivity: 82%
specificity 57%

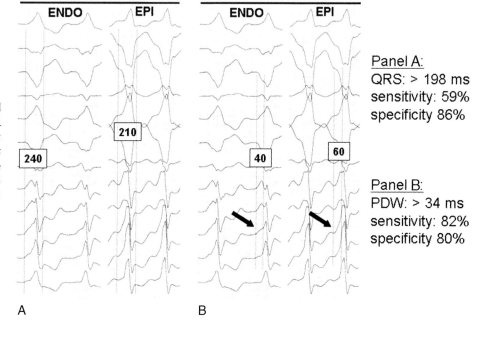

FIGURE 30–12. ECG obtained during endocardial and epicardial spontaneous VT. **A,** QRS duration; **B,** a pseudo delta wave. *Arrows* indicate pseudo delta wave (PDW). From top to bottom ECG leads I, II, III, aVR, aVL, aVF, and V1-V6.

Panel A:
QRS: > 198 ms
sensitivity: 59%
specificity 86%

Panel B:
PDW: > 34 ms
sensitivity: 82%
specificity 80%

TABLE 30-1

Findings Suggestive of Epicardial Ventricular Tachycardia

Finding	Definition
Surface electrocardiogram	
QRS duration ≥198 msec	Total QRS duration
Pseudo delta wave >34 msec*	Earliest ventricular activation to earliest fast deflection in any precordial lead
Intrinsicoid deflection time ≥85 msec*	Interval from earliest ventricular activation to nadir of the first S wave in any precordial lead
RS complex duration ≥121 msec*	Interval from earliest ventricular activation to peak of R wave in lead V_2
Delayed maximal peak deflection index ≥0.54**	Interval from earliest ventricular activation to peak of R or nadir S wave divided by total QRS duration
Intracardiac recordings	
Absence of early endocardial activation sites	
Diffuse area of earliest endocardial activation	
Poor endocardial pace maps	
Failed ablation at best endocardial sites	

*Berruezo A, Mont L, Nava S, et al.: Electrocardiographic recognition of the epicardial origin of ventricular tachycardias. Circulation 109:1842-1847, 2004.
**Diagnosis based on smallest ratio in any precordial lead.

pericardial space is easily and safely performed in the electrophysiology laboratory by an electrophysiologist. This approach may improve the results of the catheter ablation procedure.

References

1. Morady F: Catheter ablation of supraventricular arrhythmias: State of the art. Heart Rhythms 1:67C-84C, 2004.
2. Stevenson WG: Catheter ablation of monomorphic ventricular tachycardia. Curr Opin Cardiol 20:42-47, 2005.
3. Jais P, Sanders P, Hsu LF, et al.: Catheter ablation for atrial fibrillation. Heart 91:7-9, 2005.
4. Pappone C, Santinelli V: The who, what, why, and how-to guide for circumferential pulmonary vein ablation. J Cardiovasc Electrophysiol 15:1226-1230, 2004.
5. Hsu LF, Jais P, Sanders P, et al.: Catheter ablation for atrial fibrillation in congestive heart failure. N Engl J Med 351:2373-2383, 2004.
6. Klein LS, Shih HT, Hackett FK, et al.: Radiofrequency catheter ablation of ventricular tachycardia in patients without structural heart disease. Circulation 85:1666-1674, 1992.
7. Tchou P, Jazayeri M, Denker S, et al.: Transcatheter electrical ablation of the right bundle branch: A method of treating macroreentrant ventricular tachycardia due to bundle branch reentry. Circulation 78:246-257, 1988.
8. Littmann L, Svenson RH, Gallagher JJ, et al.: Functional role of the epicardium in postinfarction ventricular tachycardia: Observations derived from computerized epicardial activation mapping, entrainment, and epicardial laser photoablation. Circulation 83:1577-1591, 1991.
9. Cassidy DM, Vassallo JA, Miller JM, et al.: Endocardial catheter mapping in patients in sinus rhythm: Relationship to underlying heart disease and ventricular arrhythmias. Circulation 73;645-652, 1986.
10. Perlman RL, Miller J, Kindwall KE, et al.: Abnormal epicardial and endocardial electrograms in patients with idiopathic dilated cardiomyopathy: Relationship to arrhythmias [abstract]. Circulation 82(Suppl III):III-708, 1990.
11. Svenson RH, Littmann L, Gallagher JJ, et al.: Termination of ventricular tachycardia with epicardial laser photocoagulation: A clinical comparison with patients undergoing successful endocardial photocoagulation alone. J Am Coll Cardiol 15:163-170, 1990.
12. Sosa E, Scanavacca M, d'Avila A: Catheter ablation of the left ventricular outflow tract tachycardia from the left atrium. J Interv Card Electrophysiol 7:61-63, 2002.
13. Hachiya H, Aonuma K, Yamauchi Y, et al.: Successful radiofrequency catheter ablation from the supravalvular region of the aortic valve in a patient with outflow tract ventricular tachycardia. Jpn Circ J 64:459-463, 2000.
14. de Paola AA, Melo WD, Tavora MZ, Martinez EE: Angiographic and electrophysiological substrates for ventricular tachycardia mapping through the coronary veins. Heart 79:59-63, 1998.
15. Sosa E, Scanavacca M, d'Avila A, Pilleggi F: A new technique to perform epicardial mapping in the electrophysiology laboratory. J Cardiovasc Electrophysiol 7:531-536, 1996.
15a. Sosa E and Scanavacca M. Epicardial mapping and ablation techniques to control ventricular tachycardia. J Cardiovasc Electrophysiol 16:449-452, 2005.
16. Sosa E, Scanavacca M: Epicardial mapping and ablation techniques to control ventricular tachycardia. J Cardiovasc Electrophysiol 16:449-452, 2005.
17. Swarup V, Morton JB, Arruda M, Wilber DJ: Ablation of epicardial macroreentrant ventricular tachycardia associated with idiopathic nonischemic dilated cardiomyopathy by a percutaneous transthoracic approach. J Cardiovasc Electrophysiol 13:1164-1168, 2002.
18. Ouyang F, Bansch D, Schaumann A, et al.: Catheter ablation of subepicardial ventricular tachycardia using electroanatomic mapping. Herz 28:591-597, 2003.
19. Soejima K, Stevenson WG, Sapp JL, et al.: Endocardial and epicardial radiofrequency ablation of ventricular tachycardia associated with dilated cardiomyopathy: the importance of low-voltage scars. J Am Coll Cardiol 43:1834-1842, 2004.
20. Soejima K, Stevenson WG: Catheter ablation of ventricular tachycardia in patients with ischemic heart disease. Curr Cardiol Rep 5:364-368, 2003.
21. Schweikert RA, Saliba WI, Tomassoni G, et al.: Percutaneous pericardial instrumentation for endo-epicardial mapping of previously failed ablations. Circulation 108:1329-1335, 2003.
22. Sosa E, Scanavacca M, D'Avila A, et al.: Radiofrequency catheter ablation of ventricular tachycardia guided by nonsurgical epicardial mapping in chronic Chagasic heart disease. Pacing Clin Electrophysiol 22(1 Pt 1):128-130, 1999.
23. Sosa E, Scanavacca M, d'Avila A, et al.: Nonsurgical transthoracic epicardial catheter ablation to treat recurrent ventricu-

lar tachycardia occurring late after myocardial infarction. J Am Coll Cardiol 35:1442-1449, 2000.

24. Sosa E, Scanavacca M, d'Avila A: Transthoracic epicardial catheter ablation to treat recurrent ventricular tachycardia. Curr Cardiol Rep 3:451-458, 2001.

25. Sosa E, Scanavacca M, d'Avila A, et al.: Nonsurgical transthoracic mapping and ablation in a child with incessant ventricular tachycardia. J Cardiovasc Electrophysiol 11:208-210, 2000.

26. Brugada J, Berruezo A, Cuesta A, et al.: Nonsurgical transthoracic epicardial radiofrequency ablation: An alternative in incessant ventricular tachycardia. J Am Coll Cardiol 41:2036-2043, 2003.

27. d'Avila A, Gutierrez P, Scanavacca M, et al.: Effects of radiofrequency pulses delivered in the vicinity of the coronary arteries: Implications for nonsurgical transthoracic epicardial catheter ablation to treat ventricular tachycardia. Pacing Clin Electrophysiol 25:1488-1495, 2002.

28. Miranda RC: Estudo dos efeitos das aplicações de radiofrequencia sobre as artérias coronárias, grandes artérias da base, esôfago e brônquio de suínos. Tese (doutorado), São Paulo, 1999.

29. d'Avila A, Dias R, Scanavacca M, Sosa E: Epicardial fat tissue does not modify amplitude and duration of the epicardial electrograms and/or ventricular stimulation threshold [abstract]. Eur J Cardiol 23:5, 2002.

30. d'Avila A, Houghtaling C, Gutierrez P, et al.: Catheter ablation of ventricular epicardial tissue: A comparison of standard and cooled-tip radiofrequency energy. Circulation 109:2363-2369, 2004.

31. d'Avila A, Holmvang G, Houghtaling C, et al.: Focal and linear endocardial and epicardial catheter-based cryoablation of normal and infarcted ventricular tissue. Heart Rhythms 1:1S, 2004.

32. d'Avila A, Scanavacca M, Sosa E, et al.: Pericardial anatomy for the interventional electrophysiologist. J Cardiovasc Electrophysiol 14;422-430, 2003.

33. Sosa E, Scanavacca M, D'Avila A, et al.: Nonsurgical transthoracic epicardial approach in patients with ventricular tachycardia and previous cardiac surgery. J Interv Card Electrophysiol 10:281-288, 2004.

34. Rumbak M, Chokshi SK, Abel N, et al.: Left phrenic nerve paresis complicating catheter radiofrequency ablation for Wolf-Parkinson-White syndrome. Am Heart J 132;1281-1285, 1996.

35. Durnate ME, Vecchio D, Ruggiero G: Right diaphragm paralysis following cardiac ablation for inappropriate sinus tachycardia. Pacing Clin Electrophysiol 26:783-784, 2003.

36. Lee BK, Choi KJ, Rhee KS, et al.: Right phrenic nerve injury following electrical disconnection of the right superior pulmonary vein. Pacing Clin Electrophysiol 27:1444-1446, 2004.

37. Berruezo A, Mont L, Nava S, et al.: Electrocardiographic recognition of the epicardial origin of ventricular tachycardias. Circulation 109:1842-1847, 2004.

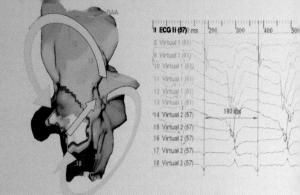

31

Ablation of Ventricular Tachycardia with Congenital Heart Disease

George F. Van Hare

Key Points

- The mechanism of ventricular tachycardia with congenital heart disease is macroreentry related to surgical scars.

- Diagnosis is based on inducibility and entrainment mapping.

- Ablation targets include specific isthmuses of ventricular myocardium related to surgical and anatomic lines of block.

- Electroanatomic mapping is helpful, and cooled radiofrequency ablation may be helpful.

- The success rate is approximately 64% acutely.

Ventricular tachycardia (VT) and its relationship to sudden death remain difficult management issues in patients who have previously undergone surgical repair of significant congenital heart defects. For the most part, the initial life-threatening hemodynamic problems in these patients have been successfully palliated or repaired by surgery, often years or decades previously. Although atrioventricular block has been implicated in the etiology of sudden death in a few patients, and atrial flutter with rapid conduction is certainly involved in the sudden death of those patients with extensive atrial surgery,[1,2] VT is an important contributor. Clinicians have observed the frequent occurrence of premature ventricular contractions and nonsustained and sustained ventricular arrhythmias in patients who have undergone complete repair of tetralogy of Fallot and related defects such as double-outlet right ventricle, and VT has been implicated in the etiology of sudden death in this patient group. Indeed, it has been reported that postoperative tetralogy of Fallot is the single most common condition in sudden death among children between the ages of 1 and 16 years,[3] although the risk of sudden death is also elevated in aortic stenosis, coarctation, and transposition.[4]

Pathophysiology

SUBSTRATE

By far the most information concerning patients with VT and congenital heart disease pertains to tetralogy of Fallot. Ventricular arrhythmias occur much more rarely in patients with other lesions.[5] However, for the purposes of management, tetralogy of Fallot can be viewed as a model for other lesions, when patients with other lesions present with ventricular arrhythmias in the setting of ventriculotomy and/or right ventricular dysfunction. Surgery and chronic pressure/volume overload in these patients lead to myocardial scarring and fibrosis that are common substrates for VT in congenital heart disease.

Controversy still exists regarding the role of various risk factors for the occurrence of ventricular arrhythmias and sudden death, the exact relationship between ventricular arrhythmias and sudden death, the role of electrophysiologic study and other procedures for risk stratification, and, ultimately, the appropriate management of postoperative VT. It is only recently that major advances in understanding of the roles of antiarrhythmic agents and implantable cardioverter defibrillators in patients with coronary disease have been made, through the conduction of large multicenter trials.[6] One can understand the much greater challenge of answering similar questions in this much smaller patient population. Indeed, as Bricker[7] pointed out, sufficient numbers of operated patients may not be available to perform an adequately powered cohort study to sort out the various likely predictors of sudden death.

PERTINENT ANATOMY

An extensive review of congenital heart disease anatomy and surgical techniques is beyond the scope of this chapter. However, one must consider the changes in surgical technique that have taken place over the years to understand how patient age, age at repair, and method of repair may interact to increase the risk of arrhythmias. The first complete repair of tetralogy of Fallot was performed in 1954 by Dr. W. C. Lillehei, and starting in the 1960s, complete repair became quite common. Although infants were operated on from the beginning, the mortality rate was high, and it was more common for patients to undergo repair later, often as late as the second or even third decade of life. Starting in the 1970s, due to improvements in both surgical technique and postoperative care, several centers chose to perform primary repair in infancy, with good results, and this is now the current practice at almost all centers.

Unoperated patients with tetralogy of Fallot have a ventricular septal defect with some degree, usually severe, of right ventricular outflow tract (RVOT) obstruction, leading to chronic cyanosis. The placement of a systemic-to-pulmonary artery shunt as a palliative procedure adds the element of potential left ventricular volume overload. Correction of the defect involves patch closure of the ventricular septal defect with relief of right ventricular obstruction. In almost all patients, this requires resection of a large amount of right ventricular muscle, and early in the experience, this was not done through the tricuspid valve but required a ventriculotomy. Finally, the pulmonary annulus is usually small, and repair with a transannular patch leads to chronic pulmonic insufficiency, which may be very severe if associated with downstream obstruction due to significant pulmonary arterial stenosis.

It has been hypothesized that ventricular arrhythmias are caused by the effect of years of chronic cyanosis, followed by the placement of a ventriculotomy, with elevation of right ventricular pressures due to inadequate relief of obstruction and severe pulmonic regurgitation with right ventricular dysfunction.[8-10] Such factors as wall stress and chronic cyanosis, coupled with the passage of time, may lead to myocardial fibrosis and result in the substrate for reentrant ventricular arrhythmias. This hypothesis is supported by histologic studies of the hearts of patients with tetralogy of Fallot who died suddenly, which have shown such extensive fibrosis.[11] It is also supported by the observation that fractionated electrograms and late potentials may be recorded from the right ventricle at electrophysiologic study, suggesting the presence of slow conduction.[12] Whereas there is a 5% incidence of coronary artery abnormalities in tetralogy of Fallot, putting the left anterior descending coronary artery or other large branches at risk at the time of complete repair, such potential damage has never been implicated in the etiology of ventricular arrhythmias or of sudden death.

MECHANISM

Careful electrophysiologic studies in patients with clinical VT after tetralogy surgery have supported the concept that the mechanism of tachycardia is macroreentry involving the RVOT, either at the site of anterior right ventriculotomy or at the site of a ventricular septal defect patch. Transient entrainment can often be documented, with constant fusion at the paced cycle length and progressive fusion at decreasing cycle lengths, and the evaluation of postpacing intervals strongly suggests that sites in the RVOT are part of a macroreentrant circuit (Fig. 31–1).

Anatomically, one may imagine several long circuits that might support macroreentry based on congenital and surgical anatomy, and there have been several circuits described in patients with tetralogy of Fallot after surgery. Whereas the simplest notion is a circuit that rotates around an RVOT patch, this is possible only if the patch does not extend all the way to the pulmonic annulus, as a transannular patch would. The best delineated putative circuit was described by Horton et al.,[14] who used pacing techniques to document the importance of the right ventricular isthmus between the tricuspid annulus and the RVOT patch. Notably, they did not map the entire circuit in their two patients, and so the rest of the circuit is unknown. Their patients both had transannular patches, so there was no possible isthmus between the RVOT patch and the pulmonic annulus. Presumably, the circuit also involved the interventricular septum. Others, notably Downar et al.,[13] have mapped VT intraoperatively and have found reentry involving the RVOT in all patients, but they only identified sites of earliest ventricular activation, rather than the entire circuit. They noted early sites located in the septum, free wall, and parietal band.

Diagnostic Criteria

SURFACE ELECTROCARDIOGRAM

The criteria for the diagnosis of VT are the same as for other forms of macroreentrant tachycardia (Table 31–1). There is a wide-complex tachycardia, often with atrioventricular dissociation. Despite the fact that most patients with tetralogy of Fallot have macroreentry arising from the RVOT, the QRS morphology is often not indicative of this location. As described by Horton et al.,[14] QRS morphology of VT

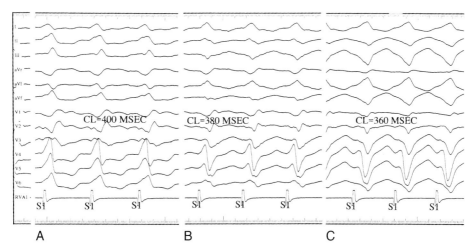

FIGURE 31–1. Tracings at electrophysiologic study of a 35-year-old man who was status post repair of tetralogy of Fallot at 11 years of age. Ventricular tachycardia was induced by ventricular extrastimulation, with a tachycardia cycle length of 435 milliseconds. Entrainment pacing is performed at (**A**) 400 milliseconds, (**B**) 380 milliseconds, and (**C**) 360 milliseconds. Note that there is progressive fusion at faster paced cycle lengths. CL, cycle length; MSEC, milliseconds.

TABLE 31-1
Keys to Diagnosis
Document ventricular macroreentry via entrainment (see Chapter 27)
Identify surgical and anatomic lines of block

arising from the RVOT mainly depends on the direction of rotation (clockwise versus counterclockwise) around the circuit, which involves the isthmus of tissue in the right ventricle between the tricuspid annulus and the RVOT patch (Fig. 31–2). They described a clockwise rotation giving rise to a negative QRS in lead I and biphasic QRS in V_1, whereas a counterclockwise rotation produces upright R waves in lead I and an entirely negative QRS ("left bundle morphology") in V_1.

INTRACARDIAC ELECTROGRAMS

As far as is known , there are no specific intracardiac electrogram features in patients with congenital heart disease. Low-amplitude and fractionated late potentials have been described, but it is uncertain whether these electrograms are involved in the substrate for VT. Still, Biblo and Carlson[15] used such mid-diastolic potentials to successfully ablate VT in a patient with tetralogy of Fallot in 1993. In addition, Stevenson et al.,[16] as well as Rostock et al.,[17] emphasized the usefulness of voltage maps for delineating the tachycardia circuit in such patients (see later discussion), and such maps depend on the presence of low-amplitude signals in association with myocardial scarring or patch material as barriers that support macroreentry.

DIAGNOSTIC MANEUVERS

The principal diagnostic maneuver that is useful in such cases is entrainment mapping, to prove the macroreentrant nature of the tachycardia. Entrainment, of course, depends on the presence of an excitable gap, which might not exist in tachycardias that are very rapid. Such rapid tachycardias may not be tolerated hemodynamically. Furthermore, in one form of concealed entrainment, pacing close to the exit site from a zone of slow conduction does not allow one to satisfy any of the criteria for entrainment. This problem occurs, despite the existence of a macroreentrant tachycardia, because of the lack of surface electrocardiogram fusion, as was pointed out by Waldo and Henthorn.[18] Therefore, the inability to demonstrate manifest entrainment does not rule out a macroreentrant mechanism.

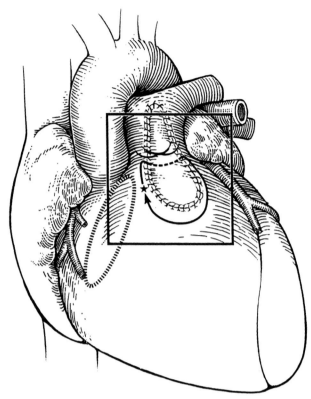

FIGURE 31–2. Right ventricle and right ventricular outflow tract with transannular patch across outflow tract and pulmonic valve. The location of the tricuspid valve annulus is shown with hatched markings. The proposed macroreentrant circuit (**inset**) for ventricular tachycardia involves clockwise or counterclockwise activation between the patch and tricuspid annulus. The *arrow* demonstrates a hypothetical pathway for the remainder of the circuit. *(From Horton RP, Canby RC, Kessler DJ, et al.: Ablation of ventricular tachycardia associated with tetralogy of Fallot: Demonstration of bidirectional block. J Cardiovasc Electrophysiol 8:432-435, 1997, with permission.)*

Mapping and Ablation

STRATEGIES FOR BASIC MAPPING

Because most evidence supports the concept of macroreentry as the mechanism of such well-tolerated VT, the use of entrainment pacing and mapping techniques is desirable (Table 31–2). Several investigators have reported successful procedures using radiofrequency energy.[14,19,20] Stevenson et al.,[16] in particular reported the utility of voltage maps to identify areas of scar in the right ventricle.

Although well-tolerated VT can be mapped in the electrophysiology laboratory, many patients have ventricular dysfunction and/or rapid VT rates and will not tolerate this. Several investigators have reported intraoperative mapping and ablation.[13,21-23] In particular, Downar et al.[13] used intraoperative

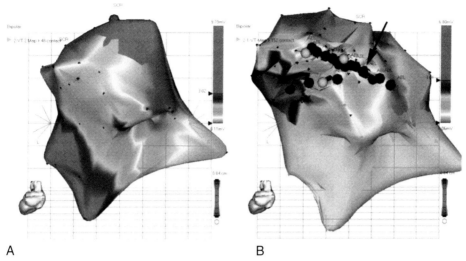

FIGURE 31-3. A, CARTO voltage map during sinus rhythm in a modified posterior anterior view showing an area of low amplitude signals at the posterior wall of the right ventricular outflow tract confined to the presumed insertion of the homograft. **B,** CARTO voltage map during ventricular tachycardia focused on the previously identified area of interest. A y-shaped ablation line was produced crossing the border zone between the presumed scar region and normal amplitude myocardium. Target sites demonstrating perfect entrainment mapping are depicted by *white spots*. *(From Rostock T, Willems S, Ventura R, et al.: Radiofrequency catheter ablation of a macroreentrant ventricular tachycardia late after surgical repair of tetralogy of Fallot using the electroanatomic mapping [CARTO]. Pacing Clin Electrophysiol 27:801-804, 2004, with permission.)*

TABLE 31-2
Targets for Ablation
Sites of early ventricular activation
Sites of concealed entrainment
Anatomic isthmuses between surgical and structural lines of block

mapping of the RVOT in the beating heart, employing an endocardial electrode balloon and a simultaneous epicardial electrode shock array. Ablation was carried out by cryotherapy lesions during normothermic cardiopulmonary bypass with the heart beating, or during anoxic arrest, with good success in three patients.

USE OF SPECIALIZED MAPPING SYSTEMS

Electroanatomic mapping of the arrhythmia circuit may be feasible if the tachycardia is inducible and is slow enough to be mapped completely. The CARTO system (Biosense Webster, Baldwin Park, Calif.) allows the construction of isochronal and propagation maps. As with other arrhythmias, the process of construction of an electroanatomic map may be time-consuming and difficult. An additional available modality provided by the CARTO system is the ability to construct three-dimensional voltage maps to better identify the anatomic barriers. For example,

Stevenson et al.[16] demonstrated the use of these modalities in the successful mapping and ablation of right ventricular reentrant tachycardia in an adult patient after repair of tetralogy of Fallot. They pointed out the usefulness of tagged ablation sites in constructing a broad line of block between the ventriculotomy scar and the tricuspid annulus. Subsequently, Rostock et al.[17] reported a procedure in a 36-year-old patient after surgical repair of tetralogy by use of a homograft conduit, using similar mapping methods. They used a combination of entrainment mapping and voltage maps constructed in sinus rhythm, using the CARTO system (Fig. 31-3). They defined an area of scar by the recording of electrogram amplitudes of less than 0.5 mV, and created a Y-shaped incision blocking conduction of impulses between the RVOT and the homograft.

TARGETS FOR ABLATION

Appropriate targets for ablation may be determined by relatively simple means, such as sites of early ventricular activation that precede surface QRS during tachycardia. Given the macroreentrant nature of these rhythms, however, it makes sense to consider the entire circuit and to focus on sites that are found to be in the circuit by entrainment mapping techniques, and where barriers can be connected by a series of lesions with the effect of bridging the isthmus and creating bidirectional block. These techniques, of course, are well developed in the ablation of typical atrial flutter, as well as in the ablation of postsurgical intra-atrial reentrant tachycardia. One of the best demonstrations of these concepts was the report by Horton et al.[14] in which two patients were found to have VT involving the isthmus between the RVOT patch and the tricuspid annulus (see Fig. 31–1). The important contribution made by this case report was the demonstration of a clear method for documenting isthmus block in both clockwise and counterclockwise directions. This capability provides a better criterion for ablation success than simple noninducibility. Horton et al.[14] demonstrated that the creation of a line of block between the tricuspid annulus and RVOT patch is associated with a characteristic alteration in the paced QRS morphology, as well as a clear change in the order of ventricular activation with pacing from specific sites (Figs. 31–4 and 31–5). Although it is not clear how many patients might be candidates for this approach due to anatomic variations, it does hold the promise of allowing ablation procedures, most of which can be performed without needing to map or ablate during VT.

ALTERNATE ENERGY SOURCES

There are, to date, no reports of the use of alternative energy sources in ablation of VT in patients with congenital heart disease. Both modalities, however, offer specific potential advantages in particular patients and clinical scenarios. First, the potential for irrigated-tip or cooled-tip radiofrequency ablation to penetrate the myocardium more deeply is clearly a potential advantage when working in the right ventricle, which may well be thick due to the chronic pressure overload and pulmonic insufficiency that often exist in such patients. Second, as Morwood et

al.[24] noted, occasionally the tachycardia circuit involves regions remarkably close to the site where the His bundle potential is recorded. In such a situation, one might imagine the utility of cryoablation, in which "ice mapping" of lesions is possible, to avoid inadvertent complete atrioventricular block.

SUCCESS AND RECURRENCE RATES

Most reports of ablation of VT in patients with congenital heart disease are single-center reports that involve one or two procedures. A listing of reported ablations in patients with tetralogy of Fallot or other congenital heart disease is found in Table 31–3. This includes one case, in 1986, in which DC ablation was attempted, as well as a number of other cases in which radiofrequency energy was used. Most procedures are reported as successful. The total success rate derived from these reports, 93%, should be treated with a great deal of caution, however. Centers that succeed in ablating this substrate are clearly more likely to report their results than are centers that have failed, and such "reporting bias" has the potential to skew the impression of expected results.

Somewhat more useful are reports of multiple cases from a single center, in which a large time frame is used and patients are included consecutively. Morwood et al.[24] recently reported the experience at the Children's Hospital in Boston with ablation for VT in young patients. They reported that, of 97 consecutive ablation procedures for VT over 13 years, 20 were in patients with congenital heart disease. In 8 of these patients, mapping and/or ablation was not considered to be feasible due to tachycardia noninducibility, tachycardia rate, hemodynamic instability,

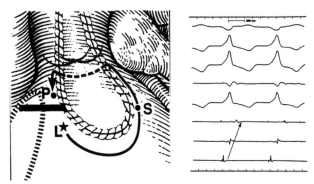

FIGURE 31–4. Location of the radiofrequency catheter ablation lesion (*solid line*), extending from the patch to the tricuspid valve annulus. This linear lesion results in bidirectional block and cure of the tachycardia. When pacing from the lateral (L) margin of the patch, there is clockwise block; activation moves counterclockwise around the patch to the septal (S) margin and finally to the pulmonic (P) margin. The surface electrograms (leads I, II, III, V1 and V6) and local electrograms are shown.

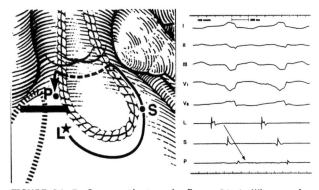

FIGURE 31–5. Same patient as in figure 31–4. When pacing from the pulmonic (P) margin on the other side of the lesion, there is counterclockwise block; activation proceeds in a clockwise direction to the septal (S) and the lateral (L) margins. Local electrograms demonstrate this sequence of activation (*straight arrows*). The bidirectional block is in distinction from the normal bidirectional conduction and clockwise ventricular tachycardia seen prior to ablation.

TABLE 31-3

Ablation in Patients with Tetralogy of Fallot or Other Congenital Heart Disease

Authors, Year (Ref. No.)	Method	No. of Procedures	No. Successful
Oda et al., 1986 (28)	DC	1	1
Burton et al., 1993 (29)	RF	2	2
Goldner et al., 1994 (30)	RF	1	1
Biblo and Carlson, 1994 (15)	RF	1	1
Chinushi et al., 1995 (31)	RF	1	1
Gonska et al., 1996 (19)	RF	16	15
Horton et al., 1997 (14)	RF	2	2
Papagiannis et al., 1998 (20)	RF	1	1
Stevenson et al., 1998 (16)	RF/CARTO	1	1
Saul and Alexander, 1999 (32)	RF	2	2
Fukuhara et al., 2000 (33)	RF	1	1
Arenal et al., 2003 (34)	RF/CARTO	1	1
Rojel et al., 2003 (35)	RF	2	2
Morwood et al., 2004 (24)	RF	12	10
Rostock et al., 2004 (17)	RF/CARTO	1	1
Total reported procedures		45	42 (93%)

CARTO, CARTO electroanatomic mapping system (Biosense Webster, Baldwin Park, Calif.); DC, direct current; RF, radiofrequency ablation.

or location close to the His bundle. Ablation was attempted in the other 12 patients, with acute success in 10 (80%). Four of these 10 patients (40%) had experienced recurrence at last follow-up.

Another source for data concerning ablations in the pediatric population is the ongoing Pediatric Radiofrequency Ablation Registry. Since 1991, pedi-

atric electrophysiologists at almost 50 centers have periodically reported their acute results to the registry.[25-27] A recent analysis of data from both the early and the late registry experience found a total of 74 procedures in patients with congenital heart disease for whom ablation of VT was attempted (D.L. Fairbrother et al., unpublished data). Of the VTs in these patients, 50/74 (68%) were mapped to a morphologically right ventricle, and 24/74 (32%) were mapped to a left ventricle. The initial success rate for these ablation attempts was only 47/74, or 64%. These multicenter data highlight the difficulties in arriving at benchmarks for ablation success when one relies on single-center reports involving very few patients.

Complications

In general, complications of radiofrequency ablation for VT are rarely reported. Overall complication rates in this population have been estimated to be approximately 3%.[24,25,27] Specific reported complications are similar to those reported for other types of ablation, including hematomas and second-degree atrioventricular block.

Troubleshooting the Difficult Case

Because ablation of VT is only rarely attempted and so little is known about the substrate and the best methods for ablation, in truth all such cases can be thought of as difficult cases. That is, there is not really any case that would qualify as a "routine" case. Therefore, it is difficult to provide any additional advice concerning the approach to a "difficult" case than what has already been provided (Table 31–4). Perhaps the only thing to say is that each case of VT in a patient with congenital heart disease should be approached in a comprehensive fashion. One must start with a detailed knowledge of the congenital heart anatomy and perform a careful review of the details of the surgical repair that was performed, using the dictated operative report if possible. All imaging studies available should be reviewed, such as echocardiogram and angiogram, because they may provide more information concerning the underlying anatomy. In the laboratory, if sustained VT is inducible and is sufficiently well tolerated, entrainment should be performed in an attempt to make a

TABLE 31-4

Troubleshooting the Difficult Case

Problem	Causes	Solutions
Complex cardiovascular anatomy	Congenital heart disease and previous surgery	Thorough review of records and imaging studies
Hemodynamically unstable ventricular tachycardia	Rapid rate	Slow with antiarrhythmic drugs Pace mapping Noncontact mapping
Unable to terminate with ablation	Dense scar Broad channel	Cooled radiofrequency ablation Create linear lesions

diagnosis of a macroreentrant tachycardia. Should the tachycardia be stable, entrainment mapping can be performed, searching for sites at which the post-pacing interval is equivalent to the tachycardia cycle length, indicating that the site is in the macroreentrant circuit. In any case, electroanatomic mapping is an important adjunct, particularly with the use of voltage mapping to identify the scars and other important anatomic details. Lesions may be planned to connect surgical scars and/or anatomic barriers. It seems important that a complete line of block should be created, and the method of Horton et al.[14] is attractive. Alternatively, one might consider documentation of the line of block by the use of repeat electroanatomic mapping.

In the final analysis, as discussed earlier, it is by no means certain that successful ablation of a VT circuit in a patient with congenital heart disease will in any way decrease or eliminate the risk of sudden death, so many patients will be appropriate candidates for implantation of implantable cardioverter defibrillators, most prominently those with strong risk factors for sudden death such as severe right ventricular dilation and dysfunction, or pulmonic insufficiency.

References

1. Harrison DA, Siu SC, Hussain F, et al.: Sustained atrial arrhythmias in adults late after repair of tetralogy of Fallot. Am J Cardiol 87:584-588, 2001.
2. Li W, Somerville J: Atrial flutter in grown-up congenital heart (GUCH) patients: Clinical characteristics of affected population. Int J Cardiol 75:129-137; discussion 138-139, 2000.
3. Garson A Jr, McNamara DG: Sudden death in a pediatric cardiology population, 1958 to 1983: Relation to prior arrhythmias. J Am Coll Cardiol 5:134B-137B, 1985.
4. Silka MJ, Hardy BG, Menashe VD, Morris CD: A population-based prospective evaluation of risk of sudden cardiac death after operation for common congenital heart defects. J Am Coll Cardiol 32:245-251, 1998.
5. Vetter VL, Horowitz LN: Electrophysiologic residua and sequelae of surgery for congenital heart defects. Am J Cardiol 50:588-604, 1982.
6. The Antiarrhythmics versus Implantable Defibrillators (AVID) Investigators. A comparison of antiarrhythmic-drug therapy with implantable defibrillators in patients resuscitated from near-fatal ventricular arrhythmias. N Engl J Med 337:1576-1583, 1997.
7. Bricker JT: Sudden death and tetralogy of Fallot: Risks, markers, and causes. Circulation 92:158-159, 1995.
8. Zahka KG, Horneffer PJ, Rowe SA, et al.: Long-term valvular function after total repair of tetralogy of Fallot: Relation to ventricular arrhythmias. Circulation 78:III14-III19, 1988.
9. Gatzoulis MA, Till JA, Somerville J, Redington AN: Mechano-electrical interaction in tetralogy of Fallot: QRS prolongation relates to right ventricular size and predicts malignant ventricular arrhythmias and sudden death. Circulation 92:231-237, 1995.
10. Gatzoulis MA, Till JA, Redington AN: Depolarization-repolarization inhomogeneity after repair of tetralogy of Fallot: The substrate for malignant ventricular tachycardia? Circulation 95:401-404, 1997.
11. Deanfield JE, Ho SY, Anderson RH, et al.: Late sudden death after repair of tetralogy of Fallot: A clinicopathologic study. Circulation 67:626-631, 1983.
12. Zimmermann M, Friedli B, Adamec R, Oberhansli I: Ventricular late potentials and induced ventricular arrhythmias after surgical repair of tetralogy of Fallot. Am J Cardiol 67:873-878, 1991.
13. Downar E, Harris L, Kimber S, et al.: Ventricular tachycardia after surgical repair of tetralogy of Fallot: Results of intraoperative mapping studies. J Am Coll Cardiol 20:648-655, 1992.
14. Horton RP, Canby RC, Kessler DJ, et al.: Ablation of ventricular tachycardia associated with tetralogy of Fallot: Demonstration of bidirectional block. J Cardiovasc Electrophysiol 8:432-435, 1997.
15. Biblo LA, Carlson MD: Transcatheter radiofrequency ablation of ventricular tachycardia following surgical correction of tetralogy of Fallot. Pacing Clin Electrophysiol 17:1556-1560, 1994.
16. Stevenson WG, Delacretaz E, Friedman PL, Ellison KE: Identification and ablation of macroreentrant ventricular tachycardia with the CARTO electroanatomical mapping system. Pacing Clin Electrophysiol 21:1448-1456, 1998.
17. Rostock T, Willems S, Ventura R, et al.: Radiofrequency catheter ablation of a macroreentrant ventricular tachycardia late after surgical repair of tetralogy of Fallot using the electroanatomic mapping (CARTO). Pacing Clin Electrophysiol 27:801-804, 2004.
18. Waldo AL, Henthorn RW: Use of transient entrainment during ventricular tachycardia to localize a critical area in the reentry

circuit for ablation. Pacing Clin Electrophysiol 12:231-244, 1989.

19. Gonska BD, Cao K, Raab J, et al.: Radiofrequency catheter ablation of right ventricular tachycardia late after repair of congenital heart defects. Circulation 94:1902-1908, 1996.

20. Papagiannis J, Kanter RJ, Wharton JM: Radiofrequency catheter ablation of multiple haemodynamically unstable ventricular tachycardias in a patient with surgically repaired tetralogy of Fallot. Cardiol Young 8:379-382, 1998.

21. Ressia L, Graffigna A, Salerno-Uriarte JA, Vigano M: The complex origin of ventricular tachycardia after the total correction of tetralogy of Fallot. G Ital Cardiol 23:905-910, 1993.

22. Frank G, Schmid C, Baumgart D, et al.: Surgical therapy of life-threatening tachycardic cardiac arrhythmias in children. Monatsschrift Kinderheilkunde 137:269-274, 1989.

23. Lawrie GM, Pacifico A, Kaushik R: Results of direct surgical ablation of ventricular tachycardia not due to ischemic heart disease. Ann Surg 209:716-727, 1989.

24. Morwood JG, Triedman JK, Berul CI, et al.: Radiofrequency catheter ablation of ventricular tachycardia in children and young adults with congenital heart disease. Heart Rhythm 1:301-308, 2004.

25. Kugler JD, Danford DA, Deal BJ, et al.: Radiofrequency catheter ablation for tachyarrhythmias in children and adolescents. The Pediatric Electrophysiology Society. N Engl J Med 330:1481-1487, 1994.

26. Van Hare GF, Carmelli D, Smith WM, et al.: Prospective assessment after pediatric cardiac ablation: Design and implementation of the multicenter study. Pacing Clin Electrophysiol 25:332-341, 2002.

27. Van Hare GF, Javitz H, Carmelli D, et al.: Prospective assessment after pediatric cardiac ablation: Demographics, medical profiles, and initial outcomes. J Cardiovasc Electrophysiol 15:759-770, 2004.

28. Oda H, Aizawa Y, Murata M, et al.: A successful electrical ablation of recurrent sustained ventricular tachycardia in a postoperative case of tetralogy of Fallot. Jpn Heart J 27:421-428, 1986.

29. Burton ME, Leon AR: Radiofrequency catheter ablation of right ventricular outflow tract tachycardia late after complete repair of tetralogy of Fallot using the pace mapping technique. Pacing Clin Electrophysiol 16:2319-2325, 1993.

30. Goldner BG, Cooper R, Blau W, Cohen TJ: Radiofrequency catheter ablation as a primary therapy for treatment of ventricular tachycardia in a patient after repair of tetralogy of Fallot. Pacing Clin Electrophysiol 17:1441-1446, 1994.

31. Chinushi M, Aizawa Y, Kitazawa H, et al.: Successful radiofrequency catheter ablation for macroreentrant ventricular tachycardias in a patient with tetralogy of Fallot after corrective surgery. Pacing Clin Electrophysiol 18:1713-1716, 1995.

32. Saul JP, Alexander ME: Preventing sudden death after repair of tetralogy of Fallot: Complex therapy for complex patients. J Cardiovasc Electrophysiol 10:1271-1287, 1999.

33. Fukuhara H, Nakamura Y, Tasato H, et al.: Successful radiofrequency catheter ablation of left ventricular tachycardia following surgical correction of tetralogy of Fallot. Pacing Clin Electrophysiol 23:1442-1445, 2000.

34. Arenal A, Glez-Torrecilla E, Ortiz M, et al.: Ablation of electrograms with an isolated, delayed component as treatment of unmappable monomorphic ventricular tachycardias in patients with structural heart disease. J Am Coll Cardiol 41:81-92, 2003.

35. Rojel U, Cuesta A, Mont L, Brugada J: Radiofrequency ablation of late ventricular tachycardia in patients with corrected Tetralogy of Fallot. Arch Cardiol Mex 73:275-279, 2003.

Miscellaneous Topics

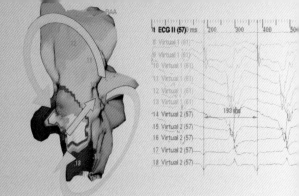

PART VIII

32

Complications Associated with Radiofrequency Catheter Ablation of Cardiac Arrhythmias

Tayseer Chowdhry • *Hugh Calkins*

Key Points

- Complications may result from any aspect of the diagnostic electrophysiologic study and ablation procedure.

- The risk of stroke is highest during catheter ablation of atrial fibrillation (AF).

- The risks of radiation exposure are cumulative and usually occur days to weeks after an ablation procedure. Children are at greatest risk of radiation injury.

- The precise types of risk and incidence of risk vary greatly depending on the ablation target. Catheter ablation of AF and of nonidiopathic VT is associated with the greatest risk.

- Because catheter ablation procedures are typically used for patients without life-threatening conditions, it is particularly important to make every effort to minimize risk.

For most cardiac arrhythmias, medical therapy with antiarrhythmic drugs is not completely effective. In addition to poor or sporadic efficacy, such drugs can be associated with a number of bothersome side effects, proarrhythmia, cost, and inconvenience. It is for this reason that nonpharmacologic interventions, initially using a surgical approach and more recently with catheter ablation, have played an increasingly important role in the management of cardiac arrhythmias.

Over the past two decades, radiofrequency (RF) catheter ablation has evolved from a highly experimental technique to first-line therapy for many cardiac arrhythmias. During the 4-year period from 1989 through 1992, the number of patients undergoing catheter ablation procedures in the United States increased more than 30-fold, from an estimated 450 procedures in 1989 to 15,000 procedures in 1993.[1] A great deal of information has been published that has focused on the acute and long-term efficacy of RF catheter ablation procedures. Perhaps of equal importance in determining the ultimate clinical role of a particular procedure are the type and incidence of complications. The purpose of this chapter is to provide an update regarding current understanding of the risks and complications that can occur during catheter ablation procedures. Particular attention is focused on defining the risks associated with catheter ablation of atrial fibrillation (AF) and identifying those techniques that may reduce the incidence of complications.

for a particular arrhythmia, data are presented from the largest and most recent single-center clinical studies. The results of four multicenter surveys of patients who underwent catheter ablation have been published.[1-4] The 1995 North American Society of Pacing and Electrophysiology (NASPE) survey retrospectively reviewed the results of approximately 37,000 catheter ablation procedures performed in 157 U. S. centers between 1989 and 1993.[1] The Multicenter European Radiofrequency Survey (MERFS) focused on complications related to catheter ablation, surveying the ablation results at 68 European institutions between 1987 and 1992.[2] The 1998 NASPE Registry prospectively enrolled 3357 patients who underwent catheter ablation procedures at 68 institutions in the United States.[3] The 2001 Spanish Registry on Catheter Ablation reviewed the results of 4374 catheter ablation procedures in 41 centers.[4] The 2002 Spanish Registry on Catheter Ablation reviewed the results of 4970 catheter ablation procedures in 4755 patients at 42 centers.[5] In addition, two prospective multicenter clinical trials focusing on the efficacy and safety of RF catheter ablation of accessory pathways (APs), atrioventricular nodal reentrant tachycardia (AVNRT), and the atrioventricular (AV) junction, as well as ventricular tachycardia (VT), have been published.[6,7] There have also been two multicenter studies on catheter ablation of atrial flutter.[8,9] This review pays particular attention to these seven studies. We have also included data from several of the largest trials of catheter ablation of AF.

Prior Studies of Complications during Catheter Ablation Procedures

Information concerning the type and incidence of complications during catheter ablation procedures can be derived from single-center experiences, registry data, and prospective multicenter clinical studies. Among these various sources, data obtained as part of a prospective multicenter clinical trial is generally the most relevant to clinical practice. Registry data is also a very useful source of complication data. In contrast, information derived from a single center may be unique to that center and therefore is less likely to reflect the types and incidence of anticipated complications when RF catheter ablation is applied on a widespread basis. For this reason, the data presented in this review have been obtained primarily from multicenter experiences and from registry information. If this type of data is unavailable

Types and Classification of Complications

There are a large number of potential complications that may occur during or after a catheter ablation procedure. These complications may be subdivided into major and minor complications. Major complications are defined as those that result in permanent injury or death, require an intervention for treatment, or prolong the duration of hospitalization. All other complications are generally referred to as minor complications.

The complications that occur during RF catheter ablation procedures can result from any aspect of the procedure, including (1) placement of a peripheral intravenous catheter, (2) conscious sedation and/or anesthesia, (3) radiation exposure resulting from fluoroscopy, (4) obtaining vascular access, (5) intravascular and intracardiac catheter manipulation, (6) cardioversion, and (7) delivery of RF energy.

Intravascular and intracardiac catheter manipulation can lead to several possible complications, including cardiac tamponade, vessel perforation, aortic dissection, traumatic valve damage, coronary artery dissection, and thromboembolism. Complications that may be directly associated with delivery of RF energy include inadvertent AV block, coronary artery spasm or occlusion, thromboembolism, or myocardial perforation. It is notable that the great majority of complications that occur during catheter ablation procedures are not directly attributable to the delivery of RF energy.

Thromboembolism and Catheter Ablation

Other than death, perhaps one of the most feared complications that may result from catheter ablation procedures is the development of a stroke. Recent studies that have evaluated thrombin-antithrombin III and D-dimer levels before and during electrophysiology testing and catheter ablation have provided evidence that sheath placement and placement of catheters result in a prothrombotic state.[10] Despite this, the risk of stroke associated with catheter ablation procedures for most arrhythmias has been small. Perhaps the most notable exception is catheter ablation of AF. The stroke risks associated with catheter ablation of AF are discussed later in this chapter. Zhou et al.[11] recently reviewed the published literature on thromboembolic complications of catheter ablation and found that the overall incidence was 0.6%.

The 1995 NASPE survey reported 8 (0.15%) cerebrovascular accidents (CVAs) among 5427 patients who underwent catheter ablation of APs, 2 (0.10%) CVAs among 2084 patients who underwent catheter ablation of the AV junction (both used a left-sided approach), no CVAs among 5423 patients who underwent ablation of AVNRT, and 3 systemic emboli (0.36%) among 844 patients who underwent catheter ablation of non-idiopathic VT.[1] In MERFS, Hindricks reported thromboembolic complications in 33 (0.8%) of 4398 patients, including cerebral embolism (0.4%), pulmonary embolism (0.2%), arterial thrombosis (0.5%), and peripheral arterial embolism (0.06%).[2,11] A more recent registry reported a lower incidence of thromboembolic complications, with only 1 CVA among the 3357 ablation procedures that were reported in the 1998 NASPE survey.[3] In the 2002 Spanish Registry on Catheter Ablation, Alvarez Lopez et al.[5] reported 1 case of pulmonary embolism

(0.07%) resulting in 1 death among 4755 patients. This lower incidence of thromboembolic complications may reflect, at least in part, the greater use of closed-loop temperature control, which has been shown to decrease the incidence of coagulum formation, from 2.2% with power control alone to 0.8% of RF applications with temperature control ($P < .01$).[12] However, systemic embolism can occur without temperature rise or coagulum formation.[13]

The risk of stroke associated with catheter ablation of AF is far greater than the risk with other types of catheter ablation procedures. The risk of stroke associated with catheter ablation of AF ranges from 0.0% to 6.0%.[14-18] For example, Vasamreddy et al.[15] reported 2 strokes among 70 patients who underwent AF ablation using a circumferential approach. A major focus of electrophysiologists today is to reduce this risk of stroke. A number of different approaches are used, including careful attention to anticoagulation before and after the ablation procedure. Transesophageal echocardiography (TEE) is commonly performed for patients who are in AF at the time of the ablation procedure. During AF ablation procedures, heparin is administered to maintain the activated clotting time (ACT) greater than 300 seconds.

Radiation Exposure

Although electrophysiologists are aware of the acute risks associated with catheter ablation procedures, the long-term risks that result from radiation exposure received by patients and electrophysiologists are less well recognized. There have been several case reports of serious x-ray–induced skin injuries during fluoroscopy-guided interventional procedures.[19] Because radiation can be neither felt nor seen and its detrimental effects may not appear until decades later, these hidden risks of catheter ablation are easily ignored. As the number, complexity, and duration of catheter ablation procedures increase, the radiation-related risks of these procedures increase in importance.

Several studies have evaluated fluoroscopy time during catheter ablation procedures. Calkins et al.[20] reported a fluoroscopy time of 44 ± 40 minutes during catheter ablation of APs; Lindsay et al.[21] reported a fluoroscopy time of 50 ± 31 minutes during catheter ablation of AVNRT or APs; Park et al.[22] reported a fluoroscopy time of 47 ± 31 minutes during catheter ablation of a wide variety of ablation targets; and Macle et al.[23] reported a fluoroscopy time of 57 ± 30 minutes for paroxysmal AF, 20 ± 10 minutes for common atrial flutter, and 22 ± 21 minutes for APs.

Fluoroscopy uses x-radiation generated with kilovoltages typically between 65 and 100 kVp to image the heart and guide catheter placement. These x-rays have low penetrating power; as a result, the maximum dose of radiation is delivered at the skin surface. To date, a number of studies have evaluated the radiation exposure received by patients during catheter ablation procedures. Despite differences in the techniques used to estimate patient radiation exposure, the estimates in these studies are remarkably consistent.[20-24] In the study by Calkins et al.,[20] the sites receiving the largest amount of radiation was the ninth thoracic vertebral body posteriorly, with a median exposure of 7.26 rem. The mean entrance radiation dose received by the skin on the back in another trial was 1.3 ± 1.3 Sv. The threshold dose of radiation needed to cause the earliest sign of radiation injury (2 Sv) was exceeded by 19% of patients.[24] The absence of any clinical reports of skin erythema by patients in these studies may reflect a lack of awareness of this complication and the absence of formal follow-up to ascertain the effects of radiation, which may not appear for 2 to 3 weeks,[25] or the fact that the estimates of radiation exposure in these studies represent an upper limit of radiation dose. Children receive less radiation exposure than adults, and women receive less than men. Patients undergoing successful ablation procedures receive less radiation exposure than those in whom catheter ablation fails, and patients undergoing ablation of APs receive more radiation than those undergoing ablation of AVNRT or the AV junction.[24] The mean peak skin dose received by patients undergoing AF ablation was more than threefold greater than that received by patients undergoing catheter ablation of atrial flutter or AVNRT.[26] The amount of radiation received by patients during an RF catheter ablation procedure is greater than the amount previously reported during diagnostic catheterization procedures but similar to prior reports of radiation exposure during percutaneous transluminal coronary angioplasty (PTCA) procedures.

The risk of a fatal malignancy resulting from the radiation received during catheter ablation procedures has been estimated to be approximately 1 per thousand patients per hour of fluoroscopy.[20,24] The significance of this risk must be considered in terms of the baseline 20% lifetime risk of a fatal malignancy in the general population. Because the risk of a fatal malignancy resulting from radiation exposure is age dependent, being greater in children than in adults, the risk for a child younger than 14 years of age is approximately twice that of a 35-year-old patient. The risk of a genetic disorder resulting from 1 hour of fluoroscopy was estimated to be 5 per 1 million live births for men and 20 per 1 million live births for women.[20] The risk of cancer development must be considered whenever radiation is applied. This is of particular concern after procedures such as catheter ablation of AF that require prolonged fluoroscopy times. The organs that contribute most to the total risk are the lungs, stomach, and active bone marrow, as well as breast tissue in females. Despite the prolonged fluoroscopy durations, the risk of fatal malignancy resulting from catheter ablation of AF, and by extrapolation from all other catheter ablations, is low.

Another risk of catheter ablation procedures is the risk of radiation exposure to the operator. The amount of radiation received by catheter operators during RF catheter ablation procedures is small and well below the occupational radiation exposure limits, which have been established by the National Council of Radiation Protection (NCRP).[20,27] The dose limit for whole body irradiation is based on the tolerable risk to an individual of stochastic effects. Dose limits for extremities and for the lens of the eye are based on the dose thresholds at which deterministic effects occur after prolonged exposure. Of particular concern is radiation exposure to the lens of the eye. Several cases of ophthalmologically confirmed lens injuries caused by occupational exposure to radiation during interventional radiologic procedures have been reported. The doses to the eye ranged from 450 to 900 mSv per year, which exceeds the threshold for lens opacities.[28] The mean equivalent doses to the cardiologists' left hand and forehead were 0.24 mSv and 0.05 mSv, respectively, per RF ablation procedure. The effective dose to the cardiologists was less than 0.15 mSv per month.[29]

Because of long fluoroscopy times, radiation exposure is a major concern during catheter ablation of AF. Lickfett et al.[26] recently compared fluoroscopy times and radiation exposure during catheter ablation of AF, atrial flutter, and AVNRT. Their study included 15 patients with AF, 5 with atrial flutter, and 5 with AVNRT who underwent a fluoroscopic-guided procedure on a biplane x-ray system operated at a low frame pulsed fluoroscopy rate (7.5 fps). Radiation exposure was measured directly with 50 to 60 thermoluminescent dosimeters (TLDs). The positions of TLDs within the radiation field were verified by the exposure of direct film. Peak skin doses, effective radiation doses, and risk of fatal malignancies were all computed. Mean fluoroscopy durations for AF procedures were 67.8 ± 21 minutes in the right anterior oblique (RAO) view and 61.9 ± 16.6 minutes in the left anterior oblique (LAO) projection, significantly different from the durations required for atrial flutter or AVNRT. The mean peak skin doses measured with the TLDs were 1.0 ± 0.5 Gy in RAO projection and 1.5 ± 0.4 Gy in LAO. The lifetime risk of excess fatal malignancies normalized to 60 minutes of fluoroscopy was 0.07% for female and 0.1% for male patients. The relatively small amounts of radiation exposure to the patients in this study, despite the prolonged fluoroscopy durations, can be attributed in large measure to the use of very low frame pulsed fluoroscopy, the avoidance of magnification, and optimal adjustments of the fluoroscopy exposure rates. The resulting lifetime risk of fatal malignancy is within the range previously reported for standard supraventricular arrhythmia types. Basic measures to reduce X-ray exposure are listed in Table 32–1.

Complications Associated with Catheter Ablation of Supraventricular Arrhythmias

ACCESSORY PATHWAYS

The efficacy of catheter ablation of AP is approximately 95% in most series.[1-3,6] Complications associated with catheter ablation of APs include complete AV block, coronary artery injury, valvular perforation and/or damage, pericardial effusion, cardiac tamponade, hematoma formation, CVA or transient ischemic attack (TIA), venous thrombosis, and death.

Table 32–2 summarizes the type and incidence of major complications during catheter ablation of APs.

The procedure-related mortality rate has ranged from 0% to 0.2%. The MERFS reported data from 2222 patients who underwent catheter ablation of an AP.[2] The overall complication rate was 4.4%, including 3

TABLE 32-1
Basic Measures to Limit Fluoroscopic Exposure

Equipment
  Pulsed fluoroscopy
  Last image hold/image looping
  Digital cine acquisition
  Non-fluoroscopic catheter navigation systems

Operator Dependent
  Minimize use of magnification
  Collimate beam
  Shielding above and below table
  Image intensifier as close as possible to patient
  Limit cine runs

Operator Shielding
  2 piece wrap around lead
  Aprons–minimize arm hole size, coverage to mid-thigh
  Thyroid and eye protection with temple shields
  Direct beam away from operator
  Inspection of lead at least yearly

TABLE 32-2
Complications Associated with Catheter Ablation of Accessory Pathways

Complications	MERFS (N = 2222)	NASPE 1995 (N = 5427)	NASPE 1998 (N = 654)	Calkins et al.* (N = 500)
Complete AV block	14 (0.63%)	9 (0.17%)	2 (0.3%)	5 (1%)
Valve damage	1 (0.05%)	6[†](0.11%)	0 (0%)	+
Coronary artery injury/occlusion	0 (0%)	3 (0.06%)	1 (0.16%)	1 (0.2%)
Tamponade	16 (0.72%)	7 (0.13%)	7 (1.1%)	+
Venous thrombosis	4 (0.18%)	—[‡]	0 (0%)	+
Pulmonary embolism	2 (0.09%)	—[‡]	1 (0.16%)	+
Arterial thrombosis	4 (0.18%)	0 (0%)	0 (0%)	+
CVA/TIA	11 (0.49%)	8 (0.15%)	0 (0%)	1 (0.2%)[§]
Bleeding at puncture site/vascular injury	7 (0.32%)	3 (0.06%)	13 (1.99%)[¶]	+
Death	3 (0.13%)	4 (0.08%)	0 (0.00%)	1 (0.2%)

*Calkins H, Yong P, Miller JM, et al.: Catheter ablation of accessory pathways, atrioventricular nodal reentrant tachycardia, and the atrioventricular junction: Final results of a prospective, multicenter clinical trial. The Atakr Multicenter Investigators Group [see comments]. Circulation 99:262-270, 1999.
[†]Aortic valve perforations in 4 and mitral valve damage in 2.
[‡]Reported but no number specified.
[§]Left-side AP with trans-septal approach.
[¶]Twelve left free wall APs and 1 septal AP.
+, Complications were presented for all arrhythmias and were not all categorized based on the target arrhythmia; AP, accessory pathway; AV, atrioventricular; CVA, cerebrovascular accident; MERFS, Multicenter European Radiofrequency Survey; NASPE, North American Society of Pacing and Electrophysiology; TIA, transient ischemic attack.

deaths (0.13%). In the 1995 NASPE survey,[1] of the 5427 patients who underwent catheter ablations of an AP, a total of 99 (1.82%) had significant complications, including 4 procedure-related deaths (0.08%). The 1998 NASPE registry included 654 patients with APs[3]; there were no procedure-related deaths. Calkins et al.[6] reported the only data available from a multicenter clinical trial. They studied 1050 patients who underwent catheter ablation of an AP, AVNRT, or the AV junction. Among the 500 patients undergoing ablation of an AP in this series, there was 1 death (0.2%). This patient died of a dissected left main coronary artery during an attempt at catheter ablation of a left free wall AP. In the 2001 Spanish Registry,[4] 1084 patients underwent catheter ablation of APs, with a success rate of 93%. Major complications occurred in 17 patients (1.6%), the most frequent being vascular arterial complications (9 patients). There were no deaths. In the 2002 Spanish Registry,[5] 1416 procedures of catheter ablation were done in 1350 patients. Major complications occurred in 12 patients (0.9%).

The two most common types of major complications that have been reported during catheter ablation of APs are inadvertent complete AV block and cardiac tamponade. The incidence of inadvertent complete AV block ranges from 0.17% to 1.0%.[1-3,6] Most instances of complete AV block occur in the setting of ablation of septal and posteroseptal APs. Cryoablation has recently received approval from the U.S. Food and Drug Administration for catheter ablation of supraventricular arrhythmias. A potential advantage of cryoablation is that it may be associated with a lower risk of inadvertent AV block.[30] Several small case series have reported the safe and successful ablation of anterospetal, midseptal, and parahisian APs with cryoablation.[30,31] Despite these results, the need for cryoablation for APs in this region must be considered unproven. It is hoped that further data will emerge to help better define its clinical role. The frequency of cardiac tamponade as a result of the ablation of APs varies between 0.13% and 1.1%.[1-3,6]

ATRIOVENTRICULAR NODAL REENTRANT TACHYCARDIA

Catheter ablation of AVNRT is performed by targeting the slow pathway. The ablation catheter is directed into the low right ventricle, near the posterior septum, and is then withdrawn until an electrogram is recorded with a small atrial electrogram and a large ventricular electrogram. Specific ablation sites along the posterior portion of the tricuspid annulus can be selected based on the appearance of the local atrial electrogram or based strictly on anatomic factors.[32-34] Junctional beats occurring during the application of RF energy are a marker for successful ablation. Catheter ablation of AVNRT is effective in more than 95% of patients.[1-3,6,32,34] The incidence of AV block is 1% or less.

Complications associated with catheter ablation of AVNRT include complete AV block, pneumothorax, tamponade, pulmonary emboli, CVA/TIA, and significant bleeding and vessel injury. There were no reported deaths from ablation of AVNRT in MERFS, the 1995 NASPE survey, the 1998 NASPE registry, or the study by Calkins.[1-3,6]

Table 32–3 details the complications associated with catheter ablation of AVNRT. The most common type of major complication is inadvertent complete AV block. In the 1995 NASPE survey,[1] 6 (0.11%) of 5423 patients who underwent catheter ablation for AVNRT developed complete AV block. On the other hand, 41 (5.07%) of 815 patients in MERFS[2] developed complete heart block. The difference in results between these two retrospective surveys can be attributed to a higher incidence of complete AV block with the anterior approach (6.2%), compared with the posterior approach (2.0%). In the 1998 NASPE registry,[3] 9 (0.74%) of 1197 patients who underwent ablation for AVNRT developed complete heart block. In the study by Calkins et al.,[6] complete AV block occurred in 5 (1.3%) of 373 patients who had the catheter ablation procedure for AVNRT. Delise et al.[35] compiled the results of a 10-year multicenter study on the risks of intraprocedural atrioventricular block. From February 1990 to December 2000, 510 patients were enrolled for AVNRT. Intraprocedural second- and third-degree AV block occurred in 20 patients. The block was transient in 14 patients, 4 with second-degree AV block, and 10 with third-degree AV block. Persistent AV block occurred in 6 patients, including 2 with second-degree block and 4 with third-degree block. Transient late AV block occurred in 1 patient. One patient with transient intraprocedural third-degree AV block developed a persistent late third-degree AV block 2 days after the procedure. Another patient who had transient acute third-degree AV block developed a persistent late second-degree AV block. Chronic second- or third-degree AV block occurred in 7 of the patients. A pacemaker was implanted for permanent third-degree AV block in 5 patients. Two of the patients with second-degree AV block did not require a pacemaker because they had a good heart rate at rest and during effort.

A number of techniques have been described to reduce the likelihood of inadvertent AV block. Several authors have reported that the likelihood of developing AV block increases as the ablation catheter nears the His bundle. However, AV block has been reported even when RF energy was delivered at the level of the coronary sinus ostium. It is critical

TABLE 32-3

Complications Associated with Catheter Ablation of AVNRT

Complications	MERFS (N = 815)	NASPE 1995 (N = 5423)	NASPE 1998 (N = 1197)	Calkins et al.* (N = 373)
Complete AV block	41 (5.07%)	6 (0.11%)	9 (0.74%)	5 (1.3%)
Pneumothorax	0 (0%)	5 (0.09%)	1 (0.08%)	+
Tamponade or pericarditis	2 (0.24%)	18 (0.33%)	0 (0%)	+
Venous thrombosis	9 (1.11%)	5 (0.09%)	1 (0.08%)	
Pulmonary emboli	2 (0.24%)	0 (0%)	1 (0.08%)	+
CVA/TIA	1 (0.12%)	0 (0%)	0 (0%)	+
Bleeding at puncture site/vascular injury	2 (0.24%)	3 (0.06%)	6 (0.49%)	+
Death	0 (0%)	0 (0%)	0 (0%)	0 (0%)

*Calkins H, Yong P, Miller JM, et al.: Catheter ablation of accessory pathways, atrioventricular nodal reentrant tachycardia, and the atrioventricular junction: Final results of a prospective, multicenter clinical trial. The Atakr Multicenter Investigators Group [see comments]. Circulation 99:262-270, 1999.

+, Complications were presented for all arrhythmias and were not all categorized based on the target arrhythmia; AV, atrioventricular; CVA, cerebrovascular accident; MERFS, Multicenter European Radiofrequency Survey; NASPE, North American Society of Pacing and Electrophysiology; TIA, transient ischemic attack.

that AV conduction be continuously monitored during an application of RF energy. If AV block occurs, the application should be terminated immediately. If a junctional rhythm develops during an application of RF energy, as is often the case, ventricle-to-atrium (VA) conduction can be monitored. The development of VA block in association with a junctional rhythm is an indication of damage to the fast pathway and should prompt immediate termination of the application. We have employed an even more conservative approach, discontinuing RF energy delivery whenever a junctional rhythm is observed. Once AV conduction is confirmed, RF energy is reapplied to the same site. Longer and longer applications of RF energy are delivered until eventually no junctional rhythm is observed. With this technique, no patients have developed AV block during catheter ablation of AVNRT.

Cryoablation has made great strides in the treatment of AVNRT, due in part to a novel feature, ice mapping. Ice mapping is the ability to test the functionality of a potential ablation site before a permanent lesion is created. It is a fully reversible process. This process is accomplished by cooling the tissue to mild temperatures (0°C to −10°C). Skanes et al.[30] demonstrated successful ice mapping of the slow pathway during AVNRT and AP conduction. Eighteen patients with typical AVNRT underwent cryoablation. Reversible loss of slow pathway conduction during cryothermy (ice mapping) was demonstrated in 11 of 12 patients. Riccardi et al.[36] performed cryothermal ablation of AVNRT in 32 patients. Slow

pathway ablation guided by a slow pathway potential was successfully performed in 31 of the patients, with a mean of 2.6 ± 1.0 cryoapplications. No complications occurred in any patients. Lowe et al.[37] performed cryoablation procedures in 14 patients with AVNRT. Cryoablation was successful in 11 patients and was painless in all patients, with overall procedural discomfort being significantly less than for patients treated with RF. Cryothermy is a painless and safe alternative to RF.[37] It is particularly useful for catheter ablation of patients with pathways close to the AV node. Inadvertent cooling of the AV node results in fully reversible prolongation of the PR interval as well as AV block.[30] Therefore, inadvertent AV block as a complication of ablation should be eliminated with this technology.

ATRIOVENTRICULAR JUNCTION

Catheter ablation of the AV junction is usually reserved for atrial arrhythmias that cannot be controlled with pharmacologic therapy and that result in a rapid ventricular response. The procedure is performed by positioning a steerable ablation catheter across the tricuspid annulus to record the largest His bundle electrogram associated with the largest atrial electrogram. A second electrode catheter is placed at the apex of the right ventricle for temporary pacing. Once an appropriate target site is identified, RF energy is delivered for 30 to 60 seconds. If this is unsuccessful, a left-sided approach can be used.[38] The efficacy of catheter ablation of the AV junction approaches 100%.[6,38-40] After catheter ablation of the AV junction, a permanent rate-responsive pacemaker is inserted.

Complications associated with catheter ablation of the AV junction include pneumothorax, tamponade, arterial and/or venous thrombosis, and sudden death. Sudden cardiac death, occurring early or late after catheter ablation of the AV junction, is by far the most feared complication of this procedure The MERFS reported data from 900 patients who underwent catheter ablation of the AV junction.[2] The overall complication rate was 3.2%, including 1 sudden death that occurred 7 days after catheter ablation (0.11%). In the 1995 NASPE survey,[1] 3 (0.15%) of the 2084 patients who underwent catheter ablation for AV junction developed polymorphic VT or a cardiac arrest after the procedure. The 1998 NASPE registry included 646 patients with AV junction ablation[3]; there was 1 sudden death (0.15%) that resulted from pacemaker malfunction 3 hours after the procedure. In a prospective multicenter trial by Calkins et al.,[6] 2 (1.65%) of the 121 patients undergoing AV junction ablation and pacemaker implantation died suddenly within 30 days after the ablation procedure. Table 32–4 summarizes and categorizes the rates of complications associated with catheter ablation of the AV junction.

Recent studies have demonstrated that the risk of sudden death after catheter ablation of the AV junction

can be reduced by an increased rate of ventricular pacing. Geelen et al. reported a 6% incidence of ventricular fibrillation or sudden death within 1 month after RF ablation of the AV junction when pacing rates were set to 60 beats per minute for the first 1 to 3 months after the procedure, compared with no incidence of sudden cardiac death when pacing rates were programmed to 90 bpm for the first 1 to 3 months and subsequently reduced to 70 bpm.[41,42] Based on the results of these and other studies, a general consensus exists that patients who undergo ablation of the AV junction should be paced at 90 bpm for at least 1 month after the catheter ablation procedure.

INAPPROPRIATE SINUS TACHYCARDIA

The clinical presentation for patients with inappropriate sinus tachycardia is an elevated resting heart rate (>100 bpm) or an exaggerated increase in heart rate in response to exercise, or both, in the absence of identifiable causes for sinus tachycardia. Man et al.[43] studied 29 consecutive patients with drug-refractory inappropriate sinus tachycardia who underwent catheter ablation and reported an acute success rate of 76%. Two complications (7%) were noted. One patient had a near-syncope with sinus pauses up to 4 seconds in duration, and another patient developed right hemidiaphragm paralysis after catheter ablation. In the 1998 NASPE registry,[3] there were a total

TABLE 32–4

Complications Associated with Catheter Ablation of the Atrioventricular Junction

Complications	MERFS (N = 900)	NASPE 1995 (N = 2084)	NASPE 1998 (N = 646)	Calkins et al.* (N = 121)
Tamponade	1 (0.11%)	2 (0.1%)	0 (0%)	+
Venous thrombosis	9 (1.00%)	0 (0%)	0 (0%)	+
Pulmonary emboli	2 (0.22%)	0 (0%)	0 (0%)	1 (0.82%)
Significant TR	1 (0.11%)	0 (0%)	1 (0.15%)	+
Bleeding at puncture site/ vascular injury	0 (0%)	0 (0%)	2 (0.30%)	+
CVA/TIA	0 (0%)	2[†] (0.1%)	0 (0%)	1[†] (0.82%)
Myocardial infarction	0 (0%)	1 (0.05%)	0 (0%)	0 (0%)
Sudden death/polymorphic VT	1 (0.11%)	3 (0.15%)	1[‡] (0.15%)	2 (1.65%)
Death (total)	1 (0.11%)	4 (0.2%)	1 (0.15%)	2 (1.65%)

*Calkins H, Yong P, Miller JM, et al.: Catheter ablation of accessory pathways, atrioventricular nodal reentrant tachycardia, and the atrioventricular junction: Final results of a prospective, multicenter clinical trial. The Atakr Multicenter Investigators Group [see comments]. Circulation 99:262-270, 1999.

[†]All associated with left-sided approach.

[‡]Death due to pacemaker malfunction.

+, Complications were presented for all arrhythmias and were not all categorized based on the target arrhythmia; CVA, cerebrovascular accident; MERFS, Multicenter European Radiofrequency Survey; NASPE, North American Society of Pacing and Electrophysiology; TIA, transient ischemic attack; TR, tricuspid regurgitation; VT, ventricular tachycardia.

of 40 patients who underwent catheter ablation of inappropriate sinus tachycardia. The acute success rate was 71.4%, and there were 2 complications (5%). The first was inadvertent complete heart block, and the second was damage to a previously implanted pacemaker. More recently, Marrouche et al.[44] studied the usefulness of three-dimensional nonfluoroscopic mapping in 39 patients with debilitating inappropriate sinus tachycardia. The sinus node was successfully modified in all patients (100%). The heart rate dropped from a mean of 99 ± 14 bpm to 72 ± 8 bpm. Twenty-one percent of the patients experienced recurrence of inappropriate sinus tachycardia and were successfully reablated. No complications occurred.

ATRIAL FLUTTER

Atrial flutter is an atrial arrhythmia characterized by a regular rate, a uniform morphology, and a rate greater than 240 bpm. Atrial flutter can be categorized as isthmus-dependent, non–isthmus-dependent, or atypical.[45,46] Isthmus-dependent and non–isthmus-dependent atrial flutters can be cured with catheter ablation. In isthmus-dependent flutter, the lesions are placed in one or more lines across the isthmus, from the tricuspid annulus to the inferior vena cava.[47] In non–isthmus-dependent flutter, the slow conduction zone is identified with entrainment mapping and subsequently ablated.

Catheter ablation of typical atrial flutter is performed with the use of a deflectable ablation catheter positioned in the inferior right atrium, usually via the right femoral vein. The end point for this procedure is demonstration of bidirectional conduction block through the isthmus after the procedure.[48,49] Use of this strategy has led to an acute success rate of 100% and a recurrence rate of approximately 7% in three published series.[48-50] In some cases of typical atrial flutter, achieving bidirectional isthmus block is challenging. In these situations, cooled-tip RF ablation may be useful, because it creates deeper lesions.[51,52] More recently, the use of ablation catheters with 8- to 10-mm distal tips and RF generators capable of delivering 100 W of power has been associated with very high success rates and short procedure times. Calkins' group[52] noted a success rate of 88%. The mean procedural time was 2.1 ± 1 hours, the mean fluoroscopy time was 34 ± 24 minutes, and the mean time required for ablation was 49 ± 48 minutes. At the present time, almost all flutter ablation procedures are performed either with irrigated-tip ablation catheters or with high-power RF generators coupled with 8- or 10-mm-tip ablation electrodes.

The complications associated with catheter ablation of atrial flutter, including complete AV block, tamponade, bleeding/hematoma, and hemopneu-

mothorax, are similar to those associated with other catheter ablation procedures. Catheter ablation of atrial flutter is notable, however, because of the infrequency with which complications occur. There have been no deaths reported during catheter ablation of atrial flutter.[1,3,53,54] The 1995 NASPE survey[1] reported that, among 570 patients undergoing atrial flutter ablation, the overall complication rate was 0.4%. Complete heart block occurred in 1 patient. The 1998 NASPE registry[3] included 477 patients who underwent atrial flutter ablation. One patient developed tamponade (0.21%), 1 developed a hemopneumothorax (0.21%), 2 developed complete AV block (0.42%), and 3 developed bleeding and/or hematoma at the site of vascular access (0.63%). There were no deaths. MERFS[2] did not specifically examine the frequency with which complications developed during catheter ablation of atrial flutter.

Two recently published multicenter studies have discussed the safety and efficacy of catheter ablation of atrial flutter. Feld et al.[8] noted a complication rate of 3.6% in 169 patients. They observed six major adverse events, including 1 patient each with pulmonary embolism, bilateral lower extremity ischemia due to systemic thromboembolism, deep venous thrombosis, right groin hematoma, cerebral embolus with resolution of neurologic findings, cerebral infarct (thrombotic) 5 days after the procedure with persistent mild aphasia, and a fractured femur. The fractured femur was accidental and unrelated to the procedure itself. The cerebral embolus and cerebral infarct were associated with a left atrial ablation procedure and intracranial stenosis of right and left middle cerebral arteries, respectively. Calkins et al.[9] had a complication rate of 2.7%. They noted four significant device- or procedure-related complications occurring within 1 week after the procedure, among 150 ablated patients. The complications were a small pericardial effusion, ongoing right-sided pleural effusion that was present at baseline, ventricular fibrillation during RF energy delivery, and a large groin hematoma (1 patient each). In addition to these four significant complications, three patients developed second-degree skin burns at the edge of the dispersive pad. This was subsequently remedied in the next 105 patients through the use of a dual dispersive pad system. In addition to this registry and multicenter information, there have been many small studies of patients undergoing ablation of atrial flutter that also reported a very low incidence of complications.[53-57]

ATRIAL TACHYCARDIA

In the 1998 NASPE registry,[3] catheter ablation of ectopic atrial tachycardia was performed in 216 patients, with an overall success rate of 73.0%. Complications included cardiac tamponade in 2 patients, damage to the pacemaker lead in 1 patient, transient AV block in 1 patient, aspiration pneumonia in 1 patient, and right atrial to aortic fistula in 1 patient. In the 2001 Spanish Registry,[4] 137 procedures of catheter ablation for focal atrial tachycardia were performed in 124 patients, with an overall success rate of 82%. Successful results were obtained in 83% of the tachycardias located in the right atrium, compared with 71% of the tachycardias located in the left atrium. No complications were listed.

ATRIAL FIBRILLATION

Catheter ablation of AF has made enormous strides since the identification of pulmonary veins (PVs) as an important trigger of AF by Haissaguerre et al.[58,59] The strategies employed for AF ablation have evolved from focal ablation targeting arrhythmogenic triggers[14,58-61] to empiric isolation of PVs that demonstrate PV potentials.[60-65]

Ectopic beats originating from PVs can trigger paroxysmal AF. This type of "focal" AF can be cured with catheter ablation in 50% to 70% of patients.[14,65-67] In one series of 90 patients,[66] complications included air embolism in 5 patients, hemopericardium requiring percutaneous drainage in 1, TIA in 2, and PV stenosis in 6. In another series of 79 patients,[14] the complications included a TIA in 2 patients and hemothorax and hemopericardium requiring intervention in 1 patient.

The complications associated with catheter ablation of AF are numerous. Vasamreddy et al.[15] reported complications in 6 (8%) of 75 patients. The most significant complications were pericardial tamponade (2 patients), mitral valve injury requiring replacement (1), CVAs (2), and complete but asymptomatic PV stenosis (1). Other complications that arose were mild PV stenosis (<50%) in 3 patients; moderate PV stenosis (50% to 70%) in 2 patients; and cough, groin bleeding requiring transfusion, and pseudoaneurysm in the groin in 1 patient each. Pappone et al.[68] reported the results of catheter ablation in 251 patients. Transient, advanced, complete AV block or systolic hypotension occurred in 30 patients during RF delivery, particularly around the superolateral PV. They also reported cardiac tamponade requiring pericardiocentesis in 2 patients and minor pericardial effusion that was managed medically in 2 patients. Bhargava et al.[69] reported the results of PV isolation in 323 patients. Three strokes occurred during the procedure in patients older than 60 years of age. They also noted cardiac tamponade requiring pericardiocentesis (2 patients), coronary sinus perforation requiring open heart surgery (1), severe PV stenosis (2), and mild confusion and facial droop after the procedure (1). Hoff et al.[70] performed catheter ablation for AF in 72 patients. Complications included drainage of pericardial effusion, cerebral embolus with partial visual impairment, and an asymptomatic PV stenosis (1 patient each). Schwartzman et al.[71] performed catheter ablation in 112 patients. There were 7 complications, including femoral pseudoaneurysm (3 patients), arteriovenous fistula (2), femoral blood loss requiring transfusion (1), and transient postoperative noncardiogenic pulmonary edema (1). Finally, in a German study, Ernst et al.[72] reported 5 complications in 84 patients. These complications were stroke (1 patient), TIA (1), total occlusion of a PV (1), and acute tamponade (2).

Among these complications, perhaps one of the most feared is PV stenosis.[73,74] The reported rate of PV stenosis ranges from 3% to 42%. Purerfellner et al.[75] recently documented the incidences of PV stenosis in 57 of their patients, including 115 targeted PVs. Compared with baseline, 7 (6.08%) of the 115 PVs showed mild PV stenosis (luminal diameter reduction of 20% to 49%), and 2 (1.73%) showed severe stenosis (luminal diameter reduction >90%). Luminal narrowing occurred most frequently in the left inferior PV (6/9). Mildly stenosed PVs showed their maximal luminal regression within the 3-month follow-up period. Two of two PVs with narrowing greater than 50% at 3 months progressed to high-grade stenosis. Saad et al.[76] documented the incidence of PV stenosis in 355 of their patients. Severe PV stenosis was detected in 18 patients (5%). Eight of these patients reported shortness of breath, 7 reported cough, and 5 reported hemoptysis. Radiologic abnormalities were present in 9 patients and led to diagnoses of pneumonia in 4 patients, lung cancer in 1, and pulmonary embolism in 2. Recent data suggest that limiting the RF power to 30 W, limiting the temperature of the ablation electrode to 50° C, and limiting ablation to the most proximal portion of the PV can minimize the probability of developing PV stenosis.[59-61] Purerfellner et al.[75] made a similar conclusion, saying that occurrence of stenosis tended to be related to the amount of energy delivered.

It is important to note that the techniques used for catheter ablation of AF are continuing to evolve rapidly. As mentioned, one of the biggest fears of performing RF catheter ablation of AF is PV stenosis. Cryoablation is expected to produce minimal PV stenosis due to the lack of endothelial disruption and lack of hyperthermic injury with this procedure.[31] Initial data confirm this hypothesis. Tse et al.[77] evaluated the efficacy and safety of PV isolation using transvenous cryoablation for the treatment of AF. They performed the procedure on 52 patients, completely isolating all targeted PVs in 49 (94%). Of 152 PVs targeted, 147 (97%) were successfully isolated. At

3 and 12 months after the procedure, computed tomography scans showed no evidence of PV stenosis associated with cryoablation in any patient.[77] Catheter ablation of AF should be regarded as a second-line defense and reserved for only symptomatic patients for whom treatment with pharmacologic therapy has failed.

An even more worrisome complication associated with catheter ablation of AF is esophageal injury. A recent study[78] reported that two patients developed an atrioesophageal fistula after catheter ablation of AF using the circumferential approach. One patient died, and the other developed severe thromboembolic complications. It was estimated that the probability of this complication is approximately 0.1%. Modifications have been suggested to reduce this risk, including reducing the target temperature to 52°C and the power to 50 W when ablating in the posterior left atrium.

Complications Associated with Catheter Ablation of Ventricular Tachycardia

IDIOPATHIC VENTRICULAR TACHYCARDIA

Idiopathic VT is defined as VT that occurs in patients without structural heart disease, metabolic abnor-

malities, or the long QT syndrome.[79,80] In the United States, idiopathic VT typically arises in the outflow tract of the right ventricle (RVOT). A recent review of the results of catheter ablation of idiopathic VT arising in the RVOT reported an acute success rate of 93% (range, 85% to 100%) with the mean recurrence rate of 7%.[79] Complications included death from a perforated outflow tract in 1 patient (1%) and persistent right bundle branch block in 2 patients (2%). In the 1998 NASPE registry,[3] 82 (85.7%) of 98 patients had successful catheter ablation for RVOT VT. In the 2001 Spanish Registry,[4] 90 (78%) of 125 patients had successful catheter ablation in 30 centers. The RVOT was the most frequent location (76%), followed by fascicular (14%), left ventricular outflow tract (4%), and other locations (6%). Pericardial effusion in one patient was the only major complication (0.8%). The complications associated with catheter ablation of VT were not categorized based on the specific type of VT.[3] Table 32–5 summarizes the overall complications that can occur during catheter ablation of all types of VT.

NONIDIOPATHIC VENTRICULAR TACHYCARDIA

To date, only one published prospective multicenter clinical trial has evaluated the safety and efficacy of catheter ablation of nonidiopathic VT.[7] Catheter ablation was acutely successful, as defined by elimination of all mappable VTs in 106 (75%) of 146 patients who participated in the clinical trial. Sixteen patients

TABLE 32–5

Complications Associated with Radiofrequency Ablation of Ventricular Tachycardia

Complications	MERFS (N = 320)	NASPE 1995 (N = 844)	NASPE 1998 (N = 201)	Calkins et al.* (N = 146)
Complete AV block	1 (0.31%)	1 (0.12%)	+	2 (1.4%)
Valve damage	+	+	+	1 (0.7%)
Peripheral embolism	2 (0.63%)	3 (0.36%)	+	+
Tamponade	1 (0.31%)	6 (0.71%)	2 (1.0%)	4 (2.7%)
Arterial thrombosis	1 (0.31%)	1 (0.12%)	+	+
CVA/TIA	4 (1.26%)	+	+	4 (2.7%)
Pulmonary embolism	2 (0.63%)	+	+	+
Bleeding at puncture site/vascular injury	2 (0.63%)	+	+	1 (0.7%)
Death	1 (0.31%)	0 (0%)	3† (1.5%)	4 (2.7%)‡

*Calkins H, Epstein A, Packer D, et al.: Catheter ablation of ventricular tachycardia in patients with structural heart disease using cooled radiofrequency energy: Results of a prospective multicenter study. Cooled RF Multi Center Investigators Group. J Am Coll Cardiol 35:1905-1914, 2000.

†During the follow-up.

‡One from left main occlusion, 1 from tamponade, 1 from CVA and cerebral herniation, 1 from aortic valve perforation.

+, data not provided; AV, atrioventricular; CVA, cerebrovascular accident; MERFS, Multicenter European Radiofrequency Survey; NASPE, North American Society of Pacing and Electrophysiology; TIA, transient ischemic attack.

(10.8%) had a major complication, including death (2.7%), myocardial infarction (0.7%), tamponade (2.7%), complete AV block (1.4%), CVA/TIA (2.7%), and valve injury (0.7%).

In addition to this prospective multicenter clinical trial, data regarding the safety of catheter ablation of VT was also examined in the MERFS and in the two NASPE registries. These studies did not subdivide patients based on whether they were undergoing catheter ablation of idiopathic versus nonidiopathic VT. In the 1995 NASPE survey,[1] 170 (66%) of 257 patients who underwent catheter ablation for VT associated with coronary artery disease had successful ablation. In the 1998 NASPE registry,[3] acute success of catheter ablation for VT associated with coronary artery disease was achieved in 31 (58.5%) of 53 patients.[3] Table 32–4 summarizes the complications associated with catheter ablation of VT.

The 2001 Spanish Registry[4] subdivided patients based on whether they had VT associated with postinfarction scar or macroreentrant VT not associated with postinfarction scar. In the former group, the substrate was treated in 24 centers, including 125 procedures in 99 patients. The procedure was successful in 70 patients (71%), and complications appeared in 4 patients (4%): 2 arterial vascular complications, 1 heart failure, and 1 death after a procedure.[55] Among those with macroreentrant VT not associated with postinfarction scar, 48 procedures were performed in 43 patients in 16 centers. Fifteen VTs caused by a bundle branch-branch reentry mechanism were treated; 17 patients had dilated idiopathic cardiomyopathy, and 12 patients had an arrhythmogenic right ventricular dysplasia. The procedure was successful in 29 patients (67%). Complications occurred in 2 patients (5%), including 1 arterial vascular complication and 1 AV block.

Selected Issues

CATHETER ABLATION IN THE ELDERLY

The safety and efficacy of RF catheter ablation in the elderly has been evaluated in several studies.[3,81,82] Epstein et al.,[81] for example, reported on the efficacy and safety of catheter ablation for the treatment of supraventricular tachycardias in 68 patients who were older than 70 years of age. The success rate was 98.5%, and the complication rate was 7.4%, similar to those in a younger population. Other studies have reported similar findings.[3,81] Da Costa et al.[83] studied the safety and efficacy of catheter ablation of atrial flutter in elderly patients. They compared the results of 61 patients older than 75 years of age with those of 187 patients younger than age 75. Da Costa's group also found that catheter ablation of atrial flutter in very elderly patients is a reasonable approach regarding feasibility, effectiveness, and low procedural risks.[83]

CATHETER ABLATION IN PEDIATRIC PATIENTS

The Pediatric Radiofrequency Ablation Registry reported the outcome of catheter ablation in 652 patients.[83] The median age was 13.5 years, with 41% of patients younger than 13 and 8% younger than 4 years of age. Major complications occurred in 35 patients (4.8%). Independent risk factors for complications, which were identified by multivariate analysis, included a body weight of less than 15 kg and the number of ablation procedures performed at a medical center. The complication rate among children weighing less than 15 kg was 10%. The results of this study suggest that catheter ablation procedures should be avoided in very small children unless other therapeutic options do not exist.

Torres et al.[85] looked at the treatment of supraventricular arrhythmias in 203 patients younger than 18 years of age. The presence of an AP caused the tachyarrhythmia in 181 patients (89.1%) with a total of 187 APs; AV nodal reentry caused the arrhythmia in 18 patients (8.8%), and atrial flutter was the cause in only 4 patients (1.9%). These researchers were able to eliminate the AP in 171 patients (91.4%). A total of 23 patients showed a recurrence of the tachycardia, and there were complications in 4 patients (2.1%). The procedure successfully treated the AV nodal reentry in all 18 cases, with ablation of the slow pathway in 17 cases and ablation of the fast pathway in only 1 patient. One patient showed total AV block, and there was recurrence of the arrhythmia in 3 cases (16.6%). The procedure was successful in all 4 cases of atrial flutter, with 1 recurrence (25%). Overall, the RF catheter ablation procedures were successful in 193 patients (95%), with recurrence of the arrhythmia in 27 cases (13.3%) and with complications in only 5 patients (2.6%).[85] The results of this study suggest that catheter ablation is a safe and effective procedure for the treatment of supraventricular tachyarrhythmia in children.

Celiker et al.,[87] in a Turkish study, reported the outcome of catheter ablation in 73 pediatric patients with tachyarrhythmia, ranging from 2 to 21 years of age. The median age was 11 years. Procedure-related complications occurred in 8 patients (11%), and the overall final success rate for all diagnoses (60 patients) was 82%. These results suggest that RF catheter ablation has a good success rate and a low risk of complications in pediatric patients.

Conclusion

In conclusion, RF catheter ablation is a highly effective approach to the treatment of cardiac arrhythmias. Success rates of greater than 90% with complication rates of less than 3% should be anticipated for catheter ablation of AVNRT, APs, atrial flutter, idiopathic VT, and the AV junction. For these arrhythmias, the safety and efficacy profile of catheter ablation suggests that it should be considered as an alternative to pharmacologic therapy. In contrast, the safety and efficacy of RF catheter ablation is less than 90% and the incidence of complications is generally greater than 3% during attempts at catheter ablation of AF and nonidiopathic VT, and also for catheter ablation in very small children. This safety and efficacy profile suggests that the appropriate role of catheter ablation for these arrhythmias is as a second-line therapy, after attempts at pharmacologic therapy have failed. With greater attention to detail and implementation of some of the techniques described here, the probability of developing a complication can be minimized. The precise role of cryoablation will become better defined in the years ahead.

References

1. Scheinman MM: NASPE survey on catheter ablation. Pacing Clin Electrophysiol 18:1474-1478, 1995.
2. Hindricks G: The Multicentre European Radiofrequency Survey (MERFS): Complications of radiofrequency catheter ablation of arrhythmias. The Multicentre European Radiofrequency Survey (MERFS) investigators of the Working Group on Arrhythmias of the European Society of Cardiology [see comments]. Eur Heart J 14:1644-1653, 1993.
3. Scheinman MM, Huang S: The 1998 NASPE prospective catheter ablation registry. Pacing Clin Electrophysiol 23:1020-1028, 2000.
4. Álvarez Lopez M, Merino JL: Spanish Registry on Catheter Ablation: 1st Official Report of the Working Group on Electrophysiology and Arrhythmias of the Spanish Society of Cardiology (Year 2001). Rev Esp Cardiol 55:1273-1285, 2002.
5. Álvarez Lopez M, Merino JL: Spanish Registry on Catheter Ablation. II Official Report (2002). Cirugía Cardiovascular 1:83-96, 2004.
6. Calkins H, Yong P, Miller JM, et al.: Catheter ablation of accessory pathways, atrioventricular nodal reentrant tachycardia, and the atrioventricular junction: Final results of a prospective, multicenter clinical trial. The Atakr Multicenter Investigators Group [see comments]. Circulation 99:262-270, 1999.
7. Calkins H, Epstein A, Packer D, et al.: Catheter ablation of ventricular tachycardia in patients with structural heart disease using cooled radiofrequency energy: Results of a prospective multicenter study. Cooled RF Multi Center Investigators Group. J Am Coll Cardiol 35:1905-1914, 2000.
8. Feld G, Wharton M, Plumb V, et al., and EPT-1000 XP Cardiac Ablation System Investigators: Radiofrequency catheter ablation of type 1 atrial flutter using large-tip 8- or 10-mm electrode catheters and a high-output radiofrequency energy generator: Results of a multicenter safety and efficacy study. J Am Coll Cardiol 43:1466-1472, 2004.
9. Calkins H, Canby R, Weiss R, et al., for the 100W Atakr II Investigator Group: Results of catheter ablation of typical atrial flutter. Am J Cardiol 94:437-442, 2004.
10. Lee DS, Dorian P, Downar E, et al.: Thrombogenicity of radiofrequency ablation procedures: What factors influence thrombin generation? Europace 3:195-200, 2001.
11. Zhou L, Keane D, Reed G, Ruskin J: Thromboembolic complications of cardiac radiofrequency catheter ablation: A review of the reported incidence, pathogenesis and current research directions. J Cardiovasc Electrophysiol 10:611-620, 1999.
12. Calkins H, Prystowsky E, Carlson M, et al.: Temperature monitoring during radiofrequency catheter ablation procedures using closed loop control. Atakr Multicenter Investigators Group. Circulation 90:1279-1286, 1994.
13. Epstein MR, Knapp LD, Martindill M, et al.: Embolic complications associated with radiofrequency catheter ablation. Atakr Investigator Group. Am J Cardiol 77:655-658, 1996.
14. Chen SA, Hsieh MH, Tai CT, et al.: Initiation of atrial fibrillation by ectopic beats originating from the pulmonary veins: Electrophysiological characteristics, pharmacological responses, and effects of radiofrequency ablation. Circulation 100:1879-1886, 1999.
15. Vasamreddy C, Lickfett L, Jayam V, et al.: Predictors of recurrence following catheter ablation of atrial fibrillation using an irrigated-tip ablation catheter. J Cardiovasc Electrophysiol 15:1-6, 2004.
16. Kok LC, Mangrum JM, Haines DE, Mounsey JP: Cerebrovascular complication associated with pulmonary vein ablation. J Cardiovasc Electrophysiol 13:764-767, 2002.
17. Bombeli T, Mueller M, Haeberli A: Anticoagulant properties of the vascular endothelium. Thromb Haemost 77:408-423, 1997.
18. Cauchemez B, Extramiana F, Cauchemez S, et al.: High-flow perfusion of sheaths for prevention of thromboembolic complications during complex catheter ablation in the left atrium. J Cardiovasc Electrophysiol 15:276-283, 2004.
19. Rosenthal LS, Beck TJ, Williams J, et al.: Acute radiation dermatitis following radiofrequency catheter ablation of atrioventricular nodal reentrant tachycardia. Pacing Clin Electrophysiol 20:1834-1839, 1997.
20. Calkins H, Niklason L, Sousa J, et al.: Radiation exposure during radiofrequency catheter ablation of accessory atrioventricular connections [see comments]. Circulation 84:2376-2382, 1991.
21. Lindsay BD, Eichling JO, Ambos HD, Cain ME: Radiation exposure to patients and medical personnel during radiofrequency catheter ablation for supraventricular tachycardia. Am J Cardiol 70:218-223, 1992.
22. Park TH, Eichling JO, Schechtman KB, et al.: Risk of radiation induced skin injuries from arrhythmia ablation procedures. Pacing Clin Electrophysiol 19:1363-1369, 1996.
23. Macle L, Weerasooriya R, Jais P, et al. Radiation exposure during radiofrequency catheter ablation for atrial fibrillation. Pacing Clin Electrophysiol 26:288-291, 2003.
24. Rosenthal LS, Mahesh M, Beck TJ, et al.: Predictors of fluoroscopy time and estimated radiation exposure during radiofrequency catheter ablation procedures. Am J Cardiol 82:451-458, 1998.
25. Wagner LK, Eifel PJ, Geise RA: Potential biological effects following high X-ray dose interventional procedures. J Vasc Interv Radiol 5:71-84, 1994.
26. Lickfett L, Mahesh M, Vasamreddy C, et al.: Radiation exposure during catheter ablation of atrial fibrillation. Circulation 110:3003-3010, 2004.

27. National Council on Radiation Protection and Measurements: Limitation on Exposure to Ionizing Radiation. NRCP Report No. 116. Bethesda, Md.: NCRP, 1993.

28. Vano E, Gonzalez L, Beneytez F, Moreno F: Lens injuries induced by occupational exposure in non-optimized interventional radiology laboratories. Br J Radiol 71:728-733, 1998.

29. McFadden SL, Mooney RB, Shepherd PH: X-ray dose and associated risks from radiofrequency catheter ablation procedures. Br J Radiol 75:253-265, 2002.

30. Skanes AC, Dubuc M, Klein GJ, et al.: Cryothermal ablation of the slow pathway for the elimination of atrioventricular nodal reentrant tachycardia. Circulation 102:2856-2860, 2000.

31. Skanes AC, Yee R, Krahn AD, Klein GJ: Cryoablation of atrial arrhythmias. Card Electrophysiol Rev 6:383-388, 2002.

32. Langberg JJ, Leon A, Borganelli M, et al.: A randomized, prospective comparison of anterior and posterior approaches to radiofrequency catheter ablation of atrioventricular nodal reentry tachycardia. Circulation 87:1551-1556, 1993.

33. Lee MA, Morady F, Kadish A, et al.: Catheter modification of the atrioventricular junction with radiofrequency energy for control of atrioventricular nodal reentry tachycardia. Circulation 83:827-835, 1991.

34. Kottkamp H, Hindricks G, Willems S, et al.: An anatomically and electrogram-guided stepwise approach for effective and safe catheter ablation of the fast pathway for elimination of atrioventricular node reentrant tachycardia [see comments]. J Am Coll Cardiol 25:974-981, 1995.

35. Delise P, Sitta N, Zoppo F, et al.: Radiofrequency ablation of atrioventricular nodal reentrant tachycardia: The risk of intraprocedural, late and long-term atrioventricular block. The Veneto Region multicenter experience. Ital Heart J 3:715-720, 2002.

36. Riccardi R, Gaita F, Caponi D, et al.: Percutaneous catheter cryothermal ablation of atrioventricular nodal reentrant tachycardia: Efficacy and safety of a new ablation technique. Ital Heart J 4:35-43, 2003.

37. Lowe MD, Meara M, Mason J, et al.: Catheter cryoablation of supraventricular arrhythmias: A painless alternative to radiofrequency energy. Pacing Clin Electrophysiol 26:500-503, 2003.

38. Sousa J, el-Atassi R, Rosenheck S, et al.: Radiofrequency catheter ablation of the atrioventricular junction from the left ventricle. Circulation 84:567-571, 1991.

39. Morady F, Calkins H, Langberg JJ, et al.: A prospective randomized comparison of direct current and radiofrequency ablation of the atrioventricular junction. J Am Coll Cardiol 21:102-109, 1993.

40. Trohman RG, Simmons TW, Moore SL, et al.: Catheter ablation of the atrioventricular junction using radiofrequency energy and a bilateral cardiac approach. Am J Cardiol 70:1438-1443, 1992.

41. Hamdan MH, Page RL, Sheehan CJ, et al.: Increased sympathetic activity after atrioventricular junction ablation in patients with chronic atrial fibrillation. J Am Coll Cardiol 36:151-158, 2000.

42. Geelen P, Brugada J, Andries E, Brugada P: Ventricular fibrillation and sudden death after radiofrequency catheter ablation of the atrioventricular junction. Pacing Clin Electrophysiol 20:343-348, 1997.

43. Man KC, Knight B, Tse HF, et al.: Radiofrequency catheter ablation of inappropriate sinus tachycardia guided by activation mapping. J Am Coll Cardiol 35:451-457, 2000.

44. Marrouche NF, Beheiry S, Tomassoni G, et al.: Three-dimensional nonfluoroscopic mapping and ablation of inappropriate sinus tachycardia: Procedural strategies and long-term outcome. J Am Coll Cardiol 39:1046-1054, 2002.

45. Kalman JM, Olgin JE, Saxon LA, et al.: Activation and entrainment mapping defines the tricuspid annulus as the anterior barrier in typical atrial flutter [see comments]. Circulation 94:398-406, 1996.

46. Nakagawa H, Lazzara R, Khastgir T, et al.: Role of the tricuspid annulus and the eustachian valve/ridge on atrial flutter: Relevance to catheter ablation of the septal isthmus and a new technique for rapid identification of ablation success [see comments]. Circulation 94:407-424, 1996.

47. Poty H, Saoudi N, Abdel Aziz A, et al.: Radiofrequency catheter ablation of type 1 atrial flutter: Prediction of late success by electrophysiological criteria. Circulation 92:1389-1392, 1995.

48. Poty H, Saoudi N, Nair M, et al.: Radiofrequency catheter ablation of atrial flutter. Further insights into the various types of isthmus block: Application to ablation during sinus rhythm. Circulation 94:3204-3213, 1996.

49. Tai CT, Chen SA, Chiang CE, et al.: Long-term outcome of radiofrequency catheter ablation for typical atrial flutter: Risk prediction of recurrent arrhythmias. J Cardiovasc Electrophysiol 9:115-121, 1998.

50. Tai CT, Chen SA, Chiang CE, et al.: Electrophysiologic characteristics and radiofrequency catheter ablation in patients with clockwise atrial flutter. J Cardiovasc Electrophysiol 8:24-34, 1997.

51. Jais P, Haissaguerre M, Shah DC, et al.: Successful irrigated-tip catheter ablation of atrial flutter resistant to conventional radiofrequency ablation. Circulation 98:835-838, 1998.

52. Wu RC, Berger R, Calkins H: Catheter ablation of atrial flutter and macroreentrant atrial tachycardia. Curr Opin Cardiol 17:58-64, 2002.

53. Feld GK, Fleck RP, Chen PS, et al.: Radiofrequency catheter ablation for the treatment of human type 1 atrial flutter: Identification of a critical zone in the reentrant circuit by endocardial mapping techniques [see comments]. Circulation 86:1233-1240, 1992.

54. Cauchemez B, Haissaguerre M, Fischer B, et al.: Electrophysiological effects of catheter ablation of inferior vena cava-tricuspid annulus isthmus in common atrial flutter. Circulation 93:284-294, 1996.

55. Cosio FG, Lopez-Gil M, Goicolea A, et al.: Radiofrequency ablation of the inferior vena cava-tricuspid valve isthmus in common atrial flutter. Am J Cardiol 71:705-709, 1993.

56. Fischer B, Haissaguerre M, Garrigues S, et al.: Radiofrequency catheter ablation of common atrial flutter in 80 patients. J Am Coll Cardiol 25:1365-1372, 1995.

57. Schwartzman D, Callans DJ, Gottlieb CD, et al.: Conduction block in the inferior vena caval-tricuspid valve isthmus: Association with outcome of radiofrequency ablation of type I atrial flutter. J Am Coll Cardiol 28:1519-1531, 1996.

58. Jais P, Haissaguerre M, Shah DC, et al.: A focal source of atrial fibrillation treated by discrete radiofrequency ablation. Circulation 95:572-576, 1997.

59. Haissaguerre M, Jais P, Shah DC, et al.: Spontaneous initiation of atrial fibrillation by ectopic beats originating in the pulmonary veins. N Engl J Med 339:659-666, 1998.

60. Gerstenfeld EP, Guerra P, Sparks PB, et al.: Clinical outcome after radiofrequency catheter ablation of focal atrial fibrillation triggers. J Cardiovasc Electrophysiol 12:900-908, 2001.

61. Marrouche NF, Dresing T, Cole C, et al.: Circular mapping and ablation of the pulmonary vein for treatment of atrial fibrillation: Impact of different catheter technologies. J Am Coll Cardiol 40:464-474, 2002.

62. Pappone C, Rosanio S, Oreto G, et al.: Circumferential radiofrequency ablation of pulmonary vein ostia: A new anatomic approach for curing atrial fibrillation. Circulation 102:2619-2628, 2000.

63. Mangrum JM, Mounsey JP, Kok LC, et al.: Intracardiac echocardiography-guided, anatomically based radiofrequency ablation of focal atrial fibrillation originating from pulmonary veins. J Am Coll Cardiol 39:1964-1972, 2002.

64. Oral H, Knight BP, Tada H, et al.: Pulmonary vein isolation for paroxysmal and persistent atrial fibrillation. Circulation 105:1077-1081, 2002.

65. Macle L, Jais P, Weerasooriya R, et al.: Irrigated-tip catheter ablation of pulmonary veins for treatment of atrial fibrillation. J Cardiovasc Electrophysiol 13:1067-1073, 2002.

66. Ouyang F, Antz M, Ernst S, et al.: Recovered pulmonary vein conduction as a dominant factor for recurrent atrial tachyarrhythmias after complete circular isolation of the pulmonary veins: lessons from double Lasso technique. Circulation. 111(2):127-135, 2005.

67. Haissaguerre M, Jais P, Shah DC, et al.: Electrophysiological end point for catheter ablation of atrial fibrillation initiated from multiple pulmonary venous foci. Circulation 101:1409-1417, 2000.

68. Chen SA, Hsieh MH, Tai CT, et al.: Initiation of atrial fibrillation by ectopic beats originating from the pulmonary veins: Electrophysiological characteristics, pharmacological responses, and effects of radiofrequency ablation. Circulation 100:1879-1886, 1999.

69. Pappone C, Oreto G, Rosanio S, et al.: Atrial electroanatomic remodeling after circumferential radiofrequency pulmonary vein ablation: Efficacy of an anatomic approach in a large cohort of patients with atrial fibrillation. Circulation 104:2539-2544, 2001.

70. Bhargava M, Marrouche NF, Martin DO, et al.: Impact of age on the outcome of pulmonary vein isolation for atrial fibrillation using circular mapping technique and cooled-tip ablation catheter: A retrospective analysis. J Cardiovasc Electrophysiol 15:8-13, 2004.

71. Hoff PI, Chen J, Erga KS, et al.: Curative treatment of paroxysmal atrial fibrillation with radiofrequency ablation. Tidsskr Nor Laegeforen 124:625-628, 2004.

72. Schwartzman D, Bazaz R, Nosbisch J: Catheter ablation to suppress atrial fibrillation: Evolution of technique at a single center. J Interv Card Electrophysiol 9:295-300, 2003.

73. Ernst S, Ouyang F, Lober F, et al.: Catheter-induced linear lesions in the left atrium in patients with atrial fibrillation: an electroanatomic study. J Am Coll Cardiol 42:1271-1282, 2003.

74. Taylor GW, Kay GN, Zheng X, et al.: Pathological effects of extensive radiofrequency energy applications in the pulmonary veins in dogs. Circulation 101:1736-1742, 2000.

75. Robbins IM, Colvin EV, Doyle TP, et al.: Pulmonary vein stenosis after catheter ablation of atrial fibrillation. Circulation 98:1769-1775, 1998.

76. Purerfellner H, Cihal R, Aichinger J, et al.: Pulmonary vein stenosis by ostial irrigated-tip ablation: Incidence, time course, and prediction. J Cardiovasc Electrophysiol 14:165-167, 2003.

77. Saad EB, Marrouche NF, Saad CP, et al.: Pulmonary vein stenosis after catheter ablation of atrial fibrillation: Emergence of a new clinical syndrome. Ann Intern Med 138:634-638, 2003.

78. Tse HF, Reek S, Timmermans C, et al.: Pulmonary vein isolation using transvenous catheter cryoablation for treatment of atrial fibrillation without risk of pulmonary vein stenosis. J Am Coll Cardiol 42:752-758, 2003.

79. Pappone C, Oral H, Santinelli V, et al.: Atrio-esophageal fistula as a complication of percutaneous transcatheter ablation of atrial fibrillation. Circulation 109:2724-2726, 2004.

80. Calkins H: Role of invasive EP testing in the evaluation and management of right ventricular outflow tract tachycardias. Cardiac EP Rev 4:71-75, 2000.

81. Wen MS, Yeh SJ, Wang CC, et al.: Radiofrequency ablation therapy in idiopathic left ventricular tachycardia with no obvious structural heart disease. Circulation 89:1690-1696, 1994.

82. Epstein LM, Chiesa N, Wong MN, et al.: Radiofrequency catheter ablation in the treatment of supraventricular tachycardia in the elderly. J Am Coll Cardiol 23:1356-1362, 1994.

83. Zado ES, Callans DJ, Gottlieb CD, et al.: Efficacy and safety of catheter ablation in octogenarians. J Am Coll Cardiol 35:458-462, 2000.

84. Da Costa A, Zarqane-Sliman N, Romeyer-Bouchard C, et al.: Safety and efficacy of radiofrequency ablation of common atrial flutter in elderly patients: A single center prospective study. Pacing Clin Electrophysiol 26:1729-1734, 2003.

85. Kugler JD, Danford DA, Deal BJ, et al.: Radiofrequency catheter ablation for tachyarrhythmias in children and adolescents. The Pediatric Electrophysiology Society. N Engl J Med 330:1481-1487, 1994.

86. Torres Iturralde P, Garrido Garcia LM, Cordero A, et al.: Radiofrequency ablation in the treatment of supraventricular arrhythmias in pediatrics: Experience with 203 consecutive patients. Arch Inst Cardiol Mex 68:27-36, 1998.

87. Celiker A, Kafali G, Karagoz T, et al.: The results of electrophysiological study and radio-frequency catheter ablation in pediatric patients with tachyarrhythmia. Turk J Pediatr 45:209-216, 2003.

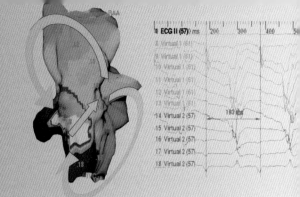

33

Trans-septal Catheterization

Westby G. Fisher • Alexander S. Ro

Key Points

- Safe trans-septal catheterization requires thorough familiarity with cardiac anatomy and the trans-septal apparatus.

- Contraindications to trans-septal catheterization include left atrial thrombus, severe bleeding diathesis, atrial septal closure devices, significant anatomic abnormalities and uncooperative patient.

- Intracardiac echocardiography minimizes complications and greatly facilitates difficult cases.

- The risks of complications is inversely related to operator expertise.

Trans-septal catheterization has gained widespread acceptance in the electrophysiology community as a viable approach for ablation of left-sided arrhythmias. With growing interest in pulmonary vein isolation for atrial fibrillation as well as the ability to map and ablate focal left atrial tachycardias, it is likely that experience with this technique will become an indispensable skill for any interventional electrophysiologist. First introduced in 1958 by Ross et al.[1] and Cope,[2] trans-septal catheterization was seen as an alternative method to retrograde transaortic measurement of left-sided pressures. Despite subsequent modifications in the technique by Braunwald,[3] Brockenbrough et al.,[4] and Mullins,[5] its popularity quickly declined because of fear of cardiac perforation and the use of pulmonary artery flotation catheters as a surrogate for left atrial pressures. The advent of percutaneous mitral valve commissurotomy renewed interest in the procedure in the 1980s. However, its use remained restricted to a limited number of interventional cardiologists in high-volume cardiac catheterization laboratories.

With the development of radiofrequency catheter ablation, resurgence of trans-septal catheterization developed as an alternative approach to left-sided accessory pathway ablation. Studies comparing trans-septal to retrograde approaches for left-sided accessory pathway ablation have suggested at least comparable success and fewer complications with the trans-septal approach.[6,7] The trans-septal approach to accessory pathway ablation provides a nonobstructive path from the right atrium to the mitral valve annulus and avoids arterial system complications such as femoral arteriovenous fistula, femoral artery pseudoaneurysm, iliofemoral thrombotic occlusion, papillary muscle disruption, aortic dissection, and aortic valvular perforation.[8]

Trans-septal catheterization will continue to play a significant role in the field of electrophysiology. Lack of familiarity with the technique, however, makes performing the procedure a formidable task for many. Ultimately, the most important predictor for the likelihood of a successful procedure is operator experience. With recent refinements in the technique, newer imaging modalities, and the understanding of anatomic landmarks reliably gained from electrode catheters in the heart, it is hoped that the procedure will become more accepted by electrophysiologists and associated with less apprehension and fear.

This chapter reviews the anatomy of the interatrial septum and vital surrounding structures; the technique of trans-septal catheterization, including setup and adjunctive tools that we commonly use in our laboratory; and potential complications and pitfalls that should be avoided. The use of intracardiac echocardiography (ICE) during trans-septal catheterization is also reviewed, as are more complicated variations of the trans-septal technique used to gain access to the left atrium with two sheaths.

Anatomy

A thorough understanding of anatomy for both right and left atria and the interatrial septum is vital for a successful and safe trans-septal catheterization.[9] The right atrium lies rightward, superior, and anterior to the left atrium. Its free wall has a smooth posterior portion and a muscular anterolateral portion, and its floor is the orifice of the tricuspid valve. In contrast, the left atrium lies leftward, posterior, and inferior to the right atrium at the base of the heart. The interatrial septum lies between the two and is bounded anteriorly by the sinus of Valsalva and posteriorly by pericardium. Access to the left atrium from the right side is obtained through the fossa ovalis via either a needle puncture or a patent foramen ovale (Fig. 33–1). The fossa ovalis lies in the posterior aspect of the intra-atrial septum and is bounded superiorly by the limbus, an arch-shaped outer muscular rim.

The fossa ovalis comprises roughly 25% to 30% of the total septal area and is usually the thinnest portion of the septum. The diameter of the fossa can vary dramatically from patient to patient. In one series of older children and adults aged 10 to 70 years, fossa areas ranged from 97 to 490 mm^2 (average, 240 mm^2).[10] The membrane consistency varies as well, usually becoming thicker and more fibrotic with age. From an embryologic standpoint, the interatrial septum arises from the development of two membranes in succession that separate the primitive left and right atria. The septum primum grows ventrally from the dorsal cranial wall, followed by the septum secundum, which grows from the ventral cranial wall. The fossa ovalis is the remnant of the foramen ovale, which acts as the communication between the two atria that allows well-oxygenated blood to move from the inferior vena cava to the left side of the heart during fetal life. In 20% of patients, this opening remains patent, allowing for access to the left heart without the use of a needle puncture.

Most complications that arise from trans-septal catheterization occur as a result of inadvertent puncture of adjacent structures to the interatrial septum and fossa ovalis. As stated earlier, the interatrial septum is bounded posteriorly by the pericardium. The aortic root lies superior and anterior to the fossa ovalis, whereas the ostium of the coronary sinus (CS) lies inferior to the fossa ovalis and posterior to the tricuspid valve orifice. In pathologic hearts, there fre-

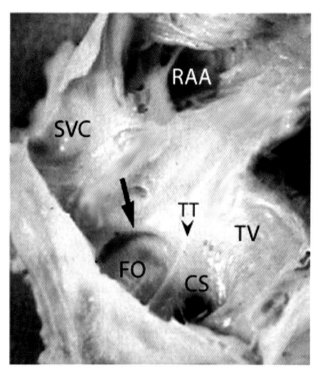

FIGURE 33–1. Right atrial septal anatomy. A post-mortem right atrium opened to expose the septal wall of the right atrium is seen. Note the right atrial free wall was incised and the superior portion of the atrium lifted superiorly to expose the endocardium of the right atrial appendage (RAA). The posterior aspect of the atrium lies to the left and the anterior aspect of the atrium to the right. Note the fossa ovalis (FO) occupies a significant portion of the right atrial septum. The superior limbus of the fossa ovalis (*larger arrow*) is clearly demonstrated. CS, coronary sinus os; SVC, superior vena cava; TT, Tendon of Todaro; TV, tricuspid valve.

quently is distortion of the atrial and interatrial septum anatomy, which can significantly alter the proximity of these structures. The septum tends to lie more horizontal in patients with left atrial enlargement, and it can be more vertical in patients with aortic valve disease or a dilated aortic root. Varying degrees of kyphoscoliosis can also alter intrathoracic cardiac rotation. In addition, prior open heart surgery can result in a thickened fossa ovalis, because surgeons occasionally must oversew the fossa in patients with a patent foramen ovale to ensure evacuation of air from the left atrium before terminating cardiopulmonary bypass. Because fluoroscopy allows only indirect assessment of the location of the fossa ovalis without good visual representation of these critical anatomic landmarks, advancement of the trans-septal needle using earlier, fluoroscopically-guided techniques was frequently associated with unpredictable outcomes. More recently, the introduction of ICE has added greatly to the appreciation of the anatomic variability and location of the fossa ovalis.[11-13] ICE has permitted many more electro-

physiologists to gain acceptable confidence to perform the procedure and its use adds valuable early insight to the development of pericardial effusion or, in the case of pulmonary vein isolation procedures, accelerated pulmonary venous flows indicative of impending stenosis.

PROCEDURAL PREPARATION

The Laboratory Facilities and Staff

Although complications are rare, trans-septal catheterization must be performed by doctors and laboratory personnel familiar with the administration of conscious sedation and the associated monitoring required, including electrocardiographic, hemodynamic, and pulse oximetry or end-tidal carbon dioxide measurements. Equipment for treatment of cardiovascular emergencies such as pericardial tamponade should also be readily available. With the close attention to administrative cost-saving measures at interventional laboratories, pressure to limit personnel performing this procedure exists. A minimum of four personnel should be present when trans-septal catheterization is performed: (1) the physician performing the procedure, (2) the nurse or anesthesiologist to monitor vital signs and monitor conscious sedation, (3) a circulator to bring equipment, and (4) an individual to call for help, if needed. Any fewer personnel might delay the rapid response required to manage acute tamponade occurring in the anticoagulated patient after trans-septal catheterization.

Protamine Sulfate

Although it happens rarely, the operator must be prepared to deal with acute pericardial tamponade should cardiac perforation occur during the trans-septal process. In the setting of significant systemic anticoagulation with heparin, tamponade can develop rapidly, and anticoagulation must be reversed expeditiously. Familiarity with protamine sulfate, an antidote to heparin, must be gained before proceeding with trans-septal catheterization.

Protamine sulfate is itself a mild anticoagulant, but when it is given with heparin (which is strongly acidic), a stable, noncoagulating salt is created that inactivates the anticoagulant effect of heparin. On average, 1 mg of protamine will reverse approximately 90 USP units of heparin derived from beef lung or 115 USP units of heparin derived from porcine intestinal mucosa. Usually it is advised that no more than 50 mg of protamine be given over 10 minutes. Rapid administration of protamine can result in severe hypotension, anaphylactoid reactions, and respiratory compromise. Typically, no more than 100 mg of protamine should be administered acutely. Because protamine sulfate can cause anaphylaxis, medications should also be available to deal with this emergency.

Imaging Equipment

The importance of adequate (and preferably biplane) fluoroscopic equipment cannot be overstated. One must be able to visualize relatively small structures, such as the tip of the trans-septal needle within the dilator of a long vascular trans-septal sheath in obese patients. The ability to alter the angulation of the acquired fluoroscopic images to the right anterior oblique (RAO) or left anterior oblique (LAO) view should be present, because imaging in multiple planes provides added assurance of needle location before the trans-septal puncture.

Some centers routinely perform transesophageal echocardiography (TEE) to facilitate trans-septal catheterization with real-time echocardiography. Transthoracic echocardiography has limited utility in facilitating trans-septal catheterization because of the difficulty in reliably imaging the fossa ovalis and the trans-septal needle.[14] TEE can readily image the fossa ovalis and needle assembly, but it requires a second operator and greater degrees of sedation and is not practical for long procedures. More recently, ICE has been employed to facilitate trans-septal catheterization.[11-13] With this technology, a single operator can perform the procedure painlessly and continuously without sedation during invasive left atrial procedures, adding greatly to the safety of trans-septal procedures.

A totally venous access approach to trans-septal procedures is now commonly used in experienced electrophysiology laboratories.[15] Because electrophysiologic catheters are placed in strategic anatomic locations defined by their recorded electrograms, electrophysiologic recording equipment is required. Alternatively, if the laboratory is more comfortable with an arteriovenous approach—that is, an approach requiring arterial placement of a pigtail catheter—then hemodynamic pressure recording equipment (e.g., pressure transducers, pressurized heparinized saline infusions, tubing) is required.

Finally, machines that can perform activated clotting time (ACT) measurements after the trans-septal catheterization and heparinization should be readily available and calibrated before the procedure.

Patient Preparation

Patients undergoing trans-septal catheterization must tolerate lying flat for the procedure and be psychologically capable of following directions if minimal sedation is used. Blood dyscrasias such as coagulopathies or thrombocytopenia should be evaluated before enlisting the patient for this procedure. Other contraindications to the procedure must also be considered (Table 33–1). Echocardiographic evaluation of the left atrium to exclude pathologic masses or anatomic variants should also be obtained. Preprocedure TEE should be considered in patients who are at high risk for atrial or left ventricular thrombus.

Trans-septal Sheaths and Dilators

When assembling the sheaths and needles to perform trans-septal catheterization, it is important for the electrophysiologist or interventionalist to be familiar with the relative lengths and diameters of the equipment. At the time of this writing, most adult trans-septal sheaths are 59 to 63 cm in length with dilators 67 cm in length (Figs. 33–2 and 33–3). These dilators accommodate a Brockenbrough needle 71 cm in length. It should be noted that left-sided sheath dilators typically can only accommodate a guide wire of 0.032 inch or smaller, although plans to develop dilators capable of accommodating larger guide wires are being considered.

In rare circumstances, specialty trans-septal sheaths exist for procedures in extremely large patients, for specialized ablation catheter angulations, and for placement of multiple catheters through one trans-septal puncture (Figs. 33–3 and 33–4). These sheaths are longer (73 cm) and are equipped with one or more hemostatic valves and longer dilators; they therefore require an 89-cm Brockenbrough needle if placed primarily during the

TABLE 33–1
Contraindications to Trans-septal Catheterization
Absolute contraindications
Presence of left atrial thrombus
Severe bleeding diathesis
Presence of significant anatomic anomalies (e.g., severe kyphoscolosis, pneumonectomy)
Non-hemodynamically stable patient
Patient unable to remain still during the procedure or intolerant to sedation
Preexisting percutaneous septal closure devices implanted
Relative contraindications
Prior interatrial septal surgery

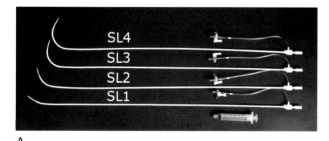

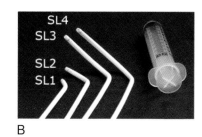

FIGURE 33–2. Trans-septal sheath designs—compound curvatures. Multiple trans-septal sheaths have been developed to provide improved catheter delivery in various portions of the left atrium. Longer distal curvatures are typically best for more inferoposterior aspects of the left atrium whereas shorter curvatures reach the upper left atrium more efficiently. St. Jude Medical's Daig SL sheaths (Minnetonka, MN) not only have varying lengths of curvature in one plane (**A**), but provide a second plane of curvature (SL1 through SL4) designed to orient the ablation catheter slightly anteriorly in close proximity to the mitral annulus (**B**).

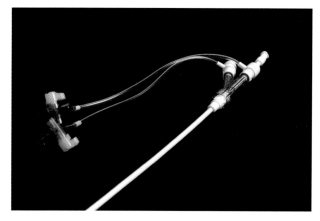

FIGURE 33–3. Trans-septal sheaths capable of carrying two wires through one lumen. Trans-septal sheaths are also available that can carry two small (4Fr) catheters with a single 8.5 F lumen. A Y-adapted hemostatic valve system is seen that assures air cannot be inadvertently passed into the left atrium. Because the Y-adapter adds 10 cm to the length of a conventional trans-septal sheath, a longer 89-cm Brockenbrough needle is required to perform trans-septal catheterization with this assembly.

trans-septal procedure. The operator should ensure that the length of the Brockenbrough needle corresponds to the length of the sheath and its dilator before proceeding with the trans-septal procedure.

The Brockenbrough Needle

Varying curvatures of the Brockenbrough needle have been developed to accommodate patients with varying right atrial anatomies. Although most trans-septal procedures are accomplished with a BRK (St. Jude Medical/Daig, St. Paul, Minn.) shaped Brockenbrough needle, adult patients with marked right atrial enlargement may require the enhanced curvature of the BRK-1 Brockenbrough needle to reach the interatrial septum (Fig. 33–5). For pediatric patients, a smaller BRK-2 curvature is available. The proximal end of the Brockenbrough needle contains a flange with a flat and a pointed end, replicating an arrow. The pointed tip of the arrow should always point in the plane of the curvature of the trans-septal needle. Additionally, all Brockenbrough needles are initially packaged with a thin stainless steel wire stylet (see Fig. 33–5B) that facilitates the passage of the needle into the dilator of the trans-septal sheath. Although this stylet can be discarded, we have found that

leaving it in place until the needle is just proximal to the distal end of the dilator prevents shearing of small filaments of plastic from the inner lumen of the trans-septal sheath with complex curvatures. The stylet should be removed and the lumen of the needle flushed with heparinized saline before trans-septal crossing.

TRANS-SEPTAL CATHETERIZATION

When performing trans-septal catheterization in the electrophysiology laboratory, it is our practice to always begin by placing a His bundle catheter and a CS catheter to provide these critical anatomic landmarks fluoroscopically. Electrophysiologists have long recognized that the presence of a His bundle catheter *that is recording a His bundle electrogram* always identifies the location of the most inferior aspect of the noncoronary cusp of the aorta. This obviates the need for an arterial puncture to place a pigtail catheter in the ascending aorta. One must remember that an electrophysiologic catheter that is *not* recording a His bundle electrogram cannot reliably determine the location of the aorta. Additionally, a CS catheter properly placed along the atrioventricular groove defines the intrathoracic cardiac rotation and demarcates the widest portion of the left atrium parallel and just posterior to the mitral annulus. One must ensure that the CS catheter courses near the mitral annulus, by ensuring that equal-amplitude atrial and ventricular electrograms exist throughout the course of the catheter. If not, the catheter may have inadvertently been placed in a posterolateral

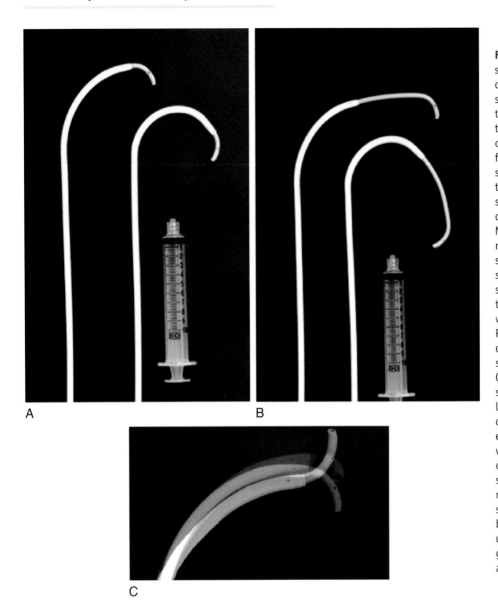

A   B

C

FIGURE   33–4. Telescoping sheath design. Another variation of trans-septal sheath demonstrates an 11Fr outer sheath through which a more conventional 8F sheath passes. The outer sheath serves as a platform from which to guide the inner sheath to different portions of the left atrium. In **A,** the outer sheath is demonstrated to have different degrees of curvature. Note the inner sheath is retracted within the outer sheath. In **B,** the inner sheath is shown extended and permits stable ablation catheter delivery to the far atrial walls in patients with left atrial enlargement. Panel **C** demonstrates the multidirectional capabilities of the sheath-within-a-sheath design. One must use care when this system is deployed within the left atrium, however, since the double sheath design is inherently stiff and unforgiving when manipulating an ablation catheter. Placement of this system within the left atrium requires a conventional trans-septal catheterization followed by a wire exchange (usually using a stiff 0.032-inch Amplatz guide wire) to place the sheath assembly within the left atrium.

branch of the CS and should be repositioned before the trans-septal catheterization is performed.

After selection of the appropriate sheath and dilator assembly and Brockenbrough needle, both the sheath and dilator should be flushed with heparinized saline. Using a modified Seldinger technique, an 8-French (F), 15-cm side-port sheath is initially placed in the right femoral vein.[16] Under fluoroscopic guidance, a 0.032-inch J wire is positioned from the right femoral venous approach retrogradely to the superior vena cava (SVC). The 8F short sheath is then removed, and the trans-septal sheath is placed over the 0.032-inch J wire into the SVC or left innominate vein. Once the sheath and dilator assembly are placed at this location, the guide wire is removed and the dilator is flushed carefully with heparinized saline to remove all evidence of bubbles. The 71-cm Brockenbrough needle and its stylet are then placed through the sheath and dilator assembly until the stylet of the needle lies just prox-

imal to the distal end of the sheath dilator (Fig. 33–6A). Because the Brockenbrough needle tapers slightly at its distal tip, care must be taken not to protrude the distal tip or needle stylet past the end of the sheath dilator to avoid inadvertent perforation of vascular structures.

Once the needle is located just proximal to the distal end of the sheath dilator, the needle is also flushed with heparinized saline, using care to first aspirate from the needle until a small amount of blood is visualized in the syringe chamber. On occasion, the sheath dilator presses against the wall of the SVC or innominate vein and aspiration from the needle is met with difficulty. In this case, small rotation of the needle is required to free the distal tip of the sheath dilator from the wall of the vessel, permitting flow of blood retrograde into the aspirating syringe. Once the blood is visualized and all bubbles have been removed from the chamber of the Brockenbrough needle, heparinized saline is flushed to clear the

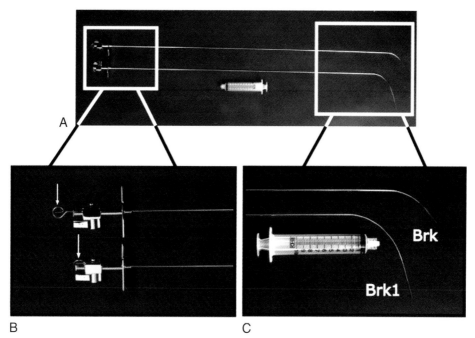

FIGURE 33–5. The Brockenbrough needle assembly. **A,** The Brockenbrough needle is typically 71 cm in length, although other long needles 89 cm in length (not shown) can be purchased for use with sheaths 73 cm in length or longer. A 10 cc syringe is shown for size comparison purposes. Note that the proximal end of the Brockenbrough needle has a hemostatic valve that contains a central thin stainless steel stylet (**B,** *arrow*) which should be removed before trans-septal crossing. **C,** Two curvatures of the Brockenbrough needle are demonstrated: BRK is used for most patients with relatively normal right atria. In the patients with marked dilation of the right atria, a BRK1 needle with its accentuated curvature will provide improved contact with the fossa ovalis.

needle of any potential source of air embolus or thrombus. The Brockenbrough needle may optionally be connected to hemodynamic measurement before trans-septal crossing with the sheath, if desired.

The LAO fluoroscopic camera view is adjusted so that the His bundle catheter is pointing directly at the image intensifier of the fluoroscopic camera in the LAO view. The RAO angulation is adjusted so that the projection of the CS catheter intersects the His bundle catheter at its midpoint and is directed perpendicular to the plane of the fluoroscopic image. Careful evaluation of the His bundle recording should be maintained to ensure an accurate anatomic reference relative to the inferior aspect of the aorta. The Brockenbrough needle and sheath assembly is withdrawn as a *single unit,* maintaining the relative positions of the needle and the sheath dilator from the SVC to the right atrium with the needle oriented in the 4 o'clock position (leftward and posterior). If the CS catheter has been placed from a superior approach, care must be used to ensure during torquing of the sheath that the CS catheter is not twisted around the sheath and needle assembly. If it is, the needle and sheath assembly should be rotated in a clockwise fashion before being withdrawn into the right atrium to free the CS catheter, and the needle should be reoriented to a 4 o'clock position. Withdrawal of the assembly from the SVC should occur in the LAO projection.

As the needle and sheath assembly is withdrawn, an initial slight leftward jump of the assembly is noted as it enters the right atrium. As it is withdrawn further, a second, more significant jump leftward occurs when the tip of the assembly approaches the level of the His bundle catheter, signifying that the assembly has fallen below the superior limbus of the fossa ovalis (see Fig. 33–6B). Once this level is located, the RAO fluoroscopic view should confirm that the assembly tip is well posterior to the site of the His bundle recording and that it is angled posterior and *parallel* to the projection of the CS catheter. This angle ensures that the assembly is not pointing posteriorly, which could allow the needle to perforate the posterior wall of the left atrium, and that it is not pointing too anteriorly, in which case the needle might enter the ascending aorta. Adjustments of angulation between 3 and 5 o'clock may be necessary, with enlarged left atria often requiring a more posterior (or 5 o'clock) angulation and vertically oriented hearts requiring a more anterior (3 o'clock) angulation of the needle.

Once the angulation of the needle and sheath assembly is confirmed, the LAO projection is visualized to perform the trans-septal crossing. The assembly is first withdrawn an additional 0.25 to 0.5 cm and then advanced to engage the limbus of the fossa ovalis (see Fig. 33–6B). At this juncture, in patients with a patent foramen ovale, the dilator of the sheath

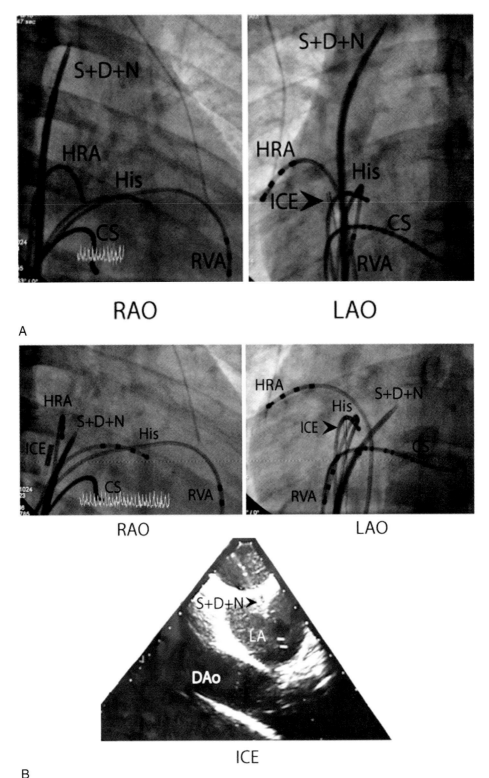

FIGURE 33–6. A, The trans-septal catheterization procedure—fluoroscopy of initial catheter placement. Forty-degree right anterior oblique (RAO) and 40-degree left anterior oblique (LAO) views are demonstrated. The sheath (S), its dilator (D), and needle (N) (S+D+N), have been placed in the left innominate vein retrograde from the right femoral venous approach. The needle is kept just proximal to the end of the sheath's dilator. Note the angulations of fluoroscopy are set so the LAO view demonstrates the His bundle catheter (His) and right ventricular apical (RVA) catheter identify the interventricular septum and are pointed toward the viewer. The RAO fluoroscopic angulation is determined by the plane where the coronary sinus (CS) catheter fluoroscopically crosses the proximal electrode of the His catheter and is oriented away from the viewer. The sheath, dilator, and needle are then withdrawn as a single unit from this position into the right atrium, maintaining the orientation of the Brockenbrough needle at approximately 4 o'clock (posterior and leftward). HRA, high right atrium; ICE, intracardiac echocardiography catheter. **B**, Trans-septal catheterization—sheath, dilator, and Brockenbrough needle at the fossa ovalis. Identical RAO and LAO fluoroscopic angulations to **A** demonstrate the sheath, dilator, and needle assembly at the level of the fossa ovalis. After withdrawing the sheath, dilator, and needle to the level of the fossa ovalis, the tip of the dilator moved distinctly leftward once the assembly reached the level of the His bundle catheter. The phased-array intracardiac echocardiographic image (ICE) at this location is also seen. Note tenting of the fossa ovalis by the dilator and needle is clearly demonstrated and the angulation of the assembly appears to be pointing toward the mid-cavity of the left atrium.

FIGURE 33–6, cont'd.
C, Trans-septal catheterization—the sheath, dilator, and Brockenbrough needle in the left atrium. Again the fluoroscopic angulations are the same as **A.** The needle was advanced slightly beyond the end of the sheath's dilator, and a palpable "pop" was noted, followed by an abrupt movement of the dilator into the left atrium. The needle has been withdrawn back into the sheath, but maintained across the septum to provide support for delivery of the sheath over the dilator and needle into the left atrium. (Catheter labels as in **A**).
D, Trans-septal catheterization—the sheath in the left atrium. RAO and LAO flouroscopic images of the sheath after it has been delivered into the left atrium and the dilator and needle withdrawn. Fluoroscopic angulations and catheter labels as in **A.**

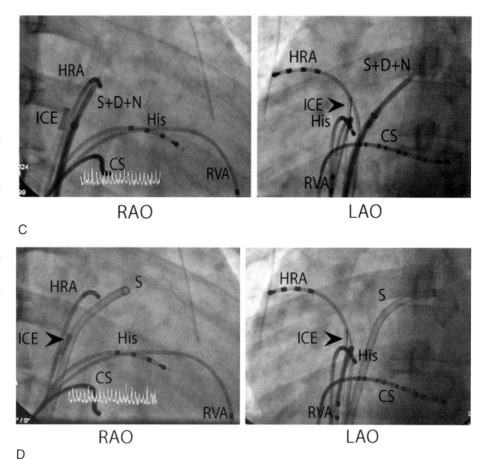

will be seen to move markedly toward the left atrium. If hemodynamic measurements are used, the left atrial pressure recording can be recorded from the trans-septal needle. Alternatively, the needle location can be confirmed by ICE (see Fig. 33–6B) or by injection of a small amount of contrast material through the trans-septal needle to confirm its left atrial location. More commonly, however, the dilator does not pass spontaneously into the left atrium. Pressure measurements taken from any trans-septal needle, if used, are usually damped or well off a 40 mm Hg scale while the needle and dilator are juxtaposed to the intra-atrial septum. Provided that the RAO and LAO projections are confirmed, the trans-septal needle can be advanced 1 to 2 mm from within the sheath dilator to enter the left atrium, and often a tactile "pop" is felt. Once the needle enters the left atrium, this position can be confirmed by a small hand contrast injection or by a pressure recording from the distal tip of the needle. The sheath dilator is then advanced over the needle assembly to enter the left atrium (see Fig. 33–6C).

Once the dilator has been placed within the left atrium, the needle is left just proximal to the end of the dilator to provide support for the more proximal aspects of the sheath to be placed over the dilator and

into the left atrium. If there is any question about the location of the needle after its advancement outside the sheath dilator, the dilator should never be advanced, to avoid catastrophic cardiac complications. A small contrast injection through the needle should be used if there is any question about its location. Puncture of the left atrium posteriorly or anteriorly *with the needle alone* has rarely resulted in significant cardiac complications. It is typically the dilation with the sheath dilator or sheath itself that can cause significant cardiac compromise. If there is aortic or pericardial staining after what is presumed to be trans-septal puncture, the needle must be removed and the dilator withdrawn; then the 0.032-inch J wire is repositioned to the SVC, and the process repeated until such time as proper trans-septal crossing is performed.

Once the dilator and sheath have been safely placed in the left atrium, the needle and dilator are removed carefully, and the sheath is aspirated to remove any evidence of thrombus or bubbles. The sheath is then carefully flushed with heparinized saline (Fig. 33–6D). Systemic heparinization is then administered. At this point, in patients requiring single trans-septal catheterization, it is our practice to place an ablation catheter into the left atrium, through the sheath, so that it lies within the pulmonary vein architecture outside the cardiac silhouette. Full curvature of the catheter is then employed, and the catheter is withdrawn from the pulmonary vein area until it falls into the body of the left atrium in a curled fashion. The ablation catheter can then be advanced carefully, with the catheter coiled so that it resembles a pig-tail catheter and has a low potential to perforate cardiac structures. Confirmation of free movement of the ablation catheter to ensure that it is positioned within the chamber of the left atrium (rather than possibly in the pericardium) is obtained by torquing the sheath clockwise and counterclockwise to document free mobility. Once this is confirmed, the patient should be immediately administered a heparin bolus (150 units/kg), followed by a continuous infusion to maintain an ACT of approximately 300 seconds. The ablation catheter curve can then be opened so that the catheter can lie on the mitral annulus or manipulated carefully to the areas of the pulmonary vein or targeted atrial tissue.

After the catheter ablation procedures, the ablation catheter and sheath are removed together by withdrawing the system back to the right atrium, and then the heparin is discontinued.

ADDITIONAL ANATOMIC CONSIDERATIONS

Just as patients have unique fingerprints, the fossa ovalis can vary in size and flexibility from patient to patient. In some, the fossa is extremely small, and localizing it can be difficult; in others, the fossa may extend above the level of the His catheter projection fluoroscopically, magnifying the concern about inadvertent perforation of the roof of the left atrium. In other cases, particularly in patients with septal aneurysms, the interatrial septum is very floppy or pliable, and the potential exists for the dilator to push the septal aneurism across the left atrium and perforate the posterior wall of the atrium. If there is a question about the size or location of the fossa ovalis or if trans-septal catheterization is difficult, either TEE or, more commonly, ICE should be used.

Adjunctive Intracardiac Ultrasound Imaging during Trans-septal Catheterization

In many centers, it is routine to perform ICE during trans-septal catheterization. Facilities that have such technology available should encourage its use. We have found cardiac ultrasound imaging to be invaluable during complicated ablation procedures, because it minimizes the risks of trans-septal catheterization while affording the advantage of continuous monitoring of the patient's pericardial space for fluid. Early identification of pericardial effusion can be made with ICE and prompt measures can be undertaken before hemodynamic compromise occurs. Perhaps the greatest assistance for the operator is in localization of the proper site of puncture during trans-septal catheterization.

In performing ICE imaging during trans-septal catheterization, two types of ultrasound catheters are available (Fig. 33–7). One is a 64-element, phased-array ultrasound system using a 10F, 9-MHz transducer (AcuNav, Seimens Acuson, Mountain View, Calif.) that images in a sector field oriented in the plane of the catheter rather than in a circumferential field of view (Fig. 33–8). The alternative ultrasound system uses a single rotating crystal ultrasound transducer based on either a 9F, 9-MHz rotating crystal or a 6.5F, 12.5-MHz ultrasound crystal (Boston Scientific CVIS, Sunnyvale, Calif.) (Fig. 33–9).

Rotating crystal transducers (see Fig. 33–9) image circumferentially for 360 degrees in the horizontal plane and view the intra-atrial septum well, but they do not have the capability to perform Doppler flow analysis and are not freely deflectable, so their imaging utility is limited. However, the 360-degree images make it relatively easy to interpret catheter orientation relative to anatomic structures. Several rotating crystal ultrasound catheter frequencies exist. Higher frequencies have better near-field resolution but penetrate for only limited distances. Ultrasound crystal frequencies greater than 12.5-MHz cannot adequately image far-field cardiac structures and therefore have limited utility during trans-septal catheterization. The ideal imaging frequency of the rotating crystal ultrasound catheter for trans-septal catheterization is 9-MHz.

It is the practice in our laboratory to use the phased-array ultrasound system during trans-septal catheterization. Although this catheter requires a steeper learning curve, the advantages of higher-resolution images, superior depth of imaging, and Doppler flow imaging capability make this a technology well suited for imaging left-sided anatomies (Fig. 33–10). The use of this catheter is accomplished by first placing an 8F sheath in the femoral vein, using a modified Seldinger technique, and then replacing it with an 11F, 23-cm sheath extending to the inferior vena cava, using an exchange guide wire approach. This sheath is then flushed with heparinized saline, and a 10F, 9 MHz deflectable ultrasound catheter is passed retrogradely to the right atrium. Once the catheter enters the right

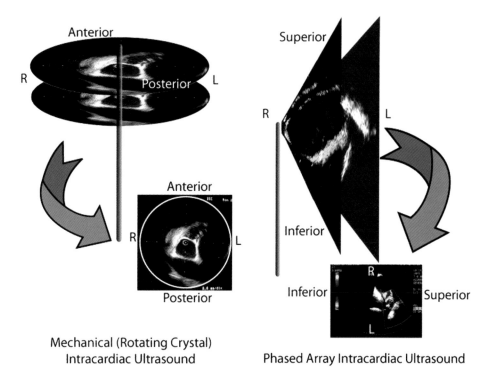

Mechanical (Rotating Crystal) Intracardiac Ultrasound

Phased Array Intracardiac Ultrasound

FIGURE 33–7. Comparison of images generated by two commercially available intracardiac echocardiographic catheters. The **left panel** demonstrates the plane of acquisition of images obtained using a mechanical rotating crystal catheter design. Since this catheter gathers echo data from a plane orthogonal to the length of the catheter in a 360-degree fashion, images demonstrate anatomy in the horizontal plane. In the **right panel**, phased array ultrasound catheters gather echo images from planes parallel to the orientation of the catheter and demonstrate only a sector of the plane. As such, only a segment of the anatomy is displayed. The anatomic detail is improved by providing 64 elements of piezoelectric crystals that are stationary and not influenced by rotational distortions. Additionally, doppler information is available to the operator to evaluate physiologic parameters of blood flow. *(See Figure 33–10.)*

atrium, it should be rotated to visualize the tricuspid valve. Clockwise torque of the catheter from this image rotates the crystal array posteriorly, so that the ascending aorta comes into view, followed by the more posterior fossa ovalis (see Fig. 33–8). It is helpful to deflect the catheter slightly away from the intra-atrial septum, so that it does not lie immediately adjacent to the interatrial septum; this provides better imaging and less interference with the trans-septal equipment. The ultrasound catheter is left in place, and the remainder of the trans-septal catheterization process is performed using both fluoroscopic and ultrasound guidance. The greatest utility of the ultrasound approach can be seen in tenting of the intra-atrial septum (see Fig. 33–6B). Care should be taken, however, to identify the tip of the *needle*, because septal tenting can be seen when the needle is against the thicker portions of the intra-atrial septum. A pitfall is to see the body of the trans-septal catheter transected by the echocardiographic beam and mistake this for the catheter tip.

Double Trans-septal Technique

In some procedures, there is an advantage to having two trans-septal sheaths placed through the intratrial septum simultaneously. The placement of a non-contact mapping balloon or basket mapping catheter through one sheath and an ablation catheter through the alternate sheath requires this approach. There are generally two approaches to this procedure: (1) perform two separate punctures of the fossa ovalis as outlined previously, or (2) place two sheaths via separate skin punctures through the same single site of the initial trans-septal puncture. Our laboratory typically performs the latter approach because of the ease of the exchange guide wire technique.

To place two sheaths through one trans-septal puncture site, after the first sheath is safely placed into the left atrium, it is flushed with heparinized saline.

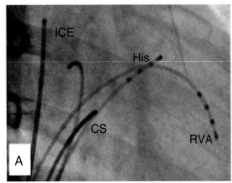

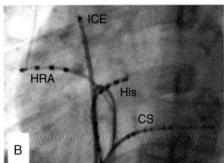

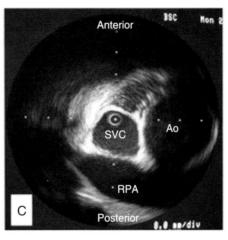

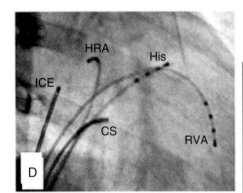

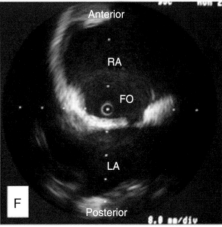

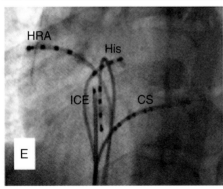

FIGURE 33–8. Example images obtained from a phased-array intracardiac echocardiographic catheter. **A,** After placing a phased array intracardiac echocardiographic (ICE) catheter into the right atrium (RA), the tricuspid valve should be identified. Clockwise rotation of the ICE catheter from this starting point will first identify the ascending aorta (Ao) (**B**). Note the His bundle catheter (His) is noted to be immediately adjacent to the non-coronary cusp of the aorta, and reliably identifies the inferior aspect of the aorta during trans-septal catheterization. Additional clockwise rotation of the catheter brings the left inferior pulmonary vein (LIPV) and portions of the left superior pulmonary vein (LSPV) into view (**C**). The descending aorta (DAO) is demonstrated immediately posterior to the LIPV. Additional rotation will identify the posterior left atrium (**D**) without the descending aorta in view. The foramen ovale (FO) is well seen in Panel **C** and **D**.

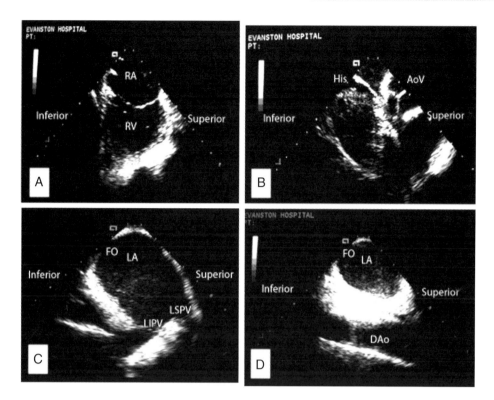

FIGURE 33–9. Example of rotating crystal intracardiac echo images. Right anterior oblique (RAO) (**A** and **D**) and left anterior oblique (LAO) (**B** and **E**) fluroscopic images demonstrating location of the intracardiac echocardiographic catheter (ICE) locations and their associated ultrasound images (**C** and **F**) are demonstrated at two different imaging planes. Panel **A** demonstrates the 40-degree RAO fluoroscopic image of the ICE catheter in the superior vena cava (SVC). Panel **B** demonstrates the same catheters as in panel **A** in the 40-degree LAO fluoroscopic projection. Panel **C** demonstrates the corresponding ICE image obtained at this level. The image has been rotated so anatomic leftward structures are to the right of the image and posterior structures are at the bottom of the image. Panels **D** and **E** are the 40-degree RAO and LAO images after the ICE catheter has been withdrawn from the SVC to lie at the level of the fossa ovalis (FO). Panel **F** demonstrates the corresponding intracardiac echocardiographic image at the level of the FO. Note the central circle within each ICE image was created by the ICE catheter itself. CS, coronary sinus catheter; His, His bundle catheter; HRA, Hight right atrium; RVA, right ventricular apical catheter.

FIGURE 33–10. Phased array intracardiac echocardiographic evaluation of pulmonary venous flows. **A,** Image of the left atrium (LA) in the plane of the left inferior pulmonary vein (LIPV) is demonstrated. **B,** Pulsed-wave doppler can be utilized to demonstrate the peak flow velocities through the pulmonary vein. Alternatively, color flow analysis of the pulmonary venous flow (**C**) can help identify blood flow direction and turbulence of flow.

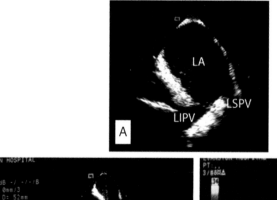

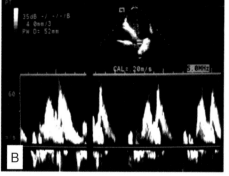

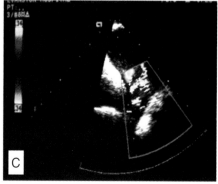

Then the dilator of the first trans-septal sheath is removed and flushed with heparinized saline. Next, an alternate 8F, 15-cm sheath, previously placed in the right femoral vein, is removed and replaced with the second trans-septal sheath, which is again placed retrograde to the SVC or left innominate vein. The dilator of this second sheath is also flushed with heparinized saline to remove all evidence of bubbles. A Brockenbrough needle is placed into the second sheath and flushed carefully with heparinized saline.

Next, a 0.032-inch guide wire is passed through the dilator of the *first* trans-septal sheath, and the guide wire and dilator are replaced back into the first trans-septal sheath, using care to pass the guide wire well into the left superior or left inferior pulmonary vein. Once the guide wire is placed well into the pulmonary vein, the first sheath and dilator are withdrawn back into the right atrium, leaving the 0.032-inch guide wire in the left atrium. The *second* sheath/dilator assembly is then withdrawn from the SVC in the same angle as the first trans-septal crossing, using the Brockenbrough needle to torque the second sheath. Once the dilator falls to the level of the existing trans-septal guide wire, the biplane orientation of the second sheath's dilator to the transseptal guide wire is adjusted until the dilator passes immediately adjacent to the guide wire into the left atrium. Needle puncture of the interatrial septum typically is not required. The second sheath and dilator are passed into the left atrium, and the Brockenbrough needle and dilator are removed. The second sheath is then flushed carefully with heparinized saline. Finally, the first sheath and dilator are advanced over the trans-septally retained guide wire, and the dilator and guide wire are removed, leaving both sheaths within the left atrium. The original sheath is again carefully flushed with heparinized saline. Heparin administration is then begun, and placement of the mapping basket or lasso catheter can begin after the ACTs exceed 300 sec.

Conclusion

Trans-septal catheterization is now routinely performed in electrophysiology laboratories to access the left atrium for a wide variety of procedural indications. Electrophysiology catheters and ICE, coupled with increased operator experience and improvements in understanding of the anatomic variables among patients, have resulted in improved safety and reliability of this approach. With appropriate care and respect for the issues involved with the procedure, trans-septal catheterization is now readily accessible and is an indispensable skill for the busy electrophysiologist.

Acknowledgments

The authors would like to thank Mr. Jonathan F. Hillebrand of Multimedia Services at Evanston Hospital, Evanston, Illinois, for his tireless efforts to secure the figures that accompany this chapter. In addition, we thank the staff of the Electrophysiology Division of Evanston Northwestern Healthcare for their exceptional professionalism and care rendered to our patients during the preparation of this manuscript.

References

1. Ross J, Braunwald E, Morrow AG: Transseptal left atrial puncture: New technique for the measurement of left atrial pressures. Am J Cardiol 3:653-655, 1959.
2. Cope C: Technique for the transseptal catheterization of the left atrium: Preliminary report. J Thorac Surg 37:482-486, 1959.
3. Braunwald E: Transseptal left heart catheterization. Circulation 37(Suppl 3):74-79, 1968.
4. Brockenbrough EC, Braunwald E, Ross J Jr: Transseptal left heart catheterization: A review of 450 studies and description of an improved technique. Circulation 25:15-21, 1962.
5. Mullins CE: Transseptal left heart catheterization: Experience with a new technique in 520 pediatric and adult patients. Pediatr Cardiol 4:239-245, 1983.
6. Lesh MD, Van Hare GF, Scheinman MM, et al.: Comparison of the retrograde and transseptal methods for left free wall accessory pathways. J Am Coll Cardiol 22:542-549, 1993.
7. Packer DL, Hammill SC, Holmes DR: Comparison of transaortic and transseptal approaches for the ablation of left-sided accessory pathways [abstract]. Circulation 86(Suppl 1):I-783, 1992.
8. Seifort MJ, Morady F, Calkins HG, Langberg JJ: Aortic leaflet perforation during radiofrequency ablation. Pacing Clin Electrophysiol 14:1582-1585, 1991.
9. Anderson RH, Becker AE: Cardiac Anatomy: An Integrated Text and Color Atlas. London: Gower Medical Publishing, 1980, pp 2.2-2.22.
10. Sweeney LJ, Rosenquist GC: The normal anatomy of the atrial septum in the human heart. Am Heart J 98:194-199, 1979.
11. Hung JS, Fu M, Yeh KH, et al.: Usefulness of intracardiac echocardiography in complex transseptal catheterization during percutaneous transvenous commissurotomy. Mayo Clin Proc 71:134-140, 1996.
12. Daoud EG, Kalbfleisch SJ, Hummel JD: Intracardiac echocardiography to guide transseptal catheterization for radiofrequency catheter ablation. J Cardiovasc Electrophysiol 10:358-363, 1999.
13. Epstein LM, Smith T, TenHoff H: Nonfluoroscopic transseptal catheterization: Safety and efficacy of intracardiac echocardiographic guidance. J Cardiovasc Electrophysiol 9:625-630, 1998.
14. Sethi KK, Mohan JC: Transseptal catheterization for the electrophysiologist: Modification with a "view." J Interv Card Electrophysiol 5:97-99, 2001.
15. Gonzalez MD, Otomo K, Shah N, et al.: Transseptal left heart catheterization for cardiac ablation procedures. J Interv Cardiac Electrophysiol 5:89-95, 2001.
16. Swartz JF, Fisher WG, Tracy CM: Ablation of left-sided atrioventricular accessory pathways via the transeptal atrial approach. In: Huang SKS (ed). Radiofrequency catheter ablation of cardiac arrhythmias: Basic concepts and clinical applications. Armonk NY: Futura Publishing, 1995, p. 255.

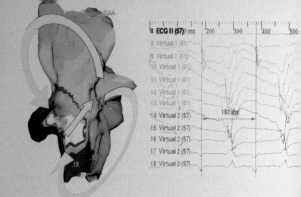

34

Special Considerations for Ablation in Pediatric Patients

J. Philip Saul

Key Points

- Children have the same variety of arrhythmia mechanisms as adults, but with a different distribution and often in different clinical settings.

- Although older children are physically similar to adults, children are not just little adults when it comes to the choice to proceed with and techniques for performing ablation.

- Ablation in infants and very small children carries a variety of special risks and should be undertaken only after failure of medical therapy and in the most experienced hands.

- The presence of structural congenital heart disease significantly complicates any ablation procedure, demanding that the operator be familiar with both the structural and electrophysiologic issues at hand, particularly if atrioventricular discordance is present.

- Atrial flutter and fibrillation are rare arrhythmias in the pediatric population in the absence of congenital heart disease.

- Atrial ectopic tachycardia, junctional ectopic tachycardia, and the permanent form of junctional reciprocating tachycardia can all manifest as incessant tachyarrhythmias with a dilated cardiomyopathy in children. Ablation therapy may be particularly helpful in such cases, if it can be performed safely.

- For ablation in children, safety should always take precedence over efficacy. Consequently, if it is appropriate, cryotherapy is often the technology of first choice.

The explosion in understanding and management of most arrhythmias in adults over the last 15 years is both reflected and amplified in the field of pediatrics. The application of procedures or devices commonly used in the management of arrhythmias in adults is often somewhat delayed in children due to technical issues related to size or lack of regulatory approval. Other issues, such as a smaller numbers of patients and a higher diversity of clinical characteristics and age, have limited the ability to perform controlled therapeutic trials, even multicenter ones. Despite these limitations, a combination of continued technical developments in the miniaturization of devices, multicenter retrospective reviews,[1,2] and the use of pharmacologic agents approved by the U.S. Food and Drug Administration for adults[3,4] has resulted in an equivalence in the armamentarium of adult and pediatric electrophysiologists. However, as is reviewed in this chapter, the parity of tools does not necessarily imply parity of disease and its management.

This chapter concentrates primarily on two categories of rhythm disorders: arrhythmias that are mechanistically similar or identical to those in adults, but whose presentation and management is complicated by the presence of young age or congenital heart disease, and arrhythmias that are either unique to pediatric patients or are observed only rarely in adults (Table 34–1). Some arrhythmias and their presentations are covered in other chapters and are mentioned here only briefly in the context of differences from the typical adult patient. Although many patients with congenital heart disease and arrhythmias are in fact adults, for the purposes of this chapter, the term *adult* will be used to refer to patients without congenital heart disease who are not usually cared for by a pediatric cardiologist.

Are Children Just Little Adults?

The notion that children are simply small adults is not entirely inaccurate, particularly when it comes to catheter ablation for some arrhythmias in relatively older and larger children, perhaps after 10 to 12 years of age. However, for many procedures, what seems like only a difference of scale can have dramatic implications, which begin with the diagnosis,[5] extend from the initial recommendation for an ablation to the technical performance of the procedure,[6] and end with the long-term risks of producing radiofrequency (RF) lesions in developing myocardium[7] and near coronary arteries.[8-12]

TABLE 34–1
Comparison of Arrhythmias in Children and Adults
Arrhythmias not typically observed in adults
Ectopic atrial tachycardia
Junctional ectopic tachycardia
Permanent junctional reciprocating tachycardia (PJRT)
Double atrioventricular nodes
Alternative presentations of arrhythmias commonly observed in adults
Atrioventricular nodal reentrant tachycardia (AVNRT)
Preexcitation syndromes in infants
Preexcitation syndromes with congenital heart disease
Ventricular tachycardia with tetralogy of Fallot
Atrial reentry with congenital heart disease
Arrhythmias with similar management in adults and children
Preexcitation syndromes after infancy
Congenital long QT syndrome
Right ventricular outflow tract (RVOT) ventricular tachycardia
Arrhythmogenic right ventricular dysplasia
Benign accelerated idioventricular rhythm

On average, children are obviously smaller than adults, resulting in smaller cardiac chambers, thinner and perhaps more fragile tissues, smaller coronary arteries, and smaller distances between structures, such as the posterior septum and the atrioventricular (AV) node, or the AV ring and the coronary arteries. Not so obviously, children may be dissimilar from adults in ways other than size. Arrhythmia mechanisms overlap but are proportionately very different.[5,13-15] Incessant arrhythmias are much more common,[16-18] probably based both on better early tolerance and on late morbidity and mortality if left untreated, which ensures that most patients will not reach adulthood with their arrhythmias. Accessory pathway (AP) locations are skewed toward the right side,[18,19] at least partially related to the simultaneous presence of structural congenital heart disease.[20-23] In addition, developing myocardium appears to have the potential for spontaneous cure of an arrhythmia[2] but also the potential for dramatic RF lesion growth with time.[7] Finally, children are generally less cooperative and tolerant than adults, a feature that necessitates special attention in all aspects of the ablation procedure. These issues are discussed in detail in this chapter, along with a review of possible solutions and the implications for management of arrhythmias treatable by RF catheter ablation in both children and adults.

ARRHYTHMIA MECHANISMS

The arrhythmias seen in pediatric patients are typically the more treatable varieties. Ventricular tachycardia is relatively rare in children, accounting for fewer than 5% of all tachycardias and only 20% of wide-complex tachycardias.[24] In addition, when ventricular tachycardia does occur in a child without structural heart disease, it is more likely than in an adult to have one of the ablatable mechanisms (see Chapters 25 through 28).[25-27] Supraventricular tachycardia (SVT), which accounts for the vast majority of arrhythmias in children, is most likely to result from a concealed or manifest accessory AV pathway (Fig. 34–1),[5] again portending well for possible catheter ablation therapy. In the absence of a history of surgery for structural congenital heart disease, APs probably underlie about 75% of all SVTs in children[5] and account for about 95% of SVTs in neonates,[28,29] compared with 30% to 40% of SVTs in adults.[14,15] Atrioventricular nodal reentrant tachycardia (AVNRT) and primary atrial tachycardias (both reentrant and automatic) each appear to account for about half of the remaining SVTs (see Fig. 34–1).[5]

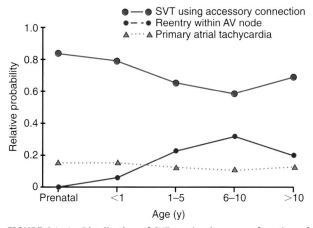

FIGURE 34–1. Distribution of SVT mechanisms as a function of age in pediatric patients. The percentage of patients with primary atrial tachycardias remains relatively constant, while there is a shift from accessory pathway mediated tachycardias to AV nodal reentry from infancy to adolescence. *(From Ko JK, Deal BJ, Strasburger JF, Benson DW Jr.: Supraventricular tachycardia mechanisms and their age distribution in pediatric patients. Am J Cardiol 69:1028-1032, 1992, with permission.)*

THE DECISION TO ABLATE: SAFETY VERSUS EFFICACY

One overriding theme in the management of arrhythmias in children compared with adults is an emphasis on safety over efficacy. Although there are few cases at any age in which safety is not an important concern, the relatively benign course of many arrhythmic conditions in childhood, the potential disruption that even therapies such as permanent pacing cause for a child, and the fact that parents are usually the decision-making surrogate for the child often lead to a different decision tree for children than for adults. Further, for some situations and technologies (e.g., the potential for coronary damage with RF energy application at the AV groove), the size of the patient and of the heart may really matter.

Ablation in patients with Wolff-Parkinson-White (WPW) syndrome is an excellent example of how decision making may be highly age dependent.[30] In this chapter, the term *WPW* will be used to describe the condition of preexcitation on the surface electrocardiogram (ECG), with or without coexisting tachycardia. Due to a variety of concerns, even the most symptomatic infant with WPW and paroxysmal SVT is only rarely a candidate for ablation.[31-33] Myocardial injury[7] and potentially severe coronary injury[8-10,34] are more likely with ablation in this age group. Further, about 40% of APs in infants spontaneously stop functioning during the first year of life,[2,35] and an additional third of patients are unlikely to have symptoms between infancy and early childhood.[36] In children older than 4 years of age who have symptomatic arrhythmias, the balance between risks and benefits clearly shifts toward ablation therapy, but usually only if the ablation can be performed safely.[30] In contrast to the situation in infants, even asymptomatic WPW patients between the ages of 10 and 18 years may be managed more aggressively than adults. Unlike asymptomatic adults older than age 28 years, who are unlikely to ever have symptoms,[37,38] the older child with a high-risk pathway is exactly the type of patient who may present with sudden arrhythmic death as their initial symptom, leading to the recommendation that such patients should undergo risk stratification, with those who are high risk being offered catheter ablation as a therapeutic option.[39] Further, the guidelines for sports participation in patients with WPW recommend risk stratification before approval for this age group.[40] Other age-dependent differences in management decisions are addressed in the discussions of individual arrhythmias.

Alternative Presentations or Management of Arrhythmias Commonly Observed in Adults

The complexity of an arrhythmia and its management may result from either the nature of the abnormal rhythm or the setting in which it occurs. The latter aspect is addressed in this section of the chapter, including AVNRT in the child, preexcitation syndromes in the infant and small child, preexcitation syndromes in the patient with congenital heart disease, and atrial reentry (flutter or fibrillation) in the pediatric patient without congenital heart disease. Atrial and ventricular tachyarrhythmias in the patient with congenital heart disease are addressed in Chapters 13 and 31, respectively.

ATRIOVENTRICULAR NODAL REENTRY TACHYCARDIA IN THE CHILD

The issue, addressed earlier, of rebalancing safety and efficacy in the decision-making process for a child is particularly important in the management of AVNRT. A number of factors that are distinctly different in children compared with adults must be taken into account. These factors are related to particular risk in children that may affect the decision to ablate, the diagnosis of dual AV nodal physiology and AVNRT, and the technical aspects of the ablation procedure.

Medical Management

No natural history data exist for the medical management of AVNRT presenting in childhood. However, at presentation AV node reentry appears easier to manage medically in children than in adults, and particularly in infants.[41]

Atrioventricular Node Physiology in Children

Based on the classic definition for dual AV node physiology—a 50-msec increase in the atrium-to-His bundle (AH) interval for a 10-msec decrement in the atrium-to-atrium (A-A) interval, many fewer pediatric[42,43] than adult[44] patients with inducible AVNRT have demonstrable dual AV nodal physiology (about 60% versus 90% to 100%, respectively). Because the mechanism of AVNRT induction is similar in children with or without demonstrable dual AV nodal physiology, the presence of two pathways must be assumed. The notion is that the difference in the baseline conduction properties of the two pathways does not reach the threshold for dual physiology in about

40% of children, suggesting that less stringent or more specific criteria may be necessary to define dual AV nodal physiology in children. For instance, the transition from fast to slow pathway conduction may occur with a change in the slope of the AH response to a change in A-A interval,[45] but without a change in AH interval that meets the 50-msec criterion.[46] In fact, a change in conduction pathway could theoretically take place without any change in the AH interval. One might speculate that the magnitude of the AH change at the transition from the fast to the slow pathway would indeed be related to heart size and therefore to age, because normal AV nodal conduction times, expressed as either the AH or the PR interval, increase with age. Younger children have also been shown to have faster conduction in the slow pathway than older children and adults.[47] Consequently, in children, the slope change of AH versus A-A is probably a more reliable and specific measure of the transition between the fast and slow pathways than AH jump criterion alone.

Decision to Ablate and Safety Issues

Once a decision has been made to perform slow pathway modification in a child, identification of appropriate locations for modification is not particularly different from that in adults (see Chapters 18 and 19). Further, the ablation technique and end points for either RF ablation or cryoablation do not vary significantly in children and adults, with the exception that a smaller catheter should generally be used in smaller children (<20 kg or so), to minimize the lesion size. With the use of such techniques, it appears that more than 95% of AVNRT can be eliminated in adults or children.[18,19,43] However, two safety issues and their implications should make a significant difference between adults and children in the decision to use RF ablation: the risk of AV block and the risk of coronary damage.

Atrioventricular Block

The possibility of ablation-induced complete heart block deserves special attention in the pediatric patient for two reasons. First, the risk of heart block is theoretically higher in smaller patients, simply due to a number of geometric differences. Because the size of an average RF lesion does not depend on patient size,[7,48,49] the typical lesion is relatively large compared with the size of the heart in a smaller patient. The smaller the patient, the closer the AV node is to the area of the slow pathway and to the posterior and anterior septum, common locations for APs. Further, the AV node itself is smaller in small hearts and therefore can be included in a typically sized lesion more easily than in an adult heart. Despite these potential problems, the reported incidence of ablation-induced complete heart block does not appear to be significantly higher in infants and children than in adults.[6,19,43,50-54] However, a second consideration is the technical details of pacing if heart block occurs. Superior vena caval thrombosis complicating transvenous pacing can occur with both single and dual chamber systems, leading most clinicians to place epicardial pacing systems in children who weigh less than 10 to 12 kg, and only single-chamber transvenous systems in patients weighing between 10 and 20 kg. For this reason, pacing may require chest surgery and may leave the patient physiologically compromised by asynchronous pacing. In addition, the pacing system in a child may need to be maintained for as many as 70 to 80 years, and its presence will almost certainly restrict the child from many competitive sports, thereby setting lifestyle limits that are of less concern for most adult patients. These issues should affect both the decision to ablate and the procedure itself when ablating near the normal AV conduction system, if either the AV node or an AP is targeted.

Coronary Artery Damage

Acute and late coronary artery injury has been reported after RF ablation for AP-mediated tachycardias in children, adults, and animals.[9,10,34,55-58] These cases have involved both left- and right-sided coronary arteries,[10,55,58] as well as a posterior descending branch of the right coronary artery during ablation of a right posteroseptal AP.[57]

Recently, we reported a case of coronary damage during slow pathway modification in a 30-month-old, 15.5-kg child with recurrent AVNRT resistant to drug therapy. Approximately 100 seconds after a fourth application of RF energy, ST elevation was noted (Fig. 34–2); it lasted about 15 minutes and was not accompanied by hemodynamic compromise or echocardiographic abnormalities. Selective coronary angiography revealed a dominant right coronary artery giving off a posterior left ventricular branch artery that had an 80% stenosis (Fig. 34–3). The vessel course was within 2 to 3 mm of where the catheter tip had been placed during the last RF application ablation. Acute management was conservative, including nitroglycerin, Solu-Medrol, and heparin. After 2 days, repeat angiography revealed some improvement, with an approximately 50% stenosis. Discharge medications included aspirin and amlodipine. Repeat selective right coronary angiography 2 months later revealed complete resolution of

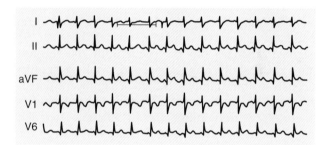

FIGURE 34–2. ST segment elevation occurring approximately 100 seconds following the last RF application for slow pathway modification in a 2.5 year old with AVNRT. *(From Blaufox AD, Saul JP: Acute coronary artery stenosis during slow pathway ablation for atrioventricular nodal reentrant tachycardia in a child. J Cardiovasc Electrophysiol 15:97-100, 2004, with permission.)*

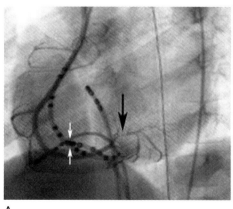
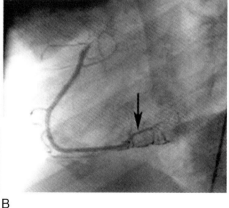

A   B

FIGURE 34–3. A, LAO projection of right coronary angiogram a few minutes after the ST segment changes in Figure 34–2 had spontaneously normalized. An approximately 80% stenosis *(arrow)* is seen in a posterior left ventricular branch off a dominant right coronary. Ablation catheter was moved away from the septum at the time of angiogram, but had been immediately adjacent to the stenosis during the RF application. **B,** Similar LAO projection of right coronary angiogram 2 months following ablation. *Arrow* marks are of prior stenosis, which is now resolved. *(From Blaufox AD, Saul JP: Acute coronary artery stenosis during slow pathway ablation for atrioventricular nodal reentrant tachycardia in a child. J Cardiovasc Electrophysiol 15:97-100, 2004, with permission.)*

narrowing (see Fig. 34–3), and repeat electrophysiologic studies with and without isuprel failed to induce any AVNRT. ST segments remained normal with the isuprel infusion. Digoxin and amlodipine were discontinued, and follow-up has been unremarkable.

Although this case is anecdotal, it reveals several important issues regarding the potential for coronary artery injury during RF ablation in children. First, coronary artery injury may occur with slow pathway ablation for AVNRT. Second, acute coronary artery injury has the potential to be missed and is probably an under-reported phenomenon. Third, infants and young children may be at particular risk. The inflammatory component of tissue injury caused by RF energy has been shown to invade layers of the right coronary artery, leading to acute narrowing, when RF energy is applied to the atrial side of the lateral tricuspid annulus in pigs.[34] Further maturation of this injury can result in significant late coronary stenosis.[59] Therefore, with RF energy application, coronary stenosis may occur acutely or be delayed. Our patient's injury was almost missed because ST segment changes did not occur until 100 seconds after the last RF application and resolved spontaneously within minutes, despite a significant persistent stenosis of the involved artery. Other instances of coronary artery injury after RF ablation were also nearly missed because of this delay.[10,58] In large retrospective and prospective studies in which there were no coordinated attempts to investigate coronary injury after RF ablation, the reported incidences of injury were 0.03% in children[19] and 0.06% to 0.1% in adults.[53] However, in a study in which coronary angiography was performed before and after RF ablation for AP-mediated tachycardias, Solomon et al.[56] reported a 1.3% incidence of coronary artery injury in 70 patients. Therefore, unless evidence for coronary artery injury is actively sought, it may go undiagnosed and under-reported.

Smaller children may be at particular risk for coronary injury, because the distance between the ablation catheter and the coronary arteries is significantly less than in adults. Although coronary blood flow probably helps reduce this risk, the flow in small coronaries in any patient may be inadequate to prevent damage. Understanding these factors is critical to preventing damage.

To absolutely minimize the chance of coronary injury in children, we make the following recommendations for patients who weigh less than 40 kg and are undergoing slow pathway modification for AVNRT (Table 34–2): (1) cryotherapy is the preferred ablation methodology; (2) in all cases in which RF energy is used, selective coronary angiography of the artery supplying the posterior septum should be per-

TABLE 34–2
Precautions for Ablation of AVNRT in Children Weighing Less Than 40 Kilograms
Cryoablation is the preferred energy modality.
If RF used, coronary angiography to visualize the region from the artery to the posterior septum should be performed.
If the coronary artery is <2-3 mm from an RF ablation site, energy should *NOT* be delivered.
After RF delivery, immediate repeat coronary angiography should be performed.
For all patients weighing <20 kg, preablation and postablation coronary angiography should be performed regardless of energy source.

AVNRT, atrioventricular nodal reentry tachycardia; RF, radiofrequency energy.

formed before ablation; (3) if a small coronary artery is within 2 to 3 mm of the expected ablation location, RF energy should not be delivered; (4) if any RF energy is delivered, acute follow-up angiography should be performed after ablation; (5) all patients weighing less than 20 kg should have preablation and postablation angiography performed regardless of the ablation technology used.

PREEXCITATION SYNDROMES IN INFANTS

There are three special considerations in infants that make management of symptoms secondary to an AP different from those in an older child or adult. First, the risk of a sustained reentrant primary atrial tachycardia, such as atrial fibrillation, is very close to zero in the small, structurally normal heart, making the risk of sudden death in infants with WPW very low.[2,60] Second, as noted earlier, AP function may spontaneously disappear by 1 year of age.[2,35] Finally, the known risks of any catheterization, combined with the specific risks of catheter ablation in this age group,[33,61-64] suggest that pharmacologic control should be aggressively pursued before ablation is attempted. This last issue deserves further discussion.

In humans, myocardial cell division probably occurs through approximately 6 months of age.[65] Although this finding could potentially protect the myocardium from long-term complications secondary to early injury, ventriculotomy scars produced in newborn puppies[66] and RF ablation lesions in immature lambs[7] appear to increase in size during subsequent development. In addition, in contrast to mature ablation scars from adult animals, late lesions from the neonatal lambs were often histologically invasive and poorly demarcated from the surrounding tissue.[7] The potential clinical importance of these results is underscored by a reported sudden death 2 weeks after an AP ablation in a 5-week-old, 3.2-kg infant.[6,61] An echocardiogram from the infant at the time of a brief resuscitation, as well as autopsy findings, revealed relatively large lesions extending into the left ventricle from the intended mitral groove ablation site (Fig. 34–4). Another heightened risk in infants is coronary artery damage due to the potentially close proximity of the coronaries to the ablation catheter and the reduced capacity for protective cooling during RF application in any small coronary artery. Although most reports of coronary damage in the literature have been limited to the posterior septum or a nondominant right coronary artery,[8,10,34] complete occlusion of the left circumflex artery was reported in a 5-week-old, 5.0-kg infant undergoing RF ablation of a left lateral AP.[9]

Despite these disturbing cases, nonpharmacologic therapy will be necessary in a small subset of infants with AP-mediated tachycardia.[63,67] Until accurate methods are available to assess lesion size in real time, alternative methodologies should be used in all infants. Early data on the effects of cryotherapy suggest that this form of energy may be much less harmful to coronary arteries, even when they are in very close contact,[68] due to the differing effects of cold and heat on connective tissue and the vascular inflammatory response. Coronary artery flow also protects the vessel through local warming during cryotherapy, similar to the way in which blood flow protects through local cooling during RF energy application. If technical or other considerations require the use of RF energy, considerable caution should be used. RF lesion size is related to catheter tip size, RF power, tip temperature, and lesion duration (see Chapter 1).[48,49] Therefore, the following technical modifications should be adopted (Table 34–3): (1) deliver energy in as atrial a location as possible; (2) use a 5-French (5F) catheter tip; (3) use *low temperature mapping* (50°C to 55°C) to identify the correct location before higher-temperature RF application[69]; (4) use a lower temperature set point of 60°C for the ablation lesion; and (5) use lesions of shorter duration (7 to 10 times the time to effect, with a maximum of 30 to 40 seconds). The future development of real-time ultrasonographic or other modality monitoring of lesion size may also help reduce the procedural risks.[70]

PREEXCITATION SYNDROMES IN PATIENTS WITH STRUCTURAL CONGENITAL HEART DISEASE

Though it is not strictly a pediatric issue, the combination of structural heart disease and arrhythmia is clearly encountered more often by pediatric electrophysiologists than by others. In agreement with previous studies,[22,71] a review of this issue in unselected patients with congenital heart disease at the Children's Hospital in Boston found that preexcitation syndromes are statistically increased in patients with Ebstein's malformation, L-transposition of the great arteries, or hypertrophic myopathy (Table 34–4).[21] Of course, preexcitation also occurs in other patients with congenital heart disease, but with an incidence not statistically higher than in the general population.

Anatomy

The association of WPW with Ebstein's anomaly and with the left-sided tricuspid valve in L-transposition

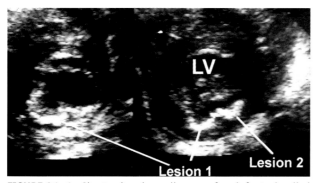

FIGURE 34–4. Short axis echocardiogram of an infant who died suddenly 2 weeks after an ablation procedure for 2 left-sided accessory pathways. Immediately after resuscitation 2 large echo dense regions were seen in the left ventricle (LV) despite radiofrequency applications being placed from an atrial approach. These echo dense lesions correlated with the findings on post mortem examinations. *(From Erickson CC, Walsh EP, Triedman JK, Saul JP: Efficacy and safety of radiofrequency ablation in infants and young children <18 months of age. Am J Cardiol 74:944-947, 1994, with permission.)*

TABLE 34–3
Precautions for Ablation of Accessory Atrioventricular Connections in Infants
Deliver energy as far on the atrial side as possible.
Use a 5F RF ablation catheter.
Use preliminary low-temperature RF delivery (50°C-55°C) before high-temperature delivery.
Limit maximal target temperature to 60°C.
Use short-duration RF delivery of 7-10 × time to effect with 30-40 sec maximal delivery.

RF, radiofrequency energy.

TABLE 34-4

Associations of Wolff-Parkinson-White (WPW) Syndrome and Congenital Heart Lesions

Lesion	No. of Patients	No. of Patients with WPW Syndrome	Prevalence (%)
Ebstein's	234	21	8.97*
L-TGA	588	8	1.36*
HCM	300	3	1.00*
Pulmonary valve disease	424	2	0.47
Tricuspid atresia	458	2	0.44
VSD-membranous	2,659	10	0.38
DORV	955	3	0.31
HLHS	666	2	0.30
MVP	1,096	3	0.27
Dextrocardia	427	1	0.23
Trisomy 21	916	2	0.22
TOF-pulmonary atresia	556	1	0.18
TOF	2,520	3	0.12
AV canal defect	2,058	2	0.09
D-TGA (all)	2,156	2	0.09
Coarctation	2,862	1	0.04*
d-TGA/IVS	704	0	0.00
Mitral atresia	417	0	0.00
Total	20,303	66	0.33

*$P < .01$ compared to general population estimate of 0.30%.

AV, atrioventricular; DORV, double-outlet right ventricle; HCM, hypertrophic cardiomyopathy; HLHS, hypoplastic left heart syndrome; IVS, intact ventricular septum; MVP, mitral valve prolapse; D-TGA, transposition of the great arteries with D-looped ventricles; L-TGA, "corrected" transposition of the great arteries; TOF, tetralogy of Fallot; VSD, ventricular septal defect.

From Children's Hospital, Boston, and New England Infant Regional Cardiac Program Computer Records.

probably has its basis in the embryology of tricuspid valve formation.[72-74] The leaflets of the AV valves normally develop through a process of undermining or delamination of the interior surface of the embryonic ventricular myocardium. Separation of the atrium from the ventricle occurs through completion of this process and encroachment of fibrous tissue from the AV sulcus. The mitral valve and the anterior leaflet of the tricuspid valve are fully delaminated early in development; however, the posterior and septal leaflets of the tricuspid valve are not even fully formed by 3 months gestation.[74] Ebstein's anomaly appears to occur when there is arrested development of tricuspid valve formation sometime between delamination of the anterior and of the posterior leaflets. The high prevalence of preexcitation combined with anatomic findings of accessory connections in a number of selected cases of Ebstein's anomaly[73,75] suggests that the arrested valve development results in remnants of muscular or specialized tissue connections that cross the AV groove. In fact, multiple pathways are common in these patients, often with a combination of a posteroseptal pathway and one or more additional free wall pathways.

Pathophysiology

The electrophysiology of the APs in patients with congenital heart disease is not particularly unique. Bidirectional, antegrade-only, and retrograde-only APs have been reported. Further, these patients have the same range of tachyarrhythmias found in patients with structurally normal hearts: orthodromic and antidromic AV reciprocating tachycardias and other SVTs (e.g., AVNRT, atrial flutter/fibrillation) with bystander participation of an antegrade conducting AP. However, the physiologic and clinical implications of the tachycardia may be markedly different in patients with congenital heart disease.

Abnormal hemodynamics, increased incidence of isolated atrial and ventricular ectopy, sometimes poor tolerance of antiarrhythmic therapy, and the need for surgical repair that accompanies congenital heart disease all contribute to an increased need for aggressive arrhythmia management in this patient population. However, abnormal anatomy and atypical conduction systems may also enhance the difficulty and risks of either surgical or catheter ablation (Fig. 34-5). Although RF catheter ablation is difficult in these patients, results have been good enough to recommend the procedure in all patients who require subsequent surgical repair to avoid postoperative arrhythmias as a complication and in most symptomatic patients older than 1 year of age who have significant structural lesions.

A review of the reported cases of RF ablation in patients with congenital heart disease revealed that most of the patients had Ebstein's malformation of a right-sided tricuspid valve.[20,53,54,76,77] However, a significant proportion had more complex anatomy, with AV valve discordance (right atrium to left ventricle, left atrium to right ventricle—S,L,L or I,D,D) and often heterotaxy. Multiple pathways are extremely

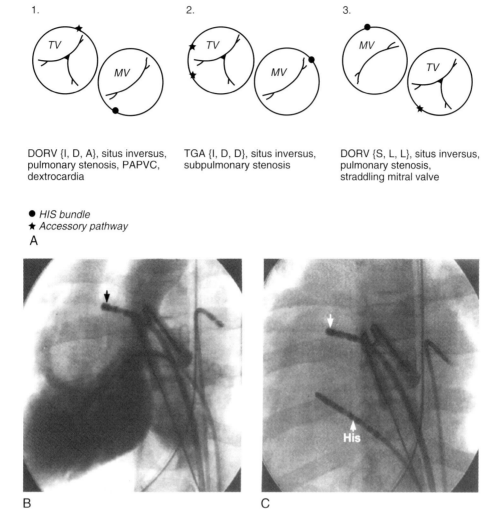

FIGURE 34–5. A, A cartoon demonstrating the locations of the mitral valve (MV), tricuspid valve (TV), the His bundle, and accessory pathways in three patients with preexcitation syndromes and atrioventricular discordance. Patient 1 corresponds with **B** and **C**. The angiogram in the anteroposterior projection (**C**) illustrates the importance of defining the anatomy of the AV valves. The decapolar catheter (*bottom white arrow* in **C**) was advanced from the left-sided inferior vena cava across the mitral valve and positioned with the second pair of electrodes at the His bundle. The mapping catheter (*black arrow* in **B**, *upper white arrow* in **C**) was advanced from the inferior vena cava across the atrial septum to the right-sided (anatomic) left atrium and positioned at the location of the accessory pathway, which in this case was at the superior and anterior portion of the left-sided tricuspid valve. The unmarked catheter is an atrial pacing catheter in the left-sided right atrium. DORV, double outlet right ventricle; PAPVC, partial anomalous pulmonary venous connection; TGA, transposition of the great arteries. *(From Saul JP, Walsh EP, Triedman JK: Mechanisms and therapy of complex arrhythmias in pediatric patients. J Cardiovasc Electrophysiol 6:1129-1148, 1995, with permission.)*

common in this group, occurring in 30% to 80% of patients,[20,54,75,76,78] compared with 5% to 10% of patients without congenital heart disease.[52-54,79,80] Like the patients with Ebstein's malformation, those with AV discordance had all of their APs associated with the tricuspid valve regardless of atrial situs, AV relationship, or valve function. This finding is in contrast to the more random location of APs reported for patients without congenital heart disease.[52-54,79-83] Hypertrophic cardiomyopathy is the exception: APs are more likely to be on the normal left-sided mitral valve.

Mapping and Ablation in Patients with Ebstein's Anomaly

Some aspects of the procedure in patients with Ebstein's malformation are of special note. First, differentiation of atrial and ventricular signals and precise localization of the AV groove can be difficult, leading to a lack of specificity for what appear to be excellent signals in predicting a successful ablation site. In fact, very early ventricular activations, which might be termed "pseudo" AP potentials can often be seen near the AV groove (Fig. 34–6). This issue is

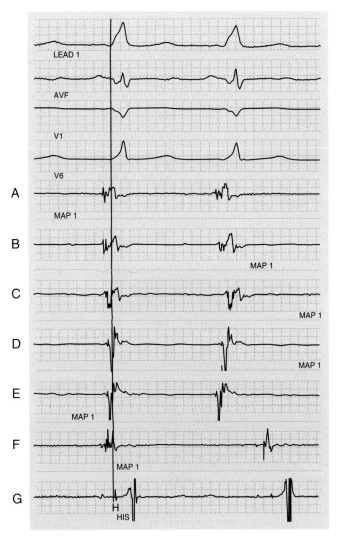

FIGURE 34–6. Electrograms near the AP in a patient with Ebstein's malformation. Electrograms *A* through *F* were recorded with the distal pair of an ablating catheter very near the point of successful ablation shown in *F*. Note early ventricular activation in *A* through *D*, despite lack of success. Electrograms in *D* and *E* were not significantly different, but *E* had transient success. *F*, the point of permanent success, probably has the earliest activation, however, the differences are much more clear in retrospect. The dark vertical line marks the point of earliest surface QRS activation for all electrograms. *G* shows the position of the atrial and HIS electrograms. Pathway location was posterior septal. *(From Saul JP: Ablation of atrioventricular accessory pathways in children with and without congenital heart disease. In Huang SK (ed.): Radiofrequency Catheter Ablation of Cardiac Arrhythmias: Basic Concepts and Clinical Applications. Mt. Kisko, N. Y.: Futura, 1994, pp 365-396, with permission.)*

particularly important for older patients who have large hearts with poorly defined AV grooves. The true AV groove is best identified by the right coronary artery. Use of a right coronary electrode wire can be considered[52,84] but may be difficult due to a diminutive right coronary artery, and the wire may need to be in place for long periods if multiple path-

ways are present. A safer and recommended alternative is continual display of the relevant coronary angiogram using a real-time biplane image storage and display system. As with any AP, searching for balanced atrial and ventricular electrograms during mapping is important. Despite these maneuvers, it may still be very difficult to define the AV groove in these patients, necessitating more test applications of the ablation modality to identify the correct location. Catheter stabilization for free wall pathways in the largest hearts is difficult and is not sufficiently improved through the use of a long sheath or a variety of approaches.[6] The overall issue of patient size is addressed later.

As expected, it appears to be impossible to approach the ventricular side of the tricuspid valve in patients with Ebstein's malformation. No specific reports have noted the use of nonstandard ablation technologies for these patients, but a few observations can be made. Coronary damage has been reported on multiple occasions in patients with Ebstein's anomaly, probably because of the thin RV wall and often diminutive right coronary artery. Consequently, despite the tendency to use higher power ablation systems with active or passive cooling for difficult cases, such technologies should be employed only if an adequate distance between the catheter tip and the artery has been documented. The definition of *adequate* here depends on the size of the nearby coronary artery: the larger the size, the safer the ablation. Further, strong consideration should be given to the use of cryotherapy, at least as a mapping tool. Safety is enhanced, and the adhesion of the catheter may be particularly useful in larger patients.

If multiple pathways are present, persistence may be the electrophysiologist's best weapon for successful ablation. In general, 80% to 90% of patients can be rendered arrhythmia free by the procedure, with relatively infrequent major complications such as permanent AV block.[18,20,54,76] However, recurrence rates have been reported to be as high as 40%, particularly if multiple pathways are present.[18,20,54,76]

Atrioventricular Discordance

Ablation procedures in patients with heterotaxy and/or AV discordance require special considerations. First, detailed echocardiography and angiography are instrumental in defining the complex anatomy of the atria, the AV ring, and the coronary sinus, so that the cameras and catheters can be positioned appropriately (see Fig. 34–5). Second, careful attention must be given to locating the normal conduction system. In virtually all patients with AV discordance, the AP has been associated with the tricuspid valve, whereas the His bundle has been associated more closely with the mitral valve. As predicted by Ho and Andersen,[85] the normal conduction axis is often located at an anterior position along the AV groove. Once the "normal" and abnormal conduction fibers are located, electrophysiologic study and RF ablation of the APs can proceed with less risk of damage to the normal conduction system.

Mapping and ablation require detailed knowledge of the anatomy and often innovative approaches. For instance, in cases of atrial inversion (right atrium on the left, or vice versa) with AV discordance (I,D,D), an atrial approach to the right-sided tricuspid valve may require a *reverse* trans-septal procedure from the left-sided inferior vena cava and right atrium to the right-sided left atrium. If present, the coronary sinus in such cases will also be reversed. AVNRT may also be present in these patients, requiring identification of the slow pathway of an AV node that is typically along the anterior mitral annulus. Clearly, the need for a detailed understanding of the anatomy in these cases cannot be overemphasized. Ablation technologies similar to those recommended for patients with Ebstein's anomaly are applicable to patients with AV discordance as well.

Patient Size and Structural Disease

One observation that is difficult to prove statistically but seems clear from our own experience is that the smaller chamber size in smaller patients with structural heart disease is a technical asset in catheter ablation. In our initial series,[20] a total of seven procedures lasting an average of 4.1 hours were required to ablate seven of nine accessory connections in six patients weighing less than 40 kg, whereas seven procedures lasting an average of 6.5 hours were used to ablate only three of seven connections in four patients who weighed more than 40 kg. Although larger patient size may be useful when the retrograde approach to left-sided accessory connections is used, smaller patient size appears to be helpful for catheter stabilization during an atrial approach, particularly in patients with structural heart disease and potentially very large hearts. Consequently, earlier intervention during childhood is preferable to waiting for near-adult size.

Recurrence Risk

The incidence of recurrence of tachycardia or preexcitation in patients who were initially successfully ablated has been reported to be as high as 40%. Although this recurrence risk is higher than the range of 8% to 12% reported in other large series,[19,53,54,79,86] the authors did note an increased risk of recurrence with right-sided pathways and with multiple pathways.[19,79,86] Both of these conditions occur with increased frequency in this patient population, and, in combination with the complex anatomy, this probably accounts for the high recurrence rate.

Summary

Based on our own observations and those in the literature, a few recommendations concerning catheter ablation in patients with congenital defects can be made: (1) an attempt should be made to carefully identify the location of the normal AV conducting system, particularly in patients with AV discordance; (2) the anatomic tricuspid valve is the most likely location for accessory connections; (3) smaller patient size may be an asset; (4) an atrial approach should probably be attempted first for connections around the tricuspid annulus (right- or left-sided); and (5) the true AV groove should be well identified, using either atrial and ventricular electrogram balance, a coronary angiogram, or, if available, a coronary mapping wire in larger patients. With these caveats in mind, it appears that, despite the difficulties of unusual anatomic landmarks and abnormally positioned conduction systems, most APs in patients with structural congenital heart disease can be safely and effectively ablated.

ATRIAL FLUTTER OR FIBRILLATION IN THE ABSENCE OF OTHER HEART DISEASE

In the pediatric patient, atrial reentry tachycardias are relatively rare in the absence of either structural or functional heart disease. The term *lone atrial flutter* or *fibrillation* has been applied here, referring to the isolated nature of the arrhythmia findings. However, both of these tachyarrhythmias are occasionally observed in pediatric patients. There are two age ranges for presentation. Perhaps the most common is during the third trimester of fetal life, when atrial flutter accounts for up to one third of fetal tachycardias,[5] often lasting through delivery and leading to ventricular dysfunction. Neonatal atrial flutter almost universally resolves without recurrence if it can be managed successfully during fetal and early neonatal life.[87] Consequently, ablation therapy for such infants should not be necessary and has never been reported.

A second presentation peak occurs during adolescence, when both atrial flutter and fibrillation may occur in the absence of any identifiable structural, hormonal, or chemical cause. Although initial management should be conservative, in contrast to the cases in infants, the arrhythmia typically recurs multiple times in this age group despite medical therapy, creating a need for ablation therapy similar to the scenario in adults. The use of catheter ablation has been reported for both flutter and fibrillation in young patients. Success rates were greater than 90% for the flutter subgroup in a relatively large series of patients in the Pediatric Ablation Registry.[88] Acute success was also recently reported in seven of eight pediatric patients with paroxysmal fibrillation who underwent either ablation of a single ectopic atrial focus or pulmonary vein electrical isolation.[89] Further, one of the cases that we included in a series of ablations for patients with ectopic atrial tachycardia (EAT) in 1992[90] was a 12-year-old boy who presented with recurrent atrial fibrillation that was permanently eliminated after ablation of a single left pulmonary vein ectopic focus.

Specific technical details for ablation of either atrial flutter or fibrillation in the larger child are not particularly different from those in adults and are not repeated here; however, the decision of when to ablate can be quite different, particularly for fibrillation. After conversion from a first episode of one of these arrhythmias, either no therapy or a drug to block the AV node response is adequate. After recurrences, the threshold for ablation of atrial flutter can be similar to that in adults. The use of ablation therapy for the rare cases of atrial fibrillation in pediatric patients is also appealing, but the high emphasis on safety over efficacy for all children mandates that a decision to use RF ablation in this age group be considered only after failure of multiple antiarrhythmic agents. Further, the technique chosen should be the most conservative in terms of safety, because complications such as pulmonary vein stenosis and stroke can be devastating to a child.

ATRIAL AND VENTRICULAR TACHYCARDIAS IN PATIENTS WITH CONGENITAL HEART DISEASE

Atrial and ventricular tachycardias in patients with congenital heart disease are covered in Chapters 13 and 31.

Arrhythmias Unique to the Pediatric Patient

A variety of issues may account for differences between adults and children in the incidence or prevalence of an arrhythmia (see Table 34–1).[5] For the arrhythmia labeled *congenital* junctional ectopic tachycardia (JET), the issue is definitional, because its congenital nature has been presumed based on presentation with incessant junctional tachycardia before

6 months of age and familial tendencies.[91,92] Patients with other incessant tachycardias, including EAT and the permanent form of junctional reciprocating tachycardia (PJRT), may present as children because they are unlikely to reach maturity with their arrhythmia due to a tendency to develop ventricular dysfunction and congestive heart failure secondary to the tachycardia.[93,94] Finally, the cardiac substrate for arrhythmia is clearly age dependent, in terms of both myocardial cellular development[95] and the presence of structural congenital heart disease.

INCESSANT ECTOPIC ATRIAL TACHYCARDIA IN THE CHILD

EAT is an uncommon rhythm disorder that accounts for 5% to 20% of SVTs in children[90,96] (see Table 34–1) but fewer than 2% of SVTs in adult series[13-15] (see Chapter 10). It involves abnormally rapid impulse generation from a single atrial focus outside the sinus node. Because the tachycardia is frequently incessant, the presentation is accompanied by a functional left ventricular myopathy in 50% to 75% of cases.[93,94,97] Although EAT may resolve spontaneously in some patients, particularly those younger than 6 months of age,[98-100] in many cases neither conventional antiarrhythmic drug therapy[16,90,97,101] nor arrhythmia surgery has been highly successful[16,83,102,103] (Table 34–5). The fact that ventricular function usually returns to normal if the arrhythmia can be controlled[93,94] has led to an aggressive search for other therapies, most notably catheter ablation.

Mechanism

Although a precise cellular mechanism of EAT has not been determined, a variety of clinical and electrophysiologic data, as well as intracellular recordings from a single operative specimen, strongly suggest a disorder of automaticity.[104] EAT is a nearly incessant tachycardia with wide fluctuations in atrial rate which often parallel the autonomic state and respond to isoproterenol in a similar way to sinus rhythm (Fig. 34–7A,B).[97] Typically, the ectopic focus rate changes gradually with a "warm-up" at initiation, and a "cool-down," sometimes associated with exit block, at termination. Programmed atrial stimulation is usually of little value in initiation of EAT, and neither atrial stimulation nor direct current (DC) cardioversion is useful for terminating it. Finally, the reset response of the EAT focus to single premature atrial stimuli can be almost identical to that of the normal sinus node (Fig. 34–7C).[97] These characteristics virtually rule out reentry as the underlying mechanism, but they do not absolutely exclude triggered activity. However, microelectrode recordings from

TABLE 34–5

Single Focus Ectopic Atrial Tachycardia

Authors, Year (Ref. No.)	PATIENTS						Mean Age at Pres (yr)	Positive Initial Drug Response†	Mean Follow-up (yr)	SPONTANEOUS RESOLUTION (NO. OF PATIENTS)‡	
	Total	Age <6 mo at Pres	CHD	Incessant (vs Repetitive)	RA*	LA*				Total	Age <6 mo at Pres
Koike et al., 1988 (115)	9	1	—	≥4	7	1	6.6§	6	2.0	3	0
Mehta et al., 1988 (100)	10	5	1	10	8	2	0.5§	9	1.7§	4	3
Garson et al., 1990 (16)	54	—	4	48	40	14	7.2	35	4.2	≤12	—
von Bernuth et al., 1992 (116)	21	8	0	14	14	7	2.0§	18	2.5§	5	3
Dhala et al., 1994 (102)	10	≤4	≤4	—	—	—	2.5§	≤4	—	0	0
Naheed et al., 1995	6	3	0	—	5	1	2.5§	6	3.1	5	—
Walsh et al., 1994 (113)	26	2	1	16	8	12	12.0	11	2.0§	0	0
Bauersfeld et al., 1995 (99)	19	19	7	—	—	—	<0.5	18	1.6	17	17
Totals	155	42/101 (42%)	17/146 (12%)	92/120 (77%)	82/119 (69%)	37/119 (31%)	—	107/155 (69%)	—	46/155 (30%)	23/32 (72%)

*Ectopic focus location by either electrocardiogram or electrophysiology study for patients reported.
†Full or partial response considered clinically successful by authors.
‡No tachycardia seen on 24-hour Holter monitoring without drug therapy.
§Median.

CHD, congenital heart disease; LA, left atrium; Pres, presentation; RA, right atrium.

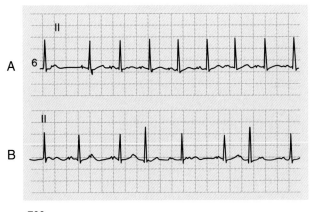

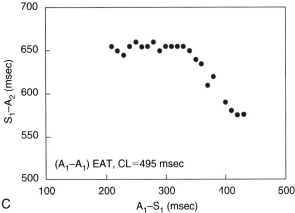

FIGURE 34–7. Surface ECG in patient with EAT at rest (**A**) and after mild exertion (**B**). (**C**) demonstrates the effect of single atrial premature stimuli (A_1-S_1) on the timing of ectopic atrial tachycardia focus discharge (S_1-A_2). The curve is similar to data generated for measurement of sinoatrial conduction time and demonstrates a clear reset zone. *(From Walsh EP: Ablation of ectopic atrial tachycardia in children. In Huang SK (ed.): Radiofrequency Catheter Ablation of Cardiac Arrhythmias: Basic Concepts and Clinical Applications. Mt. Kisko, N. Y.: Futura, 1994, pp 421-443, with permission.)*

left atrial appendage tissue obtained at the time of surgical excision of an EAT focus revealed a high resting membrane potential and spontaneous phase 4 automaticity.[104] Therefore, although it remains possible that the clinical condition of EAT may include cases caused by a triggered mechanism, at least some characteristic ones are the result of automaticity. Alternatively, the characteristics of many EATs in adults are distinctly different, with features favoring a triggered mechanism in some patients.[105,106]

The underlying cause of EAT in the pediatric patient has not been elucidated. Most cases are not associated with specific pathologic abnormalities of either noninvolved cardiac or skeletal muscle,[107] nor with resected atrial tissue near the focus.[16] Pathologic findings have been either normal or limited to non-specific fibrosis, cellular hypertrophy, and patchy fatty infiltrates, all of which may be secondary to the

tachycardia-induced myopathy.[108] Other clues to the etiology of EAT may come from the use of RF catheter therapy. First, it has been observed that EAT almost always involves a small area of tissue or a single cell, because it is eliminated within a few seconds after application of RF energy.[90,109] Second, just before successful elimination of the foci, the ectopic rate often accelerates, consistent with enhanced automaticity observed in response to RF energy in other tissue (Fig. 34–8).[110] Finally, the foci seem to cluster in a few specific areas of the right and left atrial appendages, and near or within the pulmonary venous ostia (Fig. 34–9). Of note, one of the primary differences between EAT in adult versus pediatric patients is a propensity for right-sided foci in adults,[105,106] whereas both left- and right-sided ones are seen in children (see Table 34–5).[16,90] These findings all suggest that EAT involves subtle electrical changes in otherwise normal tissue from trabeculated atria or connections between the primitive atria and the systemic veins.

Therapy

Virtually every class of antiarrhythmic agent has been used as pharmacologic therapy for EAT. Although no single class or agent appears to be universally effective, the best results have been observed with class IC and class III agents,[16,98,111,112] with amiodarone perhaps the most effective. Occasional successes have also been reported with phenytoin and β-blockers; however, in a large series of 54 young patients, a fully effective drug was found for only 50% of cases.[16] Ventricular, but rarely atrial, rate control may occasionally be achieved with either digoxin or verapamil. Also, adenosine may be useful diagnostically by inducing transient AV block, and it may cause transient EAT slowing and termination. Spontaneous resolution of EAT has also been reported after successful pharmacologic control, with rates ranging from 90% in a group of infants younger than 6 months of age[99] to 0% in a group of mostly older patients[113] and an average resolution rate from eight contemporary studies of 30% (see Table 34–5).[16,98-100,102,113-116] The wide variation in these rates appears to be due to a combination of factors but is probably most influenced by age at presentation, with 72% of the spontaneous resolutions occurring in patients who presented at before 6 months of age. Low spontaneous resolution rates were not associated with shorter follow-up duration among the eight studies (see Table 34–5). In fact, our initial experience at the Children's Hospital, Boston,[113] included no spontaneous resolutions, with a median follow-up before catheter ablation therapy of longer than 24 months, and longer than 4 years in eight patients.

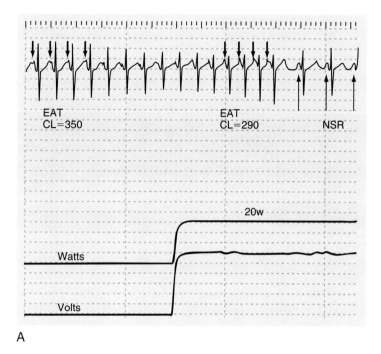

FIGURE 34–8. EAT ablation. **A,** Note how ectopic P waves (*arrows*) terminate after a brief period of acceleration. In (**B**) EAT slows briefly, then terminates. In both cases, the changes occur soon after RF application. In other cases, the ectopic focus may stop immediately at the onset of application of RF energy.

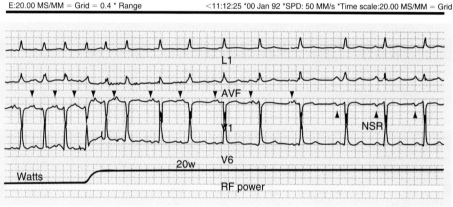

In contrast to pharmacologic therapy, RF catheter ablation for EAT arising from a single focus has been acutely successful in 90% to 100% of cases without significant complications.[19,90,106,109] Because of the high success rates of RF catheter ablation and the morbidity of drug therapy, the question of drug therapy has generally been reduced to one of whether it should be attempted at all in patients with severe ventricular dysfunction—and, if so, for how long—while waiting for spontaneous reversion to sinus rhythm.

Mapping

Most incessant EATs can be successfully mapped using a bipolar signal from the distal electrode pair of a single map/ablation catheter referenced to a single fixed intra-atrial signal. Comparison with the beginning of the surface P wave, when it can be iden-

tified, is very useful to identify timing in relation to some known measure of early atrial activation. Map signals that precede the surface P wave by more than 20 msec are most likely to indicate a successful location.[90] Although virtually all early ablation series were done with such basic mapping techniques, there are many situations in which more sophisticated mapping is useful or even necessary. Multipoint mapping can be performed with a variety of technologies and levels of sophistication.

A simple decapolar catheter, which provides four or more nearby timing points to the distal bipole, yields a great deal of directional information. Early distal timing with sequentially later timing of the proximal pairs suggests that the tip is indeed near the ectopic focus. However, even very early timing of the distal bipole when proximal timing is equivalent indicates that activation is approaching the catheter

EAT Focus Location

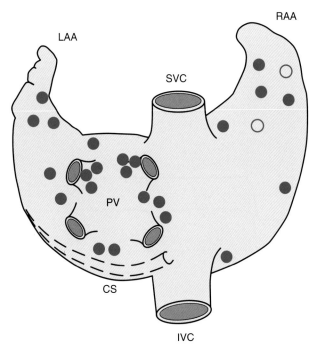

FIGURE 34–9. Location of EAT foci in the first 25 patients ablated at Children's Hospital in whom detailed mapping was possible. *Closed circles* (n = 23) indicate sites of successful ablation, and *open circles* (n = 2) indicate foci that could not be eliminated, in one case because of a broad area of fibrous dysplasia which was resected at surgery, and another patient because of multiple atrial foci of which this was only one. IVC, inferior vena cava; LAA, left atrial appendage; PV, pulmonary vein; RAA, right atrial appendage; SVC, superior vena cava. *(From Walsh EP: Ablation of ectopic atrial tachycardia in children. In Huang SK (ed.): Radiofrequency Catheter Ablation of Cardiac Arrhythmias: Basic Concepts and Clinical Applications. Mt. Kisko, N. Y.: Futura, 1994, pp 421-443, with permission.)*

from a different location. This situation often arises when an anterior right upper pulmonary vein focus is being mapped from within the high posterior right atrium. Timing may be early all along the catheter in the right atrium, but it will be early and sequential when the tip is in the right upper pulmonary vein. In such a case, ablation will be successful only when it is applied on the left atrial/pulmonary vein side of the atrial wall.

This example also highlights the value of three-dimensional (3-D) multipoint mapping, for which the available technologies have been reviewed in Chapter 8. There are a few considerations when choosing the best 3-D technology for EAT mapping, including the following: (1) some foci are intermittently active, particularly under sedation or anesthesia, making sequential activation mapping frustrating or impossible; (2) the location of right

pulmonary vein and near-septal foci may not be discernible from either the surface ECG or preliminary mapping, necessitating mapping in both the left and the right atrium; (3) some patients have multiple foci; and (4) some pediatric patients are too small for certain mapping technologies, particularly if remote areas of the left atrium must be accessed (such as ESI balloon mapping [Endocardial Solutions, St. Paul, Minn.], basket mapping, or even a 7F, relatively stiff Biosense Navistar mapping catheter [Biosense Webster, Baldwin Park, Calif.]). Given these considerations, we have found that for clearly incessant EATs sequential mapping technologies that allow simultaneous display and comparison of both the atria work well and provide the most flexibility. The CARTO system (Biosense Webster) has all these characteristics. However, for intermittent or potentially multiple foci, sequential mapping technologies may be frustrating, particularly if the focus activity is sensitive to catheter tip pressure. In such cases, a technology that allows for simultaneous single-beat mapping, such as the ESI balloon works best. However, the ESI system does not allow for simultaneous display of more than one cardiac chamber and does not lend itself to easily changing the mapping chamber. Consequently, no existing system deals with all four of the considerations noted previously. Regardless of the technology employed, if foci are intermittently active and either multilead P-wave morphologies or multipolar intra-atrial activations have been recorded during EAT, pace mapping may also be a useful adjunct to identify the focus site.

Ablation

In general, failure to eliminate EAT through catheter ablation is less dependent on the ablation technology than on obtaining a good map with early activation and the number of foci present. Because the normal atria are rarely more than 3 to 4 mm thick, most ablation technologies can easily create transmural lesions using standard settings. Therefore, techniques for creating larger lesions, such as active and passive tip cooling and high-powered generators, should rarely, if ever, be necessary. In fact, because most pediatric EAT foci are in the left atrium and often near the ostium of a pulmonary vein, less destructive ablation technologies (using lower temperature, power, and duration) or cryotherapy may be most appropriate in the child. To that end, we recently used a cryoablation catheter to successfully ablate a left atrial EAT focus in a 10-year-old boy, with no sign of EAT 15 months after the procedure.

Initial procedure failure and late recurrence tend to be associated with the presence of multiple foci or intermittent EAT during the procedure. Multiple foci portend poorly for long-term success,[16] both because of the increased difficulty in differentiating the foci during mapping and because more than one foci seems to be predictive of the emergence of other foci after the ablation procedure. Fortunately, in the pediatric population, most cases of EAT are caused by a single nonsinus focus.

Complications

Beyond the usual complications of any ablation procedure, there are few unique complications to EAT ablation. Both of these topics are covered elsewhere in this text, with the specific complications of EAT ablation covered in Chapter 10. Although, as noted earlier, some EAT foci in children are near or within a pulmonary vein (see Fig. 34–9), eliciting concerns about stenosis, clinically significant stenosis has not been reported for a pediatric case. The potential for damage to the sinus node or to the right phrenic nerve for foci that occur along the crista terminalis is addressed in Chapter 10. Most other EAT foci are not near vital structures, such as the AV node or a coronary artery.

JUNCTIONAL ECTOPIC TACHYCARDIA

In the pediatric population, unlike in adults, JET is seen in two relatively distinct settings: postoperative and congenital (Fig. 34–10).[92,117] The electrophysiologic characteristics of both varieties are similar to those of EAT,[92] suggesting they are also caused by abnormal automaticity, in this case arising from either low in the AV node or high in the His-Purkinje system. However, direct intracellular recordings have not been obtained.

The postoperative and congenital forms of JET differ primarily in their duration and response to therapy.[114,118-120] Postoperative JET is (1) strongly

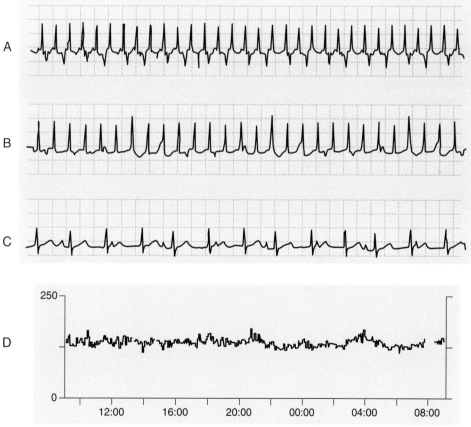

FIGURE 34–10. Junctional ectopic tachycardia in a 6 week old infant at presentation (**A**), 24 hours after intravenous amiodarone was begun (**B**), and when controlled on oral amiodarone (**C**). Note the ventricular rate of over 300 beats/minute with VA Wenckebach prior to amiodarone (**A**). After 24 hours of intravenous amiodarone, the ventricular rate decreased to approximately 260 beats/minute and there was occasional VA block (**B**). After control on amiodarone, the ventricular rate was normal at about 120-130 beats/minute (**C**). Over 24 hours (**D**), there was "normal" rate variability, but there was still junctional rhythm with occasional sinus capture throughout, as shown in (**C**). *(From Saul JP, Walsh EP, Triedman JK: Mechanisms and therapy of complex arrhythmias in pediatric patients. J Cardiovasc Electrophysiol 6:1129-1148, 1995, with permission.)*

associated with ventricular septal defect repair, either alone or at the time of repair of more complex anomalies (Table 34–6)[121]; (2) usually transient, lasting between 1 and 4 days; and (3) responds well to cooling, intravenous propafenone.[114,119,120] These observations strongly suggest that the tachycardia is a response to trauma and inflammation induced at the time of the repair. In contrast, congenital JET is (1) typically not associated with structural congenital heart disease; (2) incessant (see Fig. 34–10D); (3) has a positive family history in as many as 50% of cases; (4) anecdotally does not respond to cooling; (5) is associated with the maternal lupus anti-SSA and anti-SSB antibodies in some cases[122]; and (6) may spontaneously resolve, but over a period of months to years.[92] Both JET types may result in severe hemodynamic compromise and appear to be exacerbated by both endogenous and exogenous adrenergic stimulation,[92,120] and both arrhythmias seem to respond well to amiodarone (see Fig. 34–10C).[4]

The etiology of the congenital type, other than being "familial," is unclear. An extensive histologic evaluation was performed by Bharati et al.[123] in 2 patients who presented at or before 6 months of age. In one case, there were acute inflammatory changes at the summit of the ventricular septum and more chronic changes throughout the heart, including fibroelastosis, suggesting myocarditis. In the other, there were a variety of abnormal anatomic findings in the area of the AV node, including leftward displacement of the node and an abnormal central fibrous body. Multiple Purkinje-like tumor cells were found by Rossi et al.[124] in a third patient who did not present until 13 months of age, differentiating him slightly from the congenital group. Together these findings remain somewhat unsatisfying, because they fail to provide a unifying etiology consistent with the familial tendencies, and most patients do not present with findings of myocarditis. Recently, Dubin et al.[122] described a patient with both congenital AV block and JET, suggesting a link between the two diagnoses. The mother had Sjögren's syndrome and was strongly positive for anti-SSA and anti-SSB antibodies. Although two other families with congenital JET and positive antibodies were identified,[122] this exciting finding has not turned out to be a unifying

TABLE 34–6

Association of Postoperative Junctional Ectopic Tachycardia (JET) and Congenital Heart Lesions

Lesion	No. of Patients	No. of Patients with JET	Prevalence (%)	P Value
TOF	378	28	7.4	0.00005
VSD	285	9	3.2	0.004
TGA/VSD	57	9	15.8	0.23
Fontan	266	6	2.3	0.997
Truncus	33	4	1.2	0.824
CCAVC	177	4	2.3	0.999
PAB	111	2	1.8	0.999
HLHS	94	1	1.1	0.999
MVR	50	1	2.0	0.999
TGA/IVS	261	—	—	0.02
Coarct/Arch	375	—	—	0.0001
ASD	273	—	—	0.001
PDA	201	—	—	0.009
Systemic-PA shunt	192	—	—	0.015
Total	2753	64	2.3	—

ASD, atrial septal defect; CCAVC, complete common atrioventricular canal; coarct, coarctation; HLHS, hypoplastic left heart syndrome; IVS, intact ventricular septum; MVR, mitral valve replacement; PA, pulmonary artery; PAB, pulmonary artery band; PDA, patent ductus arteriosis; TGA, transposition of the great arteries; TOF, tetralogy of Fallot; VSD, ventricular septal defect.
From Children's Hospital, Boston, for years 1989-1994.

etiology for other cases. Thus, for most cases, JET remains an idiopathic diagnosis.

Therapy

The propensity for JET to eventually resolve spontaneously and the high theoretical risk of AV block from either catheter[125] or surgical[92] ablation of the JET focus in the AV junction suggest that JET may initially be best treated medically by minimizing adrenergic stimulation and beginning either intravenous or oral amiodarone,[4,92,126] particularly in infants. However, there are now anecdotal data from a few reports[127-132] which demonstrated that, with RF ablation, it may be possible to eliminate the JET while preserving AV conduction. Therefore, if the JET is either resistant to medical therapy, persistent after a prolonged period of control, or producing intractable hemodynamic compromise, RF ablation should probably be attempted. Because of anecdotal reports of sudden death and one case of AV block with JET, some investigators have recommended ventricular demand pacing in all patients with congenital JET,[92] but this recommendation has remained controversial.

Mapping and Ablation

The specific details in the small number of reported cases of successful JET ablation provide few overarching recommendations to use when approaching these patients. Although in most cases the region of interest has ended up in the anterior septum near the bundle of His, successful ablation in at least one case was reported in the posteroseptal region below the coronary sinus ostium, with the site identified by the use of retrograde atrial activation as a guide.[128] This region corresponds to the site used for slow pathway modification and should be associated with a low incidence of permanent AV block. However, the data presented may be most consistent with frequent paroxysms of AVNRT triggered by junctional escape beats, and other reports have not found mapping of earliest retrograde activation to be useful.[130-132] Nonetheless, because this area is generally "safe," initial attempts at ablation may be applied in the posterior septal region. If they are unsuccessful, mapping should focus on identifying the site of the earliest His potential during JET. Before ablation, the catheter should be moved very slightly posterior to that site, attempting to increase the atrial electrogram size and minimize the His activation from the distal ablation tip, similar to the methodology used in the past for fast pathway ablation. Most prior reports of successful elimination of JET without subsequent AV block have used this technique with brief, lower-power applications of RF energy. However, there is clearly a high risk of AV block in children with this technique. Recently, we had the opportunity to use cryotherapy for ablation of JET in a 10-year-old child with intermittently incessant tachycardia. Earliest His activation during tachycardia was found with retrograde mapping just under the aortic valve (Fig. 34–11). The high degree of safety of this methodology around the AV conduction system (see Chapter 4) made it ideal for both cryomapping and cryoablation, with successful elimination of the JET and preservation of the AV node, despite a catheter signal and location suggesting very close proximity to the His bundle. Although this case represents a single anecdote, the outcome observed, combined with the

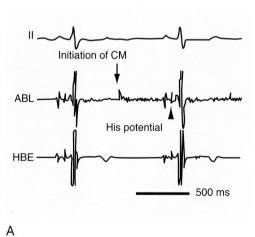

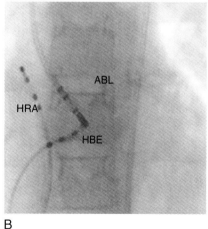

A   B

FIGURE 34–11. Successful cryoablation at location with His potential in a patient with JET. **A,** Identical His potentials are clearly seen from the ablation catheter (retrograde approach through the aortic valve) and from the His catheter (in a usual position) just prior to initiation of cryomapping (CM). **B,** Fluoroscopic images in the antero-posterior view shows the cryoablation catheter overlapping the image of the His position catheter. ABL, ablation; HBE, His bundle electrogram.

demonstrated reversibility of cryomapping applications, suggests that cryotherapy should be the treatment of first choice for ablation of JET.

PERMANENT FORM OF JUNCTIONAL RECIPROCATING TACHYCARDIA

Like EAT and JET, PJRT is an often incessant tachycardia that typically is recognized in infancy or childhood, either by detection of a rapid heart rate on a routine examination or because of the accompanying myopathy observed in many patients. First described by Coumel et al.,[133] the tachycardia is characterized by a narrow QRS rhythm with variable rates, a retrograde P-wave axis, and an RP interval that is longer than the PR interval. PJRT represents approximately 4% of the SVTs seen in infants,[96] and it accounts for 10% of pediatric patients referred for catheter ablation.[18] As is now clear from the results of electrophysiology studies, surgical[134,135] and catheter ablation results,[136-139] and anatomic data,[140,141] PJRT is caused by an orthodromic reciprocating tachycardia involving a slowly conducting concealed AP, making the name a misnomer. It is the slow and decremental retrograde conduction in the AP that leads to both the ECG characteristics and the incessant nature of the rhythm.

Therapy

As with other tachycardias caused by APs,[2] PJRT may resolve spontaneously in some patients.[142] However, in many patients PJRT is notoriously difficult to control medically. Before the era of RF catheter ablation, both surgical ablation[83,134,135] and DC catheter ablation[143-145] techniques had been used to treat PJRT, but both techniques resulted in a significant risk of AV block, as well as other complications. In addition, a false belief that the anatomic location of these APs was always posteroseptal led to a maximum success rate of only about 75%. Over the last 5 years, RF catheter ablation has proved to be a safe and highly effective technique for eliminating these fibers with virtually no risk of AV block.[136-139,146] Also, the precise AP localization provided by current mapping techniques and the demonstrated points of successful ablation have elucidated the fact that these APs are not always posteroseptal but may occur in almost any location along the AV groove (Fig. 34–12).

Mapping and Ablation

As with any other AP, the methodology for ablation of PJRT pathways depends on their location. Because many of the pathways are posteroseptal, ablation within the mouth or veins of the coronary sinus is

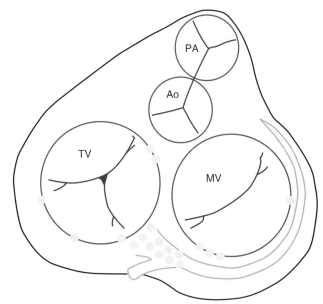

FIGURE 34–12. Schematic diagram of accessory pathway locations in patients with PJRT as identified by RF ablation. Circles represent APs causing the tachycardia. Eleven pathways were in the typical location either within or just outside the mouth of the coronary sinus, 4 were elsewhere along the tricuspid annulus, and 4 along the mitral annulus. Ao, aorta; MV, mitral valve; PA, pulmonary artery; TV, tricuspid valve. *(From Ticho BS, Walsh EP, Saul JP: Ablation of permanent junctional reciprocating tachycardia. In Huang SK (ed.): Radiofrequency Catheter Ablation of Cardiac Arrhythmias: Basic Concepts and Clinical Applications. Mt. Kisko, N. Y.: Futura, 1994, pp 397-409, with permission.)*

often necessary. Mapping should virtually always be performed during tachycardia. Electrogram characteristics, electrophysiologic techniques, and mapping techniques are somewhat different for PJRT pathways than for typical nondecremental APs. First, it is often impossible to confirm an AP as the retrograde conduction pathway using the standard technique of atrial preexcitation by a ventricular premature beat while the His is refractory, because the retrograde conduction decrements after premature ventricular stimulation. Further, the ventricle-to-atrium (VA) interval is usually long, with a long isoelectric segment between the ventricular and atrial signals, and an AP potential may be present in as many as 75% of cases (Fig. 34–13).[147] Finally, the pathways must usually be mapped and ablated in tachycardia (Fig. 34–14), because it is often not possible to achieve reliable exclusive AP conduction during ventricular pacing, due to either AV node conduction or retrograde block at any cycle length longer than that of the tachycardia. Given these constraints, more than 95% of pathways are still ablatable, but recurrence rates are higher than for typical APs, and some patients

FIGURE 34–13. Electrophysiological recordings of a single cycle of tachycardia in 8 patients with PJRT. Probable AP potentials *(arrows)* are present in strips **1** through **6**, and are identified as a rapid deflection that immediately precedes the atrial deflection. Strips **7** and **8** do not show such a potential. All recordings were made from the ablation catheter just prior to and at the location of successful ablation. After ablation the AP potential was not present and the ventricular signal did not change. Electrogram **7** was recorded with a catheter on the ventricular side of the tricuspid valve. *A* indicates atrial activation, and *V* ventricular activation. *(From Ticho BS, Saul JP, Hulse JE, et al.: Variable location of accessory pathways associated with the permanent form of junctional reciprocating tachycardia and confirmation with radiofrequency ablation. Am J Cardiol 70:1559-1564, 1992, with permission.)*

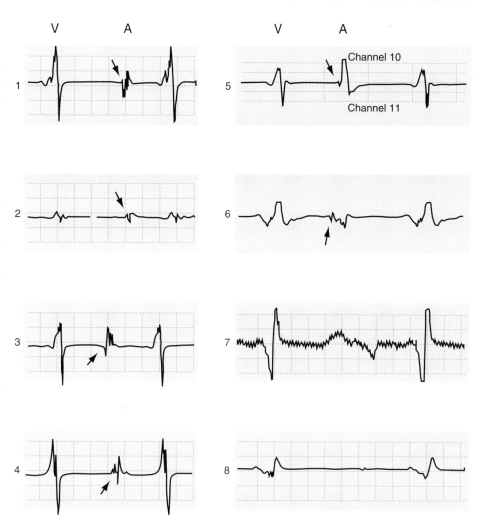

may require more than one procedure for initial success.[18,136-138,143,147]

Complications

Despite the proximity to the AV node, AV block has not been reported in the larger series of patients who have undergone RF ablation.[136-138,147] However, it is now clear that if RF energy is used to ablate posteroseptal pathways, both inside and outside the coronary sinus, there is a significant risk of coronary damage, particularly if ablation is performed near a terminating branch of the right coronary or left circumflex artery.[8] This issue and the possibility that subclinical coronary damage occurs much more often than has been previously recognized were discussed earlier in the section on AVNRT and are probably most applicable in the setting of posteroseptal PJRT pathways. In fact, Dr. Warren Jackman has often presented the unpublished case of a 15-year-old boy who was referred to him after a failed attempted ablation of a posteroseptal pathway within the mouth of the coronary sinus. A coronary angiogram performed demonstrated complete occlusion of the terminal portion of a nondominant left circumflex artery, despite the absence of any clinical or ECG changes during the first ablation attempt. Given the numerous anecdotes now available indicating high risk when RF energy is applied in close proximity to small coronary arteries,[8-10,12] we recommend the following for all pediatric patients: (1) coronary angiography should be performed before application of RF energy along the posterior AV groove, particularly near the septum, or within the coronary sinus; (2) if a small coronary artery is within 2 to 3 mm of an ablation site, cryotherapy is the preferred initial ablation choice; (3) if cryotherapy is either unavailable or ineffective, RF energy application should be minimized by reducing either catheter size, the temperature set point, or maximum power and/or duration; and (4) high energy RF application with active or passive cooled-tip technology should be entirely avoided or used with extreme caution.

Despite these safety concerns, the high efficacy and relative safety of RF ablation for PJRT, combined with the fact that pharmacologic therapy is often

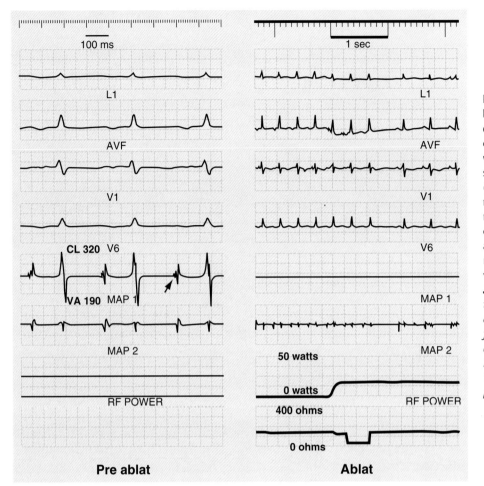

FIGURE 34-14. Electrophysiological recordings before and during transcatheter RF ablation of PJRT. The recording on the left was made during tachycardia and shows a probable AP potential (*arrow*). The recording on the right shows conversion to sinus rhythm within 2 seconds of RF energy application. Ablat, RF ablation; CL, cycle length in msec; VA, ventriculo-atrial interval in msec. *(From Ticho BS, Saul JP, Hulse JE, et al.: Variable location of accessory pathways associated with the permanent form of junctional reciprocating tachycardia and confirmation with radiofrequency ablation. Am J Cardiol 70:1559-1564, 1992, with permission.)*

ineffective, suggest that catheter ablation is reasonably appropriate as a first-line therapy for this syndrome, particularly if ventricular dysfunction is present.

DOUBLE ATRIOVENTRICULAR NODES

In hearts with normal or inverted atrial situs, but discordant AV connections (S,L,L or I,D,D), the anterosuperior ventricle is a morphologic left ventricle that carries with it the mitral valve.[148] When all four valves are well formed in such hearts, the condition is often referred to as *corrected transposition,* because the physiologic connections are all correct (i.e., systemic venous return flows to the lungs and pulmonary venous return flows to the aorta). As Anderson and others[72,85] have described, the AV node in corrected transposition is typically situated superior and anterior in the atrial wall, near the anterolateral quadrant of the mitral valve (Fig. 34–15A). The penetrating bundle then runs in the fibrous continuity between the right-sided mitral valve and the anterior cusp of the posterior great artery, eventually linking to the left bundle branch on the right side of

the ventricular septum. The right bundle branch then penetrates the ventricular septum to emerge in the inferior left-sided right ventricle. A second AV node that is often present more inferiorly, in the normal area of the triangle of Koch, can also link to the ventricular conduction fibers posteriorly, usually inferior to a ventricular septal defect. If the posterior and anterior ventricular bundle branches link together, a conduction sling (see Fig. 34–15B), sometimes referred to as a Monckeberg sling, is formed.[73-75] These anatomic findings provide the substrate for a host of different modes of ventricular excitation or preexcitation and AV reciprocating tachycardias. However, before the publication of one recent report,[149] there had been no electrophysiologic documentation of this phenomenon.

In 2001, we reported on seven of these patients, all of whom had AV discordance (2-S,L,L and 1-I,D,D) and characteristics consistent with the diagnosis of two separate AV nodes (twin or double).[150] Five of the seven patients also had a malaligned AV canal defect. The electrophysiologic findings included (1) the existence of two discrete, nonpreexcited QRS morphologies, each with an associated His-bundle electrogram

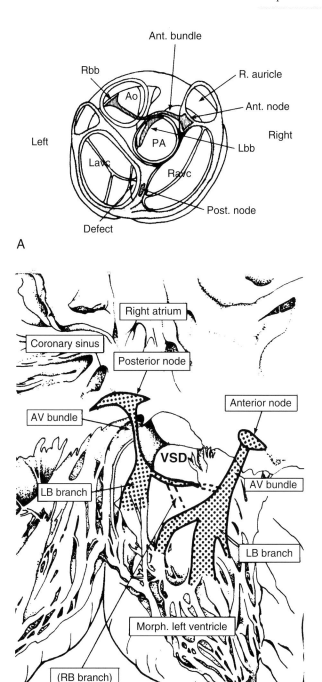

A

B

FIGURE 34–15. A, Diagram of the base of the heart and the AV conduction system in L-transposition of the great arteries (corrected) as seen from above. Note the bicommissural mitral valve on the right and the tricommissural tricuspid valve on the left. The AV node may either lie posteriorly (Post. Node) in the septum in a somewhat normal location, anteriorly on the right-sided mitral valve (Ant. Bundle), or in both places. RBB, right bundle branch; LBB, left bundle branch. (From Anderson RH, Arnold R, Wilkinson JL: The conducting system in congenitally corrected transposition. Lancet 1:1286-1288, 1973, with permission.) **B,** Diagram of the conduction system from a patient with corrected transposition in a criss-cross heart, with AV valve anatomy similar to that shown in (**A**). Note the dual conduction system with both the posterior and anterior AV nodes penetrating into the ventricles, and near connection of the conduction systems within the ventricle. *(From Symons JC, Shinebourne EA, Joseph MC, et al.: Criss-cross heart with congenitally corrected transposition: Report of a case with d-transposed aorta and ventricular preexitation. Eur J Cardiol 5:493, 1977, with permission.)*

involved two AV connections. In all cases, applications of RF energy at the site of the bidirectional pathway resulted in transient *junctional* acceleration with an identical QRS morphology to that generated by anterograde conduction over the targeted AV node, and modified or eliminated both antegrade and retrograde conduction at that site. Although there is a possibility that one or the other of these pathways was a *Mahaim-type* AV fiber, their locations and the presence of near-normal HV intervals, retrograde conduction, *orthodromic* tachycardia, and *junctional*-type acceleration during RF ablation all favor a second AV node. The precise etiology may make little difference for the medical management of such patients, but is important if damage to the best of the two conduction systems is to be avoided during ablation procedures performed before surgery in these patients with complex anatomy.

One patient with AV discordance and complete common AV canal was particularly illustrative of the features described. Two QRS morphologies were seen during *normal* rhythm, each with a normal PR interval (Fig. 34–16). One of the QRS morphologies (#1) was more typical of an endocardial cushion defect with a superior axis. At electrophysiology study, QRS morphology #1 could be produced by posterior atrial pacing and had an HV interval of about 50 msec with the His potential found posteriorly in the ventricle (Fig. 34–17). The other QRS morphology (#2) could be produced by anterior atrial pacing and had an associated HV interval (from the posterior His) of only 20 msec, but the QRS appearance did not strongly suggest preexcitation (see Fig. 34–17). The antegrade effective refractory period (ERP) of this anterior pathway was approximately 200 msec. Earliest ventricular activation was near the

and a normal His-to-ventricle (HV) interval; (2) decremental as well as adenosine-sensitive anterograde and retrograde conduction; and (3) inducible AV reciprocating tachycardia with anterograde conduction over one AV node and retrograde conduction over the other. Ventricular premature beats placed into tachycardia while the His was refractory could preexcite the atrium, indicating that the tachycardia

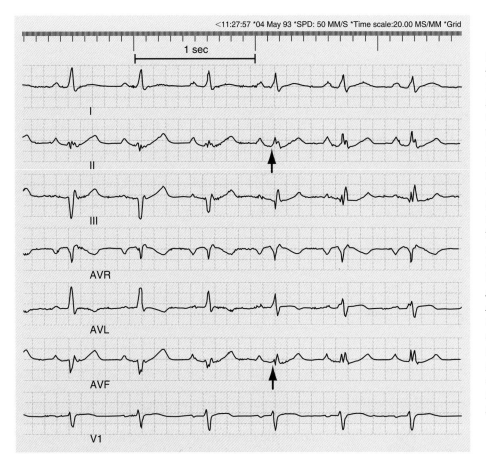

FIGURE 34–16. Six lead electrocardiogram in a patient with L-looped ventricles and common AV canal. Note spontaneously changing QRS morphology without obvious changes in the PR interval (*arrows*). The first morphology has a superior axis consistent with non-preexcited rhythm from a posterior location as in common AV canal. The other morphology was presumed to be from a second anterior AV node as per the electrophysiologic study findings (see Figure 34–15 and text). *(From Saul JP: Ablation of atrioventricular accessory pathways in children with and without congenital heart disease. In Huang SK (ed.): Radiofrequency Catheter Ablation of Cardiac Arrhythmias: Basic Concepts and Clinical Applications. Mt. Kisko, N. Y.: Futura, 1994, pp 365-396, with permission.)*

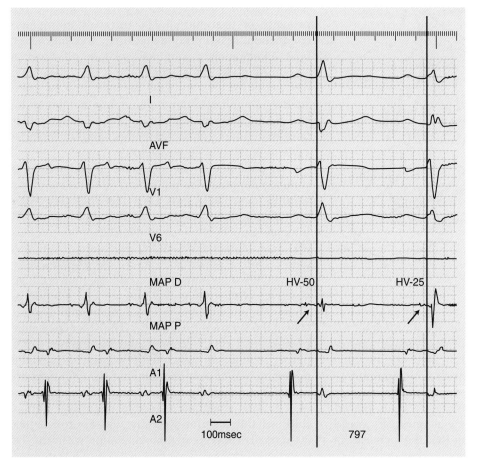

FIGURE 34–17. Intracardiac recordings in same patient as Figure 34–16 with L-loop ventricles and common AV canal. Note HV interval of 50 msec during the tachycardia and the first sinus beat after spontaneous termination. QRS morphologies for the tachycardia and this beat were identicle. Also note shorter HV interval of 25 msec during the last beat which is the anterior AV node QRS morphology. *(From Saul JP: Ablation of atrioventricular accessory pathways in children with and without congenital heart disease. In Huang SK (ed.): Radiofrequency Catheter Ablation of Cardiac Arrhythmias: Basic Concepts and Clinical Applications. Mt. Kisko, N. Y.: Futura, 1994, pp 365-396, with permission.)*

septal remnant regardless of QRS morphology. A regular tachycardia involving (1) QRS morphology #1 (see Fig. 34–17), (2) a 1:1 A/V relation, (3) a minimum VA interval of 70 msec, and (4) earliest retrograde atrial activation at the left anterior AV groove near the midline (tricuspid side of common valve) could be reproducibly induced with ventricular pacing. Ventricular premature beats placed into tachycardia while the His was refractory could pre-excite the atrium, indicating that the tachycardia involved two AV connections. Retrograde VA conduction was all via the anterior pathway, was decremental, and had an ERP of 230 msec. Application of RF energy near the point of earliest retrograde conduction (anterior and to the left) resulted in transient junctional acceleration of QRS rhythm #2, followed by a sudden change to a regular slower rhythm of QRS #1 (Fig. 34–18). After RF application, VA conduction was eliminated and tachycardia was noninducible. These findings illustrate the following important features: (1) there were two antegrade conduction pathways, one posteroseptal and one anterospetal; (2) both pathways were on the left (tricuspid) side of the common AV ring; (3) both pathways had slow conduction properties; (4) retrograde conduction occurred over only the anterior pathway;

and (5) tachycardia was *orthodromic*, antegrade posterior and retrograde anterior.

Clearly, an extensive understanding of the anatomy and electrophysiology should be obtained in such patients before proceeding to mapping and ablation. Further, lack of clarity in defining the anatomy of AV conduction in these patients suggests that ablation should first be undertaken using cryotherapy, proceeding to RF energy only if cryotherapy is unsuccessful or after a recurrence. The one caveat to this recommendation is that low-power RF application may be helpful in identifying the location of the anterior and posterior AV nodes through their acceleration response when heated.

General Consideration of Risk in the Pediatric Patient

OTHER COMPLICATIONS

A distinct risk of vascular injury, secondary to thrombus or embolus formation, exists with any catheterization in smaller children but is particularly present

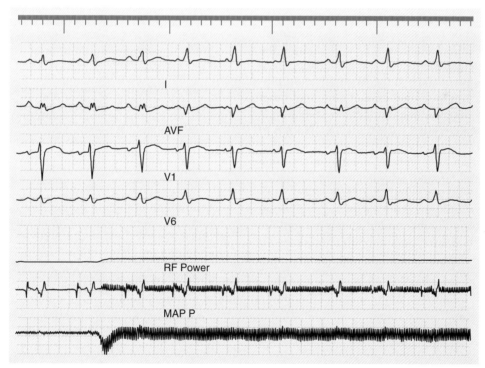

FIGURE 34–18. Response to RF ablation at the location of the anterior AV node in the same patient as Figures 34–16 and 34–17. Within one second after application of RF energy, the PR interval shortened, presumably due to junctional acceleration. Approximately one second later, the junctional acceleration stopped, and the PR interval lengthened with a change in QRS morphology consistent with loss of the morphology associated with the anterior AV node that had a shorter HV interval. *(From Saul JP: Ablation of atrioventricular accessory pathways in children with and without congenital heart disease. In Huang SK (ed.): Radiofrequency Catheter Ablation of Cardiac Arrhythmias: Basic Concepts and Clinical Applications. Mt. Kisko, N. Y.: Futura, 1994, pp 365-396, with permission.)*

with any interventional or prolonged diagnostic catheterization.[151] Therefore, it is not surprising that vascular complications, including microembolism to the foot[146] and arterial occlusion,[152] have been reported with catheter ablation. Of note, however, the incidence of these problems appears to be quite low, even in the smallest patients, probably because of meticulous heparinization, a tendency not to use the retrograde arterial approach in most pediatric centers, and the current availability of smaller diagnostic and ablation catheters. Production of new,[153] or increased[6] valvar regurgitation has been reported in pediatric patients after use of the retrograde arterial approach, providing an additional reason to avoid this approach in smaller patients. The risk of acute coronary damage was addressed earlier, but it should also be noted that only limited data in humans are available, and no data on late coronary function have been reported in animals, children, or adults.

SEDATION AND ANESTHESIA

The pain and discomfort of an RF ablation procedure do not appear to be very much higher than for a typical diagnostic catheterization, even accounting for the pain some patients feel during the actual RF application. Therefore, general anesthesia is by no means necessary. However, we began using general or near-general anesthesia for most patients early in our experience, for two reasons. First and foremost, uncontrolled patient movement that dislodges the catheter may inadvertently occur at a critical point in the procedure, particularly if the RF application produces pain. In fact, our only case of complete heart block occurred in part as the result of untimely movement of an uncooperative patient during ablation of a midseptal AP, leading us to replace heavy, often disorienting sedation with general anesthesia for most younger patients. Second, after beginning the use of general anesthesia, we found that even older, cooperative children and young adults find a long procedure much more tolerable under anesthesia and are more willing to return for follow-up procedures, if needed.

Summary

Children are usually smaller than adults, but in general ablation techniques used in adults should not simply be miniaturized to fit the size of the pediatric patient. Multiple factors, including the distribution of arrhythmia mechanisms, ongoing myocardial development, and potentially increased risk of vascular

injury and AV node damage, as well as the effects of smaller cardiac size, should all influence the ablation technique. An overriding theme in the child should be that safety takes precedence over efficacy. Therefore, variations of technique should be applied to the decision to ablate, the energy source and its delivery, the catheter approach to the heart and the AV ring, and the follow-up. For instance, because of its strong safety profile, despite lower efficacy, the use of cryotherapy may be even better suited to ablation in children than in adults. Attention to these factors is probably most important in infants, a group who differ both quantitatively and qualitatively from adults. In addition, the pediatric patient is obviously more likely than an adult to have the simultaneous presence of structural congenital heart disease, which in itself has a variety of implications for the decision to ablate and the procedure technique. On the other hand, there are numerous similarities between adult and pediatric patients. Specifically, regardless of age, it seems clear that a variety of techniques and approaches are necessary to successfully ablate APs in all locations around the AV groove.

References

1. Garson A Jr, Dick M 2nd, Fournier A, et al.: The long QT syndrome in children: An international study of 287 patients [see comments]. Circulation 87:1866-1872, 1993.
2. Deal BJ, Keane JF, Gillette PC, Garson A Jr: Wolff-Parkinson-White syndrome and supraventricular tachycardia during infancy: Management and follow-up. J Am Coll Cardiol 5:130-135, 1985.
3. Musto B, D'Onofrio A, Cavallaro C, Musto A: Electrophysiological effects and clinical efficacy of propafenone in children with recurrent paroxysmal supraventricular tachycardia. Circulation 78:863-869, 1988.
4. Perry JC, Fenrich AL, Hulse JE, et al.: Pediatric use of intravenous amiodarone: Efficacy and safety in critically ill patients from a multicenter protocol. J Am Coll Cardiol 27:1246-1250, 1996.
5. Ko JK, Deal BJ, Strasburger JF, Benson DW Jr.: Supraventricular tachycardia mechanisms and their age distribution in pediatric patients. Am J Cardiol 69:1028-1032, 1992.
6. Saul JP, Hulse JE, De W, et al.: Catheter ablation of accessory atrioventricular pathways in young patients: Use of long vascular sheaths, the transseptal approach and a retrograde left posterior parallel approach. J Am Coll Cardiol 21:571-583, 1993.
7. Saul JP, Hulse JE, Papagiannis J, et al.: Late enlargement of radiofrequency lesions in infant lambs: Implications for ablation procedures in small children. Circulation 90:492-499, 1994.
8. Blaufox AD, Saul JP: Acute coronary artery stenosis during slow pathway ablation for atrioventricular nodal reentrant tachycardia in a child. J Cardiovasc Electrophysiol 15:97-100, 2004.
9. Paul T, Kakavand B, Blaufox AD, Saul JP: Complete occlusion of the left circumflex coronary artery after radiofrequency catheter ablation in an infant. J Cardiovasc Electrophysiol 14:1004-1006, 2003.

10. Bertram H, Bokenkamp R, Peuster M, et al.: Coronary artery stenosis after radiofrequency catheter ablation of accessory atrioventricular pathways in children with Ebstein's malformation. Circulation 103:538-543, 2001.

11. Hope EJ, Haigney MC, Calkins H, Resar JR: Left main coronary thrombosis after radiofrequency ablation: Successful treatment with percutaneous transluminal angioplasty. Am Heart J 129:1217-1219, 1995.

12. Nakagawa H, Chandrasekaren K, Pitha J, Yamanashi W: Early detection of coronary artery injury produced by radiofrequency ablation within the coronary sinus using intravascular ultrasound imaging. Circulation 92:I-610, 1995.

13. Rodriguez LM, de Chillou C, Schlapfer J, et al.: Age of onset and gender of patients with different types of supraventricular tachycardias. Am J Cardiol 70:1213-1215, 1992.

14. Josephson ME, Wellens HJJ: Differential diagnosis of supraventricular tachycardia. Cardiol Clin 8:441-442, 1990.

15. Wellens HJJ, Brugada P: Mechanisms of supraventricular tachycardia. Am J Cardiol 62:10D-15D, 1988.

16. Garson A Jr, Smith RT, Moak JP, et al.: Atrial automatic ectopic tachycardia in children. In Touboul P, Waldo AL (eds.): Atrial Arrhythmias: Current Concepts and Management. St. Louis: Mosby Year Book, 1990, pp 282-287.

17. Silka MJ, Gillette PC, Garson A Jr, Zinner A: Transvenous catheter ablation of a right atrial automatic ectopic tachycardia. J Am Coll Cardiol 5:999-1001, 1985.

18. Tanel RE, Walsh EP, Triedman JK, et al.: Five-year experience with radiofrequency catheter ablation: Implications for management of arrhythmias in pediatric and young adult patients. J Pediatr 131:878-887, 1997.

19. Kugler JD, Danford DA, Deal BJ, et al.: Radiofrequency catheter ablation for tachyarrhythmias in children and adolescents. The Pediatric Electrophysiology Society. N Engl J Med 330:1481-1487, 1994.

20. Levine JC, Walsh EP, Saul JP: Radiofrequency ablation of accessory pathways associated with congenital heart disease including heterotaxy syndrome. Am J Cardiol 72:689-693, 1993.

21. Saul JP, Walsh EP, Triedman JK: Mechanisms and therapy of complex arrhythmias in pediatric patients. J Cardiovasc Electrophysiol 6:1129-1148, 1995.

22. Schiebler GL, Adams P Jr, Anderson RC: The Wolff-Parkinson-White syndrome in infants and children: A review and a report of 28 cases. Pediatrics 24:585-603, 1959.

23. Dick M 2nd, Behrendt DM, Byrum CJ, et al.: Tricuspid atresia and the Wolff-Parkinson-White syndrome: Evaluation methodology and successful surgical treatment of the combined disorders. Am Heart J 101:496-500, 1981.

24. Benson DW, Smith WM, Dunnigan A: Mechanisms of regular wide QRS tachycardia in infants and children. Am J Cardiol 49:1776-1788, 1982.

25. Morady F, Kadish AH, DiCarlo L, et al.: Long-term results of catheter ablation of idiopathic right ventricular tachycardia. Circulation 82:2093-2099, 1990.

26. Klein LS, Shih HT, Hackett K, et al.: Radiofrequency catheter ablation of ventricular tachycardia in patients without structural heart disease. Circulation 85:1666-1674, 1992.

27. Laohakunakorn P, Paul T, Knick B, et al.: Ventricular tachycardia in nonpostoperative pediatric patients: Role of radiofrequency catheter ablation. Pediatr Cardiol 24:154-160, 2003.

28. Weindling SN, Walsh EP, Saul JP: Management of supraventricular tachycardia in infants. J Am Coll Cardiol 21:294a, 2000.

29. Benson DW Jr, Dunnigan A, Benditt DG, et al.: Transesophageal study of infant supraventricular tachycardia: Electrophysiologic characteristics. Am J Cardiol 52:1002-1006, 1983.

30. Friedman RA, Walsh EP, Silka MJ, et al.: NASPE Expert Consensus Conference. Radiofrequency catheter ablation in children with and without congenital heart disease: Report of the writing committee. North American Society of Pacing and Electrophysiology [review, 127 refs]. Pacing Clin Electrophysiol 25:1000-1017, 2002.

31. Blaufox AD, Denslow S, Felix GL, Saul JP, and Participating Members of the Pediatric Electrophysiology Society: Radiofrequency catheter ablation in Registry infants: When is it done and how do they fare? Circulation 102:II-698, 2000.

32. Blaufox AD, Paul T, Saul JP: Radiofrequency catheter ablation in small children: Relationship of complications to application dose. Pacing Clin Electrophysiol 27:224-229, 2004.

33. Blaufox AD, Felix GL, Saul JP, and Pediatric Catheter AR: Radiofrequency catheter ablation in infants </ = 18 months old: When is it done and how do they fare? Short-term data from the pediatric ablation registry. Circulation 104:2803-2808, 2001.

34. Paul T, Bokenkamp R, Mahnert B, Trappe HJ: Coronary artery involvement early and late after radiofrequency current application in young pigs. Am Heart J 133:436-440, 1997.

35. Benson DW Jr, Dunnigan A, Benditt DG: Follow-up evaluation of infant paroxysmal atrial tachycardia: Transesophageal study. Circulation 75:542-549, 1987.

36. Perry JC, Garson A Jr: Supraventricular tachycardia due to Wolff-Parkinson-White syndrome in children: Early disappearance and late recurrence [see comments]. J Am Coll Cardiol 16:1215-1220, 1990.

37. Klein GJ, Yee R, Sharma AD: Longitudinal electrophysiologic assessment of asymptomatic patients with the Wolff-Parkinson-White electrocardiographic pattern [see comment]. N Engl J Med 320:1229-1233, 1989.

38. Zardini M, Yee R, Thakur RK, Klein GJ: Risk of sudden arrhythmic death in the Wolff-Parkinson-White syndrome: Current perspectives. Pacing Clin Electrophysiol 17:966-975, 1994.

39. Bromberg BI, Lindsay BD, Cain ME, Cox JL: Impact of clinical history and electrophysiologic characterization of accessory pathways on management strategies to reduce sudden death among children with Wolff-Parkinson-White syndrome. J Am Coll Cardiol 27:690-695, 1996.

40. Zipes DP, Garson A Jr: 26th Bethesda conference: Recommendations for determining eligibility for competition in athletes with cardiovascular abnormalities. Task Force 6: Arrhythmias [review, 35 refs]. Med Sci Sports Exerc 26(Suppl):S276-S283, 1994.

41. Gross GJ, Epstein MR, Walsh EP, Saul JP: Characteristics, management and mid-term outcome in infants with atrioventricular nodal reentry tachycardia. Am J Cardiol 82:956-960, 1998.

42. Silka MJ, Kron J, Halperin BD, McAnulty JH: Mechanisms of AV node reentrant tachycardia in young patients with and without dual AV node physiology. Pacing Clin Electrophysiol 17:2129-2133, 1994.

43. Van Hare GF, Chiesa NA, Campbell RM, et al., and Pediatric Electrophysiology Society: Atrioventricular nodal reentrant tachycardia in children: Effect of slow pathway ablation on fast pathway function [comment]. J Cardiovasc Electrophysiol 13:203-209, 2002.

44. Rosen KM, Bauernfeind RA, Swiryn S, et al.: Dual AV nodal pathways and AV nodal reentrant paroxysmal tachycardia. Am Heart J 101:691-695, 1981.

45. Denes P, Wu D, Dhingra R, et al.: Dual atrioventricular nodal pathways: A common electrophysiological response. Br Heart J 37:1069-1076, 1975.

46. Blaufox AD, Saul JP: Influences on fast and slow pathway conduction in children: Does the definition of dual atrioventricular node physiology need to be changed? [comment]. J Cardiovasc Electrophysiol 13:210-211, 2002.

47. Blaufox AD, Rhodes JF, Fishberger SB: Age related changes in dual AV nodal physiology. Pacing Clin Electrophysiol 23:477-480, 2000.

48. Haines DE: The biophysics of radiofrequency catheter ablation in the heart: The importance of temperature monitoring. Pacing Clin Electrophysiol 16:586-591, 1993.

49. Haines DE, Watson DD, Verow AF: Electrode radius predicts lesion radius during radiofrequency energy heating: Validation of a proposed thermodynamic model. Circ Res 67:124-129, 1990.

50. Dick M 2nd, O'Connor KB, Serwer GA, et al.: Use of radiofrequency current to ablate accessory connections in children. Circulation 84:2318-2324, 1991.

51. Schaffer MS, Silka MJ, Ross BA, Kugler JD: Inadvertent atrioventricular block during radiofrequency catheter ablation: Results of the Pediatric Radiofrequency Ablation Registry. Pediatric Electrophysiology Society. Circulation 94:3214-3220, 1996.

52. Lesh MD, Van Hare GF, Schamp DJ, et al.: Curative percutaneous catheter ablation using radiofrequency energy for accessory pathways in all locations: Results in 100 consecutive patients. J Am Coll Cardiol 19:1303-1309, 1992.

53. Calkins H, Langberg J, Sousa J, et al.: Radiofrequency catheter ablation of accessory atrioventricular connections in 250 patients: Abbreviated therapeutic approach to Wolff-Parkinson-White syndrome. Circulation 85:1337-1346, 1992.

54. Jackman WM, Wang XZ, Friday KJ, et al.: Catheter ablation of accessory atrioventricular pathways (Wolff-Parkinson-White syndrome) by radiofrequency current [see comments]. N Engl J Med 324:1605-1611, 1991.

55. Benito F, Sanchez C: Radiofrequency catheter ablation of accessory pathways in infants. Heart 78:160-162, 1997.

56. Solomon AJ, Tracy CM, Swartz JF, et al.: Effect on coronary artery anatomy of radiofrequency catheter ablation of atrial insertion sites of accessory pathways. J Am Coll Cardiol 21:1440-1444, 1993.

57. Khanal S, Ribeiro PA, Platt M, Kuhn MA: Right coronary artery occlusion as a complication of accessory pathway ablation in a 12-year-old treated with stenting. Cathet Cardiovasc Interv 46:59-61, 1999.

58. Chatelain P, Zimmermann M, Weber R, et al.: Acute coronary occlusion secondary to radiofrequency catheter ablation of a left lateral accessory pathway. Eur Heart J 16:859-861, 1995.

59. Bokenkamp R, Wibbelt G, Sturm M, et al.: Effects of intracardiac radiofrequency current application on coronary artery vessels in young pigs. J Cardiovasc Electrophysiol 11:565-571, 2000.

60. Mantakas ME, McCue CM, Miller WW: Natural history of Wolff-Parkinson-White syndrome in infants and children: A review and a report of 28 cases. Am J Cardiol 41:1097-1103, 1978.

61. Erickson CC, Walsh EP, Triedman JK, Saul JP: Efficacy and safety of radiofrequency ablation in infants and young children <18 months of age. Am J Cardiol 74:944-947, 1994.

62. Kugler JD: Radiofrequency catheter ablation for supraventricular tachycardia: Should it be used in infants and small children? [editorial; comment]. Circulation 90:639-641, 1994.

63. Case CL, Gillette PC, Oslizlok PC, et al.: Radiofrequency catheter ablation of incessant, medically resistant supraventricular tachycardia in infants and small children. J Am Coll Cardiol 20:1405-1410, 1992.

64. Case CL, Gillette PC: Indications for catheter ablation in infants and small children with reentrant supraventricular tachycardia [letter]. J Am Coll Cardiology 27:1551-1552, 1996.

65. Zak R: Development and proliferative capacity of cardiac muscle cells. Circ Res 35(Suppl II):17-26, 1974.

66. Denfield SW, Kearney DL, Michael L, et al.: Developmental differences in canine cardiac surgical scars. Am Heart J 126:382-389, 1993.

67. Erickson CC, Carr D, Greer GS, et al.: Emergent radiofrequency ablation of the AV node in a neonate with unstable, refractory supraventricular tachycardia. Pacing Clin Electrophysiol 18:1959-1962, 1995.

68. Finelli A, Rewcastle JC, Jewett MA: Cryotherapy and radiofrequency ablation: Pathophysiologic basis and laboratory studies [review, 48 refs]. Curr Opin Urol 13:187-191, 2003.

69. Cote JM, Epstein MR, Triedman JK, et al.: Low-temperature mapping predicts site of successful ablation while minimizing myocardial damage. Circulation 94:253-257, 1996.

70. Chu E, Fitzpatrick AP, Chin MC, et al.: Radiofrequency catheter ablation guided by intracardiac echocardiography. Circulation 89:1301-1305, 1994.

71. Schiebler GL, Adams P Jr, Anderson RC, et al.: Clinical study of twenty-three cases of Ebstein's anomaly of the tricuspid valve. Circulation 19:187, 1959.

72. Anderson RH, Becker AE, Arnold R, Wilkinson JL: The conducting tissues in congenitally corrected transposition. Circulation 50:911-923, 1974.

73. Symons JC, Shinebourne EA, Joseph MC, et al.: Criss-cross heart with congenitally corrected transposition: Report of a case with d-transposed aorta and ventricular preexcitation. Eur J Cardiol 5:493, 1977.

74. Van Mierop LHS, Kutsche LM, Victoria BF: Ebstein's anomaly. In Adams FH, Emmanouilides GC, Riemenschneider TA (eds.): Heart Disease in Infants, Children and Adolescents. Baltimore: Williams & Wilkins, 1989, pp 361-363.

75. Lev M, Gibson S, Miller RA: Ebstein's disease with Wolff-Parkinson-White syndrome: Report of a case with a histopathologic study of possible conduction pathways. Am J Cardiol 49:724-741, 1955.

76. Van Hare GF, Lesh MD, Stanger P: Radiofrequency catheter ablation of supraventricular arrhythmias in patients with congenital heart disease: Results and technical considerations. J Am Coll Cardiol 22:883-890, 1993.

77. Kuck KH, Schluter M, Geiger M, et al.: Radiofrequency current catheter ablation of accessory atrioventricular pathways. Lancet 337:1557-1561, 1991.

78. Smith WM, Gallagher JJ, Kerr CR, et al.: The electrophysiologic basis and management of symptomatic recurrent tachycardia in patients with Ebstein's anomaly of the tricuspid valve. Am J Cardiol 49:1223-1234, 1982.

79. Twidale N, Wang X, Beckman KJ, et al.: Factors associated with recurrence of accessory pathway conduction after radiofrequency catheter ablation. Pacing Clin Electrophysiol 14:2042-2048, 1991.

80. Gallagher JJ, Pritchett ELC, Sealy WC, et al.: The preexcitation syndromes. Prog Cardiovasc Dis 20:285-327, 1978.

81. Cox JL, Gallagher JJ, Cain ME: Experience with 118 consecutive patients undergoing operation for the Wolff-Parkinson-White syndrome. J Thorac Cardiovasc Surg 90:490-501, 1985.

82. Gillette PC, Garson A Jr, Kugler JD, et al.: Surgical treatment of supraventricular tachycardia in infants and children. Am J Cardiol 46:281-284, 1980.

83. Ott DA, Gillette PC, Garson A Jr: Surgical management of refractory supraventricular tachycardia in infants and children. J Am Coll Cardiol 5:124-129, 1985.

84. Weston LT, Hull RW, Laird JR: A prototype coronary electrode catheter for intracoronary electrogram recording. Am J Cardiol 70:1492-1493, 1992.

85. Ho SY, Anderson RH: Embryology and anatomy of the normal and abnormal conduction system. In Gillette PC, Garson A Jr: Pediatric Arrhythmias: Electrophysiology and Pacing. Philadelphia: Saunders, 1990, pp 2-27.

86. Langberg JJ, Calkins H, Kim YN, et al.: Recurrence of conduction in accessory atrioventricular connections after initially successful radiofrequency catheter ablation. J Am Coll Cardiol 19:1588-1592, 1992.

87. Dunnigan A, Benson DW, Benditt DG: Atrial flutter in infancy: Diagnosis, clinical features, and treatment. Pediatrics 75:725-729, 1985.

88. Kugler JD, Danford DA, Houston K, Felix G: Radiofrequency catheter ablation for paroxysmal supraventricular tachycardia in children and adolescents without structural heart disease. Pediatric EP Society, Radiofrequency Catheter Ablation Registry. Am J Cardiol 80:1438-1443, 1997.

89. Nanthakumar K, Lau YR, Plumb VJ, et al.: Electrophysiological findings in adolescents with atrial fibrillation who have structurally normal hearts. Circulation 110:117-123, 2004.

90. Walsh EP, Saul JP, Hulse JE, et al.: Transcatheter ablation of ectopic atrial tachycardia in young patients using radiofrequency current [see comments]. Circulation 86:1138-1146, 1992.

91. Garson A Jr, Gillette PC: Junctional ectopic tachycardia in children: Electrocardiography, electrophysiology and pharmacologic response. Am J Cardiol 44:298-302, 1979.

92. Villain E, Vetter VL, Garcia JM, et al.: Evolving concepts in the management of congenital junctional ectopic tachycardia: A multicenter study [see comments] [review]. Circulation 81:1544-1549, 1990.

93. Fishberger SB, Colan SD, Saul JP, et al.: Myocardial mechanics before and after ablation of chronic tachycardia. Pacing Clin Electrophysiol 19:42-49, 1996.

94. Gillette PC, Smith RT, Garson A Jr, et al.: Chronic supraventricular tachycardia: A curable cause of congestive cardiomyopathy. JAMA 253:391-392, 1985.

95. Rakusan K: Cardiac growth, maturation and aging. In Zak R (ed.): Growth of the Heart in Health and Disease. New York: Raven Press, 1984, pp 131-164.

96. Weindling SN, Saul JP, Walsh EP: Efficacy and risks of medical therapy for supraventricular tachycardia in neonates and infants. Am Heart J 131:66-72, 1996.

97. Walsh EP: Ablation of ectopic atrial tachycardia in children. In Huang SK (ed.): Radiofrequency Catheter Ablation of Cardiac Arrhythmias: Basic Concepts and Clinical Applications. Mt. Kisko, N. Y.: Futura, 1994, pp 421-443.

98. Naheed ZJ, Strasburger JF, Benson DW Jr, Deal BJ: Natural history and management strategies of automatic atrial tachycardia in children. Am J Cardiol 75:405-407, 1995.

99. Bauersfeld U, Gow RM, Hamilton RM, Izukawa T: Treatment of atrial ectopic tachycardia in infants <6 months old. Am Heart J 129:1145-1148, 1995.

100. Mehta AV, Sanchez GR, Sacks EJ, et al.: Ectopic automatic atrial tachycardia in children: Clinical characteristics, management and follow-up. J Am Coll Cardiol 11:379-385, 1988.

101. Kunze KP, Kuck KH, Schluter M, Bleifeld W: Effect of encainide and flecainide on chronic ectopic atrial tachycardia. J Am Coll Cardiol 7:1121-1126, 1986.

102. Dhala AA, Case CL, Gillette PC: Evolving treatment strategies for managing atrial ectopic tachycardia in children. Am J Cardiol 74:283-286, 1994.

103. Garson A Jr, Gillette PC, Titus JL, et al.: Surgical treatment of ventricular tachycardia in infants. N Engl J Med 310:1443-1445, 1984.

104. de Bakker JM, Hauer RN, Bakker PF, et al.: Abnormal automaticity as mechanism of atrial tachycardia in the human heart—Electrophysiologic and histologic correlation: A case report. J Cardiovasc Electrophysiol 5:335-344, 1994.

105. Kay GN, Chong F, Epstein AE, et al.: Radiofrequency ablation for treatment of primary atrial tachycardias [see comments]. J Am Coll Cardiol 21:901-909, 1993.

106. Tracy CM, Swartz JF, Fletcher RD, et al.: Radiofrequency catheter ablation of ectopic atrial tachycardia using paced activation sequence mapping [see comments]. J Am Coll Cardiol 21:910-917, 1993.

107. Dunnigan A, Pierpont ME, Smith SA, et al.: Cardiac and skeletal myopathy associated with cardiac dysrhythmias. Am J Cardiol 53:731-737, 1994.

108. Spinale FG, Fulbright BM, Mukherjee R, et al.: Relation between ventricular and myocyte function with tachycardia-induced cardiomyopathy. Circ Res 71:174-187, 1992.

109. Lesh MD, Van Hare GF, Epstein LM, et al.: Radiofrequency catheter ablation of atrial arrhythmias: Results and mechanisms. Circulation 89:1074-1089, 1994.

110. Nath S, Lynch C 3rd, Whayne JG, Haines DE: Cellular electrophysiological effects of hyperthermia on isolated guinea pig papillary muscle: Implications for catheter ablation. Circulation 88(Pt 1):1826-1831, 1993.

111. Evans VL, Garson A Jr, Smith RT, et al.: Ethmozine (moricizine HCl): A promising drug for "automatic" atrial ectopic tachycardia. Am J Cardiol 60:83F-86F, 1987.

112. Tanel RE, Walsh EP, Lulu JA, Saul JP: Sotalol for refractory arrhythmias in pediatric and young adult patients: Initial efficacy and long-term outcome. Am Heart J 130:791-797, 1995.

113. Walsh EP, Saul JP, Triedman JK, et al.: Natural and unnatural history of ectopic atrial tachycardia: One institution's experience. Pacing Clin Electrophysiol 17:746, 1994.

114. Balaji S, Sullivan I, Deanfield J, James I: Moderate hypothermia in the management of resistant automatic tachycardias in children. Br Heart J 66:221-224, 1991.

115. Koike K, Hesslein PS, Finlay CD, et al.: Atrial automatic tachycardia in children. Am J Cardiol 61:1127-1130, 1988.

116. von Bernuth G, Engelhardt W, Kramer HH, et al.: Atrial automatic tachycardia in infancy and childhood. Eur Heart J 13:1410-1415, 1992.

117. Gillette PC: Diagnosis and management of postoperative junctional ectopic tachycardia. Am Heart J 118:192-194, 1989.

118. Sholler GF, Walsh EP, Saul JP, et al.: Evaluation of a staged treatment protocol for postoperative rapid junctional ectopic tachycardia. Circulation 78:II-597, 1988.

119. Bash SE, Shah JJ, Albers WH: Hypothermia for the treatment of postsurgically accelerated junctional ectopic tachycardia. J Am Coll Cardiol 10:1095-1099, 1987.

120. Till JA, Rowland E: Atrial pacing as an adjunct to the management of post-surgical His bundle tachycardia. Br Heart J 66:225-229, 1991.

121. Walsh EP, Saul JP, Sholler GF, et al.: Evaluation of a staged treatment protocol for rapid automatic junctional tachycardia after operation for congenital heart disease. J Am Coll Cardiol 29:1046-1053, 1997.

122. Dubin AM, Cuneo B, Strasburger J, et al.: Congenital junctional tachycardia and congenital complete AV block: A shared etiology? Heart Rhythm 2:313-315, 2005.

123. Bharati S, Moskowitz WB, Scheinman M, et al.: Junctional tachycardias: Anatomic substrate and its significance in ablative procedures. J Am Coll Cardiol 18:179-186, 1991.

124. Rossi L, Piffer R, Turolla E, et al.: Multifocal Purkinje-like tumor of the heart: Occurrence with other anatomic abnormalities in the atrioventricular junction of an infant with junctional tachycardia, Lown-Ganong-Levine syndrome, and sudden death. Chest 87:340-345, 1985.

125. Gillette PC, Garson A Jr, et al.: Junctional automatic ectopic tachycardia: New proposed treatment by transcatheter His bundle ablation. Am Heart J 106:619-623, 1983.

126. Figa FH, Gow RM, Hamilton RM, Freedom RM: Clinical efficacy and safety of intravenous amiodarone in infants and children. Am J Cardiol 74:573-577, 1994.

127. Balaji S, Gillette PC, Case CL: Successful radiofrequency ablation of permanent junctional reciprocating tachycardia in an 18-month-old child. Am Heart J 127:1420-1421, 1994.

128. Ehlert FA, Goldberger JJ, Deal BJ, et al.: Successful radiofrequency energy ablation of automatic junctional tachycardia preserving normal atrioventricular nodal conduction. Pacing Clin Electrophysiol 16:54-61, 1993.

129. Rychik J, Marchlinski FE, Sweeten TL, et al.: Transcatheter radiofrequency ablation for congenital junctional ectopic tachycardia in infancy. Pediatr Cardiol 18:447-450, 1997.

130. Van Hare GF, Velvis H, Langberg JJ: Successful transcatheter ablation of congenital junctional ectopic tachycardia in a ten-month-old infant using radiofrequency energy. Pacing Clin Electrophysiol 13:730-735, 1990.

131. Young ML, Mehta MB, Martinez RM, et al.: Combined alpha-adrenergic blockade and radiofrequency ablation to treat junctional ectopic tachycardia successfully without atrioventricular block. Am J Cardiol 71:883-885, 1993.

132. Fishberger SB, Rossi AF, Messina JJ, Saul JP: Successful radiofrequency catheter ablation of congenital junctional ectopic tachycardia with preservation of atrioventricular conduction in a 9-month-old infant. Pacing Clin Electrophysiol 21:2132-2135, 1998.

133. Coumel P, Cabrol C, Fabiato A, et al.: Tachycardie permanente par rythme reciproque. Arch Mal Coeur 60:1830-1864, 1967.

134. O'Neill BJ, Klein GJ, Guiraudon GM, et al.: Results of operative therapy in the permanent form of junctional reciprocating tachycardia. Am J Cardiol 63:1074-1079, 1989.

135. Gallagher JJ, Sealy WC: The permanent form of junctional reciprocating tachycardia: Further elucidation of the underlying mechanism. Eur J Cardiol 8:413-430, 1978.

136. Ticho BS, Saul JP, Hulse JE, et al.: Variable location of accessory pathways associated with the permanent form of junctional reciprocating tachycardia and confirmation with radiofrequency ablation. Am J Cardiol 70:1559-1564, 1992.

137. Ticho BS, Walsh EP, Saul JP: Ablation of permanent junctional reciprocating tachycardia. In Huang SK (ed.): Radiofrequency Catheter Ablation of Cardiac Arrhythmias: Basic Concepts and Clinical Applications. Mt. Kisko, N. Y.: Futura, 1994, pp 397-409.

138. Gaita F, Haissaguerre M, Giustetto C, et al.: Catheter ablation of permanent junctional reciprocating tachycardia with radiofrequency current. J Am Coll Cardiol 25:648-654, 1995.

139. Gaita F, Antonio M, Riccardi R, et al.: Cryoenergy catheter ablation: A new technique for treatment of permanent junctional reciprocating tachycardia in children. J Cardiovasc Electrophysiol 15:263-268, 2004.

140. Critelli G, Gallagher JJ, Monda V, et al.: Anatomic and electrophysiologic substrate of the permanent form of junctional reciprocating tachycardia. J Am Coll Cardiol 4:601-610, 1984.

141. Guarnieri T, German LD, Gallagher JJ: The long R-P' tachycardias [review]. Pacing Clin Electrophysiol 10:103-117, 1987.

142. Lindinger A, Heisel A, von Bernuth G, et al.: Permanent junctional re-entry tachycardia: A multicentre long-term follow-up study in infants, children and young adults. Eur Heart J 19:936-942, 1998.

143. Morady F, Scheinman MM, Kou WH, et al.: Long-term results of catheter ablation of a posteroseptal accessory atrioventricular connection in 48 patients. Circulation 79:1160-1170, 1989.

144. Chien WW, Cohen TJ, Lee MA, et al.: Electrophysiological findings and long-term follow-up of patients with the permanent form of junctional reciprocating tachycardia treated by catheter ablation. Circulation 85:1329-1336, 1992.

145. Smith RT Jr, Gillette PC, Massumi A, et al.: Transcatheter ablative techniques for treatment of the permanent form of junctional reciprocating tachycardia in young patients. J Am Coll Cardiol 8:385-390, 1986.

146. Van Hare GF, Lesh MD, Scheinman M, Langberg JJ: Percutaneous radiofrequency catheter ablation for supraventricular arrhythmias in children. J Am Coll Cardiol 17:1613-1620, 1991.

147. Haissaguerre M, Montserrat P, Warin JF, et al.: Catheter ablation of left posteroseptal accessory pathways and of long RP' tachycardias with a right endocardial approach. Eur Heart J 12:845-859, 1991.

148. Van Praagh R: Segmental approach to diagnosis. In Fyler DC (ed.): Nadas' Pediatric Cardiology. Philadelphia: Hanley & Belfus, 1992, pp 27-35.

149. Walsh EP, Saul JP, Triedman JK, et al.: Ablation of the "second conducting system": Mahaim fibers and "double AV nodes" in congenital heart disease. Circulation 90:I-100, 1994.

150. Epstein MR, Saul JP, Weindling SN, et al.: Atrioventricular reciprocating tachycardia involving twin atrioventricular nodes in patients with complex congenital heart disease. J Cardiovasc Electrophysiol 12:671-679, 2001.

151. Fellows KE, Radtke WAK, Keane JF, Lock JE: Acute complications of catheter therapy for congenital heart disease. Am J Cardiol 60:679-683, 1987.

152. Schluter M, Kuck KH: Radiofrequency current for catheter ablation of accessory atrioventricular connections in children and adolescents: Emphasis on the single-catheter technique. Pediatrics 89:930-935, 1992.

153. Minich LL, Snider AR, McDonald D: Doppler detection of valvular regurgitation after radiofrequency ablation of accessory connections. Am J Cardiol 70:116-117, 1992.

154. Saul JP: Ablation of atrioventricular accessory pathways in children with and without congenital heart disease. In Huang SK (ed.): Radiofrequency Catheter Ablation of Cardiac Arrhythmias: Basic Concepts and Clinical Applications. Mt. Kisko, N. Y.: Futura, 1994, pp 365-396.

155. Anderson RH, Arnold R, Wilkinson JL: The conducting system in congenitally corrected transposition. Lancet 1:1286-1288, 1973.

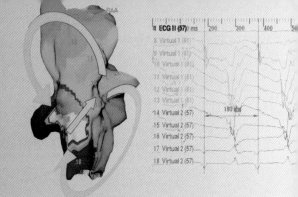

Subject Index

Page numbers followed by *f* indicate figures; page numbers followed by *t* indicate tables.